ADA/PDR Guide to

DENTAL
THERAPEUTICS

Fourth Edition

American Dental Association
www.ada.org

211 East Chicago Avenue
Chicago, Illinois 60611-2678

THOMSON
PDR

ADA/PDR Guide to
DENTAL THERAPEUTICS
Fourth Edition

American Dental Association

ADA Publishing Division
211 East Chicago Avenue
Chicago, IL 60611-2678
Phone: 312-440-2500
E-mail: adapub@ada.org
Website: http://www.ada.org

PDR Publishing Staff
Director, Editorial Services: Bette LaGow
Manager, Professional Services: Michael DeLuca, PharmD, MBA
Drug Information Specialists: Majid Kerolous, PharmD; Cathy Kim, PharmD; Nermin Shenouda, PharmD
Project Editor: Lori Murray
Production Editor: Elise Philippi
Index Editor: Caryn Sobel
Manager, Production Purchasing: Thomas Westburgh
Production Design Supervisor: Adeline Rich
Senior Electronic Publishing Designer: Livio Udina
Electronic Publishing Designers: Deana DiVizio, Carrie Faeth, Monika Popowitz
Production Associate: Joan K. Akerlind

Thomson PDR
Executive Vice President, PDR: Kevin D. Sanborn
Senior Vice President, PDR Sales: Roseanne McCauley
Vice President, Product Management: William T. Hicks
Vice President, PDR Services: Brian Holland
Senior Director, New Business Development: Michael Bennett
Director of Trade Sales: Bill Gaffney
Senior Manager, Direct Marketing: Amy Cheong
Promotion Manager: Linda Levine
Senior Director, Client Services: Stephanie Struble
Director of Operations: Robert Klein
Director of Finance: Mark S. Ritchin

The American Dental Association (ADA) and Thomson PDR (together the "Publishers") publish and present this book to you. The editor and authors of the *ADA/PDR Guide to Dental Therapeutics* have used care to confirm that the drugs and treatment schedules set forth in this book are in accordance with current recommendations and practice at the time of publication. This guide does not, however, constitute policy of the ADA, establish a standard of care or restrict a dentist's exercise of professional judgment. As the science of dental therapeutics evolves, changes in drug treatment and use become necessary. The reader is advised to consult the package insert for each drug to consider and adopt all safety precautions before use, particularly with new and infrequently used drugs. The reader is responsible for ascertaining the U.S. Food and Drug Administration clearance of each drug and device used in his or her practice.

The treatment and pharmacotherapy discussed in this book should be undertaken only within the bounds of applicable federal and state laws, including those pertaining to privacy and confidentiality, such as the Health Insurance Portability and Accountability Act and similar state laws. This book does not provide legal advice, and readers must consult with their own attorneys for such advice.

The Publishers, editor and authors disclaim all responsibility for any liability, loss, injury or damage resulting directly or indirectly from the reader's use and application of the information in this book and make no representations or warranties with respect to such information, including the products described herein.

The Publishers, editor and authors have produced this book in their individual capacities and not on behalf or in the interest of any pharmaceutical companies or state or federal agencies. Many of the proprietary names of the products listed in this book are trademarked and registered in the U.S. Patent Office. It should be understood that by making this material available, the Publishers are not advocating the use of any product described herein, nor are the Publishers responsible for misuse of a product due to typographical error. Additional information on any product may be obtained from the manufacturer.

Officers of Thomson Healthcare, Inc.: *President and Chief Executive Officer:* Bob Cullen; *Chief Financial Officer:* Paul Hilger; *Chief Medical Officer:* Rich Klasco, MD, FACEP; *Chief Strategy Officer:* Vincent A. Chippari; *Executive Vice President, Medstat:* Carol Diephuis; *Executive Vice President, Micromedex:* Jeff Reihl; *Executive Vice President, PDR:* Kevin D. Sanborn; *Senior Vice President, Technology:* Michael Karaman; *Vice President, Finance:* Joseph Scarfone; *Vice President, Human Resources:* Pamela M. Bilash; *Vice President, Planning and Business Development:* Ray Zoeller; *Vice President, Product Strategy:* Anita Brown; *Vice President, Strategic Initiatives:* Timothy Murray

ISBN: 1-56363-604-2   P063

Maria Salnik
M.S. Candidate Research Assistant
Complementary and Alternative Medicine Masters Program
Department of Physiology and Biophysics
Georgetown University
Washington, D.C.

Sol Silverman Jr., M.A., D.D.S.
Professor of Oral Medicine
University of California, San Francisco
School of Dentistry
San Francisco, California

Martha Somerman, D.D.S., Ph.D.
Dean and Professor of Periodontics
University of Washington
School of Dentistry
Seattle, Washington

Eric T. Stoopler, D.M.D.
Assistant Professor of Oral Medicine
Director, Oral Diagnosis and
  Emergency Care Clinics
University of Pennsylvania School of Dental Medicine
Philadelphia, Pennsylvania

Lakshmanan Suresh, D.D.S., M.S.
Assistant Director of Oral Pathology and Immunopathology
IMMCO Diagnostics, Inc.
Buffalo, New York

Leonard S. Tibbetts, D.D.S., M.S.D.
Private Practitioner
Arlington, Texas
Visiting Assistant Professor of Periodontics
University of Washington
Seattle, Washington

Clay Walker, Ph.D.
Professor of Oral Biology
Department of Oral Biology and Periodontal
  Disease Research Clinics
College of Dentistry
University of Florida
Gainesville, Florida

John A. Yagiela, D.D.S., Ph.D.
Professor and Chair
Division of Diagnostic and Surgical Sciences
School of Dentistry
Professor, Department of Anesthesiology
School of Medicine
University of California, Los Angeles
Los Angeles, California

TABLE OF CONTENTS

SECTION III. DRUG ISSUES IN DENTAL PRACTICE

APPENDICES

FOREWORD

Dentists are prescribing more medications today than ever before. Patients seeking dental care are using a wide range of medications for medical problems. And both dentists and patients have choices to make about the variety of nonprescription products available for treating various disorders of the mouth.

Dentists are vocal about their need for a quick and accurate drug reference that is more than a dictionary and yet not a textbook of pharmacology. In response, the ADA published the first edition of the *ADA Guide to Dental Therapeutics* in 1998. The guide was based on what dentists told us they needed to make their practices complete: concise and accurate information about the medications they use, information based on the science of pharmacology and organized by drug category in an easy-to-use tabular format. This fourth edition marks the collaboration of the ADA and the *Physicians' Desk Reference®*, making it the most comprehensive dental drug reference of its kind—the only one complete enough to bear the ADA name.

For this latest edition, every chapter has been updated and now features two comprehensive drug tables at the end, one with prescribing information and the other with drug interactions. When applicable, the chapters also contain tables with other pertinent pharmacologic information.

As a practical chairside resource, the guide offers easy access to crucial information about the drugs prescribed for and taken by dental patients—nearly 1,000 generic drugs and 3,000 brand-name drugs in all. Every practicing dentist, dental educator, dental student and member of the dental team can profit from using this book. In addition, it serves as a useful resource in preparing for various board examinations.

A major strength of this book is that it was written by both academicians and clinicians in a team approach. Writers were selected because of their expertise and reputations in dental therapeutics. The content is as up to the minute as possible and is scheduled to be updated every two to three years. Readers and reviewers of earlier editions gave us their comments, many of which were incorporated into this fourth edition. I encourage you to send us your comments so that the fifth edition can grow even more than the fourth.

The ADA Council on Scientific Affairs has reviewed all the material in this book, which is the only one of its kind that identifies medications—both prescription and nonprescription—that carry the ADA Seal of Acceptance. This Seal is designed to help the public and dental professionals make informed decisions about dental products. Backed by the knowledge of the Council, it provides an assurance that all products have met the ADA's standards of efficacy, safety and truth in advertising. Knowing which products carry the ADA Seal will enable all members of the dental team to select professional products knowledgeably and to discuss various toothpastes, mouthrinses and other nonprescription medications with their patients.

KEY FEATURES

The guide is unlike any other drug book available, offering a host of benefits to the practicing dentist:

- clear, well-organized tables that offer rapid access to information on more than 900 drugs used in dentistry, including therapeutic products that carry the ADA Seal of Acceptance;
- crucial data on dosage, interactions, precautions and adverse effects at the reader's fingertips;
- brief but informative descriptions of drug categories that bridge the gap between drug handbooks and pharmacology texts;
- information on more than 3,000 drugs used in medicine, enabling dentists to communicate knowledgeably with other medical professionals about patients' medications and their dental side effects;
- an evidence-based overview of herbs and dietary supplements;
- a one-of-a-kind chapter on oral manifestations of systemic agents;
- an appendix on drugs that cause photosensitivity;
- other appendices covering drug-related issues that affect dental practice: substance abuse, tobacco-use cessation, infection control, and many others.

DRUGS USED IN DENTISTRY

This book is arranged in three sections. The first focuses on drugs prescribed primarily by dentists, so that the practitioner can readily prescribe them with a full understanding of their actions, adverse effects and interactions. It contains drug information essential to solving patients' dental problems. Dentists will be able to quickly locate dosages and information of clinical significance (interactions, adverse effects, precautions and contraindications). Drugs and products that have received the ADA Seal of Acceptance are identified with a star ★.

In Section I, each chapter is organized by:
- description of the general category of drugs and the accepted indications;
- listings of specific drugs by generic and brand name—including adult and child dosages, forms and strengths;
- special dental considerations—drug interactions, pertinent laboratory value alterations, drug cross-sensitivities and effects on pregnant and nursing women, children, elderly patients and other patients with special needs;
- adverse effects and precautions, arranged by drug class or body system;
- pharmacology;
- information for patient/family consultation.

If any of these categories or subcategories does not appear (for instance, laboratory value alterations), it is because it did not pertain to the particular type of drug or because there was no such information available.

In each chapter in Section I, the prescribing information table (which appears at the end of the chapter text) is based on the assumption that the dentist has determined—through taking a health history and interviewing the patient—that the patient is in general good health and is not taking any medications that may interact with the drug in question. For quick reference, drug interactions are detailed in a separate table that also appears at the end of each chapter.

This book includes all ADA-accepted products in the various categories discussed. However, in some cases we have included only a representative sampling of products in a category—ADA-accepted or not. Inclusion of a particular product in no way indicates that it is superior to others.

DRUGS USED IN MEDICINE

Increasingly, dental patients are taking one or more prescription drugs. To assist the dentist, the second section of the book focuses on drugs prescribed primarily by physicians. It presents drug information in a more abbreviated form, emphasizing each drug's effect on dental diagnosis and treatment planning. The information here will help the dentist interact effectively with the patient's physician about the patient's medications, particularly when a modification of drug therapy is in question. Helpful dosage ranges enable dentists to anticipate potential side effects in patients at the upper end of the dosage range.

DRUG ISSUES IN DENTAL PRACTICE

The book's third section focuses on issues related to dental pharmacology that affect the dentist's practice, including legal considerations of using drugs in dentistry and information on herbs and dietary supplements. As part of the community of practitioners interested in patients as people and not just as "teeth and gums," dentists can use the information discussed here as building blocks for a successful and expanding practice. A highlight of this section is the chapter on oral manifestations of systemic medications. The topics presented in Section III are not addressed in most dental drug handbooks.

APPENDICES AND INDEX

The book features several appendices covering a broad range of topics, including a new section on bisphosphonate-associated osteonecrosis of the jaw. The comprehensive index at the back of the book is designed to help you find information quickly and easily.

ACKNOWLEDGMENTS

I wish to acknowledge the pioneering efforts of contributors to the ADA's Accepted Dental Therapeutics (which ceased publication in 1984), who laid the foundation for this book. I also wish to thank the authors, who applied their time and their broad talents generously to this task. I am grateful to my dean, Richard N. Buchanan, D.M.D., and to my wife, Marilyn, both of whom gave me the time and support needed to serve as editor. The authors and I thank the following people, who lent us their editorial or administrative assistance: Christine Chico, B.S., and Clifford Whall, Ph.D. from the ADA Council on Scientific Affairs; Jerome Bowman of the ADA Council on Legal Affairs, and my secretary Judy Dorsheimer. Finally, a special thanks is due to Carolyn B. Tatar, Senior Manager, Product Development of the American Dental Association and to my staff for helping me through the months of preparation; and especially to Lori Murray, Bette LaGow, Bill Gaffney and Mike Bennett of Thomson PDR for their patience, persistence, and devotion to excellence. The combined efforts of all these people as well as our chapter authors helped make this a dental therapeutics book of true distinction.

Sebastian G. Ciancio, D.D.S.
University at Buffalo
State University of New York
August 2006

HOW TO USE THIS BOOK

The fourth edition of the *ADA/PDR Guide to Dental Therapeutics* features a new table format designed to help you find the information you need as quickly and easily as possible. Book chapters are divided into three parts, allowing you to go directly to a particular therapeutic category:

I.   **Drugs Used in Dentistry**
II. **Drugs Used in Medicine: Treatment and Pharmacological Considerations for Dental Patients Receiving Medical Care**
III. **Drug Issues in Dental Practice**

Chapter text is organized by drug or product class. Each section includes general pharmacological information and special dental considerations. Suggested references and further readings are given at the end of each section or chapter, where applicable.

Drug tables are organized by therapeutic drug class. Within each class, products are listed alphabetically. **For ease of use, all tables are located at the end of each chapter.** For definitions of the abbreviations used in these tables, see the key at the end of this discussion.

Tables with prescribing information appear first and give pertinent details on the following:

- **Generic name:** Listed in bold, with brand names appearing in parentheses. Controlled substances are marked with their corresponding classification (eg, CII) after the generic name. Appendix A gives definitions of these classifications. In addition, products bearing the ADA Seal of Acceptance are marked with a star (★) after the name.
- **Drug forms and strengths:** Indicates whether the drug comes as a tablet, capsule, injection, etc. Scored tablets are noted with an asterisk.
- **Dosage:** Highlights adult and pediatric dosages in bold italics. Dosages are arranged according to each drug's indication, shown in bold type. Special dosing considerations—maximum dose, titration, dosage reductions for special patient groups—are also highlighted in bold.
- **Warnings/precautions and contraindications:** Lists crucial warnings and precautions first (denoted with **W/P**), followed by contraindications (denoted with **Contra**) and pregnancy/nursing information (denoted with **P/N**). Pregnancy categories (eg, Category C) are defined in Appendix B. Where applicable, "black box" warnings—that is, those that require special vigilance—are highlighted in bold type.
- **Adverse effects:** Lists the most common side effects occurring in ≥3% of patients as noted in the manufacturer's package insert. Dental-related side effects are noted in bold.

Tables with drug interactions appear after the prescribing information. These are also organized alphabetically by therapeutic class and generic name. Please keep in mind that the chance of an interaction varies among patients, and that previously undocumented drug interactions are always a possibility.

Other pharmacological tables are also included at the end of each chapter as necessary. These may include overall class definitions or special dental-related information.

APPENDIXES AND INDEX

These appear at the end of the book. Appendix topics are outlined in the Table of Contents. The comprehensive alphabetical Index contains all brand and generic names as well as general subject and chapter entries. Information appearing in a table is denoted with a "t" after the page number. Products with the ADA Seal are denoted with a star (★).

KEY TO ABBREVIATIONS USED IN THIS BOOK

ac	before meals		inh	inhaler
ACTH	adrenocorticotropan hormone		inj	injection
ADHD	attention deficit hyperactivity disorder		INR	international normalized ratio
			IOP	intraocular pressure
AED	anti-epileptic drug		IPPB	intermittent positive pressure breathing
ANC	absolute neutrophil count		IU	international unit
ASA	acetylsalicylic acid (aspirin)		IV	intravenous
AST	aspartate aminotransferase		KOH	potassium hydroxide
AUC	area under the concentration-time curve		LFT	liver function test
bid	twice a day		lot	lotion
BMD	bone mineral density		loz	lozenge
BMT	bone marrow transplantation		maint	maintenance dose
BP	blood pressure		MAOI	monoamine oxidase inhibitor
BUN	blood urea nitrogen		MDI	metered dose inhaler
BZD	benzodiazepine		MI	myocardial infarction
CAD	coronary artery disease		MIU	million international units
cap	capsule		MDD	minimum daily dose
CAPD	continuous ambulatory peritoneal dialysis		MMD	major mood disorder
			NG	nasogastric
CBC	complete blood count		NMS	neuroleptic malignant syndrome
CHF	chronic heart failure		NSAID	nonsteroidal anti-inflammatory drug
CML	chronic myeloid leukemia		NYHA	New York Heart Association
CMV	cytomegalovirus		OCD	obsessive-compulsive disorder
CNS	central nervous system		oint	ointment
Contra	contraindications		OSAHS	obstructive sleep apnea/ hypopnea syndrome
COPD	chronic obstructive pulmonary disorder		OTC	over the counter
			P/N	pregnancy category rating and nursing considerations
CPK	creatine phosphokinase			
CrCl	creatinine clearance		pc	after meals
cre	cream		PE	pulmonary embolism
CSF	cerebrospinal fluid		PKU	phenylketonuria
CV	cardiovascular		PO	by mouth
CVD	cardiovascular disorder		PT	prothrombin time
DM	diabetes mellitus		PTT	partial thromboplastin time
DSST	Digital Symbol Substitution Test		q4-6h	every 4 to 6 hours
DVT	deep vein thrombophlebitis		q6h	every 6 hours
ECG	electrocardiogram/electrocardiograph		q8h	every 8 hours
EEG	electroencephalogram		q12h	every 12 hours
EIAED	enzyme-inducing anti-epileptic drug		qam	every morning
EIB	exercise-induced bronchospasm		qd	every day
EPS	extrapyramidal syndrome		qhs	every night at bedtime
ESRD	end-stage renal disease		qid	four times daily
ETFN	empiric therapy in febrile neutropenia		qod	every other day
FBG	fasting blood glucose		qow	every other week
FBS	fasting blood sugar		qpm	every evening
FSH	follicle-stimulating hormone		SC/SQ	subcutaneous
GH	growth hormone		SCr	serum creatinine
GHD	growth hormone deficiency		SIADH	syndrome of inappropriate antidiuretic hormone
GI	gastrointestinal			
HBV	hepatitis B virus		SLE	systemic lupus erythematosus
hCG	human chorionic gonadotropin		sol	solution
Hct	hematocrit		SSRI	selective serotonin reuptake inhibitor
HCV	hepatitis C virus		sup	suppository
HDL	high-density lipoprotein		sus	suspension
HFA	hydrofluoroalkane		SWSD	shift work sleep disorder
hFSH	human follicle-stimulating hormone		syr	syrup
hgb	hemoglobin		tab	tablet
HIV	human immunodeficiency virus		TB	tuberculosis
HPA	hypothalamic-pituitary-adrenal		tbs	tablespoon
HR	heart rate		TCA	tricyclic antidepressants
hs	at bedtime		TIA	transient ischemic attack
HSCT	hematopoietic stem cell transplantation		tid	three times per day
			tiw	three times per week
HSV	herpes simplex virus		ULN	upper limit of normal range
HTN	hypertension		UTI	urinary tract infection
ICU	intensive care unit		W/P	warnings/precautions
IgE	immunoglobulin type E		WBC	white blood cell count
IM	intramuscular			

Section I.

Drugs Used in Dentistry

Chapter 1

Injectable and Topical Local Anesthetics

John A. Yagiela, D.D.S., Ph.D.

Injectable Local Anesthetics

Local anesthetics reversibly block neural transmission when applied to a circumscribed area of the body. Cocaine, the first local anesthetic (introduced in 1884), remains an effective topical agent, but it proved too toxic for parenteral use. Procaine, introduced in 1904, was the first practical local anesthetic for injection and contributed greatly to breaking the historic connection between dentistry and pain.

Vasoconstrictors are agents used in local anesthetic solutions to retard systemic absorption of the local anesthetic from the injection site. Although not active themselves in preventing neural transmission, vasoconstrictors such as epinephrine and related adrenergic amines can significantly increase the duration and even the depth of anesthesia. The vasoconstriction they produce also may be useful in reducing bleeding during intraoral procedures.

Chemistry and classification. Injectable local anesthetics consist of amphiphilic molecules; that is, they can dissolve in both aqueous and lipid environments. A lipophilic ring structure on one end of the molecule confers fat solubility, and a secondary or tertiary amino group on the other permits water solubility. Local anesthetics intended for injection are prepared commercially as the hydrochloride salt.

Two major classes of injectable local anesthetics are recognized: esters and amides. They are distinguished by the type of chemical bond joining the two ends of the drug molecules. Early local anesthetics, such as cocaine and procaine, were esters. Most local anesthetics introduced since 1940 have been amides.

The use of injectable local anesthetics in dentistry is almost exclusively limited to amide-type drugs. In fact, no ester agent is currently being marketed in dental cartridge form in the United States. Given the number of local anesthetic injections administered in dentistry (conservatively estimated at more than 300 million in the United States annually), a drug with a minimal risk of allergy is desirable. Amide anesthetics offer a significantly lower risk of allergy than ester anesthetics. Conversely, amides also have a somewhat greater risk of systemic toxicity than do esters. However, as toxic reactions usually are dose-related, adherence to proper injection techniques—including the use of minimal volumes of anesthetic—minimizes this risk. Amide formulations have also proved more effective than esters for achieving intraoral anesthesia. Thus, amide local anesthetics, as used in dentistry, offer the fewest overall risks and the greatest clinical benefits.

Selecting a local anesthetic. The selection of a local anesthetic for use in a dental procedure is based on four criteria:

• duration of the dental procedure;
• requirement for hemostasis;
• requirement for postsurgical pain control;
• contraindication(s) to specific anesthetic drugs or vasoconstrictors.

Duration. Local anesthetic formulations intended for use in dentistry are categorized by their expected duration of pulpal anesthesia as short-, intermediate- and long-acting drugs.

- Short-acting drugs, which typically provide pulpal and hard tissue anesthesia for up to 30 minutes after submucosal infiltration: 2% lidocaine, 3% mepivacaine and 4% prilocaine.
- Intermediate-acting agents, which provide up to 70 minutes of pulpal anesthesia: 4% articaine with 1:100,000 or 1:200,000 epinephrine, 2% lidocaine with 1:50,000 or 1:100,000 epinephrine, 2% mepivacaine with 1:20,000 levonordefrin and 4% prilocaine with 1:200,000 epinephrine.
- Long-acting drugs, which last up to 8 hours after nerve block anesthesia: 0.5% bupivacaine with 1:200,000 epinephrine.

For most clinical situations, an intermediate-acting formulation is appropriate. These agents are highly effective and have durations of action that can accommodate most intraoral procedures. The 4% prilocaine and 3% mepivacaine solutions, however, may be preferred for maxillary supraperiosteal injections when there is a need for pulpal anesthesia of only short duration. (The 2% lidocaine plain formulation cannot be recommended because pulpal anesthesia is not consistently achieved.) Long-acting local anesthetics are helpful for providing anesthesia of extended duration. Unfortunately, pulpal anesthesia after supraperiosteal injection is less reliable than with the intermediate-acting drugs, because the highly lipophilic long-acting drugs do not readily reach the superior dental nerve plexus.

Hemostasis. Lidocaine with epinephrine is the formulation usually administered to achieve temporary hemostasis in tissues undergoing treatment. Although the 1:50,000 strength of epinephrine provides little benefit over the 1:100,000 concentration with regard to the duration of local anesthesia, it can significantly decrease bleeding associated with periodontal tissue when given by local infiltration.

Postsurgical pain control. The bupivacaine formulation can help the surgical patient remain pain-free for up to 8 hours after treatment. This agent may be administered before the procedure to provide local anesthesia intraoperatively or afterward to maximize the duration of postsurgical pain relief.

Contraindications. True allergy is the only absolute contraindication to the use of any local anesthetic formulation. Although there is little evidence of cross-allergenicity among the amides, it is probably prudent to avoid amides with the greatest molecular similarity to the putative allergen. Lidocaine is most similar to prilocaine in structure, whereas mepivacaine is most similar to bupivacaine. Articaine is identical in structure to prilocaine except that it contains a thiophene group instead of the typically substituted benzene ring. If a sulfite preservative is the allergen, then the 3% mepivacaine and 4% prilocaine solutions without vasoconstrictor are the formulations of choice because they are free of sulfites.

These plain solutions also are indicated when the use of epinephrine and levonordefrin is not recommended. However, formulations containing 1:200,000 epinephrine may be considered when modest doses of vasoconstrictor are permissible and when the plain solutions might not provide anesthesia of sufficient depth or duration. (Specific contraindications and restrictions to vasoconstrictors are reviewed later in this chapter.)

Accepted Indications

Injectable local anesthetics are used to provide local or regional analgesia for surgical and other dental procedures.

They are also used for diagnostic or other therapeutic purposes via routes of administration specified in product labeling.

General Dosing Information

General dosing information is provided in Table 1.1. In addition, standard textbooks provide information on the appropriate dosage (both concentration and injection volume) of local anesthetic to be used for specific injection techniques and dental procedures. The dosage depends on:

- the specific anesthetic technique and operative procedure;
- tissue vascularity in the area of injection;
- individual patient response.

In general, the dentist should administer the lowest concentration and volume of anesthetic solution that provide adequate anesthesia.

Maximum Recommended Doses

Table 1.1 lists the maximum recommended doses for local anesthetic formulations per procedure or appointment, as approved by the U.S. Food and Drug Administration (FDA). Additional anesthetic may be administered only after sufficient time is allowed for elimination of the initial dose.

Dosage Adjustments

The actual maximum dose for each patient must be individualized depending on his or her size, age and physical status; other drugs he or she may be taking; and the anticipated rate of absorption of the local anesthetic from the injected tissues. Reduced maximum doses are often indicated for pediatric and geriatric patients, patients who have serious illness or disability and patients who have medical conditions or are taking drugs that alter responses to local anesthetics or vasoconstrictors.

Table 1.1 presents specific limits for local anesthetic doses in pediatric patients.

Vasoconstrictors

A vasoconstrictor added to a local anesthetic may significantly prolong the anesthetic's duration of action by reducing blood flow around the injection site. This, in turn, may reduce the local anesthetic's peak plasma concentration and the risk of adverse systemic reactions.

Repeated injection of vasoconstrictors in local anesthetics also may decrease blood flow sufficiently to cause anoxic injury in the local tissue, leading to delayed wound healing, edema or necrosis. The use of local anesthetic solutions containing vasoconstrictors may be restricted or contraindicated in patients who have advanced cardiovascular disease or who are taking medications that increase the activity of the vasoconstrictor.

Although there are no officially recognized maximum doses for vasoconstrictors when administered with local anesthesia, it is widely accepted that vasoconstrictor usage be minimized in patients with increased risk of vasoconstrictor toxicity. Because plasma concentrations of epinephrine measured in subjects performing normal activities of daily living are comparable to those achieved by the intraoral injection of two cartridges of lidocaine with 1:100,000 epinephrine (about 0.04 mg epinephrine) in reclining subjects, it is assumed that this dosage should be safe in the ambulatory patient with cardiovascular disease. Slow, careful injection with frequent aspiration attempts and avoidance of the 1:50,000 epinephrine formulation are additional precautions to take for the patient with reduced vasoconstrictor tolerance.

Special Dental Considerations

Drug Interactions of Dental Interest

Drug interactions and related problems involving local anesthetics and vasoconstrictors (Table 1.2) are potentially of clinical significance in dentistry.

Laboratory Value Alterations

- Pancreatic function tests using bentiromide are altered by ester local anesthetics or lidocaine.

Cross-Sensitivity

Table 1.3 describes potential cross-sensitivity considerations.

Special Patients

Pregnant and nursing women

Local anesthetics readily cross the placenta and enter the fetal circulation. Although retrospective investigations of pregnant women receiving local anesthesia during the first trimester of pregnancy have found no evidence of fetal toxicity, animal investigations indicate a potential for birth defects—albeit at enormous doses—with some local anesthetics.

Considerations of risk/benefit suggest that purely elective treatment be delayed until after delivery and that other dental care be performed, if possible, during the second trimester. Lidocaine and, probably, other local anesthetics are distributed into breast milk; again, however, no problems with injected local anesthetics have been documented in humans.

Table 1.1 lists the FDA pregnancy risk category classifications for injectable local anesthetics used in dentistry.

Pediatric, geriatric and other special patients

Although there are some data to suggest that adverse reactions to local anesthetics may be more prevalent in pediatric and geriatric populations, studies involving mepivacaine and other local anesthetics have found no age-specific problem that would limit use. However, overdosage is more likely to occur in young children because of their small size and the commensurately low margin for error. Increased variability of response to the local anesthetic or vasoconstrictor is likely to be encountered in elderly patients and in those with significant medical problems. Lower maximum doses in these patients provide an extra margin of safety.

Local anesthetics are less effective than normal in the presence of inflammation or infection. Strategies that may assist the clinician in achieving pain control include the use of nerve block techniques proximal to the affected tissue and intraosseous anesthesia.

Patient Monitoring: Aspects to Watch

- State of consciousness
- Respiratory status
- Cardiovascular status

Adverse Effects and Precautions

The incidence of adverse reactions to local anesthetic agents is low. Many reactions (headache, palpitation, tremor, nausea, dyspnea, hyperventilation syndrome, syncope) result from the perceived stress of injection and are not caused by the agents themselves. Toxic systemic reactions generally are associated with high plasma concentrations of the local anesthetic or vasoconstrictor, or both, after an accidental intravascular injection, administration of drug in a manner that causes rapid absorption, administration of a true overdosage or selection of a drug formulation inappropriate for the specific patient. Idiosyncratic and allergic reactions account for a small minority of adverse responses. In addition, a small subset of asthmatic patients intolerant of inhaled or dietary sulfites may develop bronchospasm after injection of local anesthetic solutions containing sulfite antioxidants.

Systemic reactions to local anesthetics may occur immediately on administration or may be delayed for up to 30 minutes or more. Oxygen, resuscitative equipment and drugs necessary to treat systemic emergencies must be immediately available whenever a local anesthetic is administered. Table 1.1 lists adverse effects for injectable local anesthetics and vasoconstrictors.

Pharmacology

Local Anesthetics

Local anesthetics bind to sodium channels in the nerve membrane and prevent the entry of sodium ions in response to the membrane's depolarization. Propagation of the action potential is inhibited in the area of injection, and nerve conduction fails when an adequate length of nerve is exposed to a sufficient concentration of local anesthetic. Nerve conduction is restored as the anesthetic diffuses away from the injection site and is absorbed into the systemic circulation. Systemic effects, should they occur, are largely the result of the local anesthetic's inhibiting other excitable tissues. Systemic reactions are minimized when metabolism of the local anesthetic is able to inactivate the drug as it is absorbed into the bloodstream.

The rate of absorption of a local anesthetic is governed by several factors, including the drug, its concentration and dose, the vascularity of the injection site and the presence of a vasoconstrictor. Generally, peak concentrations are achieved in 10 to 30 minutes.

Most amide anesthetics are metabolized in the liver. Prilocaine is unusual in that it is metabolized in the kidneys to some extent.

Most esters are hydrolyzed by plasma esterase to inactive products; some metabolism also occurs in the liver. Although classified as an amide local anesthetic, articaine is largely inactivated by carboxyesterase enzymes, which cleave a vital ester side chain from the drug.

Small amounts of local anesthetics (2%-20%) and the various metabolites eventually are excreted into the urine.

Vasoconstrictors

Epinephrine, levonordefrin and other adrenergic amine vasoconstrictors help retard absorption of the local anesthetic by stimulating α-adrenergic receptors in the local vasculature. The resultant reduction in tissue blood flow gives the local anesthetic more time to reach its site of action in the nerve membrane.

Systemic effects of vasoconstrictors are associated with stimulation of both α- and β-adrenergic receptors. The intensity and duration of these effects parallel the rate of absorption of the vasoconstrictor from the injection site. Stimulation of β receptors results in cardiac stimulation and vasodilation in skeletal muscle (β_2 receptors only). Stimulation of α receptors causes constriction of resistance arterioles throughout the body as well as capacitance veins in the legs and abdomen, which increases peripheral vascular resistance and venous return to the heart. Both α- and β-receptor effects contribute to the potential for cardiac dysrhythmias.

The adrenergic vasoconstrictors used in dentistry are quickly inactivated (plasma half-life of 1-2 minutes) by the enzyme catechol-O-methyltransferase. Additional metabolism of epinephrine by monoamine oxidase may occur, and the products are then excreted in the urine.

Patient Advice

- Injury to the anesthetized tissues may occur without any resulting sensation.
- To prevent injury, patients should not test for anesthesia by biting the lip or tongue, nor should they eat or chew anything until the anesthetic effect has dissipated.
- Children should be warned not to bite their lip or tongue and be monitored by their parents to prevent injury.

Suggested Readings

Malamed SF. Handbook of local anesthesia. 5th ed. St. Louis: Mosby; 2004.

Malamed SF, Gagnon S, Leblanc D. Efficacy of articaine: a new amide local anesthetic. JADA 2000;131(5):635–42.

Moore PA. Adverse drug interactions associated with local anesthetics, sedatives and anxiolytics. JADA 1999;130(4):541–54.

Yagiela JA. Adverse drug interactions in dental practice: interactions associated with vasoconstrictors. JADA 1999;130(5):701–9.

Yagiela JA. Local anesthetics. In Yagiela JA, Dowd FJ, Neidle EA, eds. Pharmacology and therapeutics for dentistry. 5th ed. St. Louis: Mosby; 2004.

Topical Local Anesthetics

Topical local anesthetic preparations used on oral mucosa differ in several respects from injectable preparations. Topical agents are selected for their ability to penetrate the oral mucosa and depend on diffusion to reach their site of action. Many of the anesthetics effective for nerve block or infiltration do not cross the mucosa adequately and, therefore, are not used for topical anesthesia.

In contrast to their injectable counterparts, topical ester-type agents are important for producing anesthesia, and some drugs used for mucosal anesthesia are neither esters nor amides. Life-threatening allergic reactions are extremely unlikely with topical anesthetics, regardless of type, and the inclusion of paraben preservatives in some topical amide formulations reduces the disparity in risk of allergy among these preparations.

Topical anesthetics are manufactured in a variety of forms. Gels, viscous gels and ointments are best used to limit the area of coverage of the topical anesthetic; aerosol sprays and solution rinses are best used for widespread application; lozenges, pastes and film-forming gels are specifically formulated to provide prolonged pain relief.

Several drugs used as topical anesthetics are so insoluble in water that they cannot be prepared in aqueous solutions. They are soluble in alcohol, propylene glycol, polyethylene glycol, volatile oils and other vehicles suitable for surface application. Included in this group of anesthetics are benzocaine and lidocaine bases. The poor water solubility of benzocaine in particular makes it safe for topical use on abraded or lacerated tissue.

To facilitate diffusion, the concentration of anesthetic used for surface application usually is much higher than that of injectable preparations. As a consequence, the potential toxicity of these preparations can be significant if large quantities are absorbed or even ingested. Systemic absorption of some topical anesthetics applied to the mucosa can be rapid, and blood concentrations approaching those with intravenous infusion may be achieved with tetracaine, depending on the area of coverage and method of application.

The rate of onset for topical anesthesia varies from 30 seconds to 5 minutes, depending on the anesthetic agent. Optimum effectiveness may be delayed, depending on the preparation. The mucosa should be dried before application to improve local uptake. The duration of topical anesthesia is generally shorter than with injected anesthesia. Table 1.4 indicates the approximate durations of action of the various topical anesthetics for mucosal anesthesia.

An occlusive dressing preventing the loss of agent can extend the duration; removing the residual agent and rinsing the mouth can shorten it. Topical preparations do not contain adrenergic vasoconstrictors.

Generally, mucosal anesthesia is only about 2 mm deep and is poor or nonexistent in the hard palate. Lidocaine and prilocaine prepared together in a eutectic mixture have been shown to improve anesthetic depth; however, the only preparation currently available for intraoral use is approved only for anesthesia of periodontal pockets. Given the trade name Oraqix, this lidocaine and prilocaine periodontal gel is marketed in special cartridge form and is applied into the pocket. Anesthesia begins in 30 seconds and lasts for about

20 minutes. A mucoadhesive patch containing lidocaine—DentiPatch Lidocaine Transoral Delivery System—also has shown increased efficacy as a topical anesthetic agent. The patch is applied directly to the mucosa in the area where anesthesia is desired so that the lidocaine's effect is maximized and the flow and dilution of the medication are limited. Anesthesia begins in 2.5 minutes, but the patch can be left in place for up to 15 minutes to increase the effect. Site-specific topical anesthesia additionally can be obtained with the use of a solid gel patch containing 18% benzocaine (Topicale GelPatch). The patch can be trimmed and shaped to fit the intended target. Anesthesia begins in about 30 seconds and is maintained as the patch dissolves during the next 20 minutes.

Accepted Indications

Topical local anesthetics are used to provide mucosal analgesia before local anesthetic injection; to facilitate dental examination, including pocket probing, the taking of radiographs, periodontal pocket scaling and other relatively noninvasive dental procedures by minimizing pain and the gag reflex; and to provide temporary symptomatic relief of toothache, oral lesions and wounds, as well as irritation caused by dentures and other appliances.

Additional uses for diagnostic and therapeutic purposes are described in product labeling.

General Dosing Information

The dosage of topical anesthetics depends on the anesthetic preparation selected, the area to be anesthetized, the ability to maintain the anesthetic agent on the area of application, the vascularity of the administration site and the patient's age, size and health status. Physical removal of the anesthetic and rinsing of the mouth once the need for topical anesthesia has passed preclude further absorption of the drug.

Maximum Recommended Doses

Table 1.5 lists the usual dose and the maximum recommended dose for topical anesthetic formulations per application and, where appropriate or available, the application interval.

Dosage Adjustments

The actual maximum dose for each patient must be individualized depending on his or her size, age and physical status; other drugs he or she may be taking; and the anticipated rate of absorption of the topical anesthetic from the application site. Reduced maximum doses are often indicated for pediatric and geriatric patients, people who have serious illness or disability and patients who have medical conditions or are taking drugs that alter responses to topical anesthetics.

Specific limits for topical anesthetic use in pediatric patients appear in Table 1.5.

Special Dental Considerations

Drug Interactions of Dental Interest

Drug interactions and related problems involving topical anesthetics are in general the same as those listed in Table 1.2. Interactions specific to cocaine are not included, since this drug is rarely used in dentistry.

Cross-Sensitivity

The potential for cross-sensitivity of topical local anesthetics is addressed in Table 1.3.

Special Patients

Pregnant and nursing women

Once absorbed into the systemic circulation, topical anesthetics can cross the placenta to enter the fetal circulation. Table 1.5 includes the FDA pregnancy category classifications for topical anesthetics used in dentistry. Considerations of risk/benefit suggest that purely elective treatment should be delayed until after delivery and that other dental care should be performed, if possible, during the second trimester. Lidocaine and probably other topical anesthetics are distributed into breast milk, but no problems have been documented in humans, except with cocaine. Cocaine intake by infants during nursing has led to overt toxicity, including convulsions and cardiovascular derangements.

Pediatric, geriatric and other special patients

Adverse reactions to topical anesthetics are rare in dentistry but may be more prevalent in pediatric and geriatric populations. Overdosage is more likely to occur in young children because of their small size and the commensurately low margin for error. Methemoglobinemia with use of benzocaine is largely limited to young children. Increased variability of response to local anesthetics is likely to be encountered in elderly patients and in those with significant medical problems. Lower maximum doses in these patients provides an extra margin of safety.

Patient Monitoring: Aspects to Watch

- State of consciousness
- Respiratory status
- Cardiovascular status

Adverse Effects and Precautions

Systemic reactions may occur when local anesthetics are applied topically. Systemic absorption of these agents should be minimized by limiting the concentration of the drug, the area of application, the total amount of agent applied and the time of exposure for drugs that can be removed once the effect has been achieved. To minimize absorption, spe-

cial caution is needed when applying topical agents to severely traumatized mucosa or to areas of sepsis.

Several topical anesthetic preparations are marketed in pressurized spray containers. It is difficult to control the amount of drug expelled with unmetered spray devices and to confine the agent to the desired site. Thus, a patient inadvertently may inhale sufficient quantities of the aerosol spray to provoke an adverse reaction. Therefore, caution is advised when using any spray device, and metered spray devices are preferred because they dispense a set amount of drug.

Adverse effects and precautions for topical anesthetics are included in Table 1.5.

Pharmacology

Topical local anesthetics provide anesthesia by anesthetizing the free nerve endings in the mucosa. The mechanism of action is identical to that described in the previous section for injectable local anesthetics. Cocaine, however, has a distinct pharmacology. In addition to its local anesthetic action, cocaine blocks the reuptake of released adrenergic neurotransmitters (norepinephrine, dopamine) back into the nerve terminal. This action gives cocaine its vasoconstrictor and CNS-stimulant properties, as well as its addictive potential and increased risk of cardiovascular toxicity.

The rate of absorption of a topical anesthetic depends on the dose administered, the duration of exposure, the area of coverage, the mucosa's permeability, the mucosa's intactness and the vascularity of the tissue. Benzocaine is unique in its poor solubility in water and is the least absorbed into the bloodstream.

A considerable portion of topical anesthetics administered intraorally is swallowed. Although absorption from the gastrointestinal tract occurs, extensive metabolism of the drug in the hepatic-portal system prevents toxic blood concentrations except with excessive doses. The metabolic fate and excretion of these drugs is covered in the first part of this chapter, in the section on injectable local anesthetics.

Patient Advice

- Injury to the anesthetized tissues may occur without any resulting sensation.
- To prevent pulmonary aspiration, patients who have undergone topical anesthesia of the pharynx should use caution when eating or drinking until normal sensation has returned.
- To prevent injury, patients should not test for anesthesia by biting the lip or tongue, nor should they eat or chew anything until the anesthetic effect has dissipated.

- Children should be warned not to bite their lips or tongue and be monitored by their parents to prevent injury.
- Patients using topical anesthetics to manage toothache, intraoral conditions or ill-fitting dental appliances should seek professional dental care for definitive treatment.

Suggested Readings

Hersh EV, Houpt MI, Cooper SA, et al. Analgesic efficacy and safety of an intraoral lidocaine patch. JADA 1996;127(11):1626-34.

Magnusson I, Jeffcoat MK, Donaldson D, Otterbom IL, Henriksson J. Quantification and analysis of pain in nonsurgical scaling and/or root planing. JADA 2004;135(12):1747-54.

Malamed SF. Handbook of local anesthesia. 5th ed. St. Louis: Mosby; 2004.

Meechan JG. Intra-oral topical anaesthetics: a review. J Dent 2000;28(1):3-14.

Table 1.1: PRESCRIBING INFORMATION FOR INJECTABLE LOCAL ANESTHETICS

NAME	FORM/ STRENGTH	DOSAGE	WARNINGS/PRECAUTIONS & CONTRAINDICATIONS	ADVERSE EFFECTS
Articaine Hydrochloride w/ Epinephrine (Septocaine★, Zorcaine)	**Sol, Inj:** (Articaine-Epinephrine) 4%-1:100,000/1.7mL	***Adults:* Submucosal Infiltration:** 0.5-2.5mL. **Nerve Block:** 0.5-3.4mL. **Oral Surgery:** 1-5.1mL. **Max:** 7mg/kg (0.175mL/kg) or 3.2mg/lb (0.0795mL/lb). ***Pediatrics:* ≥4 yrs: Submucosal Infiltration/Nerve Block/Oral Surgery:** Up to 7mg/kg (0.175mL/kg) or 3.2mg/lb (0.0795mL/lb).	**W/P:** Avoid intravascular injection; aspirate needle before use. Intravascular injection is associated with convulsions, followed by CNS or cardiorespiratory depression and coma progressing to respiratory arrest. CNS or cardiovascular effects may also occur with systemic absorption. Epinephrine can cause local tissue necrosis or systemic toxicity. Multiple injections at same tissue site increase likelihood of local tissue damage. Cardiovascular toxicity is more likely in patients with pre-existing cardiac defects, disease or dysrhythmias; peripheral vascular disease; hypokalemia; or uncontrolled hypertension, pheochromocytoma or thyroid disease. **Contra:** Known hypersensitivity to amide local anesthetics or sulfite preservatives. **P/N:** Category C, caution in nursing.	Confusion, restlessness, anxiety, dizziness, tinnitus, blurred vision, tremors, convulsions, nausea, vomiting, chills, unconsciousness, respiratory depression and arrest, hypotension, bradycardia, tachycardia, ventricular dysrhythmias, palpitation, angina pectoris, cardiac arrest, urticaria, pruritus, erythema, bronchospasm, anaphylaxis, facial edema, trismus, headache, infection, pain, local tissue damage, long-lasting paresthesia.
Bupivacaine Hydrochloride w/ Epinephrine (Marcaine w/ Epinephrine★)	**Sol, Inj:** (Bupivacaine-Epinephrine) 0.5%-1:200,000/1.8mL	***Adults:*** Individualize dose. Dosage varies depending on procedure, area to be anesthetized, vascularity of tissues, and patient tolerance and physical condition. **Single Dose Max:** 90mg (225mg for nondental uses). **Elderly/Debilitated/Cardiac or Liver Disease:** Reduce dose. ***Pediatrics:* ≥12 yrs:** Individualize dose. Dosage varies depending on procedure, area to be anesthetized, vascularity of tissues, and patient tolerance and physical condition.	**W/P:** Avoid intravascular injection; aspirate needle before use. Acidosis, cardiac arrest, and death reported from delay in toxicity management. Monitor cardiovascular and respiratory vital signs and state of consciousness after each injection. Caution with hepatic disease and impaired cardiovascular function. Epinephrine can cause local tissue necrosis or systemic toxicity. Multiple injections at same tissue site increase likelihood of local tissue damage. Cardiovascular toxicity is more likely in patients with pre-existing cardiac defects, disease or dysrhythmias; peripheral vascular disease; hypokalemia; or uncontrolled hypertension, pheochromocytoma or thyroid disease. Patients should be warned about inadvertent trauma to oral tissues and advised not to chew solid food while anesthetized. **Contra:** Known hypersensitivity to amide local anesthetics or sulfite preservatives. **P/N:** Category C, not for use in nursing.	Confusion, restlessness, anxiety, dizziness, tinnitus, blurred vision, tremors, convulsions, nausea, vomiting, chills, unconsciousness, respiratory depression and arrest, hypotension, bradycardia, tachycardia, ventricular dysrhythmias, palpitation, angina pectoris, myocardial depression, cardiac arrest, urticaria, pruritus, erythema, bronchospasm, anaphylaxis, facial edema, trismus, local tissue damage.
Lidocaine Hydrochloride (Xylocaine★)	**Sol, Inj:** 2%/1.8mL	***Adults:*** Dosage varies depending on procedure, area to be anesthetized, vascularity of tissues, and patient tolerance and physical condition. **Max:** 4.5mg/kg (2mg/lb) or total dose of 300mg. **Children/Elderly/Debilitated/Cardiac or Liver Disease:** Reduce dose. ***Pediatrics:* >3 yrs: Max:** 4.5mg/kg (2mg/lb).	**W/P:** Avoid intravascular injection; aspirate needle before use. Acidosis, cardiac arrest, and death reported from delay in toxicity management. Use lowest effective dose. Reduce dose with debilitated, elderly, acutely ill, and children. Monitor cardiovascular and respiratory vital signs and state of consciousness after each injection. Caution with hepatic disease and cardiovascular disorders. **Contra:** Known hypersensitivity to amide local anesthetics. **P/N:** Category B, caution in nursing.	Confusion, restlessness, anxiety, dizziness, tinnitus, blurred vision, tremors, convulsions, nausea, vomiting, chills, unconsciousness, respiratory depression and arrest, hypotension, bradycardia, ventricular dysrhythmias, cardiac arrest, urticaria, pruritus, erythema, anaphylaxis, facial edema, trismus.

★indicates a drug bearing the ADA Seal of Acceptance.   †Generic manufacturer.

NAME	FORM/ STRENGTH	DOSAGE	WARNINGS/PRECAUTIONS & CONTRAINDICATIONS	ADVERSE EFFECTS
Lidocaine Hydrochloride w/ Epinephrine (Lignospan Standard★, Lignospan Forte★, Octocaine 50★, Octocaine 100★, Xylocaine w/ Epinephrine★, Darby Lidocaine HCl w/ Epinephrine★†, Henry Schein Lidocaine HCl w/ Epineph- rine★†)	**Sol, Inj:** (Lidocaine-Epinephrine) 2%-1:50,000/1.8mL; 2%-1:100,000/1.8mL	**Adults:** Dosage varies depending on procedure, area to be anesthetized, vascularity of tissues, and patient tolerance and physical condition. **Max:** 7mg/kg (3.2 mg/lb) or total dose of 500mg. **Children/Elderly/ Debilitated/Cardiac or Liver Disease:** Reduce dose. **Pediatrics: >3 yrs: Max:** 7mg/kg (3.2 mg/lb).	**W/P:** Avoid intravascular injection; aspirate needle before use. Acidosis, cardiac arrest, and death reported from delay in toxicity management. Use lowest effective dose. Reduce dose with debilitated, elderly, acutely ill, and children. Multiple injections at same tissue site increase likelihood of local tissue damage. Epinephrine can cause local tissue necrosis or systemic toxicity. Multiple injections at same tissue site increase likelihood of local tissue damage. Cardiovascular toxicity is more likely in patients with pre-existing cardiac defects, disease or dysrhythmias; peripheral vascular disease; hypokalemia; or uncontrolled hypertension, pheochromocytoma or thyroid disease. Monitor cardiovascular and respiratory vital signs and state of consciousness after each injection. Caution with hepatic disease and cardiovascular disorders. **Contra:** Known hypersensitivity to amide local anesthetics or sulfite preservatives. **P/N:** Category B, caution in nursing.	Confusion, restlessness, anxiety, dizziness, tinnitus, blurred vision, tremors, convulsions, nausea, vomiting, chills, unconsciousness, respiratory depression and arrest, hypotension, bradycardia, tachycardia, ventricular dysrhythmias, palpitation, angina pectoris, cardiac arrest, urticaria, pruritus, erythema, bronchospasm, anaphylaxis, facial edema, trismus, local tissue damage.
Mepivacaine Hydrochloride (Carbocaine 3%★, Isocaine 3%★, Polocaine 3%★, Scandonest 3% Plain★, Darby Dental Supply Mepivacaine HCl★†, Henry Schein† Mepivacaine HCl★†)	**Sol, Inj:** 3%/1.8mL	**Adults:** Dose varies with anesthetic procedure, area to be anesthetized, vascularity of tissues, number of neuronal segments to be blocked, depth of anesthesia and degree of muscle relaxation required, and duration of anesthesia required. **Max:** 6.6mg/kg or total dose of 400mg. **Pediatrics:** Dose not to exceed 5-6mg/kg.	**W/P:** Aspiration for blood should be done prior to injection of initial and all subsequent doses to avoid intravascular injection. Use with caution if inflammation and/or sepsis in region of proposed injection. Avoid injecting mepivacaine too rapidly or into intravascular spaces (systemic toxicity could result). Use with caution in patients with hepatic disease. **Contra:** Hypersensitivity to amide-type anesthetics. **P/N:** Category C, caution in nursing.	Lightheadedness, nervousness, euphoria, confusion, dizziness, drowsiness, tinnitus, blurred vision, vomiting, heat/cold sensations, twitching, tremors, convulsions, respiratory depression, bradycardia, ventricular dysrhythmias, hypotension, urticaria, edema, anaphylaxis, trismus.
Mepivacaine Hydrochloride w/ Levonordefrin (Carbocaine w/ NeoCobefrin, Isocaine w/ Levonordefrin★, Scandonest L★, Polocaine w/ Levonorde-frin★, Darby Dental Supply Mepivacaine HCl w/ Levo-nordefrin★†, Henry Schein Mepivacaine HCl w/ Levonorde-frin★†)	**Sol, Inj:** (Mepivacaine-Levonordefrin) 2%-1:20,000/1.8mL	**Adults:** Dose varies with anesthetic procedure, area to be anesthetized, vascularity of tissues, number of neuronal segments to be blocked, depth of anesthesia and degree of muscle relaxation required, and duration of anesthesia required. **Max:** 6.6mg/kg or total dose of 400mg. **Pediatrics:** Dose not to exceed 5-6mg/kg.	**W/P:** Aspiration for blood should be done prior to injection of initial and all subsequent doses to avoid intravascular injection. Use with caution if inflammation and/or sepsis in region of proposed injection. Levonordefrin can cause local tissue necrosis or systemic toxicity. Multiple injections at same tissue site increase likelihood of local tissue damage. Cardiovascular toxicity is more likely in patients with pre-existing cardiac defects, disease or dysrhythmias; peripheral vascular disease; hypokalemia; or uncontrolled hypertension, pheochromocytoma or thyroid disease. Use with caution in patients with hepatic disease. **Contra:** Hypersensitivity to amide-type anesthetics and sulfite preservatives. **P/N:** Category C, caution in nursing.	Lightheadedness, nervousness, euphoria, confusion, dizziness, drowsiness, tinnitus, blurred vision, vomiting, heat/cold sensations, twitching, tremors, convulsions, respiratory depression, ventricular dysrhythmias, palpitation, angina pectoris, hypotension, hypertension, urticaria, edema, bronchospasm, anaphylaxis, trismus, local tissue damage.

NAME	FORM/ STRENGTH	DOSAGE	WARNINGS/PRECAUTIONS & CONTRAINDICATIONS	ADVERSE EFFECTS
Prilocaine Hydrochloride (Citanest★)	**Sol, Inj:** 4%/1.8mL	***Adults:*** **Maxillary Infiltration: Initial:** 1-2mL. **<70kg: Max:** 8mg/kg per injection. **≥70kg: Max:** 600mg (15mL) per injection. The dosage varies and depends on the physical status of the patient. Aspiration prior to injection is recommended. ***Pediatrics:*** **<10 yrs:** 40mg per procedure. **Max:** 8mg/kg.	**W/P:** Avoid intravascular injection; aspiration should be performed. Caution in patients with congenital or idiopathic methemoglobinemia, or patients with glucose-6-phosphate deficiencies, and very young patients. Use with caution in patients with severe shock or heart block. Use with caution in patients with hepatic disease. **Contra:** Congenital methemoglobinemia; hypersensitivity to amide containing anesthetics. **P/N:** Category B, caution in nursing.	Lightheadedness, nervousness, euphoria, confusion, dizziness, drowsiness, tinnitus, blurred vision, vomiting, heat/cold sensations, twitching, tremors, convulsions, respiratory depression, or idiopathic tachypnea and hypoxemia, bradycardia, ventricular dysrhythmias, hypotension, urticaria, edema, anaphylaxis, cardiac arrest, long-lasting paresthesia
Prilocaine Hydrochloride w/ Epinephrine (Citanest Forte★)	**Sol, Inj:** (Citanest-Epinephrine) 4%-1:200,000/1.8mL	***Adults:*** **Maxillary Infiltration: Initial:** 1-2mL. **<70kg: Max:** 8mg/kg per injection. **≥70kg: Max:** 600mg (15mL) per injection. The dosage varies and depends on the physical status of the patient. Aspiration prior to injection is recommended. ***Pediatrics:*** **<10 yrs:** 40mg per procedure. **Max:** 8mg/kg.	**W/P:** Avoid intravascular injection; aspiration should be performed. Caution in patients with congenital or idiopathic methemoglobinemia, or patients with glucose-6-phosphate deficiencies, and very young patients. Use with caution in patients with severe shock or heart block. Epinephrine can cause local tissue necrosis or systemic toxicity. Multiple injections at same tissue site increase likelihood of local tissue damage. Cardiovascular toxicity is more likely in patients with pre-existing cardiac defects, disease or dysrhythmias; peripheral vascular disease; hypokalemia; or uncontrolled hypertension, pheochromocytoma or thyroid disease. Use with caution in patients with hepatic disease. **Contra:** Congenital or idiopathic methemoglobinemia; hypersensitivity to amide-type anesthetics and sulfite preservatives. **P/N:** Category B, caution in nursing.	Lightheadedness, nervousness, euphoria, confusion, dizziness, drowsiness, tinnitus, blurred vision, vomiting, heat/cold sensations, twitching, tremors, convulsions, respiratory depression, tachypnea and hypoxemia, bradycardia, tachycardia, ventricular dysrhythmias, palpitation, angina pectoris, hypotension, urticaria, edema, bronchospasm, anaphylaxis, ventricular dysrhythmias, cardiac arrest, trismus, local tissue damage, long-lasting paresthesia.

★indicates a drug bearing the ADA Seal of Acceptance.   †Generic manufacturer.

Table 1.2: DRUG INTERACTIONS FOR INJECTABLE LOCAL ANESTHETICS

Articaine Hydrochloride w/ Epinephrine (Septocaine, Zorcaine)

α-adrenergic blockers (prazosin), butyrophenones (haloperidol) and phenothiazines (thioridazine)	May reduce or reverse pressor effect of epinephrine (large doses only); use vasoconstrictor cautiously.
Antidysrhythmic agents (class I)	Additive CNS and cardiac toxicity; use local anesthetic cautiously and in reduced maximum doses.
β-adrenergic blockers (nonselective)	May cause hypertension and bradycardia with vasoconstrictor; monitor patient and use vasoconstrictor cautiously.
CNS depressants (including alcohol, opioids, antidepressants, and other local anesthetics)	Additive or supraadditive CNS and respiratory depression; use local anesthetic cautiously and in reduced maximum doses.
CNS stimulants (amphetamine) and ergot derivatives (dihydroergotamine)	May cause hypertension with vasoconstrictor; monitor patient and use vasoconstrictor cautiously.
Cocaine	May increase cardiovascular responses to vasoconstrictor; avoid vasoconstrictor use in patient under influence of cocaine.
COMT inhibitors (entacapone)	Inhibition of metabolism may enhance systemic effects of vasoconstrictor; monitor patient and use vasoconstrictor cautiously.
Digoxin	May increase risk of cardiac dysrhythmias; use vasoconstrictor in consultation with physician.
Hydrocarbon inhalation anesthetics (halothane)	May cause cardiac dysrhythmias with vasoconstrictors; consult anesthesiologist about vasoconstrictor use.
Levodopa and thyroid hormones (levothyroxine)	Large doses (beyond replacement doses of thyroid hormone) may increase risk of cardiac toxicity; use vasoconstrictor cautiously.
Methyldopa and adrenergic neuron blockers (guanadrel)	May enhance systemic effects of vasoconstrictor; use vasoconstrictor cautiously.
Tricyclic (imipramine) and heterocyclic (amoxapine) antidepressants	May enhance systemic effects of epinephrine; use vasoconstrictor cautiously and in reduced maximum dosages.

Bupivacaine Hydrochloride w/ Epinephrine (Marcaine w/ Epinephrine)

α-adrenergic blockers (prazosin), butyrophenones (haloperidol) and phenothiazines (thioridazine)	May reduce or reverse pressor effect of epinephrine (large doses only); use vasoconstrictor cautiously.
Antidysrhythmic agents (class I)	Additive CNS and cardiac toxicity; use local anesthetic cautiously and in reduced maximum doses.
β-adrenergic blockers (nonselective)	May cause hypertension and bradycardia with vasoconstrictor; monitor patient and use vasoconstrictor cautiously.

Table 1.2: DRUG INTERACTIONS FOR INJECTABLE LOCAL ANESTHETICS (cont.)

Bupivacaine Hydrochloride w/ Epinephrine (cont.)

CNS depressants (including alcohol, opioids, antidepressants, and other local anesthetics)	Additive or supraadditive CNS and respiratory depression; use local anesthetic cautiously and in reduced maximum doses.
CNS stimulants (amphetamine) and ergot derivatives (dihydroergotamine)	May cause hypertension with vasoconstrictor; monitor patient and use vasoconstrictor cautiously.
Cocaine	May increase cardiovascular responses to vasoconstrictor; avoid vasoconstrictor use in patient under influence of cocaine.
COMT inhibitors (entacapone)	Inhibition of metabolism may enhance systemic effects of vasoconstrictor; monitor patient and use vasoconstrictor cautiously.
Digoxin	May increase risk of cardiac dysrhythmias; use vasoconstrictor in consultation with physician.
Hydrocarbon inhalation anesthetics (halothane)	May cause cardiac dysrhythmias with vasoconstrictors; consult anesthesiologist about vasoconstrictor use.
Levodopa and thyroid hormones (levothyroxine)	Large doses (beyond replacement doses of thyroid hormone) may increase risk of cardiac toxicity; use vasoconstrictor cautiously.
Methyldopa and adrenergic neuron blockers (guanadrel)	May enhance systemic effects of vasoconstrictor; use vasoconstrictor cautiously.
Tricyclic (imipramine) and heterocyclic (amoxapine) antidepressants	May enhance systemic effects of epinephrine; use vasoconstrictor cautiously and in reduced maximum dosages.

Lidocaine Hydrochloride (Xylocaine)

Amiodarone, β-adrenergic blockers (propranolol), cimetadine	Hepatic metabolism may be decreased; use local anesthetic cautiously, especially regarding repeat dosing.
Antidysrhythmic agents (class I)	Additive CNS and cardiac toxicity; use local anesthetic cautiously and in reduced maximum doses.
CNS depressants (including alcohol, opioids, antidepressants, and other local anesthetics)	Additive or supraadditive CNS and respiratory depression; use local anesthetic cautiously and in reduced maximum doses.

Lidocaine Hydrochloride w/ Epinephrine (Lignospan Standard, Lignospan Forte, Octocaine 50, Octocaine 100, Xylocaine w/ Epinephrine)

α-adrenergic blockers (prazosin), butyrophenones (haloperidol) and phenothiazines (thioridazine)	May reduce or reverse pressor effect of epinephrine (large doses only); use vasoconstrictor cautiously.
Amiodarone, β-adrenergic blockers, cimetadine	Hepatic metabolism may be decreased; use local anesthetic cautiously, especially regarding repeat dosing.

Lidocaine Hydrochloride w/ Epinephrine (cont.)

Antidysrhythmic agents (class I)	Additive CNS and cardiac toxicity; use local anesthetic cautiously and in reduced maximum doses.
β-adrenergic blockers (nonselective)	May cause hypertension and bradycardia with vasoconstrictor; monitor patient and use vasoconstrictor cautiously.
CNS depressants (including alcohol, opioids, antidepressants, and other local anesthetics)	Additive or supraadditive CNS and respiratory depression; use local anesthetic cautiously and in reduced maximum doses.
CNS stimulants (amphetamine) and ergot derivatives (dihydroergotamine)	May cause hypertension with vasoconstrictor; monitor patient and use vasoconstrictor cautiously.
Cocaine	May increase cardiovascular responses to vasoconstrictor; avoid vasoconstrictor use in patient under influence of cocaine.
COMT inhibitors (entacapone)	Inhibition of metabolism may enhance systemic effects of vasoconstrictor; monitor patient and use vasoconstrictor cautiously.
Digoxin	May increase risk of cardiac dysrhythmias; use vasoconstrictor in consultation with physician.
Hydrocarbon inhalation anesthetics (halothane)	May cause cardiac dysrhythmias with vasoconstrictors; consult anesthesiologist about vasoconstrictor use.
Levodopa and thyroid hormones (levothyroxine)	Large doses (beyond replacement doses of thyroid hormone) may increase risk of cardiac toxicity; use vasoconstrictor cautiously.
Methyldopa and adrenergic neuron blockers (guanadrel)	May enhance systemic effects of vasoconstrictor; use vasoconstrictor cautiously.
Tricyclic (imipramine) and heterocyclic (amoxapine) antidepressants	May enhance systemic effects of epinephrine; use vasoconstrictor cautiously and in reduced maximum dosages.

Mepivacaine Hydrochloride (Carbocaine, Polocaine)

Amiodarone, β-adrenergic blockers, cimetadine	Hepatic metabolism may be decreased; use local anesthetic cautiously, especially regarding repeat dosing.
Antidysrhythmic agents (class I)	Additive CNS and cardiac toxicity; use local anesthetic cautiously and in reduced maximum doses.
CNS depressants (including alcohol, opioids, antidepressants, and other local anesthetics)	Additive or supraadditive CNS and respiratory depression; use local anesthetic cautiously and in reduced maximum doses.

Mepivacaine Hydrochloride w/ Levonordefrin (Carbocaine w/ NeoCobefrin, Isocaine, Scandonest L, Polocaine w/ Levonordefrin)

Amiodarone, β-adrenergic blockers, cimetadine	Hepatic metabolism may be decreased; use local anesthetic cautiously, especially regarding repeat dosing.
Antidysrhythmic agents (class I)	Additive CNS and cardiac toxicity; use local anesthetic cautiously and in reduced maximum doses.

Table 1.2: DRUG INTERACTIONS FOR INJECTABLE LOCAL ANESTHETICS *(cont.)*

Mepivacaine Hydrochloride w/ Levonordefrin *(cont.)*

CNS depressants (including alcohol, opioids, antidepressants, and other local anesthetics)	Additive or supraadditive CNS and respiratory depression; use local anesthetic cautiously and in reduced maximum doses.
β-adrenergic blockers (nonselective)	May cause hypertension and bradycardia with vasoconstrictor; monitor patient and use vasoconstrictor cautiously.
CNS stimulants (amphetamine) and ergot derivatives (dihydroergotamine)	May cause hypertension with vasoconstrictor; monitor patient and use vasoconstrictor cautiously.
Cocaine	May increase cardiovascular responses to vasoconstrictor; avoid vasoconstrictor use in patient under influence of cocaine.
COMT inhibitors (entacapone)	Inhibition of metabolism may enhance systemic effects of vasoconstrictor; monitor patient and use vasoconstrictor cautiously.
Digoxin	May increase risk of cardiac dysrhythmias; use vasoconstrictor in consultation with physician.
Hydrocarbon inhalation anesthetics (halothane)	May cause cardiac dysrhythmias with vasoconstrictors; consult anesthesiologist about vasoconstrictor use.
Levodopa and thyroid hormones (levothyroxine)	Large doses (beyond replacement doses of thyroid hormone) may increase risk of cardiac toxicity; use vasoconstrictor cautiously.
Methyldopa and adrenergic neuron blockers (guanadrel)	May enhance systemic effects of vasoconstrictor; use vasoconstrictor cautiously.
Tricyclic (imipramine) and heterocyclic (amoxapine) antidepressants	May strongly enhance systemic effects of levonordefrin; avoid concurrent use.

Prilocaine Hydrochloride (Citanest Plain)

Acetaminophen, acetanilid, aniline dyes, benzocaine, chloroquine, dapsone, naphthalene, nitrates and nitrites, nitrofurantoin, nitroglycerin, nitroprusside, pamaquine, para-aminosalicylic acid, phenacetin, phenobarbital, phenytoin, primaquine, quinine, and sulfonamides	Increased risk for developing methemoglobinemia; use prilocaine in reduced maximum doses.
Amiodarone, β-adrenergic blockers, cimetadine	Hepatic metabolism may be decreased; use local anesthetic cautiously, especially regarding repeat dosing.
Antidysrhythmic agents (class I)	Additive CNS and cardiac toxicity; use local anesthetic cautiously and in reduced maximum doses.
CNS depressants (including alcohol, opioids, antidepressants, and other local anesthetics)	Additive or supraadditive CNS and respiratory depression; use local anesthetic cautiously and in reduced maximum doses.

Prilocaine Hydrochloride w/ Epinephrine (Citanest Forte)	
α-adrenergic blockers (prazosin), butyrophenones (haloperidol) and phenothiazines (thioridazine)	May reduce or reverse pressor effect of epinephrine (large doses only); use vasoconstrictor cautiously.
Acetaminophen, acetanilid, aniline dyes, benzocaine, chloroquine, dapsone, naphthalene, nitrates and nitrites, nitrofurantoin, nitroglycerin, nitroprusside, pamaquine, para-aminosalicylic acid, phenacetin, phenobarbital, phenytoin, primaquine, quinine, and sulfonamides	Increased risk for developing methemoglobinemia; use prilocaine in reduced maximum doses.
Amiodarone, β-adrenergic blockers, cimetadine	Hepatic metabolism may be decreased; use local anesthetic cautiously, especially regarding repeat dosing.
Antidysrhythmic agents (class I)	Additive CNS and cardiac toxicity; use local anesthetic cautiously and in reduced maximum doses.
β-adrenergic blockers (nonselective)	May cause hypertension and bradycardia with vasoconstrictor; monitor patient and use vasoconstrictor cautiously.
CNS depressants (including alcohol, opioids, antidepressants, and other local anesthetics)	Additive or supraadditive CNS and respiratory depression; use cautiously and in reduced maximum doses.
CNS stimulants (amphetamine) and ergot derivatives (dihydroergotamine)	May cause hypertension with vasoconstrictor; monitor patient and use vasoconstrictor cautiously.
Cocaine	May increase cardiovascular responses to vasoconstrictor; avoid vasoconstrictor use in patient under influence of cocaine.
COMT inhibitors (entacapone)	Inhibition of metabolism may enhance systemic effects of vasoconstrictor; monitor patient and use vasoconstrictor cautiously.
Digoxin	May increase risk of cardiac dysrhythmias; use vasoconstrictor in consultation with physician.
Hydrocarbon inhalation anesthetics (halothane)	May cause cardiac dysrhythmias with vasoconstrictors; consult anesthesiologist about vasoconstrictor use.
Levodopa and thyroid hormones (levothyroxine)	Large doses (beyond replacement doses of thyroid hormone) may increase risk of cardiac toxicity; use vasoconstrictor cautiously.
Methyldopa and adrenergic neuron blockers (guanadrel)	May enhance systemic effects of vasoconstrictor; use vasoconstrictor cautiously.
Tricyclic (imipramine) and heterocyclic (amoxapine) antidepressants	May enhance systemic effects of epinephrine; use vasoconstrictor cautiously and in reduced maximum dosages.

Table 1.3: LOCAL ANESTHETICS: POTENTIAL CROSS-SENSITIVITY WITH OTHER DRUGS

A PERSON WITH A SENSITIVITY TO	MAY ALSO HAVE A SENSITIVITY TO
Para-aminobenzoic acid (PABA) or paraben preservative	Procaine, chloroprocaine, benzocaine, butamben, tetracaine, other local anesthetic solutions containing paraben preservatives (as in multidose vials) other local anesthetic solutions containing paraben preservatives (as in multidose vials)
Any ester local anesthetic	Other ester local anesthetics
Any amide local anesthetic	Other amide local anesthetics (rarely)
Sulfites	Any local anesthetic with an adrenergic vasoconstrictor (sulfites are included with vasoconstrictors as antioxidants)

Table 1.4: TOPICAL ANESTHETICS: DURATION OF ACTION

DRUG	DURATION OF ANESTHETIC ACTION
Benzocaine	10-20 min
Cocaine	20-40 min
Dyclonine	20-40 min
Lidocaine	10-20 min*
Tetracaine	20-60 min

*Duration can be extended up to 45 min if lidocaine transoral delivery patch is applied for 15 min.

Table 1.5: PRESCRIBING INFORMATION FOR TOPICAL LOCAL ANESTHETICS

NAME	FORM/STRENGTH	DOSAGE	WARNINGS/PRECAUTIONS & CONTRAINDICATIONS	ADVERSE EFFECTS
Benzocaine	**Cre:** Benzocaine 5%, Orajel PM Maximum Strength 20%; **Gel:** HDA Toothache 6.5%, Baby Anbesol 7.5%, Baby Oral Pain Reliever 7.5%, Dentane 7.5%, Orajel Baby Happy Smiles Kit 7.5%, Orajel Baby Teething Medication 7.5%, Orajel 10%, Orajel Baby Nightime Teething Baby Medicine 10%, Zilactin Baby Extra Strength 10%, Zilactin-B 10%, Orajel Denture Plus 15%, Orajel Ultra Mouth Sore 15%, Americaine Anesthetic Lubricant 20%, Anbesol Maximum Strength 20%, Comfortcaine 20%, Darby Super-Dent Benzocaine Topical Anesthetic Gel★, Dentsply Benzocaine Oral Anesthetic Gel 20%★, Dentapaine 20%, Gingicaine 20%★, Hurricaine 20%★, Kank-A Soft Brush 20%, Lubricant 20%, Oral Anesthetic 20%, Orabase-B 20%★, Orajel Maximum Strength 20%, Orajel Mouth-Aid 20%, Patterson 20%★, Topex 20%★, Topicale 20%★; **Gel patch:** Topicale GelPatch 36mg/patch; **Gum:** Dent's Extra Strength Toothache 20%; **Liq:** Orasept 1.53%, Gumsol 2%, Babee Teething Lotion 2.5%, Rid-A-Pain 6.3%, Miradyne-3 (9%), Tanac Liquid 10%, Anbesol Maximum Strength 20%, Dent's Maxi-Strength Toothache Drops 20%, Gingicaine 20%★, Hurricaine 20%★, Kank-A 20%★, Topex 20%★; **Loz:** Chloraseptic Sore Throat 6 mg, Cepacol Extra Strength 10mg, Spec-T 10mg, Bi-Zets 15mg; **Oint:** Anacaine 10%, Benzodent 20%★, CoraCaine 20%★, Red Cross Canker 20%, Topicale 20%★; **Paste:** Orabase-B with Benzcocaine 20%★; **Spray:** Americaine 20%, Hurricaine 20%★, Topex 20%★; **Swab:** Orajel Baby Teething Swabs 7.5%, Dentemp's Oral Pain Relief 20%, Gingicaine One SwabStick 20%★, Hurricane 20%, Orajel Medicated Mouthsore Swab 20%, Orajel Medicated Toothache Swab 20%, Topex 20%, Zilactin Toothache Maximum Strength 20%	**(Cre) Adults:** Apply to affected area up to 4 times daily or as directed. **Pediatrics: <2 yrs:** Dose must be individualized by dentist or physician. **(Gel) Adults:** Apply to affected area up to 4 times daily or as directed. **Pediatrics: <4 mo:** Nonprescription teething products should not be used. **<2 yrs:** Dosages of all benzocaine products for children under 2 yrs should be individualized based on child's age, weight and physical status. **(Gel Patch)** Apply to affected area up to 4 times daily or as directed. **(Gum)** Clean tooth cavity by rinsing with warm water; then cut gum to fit and press into cavity. **(Liq) Adults:** Apply to affected area up to 4 times daily or as directed. **Pediatrics: <2 yrs:** Dosages for children should be individualized based on child's age, weight and physical status. **(Loz) Adults:** Dissolve 1 lozenge no more frequently than every 2 hrs. **Pediatrics: 2-12 yrs:** Varies by individual product. **(Oint) Adults:** Apply to affected area up to 4 times daily or as directed. **(Paste) Adults:** Apply to affected area up to 4 times daily or as directed. **Pediatrics: < 6 yrs:** Dose must be individualized by dentist or physician. **(Spray) Adults:** Spray should be applied for 1 sec or less for normal anesthesia. Spray in excess of 2 sec is contraindicated. **(Swab)** Apply to affected area up to 4 times daily or as directed.	**W/P:** Patients with a history of allergy to local anesthetics such as procaine, butacaine, benzocaine or other "caine" anesthetics should be instructed not to use these products. Methemoglobinemia (rare) has been reported with benzocaine-containing products, especially with unmetered spray formulations. Benzocaine sprays should not exceed 2 sec in total. Avoid contact with eyes. Patients should be instructed that fever and nasal congestion are not symptoms of teething and may indicate the presence of infection. Patient should not use for more than 7 days unless directed to. Patients should be instructed to alert dentist or physician if sore mouth symptoms do not get better in 7 days; irritation, pain, or redness does not go away; or swelling, rash or fever develops. Keep out of reach of children. **Contra:** Hypersensitivity to benzocaine/ester-type local anesthetics. **P/N:** Category C, caution in nursing.	Burning, stinging, swelling, skin rash, redness, itching, or hives in or around the mouth; methemoglobinemia, dizziness, tiredness, headache or weakness.
Benzocaine, Butambin and Tetracaine Hydrochloride	**Gel:** Cetacaine Hospital 14%/2%/2%; **Sol:** Cetacaine 14%/2%/2%★; **Spray:** Cetacaine 14%/2%/2%★	**(Gel) Adults:** Apply up to 1mL to affected area. **(Sol) Adults:** Apply up to 1mL to affected area. **(Spray) Adults:** Spray up to 1mL (or 2 sec) on affected area.	**W/P:** Patients with a history of allergy to ester local anesthetics such as procaine, butacaine, benzocaine or tetracaine should be instructed not to use these products. Methemoglobinemia (rare) has been reported with benzocaine-containing products, especially with unmetered spray formulations. Sprays should not exceed 2 sec in total. Avoid inhalation, which could result in rapid absorption and systemic toxicity.	Burning, stinging, swelling or tenderness not present before treatment; skin rash, redness, itching or hives in or around the mouth; methemoglobinemia, dizziness, tiredness, headache, weakness or

★indicates a drug bearing the ADA Seal of Acceptance.

NAME	FORM/ STRENGTH	DOSAGE	WARNINGS/PRECAUTIONS & CONTRAINDICATIONS	ADVERSE EFFECTS
Benzocaine, Butambin and Tetracaine Hydrochloride *(cont.)*			Do not exceed recommended dose. Keep out of the reach of children. Avoid contact with eyes. **Contra:** Hypersensitivity to ester-type local anesthetics. **P/N:** Category C, caution in nursing.	lightheadedness; nervousness, confusion, euphoria, dizziness, drowsiness, blurred vision, tremors, convulsions, respiratory depression, bradycardia or hypotension.
Dyclonine Hydrochloride	**Loz:** Sucrets Children's 1.2mg, Sucrets Regular Strength 2mg, Sucrets Maximum Strength 3mg; **Sol:** Dyclone 1%; **Spray:** Cepacol Sore Throat, Maximum Strength 0.1%	***Adults:*** Dissolve 1 lozenge slowly no more than once every 2 hrs up to a maximum of 10 lozenges per day. ***Pediatrics:*** **2-12 yrs:** Limit dose to 1.2 mg/lozenge. **(Sol)** ***Adults:*** Apply up to 300mg (30mL) to affected area per examination. May be used after dilution to a 0.5% concentration as a mouthwash or gargle and the excess expelled. **(Spray)** ***Adults:*** Spray up to 4 times per use no more frequently than 4 uses per day. ***Pediatrics:*** **3-12 yrs:** Spray up to 3 times per use no more frequently than 4 uses per day.	**W/P:** Reduce dose in elderly, debilitated, acutely ill. Increased likelihood for local or systemic reactions when applied to traumatized mucosa or areas with sepsis Caution with heart block and severe shock. Excessive dose or too-frequent administration may result in high plasma levels and serious adverse effects requiring resuscitative measures. Dosing not established in children under 12 yrs. **P/N:** Category C, caution in nursing.	Lightheadedness, nervousness, confusion, euphoria, dizziness, drowsiness, blurred vision, tremors, convulsions, respiratory depression, bradycardia, hypotension, edema, irritation, stinging, swelling, urticaria.
Lidocaine	**Oint:** Octacaine 5%, Xylocaine 5%★; **Patch:** DentiPatch 46.1mg; **Sol:** Zilactin-L 2.5%	**(Oint)** ***Adults:*** Apply to affected area or denture up to a maximum of 5g ointment (250mg lidocaine) in 6 hrs. ***Pediatrics:*** Limit dose to 4.5mg/kg body weight (lidocaine) or 2.5g of ointment in 6 hrs. **(Patch)** ***Adults:*** Apply single patch. **(Sol)** ***Adults:*** Apply to perioral area every 1-2 hrs with a cotton swab as needed.	**W/P:** Reduce dose in elderly, debilitated, acutely ill, and pediatrics. Caution with heart block and severe shock. Excessive dose or too-frequent administration may result in high plasma levels and serious adverse effects requiring resuscitative measures. Extreme caution if mucosa traumatized; risk of rapid systemic absorption. Overdose reported in pediatrics due to inappropriate dosing. **Contra:** Hypersensitivity amide-local anesthetics. **P/N:** Category B, caution in nursing.	Lightheadedness, nervousness, confusion, euphoria, dizziness, drowsiness, blurred vision, tremors, convulsions, respiratory depression, bradycardia, hypotension, urticaria, edema, and anaphylactoid reactions.
Lidocaine Hydrochloride	**Gel:** Xylocaine Jelly 2%; **Oral Topical Sol:** Xylocaine Viscous 2%; **Sol:** Xylocaine 4%	**(Gel)** Apply to affected area up to a maximum of 4.5mg/kg or 300mg lidocaine. **(Oral Topical Sol)** ***Adults:*** Apply to affected area or swish or gargle and then expectorate, using up to a maximum dose of 4.5mg/kg or 300mg lidocaine every 3 hrs. ***Pediatrics:*** ≤ **3 yrs:** Apply up to 1.25mL solution (25mg lidocaine) every 3 hrs. **(Sol)** Apply to affected area up to a maximum of 4.5mg/kg or 300mg lidocaine.	**W/P:** Reduce dose in elderly, debilitated, acutely ill, and pediatrics. Caution with heart block and severe shock. Excessive dose or too-frequent administration may result in high plasma levels and serious adverse effects requiring resuscitative measures. Extreme caution if mucosa traumatized; risk of rapid systemic absorption. Overdose reported in pediatrics due to inappropriate dosing. **Contra:** Hypersensitivity to amide-local anesthetics. **P/N:** Category B, caution in nursing.	Lightheadedness, nervousness, confusion, euphoria, dizziness, drowsiness, blurred vision, tremors, convulsions, respiratory depression, bradycardia, hypotension, urticaria, edema, and anaphylactoid reactions.
Lidocaine and Prilocaine Periodontal Gel (Oraqix)	**Gel:** 2.5%/2.5%	***Adults:*** Apply Oraqix on the gingival margin around selected teeth using blunt-tipped applicator included with package. Wait 30 sec, then fill periodontal pockets with Oraqix using blunt-tipped applicator until gel becomes	**W/P:** Allergic reactions, including anaphylaxis, can occur. Elevated methemoglobin levels. Patients with elevated methemoglobin levels, glucose-6-phosphate dehydrogenase deficiency or congenital or idiopathic methemoglobinemia should	Pain, soreness, irritation, numbness, vesicles, ulcerations, edema and/or redness in the treated area, headache, taste

Table 1.5: PRESCRIBING INFORMATION FOR TOPICAL LOCAL ANESTHETICS *(cont.)*

NAME	FORM/ STRENGTH	DOSAGE	WARNINGS/PRECAUTIONS & CONTRAINDICATIONS	ADVERSE EFFECTS
Lidocaine and Prilocaine Periodontal Gel *(cont.)*		visible at the gingival margin. Wait another 30 sec before starting treatment. Maximum 8.5g gel per treatment session.	not use Oraqix. Oraqix should not be used with standard dental syringes. Only use this product with the Oraqix Dispenser. **Contra:** Hypersensitivity to amide-local anesthetics. **P/N:** Category B, caution in nursing women.	alteration, nausea, fatigue, flu, respiratory infection, musculoskeletal pain and accidental injury.
Tetracaine Hydrochloride (Pontocaine)	**Sol:** 2%	***Adults:*** Apply as a a 0.25% or 0.5% topical solution or as a 0.5% nebulized spray; total dosage not to exceed 20mg.	**W/P:** Patients should be instructed not use tetracaine if they have a history of allergy to ester local anesthetics such as procaine, butacaine or benzocaine. Avoid contact with eyes. Do not exceed recommended dose. Caution with heart block and severe shock. Excessive dose or too-frequent administration may result in high plasma levels and serious adverse effects requiring resuscitative measures. Keep out of the reach of children. **Contra:** Hypersensitivity to tetracaine/ester-type local anesthetics. **P/N:** Category C, caution in nursing.	Burning, stinging, swelling or tenderness not present before treatment; skin rash, redness, itching or hives; lightheadedness, nervousness, confusion, euphoria, dizziness, drowsiness, blurred vision, tremors, convulsions, respiratory depression, bradycardia, hypotension.

Chapter 2

Conscious Sedation and Agents for the Control of Anxiety

B. Ellen Byrne, R.Ph., D.D.S., Ph.D.;
Leonard S. Tibbetts, D.D.S., M.S.D.

All types of dental care—from that rendered with no anesthesia to treatment rendered under general anesthesia—require accurate diagnosis, proper treatment and effective patient monitoring. This involves obtaining a current complete medical history, performing a comprehensive examination and a thorough pretreatment evaluation.

Providing care and ensuring the well-being of patients in the dental office is based on a continuum of techniques that are available for the management of anxiety and pain. This chapter focuses on the calming of apprehensive and/or nervous patients through the use of drugs, without causing the loss of consciousness.

Using various techniques to control anxiety and pain has been an integral part of the practice of dentistry since the profession's early years. Today, the term "conscious sedation" is used to describe the amelioration of patient anxiety, the blunting of the stress response and often some degree of amnesia produced by a combination of psychological techniques and drugs. Unfortunately, the term "intravenous sedation" means general anesthesia to much of the public and to many medical and dental professionals. When properly understood, the term "conscious sedation," coined by dentist/anesthesiologist Richard Bennett in the 1970s, does much to alleviate this misconception. Conscious sedation is a minimally depressed level of consciousness in which the patient retains the ability to independently and continuously maintain an airway—as well as to respond appropriately to physical stimulation or verbal command—that can be produced by a pharmacological or nonpharmacological method or both.

Examples of nonpharmacological methods used for anxiety and pain management are hypnosis, acupuncture, acupressure, audio-analgesia, biofeedback, electroanesthesia (transcutaneous electrical nerve stimulation) and electrosedation.

Appropriately trained dentists may use any of a number of preoperative and operative pharmacological conscious sedation techniques to achieve the goals of anxiety reduction and pain control. Such techniques may include sedation by enteral (absorption by way of the alimentary canal), inhalation (absorption into the lungs) and parenteral (introduction via subcutaneous, intramuscular, intraorbital or intravenous routes) means.

Each category of pharmacological conscious sedation has specific educational and monitoring requirements for safe, effective and efficacious patient usage, as well as specific licensing requirements mandated by regulatory agencies. The use of conscious sedation techniques in the various categories by appropriately trained dentists has a remarkable safety record. (For further information, consult the American Dental Association's Policy Statement "The Use of Conscious Sedation, Deep Sedation and General Anesthesia in Dentistry," as adopted by the ADA House of Delegates in October 1999, and the "Guidelines for Teaching the Comprehensive Control of Anxiety and Pain in Dentistry," as adopted by the ADA Council on Dental Education and Licensure in October 2002.)

Whatever the methods of conscious sedation in which dentists strive to be educationally and professionally competent, the use of a wide array of drugs for various types of conscious sedation is contraindicated without an adequately detailed working knowledge about them. In fact, using as few drugs as possible to appropriately and adequately sedate patients is advised as the dentist can become intimately familiar with a limited number of drugs, their pharmacological actions, indications, contraindications, precautions and drug interactions.

Intravenous conscious sedation induced in the dental office, for example, can be handled almost entirely by a combination of the following five drugs, which fall into these three classes:

- benzodiazepines—diazepam, midazolam;
- sedatives—pentobarbital;
- narcotic analgesics—morphine, meperidine.

Today, the most common pharmacological method of controlling anxiety with intravenous sedation is through the use of one of the benzodiazepines in combination with a narcotic analgesic. The benzodiazepines are used to reduce the apprehension and fear, as well as to provide an amnesia effect, while the narcotics produce analgesia and euphoria. The sedative pentobarbital, in combination with meperidine, can be used when there are contraindications to the use of the benzodiazepines.

Administration routes. Of the various administration routes for conscious sedation drugs, each has advantages and disadvantages.

The oral route is most commonly used, and it has the advantages of almost universal acceptance by patients, ease of administration and relative safety. Its disadvantages include its requirement of a bolus dosage of medication, based on the patient's weight and age; its long latent period; its unreliable absorption; its inability to be titrated due to the long latency period; and its prolonged duration of action.

Titration of oral medication for the purpose of sedation, therefore, is unpredictable. Repeated dosing of orally administered sedative agents may result in an alteration in the state of consciousness beyond the practitioner's intent. Except in unusual circumstances, the maximum recommended dose of an oral medication should not be exceeded.

The rectal route of administration is used in dentistry only occasionally, when patients are either unwilling or unable to take the drugs by mouth. This route's advantages and disadvantages are similar to those of oral administration.

Another option is the combined inhalation-enteral route of conscious sedation. The advantages of using this combination include greater patient acceptance and a higher degree of effectiveness than either technique offers individually. The disadvantage is that the dentist must be proficient in the pharmacology of agents used in the management of both inhalation and enteral sedation—drug interactions and incompatibilities, problems and complications—as well as in making the distinction between the conscious and unconscious state and in clinical airway management.

All other routes of drug administration bypass the gastrointestinal system. In these routes, the drugs are absorbed directly by the body from the site of administration into the cardiovascular system. This includes inhalation and parenteral routes of administration. In dentistry, nitrous oxide and oxygen sedation are synonymous with inhalation sedation. The advantages of inhalation conscious sedation with nitrous oxide and oxygen are that the observed latent period is short, the administrator can titrate the agent appropriately, actions of the agent can be quickly adjusted to decrease or increase the depth of sedation, and recovery is rapid. The disadvantage is that the nitrous oxide–oxygen combination, with no less than a 70:30 ratio, is not a very potent agent, and a certain proportion of patients will not experience the desired effect.

The subcutaneous (SC) route of administration is used primarily in pediatric dentistry. It offers advantages and disadvantages similar to those of intramuscular (IM) administration as compared with enteral administration. Compared with enteral administration, both SC and IM administrations offer more rapid onset of action, as well as a more pronounced clinical effect with the same dosage. The SC route is useful for injecting nonvolatile, water- and fat-soluble hypnotic and narcotic drugs. The relatively poor blood supply of subcutaneous tissues, however, limits the effectiveness of this technique. For the uncooperative pediatric patient, both SC and IM techniques require a short period of restraint during administration. The major disadvantage of both techniques is the inability to titrate the medications accurately, so typically a bolus dosage is administered based on the patient's age and size. It is also impossible to retrieve the dosage should overdosage occur. For this reason, proper patient monitoring is extremely important, so complications can be intercepted early.

Intravenous (IV) conscious sedation represents the most effective method of acquiring adequate and predictable sedation in virtually all patients, with the exception of disruptive patients, whose cooperation is needed for successful venipuncture. IV conscious sedation allows effective

blood levels of drugs to be achieved rapidly with titration (the incremental administration of small drug dosages over appropriate time intervals until the desired level of sedation is achieved) and rapidly enhances the action of a drug. For many IV-administered drugs, the desired and maximum clinical sedative effects are reached within 2 to 8 minutes. Some of the currently available drugs for anxiety reduction are capable of producing an amnesia effect in 80% to 90% of patients for 20 to 40 minutes after administration.

While it is possible with the use of specific antagonists to reverse the actions of some medications in conscious sedation, it is not possible to reverse the action of all drugs after they have been injected. The rapid onset of action and the pronounced clinical actions of intravenously injected drugs will result in exaggerated problems with overdosage. This means the entire dental office staff must be well-trained in the recognition and management of adverse reactions and emergencies that may accompany the drugs used so that patient safety and quality dental care are never compromised.

Records and monitoring. Written, advised, informed consent for all forms of conscious sedation is essential. The standard of care for physiological and vital-sign monitoring for the various types of conscious sedation is well-established, as is that for documentation of drugs used, dosage, adverse reactions to medications and recovery from the anesthetic.

State-of-the-art monitoring of patients' vital signs has improved dramatically in the past several years. Pulse rate, blood pressure and respiration now can be monitored either physically or electronically. Today, pulse oximetry offers a rapid and effective means of monitoring the blood oxygen saturation and pulse rate and should be used for all methods of conscious sedation, including oral conscious sedation. These methods, in combination with the old standbys of close patient observation and conversation, are the current standards of monitoring care for patients in ASA Class I and II (healthy or with mild-to-moderate systemic disease) who are undergoing any type of parenteral conscious sedation or inhalation-enteral conscious sedation. In the treatment of patients of ASA Class III (with severe systemic disease that limits activity) or higher (ranging from IV, with severe life-threatening systemic disease, to VI, clinically dead but being maintained for harvesting of organs), electrocardiogram monitoring also becomes the standard of care, in addition to the other means of monitoring.

This chapter covers the drugs most frequently used in dental conscious sedation (benzodiazepines and their antagonist flumazenil, barbiturates, opioids and their antagonist naloxone). It also addresses older, less frequently used drugs: chloral hydrate, ethchlorvynol and meprobamate.

Benzodiazepines

The benzodiazepines are among the most popular classes of drugs available today, having been used since the late 1950s for effective and safe treatment of a variety of anxiety states, as well as for epilepsy (diazepam, clonazepam) and sleep disorders (flurazepam, temazepam, triazolam). Along with their use in anxiety, the benzodiazepines have extensive clinical applications in anesthesia procedures (diazepam, midazolam) and as muscle relaxants (diazepam). In addition, triazolam is increasing in popularity as oral/sublingual premedication prescribed by dentists for anxious patients. Recent anecdotal reports suggest that incremental dosing of triazolam maybe an effective technique for producing conscious sedation in the dental setting. While showing promise, no laboratory or clinical data are available to evaluate the efficacy or safety of this approach.

Although the benzodiazepines have a wide margin of safety, they are not without adverse effects. Their time course of action is variable among patients as well as among various agents. Although all benzodiazepines are effective, there are significant differences among them. When used enterally, diazepam and flurazepam are among the most rapidly absorbed, whereas oxazepam is one of the most slowly absorbed. Use of IM routes of administration for benzodiazepines often results in erratic and poor absorption. Most of the benzodiazepines are poorly soluble in water and are not available for IV use. Diazepam and midazolam, however, are the two agents most commonly used for IV conscious sedation, and an anterograde amnesia is strongly associated with this class of drugs. The level of amnesia varies with agent and route of administration.

All benzodiazepines in use are bound 50% or more to plasma proteins. Their distribution to tissue depends on their lipid solubility.

The metabolism and excretion of the benzodiazepines are complex. Clorazepate is a pro-drug converted by metabolism to the active form; others are inactivated by metabolism; still others are biotransferred to metabolites that retain activity. Many of the metabolites of benzodiazepines have longer half-lives than the parent compound and so accumulate to a greater extent. It is important to recognize that some of these compounds have the potential for extremely long durations of action. Thus, benzodiazepine half-lives vary from a few hours to as long as a week.

The imidazopyridine sedative hypnotic zolpidem is included in this section of the chapter because, although it is structurally dissimilar to the benzodiazepines, many of its actions are explained by its action on the benzodiazepine receptor.

Antagonist. The benzodiazepines have a specific antagonist, flumazenil, that is administered intravenously. It reverses the CNS effects of benzodiazepines, including respiratory depression. Its duration of action may be as brief as 30 minutes, so treatment with it requires continuous monitoring of the patient and possibly repeated administration.

Accepted Indications

Benzodiazepines are used for the treatment of anxiety, insomnia, epilepsy, panic disorders and alcohol withdrawal. As adjuncts in anesthesia, they are used as a preanesthetic medication to produce sedation, relieve anxiety and produce anterograde amnesia.

General Dosing Information

All benzodiazepines have similar pharmacologic actions. Their different clinical uses are often based on pharmacokinetic differences and availability of clinical use data. Optimal dosage of benzodiazepines varies with diagnosis, method of administration and patient response. The minimum effective dose should be used for the shortest period of time. Prolonged enteral use (for weeks or months) may result in psychological or physical dependence. After prolonged administration, benzodiazepines should be withdrawn gradually to prevent withdrawal symptoms.

For parenteral dosing, after administration of the drug, patients should be kept under observation until they have recovered sufficiently to return home. Bolus doses and rapidly administered IV doses may result in respiratory depression, apnea, hypotension, bradycardia and cardiac arrest. When parenteral benzodiazepines are administered intravenously, equipment necessary to secure and maintain an airway should be immediately available.

Table 2.1 provides benzodiazepine dosing information.

Dosage Adjustments

Geriatric or debilitated patients, children and patients with hepatic or renal function impairment should receive a lower initial dosage, as elimination of benzodiazepines may be slower in these patients, resulting in impaired coordination, dizziness and excessive sedation.

Special Dental Considerations

Drug Interactions of Dental Interest

Table 2.2 lists possible interactions of the benzodiazepines and zolpidem with other drugs.

Cross-Sensitivity

There may be cross-sensitivity between benzodiazepines.

Special Patients

Pregnant and nursing women
See Table 2.1 for pregnancy risk categories.

Benzodiazepines are reported to increase the risk of congenital malformations when used during the first trimester; chronic use may cause physical dependence in the neonate, resulting in withdrawal symptoms and CNS depression.

Benzodiazepines and their metabolites may distribute into breast milk, thus creating feeding difficulties and weight loss in the infant.

Pediatric, geriatric and other special patients
Children (especially the very young) and geriatric patients are usually more sensitive to the CNS effects of benzodiazepines. In the neonate, prolonged CNS depression may be produced because of the newborn's inability to metabolize the benzodiazepine into inactive products. In the geriatric patient, the dosage should be limited to the smallest effective dose and increased gradually to minimize ataxia, dizziness and oversedation.

Patient Monitoring: Aspects to Watch
- Respiratory status
- Patient requests for benzodiazepines (all of which are Schedule IV controlled substances in the United States)
- Possible abuse and dependence

Adverse Effects and Precautions
Table 2.1 lists adverse effects, precautions and contraindications related to benzodiazepines.

Pharmacology
Benzodiazepines depress all levels of the CNS, resulting in mild sedation, hypnosis or coma, depending on the dose. It is believed that benzodiazepines enhance or facilitate the inhibitory neurotransmitter action of γ-aminobutyric acid (GABA). After oral administration, benzodiazepines are absorbed well from the gastrointestinal tract. After IM injection, absorption of lorazepam and midazolam is rapid and complete, whereas that of chlordiazepoxide and diazepam may be slow and erratic. Rectal absorption of diazepam is rapid. The benzodiazepines are metabolized by the liver to inactive or other active metabolites. During repeated dosing with long half-life benzodiazepines, there is accumulation of the parent compound and/or active metabolites. During repeated dosing with short to intermediate half-life benzodiazepines, accumulation is minimal.

Patient Advice
- Avoid concurrent use of alcohol and other CNS depressants.
- Until CNS effects are known, avoid activities needing good psychomotor skills.
- A responsible adult should drive the patient to and from dental appointments.
- Recurrent use of these drugs may cause physical or psychological dependence.
- Benzodiazepines may cause xerostomia, which can be countered using sugarless candy, sugarless gum or a commercially available saliva substitute.

Benzodiazepine Antagonist: Flumazenil

Accepted Indications
Flumazenil is used to reverse the pharmacological effects of benzodiazepines used in anesthesia and to manage benzodiazepine overdose.

General Dosing Information
Flumazenil selectively reverses the pharmacologic effects of benzodiazepines used in anesthesia and is used to manage benzodiazepine overdose. Flumazenil does not antagonize other CNS depressants except for zolpidem. See Table 2.1.

Special Dental Considerations

Drug Interactions of Dental Interest
Table 2.2 lists the possible interactions of flumazenil with other drugs.

Cross-Sensitivity
There may be cross-sensitivity to benzodiazepines.

Special Patients
Pregnant and nursing women
Caution should be used in administering flumazenil to a nursing woman because it is not known whether flumazenil is excreted in human milk.

Pediatric, geriatric and other special patients
Flumazenil is not recommended for use in children, either for the reversal of sedation, the management of overdose or resuscitation of newborns. Pulmonary management is advised as the treatment of choice.

The pharmacokinectics of flumazenil have been studied in elderly people and are not significantly different from those in younger patients.

Patient Monitoring: Aspects to Watch

- Respiratory status
- Patient alertness
- Possible resedation
- Possible seizure activity

Adverse Effects and Precautions

Table 2.1 lists adverse effects, precautions and contraindications related to flumazenil.

Pharmacology

Flumazenil, an imidazobenzodiazepine derivative, antagonizes the actions of benzodiazepines on the CNS. Flumazenil competitively inhibits the activity at the benzodiazepine recognition site on the benzodiazepine-GABA receptor-chloride ionophore complex. Flumazenil is a weak partial agonist in some animal models of activity, but has little or no agonist activity in humans.

The onset of reversal is usually evident 1 to 2 minutes after the injection is completed. Eighty percent response will be reached within 3 minutes, with peak effect occurring at 6 to 10 minutes. The duration and degree of reversal are related to the plasma concentration of the sedating benzodiazepine as well as the dose of flumazenil given. Resedation is possible if a large single or cumulative dose of benzodiazepine has been given in the course of a long procedure and is least likely in cases where flumazenil is administered to reverse a low dose of a short-acting benzodiazepine.

Suggested Readings

American Dental Association. Guidelines for teaching the comprehensive control of anxiety and pain in dentistry. Adopted by the ADA House of Delegates, October 2002. Available at: www.ada.org/prof/ed/guidelines/index. html. Accessed March 31, 2003.

American Dental Association. Guidelines for the use of conscious sedation, deep sedation and general anesthesia for dentists. Adopted by the ADA House of Delegates, October 2002. Available at: "www.ada.org/prof/ed/guidelines/index.html". Accessed March 31, 2003.

American Dental Association. The use of conscious sedation, deep sedation and general anesthesia in dentistry. Adopted by the ADA House of Delegates, October 1999. Available at: www.ada.org/prof/ed/guidelines/cs-useof. html. Accessed March 31, 2003.

Giangrego E. Conscious sedation: benefits and risks. JADA 1984;109:546-57.

Jackson DL, Milgrom P, Heacox GA, Kharasch ED. Pharmacokinetics and clinical effects of multidose sublingual triazolam in healthy volunteers. J Clin Psychopharmacol 2006;26(1):4-8.

Kallar SK, Dunwiddie WC. In: Wetchler BV, ed. Problems in anesthesia. Philadelphia: JB Lippincott Co.; 1988:93-100.

Malamed SF. Sedation: A guide to patient management. 3rd ed., St. Louis: Mosby; 1995.

Miller RD. Clinical Therapeutics 1992;14(Special Supplemental Section):861-995.

Barbiturates

The barbiturates were the first drugs truly effective for the management of anxiety. The barbiturates are generalized CNS depressants, depressing the cerebral cortex, the limbic system, and the reticular activating system. These actions produce reduction in anxiety level, decreased mental acuity and a state of drowsiness. Barbiturates are capable of producing any level of CNS depression, ranging from light sedation through hypnosis, general anesthesia, coma and death. IV barbiturate compounds can be infused in subhypnotic doses to produce sedation.

The barbiturates used for conscious sedation are classified as sedative hypnotics and are categorized by their duration of clinical action following an average oral dose.

Short-acting barbiturates (with 3 to 4 hour duration of action), most notably pentobarbital and secobarbital, are the barbiturates best suited for dental situations. The ultrashort-acting barbiturates are classified as general anesthetics and are contraindicated for conscious sedation. They are described in Chapter 3. The long-acting (16- to 24-hour duration of action) and the intermediate-acting (6- to 8-hour duration of action) barbiturates produce clinical levels of sedation for a period exceeding that required for the usual dental or surgical appointment. The long-acting barbiturates, such as phenobarbital, are commonly used as anticonvulsants or when long-term sedation is necessary. The intermediate-acting barbiturates occasionally are used as "sleeping pills" for some types of insomnia.

Accepted Indications

Barbiturates have been used in routine cases requiring conscious sedation to relieve anxiety, tension and apprehension; however, these agents have generally been replaced with the benzodiazepines for these treatments. Barbiturates are used as adjuncts in anesthesia to reduce anxiety and facilitate induction of anesthesia. They are also used in the treatment of epilepsy and insomnia.

General Dosing Information

IV dosage of the barbiturates must be titrated individually in all patients, particularly for patients with impaired hepatic function; a low dose should be used initially. Tolerance and physical dependence occurs with repeated administration. These agents are controlled substances in the United States and Canada. See Table 2.1.

Special Dental Considerations

Drug Interactions of Dental Interest

Possible drug interactions and/or related problems of clinical significance in dentistry are shown in Table 2.2.

Special Patients

Pregnant and nursing women

Barbiturates readily cross the placenta and increase the risk of fetal abnormalities. Use

during the third trimester may result in physical dependence and respiratory depression in newborns.

Barbiturates distribute into the breast milk and may cause CNS depression in the infant.

Patient Monitoring: Aspects to Watch

• Respiratory status

Adverse Effects and Precautions

Adverse effects and precautions related to barbiturates are listed in Table 2.2.

Pharmacology

Barbiturates can produce all levels of CNS mood alteration, from excitation to sedation, hypnosis and coma. In sufficient therapeutic doses, barbiturates induce anesthesia, and overdose can produce death. These agents depress the sensory cortex, decrease motor activity, alter cerebellar function and produce drowsiness, sedation and hypnosis. Barbiturates are respiratory depressants and the degree of respiratory depression is dose-dependent. All barbiturates exhibit anticonvulsant activity.

Barbiturates are enzyme-inducing drugs. This class of drugs can enhance the metabolism of other agents. The onset of this enzyme induction is gradual and depends on the accumulation of the barbiturate and the synthesis of the new enzyme, while offset depends on elimination of the barbiturate and decay of the increased enzyme stores.

Absorption varies depending on the route of administration: oral or rectal, 20 to 60 minutes; IM, slightly faster than oral or rectal routes; IV, immediate to 5 minutes. The sodium salts of the barbiturates are more rapidly absorbed than the free acids because they dissolve rapidly. The rate of absorption is increased if the agents are taken on an empty stomach. The barbiturates are weak acids and distribute rapidly to all tissues, with high concentrations initially in the brain, liver, lungs, heart and kidneys. The more lipid-soluble the drug, the more rapidly it penetrates all tissues of the body. The barbiturates are metabolized by the liver; phenobarbital is partially excreted unchanged in the urine.

Opioids

The term "opioid" is used in a broad sense to include both opioid agonists and opioid agonists/antagonists. The opioids are administered from their analgesic properties and are considered excellent drugs for the relief of moderate to severe pain. The parenteral dosage forms of this class of drugs are also used as general anesthesia adjuncts in conjunction with other drugs, such as the benzodiazepines, neuromuscular blocking agents and nitrous oxide for the maintenance of "balanced" anesthesia. Sufentanil, alfentanil and remifentanil are discussed in Chapter 3, as they are used most often in dentistry for deep sedation and general anesthesia. All opioid narcotic agents are classified as controlled substances in the U.S. and Canada. Opioids are classified into 3 types: agonists, antagonists and mixed agents. Agonists include codeine, fentanyl, hydrocodone, hydromorphone, levorphanol, meperidine, methadone, morphine, oxycodone and oxymorphone. Antagonists are naloxone and naltrexone. Mixed agents are buprenorphine, butorphanol, nalbuphine and pentazocine.

General Dosing Information

Narcotic drugs are used to produce mood changes, provide analgesia and elevate the pain threshold. Opioid analgesics may not provide sufficient analgesia when used with nitrous oxide for the maintenance of balance anesthesia. Narcotic agents can be used in combination with other agents such as benzodiazepines, antihistamines, ultrashort-acting barbiturates and a potent hydrocarbon inhalation anesthetic. Dosage and dosing intervals should be individualized for the patient based on duration of action of the specific drug, other medications the patient is currently taking, the patient's condition and the patient's response. See Table 2.1.

Special Dental Considerations

Drug Interactions of Dental Interest
Possible drug interactions of clinical significance in dentistry are shown in Table 2.2.

Laboratory Value Alterations
- Opioids delay gastric emptying, thereby invalidating gastric emptying studies.
- In hepatobiliary imaging, delivery of technetium Tc99m disofenin to the small bowel may be prevented because opioids may constrict sphincter of Oddi; this results in delayed visualization and resembles an obstruction in the common bile duct.
- Cerebrospinal fluid may be increased secondary to respiratory-depression–induced carbon dioxide retention.
- Plasma amylase activity may be increased.
- Plasma lipase activity may be increased.
- Serum alanine aminotransferase may be increased.
- Serum alkaline phosphatase may be increased.
- Serum aspartate aminotransferase may be increased.
- Serum bilirubin may be increased.
- Serum lactate dehydrogenase may be increased.

Cross-Sensitivity
Patients hypersensitive to fentanyl may be hypersensitive to the chemically related alfentanil or sufentanil.

Special Patients

Pregnant and nursing women
Risk-benefit must be considered because opioid analgesics cross the placenta.

Pediatric, geriatric and other special patients
Geriatric patients are more susceptible to the effects of opioids, especially respiratory depression. Clearance of opioid analgesics can be reduced in the geriatric patient, which leads to a delayed postoperative recovery. Children aged up to 2 years may be more susceptible to opioids' effects, especially respiratory depression. Paradoxical excitation is especially likely to occur in the pediatric population.

Patient Monitoring: Aspects to Watch

- Respiratory status
- State of consciousness
- Heart rate
- Blood pressure

Adverse Effects and Precautions

Table 2.1 lists adverse effects, precautions and contraindications related to opioids.

Pharmacology

Opioid analgesics bind to receptors within the central nervous system and peripheral nervous system. This interaction affects both the perception of pain and the emotional response to pain. There are at least five types of opioid receptors—mu (μ), kappa (K), sigma (σ), delta (Δ) and epsilon (ε)—located throughout the body that may be activated by exogenous or endogenous opioid-like substances (endorphins). The action of various opioids at the various receptors determine the agents' specific actions and side effects (see table above).

Based on their actions at these receptors, the commercially available opioids may be divided into three groups: pure agonists, pure antagonists and mixed agents (agonists/antagonists or partial agonists).

OPIOIDS: EFFECT ON TYPES OF NERVE RECEPTORS	
Receptor	**Effect**
mu$_1$ (μ_1)	Supraspinal analgesia.
mu$_2$ (μ_2)	Respiratory depression, bradycardia, hypothermia, euphoria, moderate sedation, physical dependence, miosis.
kappa (K)	Spinal analgesia, heavy sedation, miosis.
sigma (σ)	Dysphoria, tachycardia, tachypnea, mydriasis.
delta (Δ)	Modulation of μ receptor.
epsilon (ε)	Altered neurohumoral functions.

All opioids are respiratory depressants. By exerting a depressant action on respiratory center neurons in the medulla, they decrease respiratory rate, tidal volume and minute ventilation. They may increase arterial CO_2 tensions. All opioids affect the cardiovascular system by their actions on the autonomic nervous system. Hypotension may result from arteriolar and venous dilation as a result of either histamine release or decreased sympathetic nervous system tone. Bradycardia results from vagal stimulation. Finally, all opioids disorganize GI function, causing increased tone and muscle spasm but delayed emptying and decreased motility and secretions.

Opioid (Narcotic) Antagonist: Naloxone

Like the benzodiazepines, the opioids have a specific antagonist that reverses the pharmacologic effects caused by the opioid drugs.

Accepted Indications

Naloxone is used for the complete or partial reversal of narcotic depression, such as respiratory depression induced by opioids (including both natural and synthetic narcotics). Naloxone is also used for the diagnosis of suspected acute opioid overdose.

General Dosing Information

Varying amounts of naloxone may be needed to antagonize the effects of different agents. Lack of significant improvement of CNS depression and/or respiration after administration of an adequate dose (10 mg) of naloxone may indicate that the condition is due to a nonopioid CNS depressant. Naloxone reverses the analgesic effects of the opioid and may precipitate withdrawal symptoms in physically dependent patients. See Table 2.1 for dosage and prescribing information for naloxone.

Dosage Adjustments

Repeat dosing may be required within 1- or 2-hour intervals depending on the amount and type (short- or long-acting) of narcotic and the interval since the last administration of the narcotic. Supplemental IM doses can produce a long-lasting effect.

Special Dental Considerations

Drug Interactions of Dental Interest

Possible drug interactions of clinical significance in dentistry are shown in Table 2.2.

Special Patients

Pregnant and nursing women
Naloxone crosses the placenta and may precipitate withdrawal in the fetus as well as the mother. Breast-feeding problems in humans have not been documented.

Pediatric, geriatric and other special patients
Studies performed in pediatrics have not shown problems that would limit the usefulness of naloxone in children. Geriatric-specific problems do not seem to limit the usefulness of this medication in elderly patients.

Patient Monitoring: Aspects to Watch

- Cardiac status
- State of consciousness
- Respiratory status, oxygen saturation

Adverse Effects and Precautions

Adverse effects, precautions and contraindications related to naloxone are listed in Table 2.1.

Pharmacology

Naloxone reverses the CNS and respiratory depression associated with narcotic overdose. It also reverses postoperative opioid depression. Naloxone competes with and displaces narcotics at narcotic receptor sites.

Because of naloxone's short half-life, a continuous infusion may be required to maintain alertness. A patient should never be released soon after receiving naloxone because the ingested narcotic may have a longer half-life than naloxone, and its toxic effects—such as respiratory depression—may break through.

Chloral Hydrate

Chloral hydrate is an oral sedative-hypnotic that is used when providing dental treatment to the uncooperative preschool child.

Accepted Indications

Accepted indications for chloral hydrate are nocturnal sedation; preoperative sedation to lessen anxiety; in postoperative care and control of pain as an adjunct to opiates and analgesics.

General Dosing Information

Deaths have been associated with the use of chloral hydrate, especially in children. Repetitive dosing of chloral hydrate is not recommended owing to the accumulation of the active metabolite trichloroethylene. As with any sedation procedure, this sedative should be administered where there can be proper monitoring. Practitioners must know how to properly calculate and administer the appropriate dose. See Table 2.1.

Special Dental Considerations

Drug Interactions of Dental Interest
Drug interactions between chloral hydrate and other drugs are listed in Table 2.2.

Laboratory Value Alterations
- Chloral hydrate may interfere with the copper sulfate test for glucosuria (confirm suspected glucosuria by glucose oxidase test) and with fluorometric tests for urine catecholamines (do not administer chloral hydrate for 48 hours preceding the test).

Special Patients
Pregnant and nursing women
Chloral hydrate crosses the placenta, and chronic use of chloral hydrate during pregnancy may cause withdrawal symptoms in the neonate. In addition, chloral hydrate is distributed into breast milk; its use by nursing mothers may cause sedation in the infant.

Pediatric, geriatric and other special patients
Chloral hydrate is not recommended for use in infants and children in cases in which repeated dosing would be necessary. With repeated dosing, accumulation of trichloroethanol and trichloroacetic acid metabolites may increase the potential for excessive CNS depression.

No information is available on the relationship of age to the effects of chloral hydrate in geriatric patients. Elderly patients are more likely to have age-related hepatic function impairment and renal function impairment. Dose reduction may be required.

Patient Monitoring: Aspects to Watch
- Respiratory status
- Possible abuse and dependence
- Blood pressure

Adverse Effects and Precautions
Table 2.1 lists adverse effects, precautions and contraindications related to chloral hydrate.

Pharmacology
The mechanism of action of chloral hydrate is unknown; however, it is believed that the CNS depressant effects are due to its active metabolite, trichloroethanol. It is rapidly absorbed from the gastrointestinal tract after oral administration and is metabolized in red blood cells in the liver to the active metabolite. Its onset of action is usually within 30 minutes and its duration of action is 4-8 hours.

Patient Advice
- Swallow the capsule whole; do not chew because of unpleasant taste.
- Take with a full glass of water or juice to reduce gastric irritation.
- For syrup dose: Mix with glassful of juice or water to improve flavor and reduce gastric irritation.
- For suppository form: If too soft for insertion, chill suppository in refrigerator for 30 minutes before removing foil wrapper.

Meprobamate

Meprobamate is an antianxiety agent used for the management of anxiety disorders. It is not indicated for the treatment of anxiety or tension associated with everyday life. Prolonged use of meprobamate may decrease or inhibit salivary flow, thus contributing to the development of caries, periodontal disease, oral candidiasis and oral discomfort.

Accepted Indications
Meprobamate is used for management of anxiety disorders.

General Dosing Information

Dosing information for meprobamate is listed in Table 2.1.

Special Dental Considerations

Drug Interactions of Dental Interest

Drug interactions with meprobamate are listed in Table 2.2.

Cross-Sensitivity

Patients sensitive to other carbamate derivatives (carbromal, carisoprodol, mebutamate or tybamate) may be sensitive to this medication.

Special Patients

Pregnant and nursing women

Meprobamate crosses the placenta and has been associated with congenital malformations. It is excreted in the breast milk in a concentration of 2 to 4 times maternal plasma concentration and may cause sedation in the infant.

Pediatric, geriatric and other special patients

No pediatric-specific problems have been documented. Elderly patients are more sensitive to the effects of meprobamate.

Adverse Effects and Precautions

Adverse effects and precautions related to meprobamate are listed in Table 2.1.

Pharmacology

Mechanism of action of meprobamate is unknown. It is well absorbed from the gastrointestinal tract, with an onset of action within 1 hour.

Suggested Readings

Briggs GG, Freeman RK, Vaffe SJ. Drugs in pregnancy and lactation. 4th ed. Baltimore: Williams & Wilkins; 1994.

Jastak JT, Donaldson D. Nitrous oxide. Anesth Prog 1991;38:142-53.

Kallar SK, Dunwiddie WC. Problems in anesthesia: outpatient anesthesia. In: Wetchler BV, ed. Conscious sedation. Philadelphia: JB Lippincott Co.; 1988:93-100.

Malamed SF. Sedation: a guide to patient management. 3rd ed. St. Louis: Mosby; 1995.

Table 2.1: PRESCRIBING INFORMATION FOR CONSCIOUS SEDATION/ANTIANXIETY AGENTS

NAME	FORM/STRENGTH	DOSAGE	WARNINGS/PRECAUTIONS & CONTRAINDICATIONS	ADVERSE EFFECTS†
BARBITURATES				
Pentobarbital Sodium[CII] (Nembutal Sodium)	**Inj:** 50mg/mL	***Adults: Usual:*** 150-200mg as a single IM injection. **IV:** 100mg (commonly used initial dose for 70kg adult); if needed additional small increments may be given up to 200-500mg total dose. Rate of IV injection should not exceed 50mg/min. **Elderly/Debilitated/Renal or Hepatic Impairment:** Reduce dose. ***Pediatrics:*** 2-6mg/kg as a single IM injection. **Max:** 100mg. **IV:** Proportional reduction in dosage. Slow IV injection is essential.	**W/P:** May be habit forming; avoid abrupt cessation after prolonged use. Avoid rapid administration. Tolerance to hypnotic effect can occur. Prehepatic coma use not recommended. Use with caution in patients with chronic or acute pain, mental depression, suicidal tendencies, history of drug abuse or hepatic impairment. Monitor blood, liver and renal function. May impair mental/physical abilities. Avoid alcohol. **Contra:** History of manifest or latent porphyria. **P/N:** Category D, caution with nursing.	Agitation, confusion, hyperkinesia, ataxia, CNS depression, somnolence, bradycardia, hypotension, nausea, vomiting, constipation, headache, hypersensitivity reactions, liver damage.
Phenobarbital[CIV]	**Elixir:** 20mg/5mL; **Tab:** 15mg, 30mg, 32.4mg, 60mg, 64.8mg, 100mg	***Adults: Sedation:*** 30-120mg/day given bid-tid. **Max:** 400mg/24h. **Hypnotic:** 100-200mg. **Seizures:** 60-200mg/day. **Elderly/Debilitated/Renal or Hepatic Dysfunction:** Reduce dosage. ***Pediatrics: Seizures:*** 3-6mg/kg/day.	**W/P:** May be habit forming. Avoid abrupt withdrawal. Caution with acute or chronic pain; may mask symptoms or paradoxical excitement may occur. Cognitive deficits reported in children with febrile seizures. May cause excitement in children and excitement, depression or confusion in elderly, debilitated. Caution with hepatic dysfunction, borderline hypoadrenal function, depression. **Contra:** Respiratory disease with dyspnea or obstruction, porphyria, severe liver dysfunction. Large doses with nephritic patients. **P/N:** Category D, caution in nursing.	Drowsiness, residual sedation, lethargy, vertigo, somnolence, respiratory depression, hypersensitivity reactions, nausea, vomiting, headache.
Secobarbital Sodium[CII] (Seconal)	**Cap:** 100mg	***Adults: Hypnotic:*** 100mg hs. **Preoperatively:** 200-300mg, 1-2 hrs before surgery. **Elderly/Debilitated/Renal or Hepatic Dysfunction:** Reduce dose. ***Pediatrics: Preoperatively:*** 2-6mg/kg. **Max:** 100mg.	**W/P:** May be habit-forming; avoid abrupt cessation after prolonged use. Tolerance, psychological and physical dependence may occur with continued use. Use with caution, if at all, in patients who are mentally depressed, have suicidal tendencies, or have a history of drug abuse. In patients with hepatic damage, use with caution and initially reduce dose. Caution when administering to patients with acute or chronic pain. May impair mental and/or physical abilities. Avoid alcohol. **Contra:** History of manifest or latent porphyria, marked impairment of liver function, or respiratory disease in which dyspnea or obstruction is evident. **P/N:** Category D, caution in nursing.	Agitation, confusion, hyperkinesia, ataxia, CNS depression, somnolence, bradycardia, hypotension, nausea, vomiting, constipation, headache, hypersensitivity reactions, liver damage.

*Scored.   †Bold entries denote special dental considerations.

NAME	FORM/STRENGTH	DOSAGE	WARNINGS/PRECAUTIONS & CONTRAINDICATIONS	ADVERSE EFFECTS†
BENZODIAZEPINES				
Alprazolam[CIV] (Niravam, Xanax, Xanax XR)	**Tab, Orally Disintegrating:** (Niravam) 0.25mg*, 0.5mg*, 1mg*, 2mg*. **Tab:** (Xanax) 0.25mg*, 0.5mg*, 1mg*, 2mg*. **Tab, ER:** (Xanax XR) 0.5mg, 1mg, 2mg, 3mg	**Adults:** (Niravam) **Anxiety: Initial:** 0.25-0.5mg tid. **Titrate:** May increase every 3-4 days. **Max:** 4mg/day. **Panic Disorder: Initial:** 0.5mg tid. **Titrate:** Increase by no more than 1mg/day every 3-4 days; slower titration if ≥4mg/day. **Usual:** 1-10mg/day. Decrease dose slowly (no more than 0.5mg every 3 days). **Elderly/Advanced Liver Disease/Debilitated: Initial:** 0.25mg bid-tid. **Titrate:** Increase gradually as tolerated. **(Xanax) Anxiety: Initial:** 0.25-0.5mg tid. **Titrate:** May increase every 3-4 days. **Max:** 4mg/day. **Elderly/Advanced Liver Disease/Debilitated: Initial:** 0.25mg bid-tid. **Titrate:** Increase gradually as tolerated. **Panic Disorder: Initial:** 0.5mg tid. **Titrate:** Increase by no more than 1mg/day every 3-4 days; slower titration if ≥4mg/day. **Usual:** 1-10mg/day. Decrease dose slowly (no more than 0.5mg every 3 days). **(Xanax XR) Initial:** 0.5-1mg qd, preferably in the am. **Titrate:** Increase by no more than 1mg/day every 3-4 days. **Maint:** 1-10mg/day. **Usual:** 3-6mg/day. Decrease dose slowly (no more than 0.5mg every 3 days). **Elderly/Advanced Liver Disease/Debilitated: Initial:** 0.5mg qd.	**W/P:** Risk of dependence. Withdrawal symptoms, including seizures, reported with dose reduction or abrupt discontinuation; avoid abrupt withdrawal. Caution with impaired renal, hepatic, or pulmonary function, severe depression, obesity, elderly, and debilitated. May cause fetal harm. Hypomania/mania reported with depression. Weak uricosuric effect. Periodically reassess usefulness. **Contra:** Acute narrow angle glaucoma, untreated open angle glaucoma, concomitant ketoconazole or itraconazole. **P/N:** Category D, not for use in nursing.	Drowsiness, lightheadedness, depression, headache, confusion, insomnia, **dry mouth**, constipation, diarrhea, nausea/vomiting, tachycardia/palpitations, blurred vision, nasal congestion, sedation, somnolence, memory impairment, dysarthria, abnormal coordination, fatigue, mental impairment, ataxia, decreased libido, increased/decreased appetite, irritability cognitive disorder, dysarthria, decreased libido, confusional state, hypotension, **increased salivation**.
Chlordiazepoxide Hydrochloride[CIV] (Librium)	**Cap:** 5mg, 10mg, 25mg; **Inj:** 100mg	**Adults: Mild-Moderate Anxiety:** 5-10mg PO tid-qid. **Severe Anxiety:** 20-25mg PO tid-qid or 50-100mg IM/IV initially, then 25-50mg tid-qid as needed. **Alcohol Withdrawal:** 50-100mg IM/IV initially, may repeat in 2-4 hrs or 50-100mg PO, repeated until agitation is controlled. **Preoperative Anxiety:** 5-10mg PO tid-qid on days prior to surgery or 50-100mg IM 1 hr prior to surgery. **Max:** 300mg/24 hrs for above indications. **Elderly/Debilitated:** Reduce dose (25-50mg IM/IV) or 5mg PO bid-qid. **Pediatrics: PO: ≥6 yrs:** 5mg bid-qid. May increase to 10mg bid-tid for all conditions except acute alcohol withdrawal. **Acute alcohol withdrawal:** 50-100mg followed by repeated doses until agitation is controlled. **Max:** 300mg/day. **IM/IV: ≥12 yrs: Withdrawal Symptoms of Acute Alcoholism: Initial:** 25-50mg; repeat in 2 to 4hrs. prn. **Acute/Severe Anxiety: Initial:** 25-50mg, then 12.5-50mg tid-qid prn. **Preoperative Anxiety:** 25-50mg 1 hr prior to surgery.	**W/P:** Avoid in pregnancy. Paradoxical reactions reported in psychiatric patients and in hyperactive aggressive pediatrics. Caution with porphyria, renal or hepatic dysfunction. Reduce dose in elderly, debilitated. Avoid abrupt withdrawal after extended therapy. Observe patients up to 3 hrs after IM/IV use. **P/N:** Not for use in pregnancy, safety in nursing not known.	Drowsiness, ataxia, confusion, skin eruptions, edema, nausea, constipation, extrapyramidal symptoms, libido changes, EEG changes.
Clorazepate Dipotassium[CIV] (Tranxene-SD, Tranxene T-Tab)	**Tab:** (Tranxene T-Tab) 3.75mg*, 7.5mg*, 15mg*; **Tab, Extended Release:** (Tranxene-SD) 22.5mg, (Tranxene-SD Half Strength) 11.25mg*	**Adults: Anxiety: Initial:** (Tab) 15mg qhs. **Usual:** 30mg/day in divided doses. **Max:** 60mg/day. **Elderly/Debilitated: Initial:** 7.5-15mg/day. (Tab, Extended-Release) 22.5mg q24h, (may substitute for 7.5mg tid) or 11.25mg q24h (may substitute for 3.75mg tid). Do not use Extended-Release for initial therapy. **Alcohol Withdrawal: Day 1:** (Tab) 30mg, then 30-60mg/day. **Day 2:** 45-90mg/day.	**W/P:** Avoid with depressive neuroses or psychotic reactions. Withdrawal symptoms with abrupt withdrawal; taper gradually. Caution with known drug dependency, renal/hepatic impairment. Suicidal tendencies reported; give lowest effective dose. Monitor LFTs and blood counts periodically with long-term therapy. Use lowest effective dose in elderly.	Drowsiness, dizziness, GI complaints, nervousness, blurred vision, dry mouth, headache, mental confusion.

Table 2.1: PRESCRIBING INFORMATION FOR CONSCIOUS SEDATION/ANTIANXIETY AGENTS (cont.)

NAME	FORM/STRENGTH	DOSAGE	WARNINGS/PRECAUTIONS & CONTRAINDICATIONS	ADVERSE EFFECTS†
BENZODIAZEPINES (cont.)				
Clorazepate Dipotassium^{CIV} (cont.)		**Day 3:** 22.5-45mg/day. **Day 4:** 15-30mg. Give in divided doses. Reduce dose and continue with 7.5-15mg/day; discontinue when stable. **Max:** 90mg/day. **Antiepileptic Adjunct: Initial:** (Tab) 7.5mg tid. **Titrate:** Increase by no more than 7.5mg/week. **Max:** 90mg/day. *Pediatrics:* **>9 yrs: Anxiety: Initial:** (Tab) 15mg qhs. **Usual:** 30mg/day in divided doses. **Max:** 60mg/day. (Tab, Extended-Release) 22.5mg q24h, (may substitute for 7.5mg tid) or 11.25mg q24h (may substitute for 3.75mg tid). Do not use Extended-Release for initial therapy. **>12 yrs: Antiepileptic Adjunct: Initial:** (Tab) 7.5mg tid. **Titrate:** Increase by no more than 7.5mg/week. **Max:** 90mg/day. **9-12 yrs: Initial:** 7.5mg bid. **Titrate:** Increase by no more than 7.5mg/week. **Max:** 60mg/day.	**Contra:** Acute narrow-angle glaucoma. **P/N:** Safety in pregnancy not known, not for use in nursing.	
Diazepam^{CIV} (Valium)	**Tab:** 2mg*, 5mg*, 10mg*	*Adults:* **Anxiety:** 2-10mg bid-qid. **Alcohol Withdrawal:** 10mg tid-qid for 24 hrs. **Maint:** 5mg tid-qid. **Skeletal Muscle Spasm:** 2-10mg tid-qid. **Seizure Disorders:** 2-10mg bid-qid. **Elderly/Debilitated:** 2-2.5mg qd-bid initially; may increase gradually as needed and tolerated. *Pediatrics:* **≥6 months:** 1-2.5mg tid-qid initially; may increase gradually as needed and tolerated.	**W/P:** Monitor blood counts and LFTs in long-term use. Neutropenia and jaundice reported. Increase in grand mal seizures reported. Avoid abrupt withdrawal. Caution with kidney or hepatic dysfunction. **Contra:** Acute narrow angle glaucoma, untreated open angle glaucoma, patients <6 months. **P/N:** Not for use during pregnancy, safety in nursing not known.	Drowsiness, fatigue, ataxia, paradoxical reactions, minor EEG changes.
Estazolam^{CIV} (ProSom)	**Tab:** 1mg*, 2mg*	*Adults:* **Initial:** 1mg qhs. May increase to 2mg qhs. **Small/Debilitated/Elderly: Initial:** 0.5mg qhs.	**W/P:** Avoid abrupt withdrawal after prolonged use. Caution with depression, elderly/debilitated, renal/hepatic impairment. May cause respiratory depression. **Contra:** Pregnancy. **P/N:** Category X, not for use in nursing.	Somnolence, hypokinesia, dizziness, abnormal coordination, constipation, **dry mouth**, amnesia, paradoxical reactions.
Flurazepam Hydrochloride^{CIV} (Dalmane)	**Cap:** 15mg, 30mg	*Adults:* **Usual:** 15-30mg at bedtime. **Elderly/Debilitated: Initial:** 15mg at bedtime. *Pediatrics:* **≥15 yrs: Usual:** 15-30mg at bedtime.	**W/P:** Caution in elderly, debilitated, severely depressed, those with suicidal tendencies, hepatic/renal impairment, respiratory disease. Ataxia and falls reported in elderly and debilitated. Withdrawal symptoms after discontinuation; avoid abrupt discontinuation. **Contra:** Pregnancy. **P/N:** Not for use in pregnancy or nursing.	Confusion, dizziness, drowsiness, lightheadedness, ataxia.
Lorazepam^{CIV} (Ativan, Ativan Injection)	**Inj:** 2mg/mL, 4mg/mL. **Tab:** 0.5mg, 1mg*, 2mg	*Adults:* **(Inj) ≥18 yrs: Status Epilepticus:** 4mg IV (given slowly at 2mg/min); may repeat 1 dose after 10-15 min seizures recur or fail to cease. **Preanesthetic Sedation: Usual:** 0.05mg/kg IM; 2mg or 0.044mg/kg IV (whichever is smaller). **Max:** 4mg IM/IV. **(Tab) Initial:** 2-3mg/day given bid-tid. **Usual:** 2-6mg/day in divided doses. **Insomnia:** 2-4mg qhs.	**W/P:** (Inj) Monitor all parameters to maintain vital function. Risk of respiratory depression or airway obstruction in heavily sedated patients. May cause fetal damage during pregnancy. Increased risk of CNS and respiratory depression in elderly. Avoid with hepatic/renal failure.	Sedation, dizziness, weakness, unsteadiness, transient amnesia, memory impairment, respiratory depression/failure, hypotension, somnolence, headache, hypoventilation.

*Scored.   †Bold entries denote special dental considerations.

NAME	FORM/ STRENGTH	DOSAGE	WARNINGS/PRECAUTIONS & CONTRAINDICATIONS	ADVERSE EFFECTS†
LorazepamCIV *(cont.)*		**Elderly/Debilitated:** 1-2mg/day in divided doses. *Pediatrics:* **>12 yrs: Initial:** 2-3mg/day given bid-tid. **Usual:** 2-6mg/day in divided doses. **Insomnia:** 2-4mg qhs.	Caution with mild to moderate hepatic/renal disease. Avoid outpatient endoscopic procedures. Possible propylene glycol toxicity in renal impairment. (Tab) Avoid with primary depression or psychosis. Withdrawal symptoms with abrupt discontinuation. Careful supervision if addiction-prone. Caution with elderly, and renal or hepatic dysfunction. Monitor for GI disease with prolonged therapy. Periodic blood counts and LFTs with long-term therapy. **Contra:** Acute narrow-angle glaucoma, sleep apnea syndrome, severe respiratory insufficiency. Not for intra-arterial injection. **P/N:** (Inj) Category D, not for use in nursing. (Tab) Not for use in pregnancy or nursing.	
Midazolam HydrochlorideCIV (Versed)	**Inj:** 1mg/mL, 5mg/mL **Syrup:** 2mg/mL	*Adults:* **IV: Sedation/Anxiolysis/Amnesia Induction: <60 yrs: Initial:** 1-2.5mg IV over 2 min. **Max:** 5mg. **Titrate:** In small increments at 2 min intervals if needed. **Concomitant Narcotics/Other CNS Depressants:** Reduce by 30%. **≥60 yrs/Debilitated/Chronically Ill: Initial:** 1-1.5mg IV over 2 min. **Max:** 3.5mg. **Titrate:** In small increments at 2 min intervals if needed. **Concomitant Narcotics/Other CNS Depressants:** Reduce by 50%. **Maint:** 25% of sedation dose by slow titration. **IM: Preoperative Sedation/Anxiolysis/Amnesia: <60 yrs:** 0.07-0.08mg/kg IM up to 1 hr before surgery. **≥60 yrs/Debilitated:** 1-3mg IM. **Anesthesia Induction: Unpremedicated: <55 yrs: Initially:** 0.3-0.35mg/kg IV over 20-30 seconds. May give additional doses of 25% of initial dose to complete induction. **≥55 yrs: Initial:** 0.3mg/kg IV. **Debilitated: Initial:** 0.15-0.25mg/kg IV. **Premedicated: <55 yrs: Initial:** 0.25mg/kg IV over 20-30 seconds. **≥55 yrs: Initial:** 0.2mg/kg IV. **Debilitated:** 0.15mg/kg IV. **Maintenance Sedation: LD:** 0.01-0.05mg/kg IV. May repeat dose at 10-15 min intervals until adequate sedation. **Maint:** 0.02-0.1mg/kg/hr. Titrate to desired level of sedation using 25-50% adjustments. Infusion rate should be decreased 10-25% every few hrs to find minimum effective infusion rate. *Pediatrics:* 0.25-1mg/kg single dose. **Max:** 20mg.	**Associated with respiratory depression and respiratory arrest especially when used for sedation in noncritical care settings. Do not administer by rapid injection to neonates. Continuous monitoring required. W/P:** Agitation, involuntary movements, hyperactivity, and combativeness reported. Caution with CHF, chronic renal failure, pulmonary disease, uncompensated acute illnesses (eg, severe fluid or electrolyte disturbances), elderly or debilitated. Avoid use with shock or coma, or in acute alcohol intoxication with depression of vital signs. Contains benzyl alcohol. **Contra:** Acute narrow-angle glaucoma, untreated open-angle glaucoma, intrathecal or epidural use. **P/N:** Category D, caution in nursing.	Decreased tidal volume and/or respiratory rate, BP/HR variations, apnea, hypotension, pain and local reactions at injection site, **hiccups,** nausea, vomiting, **desaturation.**
OxazepamCIV (Serax)	**Cap:** 10mg, 15mg, 30mg; **Tab:** 15mg	*Adults:* **Anxiety: Mild-Moderate:** 10-15mg tid-qid. **Severe:** 15-30mg tid-qid. **Elderly: Initial:** 10mg tid. **Titrate:** Increase to 15mg tid-qid. **Alcohol Withdrawal:** 15-30mg tid-qid.	**W/P:** May impair mental/physical abilities. Withdrawal symptoms with abrupt discontinuation. Caution in sensitivity to hypotension, elderly. Caution with tablets in tartrazine or ASA allergy. Risk of congenital malformations; avoid in pregnancy. **Contra:** Psychoses. **P/N:** Not for use in pregnancy or nursing.	Drowsiness, dizziness, vertigo, headache, paradoxical excitement, transient amnesia, memory impairment.

Table 2.1: PRESCRIBING INFORMATION FOR CONSCIOUS SEDATION/ANTIANXIETY AGENTS (cont.)

NAME	FORM/STRENGTH	DOSAGE	WARNINGS/PRECAUTIONS & CONTRAINDICATIONS	ADVERSE EFFECTS†
BENZODIAZEPINES (cont.)				
Temazepam^{CIV} (Restoril)	**Cap:** 7.5mg, 15mg, 22.5mg, 30mg	***Adults:*** Usual: 7.5-30mg qhs. **Transient Insomnia:** 7.5mg qhs. **Elderly/Debilitated:** Initial: 7.5mg qhs.	**W/P:** Caution in elderly, debilitated, severely depressed, those with suicidal tendencies, hepatic/renal impairment, pulmonary insufficiency. Avoid abrupt discontinuation. If no improvement after 7-10 days, may indicate primary psychiatric and/or medical condition. **Contra:** Pregnancy. **P/N:** Category X, caution in nursing.	Headache, dizziness, drowsiness, fatigue, nervousness, nausea, lethargy, hangover.
Triazolam^{CIV} (Halcion)	**Tab:** 0.125mg, 0.25mg*	***Adults:*** 0.25mg qhs. **Max:** 0.5mg. **Elderly/Debilitated: Initial:** 0.125mg. **Max:** 0.25mg.	**W/P:** Worsening or failure of response after 7-10 days may indicate other medical conditions. Increased daytime anxiety, abnormal thinking and behavioral changes have occurred. May impair mental/physical abilities. Anterograde amnesia reported with therapeutic doses. Caution with baseline depression, suicidal tendencies, history of drug dependence, elderly/debilitated, renal/hepatic impairment, chronic pulmonary insufficiency, and sleep apnea. Withdrawal symptoms after discontinuation; avoid abrupt withdrawal. **Contra:** Pregnancy. With ketoconazole, itraconazole, nefazodone, medications that impair CYP3A. **P/N:** Category X, not for use in nursing.	Drowsiness, dizziness, lightheadedness, headache, nausea, vomiting, coordination disorders, ataxia.
BENZODIAZEPINE ANTAGONIST				
Flumazenil (Romazicon)	**Inj:** 0.1mg/mL	***Adults:*** **Reversal of Conscious Sedation/General Anesthesia:** Give IV over 15 seconds. **Initial:** 0.2mg. May repeat dose after 45 seconds and again at 60-second intervals up to a max of 4 additional times until reach desired level of consciousness. **Max Total Dose:** 1mg. In event of resedation, repeated doses may be given at 20-min intervals. **Max:** 1mg/dose (0.2mg/min) and 3mg/hr. **BZD Overdose:** Give IV over 30 seconds. **Initial:** 0.2mg. May repeat with 0.3mg after 30 seconds and then 0.5mg at 1-min intervals until reach desired level of consciousness. **Max Total Dose:** 3mg. In event of resedation, repeated doses may be given at 20-min intervals. **Max:** 1mg/dose (0.5mg/min); 3mg/hr. ***Pediatrics:*** >1yr: Give IV over 15 seconds. **Initial:** 0.01mg/kg (up to 0.2mg). May repeat dose after 45 seconds and again at 60-second intervals up to a max of 4 additional times until reach desired level of consciousness.	**W/P:** Caution in overdoses involving multiple drug combinations. Risk of seizures, especially with long-term BZD-induced sedation, cyclic antidepressant overdose, concurrent major sedative-hypnotic drug withdrawal, recent therapy with repeated doses of parenteral BZDs, myoclonic jerking or seizure prior to flumazenil administration. Monitor for resedation, respiratory depression, or other residual BZD effects (up to 2 hrs). Avoid use in the ICU; increased risk of unrecognized BZD dependence. Caution with head injury, alcoholism, and other drug dependencies.	Nausea, vomiting, dizziness, injection site pain, increased sweating, headache, abnormal or blurred vision, agitation.

*Scored.   †Bold entries denote special dental considerations..

NAME	FORM/ STRENGTH	DOSAGE	WARNINGS/PRECAUTIONS & CONTRAINDICATIONS	ADVERSE EFFECTS†
Flumazenil (cont.)		**Max Total Dose:** 0.05mg/kg or 1mg, whichever is lower.	Does not reverse respiratory depression/hypoventilation or cardiac depression. May provoke panic attacks with history of panic disorder. Adjust subsequent doses in hepatic dysfunction. Not for use as treatment for BZD dependence or for management of protracted abstinence syndromes. May trigger dose-dependent withdrawal syndromes. **Contra:** Patients given BZDs for life-threatening conditions (eg, control of intracranial pressure or status epilepticus), signs of serious cyclic antidepressant overdose. **P/N:** Category C, caution in nursing.	

MISCELLANEOUS

NAME	FORM/ STRENGTH	DOSAGE	WARNINGS/PRECAUTIONS & CONTRAINDICATIONS	ADVERSE EFFECTS†
Eszopiclone CIV (Lunesta)	**Tab:** 1mg, 2mg, 3mg	*Adults:*Initial: 2mg qhs. **Max:** 3mg qhs. **Elderly: Difficulty Falling Asleep: Initial:** 1mg qhs. **Max:** 2mg qhs. **Difficulty Staying Asleep: Initial/Max:** 2mg qhs. Avoid high-fat meal.	**W/P:** A variety of abnormal thinking and behavior changes have been reported to occur in association with the use of sedative/hypnotics. Some of these changes may be characterized by decreased inhibition, similar to effects produced by alcohol and other CNS depressants. Other reported behavioral changes have included bizarre behavior, agitation, hallucinations, and depersonalization. Amnesia and other neuropsychiatric symptoms may occur unpredictably. In primarily depressed patients, worsening of depression, including suicidal thinking, has been reported in association with the use of sedative/hypnotics. Rapid dose decrease or abrupt discontinuation of use of sedative/hypnotics can result in signs and symptoms similar to those associated with withdrawal from other CNS-depressant drugs. Eszopiclone, like other hypnotics, has CNS-depressant effects and because of rapid onset of action eszopiclone should only be taken immediately prior to going to bed or after the patient has gone to bed and has experienced difficulty falling asleep. Patients should be cautioned against engaging in hazardous occupations requiring complete mental alertness or motor coordination after taking eszopiclone.	Headache, **unpleasant taste**, somnolence, **dry mouth**, dizziness, infection, rash, chest pain, peripheral edema, migraine.

Table 2.1: PRESCRIBING INFORMATION FOR CONSCIOUS SEDATION/ANTIANXIETY AGENTS *(cont.)*

NAME	FORM/ STRENGTH	DOSAGE	WARNINGS/PRECAUTIONS & CONTRAINDICATIONS	ADVERSE EFFECTS†
MISCELLANEOUS *(cont.)*				
Hydroxyzine Hydrochloride (Atarax)	**Inj:** 25mg/mL, 50mg/mL; **Syrup:** 10mg/5mL; **Tab:** 10mg, 25mg, 50mg, 100mg	*Adults:* **PO: Anxiety:** 50-100mg qid. **Pruritus:** 25mg tid-qid. **Sedation:** 50-100mg. **IM: Nausea/Vomiting:** 25-100mg. **Pre-/Post-operative and Pre-/Postpartum Adjunct:** 25-100mg. **Psychiatric/Emotional Emergencies:** 50-100mg q4-6h prn. *Pediatrics:* **PO: Anxiety/Pruritus:** <6 yrs: 50mg/day in divided doses. ≥6 yrs: 50-100mg in divided doses. **Sedation:** 0.6mg/kg. **IM: Nausea/Vomiting:** 0.5mg/lb. **Pre-/Postoperative Adjunct:** 0.5mg/lb.	**W/P:** Caution in elderly. May impair mental/physical abilities. Effectiveness as an antianxiety agent for long term use (>4 months) has not been established. **Contra:** Early pregnancy. Inj is intended only for IM administration and should not, under any circumstances, be injected subcutaneously, intra-arterially, or IV. **P/N:** Not for use in pregnancy or nursing.	**Dry mouth**, drowsiness, involuntary motor activity.
Hydroxyzine Pamoate (Vistaril)	**Cap:** 25mg, 50mg, 100mg; **Sus:** 25mg/5mL [120mL, 480mL]	*Adults:* **Anxiety:** 50-100mg qid. **Pruritus:** 25mg tid-qid. **Sedation:** 50-100mg. *Pediatrics:* **Anxiety/Pruritus:** >6 yrs: 50-100mg/day in divided doses. <6 yrs: 50mg/day in divided doses. **Sedation:** 0.6mg/kg.	**W/P:** Caution in elderly. May impair mental/physical abilities. Effectiveness as an antianxiety agent for long term use (>4 months) has not been established. **Contra:** Early pregnancy. **P/N:** Safety unknown in pregnancy and is contraindicated in early pregnancy, not for use in nursing.	**Dry mouth**, drowsiness, involuntary motor activity.
Ramelteon (Rozerem)	**Tab:** 8mg	*Adults:* 8mg within 30 min of bedtime. Do not take with or after high-fat meal.	**W/P:** Sleep disturbances may be presenting manifestations of a physical and/or psychiatric disorder, initiate therapy only after careful evaluation. Do not use in severe hepatic impairment. A variety of abnormal thinking and behavior changes have been reported to occur in association with the use of hypnotics. In primarily depressed patients, worsening of depression, including suicidal ideation, has been reported in association with the use of hypnotics. May impair physical/mental abilities. Not recommended in patients with severe sleep apnea or severe COPD. Caution with alcohol. May affect reproductive hormones. **P/N:** Category C, not for use in nursing	Headache, somnolence, fatigue, dizziness, nausea, exacerbated insomnia, upper respiratory tract infection.
Zaleplon[CIV] (Sonata)	**Cap:** 5mg, 10mg	*Adults:* **Insomnia:** 10mg qhs. **Low Weight Patients:** Start with 5mg hs. **Max:** 20mg/day. **Elderly/Debilitated/Concomitant Cimetidine:** 5mg qhs. **Max:** 10mg/day. **Mild to Moderate Hepatic Dysfunction:** 5mg qhs. Take immediately prior to bedtime.	**W/P:** Monitor elderly/debilitated closely. Abnormal thinking and behavioral changes reported. Avoid abrupt withdrawal. Abuse potential exist. Caution in respiratory disorders, depression, conditions affecting metabolism or hemodynamic responses, and mild-to-moderate hepatic insufficiency. Not for use in severe hepatic impairment. May cause impaired coordination even the following day. Re-evaluate if no improvement of insomnia after 7-10 days of therapy. Contains tartrazine. **P/N:** Category C, not for use in nursing.	Headache, asthenia, nausea, dizziness, amnesia, somnolence, eye pain, dysmenorrhea, abdominal pain.

*Scored.   †Bold entries denote special dental considerations.

NAME	FORM/ STRENGTH	DOSAGE	WARNINGS/PRECAUTIONS & CONTRAINDICATIONS	ADVERSE EFFECTS†
Zolpidem Tartrate^{CIV} (Ambien, Ambien-CR)	Tab: (Ambien) 5mg, 10mg; Tab, Extended-Release: (Ambien-CR) 6.25mg, 12.5mg	**Adults: Tab: Usual:** 10mg qhs. **Elderly/Debilitated/Hepatic Insufficiency: Initial:** 5mg. Decrease dose with other CNS-depressants. **Max:** 10mg qd. Use should be limited to 7-10 days. Revaluate if patient needs to take for more than 2-3 weeks. **(Tab, ER)** 12.5mg qhs. **Elderly/Debilitated/Hepatic Insufficiency:** 6.25mg qhs. Swallow whole; do not divide, crush, or chew.	**W/P:** (Tab) Monitor elderly and debilitated patients for impaired motor performance. Caution with depression and conditions that could affect metabolism or hemodynamic responses. (Tab, ER) Use smallest possible effective dose, especially in the elderly. Abnormal thinking and behavior changes have been reported with the use of sedative/hypnotics. Caution with depression and conditions that could affect metabolism or hemodynamic responses. Signs and symptoms of withdrawal reported with abrupt discontinuation of sedative/hypnotics. Monitor elderly and debilitated patients for impaired motor and/or cognitive performance. **P/N:** (Tab) Category B; not for use in nursing. (Tab, ER) Category C, not for use in nursing.	Drowsiness, dizziness, headache, nausea, drugged feeling, dyspepsia, myalgia, confusion, dependence, somnolence, hallucinations, back pain, fatigue.

MISCELLANEOUS SEDATIVE-HYPNOTIC

NAME	FORM/ STRENGTH	DOSAGE	WARNINGS/PRECAUTIONS & CONTRAINDICATIONS	ADVERSE EFFECTS†
Chloral hydrate^{CIV}	Syr: 500mg/5mL	**Adults:** Dilute in half glass of water, fruit juice, or ginger ale. **Hypnotic: Usual:** 500mg-1g 15-30 min before bedtime. **Sedative: Usual:** 250mg tid pc. **Alcohol Withdrawal: Usual:** 500mg-1g q6h prn. **Max:** 2g/day. **Pediatrics: Hypnotic:** 50mg/kg. **Max:** 1g/dose. **Sedative:** 8mg/kg tid. **Max:** 500mg tid. **Prior to EEG:** 20-25mg/kg.	**W/P:** May be habit forming. Caution with depression, suicidal tendencies, history of drug abuse. Avoid with esophagitis, gastritis or gastric or duodenal ulcers, large doses with severe cardiac disease. May impair mental/physical abilities. Risk of gastritis, skin eruptions, parenchymatous renal damage with prolonged use. Withdraw gradually with chronic use. **Contra:** Marked hepatic or renal impairment. **P/N:** Category C, caution in nursing.	Nausea, vomiting, diarrhea, ataxia, dizziness.
Meprobamate^{CIV} (Miltown)	Tab: 200mg, 400mg	**Adults: Usual:** 1200-1600mg/day given tid-qid. **Max:** 2400mg/day. **Elderly: >65 yrs:** Start at low end of dosing range. **Pediatrics: 6-12 yrs:** 200-600mg/day given bid-tid.	**W/P:** Physical and psychological dependence reported. Avoid abrupt withdrawal after prolonged or excessive use. Increased risk of congenital malformations with use during 1st trimester of pregnancy. Caution with liver or renal dysfunction, and in elderly. May precipitate seizures in epileptic patients. Prescribe small quantities in suicidal patients. **Contra:** Porphyria, allergic or idiosyncratic reactions to carisoprodol, mebutamate, tybamate, carbromal. **P/N:** Safety in pregnancy and nursing not known.	Drowsiness, ataxia, slurred speech, vertigo, weakness, nausea, vomiting, diarrhea, tachycardia, transient ECG changes, rash, leukopenia, petechiae.

OPIOID ANTAGONIST

NAME	FORM/ STRENGTH	DOSAGE	WARNINGS/PRECAUTIONS & CONTRAINDICATIONS	ADVERSE EFFECTS†
Naloxone (Narcan)	Inj: 0.4mg/mL, 1mg/mL	**Adults: Opioid Overdose: Initial:** 0.4-2mg IV every 2-3 min. **Opioid Depression:** 0.1-0.2mg IV every 2-3 min to desired response. May repeat in 1- to 2- hr intervals. Supplemental IM doses last longer.	**W/P:** Caution in patients including newborns of mothers known or suspected of opioid physical dependence. May precipitate acute withdrawal syndrome.	Hypotension, hypertension, ventricular tachycardia and fibrillation, dyspnea, pulmonary edema, cardiac arrest,

Table 2.1: PRESCRIBING INFORMATION FOR CONSCIOUS SEDATION/ANTIANXIETY AGENTS *(cont.)*

NAME	FORM/ STRENGTH	DOSAGE	WARNINGS/PRECAUTIONS & CONTRAINDICATIONS	ADVERSE EFFECTS†
OPIOID ANTAGONIST *(cont.)*				
Natoxone *(cont.)*		**Narcan Challenge Test: IV:** 0.1-0.2mg, observe 30 secs for signs of withdrawal, then 0.6mg, observe for 20 min. SC: 0.8mg, observe for 20 min. *Pediatrics:* **Opioid Overdose: Initial:** 0.01mg/kg IV. **Inadequate Response:** Repeat 0.01mg/kg once. IM/SC in divided doses if IV route not available. **Post-op Opioid Depression:** 0.005-0.01mg IV every 2-3 min to desired response. May repeat in 1-2 hr intervals. Supplemental IM doses last longer. **Neonates: Opioid-induced Depression:** 0.01mg/kg IV/IM/SC, may repeat every 2-3 min until desired response.	Have other resuscitative measures available. Caution with cardiac, renal, or hepatic disease. Monitor patients satisfactorily responding due to extended opioid duration of action. Abrupt postoperative opioid depression reversal may result in serious adverse effects leading to death. **P/N:** Category B, caution in nursing.	nausea, vomiting, sweating, seizures, body aches, fever, nervousness.

*Scored.   †Bold entries denote special dental considerations.

Table 2.2: DRUG INTERACTIONS FOR CONSCIOUS SEDATION/ANTIANXIETY AGENTS

BARBITURATES

Pentobarbital Sodium[CII] (Nembutal Sodium)

Anticoagulants, oral	May decrease levels of oral anticoagulants. Dosage adjustments may be required for anticoagulants.
CNS depressants	May produce additive CNS depression with other CNS depressants (eg, other sedatives/hypnotics, antihistamines, tranquilizers, alcohol).
Corticosteroids	May decrease levels of corticosteroids. Dosage adjustments may be required for corticosteroids.
Doxycycline	May decrease levels of doxycycline.
Estradiol	May decrease effects of estradiol; alternative contraceptive method should be suggested.
Griseofulvin	May decrease levels of oral griseofulvin.
MAOIs	Prolonged effect with MAOIs.
Phenytoin	Variable effects on phenytoin and monitor blood levels and adjust dose appropriately.
Valproic acid	Increased levels with valproic acid, sodium valproate; monitor blood levels and adjust dose appropriately.

Phenobarbital[CIV]

Anticoagulants, oral	Decreases effects of oral anticoagulants.
CNS depressants	May be potentiated by CNS depressants.
Contraceptives, oral	Decreases effects of oral contraceptives.
Corticosteriods	Increases corticosteroid metabolism.
Doxycycline	Decreases half-life of doxycycline.
Griseofulvin	Decreases absorption of griseofulvin.
MAOIs	May be potentiated by MAOIs.
Phenytoin	May alter phenytoin metabolism.
Valproic acid	Increased levels with sodium valproate and valproic acid.

Secobarbital Sodium[CII] (Seconal)

Anticoagulants, oral	May increase metabolism and decrease response to oral anticoagulants.
CNS depressants	May cause additive depressant effects with other CNS depressants (eg, sedatives/hypnotics, antihistamines, tranquilizers, alcohol).
Corticosteroids	May enhance metabolism of exogenous corticosteroids.
Doxycycline	May shorten half-life of doxycycline for up to 2 weeks after being discontinued.
Estradiol	May decrease effect of estradiol; alternative contraceptive methods should be suggested.
Griseofulvin	May interfere with absorption of griseofulvin, decreasing its blood level.
MAOIs	Prolonged effects with MAOIs.

Table 2.2: DRUG INTERACTIONS FOR CONSCIOUS SEDATION/ANTIANXIETY AGENTS (cont.)

BARBITURATES (cont.)

Secobarbital Sodium^{CII} (Seconal) (cont.)

Phenytoin	Variable effect on phenytoin; monitor blood levels and adjust dose appropriately.
Valproic acid	Increased levels with sodium valproate and valproic acid; monitor blood levels and adjust dose appropriately.

BENZODIAZEPINES

Alprazolam^{CIV} (Niravam, Xanax, Xanax XR)

Amiodarone	Caution with amiodarone.
Anticonvulsants	Additive effects with anticonvulsants.
Antihistamines	Additive effects with antihistamines.
Carbamazepine	Decreased plasma levels with carbamazepine.
Cimetidine	Potentiated by cimetidine.
Contraceptives, oral	Potentiated by oral contraceptives.
CYP3A inhibitors	Avoid with potent CYP3A inhibitors (eg, azole antifungals).
Desipramine	Increases levels of desipramine.
Diltiazem	Caution with diltiazem.
Ergotamine	Caution with ergotamine.
Ethanol	Additive CNS depressent effects with ethanol.
Fluoxetine	Potentiated by fluoxetine.
Fluvoxamine	Potentiated by fluvoxamine.
Imipramine	Increases levels of imipramine.
Isoniazid	Caution with isoniazid.
Itraconazole	Contraindicated with concomitant itraconazole.
Ketoconazole	Contraindicated with concomitant ketoconazole.
Macrolids	Caution with macrolides.
Nefazodone	Potentiated by nefazodone.
Nicardipine	Caution with nicardipine.
Nifedipine	Caution with nifedipine.
Paroxetine	Caution with paroxetine.
Propoxyphene	Decreased plasma levels with propoxyphene.
Psychotropic agents	Additive CNS depressant effects with psychotropic agents.
Sertraline	Caution with sertraline.

BENZODIAZEPINES *(cont.)*

Chlordiazepoxide Hydrochloride[CIV] (Librium)

Alcohol	Additive effects with alcohol.
CNS depressants	Additive effects with CNS depressants.
Psychotropic agents	Avoid other psychotropic agents.

Clorazepate Dipotassium[CIV] (Tranxene T-Tab, Tranxene-SD)

Alcohol	Additive CNS depression with alcohol.
Antidepressants	Potentiated by antidepressants.
Barbiturates	Potentiated by barbiturates.
CNS depressants	Additive CNS depression with CNS depressants.
Hypnotics	Increased sedation with hypnotics.
MAOIs	Potentiated by MAOIs.
Narcotics	Potentiated by narcotics.
Phenothiazines	Potentiated by phenothiazines.

Diazepam[CIV] (Valium)

Alcohol	Avoid alcohol.
Antidepressants	Antidepressants may potentiate effects.
Barbiturates	Barbiturates may potentiate effects.
Cimetidine	Delayed clearance with cimetidine.
CNS depressants	Avoid CNS-depressants.
Flumazenil	Risk of seizure with flumazenil.
MAOIs	MAOIs may potentiate effects.
Narcotics	Narcotics may potentiate effects.
Phenothiazines	Phenothiazines may potentiate effects.

Estazolam[CIV] (ProSom)

Alcohol	Potentiated effects with alcohol.
Anticonvulsants	Potentiated effects with anticonvulsants.
Antihistamines	Potentiated effects with antihistamines.
Barbiturates	Potentiated effects with barbiturates.
CNS depressants	Potentiated effects with CNS depressants
MAOIs	Potentiated effects with MAOIs.
Narcotics	Potentiated effects with narcotics.
Phenothiazines	Potentiated effects with phenothiazines.

Table 2.2: DRUG INTERACTIONS FOR CONSCIOUS SEDATION/ANTIANXIETY AGENTS *(cont.)*

BENZODIAZEPINES *(cont.)*

Estazolam[CIV] (ProSom)

Psychotropic medications	Potentiated effects with psychotropic medications.
Smoking	Smoking may increase clearance.

Flurazepam Hydrochloride[CIV] (Dalmane)

Alcohol	Additive effects with alcohol.
CNS depressants	Additive effects with CNS depressants.

Lorazepam[CIV] (Ativan)

Alcohol	CNS-depressant effects with alcohol. Diminished tolerance to alcohol.
Barbiturates	CNS-depressant effects with barbiturates.
CNS depressants	Increased CNS-depressant effects and diminished tolerance to CNS depressants.

Midazolam Hydrochloride[CIV]

Alcohol	Avoid use with acute alcohol intoxication.
CNS depressants	Increased sedative effects with CNS depressants.
CYP450 3A4 inhibitors	Prolonged sedation with CYP450 3A4 inhibitors (eg, erythromycin, diltiazem, verapamil, ketoconazole, itraconazole, saquinavir, cimetidine).
Droperidol	Increased sedative effects with droperidol.
Fentanyl	Increased sedative effects with fentanyl. May cause severe hypotension with concomitant use of fentanyl in neonates.
Halothane	Decreases concentration of halothane required for anesthesia.
Meperidine	Increased sedative effects with meperidine.
Morphine	Increased sedative effects with morphine.
Secobarbital	Increased sedative effects with secobarbital.
Thiopental	Decreases concentration of thiopental required for anesthesia.

Oxazepam[CIV]

Alcohol	Additive effects with alcohol.
CNS depressants	Additive effects with CNS depressants.

Temazepam[CIV] (Restoril)

Alcohol	Additive CNS depressant effects with alcohol.
CNS depressants	Additive CNS depressant effects with CNS depressants.
Diphenhydramine	May be synergistic with diphenhydramine.

Triazolam[CIV] (Halcion)

Alcohol	Additive CNS depression with alcohol.
Amiodarone	Caution with amiodarone.

BENZODIAZEPINES *(cont.)*

Triazolam[CIV] (Halcion)

Anticonvulsants	Additive CNS depression with anticonvulsants.
Antihistamines	Additive CNS depression with antihistamines.
Cimetidine	Caution with cimetidine.
Contraceptives, oral	Potentiated by the coadministration of oral contraceptives.
Cyclosporine	Caution with cyclosporine.
CYP3A inhibitors	Avoid the concomitant use with inhibitors of the CYP3A (eg, ketoconazole, itraconazole, all azole-type antifungals, nefazodone).
Diltiazem	Caution with diltiazem.
Ergotamine	Caution with ergotamine.
Fluvoxamine	Caution with fluvoxamine.
Intraconazole	Contraindicated with itraconazole.
Isoniazid	Potentiated by the coadministration of isoniazid.
Ketoconazole	Contraindicated with ketoconazole.
Marcrolides	Caution with macrolides.
Nefazodone	Contraindicated with nefazodone.
Nicardipine	Caution with nicardipine.
Paroxetine	Caution with paroxetine.
Psychotropics	Additive CNS depression with psychotropics.
Ranitidine	Potentiated by the coadministration of ranitidine.
Sertraline	Caution with sertraline.
Verapamil	Caution with verapamil.

BENZODIAZEPINE ANTAGONIST

Flumazenil (Romazicon)

Neuromuscular blockers	Avoid use until neuromuscular blockade effects are reversed. Toxic effects (eg, convulsions, cardiac dysrhythmias) may occur with mixed drug overdose (eg, cyclic antidepressants).

MISCELLANEOUS

Eszopiclone[CIV] (Lunesta)

CYP3A4	Strong inhibitors of CYP3A4 may significantly increase the AUC of eszopiclone.
Ethanol	Possible additive effect on psychomotor performance with ethanol.
Olanzapine	Coadministration with olanzapine produced a decrease in DSST score.

Table 2.2: DRUG INTERACTIONS FOR CONSCIOUS SEDATION/ANTIANXIETY AGENTS *(cont.)*

MISCELLANEOUS *(cont.)*

Hydroxyzine Hydrochloride (Atarax)

Alcohol	May increase alcohol effects.
CNS depressants	Potentiates CNS depression with other CNS depressants (eg, narcotics, non-narcotic analgesics, barbiturates, alcohol).

Hydroxyzine Pamoate (Vistaril)

CNS depressants	Potentiated by CNS depressants (eg, narcotics, non-narcotic analgesics, barbiturates); reduce dose.

Ramelteon (Rozerem)

Alcohol	Additive effect with alcohol.
CYP inducers	Decreased efficacy with strong CYP inducers (rifampin).
CYP1A2 inhibitors	Do not use with strong CYP1A2 inhibitors (fluvoxamine). Caution with less strong CYP1A2 inhibitors.
CYP2C9	Caution with strong CYP2C9 inhibitors (fluconazole).
CYP3A4	Caution with strong CYP3A4 inhibitors (ketoconazole).

Zaleplon[CIV] (Sonata)

Cimetidine	Potentiated by cimetidine.
CNS depressants	Potentiates CNS depression with psychotropics (eg, thioridazine, imipramine), anticonvulsants, antihistamines, alcohol and other CNS depressants.
CYP3A4	CYP3A4 inducers (eg, rifampin, phenytoin, carbamazepine and phenobarbital) decreases levels.

Zolpidem Tartrate[CIV] (Ambien, Ambien-CR)

Alcohol	Increased effect with alcohol and other CNS depressants.
CNS depressants	Increased effect with alcohol and other CNS depressants.
Flumazenil	Flumazenil reverses effect.
Rifampin	Rifampin may decrease effects.

MISCELLANEOUS SEDATIVE-HYPNOTIC

Chloral Hydrate[CIV]

CNS depressants	Additive CNS effects with other CNS depressants (eg, paraldehyde, barbiturates, alcohol).
Coumarin anticoagulants	Reduces effectiveness of coumarin anticoagulants. May result in transient potentiation of warfarin-induced hypoprothrombinemia.
Furosemide	Use with IV furosemide may cause diaphoresis, flushes, variable BP; use alternative hypnotic.

MISCELLANEOUS SEDATIVE-HYPNOTIC *(cont.)*

Meprobamate[CIV] (Miltown)

Alcohol	Administration with alcohol has additive effects.
CNS depressants	Administration with other CNS depressants have additive effects.
Psychotropic agents	Administration with other psychotropics have additive effects.

OPIOID ANTAGONIST

Naloxone (Narcan)

Buprenorphine	Reversal of buprenorphine-induced respiratory depression may be incomplete.

Chapter 3

Analgesics: Opioids and Nonopioids

Steven Ganzberg, D.M.D., M.S.

The use of systemically acting medications to reduce pain perception is an integral part of dental practice. Analgesic medications in dentistry are indicated for the relief of acute pain, postoperative pain and chronic pain, as well as for adjunctive intraoperative pain control. In addition, these medications can be given preoperatively to decrease expected postoperative pain. There are two general categories of analgesic medications: opioid and nonopioid.

Opioid Analgesics

Accepted Indications

Moderate-to-Severe Pain

Opioid medications are generally reserved for moderate-to-severe pain. Codeine, hydrocodone, dihydrocodeine and oxycodone, in combination preparations that contain aspirin, acetaminophen or ibuprofen, are commonly prescribed to manage acute orodental and postoperative pain in dental practice. Based on the amount of drug needed to produce a specific analgesic effect, oxycodone is a more potent analgesic than these other medications, but an equianalgesic dose can be found with any of the other agents. At an equianalgesic dose, opioid side effects of sedation, nausea, vomiting, constipation, respiratory depression and pupillary constriction are relatively similar. Table 3.1 lists the commonly prescribed combination opioids, along with oral dosages and schedule of dosing.

For severe pain, opioids such as Oxycodone, morphine and hydromorphone are available without a nonsteroidal anti-inflammatory drug (NSAID) or acetaminophen.

Other accepted indications for opioids include treatment of diarrhea, cough and some types of acute pulmonary edema; as an adjunct to anesthesia and sedation; and detoxification from opioids.

Table 3.1 lists commonly prescribed opioids not in combination with other analgesics, along with oral dosages and schedule of dosing.

Cancer and Chronic Nonmalignant Pain

Long-acting opioid analgesics, such as MS Contin, Oramorph, OxyContin, methadone, levorphanol and fentanyl patches, are available for treating oral cancer pain and selected cases of chronic nonmalignant orofacial pain. These agents are not indicated for acute pain relief and should be prescribed only for people who can tolerate short-acting opioids. Only practitioners who are skilled in the management of chronic pain should prescribe these agents.

Another potentially useful agent for chronic pain management is tramadol (Ultram), which acts as a mu (μ) agonist and weak serotonin/norepinehprine reuptake blocker. The latter effect, which would be expected to be helpful for chronic pain conditions, may also produce analgesia. The intravenous use of opioid medications for intraoperative sedation is discussed in Chapter 2 and Appendix N.

General Dosing Information

Analgesic medications should be prescribed in a manner that affords the patient the greatest degree of comfort within a high margin of safety. If the dentist suspects that a patient will have pain for 24-48 hours after a dental or surgical procedure, it is prudent to prescribe either opioid or NSAID analgesics on a regularly scheduled basis for at least 24-36 hours rather than on an as-needed or prn basis. The rationale for this approach is to provide as continuous a plasma level of medication as possible. If a patient waits until an analgesic medication loses effect and then takes another dose, he or she will be in pain for an additional 30-60 minutes. Furthermore, it requires more analgesic medication to overcome pain than to maintain pain relief once it has been established. Therefore, the clinician needs knowledge of a specific analgesic's duration of action to prescribe appropriately. Likewise, it is well-established that if an NSAID or an opioid is given preoperatively or prior to loss of local anesthetic activity, pain relief can be more easily achieved with postoperative analgesics.

All opioid medications can cause tolerance, a reduced drug effect that results from continued use and the need for higher doses to produce the same effect. These medications also can cause physical dependence, the physiological state associated with discontinuation of the drug after prolonged use (withdrawal), and psychological dependence, which is an intense craving for the drug and compulsive drug-seeking behavior. Because the pain commonly encountered in dental practice is of the acute type, tolerance of and physical and psychological dependence on opioids are so rare as to be of little concern, because such drugs are used only over the short term. The dentist should use opioid medications in sufficiently large doses for high-quality management of acute pain without fear that patients will develop dependence. The one exception may be patients with a history of drug abuse. For these patients, nonopioid analgesics should be prescribed initially. It should also be appreciated that a significant portion or analgesic activity of codeine, hydrocodone and likely oxycodone occurs following hepatic metabolism by CYP 2D6, one of the cytochrome P-450 group of hepatic microsomal enzymes. As many as 10% of patients may not have a functional form of CYP 2D6, which may significantly decrease analgesic efficacy of the above agents. If adequate analgesia does not occur with one of the above agents, it may be of value to trial another opioid. Agents such as morphine and hydromorphone do not require hepatic metabolism to achieve analgesia. The majority of important drug interactions involve the possibility of sedative and gastrointestinal side effects, among others. A complete listing of these is provided in Table 3.1.

Maximum Recommended Doses

Adult

Recommended doses for the combination products are listed in Table 3.1. The combination opioid products are generally limited by the dosage of the nonopioid product (for example, 4,000 mg per day for acetaminophen or aspirin). In general, there is no maximum dose of an opioid alone if proper titration has occurred other than the dose at which side effects are not tolerated. The use of opioids not formulated as a combination product is generally reserved for the management of severe acute pain and selected chronic pains.

Pediatric

In pediatric patients, codeine with acetaminophen and hydrocodone with acetopminophen is approved for pediatric pain not responsive to acetaminophen or ibuprofen alone. The maximum dosages for codeine with acetaminophen are shown in Table 3.1. Other opioids can be considered.

Geriatric

Geriatric patients may develop exaggerated sedative effects with opioid medications. Postural hypotension may occur. Consider starting at lower dose ranges.

Dosage Adjustments

Adjust dosage based on patient response. If duration of analgesia is insufficient, a shorter period between doses (for example, q 3 h vs q 4 h) or a higher dosage (for example, 7.5 mg vs 5 mg of hydrocodone) is appropriate. If analgesia itself is insufficient, a higher dosage of pain medication is appropriate. For short-term acute pain conditions, dependence on opioids is generally not of concern and efforts should be made to provide adequate postoperative analgesia.

Dosage Forms

Opioid medications are available for oral, intravenous, intramuscular, transnasal, transmucosal or transdermal use. The dentist will likely use oral forms (capsule, tablet or elixir—see Table 3.1) or perhaps butorphanol, which is available in a nasal spray form.

Special Dental Considerations

Opioids may decrease salivary flow. Consider long-term opioid use in the differential diagnosis of caries, periodontal disease or oral candidiasis.

Drug Interactions of Dental Interest

The most common drug interactions of concern for dentistry involve the potential sedative side effects, which are exaggerated in patients taking other CNS depressants (see Table 3.2).

Cross-Sensitivity

Cross-sensitivity is possible with opioids. It is important for the dentist to distinguish whether a true allergic reaction occurred, as most opioids can produce nausea and/or vomiting and some cause histamine release.

These reactions are typically referred to as "allergic" by patients. Consider using a non-opioid analgesic in these patients. Switching to a different opioid may produce fewer side effects.

Special Patients

Opioids should be used with caution in patients with chronic obstructive pulmonary disease, such as emphysema or chronic bronchitis, owing to possible respiratory compromise. Opioids may precipitate an asthmatic episode because of their potential for histamine release. This is considerably more likely with parenteral vs oral administration of opioids. Asthmatic patients should be warned to discontinue use of oral opioids if they experience asthmatic symptoms during therapy. Combination opioid products that contain aspirin should not be prescribed to asthmatic patients. Likewise, patients with severe cardiac disease, such as advanced congestive heart failure, may not tolerate hypotensive side effects. If mentally challenged patients are prescribed opioids, they should be closely monitored by an appropriate caregiver. Opioids should be prescribed cautiously for a patient with emotional instability, suicidal ideation or attempts, or a history of substance abuse.

Pregnant and nursing women

Opioids should not be prescribed for a pregnant or nursing patient without consultation with the patient's physician.

Pediatric, geriatric and other special patients

Pediatric and geriatric patients should be considered for lower opioid dosages.

Patient Monitoring: Aspects to Watch

- Respiratory depression and sedation: the patient should contact the dentist if these side effects are observed.
- Nausea, vomiting or both.

Adverse Effects and Precautions

The majority of important drug interactions involve the possibility of sedative and gastrointestinal side effects; a more complete listing is provided in Table 3.1.

Pharmacology

Opioid medications produce analgesia by interaction at specific receptors in the central nervous system, mimicking the effect of endogenous pain-relieving peptides (for example, dynorphin, enkephalin and β-endorphin). These receptors are present in higher brain centers such as the hypothalamus and periaqueductal gray regions, as well as in the spinal cord and trigeminal nucleus. The result of this interaction is a decrease in pain transmission to higher thalamocortical centers and a corresponding decrease in pain perception. Recent evidence suggests a possible peripheral effect of opioid analgesics.

Opioids undergo hepatic transformation generally to inactive metabolites, which are excreted in the urine and/or bile. These drugs are subdivided into agonist, agonist-antagonist or antagonist compounds based on their receptor effects.

Agonists

The opioid medications typified by morphine act primarily in the CNS through varied activity on specific opioid receptor subgroups. Although there is activity at all opioid receptors, morphine and related agents—such as codeine, hydrocodone, dihydrocodeine and oxycodone, as well as meperidine and the fentanyl derivatives—provide analgesia chiefly through agonist activity at the μ receptor.

Agonist-Antagonists

Another group of opioid analgesics, the agonist-antagonists—including pentazocine, nalbuphine and butorphanol—are agonists at the kappa (κ) receptor, and antagonists at the μ receptor.

Antagonists

Specific competitive opioid antagonist medications—namely, naloxone and naltrexone—have also been developed. Naloxone's main use in dentistry is reversal of excessive opioid IV sedation. Naltrexone is used to treat former opioid abusers and recently has been used for patients with certain CNS disorders.

Patient Advice

- Avoid use of alcohol or other CNS depressant medications unless a physician or dentist gives approval.
- Inform the dentist if nausea, vomiting, excessive dry mouth, dizziness or lightheadedness, ataxia, itching, hives or difficulty in breathing occurs.
- Exercise caution when getting up suddenly from a lying or sitting position.
- Avoid driving a motor vehicle or operating heavy machinery, especially if sedative side effects are present.

Suggested Readings

Dionne RA, Snyder J, Hargreaves KM. Analgesic efficacy of flubriprofen in comparison with acetaminophen, acetaminophen plus codeine, and placebo after impacted third molar removal. J Oral Maxillofac Surg 1994;52(9):919-24.

Forbes JA, Bates JA, Edquist IA, et al. Evaluation of two opioid-acetaminophen combinations and placebo in post-operative oral surgery pain. Pharmacotherapy 1994;14(2):139-46.

Hargreaves KM, Troullos ES, Dionne RA. Pharmacologic rationale for the treatment of acute pain. Dent Clin North Am 1987;31(4):675-94.

The United States Pharmacopeial Convention, Inc. USP Dispensing Information: drug information for the health care professional. Vol. I. 23rd ed. Greenwood Village; Colo.: Thomson Micromedex; 2003.

Nonopioid Analgesics

This group of analgesics includes the nonsteroidal anti-inflammatory drugs and acetaminophen. The site of action of these drugs is both peripheral and in the CNS.

Nonsteroidal Anti-inflammatory Drugs

Although NSAIDs influence a number of systems, the primary effect is the inhibition of the synthesis of prostaglandins, which are potent vasodilators and mediators of the inflammatory response at the site of injury. By decreasing the production of peripheral prostaglandins, NSAIDs depress the inflammatory response. This decrease in prostaglandin concentration also raises the threshold for pain-conducting nerves to discharge, thus providing an analgesic effect. In the CNS, NSAIDs reduce prostaglandin formation in critical pain processing regions producing decreased pain transmission and perception. NSAIDs also reduce fever by decreasing the concentration of prostaglandins in the hypothalamus, a brain center regulating body temperature.

The NSAIDs consist of several groups of drugs, based on structure and enzyme selectivity, that have similar mechanisms of action. They are primarily indicated for relief of mild-to-moderate pain and for chronic inflammatory conditions. Although no individual NSAID has been shown to be significantly superior for pain relief in all patients, NSAIDs do differ in duration of action and particularly side-effect profile. In regard to side effects, NSAIDs can be divided into traditional agents and cyclooxygenase-2 (COX-2) inhibitors. COX-2 inhibitors affect the production of mainly proinflammatory prostaglandins and have considerably fewer gastrointestinal and impaired platelet aggregation effects. The traditional agents affect both forms of cyclooxygenase (COX-1 and COX-2) in variable proportions but generally with greater likelihood of those adverse effects mentioned above. Some traditional agents, however, have favorable COX-1/ COX-2 activity ratios and have a decreased incidence of adverse effects (for example, nabumetone, etodolac, meloxicam). For patients at increased risk of adverse effects (for example, history of peptic ulcer disease, gastroesophageal reflux disease, inflammatory bowel disease), a predominantly COX-2–active drug may be preferred. Recently, the COX-2 inhibitors have been found to increase embolic phenomena (myocardial infarction and stroke), in part due to alteration of nitric oxide and prostacyclin formation. Long term use of COX-2 inhibitors must weigh the benefit/risk profile for an individual patient. Recently CNS COX-3 has been discovered and is inhibited by acetaminophen. In regard to pain control, if one NSAID is ineffective for pain control, the dentist should keep in mind that another NSAID from a different structural group may be effective. Many NSAIDs have a ceiling dose for analgesia and require a higher dose for the anti-inflammatory effect. For instance, ibuprofen, at 400 mg taken qid, provides close to a maximum analgesic effect, but a dose of 2,400-3,200 mg per day may be required for the anti-inflammatory effect. NSAIDs with an easier dosing schedule, such as bid or tid, may provide better patient compliance and result in a more pain-free patient. Some NSAIDs may be better analgesics while others are better anti-inflammatories. Table 3.1 lists acetaminophen and traditional NSAIDs by structural group, as well as the COX-2 inhibitors. Dosing schedule and maximum daily dose are also provided.

Acetaminophen

Acetaminophen's mechanism of action is not entirely clear but likely involves inhibition of CNS COX-3. Its analgesic and antipyretic properties are similar to those of aspirin, but acetaminophen has poor peripheral anti-inflammatory action.

Accepted Indications

NSAIDs are indicated for use as analgesics for mild to moderate pain, including pain of acute dental origin or for postoperative dental pain. These drugs are also indicated for pain of inflammatory origin, especially for rheumatic conditions and primary non-rheumatic inflammatory conditions. These drugs may also be used as antipyretics (ibuprofen and naproxen) and for treatment of primary dysmenorrhea.

NSAIDs may be indicated for longer-term use in patients with chronic orofacial pain, especially pain with an inflammatory component such as temporomandibular joint synovitis. If these medications are prescribed for a longer term, appropriate laboratory studies—including CBC, renal function tests and liver function tests—should be considered. For long-term use, the COX-2 inhibitors have the advantage of fewer gastrointestinal and impaired platelet aggregation adverse effects, although renal complications and embolic phenomena must be considered. The long-term use of these agents should be undertaken only by those skilled in chronic pain management.

General Dosing Information

It appears that many NSAIDs have a ceiling effect for analgesia. For instance, lower doses of ibuprofen may provide maximum analgesic efficacy, while higher doses are required for an anti-inflammatory effect. Depending on the condition being treated, the dentist may consider higher or lower dosages. Additionally, one NSAID may be ineffective while another provides excellent pain relief. The dentist may consider switching NSAIDs, perhaps to one from a different structural category, to obtain desired results.

As a general rule, analgesic medications should be prescribed in a manner that affords the patient the greatest degree of comfort within a high margin of safety. If the dentist suspects that a patient will have pain for 24–48 hours after a surgical procedure, it is prudent to prescribe either opioid or NSAID analgesics on a regularly scheduled basis for at least 24–36 hours rather than on an as-needed basis. The rationale for this approach is to provide as continuous a plasma level of medication as possible. If a

patient waits until an analgesic medication loses effect and then takes another dose, the patient will be in pain for an additional 30–60 minutes. Further, it requires more analgesic medication to overcome pain than to maintain pain relief once it has been established. Therefore, the clinician needs knowledge of a specific analgesic's duration of action to prescribe appropriately. Likewise, it is well-established that if an NSAID is given preoperatively or prior to loss of local anesthetic activity, pain relief can be more easily achieved with postoperative analgesics. Owing to the possible gastrointestinal side effects, NSAIDs should be prescribed with meals and/or taken with a full glass of water.

Maximum Recommended Doses

Adults

See Table 3.1.

Pregnant women

NSAIDs are generally contraindicated during pregnancy. Some NSAIDs do carry Pregnancy Category B classification during the first trimester of pregnancy. Regardless, the use of NSAIDs should be considered contraindicated in dental practice for all pregnant patients, unless prescribed in consultation with the patient's obstetrician. Acetaminophen, although generally acceptable, should be prescribed in consultation with the patient's obstetrician if there are any questions about the appropriateness of its use in an individual case.

Pediatric patients

Dosages should be reduced for children. Owing to their possible gastrointestinal side effects, NSAIDs should be prescribed with meals. Ibuprofen is the only NSAID that has been approved for use as an analgesic in children over age 2, although naproxen has been approved for juvenile rheumatoid arthritis for children over age 2.

Geriatric Patients

Dosages should be reduced for elderly patients. Owing to their possible gastrointestinal side effects, NSAIDs should be prescribed with meals.

Dosage Forms

NSAIDs and acetaminophen are available for oral use except for ketorolac tromethamine, which is also available in an IV/IM preparation. Elixir, liquid and rectal preparations are available for aspirin and acetaminophen. Liquid forms of ibuprofen are also available.

Special Dental Considerations

In the differential diagnosis of appropriate conditions, dentists should take into consideration that NSAIDs may cause soreness or irritation of the oral mucosa. Although very rare, some NSAIDs may cause leukopenia and/or thrombocyopenia.

Drug Interactions of Dental Interest

Major drug interactions with NSAIDs stem from the effect of these drugs on platelet, gastrointestinal and renal function. A specific absolute contraindication is warfarin anticoagulants (Coumadin) and NSAIDs. NSAIDS may decrease the effects of antihypertensive medications and when used longer term in combination with ACE inhibitors or beta blockers, may produce renal compromise. Others involve pharmacokinetic interactions. See Table 3.2 for major drug interactions.

Laboratory Value Alterations

- There are no laboratory tests whose results are specifically altered by NSAIDs and acetaminophen.
- The effect of these drugs on platelet function will likely increase bleeding times.
- There may also be changes in renal and hepatic function, especially with long-term NSAID use.

Cross-Sensitivity

All NSAIDs and aspirin may exhibit cross-sensitivity. Any of these drugs should be used with extreme caution, if at all, in patients who have developed signs and symptoms of allergic reaction to any NSAID, including aspirin. It should also be noted that patients with a history of nasal polyps and asthma have an increased risk of sensitivity, including allergic reactions, to aspirin, particularly, but also to other NSAIDs. Celecoxib has a sulfonamide structure and should not be prescribed to patients who report sulfonamide ("sulfa") allergy.

Special Patients

Pregnant and nursing women

NSAIDs should not be prescribed by dentists for pregnant or nursing women. Acetaminophen is generally prescribed in consultation with the patient's physician.

Pediatric, geriatric and other special patients

Only acetaminophen, aspirin and ibuprofen are approved for pediatric pain relief. Naproxen has been approved for juvenile rheumatoid arthritis for children over age 2. Aspirin may cause Reye's syndrome in children infected with influenza virus. Reye's syndrome is a serious medical condition that can lead to severe hepatic and CNS disease, as well as death. Because other drugs are available that do not manifest this concern, the dentist should consider avoiding use of aspirin in all children with fever.

Geriatric patients may be more susceptible to the gastrointestinal and renal side effects of NSAIDs. Start at lower dosages and avoid longer-acting agents that may accumulate.

Patient Monitoring: Aspects to Watch

- Short-term NSAID therapy: Laboratory monitoring is generally not necessary, but patient should notify dentist of symptoms of dyspepsia, fluid retention or worsening hypertension

- Long-term NSAID therapy: As for short-term therapy and hematologic parameters, renal and hepatic function require periodic laboratory evaluation

Adverse Effects and Precautions

These drugs have numerous side effects (Table 3.1) and drug interactions (Table 3.2). For short-term use, gastrointestinal side effects such as dyspepsia, diarrhea and abdominal pain are the most common. Longer-term use can lead to gastrointestinal ulceration, bleeding or perforation. As a precaution, NSAIDs should be taken with meals and/or a full glass of water. Various drugs have been developed to counteract some of the gastrointestinal side effects of NSAIDs, and NSAIDs that have fewer gastrointestinal side effects are listed later in this section. NSAIDs are contraindicated in patients who have active peptic ulcer disease and should be prescribed with extreme caution to patients who have a history of peptic ulcer disease or a history of long-term corticosteroid use.

Renal complications can also occur as idiosyncratic reactions with short-term use or as renal failure with long-term use. These medications are metabolized by the liver and should be prescribed cautiously to people who have liver disease.

It is important to note that NSAIDs can increase bleeding through their reversible inhibition of platelet aggregation by their effect on a platelet aggregating agent, thromboxane A_2. This is the case with all NSAIDs except aspirin, which irreversibly inhibits platelet aggregation for the entire life of the platelet (11 days). If major oral surgery is planned,

- discontinue aspirin use for 5-6 days before surgery;
- for NSAIDs that require dosing of 4-6 times per day, stop NSAID use 1-2 days before surgery;

- for NSAIDs that require bid-tid dosing, stop NSAID use 2-3 days before surgery;
- for q day NSAIDs, stop NSAID use 3-4 days before surgery to avoid excessive bleeding.

Drug interactions are presented in Table 3.2. An important contraindication involves the use of aspirin in children, which can lead to Reye's syndrome. Hypersensitivity reactions, such as anaphylactoid reactions, also have occurred with NSAIDs, especially aspirin. Patients with a history of bronchospastic disease and/or nasal polyps have an increased risk of having hypersensitivity reactions. If a patient's medical history indicates that this type of reaction could be encountered, it is prudent not to prescribe another NSAID. Some patients may exhibit minor hypersensitivity reactions to one NSAID but not another. If a patient tolerates a specific NSAID without difficulty, it seems reasonable to allow him or her to continue using that agent. Medical consultation may be appropriate. A history of anaphylactoid/anaphylactic reaction to any NSAID precludes use of another NSAID.

Some NSAIDs have potentially fewer gastrointestinal complications. The following drugs may cause less gastrointestinal irritation in a patient who, for instance, has a history of peptic ulcer disease and no longer requires ulcer medication but for whom an NSAID is indicated:

- celecoxib
- etodolac
- meloxicam
- salsalate (long-term use)

Pharmacology

Although NSAIDs influence a number of systems, a primary effect is the inhibition of the metabolism of arachidonic acid, a by product of cell wall breakdown, by the enzyme cyclooxygenase. One of the derivatives of this breakdown is prostaglandins, which are potent vasodilators and mediators of the inflammatory response. By decreasing the production of peripheral prostaglandins, NSAIDs depress the inflammatory response. This decrease in prostaglandin concentration also raises the threshold for pain-conducting nerves to discharge, thus providing an analgesic effect. In the CNS, NSAIDs reduce prostaglandin formation in critical pain processing regions producing decreased pain transmission and perception. NSAIDs also reduce fever, in part by decreasing the concentration of prostaglandins in the hypothalamus, a brain center regulating body temperature.

Three forms of cyclooxygenase have now been identified and are designated COX-1, COX-2 and COX-3. COX-1 is a constitutive form of the enzyme producing "protective" prostaglandins that, for example, serves to promote renal blood flow and decrease gastric acid secretion. COX-2 is an inducible form of the enzyme whose concentration significantly increases during inflammation. Specific agents—COX-2 inhibitors—have been developed that take advantage of this distinction. Clinical trials have shown decreased gastrointestinal and clotting side effects but an increase in embolic phenomena. Celecoxib is the only currently available COX-2 inhibitor. COX-3 is a CNS form and is inhibited by acetaminophen, which may account for its lack of peripheral anti-inflammatory effects but good analgesic activity.

It is expected that short-term use of NSAIDs, such as for three or four days of acute pain management after dental surgery, is unlikely to lead to serious sequelae, including embolic phenomena, in most healthy patients. It should be noted that idiosyncratic reactions (primarily manifesting as renal complications) can occur, and gastric mucosal irritation has been reported even with very brief use of NSAIDs.

Cyclooxygenase metabolism of arachidonic acid also produces thromboxane A_2, which increases platelet aggregability. NSAIDs decrease the production of thromboxane A_2; this decreases platelet aggregation and causes an increased tendency toward bleeding. NSAID inactivation of cyclooxygenase, and thus increased bleeding tendency, is reversible for all drugs except aspirin, which binds cyclooxygenase irreversibly.

Patient Advice

- Patients should be cautioned regarding the gastrointestinal side effects of these medications.
- These medications preferably should be taken with or after meals with a full glass of water to prevent lodging of the capsule or tablet in the esophagus.
- The patient should notify the dentist of any side effects that occur after starting use of the medication.

Suggested Readings

Brandt KD. The mechanism of action of non-steroidal anti-inflammatory drugs. J Rheumatol 1991;27(supple): 120-21.

Dionne RA, Berthold CW. Therapeutic uses of non-steroidal anti-inflammatory drugs in dentistry. Crit Rev Oral Biol Med 2001;12(4):315-30.

Dionne RA, Gordon SM. Nonsteroidal anti-inflammatory drugs for acute pain control. Dent Clin North Am 1994;38(4):645-67.

Hargreaves KM, Keiser K. Development of new pain management strategies. J Dent Educ 2002;66(1):113-21.

Joris J. Efficacy of nonsteroidal antiinflammatory drugs in post-operative pain. Acta Anaesthesiol Belg 1996; 47(3):115-23.

Khan AA, Dionne RA. The COX-2 inhibitors: new analgesic and anti-inflammatory drugs. Dent Clin North Am 2002;46:679-90.

Lawton GM, Chapman PJ. Diflunisal—a long acting nonsteroidal anti-inflammatory drug. A review of its pharmacology and effectiveness in management of dental pain. Aust Dent J 1993;38(4):265-71.

Woolf CJ, Chong MS. Preemptive analgesia—treating postoperative pain by preventing the establishment of central sensitization. Anesth Analg 1993;77(2):362-79.

Table 3.1: PRESCRIBING INFORMATION FOR ANALGESICS

NAME	FORM/ STRENGTH	DOSAGE	WARNINGS/PRECAUTIONS & CONTRAINDICATIONS	ADVERSE EFFECTS[†]
ACETAMINOPHEN & COMBINATIONS				
Acetaminophen (Feverall, Tylenol, Tylenol Arthritis, Tylenol Children's, Tylenol 8 Hour, Tylenol Extra Strength, Tylenol Infants' Tylenol Junior Strength)	**Feverall: Sup:** 80mg, 120mg, 325mg, 650mg; **Tylenol: Drops: (Infants')** 80mg/0.8mL; **Sol: (Extra Strength)** 500mg/15mL; **Sus:(Children's)** 160mg/5mL; **Tab: (Regular Strength)** 325mg, **(Extra Strength)** 500mg, **(Arthritis)** 650mg; **Tab, Chewable: (Children's)** 80mg, **(Junior)** 160mg; **Tab, Extended Release: (8 hr)** 650mg	**Tylenol: Adults:** (Regular Strength) 650mg q4-6h prn. **Max:** 3900mg/day. (Extra Strength) 1000mg q4-6h prn. **Max:** 4000mg/day. **Pediatrics: Max:** 5 doses/day. **0-3 mths (6-11 lbs):** 40mg q4h prn. **4-11 mths (12-17 lbs):** 80mg q4h prn. **12-23 mths (18-23 lbs):** 120mg q4h prn. **2-3 yrs (24-35 lbs):** 160mg q4h prn. **4-5 yrs (36-47 lbs):** 240mg q4h prn. **6-8 yrs (48-59 lbs):** 320mg q4h prn. **9-10 yrs (60-71 lbs):** 400mg q4h prn. **11 yrs (72-95 lbs):** 480mg q4h prn. **12 yrs:** 640mg q4h prn. **Older Children: Regular Strength: 6-11 yrs:** 325mg q4-6h prn. **Max:** 1625mg/day. **≥12 yrs:** 650mg q4-6h prn. **Max:** 3900mg/day. **Extra Strength: 12 yrs:** 1000mg q4-6h prn. **Max:** 4000mg/day. **Feverall: Pediatrics:** Insert sup rectally. **3-11 months:** 80mg q6h. **Max:** 480mg/24hrs. **12-36 months:** 80mg q4h. **Max:** 480mg/24hrs. **3-6 yrs:** 120mg q4-6h. **Max:** 720mg/24hrs. **6-12 yrs:** 325mg q4-6h. **Max:** 2600mg/24hrs.	**W/P:** May cause hepatic damage. **P/N:** Safety in pregnancy or nursing not known.	
Acetaminophen/Aspirin/ Caffeine (Excedrin Extra Strength, Excedrin Migraine)	**Tab:** (APAP-ASA-Caffeine) 250mg-250mg-65mg	**Adults:** Take 2 tabs with water. **Max:** 2 tabs/day.	**W/P:** Children and teenagers should not use for viral illnesses. APAP and ASA may cause liver damage and GI bleeding. **P/N:** Safety in pregnancy and nursing not known.	
Acetaminophen/ Butalbital (Phrenlin, Phrenilin Forte)	**Cap: (Phrenilin Forte)** (Butalbital-APAP) 50mg-650mg; **Tab: (Phrenilin)** 50mg-325mg	**Adults: (Phrenilin Forte)** 1 cap q4h. **(Phrenilin)** 1-2 tabs q4h. **Max:** 6 caps/tabs/day. **Pediatrics: ≥12 yrs: (Phrenilin Forte)** 1 cap q4h. **(Phrenilin)** 1-2 tabs q4h. **Max:** 6 caps/tabs/day.	**W/P:** Abuse potential. Caution in elderly/debilitated, severe renal/hepatic impairment, and acute abdominal conditions. **Contra:** Porphyria. **P/N:** Category C, not for use in nursing.	Drowsiness, lightheadedness, dizziness, sedation, shortness of breath, nausea, vomiting, abdominal pain, intoxicated feeling.
Acetaminophen/ Butalbital/Caffeine (Esgic-Plus, Fioricet)	(Butalbital-APAP-Caffeine) **Cap/ Tab: (Esgic-Plus)** 50mg-500mg-40mg* ; **Tab: (Fioricet)** 50mg-325mg-40mg	**Esgic-Plus: Adults:** 1 cap/tab q4h prn. **Max:** 6 caps/tabs/day. **Pediatrics: ≥12 yrs:** 1 cap/tab q4h prn. **Max:** 6 caps/tabs/day. **Fioricet: Adults:** 1-2 tabs q4h prn. **Max:** 6 tabs/day. Not for extended use. **Pediatrics: ≥12 yrs:** 1-2 tabs q4h prn. **Max:** 6 tabs/day. Not for extended use.	**W/P:** May be habit forming. Not for extended use. Caution in elderly, debilitated, severe renal or hepatic impairment, acute abdominal conditions. Caution in mentally depressed and suicidal tendencies, history of drug abuse. **Contra:** Porphyria. **P/N:** Category C, not for use in nursing.	Drowsiness, lightheadedness, dizziness, sedation, shortness of breath, nausea, vomiting, abdominal pain, intoxicated feeling.
Acetaminophen/ Caffeine/ Pyrilamine Maleate (Midol Maximum Strength)	**Tab:** 500mg-60mg-15mg	**Adults/Pediatrics: ≥12 yrs:** 2 tabs q6h. **Max:** 8 tabs q24h.	**W/P:** May cause hepatic damage. **P/N:** Safety in pregnancy or nursing not known.	
Acetaminophen/ Diphenhydramine Citrate (Excedrin PM, Tylenol PM)	**Tab: (Excedrin PM)** 500mg-38mg; **(Tylenol PM)** 500mg-25mg	**Adults/Pediatrics: ≥12 yrs:** 2 tabs qhs.	**W/P:** May cause hepatic damage. **P/N:** Safety in pregnancy or nursing not known.	

*Scored.   †Bold entries denote special dental considerations.

NAME	FORM/ STRENGTH	DOSAGE	WARNINGS/PRECAUTIONS & CONTRAINDICATIONS	ADVERSE EFFECTS†
Acetamino- phen/ Pamabrom (Midol Teen Formula)	**Tab:** 500mg- 25mg	***Adults/Pediatrics:*** **≥12 yrs:** 2 tabs q6h. **Max:** 8 tabs q24h.	**W/P:** May cause hepatic damage. **P/N:** Safety in pregnancy or nursing not known.	
Acetamino- phen/ Pamabrom/ Pyrilamine Maleate (Midol PMS Maximum Strength, Pamprin Multi- Symptom)	**Tab:** 500mg- 25mg-15mg	***Adults/Pediatrics:*** **≥12 yrs:** 2 tabs q6h. **Max:** 8 tabs q24h.	**W/P:** May cause hepatic damage. **P/N:** Safety in pregnancy or nursing not known.	

NSAIDs

NAME	FORM/ STRENGTH	DOSAGE	WARNINGS/PRECAUTIONS & CONTRAINDICATIONS	ADVERSE EFFECTS†
Celecoxib (Celebrex)	**Cap:** 100mg, 200mg, 400mg	***Adults:*** **≥18 yrs: OA:** 200mg qd or 100mg bid. **RA:** 100-200mg bid. **AS:** 200mg qd or 100mg bid. **Titrate:** May increase to 400mg/day after 6 weeks. **FAP:** 400mg bid with food. **Acute Pain/Primary Dysmenorrhea: Day 1:** 400mg, then 200mg if needed. **Maint:** 200mg bid prn. **Moderate Hepatic Insufficiency:** Reduce daily dose by 50%.	**Increased risk of serious cardiovascular thrombotic events, MI, and stroke, which can be fatal. Increased risk of serious GI adverse events including bleeding, ulceration, and perforation of stomach lining or intestines, which can be fatal. W/P:** Monitor blood, hepatic and renal function with chronic use. Avoid with advanced renal disease, moderate to severe hepatic dysfunction and late pregnancy. Anaphylactoid reactions and angioedema reported; avoid in ASA triad. Caution with history of peptic ulcer disease and/or GI bleeding, asthma, dehydration, fluid retention, HTN, heart failure. Do not substitute for corticosteroids or treat corticosteroid insufficiency. Discontinue if hepatic disease develops. Borderline elevations of liver enzymes may occur. Fluid retention and edema reported. Renal papillary necrosis reported. **Contra:** Sulfonamide hypersensitivity. Asthma, urticaria, or allergic type reactions after ASA or NSAID use. Treatment of peri-operative pain in coronary artery bypass graft surgery. **P/N:** Category C, not for use in nursing.	Dyspepsia, diarrhea, abdominal pain, nausea, dizziness, headache, sinusitis, upper respiratory infection, rash.
Diclofenac Potassium (Cataflam)	**Tab:** 50mg	***Adults:*** **OA:** 50mg bid-tid. **Max:** 150mg/day. **RA:** 50mg tid-qid. **Max:** 200mg/day. **Pain/Primary Dysmenorrhea: Initial:** 50mg tid or 100mg on 1st dose, then 50mg on subsequent doses.	**W/P:** Risk of GI ulceration, bleeding and perforation; extreme caution with history of ulcer disease or GI bleeding. Anaphylactoid reactions may occur. Avoid with advanced kidney disease. Avoid in late pregnancy; may cause premature closure of ductus arteriosus. Anemia may occur. May cause elevations of LFTs; discontinue if liver disease develops or systemic manifestations occur. Caution with considerable dehydration or kidney disease. Renal toxicity reported with long-term use. May inhibit platelet aggregation and prolong bleeding time; monitor with coagulation disorders. Fluid retention and edema reported; caution with fluid retention, HTN, or heart failure. Avoid with aspirin-sensitive asthma and caution with asthma.	Fluid retention, dizziness, rash, nausea, abdominal cramps, LFT abnormalities, constipation, diarrhea, heartburn, tinnitus, GI ulceration, hypertension, insomnia, **stomatitis**, pruritus.

Table 3.1: PRESCRIBING INFORMATION FOR ANALGESICS *(cont.)*

NAME	FORM/ STRENGTH	DOSAGE	WARNINGS/PRECAUTIONS & CONTRAINDICATIONS	ADVERSE EFFECTS†
NSAIDs *(cont.)*				
Diclofenac Potassium *(cont.)*			**Contra:** ASA or other NSAID allergy that precipitates asthma, urticaria or allergic reactions. **P/N:** Category C, not for use in nursing.	
Diclofenac Sodium (Voltaren, Voltaren-XR)	**Tab, Delayed Release: (Voltaren)** 25mg, 50mg, 75mg; **Tab, Extended Release: (Voltaren-XR)** 100mg	***Adults:* Voltaren: OA:** 50mg bid-tid or 75mg bid. **Max:** 150mg/day. **RA:** 50mg tid-qid or 75mg bid. **Max:** 200mg/day. **AS:** 25mg qid and 25mg qhs prn. **Max:** 125mg/day. **Voltaren-XR: OA:** 100mg qd. **RA:** 100mg qd-bid.	**W/P:** Risk of GI ulceration, bleeding and perforation; extreme caution with history of ulcer disease or GI bleeding. Anaphylactoid reactions may occur. Avoid with advanced kidney disease. Avoid in late pregnancy; may cause premature closure of ductus arteriosis. Anemia may occur. May cause elevations of LFTs; discontinue if liver disease develops or systemic manifestations occur. Caution with considerable dehydration or kidney disease. Renal toxicity reported with long-term use. May inhibit platelet aggregation and prolong bleeding time; monitor with coagulation disorders. Fluid retention and edema reported; caution with fluid retention, HTN, or heart failure. Avoid with aspirin-sensitive asthma and caution with asthma. **Contra:** ASA or other NSAID allergy that precipitates asthma, urticaria, or allergic-type reactions. **P/N:** Category C, not for use in nursing.	Fluid retention, dizziness, rash, nausea, abdominal cramps, LFT abnormalities, constipation, diarrhea, heartburn, tinnitus, GI ulceration, flatulence.
Diclofenac Sodium/Misoprostol (Arthrotec)	**Tab:** (Diclofenac- Misoprostol) 50mg-0.2mg, 75mg-0.2mg	***Adults:* OA:** 50mg tid. **RA:** 50mg tid-qid. **OA/RA:** If not tolerable, give 50-75mg bid (less effective in preventing ulcers). Do not crush, chew, or divide.	**Contraindicated in pregnancy. Must have (-) pregnancy test 2 weeks before therapy. Provide oral and written hazards of misoprostol. Begin on 2nd or 3rd day of the next normal menstrual period. Use reliable contraception. W/P:** Avoid in advanced renal disease, ASA-sensitive asthma, ASA triad, hepatic porphyria. Risk of GI ulceration, bleeding, and perforation. Check Hgb or Hct if signs of anemia arise. Caution in elderly, asthma, dehydration, HTN, coagulation disorders, heart failure, or renal disease. Monitor CBC and blood chemistry periodically. Check transaminases within 4-8 weeks, then periodically. Discontinue if develop hepatic or renal disease. **Contra:** Pregnancy. ASA or other NSAID allergy that precipitates asthma, urticaria or other allergic reactions. **P/N:** Category X, not for use in nursing.	Abdominal pain, diarrhea, dyspepsia, nausea, flatulence, GI disorders.
Diflunisal (Dolobid)	**Tab:** 250mg, 500mg	***Adults:* Pain: Initial:** 1g, then 500mg q8-12h. **OA/RA:** 250-500mg bid. **Max:** 1500mg/day. ***Pediatrics:* ≥12 yrs: Pain: Initial:** 1g, then 500mg q12h or 500mg q8h. **OA/RA:** 250-500mg bid. **Max:** 1500mg/day.	**W/P:** Risk of GI ulcerations, bleeding, and perforation. Borderline LFT elevations may occur. Inhibits platelet function at high doses. May cause adverse ocular effects. May mask signs of infection. Discontinue with hypersensitivity syndrome, liver dysfunction. Caution with pre-existing infection, compromised cardiac function, HTN, fluid retention, renal dysfunction, DM, elderly. As a derivative of salicylic acid, Reye syndrome may occur.	Nausea, dyspepsia, GI pain, diarrhea, rash, headache, insomnia, dizziness, tinnitus, fatigue.

*Scored.   †Bold entries denote special dental considerations.

NAME	FORM/ STRENGTH	DOSAGE	WARNINGS/PRECAUTIONS & CONTRAINDICATIONS	ADVERSE EFFECTS†
Diflunisal *(cont.)*			**Contra:** ASA or other NSAID allergy that precipitates acute asthmatic attack, urticaria, or rhinitis. **P/N:** Category C, not for use in nursing.	
Etodolac (Lodine, Lodine XL)	**(Lodine) Cap:** 200mg, 300mg; **(Lodine XL) Tab, Extended Release:** 400mg, 500mg	**(Lodine)** *Adults:* **Acute Pain: Usual:** 200-400mg q6-8h. **Max:** 1200mg/day. **OA/RA: Usual:** 300mg bid-tid, or 400-500mg bid. **Max:** 1200mg/day. **(Lodine XL) Adults: Usual:** 400-1000mg qd. **Max:** 1200mg/day. *Pediatrics:* **6-16 yrs: Juvenile RA: >60kg:** 1000mg. **46-60kg:** 800mg. **31-45kg:** 600mg. **20-30kg:** 400mg.	**W/P:** Risk of GI ulceration, bleeding and perforation; extreme caution with history of ulcer disease or GI bleeding. Anaphylactoid reactions may occur. Caution with advanced kidney disease. Avoid in late pregnancy; may cause premature closure of ductus arteriosis. Anemia may occur. May cause elevations of LFTs; discontinue if liver disease develops or systemic manifestations occur. Renal toxicity reported with long-term use. May inhibit platelet aggregation. Fluid retention and edema reported; caution with fluid retention, HTN, or heart failure. Avoid with aspirin-sensitive asthma and caution with asthma. **Contra:** ASA or other NSAID allergy that precipitates asthma, urticaria or other allergic type reactions. **P/N:** Category C, not for use in nursing.	Dyspepsia, abdominal pain, diarrhea, flatulence, nausea, constipation, gastritis, asthenia, malaise, dizziness, GI ulcers, gross bleeding/perforation.
Fenoprofen Calcium (Nalfon)	**Cap:** 200mg, 300mg; **Tab:** 600mg	*Adults:* **RA/OA:** 300-600mg tid-qid. **Max:** 3200mg/day. **Pain:** 200mg q4-6h prn. Take with food or milk with GI upset.	**W/P:** Risk of GI ulcerations, bleeding, and perforation. Renal toxicity and hepatotoxicity reported. Caution with compromised cardiac function or HTN. Monitor auditory and liver function with prolonged use. Extreme caution in the elderly. Decreases platelet aggregation and may prolong bleeding time. **Contra:** Significantly impaired renal function. ASA or other NSAID allergy that precipitates asthma, rhinitis, or urticaria. **P/N:** Safety in pregnancy and nursing is not known.	Dyspepsia, constipation, nausea, somnolence, dizziness, vomiting, abdominal pain, headache, diarrhea.
Flurbiprofen (Ansaid)	**Tab:** 50mg, 100mg	*Adults:* **Initial:** 200-300mg/day given bid, tid or qid. **Max:** 300mg/day or 100mg/dose.	**W/P:** Risk of GI ulceration, bleeding or perforation. Caution with renal/ hepatic dysfunction; reduce dose with significant renal impairment. Borderline LFT elevations may occur. May aggravate anemia; monitor Hgb periodically. Fluid retention and edema reported; caution in HTN and cardiac decompensation. Blurred vision reported. Prolongs bleeding time. **Contra:** ASA, with ASA triad, or other NSAID allergy that precipitates acute asthmatic attack, urticaria, or rhinitis. **P/N:** Category B, not for use in nursing.	Dyspepsia, diarrhea, abdominal pain, constipation, headache, nausea, edema.
Ibuprofen (Advil, Advil Junior, Midol Cramp Formula, Motrin, Motrin Children's, Motrin IB, Motrin Infants, Motrin Junior, Motrin Migraine Pain)	**Drops: (Motrin Infants) Sus:** 50mg/1.25mL; **(Advil/Motrin Children's)** 100mg/5mL [120mL, 480mL]; **Tab:** **(Advil/Motrin Junior)** 100mg, **(Advil/Midol**	*Adults:* **Pain:** 400mg q4-6h prn. **Dysmenorrhea:** 400mg q4h prn. **RA/OA:** 300mg qid or 400mg, 600mg or 800mg tid-qid. **Max:** 3200mg/day. Take with meals/milk. **Renal Impairment:** Reduce dose. *Pediatrics:* **Fever: 6 months-12 yrs:** 5mg/kg for temp <102.5°F; 10mg/kg if temp ≥102.5°F q6-8h. **Max:** 40mg/kg/day. **Pain: 6 months-12 yrs:** 10mg/kg q6-8h. **Max:** 40mg/kg/day.	**W/P:** Risk of GI ulceration, bleeding, and perforation. Risk of anaphylactoid reactions. Caution with significantly impaired renal disease and intrinsic coagulation defects. Fluid retention/ edema reported; caution with HTN or cardiac decompensation. Discontinue use if visual changes occur. May mask diagnostic signs of detecting infectious inflammatory painful conditions. Aseptic meningitis with fever and	Nausea, epigastric pain, heartburn, dizziness, rash.

Table 3.1: PRESCRIBING INFORMATION FOR ANALGESICS (cont.)

NAME	FORM/ STRENGTH	DOSAGE	WARNINGS/PRECAUTIONS & CONTRAINDICATIONS	ADVERSE EFFECTS[†]
NSAIDs (cont.)				
Ibuprofen (cont.)	**Cramp Formula/Motrin IB** 200mg, **(Motrin)** 400mg, 600mg, 800mg	**Juvenile RA:** 30-40mg/kg/day divided into 3 or 4 doses. Milder disease may use 20mg/kg/day.	coma reported especially with SLE and related connective tissue diseases. Increased LFTs may occur; monitor for liver dysfunction. Decreases in Hgb/Hct reported. **Contra:** Syndrome of nasal polyps, angioedema, and bronchospastic reactions to ASA or other NSAIDs. **P/N:** Not recommended in pregnancy. Not for use in nursing.	
Indomethacin (Indocin)	**Cap:** 25mg, 50mg; **Sus:** 25mg/5mL [237mL]	**Adults: RA/Ankylosing Spondylitis/ OA: Initial:** 25mg PO bid-tid. **Titrate:** May increase by 25-50mg/day at weekly intervals. **Max:** 200mg/day. **Bursitis/Tendinitis:** 75-150mg/day given tid-qid for 7-14 days. **Acute Gouty Arthritis:** 50mg PO tid until pain is tolerable, then discontinue. Take with food. **Pediatrics: ≥14 yrs: RA/Ankylosing Spondylitis/OA: Initial:** 25mg PO bid-tid. **Titrate:** May increase by 25-50mg/day at weekly intervals. **Max:** 200mg/day. **Bursitis/Tendinitis:** 75-150mg/day given tid-qid for 7-14 days. **Acute Gouty Arthritis:** 50mg PO tid until pain is tolerable, then discontinue. Take with food.	**W/P:** Risk of GI ulcerations, bleeding, perforation. Discontinue with evidence of liver dysfunction, decreased renal perfusion, severe CNS adverse reactions. Caution in pre-existing infection, CHF, HTN, fluid retention, renal dysfunction, DM, elderly, psychiatric disturbances, coagulation defects. Monitor platelet, renal, hepatic, ocular function in chronic use. False (-) results with dexamethasone suppression test. **Contra:** ASA or other NSAID allergy that precipitates acute asthmatic attack, urticaria or rhinitis. Do not give suppositories with history of proctitis or recent rectal bleeding. **P/N:** Not for use in pregnancy or nursing.	Headache, dizziness, nausea, vomiting, dyspepsia, diarrhea, abdominal pain, constipation, vertigo, somnolence, depression, fatigue.
Ketoprofen (Orudis KT, Oruvail)	**Cap: (Orudis KT)** 12.5mg, **(Oruvail)** 25mg, 50mg, 75mg	**Adults: OA/RA:** 75mg tid or 50mg qid. **Max:** 300mg/day. **Pain/Dysmenorrhea:** 25-50mg q6-8h. **Max:** 300mg. **Small Patients/Debilitated/Elderly/Hepatic or Renal Dysfunction:** Reduce dose.	**W/P:** Risk of GI ulceration, bleeding, and perforation. Caution with heart failure, fluid retention, liver or renal dysfunction, hypoalbuminemia, elderly. **Contra:** ASA or other NSAID allergy that precipitates acute asthmatic attack, urticaria or allergic-type reactions. **P/N:** Category B, not for use in nursing.	Dyspepsia, nausea, abdominal pain, diarrhea, constipation, flatulence, headache, renal dysfunction, LFT abnormalities, CNS effects.
Ketorolac Tromethamine (Toradol)	**Inj:** 15mg/mL, 30mg/mL; **Tab:** 10mg	**Adults: >16 to <65 yrs: Single-Dose:** 60mg IM or 30mg IV. **Multiple-Dose:** 30mg IM/IV q6h. **Max:** 120mg/day. **Transition from IM/IV to PO:** 20mg PO single dose, then 10mg PO q4-6h. **Max:** 40mg/24 hrs. **≥65 yrs/Renal Impairment/<50kg: Single-Dose:** 30mg IM or 15mg IV. **Multiple-Dose:** 15mg IM/IV q6h. **Max:** 60mg/day. **Transition from IM/IV to PO:** 10mg PO q4-6h. **Max:** 40mg/24 hrs. **Pediatrics: 2-16 yrs: Single-Dose: IM:** 1mg/kg. **Max:** 30mg. **IV:** 0.5mg/kg. **Max:** 15mg.	**For short-term use only (up to 5 days). Not for minor or chronic pain, intrathecal or epidural administration, use during labor/delivery or nursing, preoperatively or intraoperatively when hemostasis is critical, and with other NSAIDs. Can cause GI bleeding/ulceration, peptic ulcer and hypersensitivity reactions. Adjust dose in elderly, patients <50 kg, and if elevated serum creatinine. PO is only for continuation therapy to IM/IV. Avoid with advanced renal dysfunction or risk of renal failure due to volume depletion. W/P:** Do not exceed 5 days of therapy. Risk of GI ulcerations, bleeding and perforation. Caution with renal or liver dysfunction, dehydration, heart failure, coagulation disorders, debilitated and elderly. Preoperative use prolongs bleeding. Fluid retention, edema, NaCl retention, oliguria, anaphylactic reactions, elevated BUN and serum creatinine reported. Correct hypovolemia before therapy.	Nausea, dyspepsia, GI pain, diarrhea, edema, headache, drowsiness, dizziness.

*Scored.   †Bold entries denote special dental considerations.

NAME	FORM/ STRENGTH	DOSAGE	WARNINGS/PRECAUTIONS & CONTRAINDICATIONS	ADVERSE EFFECTS†
Ketorolac Tromethamine (cont.)			**Contra:** Active or history of peptic ulcer, GI bleeding, advanced renal impairment or risk of renal failure due to volume depletion, labor/delivery, nursing mothers, ASA or NSAID allergy, preoperatively or intraoperatively when hemostasis is critical, cerebrovascular bleeding, hemorrhagic diathesis, incomplete hemostasis, if high risk of bleeding, neuraxial (epidural or intrathecal) administration, and concomitant ASA, NSAIDs or probenecid. **P/N:** Category C, not for use in nursing.	
Lansoprazole/ Naproxen (Prevacid Naprapac 375, Prevacid Naprapac 500)	**Cap, Delayed-Release: (Naproxen-Lansoprazole)** 375mg-15mg; 500mg-15mg [14 tabs Naproxen + 7 caps Lansoprazole/weekly blister card; 4 cards/pkg]	***Adults:*** Take am dosing before eating. Lansoprazole 15mg qam + Naproxen 375mg or 500mg bid in the AM and PM. **Max:** 1000mg Naproxen/day. Swallow lansoprazole whole.	**W/P:** Risk of GI ulceration, bleeding, and perforation. Monitor for visual disturbances, fluid retention/edema, Hgb levels (if initial ≤10g), and LFTs with chronic use. Acute interstitial nephritis, hematuria, proteinuria, nephrotic syndrome and severe hepatic reactions reported. Caution with impaired renal (CrCl<20ml/min) or hepatic function, elderly, heart failure, and high doses with chronic alcoholic liver disease. **Contra:** Presence or history of NSAID/ASA allergy that precipitates asthma, rhinitis, nasal polyps, hypotension. **P/N:** Category B, not for use in nursing.	Nausea, abdominal pain, constipation, heartburn, headache, dizziness, drowsiness, pruritus, skin eruptions, ecchymoses, tinnitus, edema, dyspnea.
Meclofenamate Sodium	**Cap:** 50mg, 100mg	***Adults:*** **Mild to Moderate Pain:** 50mg q4-6h. **Max:** 400mg/day. **Excessive Menstrual Blood Loss/Primary Dysmenorrhea:** 100mg tid for up to 6 days starting at onset of menstrual flow. **RA/OA:** 200-400mg/day in 3-4 divided doses. **Max:** 400mg/day. ***Pediatrics:*** **≥14 yrs: Mild to Moderate Pain:** 50mg q4-6h. **Max:** 400mg/day. **Excessive Menstrual Blood Loss/Primary Dysmenorrhea:** 100mg tid for up to 6 days starting at onset of menstrual flow. **RA/OA:** 200-400mg/day in 3-4 divided doses. **Max:** 400mg/day.	**W/P:** Risk of GI ulcerations, bleeding, and perforation. Borderline LFT elevations may occur. Renal and hepatic toxicity. Extreme caution in the elderly. If visual symptoms occur, discontinue. **Contra:** ASA or other NSAID allergy that precipitates bronchospasm, allergic rhinitis or urticaria. **P/N:** Safety in pregnancy is not known. Not for use in nursing.	Diarrhea, nausea, vomiting, abdominal pain, edema, urticaria, pruritis, headache, dizziness, tinnitus, pyrosis, flatulence, anorexia, constipation, peptic ulcer.
Mefenamic Acid (Ponstel)	**Cap:** 250mg	***Adults:*** **Acute Pain: Usual:** 500mg, then 250mg q6h prn up to 1 week. **Primary Dysmenorrhea: Usual:** 500mg, then 250mg q6h up to 3 days. Take with food. ***Pediatrics:*** **≥14 yrs: Acute Pain: Usual:** 500mg, then 250mg q6h prn, up to 1 week. **Primary Dysmenorrhea: Usual:** 500mg, then 250mg q6h up to 3 days. Take with food.	**W/P:** Risk of GI ulceration, bleeding and perforation. Anaphylactoid reactions may occur. Monitor blood, hepatic and renal function. Caution with elderly, fluid retention, HTN, and heart failure. Avoid in late pregnancy, pre-existing kidney disease, dehydration and aspirin-sensitive asthma. **Contra:** Pre-existing renal disease, active ulceration or chronic inflammation of the GI tract. Allergic-type reactions, including asthma and urticaria, after taking ASA or other NSAIDs. **P/N:** Category C, not for use in nursing.	Abdominal pain, constipation, diarrhea, dyspepsia, flatulence, gross bleeding/perforation heartburn, nausea, GI ulcers, vomiting, abnormal renal function, anemia, dizziness, edema, elevated liver enzymes, headache, increased bleeding time, pruritus, rash, tinnitus.
Meloxicam (Mobic)	**Sus:** 7.5mg/5mL; **Tab:** 7.5mg, 15mg	***Adults:*** **≥18 yrs: OA/RA: Initial/Maint:** 7.5mg qd. **Max:** 15mg/day. ***Pediatrics:*** **>2 yrs: JRA:** 0.125mg/kg qd. **Max:** 7.5mg/day.	**NSAIDs may cause an increased risk of serious cardiovascular thrombotic events, myocardial infarction, and stroke, which can be fatal. NSAIDs cause an increased risk of serious GI adverse events including bleeding,**	Abdominal pain, constipation, diarrhea, dyspepsia, nausea, vomiting, headache, anemia, arthralgia, insomnia, upper respiratory tract infection, UTI.

Table 3.1: PRESCRIBING INFORMATION FOR ANALGESICS *(cont.)*

NAME	FORM/ STRENGTH	DOSAGE	WARNINGS/PRECAUTIONS & CONTRAINDICATIONS	ADVERSE EFFECTS[†]
NSAIDs *(cont.)*				
Meloxicam *(cont.)*			ulceration, and perforation of the stomach or intestines, which can be fatal. Meloxicam is contraindicated for the treatment of peri-operative pain in the setting of coronary artery bypass graft surgery. **W/P:** Risk of GI ulceration, bleeding and perforation; extreme caution with history of ulcer disease or GI bleeding. Anaphylactoid reactions may occur. Avoid with advanced kidney disease. Serious skin adverse events may occur. Avoid in late pregnancy; may cause premature closure of ductus arteriosis. Anemia may occur. May cause elevations of LFTs; discontinue if liver disease develops or systemic manifestations occur. Caution with considerable dehydration or kidney disease. May lead to onset of new HTN or worsening of preexisting HTN. Renal toxicity reported with long-term use. May inhibit platelet aggregation and prolong bleeding time; monitor with coagulation disorders. Fluid retention and edema reported; caution with fluid retention, HTN, or heart failure. Avoid with aspirin-sensitive asthma and caution with asthma. **Contra:** ASA or other NSAID allergy that precipitates asthma, urticaria, or allergic-type. **P/N:** Category C, not for use in nursing.	
Nabumetone (Relafen)	**Tab:** 500mg, 750mg	**Adults: Initial:** 1000mg qd. **Max:** 2000mg/day.	**W/P:** Risk of GI ulceration, bleeding, perforation. Risk of renal toxicity. Caution and monitor with renal dysfunction, heart failure, hepatic dysfunction, HTN, elderly, debilitated. May induce photosensitivity. **Contra:** Allergy to ASA or other NSAID that precipitates asthma, urticaria or other allergic-type reaction. **P/N:** Category C, not for use in nursing.	Diarrhea, dyspepsia, abdominal pain, constipation, flatulence, nausea, positive stool guaiac, dizziness, headache, pruritus, rash, tinnitus, edema.
Naproxen (Aleve, Anaprox, Anaprox DS, EC Naprosyn, Naprosyn)	**(Aleve) Tab:** 220mg; **(Anaprox) Tab:** 275mg; **(Anaprox DS) Tab:** 550mg*; **(Naprosyn) Sus:** 25mg/mL; **Tab:** 250mg*, 375mg, 500mg*; **Tab, Delayed Release:** (EC-Naprosyn) 375mg, 500mg	**Anaprox/Anaprox DS: Adults: RA/OA/AS:** 275mg bid or 550mg bid. **Max:** 1650mg/day. **Acute Gout:** 825mg followed by 275mg q8h. **Pain/Dysmenorrhea/Tendinitis/Bursitis:** 550mg followed by 550mg q12h or 275mg q6-8h prn. **Max:** 1375mg Day 1, then 1100mg/day. **EC-Naprosyn/Naproxen: Adults: RA/OA/Ankylosing Spondylitis: Naprosyn:** 250, 375, or 500mg bid. **EC-Naprosyn:** 375 or 500mg bid. **Max:** 1500mg/day. **Acute Gout: Naprosyn:** 750mg followed by 250mg q8h until attack subsides. **Pain/Dysmenorrhea/Tendinitis/Bursitis: Naprosyn:** 500mg followed by 500mg q12h or 250mg q6-8h prn. **Max:** 1250mg day 1, then 1000mg/day. EC-Naprosyn should not be chewed, crushed, or broken.	**W/P:** Risk of GI ulceration, bleeding and perforation; extreme caution with history of ulcer disease or GI bleeding. Anaphylactoid reactions may occur. Avoid with advanced kidney disease. Avoid in late pregnancy; may cause premature closure of ductus arteriosis. Anemia may occur; monitor Hgb levels if initial Hgb =10g. Monitor for visual changes or disturbances. May cause elevations of LFTs; discontinue if abnormal liver tests persist/worsen, if liver disease develops, or if systemic manifestations occur. Caution with considerable dehydration or kidney disease. Impaired renal function, renal failure, acute interstitial nephritis, hematuria, proteinuria, renal papillary necrosis, and nephrotic syndrome reported. Caution with high doses in alcoholic liver disease and elderly.	Edema, drowsiness, dizziness, constipation, heartburn, abdominal pain, nausea, headache, tinnitus, dyspnea, pruritus, skin eruptions, ecchymoses.

*Scored. †Bold entries denote special dental considerations.

NAME	FORM/ STRENGTH	DOSAGE	WARNINGS/PRECAUTIONS & CONTRAINDICATIONS	ADVERSE EFFECTS†
Naproxen *(cont.)*		***Pediatrics:*** **≥2 yrs: Juvenile RA:** (Sus) 5mg/kg bid. **Max:** 15mg/kg/day.	May inhibit platelet aggregation and prolong bleeding time; monitor with coagulation disorders. Peripheral edema reported; caution with fluid retention, HTN, or heart failure. Avoid with aspirin-sensitive asthma and caution with asthma. **Contra:** History of ASA or NSAID allergy that cause symptoms of asthma, rhinitis, nasal polyps, and hypotension. **P/N:** Category C, not for use in nursing.	
Oxaprozin (Daypro)	**Tab:** 600mg*	***Adults:*** **RA:** 1200mg qd. **Max:** 1800mg/day in divided doses (not to exceed 26mg/kg/day). **OA:** 1200mg qd, give 600mg qd for low weight or milder disease. **Max:** 1800mg/day in divided doses (not to exceed 26mg/kg/day). **Renal Dysfunction/Hemodialysis: Initial:** 600mg qd. ***Pediatrics:*** **6-16yrs: Juvenile RA: ≥55kg:** 1200mg qd. **32-54kg:** 900mg qd. **22-31kg:** 600mg qd.	**W/P:** Risk of GI ulceration, bleeding, and perforation. Risk of anemia. Caution with severe hepatic dysfunction, HTN, cardiac decompensation, hemostatic defects, renal dysfunction, heart failure, elderly, diuretic therapy, or other conditions predisposing to fluid retention. May elevate liver enzymes; discontinue if develop signs of liver disease. May induce photosensitivity. False-positive tests for benzodiazepines reported. Acute interstitial nephritis, hematuria and proteinuria reported. **Contra:** Complete or partial syndrome of nasal polyps, angioedema and bronchospastic reactivity to ASA or other NSAIDs. **P/N:** Category C, caution in nursing.	Constipation, diarrhea, dyspepsia, flatulence, nausea, rash.
Piroxicam (Feldene)	**Cap:** 10mg, 20mg	***Adults:*** 20mg qd or 10mg bid. **Elderly:** Start at lower end of dosing range.	**W/P:** Risk of GI ulceration, bleeding and perforation; extreme caution with history of ulcer disease or GI bleeding. Anaphylactoid reactions may occur. Avoid with advanced kidney disease. Avoid in late pregnancy; may cause premature closure of ductus arteriosis. Anemia may occur. May cause elevations of LFTs; discontinue if liver disease develops or systemic manifestations occur. Caution with considerable dehydration or kidney disease. Renal toxicity reported with long-term use. May inhibit platelet aggregation and prolong bleeding time; monitor with coagulation disorders. Fluid retention and edema reported; caution with fluid retention, HTN, or heart failure. Avoid with aspirin-sensitive asthma and caution with asthma. **Contra:** ASA or other NSAID allergy that precipitates asthma, urticaria, or other allergic type reactions. **P/N:** Category C, not for use in nursing.	Edema, dyspepsia, elevated liver enzymes, dizziness, rash, tinnitus, renal dysfunction, **dry mouth**, weight changes.
Sulindac (Clinoril)	**Tab:** 150mg, 200mg*	***Adults:*** **OA/RA/AS: Initial:** 150mg bid. **Acute Painful Shoulder/Acute Gouty Arthritis:** 200mg bid. **Max:** 400mg/day. Give with food.	**W/P:** Risk of GI ulcerations, bleeding, and perforation. Stop therapy with unexplained fever, evidence of hypersensitivity, liver dysfunction, pancreatitis. Caution with pre-existing infection, compromised cardiac function, HTN, fluid retention, renal dysfunction, elderly. Monitor platelet, renal, hepatic, ocular function in chronic use. **Contra:** ASA or other NSAID allergy that precipitates acute asthmatic attack, urticaria, or rhinitis. **P/N:** Not for use in pregnancy and nursing.	GI pain, dyspepsia, nausea, vomiting, diarrhea, constipation, rash, dizziness, headache, tinnitus, edema.

Table 3.1: PRESCRIBING INFORMATION FOR ANALGESICS *(cont.)*

NAME	FORM/ STRENGTH	DOSAGE	WARNINGS/PRECAUTIONS & CONTRAINDICATIONS	ADVERSE EFFECTS†
NSAIDs *(cont.)*				
Tolmetin Sodium	**Cap:** (DS) 400mg; **Tab:** 200mg*, 600mg	**Adults: OA/RA: Initial:** 400mg tid. **Usual:** 200-600mg tid. **Max:** 1800mg/day. Take with antacids other than sodium bicarbonate if GI upset occurs. **Pediatrics: JRA: ≥2 yrs: Initial:** 20mg/kg/day given tid-qid. **Usual:** 15-30mg/kg/day. **Max:** 30mg/kg/day. Take with antacids other than sodium bicarbonate if GI upset occurs.	**W/P:** Risk of GI ulcerations, bleeding, and perforation. May cause adverse ocular events. Prolongs bleeding time. Risk of renal toxicity with heart failure, liver dysfunction, and elderly. Caution with compromised cardiac function, HTN, or other conditions predisposing to fluid retention. Borderline LFT elevations may occur. Decreased bio-availability with milk or food. **Contra:** ASA or other NSAID allergy that pre-cipitates asthma, rhinitis, urticaria, or allergic-type reactions. **P/N:** Category C, not for use in nursing.	Dyspepsia, GI distress, diarrhea, flatulence, vomit-ing, headache, asthenia, elevated blood pressure, dizziness, edema.

OPIOIDS

CODEINE & COMBINATIONS

NAME	FORM/ STRENGTH	DOSAGE	WARNINGS/PRECAUTIONS & CONTRAINDICATIONS	ADVERSE EFFECTS†
Acetamino-phen/ Butalbital/ Caffeine/ Codeine Phosphate^{CIII} (Fioricet w/Codeine)	**Cap:** (Butalbital-APAP-Caffeine-Codeine) 50mg-325mg-40mg-30mg	*Adults:* 1-2 caps q4h prn. **Max:** 6 caps/day. Not for extended use.	**W/P:** May be habit forming. Not for extended use. Respiratory depression and cerebrospinal fluid pressure en-hanced with head injury or intracranial lesions. Caution in elderly, debilitated, severe renal or hepatic impairment, hypothyroidism, urethral stricture, Addison's disease, BPH, and history of drug abuse. May mask signs of acute abdominal conditions. **Contra:** Porphyria. **P/N:** Category C, not for use in nursing.	Drowsiness, lightheaded-ness, dizziness, sedation, shortness of breath, nau-sea, vomiting, abdominal pain, intoxicated feeling.
Acetamino-phen/ Codeine Phosphate^{CIII} (Tylenol w/Codeine)	(Codeine-APAP) **Elixir:** (CV) 12-120mg/5mL; **Tab:** (#3, CIII) 30-300mg, (#4, CIII) 60-300mg	*Adults:* **(Tab) Usual:** 15-60mg codeine/dose and 300-1000mg APAP/dose up to q4h prn. **Max:** 60mg codeine/dose, 360mg codeine/day and 4g APAP/day. **(Elixir):** 15mL q4h prn. *Pediatrics:* **(Elixir): Usual: 7-12 yrs:** 10mL tid-qid. **3-6 yrs:** 5mL tid-qid.	**W/P:** Respiratory depressant effects may be exacerbated with head injury or increased intracranial pressure. May obscure head injuries, acute abdominal conditions. Caution in the elderly, debilitated, severe hepatic or renal dysfunction, hypothyroidism, Addison's disease, prostatic hyper-trophy or urethral stricture. Potential for physical dependence, tolerance. Tabs contain sulfites. **P/N:** Category C, caution in nursing.	Lightheadedness, dizzi-ness, sedation, shortness of breath, nausea, vomit-ing, allergic reactions, euphoria, dysphoria, constipation, abdominal pain, pruritus.
Aspirin/Butal-bital/Caffeine/ Codeine Phosphate^{CIII} (Fiorinal w/codeine)	**Cap:** (Butalbital-ASA-Caffeine-Codeine) 50mg-325mg-40mg-30mg	*Adults:* 1-2 caps q4h prn. **Max:** 6 caps/day. Not for extended use.	**W/P:** May be habit-forming. Not for extended use. Respiratory depression and cerebrospinal fluid pressure may be enhanced with head injury or intracranial lesions. Caution in elderly, debilitated, severe renal or hepatic impairment, hypothyroid-ism, urethral stricture, head injuries, elevated intracranial pressure, acute abdominal conditions, Addison's disease, prostatic hypertrophy, peptic ulcer, coagulation disorders. Caution in children with chickenpox or flu. May obscure acute abdominal conditions. Preoperative ASA may prolong bleeding time. Avoid with ASA allergy. Risk of ASA hypersensitivity with nasal polyps and asthma. **Contra:** Porphyria, peptic ulcer disease, seri-ous GI lesions, hemorrhagic diathesis. Syndrome of nasal polyps,	Drowsiness, lightheaded-ness, dizziness, sedation, shortness of breath, nau-sea, vomiting, abdominal pain, intoxicated feeling.

*Scored. †Bold entries denote special dental considerations.

NAME	FORM/ STRENGTH	DOSAGE	WARNINGS/PRECAUTIONS & CONTRAINDICATIONS	ADVERSE EFFECTS†
Aspirin/ Butalbital/ Caffeine/ Codeine PhosphateCIII *(cont.)*			angioedema and bronchospastic reactivity to ASA or NSAIDs. **P/N:** Category C, not for use in nursing.	
Aspirin/ Carisoprodol/ Codeine PhosphateCIII (Soma Compound w/codeine)	**Tab:** (Carisoprodol-Codeine-Aspirin) 200mg-16mg-325mg	***Adults:*** 1-2 tabs qid. ***Pediatrics:*** ≥12 yrs: 1-2 tabs qid.	**W/P:** First-dose idiosyncratic reactions reported (rare). Caution with liver or renal dysfunction, elderly, peptic ulcer, gastritis, addiction-prone patients and anticoagulant therapy. Contains sulfites. **Contra:** Acute intermittent porphyria, bleeding disorders. **P/N:** Category C, not for use in nursing.	Drowsiness, dizziness, vertigo, ataxia, nausea, vomiting, gastritis, occult bleeding, constipation, diarrhea, miosis.
Codeine PhosphateCII	**Inj:** 15mg/mL, 30mg/mL, 60mg/mL; **Sol:** 15 mg/5mL; **Tab:** 30mg, 60mg	***Adults:* Pain (Mild-to-Moderate):** 15-60 mg Po/IM/SC q4-6hr prn. ***Pediatrics:* Pain (Mild-to-Moderate):** ≥1 yr: 0.5mg/kg/dose (15 mg/m²) PO/IM/SC, q4-6hr prn. **Max:** 60 mg/dose. **Pain (Mild-to-Moderate):** ≥1 yr: range for injection, 0.5mg/kg (16.7 mg/m²) IM/SC q4hr to 3mg/kg/24hr (100mg/m²/24hr) IM/SC divided into 6 doses.	**W/P:** May be habit forming. Some brands contain sodium metabisulfite, which may cause allergic-type reactions, including anaphylactic symptoms and life-threatening or less severe asthmatic episodes, in certain susceptible people. Caution with acute abdominal conditions, Addison's disease, asthma, chronic obstructive pulmonary disease, concomitant central nervous system depressants, elderly or debilitated, fever, head injuries or increased intracranial pressure, hypothyroidism, preexisting respiratory depression, hypoxia, hypercapnia prostatic hypertrophy or urethral stricture, recent gastrointestinal or urinary tract surgery, reduced blood volume, seizures, severe hepatic impairment, severe renal impairment, shock, ulcerative colitis, very young children. **Contra:** During labor when delivery of premature infant is anticipated. **P/N:** Use in pregnancy in nursing is not known.	Constipation, nausea, vomiting sedation, somnolence.
Codeine SulfateCII	**Tab:** 15mg, 30mg, 60mg	***Adults:* Cough:** 10-20mg PO q4-6hr prn. **Max:** 120mg/day. **Pain (Mild-to-Moderate):** 15-60 mg PO/IM/SC q4-6hr prn. ***Pediatrics:* Cough:** 2-5 yr: 2.5-5mg PO q4-6hr prn. **Max:** 30mg/day **Cough:** 6-12 yr: 5-10 mg/dose PO q4-6hr. **Max:** 60mg/day **Pain (Mild-to-Moderate):** ≥1yr: 0.5 mg/kg/dose (15mg/m²) PO/IM/SC q4-6hr prn. **Max:** 60mg/dose. **Pain (Mild-to-Moderate):** ≥1yr: Range for injection, 0.5mg/kg (16.7mg/m²) IM/SC q4hr to 3mg/kg/24 hr (100 mg/m²/24 hr) IM/SC divided into 6 doses.	**W/P:** May be habit forming. Some brands contain sodium metabisulfite, which may cause allergic-type reactions, including anaphylactic symptoms and life-threatening or less severe asthmatic episodes, in certain susceptible people. Caution with acute abdominal conditions, Addison's disease, asthma, chronic obstructive pulmonary disease, concomitant central nervous system depressants, elderly or debilitated, fever, head injuries or increased intracranial pressure, hypothyroidism, preexisting respiratory depression, hypoxia, hypercapnia prostatic hypertrophy or urethral stricture, recent gastrointestinal or urinary tract surgery, reduced blood volume, seizures, severe hepatic, impairment, severe renal impairment, shock, ulcerative colitis, very young children. **Contra:** During labor when delivery of premature infant is anticipated. **P/N:** Use in pregnancy and in nursing is not known.	Constipation, nausea, vomiting sedation, somnolence.

Table 3.1: PRESCRIBING INFORMATION FOR ANALGESICS (cont.)

NAME	FORM/ STRENGTH	DOSAGE	WARNINGS/PRECAUTIONS & CONTRAINDICATIONS	ADVERSE EFFECTS†
OPIOIDS (cont.)				
FENTANYL				
Fentanyl[CII] (Duragesic)	**Patch:** 12.5μg/hr, 25μg/hr, 50μg/hr, 75μg/hr, 100μg/hr [5ˢ]	**Adults:** Individualize dose. Determine dose based on opioid tolerance. **Initial:** 25μg/hr for 72 hr. **Pediatrics:** >12 yrs: Individualize dose. Determine dose based on opioid tolerance. **Initial:** 25μg/hr for 72 hr.	**Life-threatening hypoventilation can occur. Contraindicated for acute or post-op pain, mild/intermittent pain responsive to PRN or non-opioids, or in doses >25μg/hr at initiation of opioid therapy. Avoid in patients <12 yrs or if <18 yrs and weigh <50kg. Only for use in opioid tolerant patients. Concomitant use with potent CYP450 3A4 inhibitors may result in an increase in fentanyl plasma concentrations which may cause potentially fatal respiratory depression. Monitor patients receiving potent CYP450 3A4 inhibitors. W/P:** Monitor patients with adverse events for at least 12 hrs after removal. Avoid exposing application site to direct external heat. Hypoventilation may occur; caution with chronic pulmonary diseases. Caution with brain tumors, bradyarrhythmias, renal/hepatic impairment. Avoid with increased intracranial pressure, impaired consciousness, or coma. May obscure clinical course of head injury. Tolerance and physical dependence can occur. **Contra:** Management of acute/post-op pain, mild/intermittent pain responsive to PRN or non-opioid therapy. Doses >25μg/hr at initiation. Hypersensitivity to adhesives. Diagnosis or suspicion of paralytic ileus. **P/N:** Category C, not for use in nursing.	Hypoventilation, hypotension, HTN, nausea, vomiting, constipation, **dry mouth**, somnolence, confusion, asthenia, sweating.
Fentanyl Citrate[CII] (Actiq, Sublimaze)	**Inj: (Sublimaze)** 50μg/mL; **Loz: (Actiq)** 0.2mg, 0.4mg, 0.6mg, 0.8mg, 1.2mg, 1.6mg	**(Actiq) Adults: Initial:** 0.2mg (consume over 15 minutes). **Titrate:** Redose 15 minutes after previous dose is completed. No more than 2 units per breakthrough pain episode. May increase to next higher available strength if several breakthrough episodes (1-2 days) require more than 1 unit per pain episode. Repeat titration for each new dose. **Max:** 4 units/day. Prescribe 6 units with each new titration. The lozenge should be sucked, not chewed, and consumed over 15 minutes. **Pediatrics: ≥16 yrs: Initial:** 0.2mg (consume over 15 minutes). **Titrate:** Redose 15 minutes after previous dose is completed. No more than 2 units per breakthrough pain episode. May increase to next higher available strength if several breakthrough episodes (1-2 days), require more than 1 unit per pain episode. Repeat titration for each new dose. **Max:** 4 units/day. Prescribe 6 units with each new titration. The lozenge should be sucked, not chewed and consumed over 15 minutes. **(Sublimaze) Adults: ≥12 yrs:** Individualize dose. **Premedication:** 50-100μg IM 30-60 minutes prior to	**May cause life-threatening hypoventilation in opioid non-tolerant patients. Only for cancer pain in opioid tolerant patients with malignancies. Keep out of reach of children and discard properly. W/P:** (Actiq) Caution with COPD, hepatic or renal dysfunction. Risk of clinically significant hypoventilation. Extreme caution with evidence of increased intracranial pressure or impaired consciousness. Can produce morphine-like dependence. Increased risk of dental decay; ensure proper oral hygiene. Caution with bradyarrhythmias, liver or kidney dysfunction. (Sublimaze) Should only be administered by persons specifically trained in the use of IV anesthetics and management of the respiratory effects of potent opioids. An opioid antagonist, resuscitative and intubation equipment and oxygen should be readily available. Fluids and other countermeasures to manage hypotension should be available with tranquilizers. Initial dose reduction recommended with narcotic analgesia for recovery. May cause muscle rigidity particularly with muscles used for respiration. Adequate facilities	Respiratory depression, circulatory depression, headache, hypotension, shock, nausea, vomiting, constipation, dizziness, dyspnea, anxiety, somnolence, laryngospasms, anaphylaxis, euphoria, miosis, bradycardia, and bronchoconstriction.

*Scored.   †Bold entries denote special dental considerations.

NAME	FORM/STRENGTH	DOSAGE	WARNINGS/PRECAUTIONS & CONTRAINDICATIONS	ADVERSE EFFECTS†
Fentanyl Citrate[CII] *(cont.)*		surgery. **Adjunct to General Anesthesia: Low Dose: Total Dose:** 2μg/kg for minor surgery. **Maint:** 2μg/kg. **Moderate Dose: Total Dose:** 2-20μg/kg for major surgery. **Maint:** 2-20μg/kg or 25-100μg IM or IV if surgical stress or lightening of analgesia. **High Dose: Total Dose:** 20-50μg/kg for open heart surgery, complicated neurosurgery, or orthopedic surgery. **Maint:** 20-50μg/kg. **Adjunct to Regional Anesthesia:** 50-100μg IM or slow IV over 1-2 minutes. **Postoperative:** 50-100μg IM, repeat q 1-2 hrs as needed. **General Anesthetic:** 50-100μg/kg with oxygen and a muscle relaxant, up to 150μg/kg may be used. *Pediatrics:* **2-12 yrs:** Individualize dose. **Induction/Maint:** 2-3μg/kg.	should be available for postoperative monitoring and ventilation. Caution in respiratory depression susceptible patients (eg, comatose patients with head injury or brain tumor). Reduce dose for elderly and debilitated patients. Caution with obstructive pulmonary disease, decreased respiratory reserve, liver and kidney dysfunction, cardiac bradyarrhythmias. Monitor vital signs routinely. **Contra:** Opioid non-tolerant patients and management of acute or postoperative pain. **P/N:** Category C, not for use in nursing.	

Hydrocodone & Combinations

NAME	FORM/STRENGTH	DOSAGE	WARNINGS/PRECAUTIONS & CONTRAINDICATIONS	ADVERSE EFFECTS†
Acetaminophen/ Hydrocodone Bitartrate[CII] (Lorcet, Lorcet Plus, Lortab, Norco, Vicodin, Vicodin ES, Vicodin HP, Zydone)	(Hydrocodone-APAP) **Cap: (Lorcet HD)**5mg-500mg; **Sol: (Lortab)** 7.5mg-500mg/15mL; **Tab: (Lorcet Plus)** 7.5mg-650mg*; **(Lorcet (10/650))** 10mg-650mg*; **(Lortab)** 2.5mg-500mg*, 5mg-500mg*, 7.5mg-500mg*, 10mg-500mg*; **(Norco)** 5mg-325mg*, 7.5mg-325mg*, 10mg-325mg*; **(Vicodin)** 5mg-500mg*; **(Vicodin HP)** 10mg-660mg*; **(Vicodin ES)** 7.5mg-750mg*; **(Zydone)** 5mg-400mg, 7.5mg-400mg, 10mg-400mg	*Adults:* **Lorcet: (Plus, 10/650)** 1 cap/tab q4-6h prn pain. **Max:** 6 tabs/caps/day. **(HD)** 1-2 caps q4-6h prn pain. **Max:** 8 caps/day. **Lortab: (2.5/500, 5/500)** 1-2 tabs q4-6h prn. **Max:** 8 tabs/day. **(7.5/500, 10/500)** 1 tab q4-6h prn. **Max:** 6 tabs/day. **(Sol)** 15mL q4-6h prn. **Max:** 90mL/day. **Norco: (5/325)** 1-2 tabs q4-6h prn pain. **(7.5/325, 10/325)** 1 tab q4-6h prn pain. **Max:** 6 tabs/day. **Vicodin:** 1-2 tabs q4-6h prn. **Max:** 8 tabs/day. **Vicodin HP:** 1 tab q4-6h prn. **Max:** 6 tabs/day. **Vicodin ES:** 1 tab q4-6h prn. **Max:** 5 tabs/day. **Zydone: (5/400):** 1-2 tabs q4-6h prn. **Max:** 8 tabs/day. **(7.5/400, 10/400):** 1 tab q4-6h prn. **Max:** 6 tabs/day. *Pediatrics:* **≥2 yrs:** Lortab: (Sol) **12-15kg:** 3.75mL. **16-22kg:** 5mL. **23-31kg:** 7.5mL. **32-45kg:** 10mL. **≥46kg:** 15mL. May repeat q4-6h prn.	**W/P:** Caution in elderly, debilitated, severe hepatic or renal dysfunction, hypothyroidism, Addison's disease, prostatic hypertrophy, urethral stricture, pulmonary disease and postoperative use. May obscure acute abdominal conditions or head injuries. May produce dose-related respiratory depression. Monitor for tolerance. Suppresses cough reflex. **P/N:** Category C, not for use in nursing.	Lightheadedness, dizziness, sedation, nausea, vomiting, constipation, rash, respiratory depression.
Hydrocodone Bitartrate/ Ibuprofen[CIII] (Reprexain, Vicoprofen)	(Hydrocodone-Ibuprofen) **Tab: Vicoprofen:** 7.5mg-200mg; **Reprexain:** 5mg-200mg*	*Adults:* **Usual:** 1 tab q4-6h prn. **Max:** 5 tabs/day. **Elderly:** Use lowest dose or longest interval. *Pediatrics:* **≥16 yrs:** **Usual:** 1 tab q4-6h prn. **Max:** 5 tabs/day.	**W/P:** May produce dose-related respiratory depression. May obscure acute abdominal conditions or head injuries. Avoid with ASA triad, late pregnancy, advanced renal disease, ASA-sensitive asthma. Caution in elderly, debilitated, dehydration, renal disease, intrinsic coagulation defects, severe hepatic dysfunction, asthma, hypothyroidism, Addison's disease, prostatic hypertrophy, urethral stricture, heart failure,	Headache, somnolence, dizziness, constipation, dyspepsia, nausea, vomiting, infection, edema, nervousness, anxiety, pruritus, diarrhea, asthenia, abdominal pain.

Table 3.1: PRESCRIBING INFORMATION FOR ANALGESICS (cont.)

NAME	FORM/STRENGTH	DOSAGE	WARNINGS/PRECAUTIONS & CONTRAINDICATIONS	ADVERSE EFFECTS†
OPIOIDS (cont.)				
Hydrocodone Bitartrate/ Ibuprofen^{CIII} *(cont.)*			HTN, ulcer disease, pulmonary disease, postoperative use. May be habit-forming. Suppresses cough reflex. Risk of GI ulceration, bleeding, perforation. Anemia, fluid retention, edema, severe hepatic reactions reported. Possible risk of aseptic meningitis, especially in SLE patients. **Contra:** ASA or other NSAID allergy that precipitates asthma, urticaria, or other allergic reaction. **P/N:** Category C, not for use in nursing.	
HYDROMORPHONE				
Hydromorphone Hydrochloride^{CII} (Dilaudid, Dilaudid HP)	**Inj:** 1mg/mL, 2mg/mL, 4mg/mL, **(HP Formulation)** 10mg/mL, 250mg; **Sol:** 1mg/mL; **Sup:** 3mg; **Tab:** 2mg, 4mg, 8mg*	***Adults.* Initial: (SC/IM/IV)** 1-2mg q4-6h prn. **(HP Inj)** 1-14mg IM/SC; adjust dose so that 3-4 hrs of pain relief is achieved. **(Sol)** 2.5-10mg q3-6h prn. **(Tab)** 2-4mg PO q4-6h prn. **(Sup)** Insert 1 rectally q6-8h prn. **Titrate:** Increase dose as needed. **Elderly:** Start at lower end of dosing range.	**W/P:** Increased respiratory depression with head injury and/or increased intracranial pressure. May mask acute abdominal conditions. Caution with elderly/debilitated, seizures, biliary tract surgery, renal/hepatic impairment, hypothyroidism, Addison's disease, BPH, and urethral stricture. May suppress cough reflex. Potential for abuse, physical/psychological dependence. Seizures reported in compromised patients receiving high doses. Dilaudid-HP should only be used in patients already receiving large doses of narcotics. 8mg tab and sol contains sulfites. **Contra:** Intracranial lesions associated with increased intracranial pressure, COPD, cor pulmonale, emphysema, kyphoscoliosis, and in status asthmaticus. (HP-Inj) Obstetrical analgesia. **P/N:** Category C, not for use in nursing.	Excessive sedation, lethargy, mental clouding, anxiety, dysphoria, nausea, vomiting, constipation, urinary retention, respiratory depression. Orthostatic hypotension and fainting reported with injection.
MEPERIDINE				
Meperidine Hydrochloride^{CII} (Demerol)	**Inj:** 25mg/mL, 50mg/mL, 75mg/mL, 100mg/mL; **Syrup:** 50mg/5mL; **Tab:** 50mg*, 100mg	***Adults.* Inj: Pain: Usual:** 50-150mg IM/SC q3-4h prn. **Preoperative: Usual:** 50-100mg IM/SC 30-90 minutes before anesthesia. **Anesthesia Support:** Use repeated slow IV injections of fractional doses (eg, 10mg/mL) or continuous IV infusion of a more dilute solution (eg, 1mg/mL). Titrate as needed. **Obstetrical Analgesia: Usual:** 50-100mg IM/SC when pain is regular, may repeat at 1- to 3- hr intervals. **Elderly:** Start at lower end of dosage range and observe. **With Phenothiazines/Other Tranquilizers:** Reduce dose by 25 to 50%). IM method preferred with repeated use. **For IV injection:** Reduce dose and administer slowly, preferably using diluted solution. **Syrup/Tab: Usual:** 50-150mg q3-4h prn. **Concomitant Phenothiazines/Other Tranquilizers:** Reduce dose by 25-50%. Dilute syrup in 1/2 glass of water.	**W/P:** May develop tolerance and dependence; abuse potential. Extreme caution with head injury, increased intracranial pressure, intracranial lesions, acute asthmatic attack, chronic COPD or cor pulmonale, decreased respiratory reserve, respiratory depression, hypoxia, and hypercapnia. Rapid IV infusion may result in increased adverse reactions. Caution with acute abdominal conditions, atrial flutter, supraventricular tachycardias. May aggravate convulsive disorders. Caution and reduce initial dose with elderly or debilitated, renal/hepatic impairment, hypothyroidism, Addison's disease, prostatic hypertrophy or urethral stricture. Severe hypotension may occur post-op or if depleted blood volume. Orthostatic hypotension may occur. May impair mental/physical abilities. Not for use in pregnancy prior to labor. May produce depression of respiration and psychophysiologic functions in	Lightheadedness, dizziness, sedation, nausea, vomiting, sweating, respiratory/circulatory depression.

*Scored.   †Bold entries denote special dental considerations.

NAME	FORM/ STRENGTH	DOSAGE	WARNINGS/PRECAUTIONS & CONTRAINDICATIONS	ADVERSE EFFECTS†
Meperidine Hydrochlorideᶜᴴ *(cont.)*		**Usual:** 50-150mg q3-4h prn. **Concomitant Phenothiazines/Other Tranquilizers:** Reduce dose by 25-50%. Dilute syrup in 1/2 glass of water. *Pediatrics:* **Inj: Pain: Usual:** 0.5-0.8mg/lb IM/SC, up to 50-150mg, q3-4h prn. **Preoperative: Usual:** 0.5-1mg/lb IM/SC, up to 50-100mg, 30-90 minutes before anesthesia. **With Phenothiazines/Other Tranquilizers:** Reduce dose by 25 to 50%. IM method preferred with repeated use. **For IV injection:** Reduce dose and administer slowly, using diluted solution. **Syrup/Tab: Usual:** 1.1-1.8mg/kg up to 50-150mg q3-4h prn. **Concomitant Phenothiazines/Other Tranquilizers:** Reduce dose by 25-50%. Dilute syrup in 1/2 glass of water.	the newborn when used as an obstetrical analgesic. **Contra:** MAOI during or within 14 days of use. **P/N:** Safety in pregnancy and nursing not known.	

METHADONE

NAME	FORM/ STRENGTH	DOSAGE	WARNINGS/PRECAUTIONS & CONTRAINDICATIONS	ADVERSE EFFECTS†
Methadone Hydrochlorideᶜᴴ (Dolophine, Methadose)	**Concentrate:** 10mg/mL; **Tab:** 5mg, 10mg; **Tab, Dispersible:** 40mg	*Adults:* **Detoxification: Initial:** 15-20mg/day (up to 40mg/day may be required). Stabilize for 2-3 days, then may decrease every 1-2 days depending on patient symptoms. **Max:** 21 days. May not repeat earlier than 4 weeks after completing previous course. **Maintenance Treatment: ≥18 yrs:** (see literature for ages 16 to <18) individualized 20-120mg/day. **Pain: Usual:** 2.5-10mg q3-4h prn.	**Only approved hospitals and pharmacies can dispense oral methadone for the treatment of narcotic addiction. Methadone can be dispensed in any licensed pharmacy when used as an analgesic. W/P:** Do not inject agent. Extreme caution if use narcotic antagonists in patients physically dependent on narcotics. Can cause respiratory depression and elevate CSF pressure. Caution with head injuries, acute asthma attacks, COPD, cor pulmonale, decreased respiratory reserve, pre-existing respiratory depression, hypoxia, or hypercapnia. Reduce initial dose in elderly, debilitated, severe hepatic or renal impairment, hypothyroidism, Addison's disease, prostatic hypertrophy, or urethral stricture. Risk of tolerance, dependence, and abuse may occur. Impairs physical and mental abilities. Ineffective in relieving anxiety. May mask symptoms of acute abdominal conditions. May produce hypotension. **P/N:** Safety in pregnancy and nursing not known.	Lightheadedness, dizziness, sedation, sweating, nausea, vomiting.

MORPHINE

NAME	FORM/ STRENGTH	DOSAGE	WARNINGS/PRECAUTIONS & CONTRAINDICATIONS	ADVERSE EFFECTS†
Morphine Sulfateᶜᴴ (Avinza, Duramorph, Kadian, MS Contin, Oramorph SR, Roxanol)	**Cap, Extended Release: (Avinza)** 30mg, 60mg, 90mg, 120mg; **(Kadian)** 20mg, 30mg, 50mg, 60mg, 100mg; 0.5mg/mL, 1mg/mL, 5mg/mL; **Sol, Concentrate: (Roxanol)** 20mg/mL	*Adults:* **Avinza: ≥18 yrs: Conversion from Other Oral Morphine Products:** Give total daily morphine dose as a single dose q24h. **Conversion from Parenteral Morphine: Initial:** Give about 3x the previous daily parenteral morphine requirement. **Conversion from Other Inj: Duramorph: Parenteral or Oral Non-Morphine Opioids: Initial:** Give 1/2 of estimated daily morphine requirement q24h. Supplement with immediate-release morphine or short-acting analgesics if needed. **Titrate:** Adjust	**(Avinza)** Swallow capsules whole or sprinkle contents on applesauce. Do not crush, chew, or dissolve capsule beads. Avoid alcohol and alcohol-containing medications; consumption of alcohol may result in the rapid release and absorption of potentially fatal dose of morphine. **(Oramorph SR)** This is a sustained release tablet. Swallow tablet whole; do not break in half, crush or chew. **W/P:** Abuse potential. Extreme caution with COPD, cor pulmonale, decreased respiratory reserve (eg, severe kyphoscoliosis),	Constipation, nausea, somnolence, vomiting, dehydration, headache, peripheral edema, diarrhea, abdominal pain, infection, UTI, flu syndrome, back pain, rash, sweating, fever, insomnia, depression, paresthesia, anorexia, dry mouth, asthenia, dyspnea.

Table 3.1: PRESCRIBING INFORMATION FOR ANALGESICS *(cont.)*

NAME	FORM/ STRENGTH	DOSAGE	WARNINGS/PRECAUTIONS & CONTRAINDICATIONS	ADVERSE EFFECTS†
OPIOIDS *(cont.)*				
Morphine Sulfate[CII] *(cont.)*	**(Roxanol)** [30mL, 120mL, 240mL], **(Roxanol-T)** [30mL, 120mL] **Tab, Extended Release: (MS Contin)** 15mg, 30mg, 60mg, 100mg, 200mg; **(Oramorph SR)** 15mg, 30mg, 60mg, 100mg	dose as frequently as every other day. **Non-Opioid Tolerant:** 30mg q24h. **Titrate:** Increase by increments ≤30mg every 4 days. The 60, 90, and 120mg caps are for opioid-tolerant patients. **Max:** 1600mg/day. Doses >1600mg/day contain a quantity of fumaric acid, which may cause renal toxicity. **Duramorph:** *Adults:* **IV: Initial:** 2-10mg/70kg. **Epidural Injection: Initial:** 5mg in lumbar region. **Titrate:** If inadequate pain relief within 1 hr, increase by 1-2mg. **Max:** 10mg/24hrs. **Continuous Epidural: Initial:** 2-4mg/24hrs. Give additional 1-2mg if needed. **Intrathecal:** 0.2-1mg single dose, do not repeat; may follow with 0.6mg/hr naloxone infusion to reduce incidence of side effects. **Kadian: Conversion from other Oral Morphine:** Give 50% of daily oral morphine dose q12h or give 100% oral morphine dose q24h. Do not give more frequently than q12h. **Conversion from Parenteral Morphine:** Oral morphine 3x the daily parenteral morphine dose may be sufficient in chronic use settings. **Conversion from Other Parenteral or Oral Opioids: Initial:** Give 50% of estimated daily morphine demand and supplement with immediate-release morphine. May sprinkle contents on small amount of applesauce or in water for gastrostomy tube. Do not chew, crush, or dissolve pellets. **MS Contin: Conversion from MSIR:** Give 1/2 of total daily MSIR dose as MS Contin q12h or give 1/3 of total daily MSIR dose as MS Contin q8h. **Conversion from Parenteral Morphine: Initial:** If daily morphine dose ≤120mg/day, give MS Contin 30mg. **Titrate:** Switch to 60mg or 100mg MS Contin. Swallow whole; do not crush, chew, or break. Taper dose; do not discontinue abruptly. **Oramorph SR:** *Adults:* **Conversion from Parenteral or Immediate Release Oral Morphine:** Daily dose determined by the daily requirement of the immediate-release formulation. A single dose is half of the daily requirement given q12h. **Initial:** 30mg is recommended if daily morphine requirement is ≤120mg. Use 15mg for low daily morphine requirements. **Titrate:** increase to 60mg or 100mg after stable dose is reached. **Roxanol: Usual:** 10-30mg q4h. During first effective pain relief, dose should be maintained for at least 3 days before any dose reduction, if respiratory activity and other vital signs are adequate. **Elderly/Very Ill/Respiratory Problems/Severe Renal and Hepatic Impairment:** Lower doses may be required.	hypoxia, hypercapnia, pre-existing respiratory depression, increased intracranial pressure, head injury. May cause orthostatic hypotension, syncope, severe hypotension with depleted blood volume. Caution with circulatory shock, biliary tract disease, severe renal/hepatic insufficiency, Addison's disease, hypothyroidism, prostatic hypertrophy, urethral stricture, elderly or debilitated, CNS depression, toxic psychosis, acute alcoholism, delirium tremens, seizure disorders. Avoid with GI obstruction. Withdrawal symptoms with abrupt discontinuation. Tolerance and physical dependence may develop. Potential for severe constipation; use laxatives, stool softeners at onset of therapy. **Contra:** Respiratory depression in the absence of resuscitative equipment, acute or severe bronchial asthma, paralytic ileus. **P/N:** Category C, not for use in nursing.	

*Scored.   †Bold entries denote special dental considerations.

NAME	FORM/ STRENGTH	DOSAGE	WARNINGS/PRECAUTIONS & CONTRAINDICATIONS	ADVERSE EFFECTS†
Morphine Sulfate Liposome^{CII} (Depodur)	**Inj:** 10mg/1mL, 15mg/1.5mL, 20mg/2mL	**Adults: ≥18 yrs: Orthopedic surgery of the Lower Extremity:** 15mg lumbar epidural administration. **Lower Abdominal/Pelvic Surgery:** 10-15mg lumbar epidural administration. **Cesarean Section:** 10mg.	**W/P:** DepoDur should be administered by or under the direction of a physician experienced in the techniques associated with epidural drug administration and familiar with patient management following epidural opiate administration, including the management of respiratory depression. May cause severe hypotension in an individual whose ability to maintain blood pressure has already been compromised by a depleted blood volume or concurrent administration of drugs such as phenothiazines or general anesthetics. Should not be administered to patients with gastrointestinal obstruction, especially paralytic ileus. **Contra:** Contraindicated in patients with respiratory depression, acute or severe bronchial asthma, and upper airway obstruction. Contraindicated in any patient who has or is suspected of having paralytic ileus. **P/N:** Category C, not for use in nursing.	Decreased oxygen saturation, hypotension, urinary retention, vomiting, constipation, nausea, pruritus, pyrexia, anemia, headache, dizziness, hypoxia, tachycardia, insomnia, flatulence.

OPIUM & COMBINATIONS

Opium ^{CII}	**Tincture:** 10%	**Adults: Diarrhea:** 10% tincture, 0.6mL PO qid. **Max:** 6mL/day. **Diarrhea:** Paregoric (2mg/5mL), 5-10mL PO 1-4 times daily. **Max:** 40mL/day. **Pediatrics: Diarrhea:** Paregoric (2mg/5mL), 0.25-0.5mL/kg PO 1-4 times daily. **Diarrhea:** 10% tincture, 0.005-0.01 mL/kg/dose PO q3-4hr.	**W/P:** May cause addiction; tolerance may develop. Caution with acute abdominal conditions (paregoric), Addison's disease (paregoric), atrial flutter and other supraventricular tachycardias (paregoric), concomitant administration of other antidiarrheal or antiperistaltic drugs, anticholinergics, antihypertensives, concomitant administration of other central nervous system depressants, narcotic analgesics, narcotic antagonists, convulsive disorders (paregoric), depleted blood volume or difficulty maintaining blood volume (paregoric), elderly and debilitated gastrointestinal hemorrhage (tincture), head injury, increased intracranial pressure, intracranial lesions cerebral arteriosclerosis (tincture) hepatic cirrhosis or liver insufficiency (tincture), hypothyroidism (paregoric), myxedema (tincture), preexisting respiratory depression, emphysema, bronchial asthma, prostatic hypertrophy or urethral stricture (paregoric), severe impairment of renal function (paregoric). **Contra:** Diarrhea caused by poisoning until toxic material is eliminated from gastrointestinal tract. Do not use in convulsive states such as those occurring in status epilepticus, tetanus, and strychnine poisoning (paregoric). **P/N:** Category C, caution in nursing.	Constipation, nausea, vomiting, asthenia, dizziness, sedation, somnolence.

OXYCODONE & COMBINATIONS

Acetaminophen/ Oxycodone Hydrochloride^{CII} (Roxicet, Percocet, Tylox)	(Oxycodone-APAP) **Cap: (Tylox)** 5mg-500mg; **Sol: (Roxicet)** 5mg-325mg/5mL [5mL, 10^s 500mL];	**Adults: Pericocet: (2.5/325):** 1-2 tabs q6h. **Max:** 12 tabs/day. **(5/325):** 1 tab q6h prn. **Max:** 12 tabs/day. **(7.5/500):** 1 tab q6h prn. **Max:** 8 tabs/day. **(10-650):** 1 tab q6h prn. **Max:** 6 tabs/day. **(7.5/325):** 1 tab q6h prn. **Max:** 8 tabs/day. **(10/325):** 1 tab	**W/P:** May cause drug dependence and tolerance; potential for abuse. Risk of respiratory depression. Capacity to elevate CSF pressure may be exaggerated with head injury, other intracranial lesions or a pre-existing increase in intracranial pressure.	Lightheadedness, dizziness, sedation, nausea, vomiting, euphoria, dysphoria, constipation, skin rash, pruritus.

Table 3.1: PRESCRIBING INFORMATION FOR ANALGESICS (cont.)

NAME	FORM/STRENGTH	DOSAGE	WARNINGS/PRECAUTIONS & CONTRAINDICATIONS	ADVERSE EFFECTS†
OPIOIDS (cont.)				
Acetamino-phen/ Oxycodone Hydrochloride^{CII} *(cont.)*	**Tab: (Roxicet)** 5mg-325mg, 5mg-500mg; **(Percocet)** 2.5mg-325mg, 5mg-325mg, 7.5mg-325mg, 7.5mg-500mg, 10mg-325mg, 10mg-650mg	q6h prn. **Max:** 6 tabs/day. Do not exceed APAP 4g/day. **Roxicet: Usual:** 5/325 tab/sol or 5/500 tab q6h prn. **Titrate:** May need to exceed usual dose based on individual response, pain severity and tolerance. **Tylox: Usual:** 1 cap q6h prn.	May obscure the diagnosis or clinical course with head injuries or with acute abdominal conditions. Caution with severe hepatic impairment, renal dysfunction, hypothyroidism, Addison's disease, prostatic hypertrophy, urethral stricture, the elderly or debilitated. **P/N:** Category C, caution in nursing.	
Aspirin/ Oxycodone Hydrochloride/ Oxycodone Terephthalate^{CII} (Percodan)	**Tab:** (Oxycodone HCl-Oxycodone Terephthalate-ASA) 4.5mg-0.38mg-325mg*	**Adults: Usual:** 1 tab q6h prn. **Max:** 12 tabs/day or ASA 4g/day.	**W/P:** May cause drug dependence and tolerance; potential for abuse. Risk of respiratory depression. Capacity to elevate CSF pressure may be exaggerated with head injury, other intracranial lesions or a pre-existing increase in intracranial pressure. May obscure the diagnosis or clinical course with head injuries or with acute abdominal conditions. Caution with severe of hepatic impairment, renal dysfunction, hypothyroidism, Addison's disease, prostatic hypertrophy, urethral stricture, peptic ulcer, coagulation abnormalities, and the elderly or debilitated. May increase the risk of developing Reye's syndrome in children and teenagers. **P/N:** Safety in pregnancy and nursing is not known.	Lightheadedness, dizziness, sedation, nausea, vomiting, euphoria, dysphoria, constipation, pruritus.
Ibuprofen/Oxy-codone Hydrochloride^{CII} (Combunox)	**Tab:** (Oxycodone-Ibuprofen) 5mg-400mg	**Adults:** 1 tab/dose. Do not exceed 4 tabs/day and 7 days.	**W/P:** May cause drug dependence and tolerance; potential for abuse. Risk of respiratory depression. May cause severe hypotension. Capacity to elevate CSF pressure may be exaggerated with head injury, other intracranial lesions or pre-existing increase in intracranial pressure. May obscure the diagnosis or clinical course with head injuries or acute abdominal conditions. Risk of GI ulceration, bleeding and perforation. Risk of anaphylactoid reactions. Caution with severe hepatic impairment, pulmonary or renal dysfunction, hypothyroidism, Addison's disease, acute alcoholism, convulsive disorders, CNS depression or coma, delirium tremens, kyphoscoliosis associated with respiratory depression, toxic psychosis, prostatic hypertrophy, urethral stricture, biliary tract disease, elderly or debilitated. **Contra:** Significant respiratory depression, acute or severe bronchial asthma, hypercarbia, paralytic ileus, or in patients who have experienced asthma, urticaria, allergic-type reactions after taking aspirin or NSAIDs. **P/N:** Category C, caution in nursing.	Nausea, vomiting, flatulence, somnolence, dizziness, diaphoresis, asthenia, fever, headache, vasodilation, constipation, diarrhea, dyspepsia.

NAME	FORM/ STRENGTH	DOSAGE	WARNINGS/PRECAUTIONS & CONTRAINDICATIONS	ADVERSE EFFECTS†
Oxycodone Hydrochlorideᶜᴵᴵ (Oxycontin, OxyIR, OxyFast, Roxicodone)	**Cap: (OxyIR)** 5mg; **Sol: (Oxy-Fast)** 20mg/mL [30mL]; **(Roxicodone)** 5mg/5mL [5mL, 40s; 500mL], (Intensol) 20mg/mL [30mL]; **Tab: (Roxicodone)** 5mg*, 15mg*, 30mg*; **Tab, Extended Release: (Oxycontin)** 10mg, 20mg, 40mg, 80mg, 160mg	**Adults: Oxycontin: ≥18 yrs: Opioid Naive:** 10mg q12h. **Titrate:** May increase to 20mg q12h, then may increase the total daily dose by 25-50% of the current dose. Increase every 1-2 days. **Conversion from Oxycodone:** Divide 24 hr oxycodone dose in half to obtain the q12h dose. Round down to appropriate tab strength. **Opioid Tolerant Patients:** May use 80mg or 160mg tabs. Discontinue other around-the-clock opioids. **With CNS depressants:** Reduce dose by 1/3 or 1/2. Swallow whole; do not break, crush, or chew. High-fat meals increase peak levels with 160mg tab. **OxyIR/OxyFast: Usual:** 5mg q6h prn for pain. May add to 30mL of juice or other liquid, applesauce, pudding, or other semi-solid foods. **Roxicodone: Initial: Opioid Naive:** 5mg to 15mg q4-6h prn. **Titrate:** Based on individual response. For chronic pain or severe chronic pain, use around the clock dosing schedule at lowest effective dose.	**For continuous analgesia. Abuse potential. 80mg and 160mg tabs are only for opioid-tolerant patients. Swallow tabs whole. W/P:** Do not break, chew, or crush tabs. Extreme caution with COPD, cor pulmonale, decreased respiratory reserve, hypoxia, hypercapnia, pre-existing respiratory depression. Caution with circulatory shock, delirium tremens, acute alcoholism, adrenocortical insufficiency, CNS depression, myxedema or hypothyroidism, BPH, severe hepatic/renal/pulmonary impairment, toxic psychosis, biliary tract disease, increased intracranial pressure, or head injury, elderly or debilitated. May cause severe hypotension. May produce drug dependence; caution in known drug abuse. May aggravate convulsive disorders and mask abdominal disorders. **Contra:** Significant respiratory depression, acute or severe bronchial asthma, hypercarbia, paralytic ileus. **P/N:** Category B, not for use in nursing.	Respiratory depression, constipation, nausea, somnolence, dizziness, vomiting, pruritus, headache, **dry mouth**, sweating, asthenia.

Propoxyphene & Combinations

NAME	FORM/ STRENGTH	DOSAGE	WARNINGS/PRECAUTIONS & CONTRAINDICATIONS	ADVERSE EFFECTS†
Acetaminophen/ Propoxyphene Napsylate ᶜᴵⱽ (Darvocet A500, Darvocet N 50, Darvocet N 100)	(Propoxyphene-APAP) **Tab: (Darvon N)** 50mg-325mg, 100mg-650mg; **(Darvocet A500)** 100mg-500mg	**Adults: (Darvon N) Usual:** 100mg propoxyphene napsylate and 650mg APAP q4h prn for pain. **Max:** 600mg propoxyphene napsylate/day. **Elderly:** Increase dosing interval. **Hepatic/Renal Impairment:** Reduce daily dose. **(Darvocet A) Usual:** 1 tab q4h prn for pain. **Max:** 6 tabs/24 hrs. **Elderly:** Increase dosing interval. **Hepatic/Renal Impairment:** Reduce daily dose.	**W/P:** Drug dependence potential. Not for suicidal or addiction-prone patients. Caution with hepatic/renal impairment, elderly. **P/N:** Not for use in pregnancy, safety not known in nursing.	Dizziness, sedation, nausea, vomiting, liver dysfunction.
Aspirin/ Caffeine/ Propoxyphene Hydrochlorideᶜᴵⱽ (Darvon Compound-65)	**Cap:** (Propoxyphene-ASA-Caffeine) 65mg-389mg-32.4mg	**Adults: Usual:** 1 cap q4h as needed for pain. **Max:** 390mg propoxyphene HCl/day. **Elderly:** Increase dose interval. **Hepatic/Renal Impairment:** Reduce daily dose.	**W/P:** Drug dependence potential. May impair mental/physical ability for operating machinery. Caution use in peptic ulcer disease, coagulation disorders, hepatic/renal impairment and the elderly. ASA may increase risk of Reye syndrome. Not for suicidal or addiction-prone patients. Do not exceed recommended dose. **Contra:** Suicidal or addiction-prone patients. **P/N:** Not for use in pregnancy, unknown use in nursing.	Dizziness, sedation, nausea, vomiting, liver dysfunction.
Propoxyphene Hydrochlorideᶜᴵⱽ (Darvon)	**Cap:** 65mg	**Adults: Usual:** 65mg q4h as needed for pain. **Max:** 390mg/day. **Elderly:** Increase dose interval. **Hepatic/Renal Impairment:** Reduce daily dose.	**W/P:** Drug dependence potential. May impair mental/physical ability for operating machinery. Caution with hepatic or renal impairment and the elderly. Not for suicidal or addiction-prone patients. Do not exceed recommended dose. **P/N:** Not for use in pregnancy, unknown use in nursing.	Dizziness, sedation, nausea, vomiting, liver dysfunction.

Table 3.1: PRESCRIBING INFORMATION FOR ANALGESICS *(cont.)*

NAME	FORM/ STRENGTH	DOSAGE	WARNINGS/PRECAUTIONS & CONTRAINDICATIONS	ADVERSE EFFECTS†
OPIOIDS *(cont.)*				
Propoxyphene Napsylate^{CIV} (Darvon-N)	**Tab:** 100mg	**Adults: Usual:** 100mg q4h prn pain. **Max:** 600mg/day. **Elderly:** Increase dose interval. **Hepatic/Renal Impairment:** Reduce daily dose.	**W/P:** Avoid in suicidal or addiction-prone patients. May produce drug dependence in higher than recommended doses. May impair mental/ physical ability. Caution with hepatic or renal impairment. Do not exceed recommended dose and limit alcohol intake. **P/N:** Safety in pregnancy and nursing not known.	Dizziness, sedation, nausea, vomiting, constipation, abdominal pain, skin rashes, lightheadedness, headache, weakness, euphoria, dysphoria, hallucination.
OPIOID AGONIST-ANTAGONISTS				
Acetaminophen/ Pentazocine Hydrochloride^{CIV} (Talacen)	**Tab:** (Pentazocine-APAP) 25mg-650mg	**Adults:** 1 tab q4h prn. Max: 6 tabs/day.	**W/P:** Contains sodium metabisulfite. Caution with head injury, increased intracranial pressure, acute CNS manifestations, MI, certain respiratory conditions, renal or hepatic dysfunction, and biliary surgery, seizure disorders and alcohol use. Potential for physical and psychological dependence. Use in patients taking long-term opioids for chronic pain may precipitate acute opioid withdrawal syndrome. **P/N:** Category C, caution in nursing.	Nausea, vomiting, constipation, abdominal distress, anorexia, diarrhea, dizziness, lightheadedness, hallucinations, sedation, euphoria, headache, confusion, disorientation, sweating, tachycardia.
Butorphanol Tartrate^{CIV} (Stadol)	**Nasal Spray:** 10mg/mL [2.5mL]	**Adults: ≥18 yrs: Initial:** 1 spray (1mg) in 1 nostril, may repeat after 60-90 minutes (after 90-120 minutes in elderly or renal/hepatic disease) and may repeat in 3-4 hrs after 2nd dose; or may use 1 spray in each nostril, may repeat after 3-4 hrs. **Renal/Hepatic Disease:** Increase dose interval to no less than 6 hrs.	**W/P:** Not for use in narcotic-dependent patients. May result in physical dependence or tolerance. Avoid abrupt cessation. Discontinue if severe HTN occurs. Caution with hepatic or renal disease, acute MI, ventricular dysfunction, or coronary insufficiency. May impair ability to operate machinery. Increased respiratory depression with CNS disease or respiratory impairment. Severe risks with head injury. Use in patients taking long-term opioids for chronic pain may precipitate acute opioid withdrawal syndrome. **Contra:** Hypersensitivity to benzethonium chloride. **P/N:** Category C, caution in nursing.	Somnolence, dizziness, nausea, vomiting, nasal congestion, insomnia.
Nalbuphine Hydrochloride (Nubain)	**Inj:** 10mg/mL, 20mg/mL	**Adults: ≥18 yrs: Pain: Initial:** 10mg/70kg IV/IM/SC q3-6h prn. Adjust according to severity, physical status and concomitant agents. **Max:** 20mg/dose or 160mg/day. **Anesthesia Adjunct:** Induction: 0.3-3mg/kg IV over 10-15 minutes. **Maint:** 0.25-0.5mg/kg IV.	**W/P:** Increased risk of respiratory depression with head injury, intracranial lesions, or pre-existing increased intracranial pressure. Only for use by specifically trained persons. Naloxone, resuscitative and intubation equipment, and oxygen should be readily available. Caution with emotionally unstable patients, narcotic abuse, impaired respiration, MI with nausea and vomiting, biliary tract surgery. May impair ability to drive or operate machinery. Caution with renal or hepatic dysfunction; reduce dose. Caution during labor and delivery; monitor newborns for respiratory depression, apnea, bradycardia, and arrhythmias. Use in patients taking long-term opioids for chronic pain may precipitate acute opioid withdrawal syndrome. **P/N:** Category B, caution in nursing.	Sedation, sweating, nausea/vomiting, dizziness/vertigo, **dry mouth,** headache, injection site reactions.

*Scored.   †Bold entries denote special dental considerations.

NAME	FORM/ STRENGTH	DOSAGE	WARNINGS/PRECAUTIONS & CONTRAINDICATIONS	ADVERSE EFFECTS†
Pentazocine Hydrochloride/ Naloxone HydrochlorideCIV (Talwin NX)	**Tab:** (Pentazocine-Naloxone) 50mg-0.5mg	***Adults:* Usual:** 1 tab q3-4h. May increase to 2 tabs q3-4h. **Max:** 12 tabs/day. **Pediatrics: ≥12 yrs: Usual:** 1 tab q3-4h. May increase to 2 tabs q3-4h. **Max:** 12 tabs/day.	**For oral use only. Severe, potentially lethal reactions may result from misuse by injection alone, or in combination with other agents. W/P:** Caution with elderly, drug dependence, head injury, increased intracranial pressure, certain respiratory conditions, acute CNS manifestations, renal or hepatic dysfunction, biliary surgery, and MI. Use in patients taking long-term opioids for chronic pain may precipitate acute opioid withdrawal syndrome. **P/N:** Category C, caution in nursing.	Hypotension, tachycardia, hallucinations, dizziness, sedation, euphoria, sweating, nausea, vomiting, constipation, diarrhea, anorexia, facial edema, dermatitis, visual problems, chills, insomnia, urinary retention, paresthesia.
Pentazocine LactateCIV (Talwin Lactate)	**Injection Solution:** 30 mg/mL	***Adults:* Labor pain:** a single 30mg/dose IM (most common); OR 20 mg/dose IV for 2-3 doses at 2-3-hr intervals, as needed, after contractions have become regular. **Pain (Moderate to Severe):** 30-60mg IV, IM or SC every 3-4 hr as needed, **Max:** 360mg/day. ***Pediatrics:* Pain (Moderate to Severe): ≥12 yr:** 30-60mg IV, IM or SC every 3-4 hr as needed. **Max:** 360mg/day.	**W/P:** Caution with acute myocardial infarction with hypertension or left ventricular failure, alcohol use should be limited, asthma, elevated intracranial pressure, emotional instability, head injury, history of drug misuse (risk of dependency), history of seizures, patients receiving narcotics, renal or hepatic impairment, respiratory depression, sulfite sensitivity (with preparations containing acetone sodium bisulfite) therapeutic doses can cause hallucinations and disorientation. Use in patients taking long-term opioids for chronic pain may precipitate acute opioid withdrawal syndrome. **P/N:** Category C, caution in nursing.	Lightheadedness, vomiting, headache, euphoria, injection site necrosis, toxic epidermal necrolysis, hallucinations, dyspnea, respiratory depression.

OPIOID ANTAGONISTS

NAME	FORM/ STRENGTH	DOSAGE	WARNINGS/PRECAUTIONS & CONTRAINDICATIONS	ADVERSE EFFECTS†
Naloxone (Narcan)	**Inj:** 0.4mg/mL, 1mg/mL	***Adults:* Opioid Overdose: Initial:** 0.4-2mg IV every 2-3 minutes up to 10mg. IM/SQ if IV route not available. **Post-op Opioid Depression:** 0.1-0.2mg IV every 2-3 minutes to desired response. May repeat in 1-2 hr intervals. Supplemental IM doses last longer. **Narcan Challenge Test:** IV: 0.1-0.2mg, observe 30 secs for signs of withdrawal, then 0.6mg, observe for 20 minutes. SQ: 0.8mg, observe for 20 minutes. ***Pediatrics:* Opioid Overdose: Initial:** 0.01mg/kg IV. Inadequate Response: repeat 0.01mg/kg once. IM/SQ in divided doses if IV route not available. **Post-op Opioid Depression:** 0.005-0.01mg IV every 2-3 minutes to desired response. May repeat in 1-2 hr intervals. Supplemental IM doses last longer. **Neonates: Opioid-induced Depression:** 0.01mg/kg IV/IM/ SQ, may repeat every 2-3 minutes until desired response.	**W/P:** Caution in patients including newborns of mothers known or suspected of opioid physical dependence. May precipitate acute withdrawal syndrome. Have other resuscitative measures available. Caution with cardiac, renal, or hepatic disease. Monitor patients satisfactorily responding due to extended opioid duration of action. Abrupt postoperative opioid depression reversal may result in serious adverse effects leading to death. **P/N:** Category B, caution in nursing.	Hypotension, hypertension, ventricular tachycardia and fibrillation, dyspnea, pulmonary edema, cardiac arrest, nausea, vomiting, sweating, seizures, body aches, fever, nervousness.
Naltrexone (ReVia)	**Tab:** 50mg	***Adults:* Alcoholism:** 50mg qd up to 12 weeks. **Opioid Dependence: Initial:** 25mg qd. Maint: 50mg qd. **Naloxone Challenge Test:** 0.2mg IV, observe for 30 seconds, then 0.6mg IV, observe for 20 minutes; or 0.8mg SC, observe for 20 minutes.	**W/P:** Hepatotoxic with excessive doses; margin of separation between safe dose and hepatotoxic dose is 5-fold or less. Only treat patients opioid-free for 7-10 days. Attempting to overcome the opiate blockade is very dangerous. More sensitive to	Nausea, headache, dizziness, nervousness, fatigue, restlessness, insomnia, vomiting, anxiety, somnolence.

Table 3.1: PRESCRIBING INFORMATION FOR ANALGESICS (cont.)

NAME	FORM/STRENGTH	DOSAGE	WARNINGS/PRECAUTIONS & CONTRAINDICATIONS	ADVERSE EFFECTS†
OPIOID ANTAGONISTS (cont.)				
Naltrexone (cont.)			lower doses of opioids after naltrexone is discontinued. Safety in ultra rapid opiate detoxification is not known. Increased risk of suicide in substance abuse patients. Severe opioid withdrawal syndromes reported with accidental ingestion in opioid-dependent patients. Monitor closely during blockade reversal. Caution in renal or hepatic impairment. Perform naloxone challenge test if question of opioid dependence. **Contra:** Acute hepatitis, hepatic failure, patients failing naloxone challenge or opioid-dependent, concomitant opioid analgesics, acute opioid withdrawal, positive urine screen for opioids, phenanthrene sensitivity. **P/N:** Category C, caution in nursing.	
OPIOID DEPENDENCE				
Buprenorphine Hydrochlorideᶜⱽ (Buprenex, Subutex)a	**Buprenex: Inj:** 0.3mg/mL; **Subutex: Tab, SL:** 2mg, 8mg	**Buprenex: *Adults:*** 0.3mg IM/IV q6h prn. Repeat if needed, 30-60 minutes after initial dose and then prn. **High Risk Patients/Concomitant CNS Depressants:** Reduce dose by approximately 50%. May use single doses ≤0.6mg IM if not at high-risk. ***Pediatrics:* ≥13 yrs:** 0.3mg IM/IV q6h prn. Repeat if needed, 30-60 minutes after initial dose and then prn. **High Risk Patients/Concomitant CNS Depressants:** Reduce dose by approximately 50%. May use single doses ≤0.6mg IM if not at high-risk. **2-12 yrs:** 2-6µg/kg IM/IV q4-6h. **Subutex: *Adults/Pediatrics:* ≥16 yrs:** Give either agent SL as a single daily dose in the range of 12-16mg/day. Hold tabs under tongue until dissolved; swallowing tabs reduces bioavailability. **Induction: Subutex:** Give at least 4 hrs after last short-acting opioid (eg, heroin) use or preferably when early signs of opioid withdrawal appear. **Maint: Suboxone: Range:** 4mg-24mg/day. **Target Dose:** 16mg/day. **Titrate:** Adjust by 2mg or 4mg to a level that maintains treatment and suppresses opioid withdrawal effects. **Hepatic Impairment:** Adjust dose and observe for precipitated opioid withdrawal. **Concomitant CNS Depressants:** Consider dose reduction.	**W/P:** Significant respiratory depression reported; caution with compromised respiratory function. May increase CSF pressure; caution with head injury, intracranial lesions. Caution with debilitated, BPH, biliary tract dysfunction, myxedema, hypothyroidism, urethral stricture, acute alcoholism, Addison's disease, CNS disease, coma, toxic psychoses, delirium tremens, elderly, pediatrics, kyphoscoliosis or hepatic/renal/pulmonary impairment. May impair mental or physical abilities. May precipitate withdrawal in narcotic-dependence. May lead to psychological dependence. **P/N:** Category C, not for use in nursing.	Nausea, dizziness, sweating, hypotension, vomiting, headache, miosis, hypoventilation.
Buprenorphine Hydrochloride/ Naloxone Hydrochlorideᶜᴵᴵᴵ (Suboxone)	**Tab, SL:** 2mg-0.5mg, 8mg-2mg	***Adults:*** Give either agent SL as a single daily dose in the range of 12-16mg/day. Hold tabs under tongue until dissolved; swallowing tabs reduces bioavailability. **Induction: Subutex:** Give at least 4 hrs after last short-acting opioid (eg, heroine) use or preferably when early signs	**W/P:** Significant respiratory depression reported with buprenorphine; caution with compromised respiratory function. Naloxone may not be effective in reversing any respiratory depression produced by buprenorphine. Cytolytic hepatitis and hepatitis with jaundice reported. Obtain LFTs prior	Headache, infection, pain (general, abdomen, back), withdrawal syndrome, constipation, nausea, insomnia, sweating, asthenia, anxiety, depression, rhinitis.

*Scored.   †Bold entries denote special dental considerations.

NAME	FORM/ STRENGTH	DOSAGE	WARNINGS/PRECAUTIONS & CONTRAINDICATIONS	ADVERSE EFFECTS†
Buprenorphine Hydrochloride/ Naloxone Hydrochloride^{CIII} *(cont.)*		of opioid withdrawal appear. **Maint: Suboxone: Range:** 4mg-24mg/day. **Target dose:** 16mg/day. **Titrate:** Adjust by 2mg or 4mg to a level that maintains treatment and suppresses opioid withdrawal effects. **Hepatic Impairment:** Adjust dose and observe for precipitated opioid withdrawal. **Concomitant CNS Depressants:** Consider dose reduction. *Pediatrics:* **≥16 yrs:** Give either agent SL as a single daily dose in the range of 12-16mg/day. Hold tabs under tongue until dissolved; swallowing tabs reduces bioavailability. **Induction: Subutex:** Give at least 4 hrs after last short-acting opioid (eg, heroin) use or preferably when early signs of opioid withdrawal appear. **Maint: Suboxone: Range:** 4mg-24mg/day. **Target dose:** 16mg/day. **Titrate:** Adjust by 2mg or 4mg to a level that maintains treatment and suppresses opioid withdrawal effects. **Hepatic Impairment:** Adjust dose and observe for precipitated opioid withdrawal. **Concomitant CNS Depressants:** Consider dose reduction.	to initiation and periodically thereafter. Acute and chronic hypersensitivity reactions reported. May increase CSF pressure; caution with head injury, intracranial lesions. May cause miosis, changes in level of consciousness, and orthostatic hypotension. Caution with elderly, debilitated, myxedema, hypothyroidism, acute alcoholism, Addison's disease, CNS depression or coma, toxic psychoses, prostatic hypertrophy, urethral stricture, delirium tremens, kyphoscoliosis, biliary tract dysfunction or severe hepatic/renal/ pulmonary impairment. Suboxone may cause opioid withdrawal symptoms. May obscure diagnosis of acute abdominal conditions. May produce dependence. **P/N:** Category C, not for use in nursing.	

SALICYLATES & COMBINATIONS

ASPIRIN & COMBINATIONS

NAME	FORM/ STRENGTH	DOSAGE	WARNINGS/PRECAUTIONS & CONTRAINDICATIONS	ADVERSE EFFECTS†
Aluminum Hydroxide/ Aspirin/Calcium Carbonate/Magnesium Hydroxide (Ascriptin, Ascriptin Maximum Strength)	**Tab:** (Aspirin) 325mg, 500mg	*Adults/Pediatrics:* **≥12 yrs:** 2 tabs q4h. **Max:** 8-12 tabs q24h.	**W/P:** Children and teenagers should not use this medicine for chicken pox or flu symptoms before a doctor is consulted about Reye's syndrome. **P/N:** Avoid in 3rd trimester of pregnancy and nursing.	Fever, hypothermia, dysrhythmias, hypotension, agitation, cerebral edema, dehydration, hyperkalemia, dyspepsia, GI bleed, hearing loss, tinnitus, problems in pregnancy.
Aspirin (Aspergum, Bayer Aspirin, Bayer Aspirin Children's, Bayer Aspirin Regimen, Bayer Genuine Aspirin, Bayer Extra Strenght, Ecotrin, Ecotrin Adult Low Strength, Ecotrin Maximum Strength, Halfprin, St. Joseph Pain Reliever)	**Tab:** (Aspergum) 227mg; **Tab:** (Genuine Bayer Aspirin) 325mg; **Tab: (Bayer Extra Strength)** 500mg; **Tab: (Bayer Aspirin Regimen with Calcium)** 81mg; **Tab, Chewable: (Bayer Aspirin Children's)** 81mg; **Tab, Delayed Release: (Bayer Aspirin Regimen)** 81mg, 325mg; **Tab, Delayed Release: (Ecotrin)** 81mg, 325mg, 500mg;	*Adults:* **Ischemic Stroke/TIA:** 50-325mg qd. **Suspected Acute MI: Initial:** 160-162.5mg qd as soon as suspect MI. **Maint:** 160-162.5mg qd for 30 days post-infarction, consider further therapy for prevention/recurrent MI. **Prevention or Recurrent MI/Unstable Angina/Chronic Stable Angina:** 75-325mg qd. **CABG:** 325mg qd, start 6 hrs post-surgery. Continue for 1 year. **PTCA: Initial:** 325mg, 2 hrs pre-surgery. **Maint:** 160-325mg qd. **Carotid Endarterectomy:** 80mg qd to 650mg bid, start pre-surgery. **RA: Initial:** 3g qd in divided doses. Increase for anti-inflammatory efficacy to 150-300μg/mL plasma salicylate level. **Spondyloarthropathies:** Up to 4g/day in divided doses. **OA:** Up to 3g/day in divided doses. **Arthritis/SLE Pleurisy:**	**W/P:** Increased risk of bleeding with heavy alcohol use (≥3 drinks/day). May inhibit platelet function; can adversely affect inherited (hemophilia) or acquired (hepatic disease, vitamin K deficiency) bleeding disorders. Monitor for bleeding and ulceration. Avoid in history of active peptic ulcer, severe renal failure, severe hepatic insufficiency, and sodium restricted diets. Associated with elevated LFTs, BUN, and serum creatinine; hyperkalemia; proteinuria; and prolonged bleeding time. Avoid 1 week before and during labor. **Contra:** NSAID allergy, viral infections in children or teenagers, syndrome of asthma, rhinitis, and nasal polyps. **P/N:** Avoid in 3rd trimester of pregnancy and nursing.	Fever, hypothermia, dysrhythmias, hypotension, agitation, cerebral edema, dehydration, hyperkalemia, dyspepsia, GI bleed, hearing loss, tinnitus, problems in pregnancy.

Table 3.1: PRESCRIBING INFORMATION FOR ANALGESICS (cont.)

NAME	FORM/ STRENGTH	DOSAGE	WARNINGS/PRECAUTIONS & CONTRAINDICATIONS	ADVERSE EFFECTS†
SALICYLATES & COMBINATIONS (cont.)				
Aspirin (cont.)	**(Halfprin)** 81mg, 162mg; **Tab: (St. Joseph)** 81mg	**Initial:** 3g/day in divided doses. Increase for anti-inflammatory efficacy to 150-300μg/mL plasma salicylate level. **Pain:** 325-650mg q4-6h. **Max:** 4g/day.		
Aspirin/Butal-bital/Caffeine (Fiorinal)	Cap/Tab: (Butalbital-ASA-Caffeine) 50mg-325mg-40mg	**Adults:** 1-2 caps or tabs q4h prn. **Max:** 6 caps or tabs/day. Not for extended use.	**W/P:** May be habit-forming. Not for extended use. Caution in elderly, debilitated, severe renal or hepatic impairment, hypothyroidism, urethral stricture, head injuries, elevated intra-cranial pressure, acute abdominal conditions, Addison's disease, prostatic hypertrophy, peptic ulcer, coagulation disorders. Avoid with ASA allergy. Risk of ASA hypersensitivity with nasal polyps and asthma. Caution in children with chickenpox or flu. Preoperative ASA may prolong bleeding time. **Contra:** Porphyria, peptic ulcer disease, serious GI lesions, hemorrhagic diathesis. Syndrome of nasal polyps, angioedema and bronchospastic reactivity to ASA or NSAIDs. **P/N:** Category C, not for use in nursing.	Drowsiness, lightheaded-ness, dizziness, sedation, shortness of breath, nau-sea, vomiting, abdominal pain, intoxicated feeling.
Aspirin/Caf-feine (Alka-Seltzer Morning Relief, Anacin, Anacin Maximum Strength)	**Tab: (Alka-Seltzer Morning Relief)** 500mg-65mg; **(Anacin)** 400mg-32mg, 500mg-32mg	**Adults/Pediatrics:** ≥12 yrs: 2 tabs q6h. **Max:** 8 tabs q24h.	**W/P:** Children and teenagers should not use this medicine for chicken pox or flu symptoms before a doctor is consulted about Reye's syndrome. **P/N:** Avoid in 3rd trimester of preg-nancy and nursing.	Fever, hypothermia, dys-rhythmias, hypotension, agitation, cerebral edema, dehydration, hyperkalemia, dyspepsia, GI bleeding, hearing loss, tinnitus, problems in pregnancy.
Aspirin/ Calcium Carbonate (Bayer Plus Extra Strength)	Tab: (Aspirin) 500mg	**Adults/Pediatrics:** ≥12 yrs: 2 tabs q4h. **Max:** 8 tabs q24h.	**W/P:** Children and teenagers should not use this medicine for chicken pox or flu symptoms before a doctor is consulted about Reye's syndrome. **P/N:** Avoid in 3rd trimester of preg-nancy and nursing.	Fever, hypothermia, dys-rhythmias, hypotension, agitation, cerebral edema, dehydration, hyperkalemia, dyspepsia, GI bleed, hearing loss, tinnitus, problems in pregnancy.
Aspirin/Cal-cium Carbon-ate/Magnesium Carbonate/ Magnesium Oxide (Bufferin, Bufferin Extra Strength)	Tab: (Aspirin) 325mg, 500mg	**Adults/Pediatrics:** ≥12 yrs: 2 tabs q4h. **Max:** 8-12 tabs q24h.	**W/P:** Children and teenagers should not use this medicine for chicken pox or flu symptoms before a doctor is consulted about Reye's syndrome. **P/N:** Avoid in 3rd trimester of preg-nancy and nursing.	Fever, hypothermia, dys-rhythmias, hypotension, agitation, cerebral edema, dehydration, hyperkalemia, dyspepsia, GI bleed, hearing loss, tinnitus, problems in pregnancy.
Aspirin/Citric Acid/Sodium Bicarbonate (Alka-Seltzer, Alka Seltzer Extra Strength)	Tab: (Aspirin) 325mg	**Adults/Pediatrics:** ≥12 yrs: 2 tabs q4h. **Max:** 8-12 tabs q24h.	**W/P:** Children and teenagers should not use this medicine for chicken pox or flu symptoms before a doctor is consulted about Reye's syndrome. **P/N:** Avoid in 3rd trimester of preg-nancy and nursing.	Fever, hypothermia, dys-rhythmias, hypotension, agitation, cerebral edema, dehydration, hyperkalemia, dyspepsia, GI bleed, hearing loss, tinnitus, problems in pregnancy.

*Scored.   †Bold entries denote special dental considerations.

NAME	FORM/ STRENGTH	DOSAGE	WARNINGS/PRECAUTIONS & CONTRAINDICATIONS	ADVERSE EFFECTS†
MAGNESIUM SALICYLATE				
Magnesium Salicylate (Doan's Regular, Doan's Extra Strength)	**Tab:** 377mg, 500mg	**Adults/Pediatrics: ≥12 yrs:** 2 tabs q4h. **Max:** 8-12 tabs q24h.	**W/P:** Children and teenagers should not use this medicine for chicken pox or flu symptoms before a doctor is consulted about Reye's Syndrome. **P/N:** Caution in pregnancy and nursing.	
SALSALATE				
Salsalate (Salflex)	**Tab:** 500mg, 750mg*	**Adults: Usual:** 1000mg tid or 1500mg bid.	**W/P:** Competes with thyroid hormone for binding to plasma proteins. Reye's syndrome may develop in viral infections (eg, chickenpox, influenza). Caution in chronic renal impairment and peptic ulcer. Bronchospasm reported with ASA-sensitivity. Monitor salicylic acid levels and urinary pH periodically with long-term therapy. **P/N:** Category C, caution in nursing.	Tinnitus, nausea, heartburn, rash, vertigo, hearing impairment.
TRAMADOL				
Acetaminophen/ Tramadol Hydrochloride (Ultracet)	**Tab:** (Tramadol-APAP) 37.5mg-325mg	**Adults:** 2 tabs q4-6h prn for 5 days or less. **Max:** 8 tabs/24hrs. **CrCl <30mL/min: Max:** 2 tabs q12h.	**W/P:** Seizures and anaphylactic reactions reported. May complicate acute abdominal conditions. Caution with risk of respiratory depression, increased intracranial pressure, or head injury. Avoid abrupt withdrawal. Caution in elderly. Avoid use in opioid-dependent patients and with hepatic impairment. **Contra:** Acute alcohol intoxication, hypnotics, narcotics, centrally-acting analgesics, opioids or psychotropics. **P/N:** Category C, not for use in nursing.	Constipation, diarrhea, nausea, somnolence, anorexia, increased sweating, dizziness.
Tramadol Hydrochloride (Ultram)	**Tab:** 50mg*	**Adults: ≥16 yrs: Initial:** 25mg every am. **Titrate:** Increase by 25mg every 3 days to 25mg qid, then increase by 50mg every 3 days to 50mg qid. **Usual:** 50-100mg q4-6h as needed. **Max:** 400mg/day. **Elderly:** Start at low end of dosing range. **≥75 yrs:Max:** 300mg/day. **CrCl <30mL/min:** Dose q12h. **Max:** 200mg/day. **Cirrhosis:** 50mg q12h. Concomitant carbamazepine (up to 800mg/day): May need 2x the recommended dose of tramadol. **Pediatrics: ≥16 yrs: Initial:** 25mg every am. **Titrate:** Increase by 25mg every 3 days to 25mg qid, then increase by 50mg every 3 days to 50mg qid. **Usual:** 50-100mg q4-6h as needed. **Max:** 400mg/day. **Elderly:** Start at low end of dosing range. **>75 yrs: Max:** 300mg/day. **CrCl <30mL/min:** Dose q12h. **Max:** 200mg/day. **Cirrhosis:** 50mg q12h. **Concomitant carbamazepine (up to 800mg/day):** May need 2x the recommended dose of tramadol.	**W/P:** Seizures and anaphylactoid reactions reported. Do not use in opioid-dependent patients. Caution if at risk for respiratory depression, or with increased intracranial pressure or head trauma. May complicate acute abdominal conditions. Do not discontinue abruptly. Adjust dose with renal or hepatic impairment. **Contra:** Acute alcohol intoxication, hypnotics, narcotics, centrally-acting analgesics, opioids or psychotropics. **P/N:** Category C, not for use in nursing.	Dizziness, nausea, constipation, headache, somnolence, vomiting, nervousness, sweating, asthenia, dyspepsia, **dry mouth**, diarrhea, CNS stimulation, pruritus.

Table 3.2: DRUG INTERACTIONS FOR ANALGESICS

ACETAMINOPHEN & COMBINATIONS

Acetaminophen (Feverall, Tylenol, Tylenol Arthritis, Tylenol Children's, Tylenol 8 Hour, Tylenol Extra Strength, Tylenol Infants' Tylenol Junior Strength, Tylenol Sore Throat)

Alcohol	Concurrent use of alcohol and acetaminophen may increase risk of hepatotoxicity.

Acetaminophen/Aspirin/Caffeine (Excedrin Extra Strength, Excedrin Migraine)

Alcohol	Concurrent use of alcohol and acetaminophen may increase risk of hepatotoxicity.
Anticoagulant	May increase risk of bleeding with aspirin.
Celecoxib	May increase risk of gastrointestinal bleeding with aspirin.
Clopidogrel	May increase risk of bleeding with aspirin.
Corticosteroids	Concomitant use of aspirin and corticosteroids increases the risk of gastrointestinal ulceration.
Ginkgo	May increase risk of bleeding with aspirin.
Ketorolac	Enhanced gastrointestinal adverse effects (peptic ulcers, gastrointestinal bleeding and/or perforation) and possible increase in serum ketorolac levels.
SSRI	Combined use of selective serotonin reuptake inhibitors and NSAIDs has been associated with an increased risk of bleeding.

Acetaminophen/Butalbital (Phrenlin, Phrenilin Forte)

Alcohol	Concurrent use of alcohol may increase risk of hepatotoxicity and CNS depression.
Alprazolam	Additive CNS and respiratory depressant effects with butalbital.
Anileridine	Additive respiratory depression with butalbital.
Anticoagulant	Decreased anticoagulant effectiveness with butalbital.
CNS depressant	CNS depressants may cause additive depressant effects with butalbital.

Acetaminophen/Butalbital/Caffeine (Esgic-Plus, Fioricet)

Alcohol	May enhance CNS depressant effects of alcohol.
Anesthetics	May enhance CNS depressant effects of general anesthetics.
CNS depressants	May enhance CNS depressant effects of other CNS depressants.
MAOIs	Enhanced CNS effects with MAOIs.
Narcotic analgesics	May enhance CNS depressant effects of other narcotic analgesics.
Sedative hypnotics	May enhance CNS depressant effects of sedative hypnotics.
Tranquilizers	May enhance CNS depressant effects of tranquilizers.

Acetaminophen/Caffeine/Pyrilamine Maleate (Midol Maximum Strength)

Alcohol	Concurrent use of alcohol and acetaminophen may increase risk of hepatotoxicity.

Acetaminophen/Diphenhydramine Citrate (Excedrin PM, Tylenol PM)

Alcohol	Concurrent use of alcohol and acetaminophen may increase risk of hepatotoxicity.

ACETAMINOPHEN & COMBINATIONS *(cont.)*

Acetaminophen/Diphenhydramine Citrate (Excedrin PM, Tylenol PM)

Metoprolol	An increased risk of metoprolol toxicity (bradycardia, fatigue, bronchospasm) with diphenhydramine.

Acetaminophen/Magnesium Salicylate/Pamabrom (Pamprin Maximum Pain Relief)

Alcohol	Concurrent use of alcohol and acetaminophen may increase risk of hepatotoxicity.

Acetaminophen/Pamabrom (Midol Teen Formula)

Alcohol	Concurrent use of alcohol and acetaminophen may increase risk of hepatotoxicity.

Acetaminophen/Pamabrom/Pyrilamine Maleate (Midol PMS Maximum Strength, Pamprin Multi-Symptom)

Alcohol	Concurrent use of alcohol and acetaminophen may increase risk of hepatotoxicity.

Acetaminophen/Phenyltoloxamine Citrate (Percogesic)

Alcohol	Concurrent use of alcohol and acetaminophen may increase risk of hepatotoxicity.

NSAIDs

Celecoxib (Celebrex)

ACEIs	Decrease effects of ACEIs.
Anticoagulants	Monitor oral anticoagulants; reports of serious bleeding, some fatal, with warfarin.
ASA	Celecoxib is not a substitute for ASA for cardiovascular prophylaxis; may use with low-dose ASA but may increase GI complications.
CYP2C9 inhibitors	Caution with CYP2C9 inhibitors.
Drugs metabolized by CYP2D6	Caution with drugs metabolized by CYP2D6.
Fluconazole	Increased levels with fluconazole.
Furosemide	Decrease effects of furosemide.
Lithium	Monitor lithium.
Thiazides	Decrease effects of thiazides.

Diclofenac Potassium (Cataflam)

ACE-inhibitors	May diminish antihypertensive effect of ACE-inhibitors.
ASA	Increased adverse effects with ASA; avoid use.
Cyclosporine	May increase nephrotoxicity of cyclosporine; caution when co-administering.
Diclofenac products	Avoid with other diclofenac products.
Furosemide	May reduce natriuretic effect of furosemide; monitor for renal failure.
Lithium	May increase lithium levels; monitor for toxicity.
Methotrexate	May enhance methotrexate toxicity; caution when co-administering.

Table 3.2: DRUG INTERACTIONS FOR ANALGESICS *(cont.)*

NSAIDs *(cont.)*

Diclofenac Potassium (Cataflam)

Thiazides	May reduce natriuretic effect of thiazides; monitor for renal failure.
Warfarin	Synergistic effects on GI bleeding with warfarin.

Diclofenac Sodium (Voltaren, Voltaren-XR)

ACE inhibitors	May diminish antihypertensive effect of ACE inhibitors.
ASA	Increased adverse effects with ASA; avoid use.
Cyclosporine	May increase nephrotoxicity of cyclosporine; caution when co-administering.
Diclofenac products	Avoid with other diclofenac products.
Furosemide	May reduce natriuretic effect of furosemide; monitor for renal failure.
Lithium	May increase lithium levels; monitor for toxicity.
Methotrexate	May enhance methotrexate toxicity; caution when co-administering.
Thiazides	May reduce natriuretic effect of thiazides; monitor for renal failure.
Warfarin	Synergistic effects on GI bleeding with warfarin.

Diclofenac Sodium/Misoprostol (Arthrotec)

Antacids	Avoid magnesium-containing antacids.
Anticoagulants	Caution with anticoagulants; may have synergistic GI bleeding effects with warfarin.
Antihypertensives	May decrease effects of antihypertensives.
Aspirin and other NSAIDs	Avoid aspirin and other NSAIDs.
Cyclosporine	Monitor for cyclosporine toxicity.
Digoxin	Monitor for digoxin toxicity.
Diuretics	May decrease effects of diuretics.
Hypoglycemics, oral	May alter response to oral hypoglycemics.
Insulin	May alter response to insulin.
Lithium	Monitor for lithium toxicity.
Methotrexate	Monitor for methotrexate toxicity.
Phenobarbital	Monitor for phenobarbital toxicity.
Potassium	Increased serum potassium with K$^+$-sparing diuretics.
Salicylates	Avoid salicylates.

Diflunisal (Dolobid)

Acetaminophen	Increased plasma levels of acetaminophen.
Antacids	May reduce plasma levels.

NSAIDs *(cont.)*

Diflunisal (Dolobid)

Anticoagulants, oral	May prolong PT with oral anticoagulants.
Aspirin	Decreased plasma levels with aspirin.
Cyclosporine	May potentiate cyclosporine toxicities.
Furosemide	Decreases hyperuricemic effect of urosemide.
HCTZ	Decreases hyperuricemic effect of HCTZ.
Hepatotoxic drugs	Caution with hepatotoxic drugs.
Methotrexate	May potentiate methotrexate toxicities.
Nephrotoxic drugs	Caution with nephrotoxic drugs.
NSAIDs	Avoid other NSAIDs.

Etodolac (Lodine, Lodine XL)

ACE inhibitors	May decrease antihypertensive effects with ACE inhibitors.
Aspirin	Avoid with aspirin; increased adverse effect potential.
Cyclosporine	May enhance nephrotoxicity associated with cyclosporine.
Digoxin	May elevate digoxin serum levels.
Diuretics	May increase risk of renal toxicity.
Furosemide	May reduce natriuretic effect of furosemide.
Lithium	May elevate lithium serum levels.
Methotrexate	May elevate methotrexate serum levels.
Phenylbutazone	Avoid with phenylbutazone.
Thiazides	May reduce natriuretic effect of thiazides.
Warfarin	Caution with warfarin.

Fenoprofen Calcium (Nalfon)

Aspirin	May decrease effects.
Chronic phenobarbital	May decrease effects.
Coumarin-type anticoagulants	May prolong PT with coumarin-type anticoagulants.
Hydantoins	May potentiate hydantoins.
Loop diuretics	May cause resistance to the effects of loop diuretics.
Salicylates	Avoid salicylates.
Sulfonamides	May potentiate sulfonamides.
Sulfonylureas	May potentiate sulfonylureas.

Table 3.2: DRUG INTERACTIONS FOR ANALGESICS *(cont.)*

NSAIDs *(cont.)*

Flurbiprofen (Ansaid)

Anticoagulants	Caution with anticoagulants; serious bleeding reported.
Aspirin	Aspirin is not recommended.
β-blockers	May decrease hypotensive effects of β-blockers.
Diuretics	May decrease diuretic effects.

Ibuprofen (Advil, Advil Junior, Midol Cramp Formula, Motrin, Motrin Children's, Motrin IB, Motrin Infants, Motrin Junior, Motrin Migraine Pain)

Anticoagulants	Use caution with anticoagulants.
Aspirin	Avoid use with aspirin.
Furosemide	May decrease the natriuretic effects of furosemide.
Lithium	Decrease lithium clearance; monitor for toxicity.
Methotrexate	May enhance methotrexate toxicity.
Thiazides	May decrease the natriuretic effects of thiazides.

Indomethacin (Indocin, Indocin SR)

Anticoagulants	Caution with anticoagulants.
Antihypertensives	Caution with antihypertensives.
β-blockers	Decreased effects of β-blockers.
Captopril	Decreased effects of captopril.
Cyclosporine	Increases toxicity of cyclosporine.
Diflunisal	Avoid diflunisal.
Digoxin	Increases toxicity of digoxin.
Diuretics	Decreased effects of diuretics.
Lithium	Increases toxicity of lithium.
Methotrexate	Increases toxicity of methotrexate.
NSAIDs	Avoid other NSAIDs.
Potassium-sparing diuretics	May cause hyperkalemia.
Probenecid	Probenecid increases levels.
Salicylates	Avoid salicylates.
Triamterene	Avoid triamterene.

Ketoprofen (Orudis KT, Oruvail)

Anticoagulants	Monitor anticoagulants.
Aspirin	Avoid aspirin.

NSAIDs *(cont.)*

Ketoprofen (Orudis KT, Oruvail)

Diuretics	Renal toxicity potentiated by diuretics.
Lithium	Increases levels of lithium.
Methotrexate	Increases levels of methotrexate.
Probenecid	Avoid probenecid.

Ketorolac Tromethamine (Toradol)

ACE inhibitors	May increase risk of renal impairment with ACE inhibitors.
Alprazolam	Hallucinations reported with alprazolam.
Anticoagulants	May increase risk of bleeding with anticoagulants.
Aspirin	Avoid aspirin.
Carbamazepine	May increase seizures with carbamazepine.
Fluoxetine	Hallucinations reported with fluoxetine.
Furosemide	May reduce diuretic response to furosemide.
Lithium	Increased lithium levels.
Methotrexate	Increased methotrexate levels.
Morphine	Do not mix in the same syringe as morphine.
Muscle relaxants, nondepolarizing	May have adverse effects with nondepolarizing muscle relaxants.
NSAIDs	Avoid NSAIDs.
Phenytoin	May increase seizures with phenytoin.
Probenecid	Avoid probenecid.
Salicylates	Increased serum levels with salicylates.
Thiothixene	Hallucinations reported with thiothixene.

Lansoprazole/Naproxen (Prevacid Naprapac 375, Prevacid Naprapac 500)

ACE inhibitors	May potentiate renal disease with ACE inhibitors.
Aspirin	Avoid other forms of aspirin; decreased plasma levels with aspirin.
Furosemide	May antagonize natriuretic effect of furosemide.
Hydantoin	Monitor for toxicity with hydantoin.
Lansoprazole	May alter absorption of pH-dependent drugs (eg, ketoconazole, ampicillin, iron, digoxin).
Lithium	Decreases renal clearance of lithium.
Methotrexate	Decreases renal clearance of methotrexate.
Naproxen	Avoid other forms of naproxen; may displace other albumin-bound drugs.

Table 3.2: DRUG INTERACTIONS FOR ANALGESICS *(cont.)*

NSAIDs *(cont.)*

Lansoprazole/Naproxen (Prevacid Naprapac 375, Prevacid Naprapac 500)

Probenecid	Increased levels and half-life with probenecid.
Propranolol	May decrease antihypertensive effects of propranolol and other β-blockers.
Sucralfate	Take lansoprazole 30 minutes prior to sucralfate.
Sulfonamide	Monitor for toxicity with sulfonamide.
Sulfonylureas	Monitor for toxicity with sulfonylureas.
Warfarin	Caution with warfarin.

Meclofenamate Sodium

Aspirin	May lower levels.
Warfarin	Enhanced effects of warfarin.

Mefenamic Acid (Ponstel)

ACE inhibitors	Decrease effects of ACE inhibitors; monitor for renal toxicity.
Aspirin	May increase adverse effects; avoid use.
CYP2C9 inhibitors	Caution with CYP2C9 inhibitors, including fluconazole, lovastatin and trimethoprim.
Furosemide	Decrease effects of furosemide; monitor for renal toxicity.
Lithium	Increase in lithium levels.
Magnesium hydroxide	May increase mefenamic acid levels.
Methotrexate	May enhance methotrexate toxicity.
Anticoagulants, oral	May prolong PT with oral anticoagulants.
Thiazides	Decrease effects of thiazides; monitor for renal toxicity.
Warfarin	May increase GI bleeding.

Meloxicam (Mobic)

ACE inhibitors	May decrease antihypertensive effects of ACE inhibitors.
Aspirin	Potentiates GI bleeds with aspirin; avoid concomitant use.
Cholestyramine	Increased clearance with cholestyramine.
Frosemide	May decrease natriuretic effects of furosemide.
Lithium	Decreased lithium clearance/increased serum levels.
Methotrexate	Caution with methotrexate.
Thiazides	May decrease natriuretic effects of thiazides.
Warfarin	Monitor PT/INR with warfarin.

NSAIDs *(cont.)*

Nabumetone (Relafen)

Diuretics	Nephrotoxicity risk with diuretics.
Protein-bound drugs	Caution with other protein-bound drugs.
Warfarin	Caution with warfarin.

Naproxen (Aleve, Anaprox, Anaprox DS, EC Naprosyn, Naprosyn)

ACE inhibitors	May diminish antihypertensive effect and potentiate renal disease with ACE inhibitors.
Aspirin	Decreased plasma levels with aspirin.
Cyclosporine	May increase nephrotoxicity of cyclosporine; caution when co-administering.
EC-Naprosyn	Avoid with other products containing naproxen, H_2-blockers, sucralfate, or intensive antacid therapy.
Furosemide	May reduce natriuretic effect of furosemide; monitor for renal failure.
Hydantoins	Observe for dose adjustment with hydantoins.
Lithium	May increase lithium levels; monitor for toxicity.
Methotrexate	May reduce tubular secretion of methotrexate; monitor for toxicity.
Naprosyn	Avoid with other products containing naproxen.
Probenecid	May increase half-life.
Propranolol	May reduce antihypertensive effects of propranolol and other β-blockers.
Sulfonamides	Observe for dose adjustment with sulfonamides.
Sulfonylureas	Observe for dose adjustment with sulfonylureas.
Thiazides	May reduce natriuretic effect of thiazides; monitor for renal failure.
Warfarin	Synergistic effects on GI bleeding with warfarin.

Oxaprozin (Daypro)

Anticoagulants	Caution with oral anticoagulants.
Aspirin	Avoid with aspirin.
β-blockers	Monitor BP with β-blockers.

Piroxicam (Feldene)

ACE inhibitors	May decrease antihypertensive effects of ACE inhibitors.
Aspirin	Diminished effect with aspirin and may increase adverse effects.
Furosemide	May reduce natriuretic effect of furosemide.
Lithium	May increase lithium levels; monitor for toxicity.
Methotrexate	May increase methotrexate levels; monitor for toxicity.

Table 3.2: DRUG INTERACTIONS FOR ANALGESICS (cont.)

NSAIDs (cont.)

Piroxicam (Feldene)

Protein-bound drugs	May displace other protein-bound drugs.
Thiazides	May reduce natriuretic effect of thiazides.
Warfarin	Synergistic GI bleeding effects with warfarin.

Sulindac (Clinoril)

Aspirin	Avoid aspirin and other NSAIDS.
Cyclosporine	Increases cyclosporine toxicities.
Diflunisal	Diflunisal decreases plasma levels.
DMSO	Avoid DMSO.
Methotrexate	Increases methotrexate toxicities.
Probenecid	Probenecid increases plasma levels.

Tolmetin Sodium

Diuretics	Risk of renal toxicity with diuretics.
Methotrexate	May enhance methotrexate toxicity.
Warfarin	Increased PT and bleeding with warfarin.

OPIOIDS

Acetaminophen/Butalbital/Caffeine/Codeine Phosphate[CIII] (Fioricet w/Codeine)

Alcohol	May enhance CNS depressant effects of alcohol.
CNS depressants	May enhance CNS depressant effects of other CNS depressants.
General anesthetics	May enhance CNS depressant effects of general anesthetics.
MAOIs	Enhanced CNS effects with MAOIs.
Narcotic analgesics	May enhance CNS depressant effects of other narcotic analgesics.
Sedative hypnotics	May enhance CNS depressant effects of sedative hypnotics.
Tranquilizers	May enhance CNS depressant effects of tranquilizers.

Acetaminophen/Codeine Phosphate[CIII] (Tylenol w/Codeine)

Alcohol	Additive CNS depression with alcohol.
Antianxiety agents	Additive CNS depression with antianxiety agents.
Anticholinergics	May produce paralytic ileus.
Antipsychotics	Additive CNS depression with antipsychotics.
CNS depressants	Additive CNS depression with other CNS depressants.
Narcotic analgesics	Additive CNS depression with narcotic analgesics.

OPIOIDS *(cont.)*

Aspirin/Butalbital/Caffeine/Codeine Phosphate[CIII] (Fiorinal w/codeine)

6-MP	May cause bone marrow toxicity, blood dyscrasias with 6-MP.
Alcohol	Additive CNS depression with alcohol.
Anticoagulants	May enhance effects of anticoagulants.
Antidiabetic agents	May cause hypoglycemia with oral antidiabetic agents.
CNS depressants	Additive CNS depression with other CNS depressants.
Corticosteroids	Withdrawal of corticosteroids may cause salicylism with chronic ASA use.
General anesthetics	Additive CNS depression with general anesthetics.
Insulin	May cause hypoglycemia with insulin.
MAOIs	CNS effects enhanced by MAOIs.
Methotrexate	May cause bone marrow toxicity, blood dyscrasias with methotrexate.
Narcotic analgesics	Additive CNS depression with other narcotic analgesics.
NSAIDs	Increased risk of peptic ulceration, bleeding with NSAIDs.
Sedatives/hypnotics	Additive CNS depression with sedatives/hypnotics.
Tranquilizers	Additive CNS depression with tranquilizers (eg, chloral hydrate).
Uricosuric agents	Decreased effects of uricosuric agents (eg, probenecid, sulfinpyrazone).

Aspirin/Carisoprodol/Codeine Phosphate[CIII] (Soma Compound w/codeine)

Alcohol	Additive effects with alcohol; increases GI bleeding risk with alcohol.
Antacids	Antacids decrease plasma levels.
Anticoagulants	Increases bleeding risk with anticoagulants.
Antidiabetic agents	Enhances methotrexate toxicity and hypoglycemia with oral antidiabetics.
CNS depressants	Additive effects with other CNS depressants.
Corticosteroids	Corticosteroids decrease plasma levels.
Probenecid	Antagonizes uricosuric effects of probenecid.
Psychotropic drugs	Additive effects with psychotropic drugs.
Sulfinpyrazone	Antagonizes uricosuric effects of sulfinpyrazone.
Urine acidifiers	Potentiated by urine acidifiers (eg, ammonium chloride).

Codeine Phosphate[CII]

Alcohol	Increased sedation, synergistic CNS depression.
CNS depressants	May enhance CNS and respiratory depressant effects.
Opioid agonist/ antagonist	Precipitation of withdrawal symptoms (abdominal cramps, nausea, vomiting, lacrimation, rhinorrhea, anxiety, restlessness, elevation of temperature or piloerection).

Table 3.2: DRUG INTERACTIONS FOR ANALGESICS *(cont.)*

OPIOIDS *(cont.)*

Codeine Sulfate[CII]

Alcohol	Increased sedation, synergistic CNS depression.
CNS depressants	May enhance CNS and respiratory depressant effects.
Opioid agonist/ antagonist	Precipitation of withdrawal symptoms (abdominal cramps, nausea, vomiting, lacrimation, rhinorrhea, anxiety, restlessness, elevation of temperature or piloerection).

Fentanyl[CII] (Duragesic)

CNS depressants	Concomitant use with CNS depressants (opioids, sedatives, hypnotics, tranquilizers, general anesthetics, phenothiazines, skeletal muscle relaxants, alcohol) may cause respiratory depression, hypotension, profound sedation, or potentially coma or death.
CYP3A4 inducers	May increase clearance with CYP3A4 inducers (eg, rifampin, carbamazepine, phenytoin).
MAOI	Avoid use within 14 days of MAOI.

Fentanyl Citrate[CII] (Actiq, Sublimaze)

β-blockers	Appropriate monitoring and availability of β-blockers for the treatment of hypertension is indicated.
CNS depressants	Increased depressant effects with other CNS depressants, including opioids, sedatives, hypnotics, general anesthetics, phenothiazines, tranquilizers, skeletal muscle relaxants, sedating antihistamines, potent inhibitors of CYP3A4 (eg, erythromycin, ketoconazole, itraconazole, certain protease inhibitors), alcohol. Additive or potentiating effects with other CNS depressants (eg, barbiturates, tranquilizers, narcotics, general anesthetics). Reduce dose of other CNS depressants.
Conduction anesthesia	Alteration of respiration with certain forms of conduction anesthesia (eg, spinal anesthesia, some peridural anesthesia).
MAO inhibitors	Severe and unpredictable potentiation by MAO inhibitors has been reported. Avoid within 14 days of MAO inhibitors.
Neuroleptics	Elevated blood pressure, with and without pre-existing hypertension, slower normalcy of EEG patterns with neuroleptics. Extreme caution with neuroleptics in the presense of risk factors for development of prolonged QT syndrome and torsade de pointes; ECG monitoring indicated.
Nitrous oxide	Reports of cardiovascular depression with nitrous oxide.
Tranquilizers	Decreased pulmonary arterial pressure and hypotension with tranquilizers.
Vasodilators	Appropriate monitoring and availability of vasodilators for the treatment of hypertension is indicated.

HYDROCODONE & COMBINATIONS

Acetaminophen/Hydrocodone Bitartrate[CIII] (Lorcet, Lorcet Plus, Lortab, Norco, Vicodin, Vicodin ES, Vicodin HP, Zydone)

Alcohol	Additive CNS depression with alcohol.

OPIOIDS *(cont.)*

Acetaminophen/Hydrocodone Bitartrate[CIII] (Lorcet, Lorcet Plus, Lortab, Norco, Vicodin, Vicodin ES, Vicodin HP, Zydone)

Antianxiety agents	Additive CNS depression with antianxiety agents.
Antihistamines	Additive CNS depression with antihistamines.
Antipsychotics	Additive CNS depression with antipsychotics.
CNS depressants	Additive CNS depression with other CNS depressants.
MAOIs	Increased effect of antidepressant or hydrocodone with MAOIs.
Narcotic analgesics	Additive CNS depression with other narcotic analgesics.
TCAs	Increased effect of antidepressant or hydrocodone with TCAs.

Hydrocodone Bitartrate/Ibuprofen[CIII] (Vicoprofen)

ACE inhibitors	May decrease effects of ACE inhibitors.
Alcohol	Additive CNS depression with alcohol.
Antianxiety agents	Additive CNS depression with antianxiety agents.
Anticholinergics	May produce paralytic ileus with anticholinergics.
Antihistamines	Additive CNS depression with antihistamines.
Antipsychotics	Additive CNS depression with antipsychotics.
Aspirin	Avoid with aspirin.
CNS depressants	Additive CNS depression with CNS depressants.
Furosemide	May decrease effects of furosemide.
Lithium	Monitor for lithium toxicity.
MAOIs	Increased effect of antidepressant or hydrocodone with MAOIs.
Methotrexate	May enhance methotrexate toxicity.
Narcotics	Additive CNS depression with other narcotics.
TCAs	Increased effect of antidepressant or hydrocodone with TCAs.
Thiazide diuretics	May decrease effects of thiazide diuretics.
Warfarin	Risk of serious GI bleeding with warfarin.

Hydromorphone Hydrochloride[CII] (Dilaudid, Dilaudid HP)

Alcohol	Additive CNS depression with alcohol.
CNS depressants	Additive CNS depression with other CNS depressants.
General anesthetics	Additive CNS depression with general anesthetics.
Narcotic analgesics	Additive CNS depression with other narcotic analgesics.
Neuromuscular-blocking agents	Additive CNS depression with neuromuscular blocking agents.

Table 3.2: DRUG INTERACTIONS FOR ANALGESICS (cont.)

OPIOIDS (cont.)

Hydromorphone Hydrochloride[CII] (Dilaudid, Dilaudid HP)

Phenothiazines	Additive CNS depression with phenothiazines.
Sedative hypnotics	Additive CNS depression with sedative hypnotics.
TCAs	Additive CNS depression with TCAs.
Tranquilizers	Additive CNS depression with tranquilizers.

Meperidine Hydrochloride[CII] (Demerol)

Acyclovir	Caution with acyclovir.
Cimetidine	Caution with cimetidine.
CNS depressants	Caution and reduce dose with other CNS depressants (eg, narcotics, anesthetics, phenothiazines, tranquilizers, sedative-hypnotics, TCAs, alcohol).
Mixed agonist/ antagonist analgesics (eg, pentazocine, nalbuphine, butorphanol, buprenorphine)	May reduce analgesic effects and/or precipitate withdrawal symptoms.
Phenytoin	May enhance hepatic metabolism.
Ritonavir	Increased levels with ritonavir; avoid concurrent administration.
Skeletal-muscle relaxants	May enhance neuroblocking action of skeletal muscle relaxants.

Methadone Hydrochloride[CII] (Dolophine, Methadose)

CNS depressants	Caution and reduce dose with CNS depressants (eg, tranquilizers, sedative-hypnotics, phenothiazines, TCAs, alcohol).
MAOIs	May cause severe reactions.
Pentazocine	May precipitate withdrawal.
Rifampin	Decreased serum levels with rifampin.

Morphine Sulfate[CII] (Avinza, Duramorph, Kadian, MS Contin, Oramorph SR, Roxanol)

Acidifying agents	Antagonized by acidifying agents.
Alcohol	Additive effects with alcohol.
Alkalizing agents	Potentiated by alkalizing agents.
Chlorpromazine	Analgesic effect potentiated by chlorpromazine.
Cimetidine	Monitor for increased respiratory and CNS depression with cimetidine.

OPIODS *(cont.)*

Morphine Sulfate^CII (Avinza, Duramorph, Kadian, MS Contin, Oramorph SR, Roxanol)

CNS depressants	Increased risk of respiratory depression, hypotension, profound sedation, or coma with CNS depressants (eg, sedatives, barbiturates, hypnotics, general anesthetics, antiemetics, chloral hydrate, glutethimide, MAOIs such as procarbazine, phenothiazines, tranquilizers, β-blockers such as propranolol, furazolidone, other narcotics, TCAs, antihistimines, alcohol, or psychotropics); reduce initial dose of one or both agents by 50%.
Coumarin	May increase anticoagulant activity of coumarin and other anticoagulants.
General anesthetics	Risk of hypotension with general anesthetics.
Illicit drugs	Additive effects with illicit drugs that cause CNS depression.
MAOIs	Avoid within 14 days of MAOI use; may reduce diuretic effects.
Methocarbamol	Analgesic effect potentiated by methocarbamol.
Mixed agonist/ antagonists	Avoid with mixed agonist/antagonists (eg, pentazocine, nalbuphine, butorphanol, buprenorphine); mixed agonist/antagonists may reduce analgesic effects or precipitate withdrawal symptoms.
Neuroleptics	May increase respiratory depression, hypotension, sedation, and coma.
Opioids	Additive effects with other opioids.
Phenothiazines	Risk of hypotension with phenothiazines.
Psychotropics	Psychotropics potentiate CNS depression. Neuroleptics may increase respiratory depression.
Skeletal-muscle relaxants	May enhance neuromuscular blocking action and increase respiratory depression with skeletal-muscle relaxants.

Morphine Sulfate Liposome^CII (Depodur)

Alcohol	Additive effects with alcohol.
Cimetidine	Monitor for increased respiratory and CNS depression with cimetidine.
CNS depressants	Increased risk of respiratory depression, hypotension, profound sedation, or coma with CNS depressants (eg, sedatives, barbiturates, hypnotics, general anesthetics, antiemetics, chloral hydrate, glutethimide, MAOIs such as procarbazine, phenothiazines, tranquilizers, β-blockers such as propranolol, furazolidone, other narcotics, TCAs, antihistimines, alcohol, or psychotropics); reduce initial dose of one or both agents by 50%.
MAOIs	Avoid within 14 days of MAOI use; may reduce diuretic effects.
Mixed agonist/ antagonists	Avoid with mixed agonist/antagonists (eg, pentazocine, nalbuphine, butorphanol, buprenorphine); mixed agonist/antagonists may reduce analgesic effects or precipitate withdrawal symptoms.
Opioids	Additive effects with other opioids.

Table 3.2: DRUG INTERACTIONS FOR ANALGESICS *(cont.)*

OPIODS *(cont.)*

OXYCODONE & COMBINATIONS

Acetaminophen/Oxycodone Hydrochloride^{CII} (Roxicet, Percocet, Tylox)

Alcohol	Additive CNS depression with alcohol; reduce dose of one or both agents.
Anticholinergics	May produce paralytic ileus with anticholinergics.
CNS depressants	Additive CNS depression with other CNS depressants; reduce dose of one or both agents.
General anesthetics	Additive CNS depression with general anesthetics; reduce dose of one or both agents.
Narcotic analgesics	Additive CNS depression with narcotic analgesics; reduce dose of one or both agents.
Phenothiazines	Additive CNS depression with phenothiazines; reduce dose of one or both agents.
Sedatives-hypnotics	Additive CNS depression with sedatives-hypnotics; reduce dose of one or both agents.
Tranquilizers	Additive CNS depression with tranquilizers; reduce dose of one or both agents.

Aspirin/Oxycodone Hydrochloride/Oxycodone Terephthalate ^{CII} (Percodan)

Aspirin	May enhance effect of anticoagulants and inhibit effects of uricosuric agents.
CNS depressants	Additive CNS depression with other CNS depressants (including alcohol).
General anesthetics	Additive CNS depression with general anesthetics.
Opioid analgesics	Additive CNS depression with other opioid analgesics.
Phenothiazines	Additive CNS depression with phenothiazines.
Sedative-hypnotics	Additive CNS depression with sedative-hypnotics.
Tranquilizers	Additive CNS depression with tranquilizers.

Ibuprofen/Oxycodone Hydrochloride^{CII} (Combunox)

IBUPROFEN

ACE inhibitors	May diminish antihypertensive effect of ACE inhibitors.
Anticoagulants	Use caution with anticoagulants.
Aspirin	Avoid use with aspirin.
Furosemide	May decrease natriuretic effect of furosemide.
Lithium	Decreases lithium clearance; monitor for toxicity.
Methotrexate	May enhance methotrexate toxicity.
Thiazides	May decrease natriuretic effect of thiazides.

OXYCODONE

Anticholinergics	Concurrent use with anticholinergics may produce paralytic ileus.
CNS depressants	Respiratory depression, hypotension and profound sedation with other CNS depressants (eg, narcotics, tranquilizers, sedatives, anesthetics, phenothiazines, alcohol).

OPIODS *(cont.)*

OXYCODONE *(cont.)*

MAO inhibitors	Do not use with, or within 14 days of discontinuing, MAO inhibitors.
Mixed agonist/antagonist analgesics	May reduce the analgesic effect and/or cause withdrawal.
Skeletal-muscle relaxants	May enhance skeletal-muscle relaxant effects and increase respiratory depression.

Oxycodone Hydrochloride[CII] (Oxycontin, OxyIR, Oxyfast, Roxicodone)

CYP2D6 inhibitors	May interact with CYP2D6 inhibitors (eg, amiodarone, quinidine, polycyclic antidepressants).
CNS depressants	Respiratory depression, hypotension and profound sedation with other CNS depressants (eg, anesthetics, narcotic analgesics, phenothiazines, tranquilizers, sedative-hypnotics, alcohol); reduce dose.
MAOIs	Avoid within 14 days of MAOIs.
Mixed agonist/ antagonist analgesics	May reduce the analgesic effect and/or cause withdrawal.
Phenothiazines	Risk of severe hypotension with phenothiazines or other agents that compromise vasomotor tone.
Skeletal-muscle relaxants	May enhance skeletal-muscle relaxant effects and increase respiratory depression.

PROPOXYPHENE & COMBINATIONS

Acetaminophen/Propoxyphene Napsylate[CIV] (Darvocet A500, Darvocet N 50, Darvocet N 100)

Alcohol	Additive CNS-depressant effects with alcohol.
Anticonvulsants	Increases plasma levels of anticonvulsants.
Antidepressants	Additive CNS-depressant effects with antidepressants. Increases plasma levels of antidepressants.
Carbamazepine	Severe neurologic signs, including coma, reported with carbamazepine.
Coumarins	Increases plasma levels of coumarins.
Muscle relaxants	Additive CNS-depressant effects with muscle relaxants.
Sedatives	Additive CNS-depressant effects with alcohol, sedatives.
Tranquilizers	Additive CNS-depressant effects with alcohol, sedatives, tranquilizers.

Aspirin/Caffeine/Propoxyphene Hydrochloride[CIV] (Darvon Compound-65)

Alcohol	Caution with excess alcohol use.
Anticoagulants	Enhances anticoagulant effects.

Table 3.2: DRUG INTERACTIONS FOR ANALGESICS *(cont.)*

OPIODS *(cont.)*

Aspirin/Caffeine/Propoxyphene Hydrochloride[CIV] (Darvon Compound-65)

Anticonvulsants	Increases plasma levels of anticonvulsants.
Antidepressants	Caution with antidepressants; increases plasma levels of antidepressants.
Carbamazepine	Severe neurologic signs, including coma reported with carbamazepine.
CNS depressants	Additive CNS-depressant effect with other CNS depressants, including alcohol.
Coumarins	Increases plasma levels of coumarins.
Tranquilizers	Caution with tranquilizers.
Uricosuric agents	Inhibits effect of uricosuric agents.

Propoxyphene Hydrochloride[CIV] (Darvon)

Alcohol	Caution with excess alcohol use.
Anticonvulsants	Increases plasma levels of anticonvulsants.
Antidepressants	Caution with antidepressants; increases plasma levels of antidepressants.
Carbamazepine	Severe neurologic signs, including coma, reported with carbamazepine.
CNS depressants	Additive CNS-depressant effect with other CNS depressants, including alcohol.
Coumarins	Increases plasma levels of coumarins.
Tranquilizers	Caution with tranquilizers.

Propoxyphene Napsylate[CIV] (Darvon-N)

Alcohol	Caution with excess alcohol use.
Anticonvulsants	Increases plasma levels of anticonvulsants.
Antidepressants	Caution with antidepressants; increases plasma levels of antidepressants.
Carbamazepine	Severe neurologic signs, including coma reported with carbamazepine.
CNS depressants	Additive CNS-depressant effect with other CNS depressants, including alcohol.
Tranquilizers	Caution with tranquilizers.
Warfarin-like drugs	Increases plasma levels of warfarin-like drugs.

OPIOID AGONIST-ANTAGONISTS

Acetaminophen/Pentazocine Hydrochloride[CIV] (Talacen)

Alcohol	Increased CNS depressant effects with alcohol.
Narcotics	Withdrawal symptoms with narcotics.

Butorphanol Tartrate[CIV] (Stadol)

Alcohol	Increased CNS depression and respiratory depression with alcohol.
Antihistamines	Increased CNS depression and respiratory depression with antihistamines.
Barbiturates	Increased CNS depression and respiratory depression with barbiturates.

OPIOID AGONIST-ANTAGONISTS *(cont.)*

Butorphanol Tartrate[CIV] (Stadol)

Drugs that affect hepatic metabolism	May be potentiated by other drugs that affect hepatic metabolism.
Erythromycin	May be potentiated by erythromycin.
Nasal vasoconstrictors	Decreased absorption rate with nasal vasoconstrictors (eg, oxymetazoline).
Sumatriptan nasal spray	Diminished analgesic effect if administered shortly after sumatriptan nasal spray.
Theophylline	May be potentiated by theophylline.
Tranquilizers	Increased CNS depression and respiratory depression with tranquilizers.

Nalbuphine Hydrochloride (Nubain)

CNS depressants	Possible additive effects with other CNS depressants.
General anesthetics	Possible additive effects with general anesthetics.
Hypnotics	Possible additive effects with hypnotics.
Ketorolac	Incompatible with ketorolac.
Nafcillin	Incompatible with nafcillin.
Narcotic analgesics	Possible additive effects with narcotic analgesics.
Phenothiazines	Possible additive effects with phenothiazines.
Sedatives	Possible additive effects with sedatives.
Tranquilizers	Possible additive effects with tranquilizers.

Pentazocine Hydrochloride/Naloxone Hydrochloride (Talwin NX)

Alcohol	Increased CNS depressant effects with alcohol.
Narcotics	Withdrawal symptoms with narcotics.

Pentazocine Lactate (Talwin Lactate)

Ethanol	Increased sedation.
Methohexital	CNS depression.
Opioid analgesic	Concomitant administration of an opioid analgesic and an opioid agonist/antagonist may result in withdrawal symptoms.
Selegiline	May cause central nervous system (CNS) toxicity (serotonin syndrome).
Sibutramine	Increased risk of serotonin syndrome.
Thiopental	CNS depression.

OPIOID ANTAGONISTS

Naltrexone (ReVia)

Analgesics	Antagonizes analgesic agents.

Table 3.2: DRUG INTERACTIONS FOR ANALGESICS *(cont.)*

OPIOID ANTAGONISTS *(cont.)*

Naltrexone (ReVia)

Antidiarrheal agents	Antagonizes antidiarrheal agents.
Disulfiram	Do not use with disulfiram unless benefits outweigh risk of hepatotoxicity.
Opioid-containing agents	Antagonizes opioid-containing cough and cold agents.
Thioridazine	Lethargy and somnolence reported with thioridazine.

Naloxone (Narcan)

Buprenorphine	Reversal of buprenorphine-induced respiratory depression may be incomplete.
Cardiovascular agents	Caution using drugs with potential adverse cardiac effects.

OPIOID DEPENDENCE

Buprenorphine Hydrochloride[CV] (Buprenex, Subutex)

Antihistamines	Increased CNS depression with antihistamines.
Benzodiazepines	Increased CNS depression with benzodiazepines.
CNS depressants	Caution with CNS depressants.
CYP3A4 inducers	Increased clearance with CYP3A4 inducers (eg, rifampin, carbamazepine, phenytoin).
CYP3A4 inhibitors	Decreased clearance with CYP3A4 inhibitors (eg, macrolides, azole antifungals, protease inhibitors).
Diazepam	Respiratory and cardiovascular collapse reported with diazepam.
General anesthetics	Increased CNS depression with general anesthetics.
MAOIs	Caution with MAOIs.
Narcotic analgesics	Increased CNS depression with other narcotic analgesics.
Phenothiazines	Increased CNS depression with phenothiazines.
Respiratory depressants	Caution with respiratory depressants.
Sedative-hypnotics	Increased CNS depression with sedative-hypnotics.
Tranquilizers	Increased CNS depression with other tranquilizers.

Buprenorphine Hydrochloride/Naloxone Hydrochloride[CIII] (Suboxone)

Benzodiazepines	May increase risk of CNS depression; consider dose reduction of one or both agents.
CYP3A4 inducers	Monitor closely with CYP3A4 inducers (eg, phenobarbital, carbamazepine, phenytoin, rifampicin).
CYP3A4 inhibitors	May need dose reduction with CYP3A4 inhibitors (eg, azole antifungals, macrolides and HIV protease inhibitors).
General anesthetics	May increase risk of CNS depression; consider dose reduction of one or both agents.

OPIOID DEPENDENCE *(cont.)*

Buprenorphine Hydrochloride/Naloxone Hydrochloride[CIII] (Suboxone)

Other CNS depressants (including alcohol)	May increase risk of CNS depression; consider dose reduction of one or both agents.
Other narcotic analgesics	May increase risk of CNS depression; consider dose reduction of one or both agents.
Other tranquilizers	May increase risk of CNS depression; consider dose reduction of one or both agents.
Phenothiazines	May increase risk of CNS depression; consider dose reduction of one or both agents.
Sedative/hypnotics	May increase risk of CNS depression; consider dose reduction of one or both agents.

SALICYLATES & COMBINATIONS

Aluminum Hydroxide/Aspirin/Calcium Carbonate/Magnesium Hydroxide (Ascriptin, Ascriptin Maximum Strength)

ACE inhibitors	Diminished hypotensive and hyponatremic effects of ACE inhibitors.
Acetazolamide	May increase levels of acetazolamide.
β-blockers	Decreased hypotensive effects of β-blockers.
Diuretics	Decreased diuretic effects with renal or cardiovascular disease.
Heparin	Increased bleeding risk with heparin.
Hypoglycemic agents	Increased effects of hypoglycemic agents.
Methotrexate	Decreased methotrexate clearance; increased risk of bone marrow toxicity.
NSAIDs	Avoid NSAIDs.
Phenytoin	Decreased levels of phenytoin.
Uricosuric agents	Antagonizes uricosuric agents.
Valproic acid	May increase levels of valproic acid.
Warfarin	Increased bleeding risk with warfarin.

Aspirin (Aspergum, Bayer Aspirin, Bayer Aspirin Children's, Bayer Aspirin Regimen, Bayer Genuine Aspirin, Bayer Extra Strenght, Ecotrin, Ecotrin Adult Low Strength, Ecotrin Maximum Strength, Halfprin, St. Joseph Pain Reliever)

ACE inhibitors	Diminished hypotensive and hyponatremic effects of ACE inhibitors.
Acetazolamide	May increase levels of acetazolamide.
β-blockers	Decreased hypotensive effects of β-blockers.
Diuretics	Decreased diuretic effects with renal or cardiovascular disease.
Heparin	Increased bleeding risk with heparin.
Hypoglycemic agents	Increased effects of hypoglycemic agents.

Table 3.2: DRUG INTERACTIONS FOR ANALGESICS *(cont.)*

SALICYLATES & COMBINATIONS *(cont.)*

Aspirin (Aspergum, Bayer Aspirin, Bayer Aspirin Children's, Bayer Aspirin Regimen, Bayer Genuine Aspirin, Bayer Extra Strength, Ecotrin, Ecotrin Adult Low Strength, Ecotrin Maximum Strength, Halfprin, St. Joseph Pain Reliever)

Methotrexate	Decreased methotrexate clearance; increased risk of bone marrow toxicity.
NSAIDs	Avoid NSAIDs.
Phenytoin	Decreased levels of phenytoin.
Uricosuric agents	Antagonizes uricosuric agents.
Valproic acid	May increase levels of valproic acid
Warfarin	Increased bleeding risk with warfarin.

Aspirin/Butalbital/Caffeine (Fiorinal)

6-MP	May cause bone marrow toxicity and blood dyscrasias with 6-MP.
Alcohol	Additive CNS depression with alcohol.
Anticoagulants	May enhance effects of anticoagulants.
CNS depressants	Additive CNS depression with other CNS depressants.
Corticosteroids	Withdrawal of corticosteroids may cause salicylism with chronic ASA use.
General anesthetics	Additive CNS depression with general anesthetics.
Insulin	May cause hypoglycemia with insulin.
MAOIs	CNS effects enhanced by MAOIs.
Methotrexate	May cause bone marrow toxicity and blood dyscrasias with methotrexate.
Narcotic analgesics	Additive CNS depression with other narcotic analgesics.
NSAIDs	Increased risk of peptic ulceration and bleeding with NSAIDs.
Antidiabetic agents	May cause hypoglycemia with oral antidiabetic agents.
Sedatives/hypnotics	Additive CNS depression with sedatives/hypnotics.
Tranquilizers	Additive CNS depression with tranquilizers (eg, chloral hydrate).
Uricosuric agents	Decreased effects of uricosuric agents (eg, probenecid, sulfinpyrazone).

Aspirin/Caffeine (Alka-Seltzer Morning Relief, Anacin, Anacin Maximum Strength)

ACE inhibitors	Diminished hypotensive and hyponatremic effects of ACE inhibitors.
Acetazolamide	May increase levels of acetazolamide.
β-blockers	Decreased hypotensive effects of β-blockers.
Diuretics	Decreased diuretic effects with renal or cardiovascular disease.
Heparin	Increased bleeding risk with heparin.
Hypoglycemic agents	Increased effects of hypoglycemic agents.
Methotrexate	Decreased methotrexate clearance; increased risk of bone marrow toxicity.

SALICYLATES & COMBINATIONS (cont.)

Aspirin/Caffeine (Alka-Seltzer Morning Relief, Anacin, Anacin Maximum Strength)

NSAIDs	Avoid NSAIDs.
Phenytoin	Decreased levels of phenytoin.
Uricosuric agents	Antagonizes uricosuric agents.
Valproic acid	May increase levels of valproic acid.
Warfarin	Increased bleeding risk with warfarin.

Aspirin/Calcium Carbonate (Bayer Plus Extra Strength)

ACE inhibitors	Diminished hypotensive and hyponatremic effects of ACE inhibitors.
Acetazolamide	May increase levels of acetazolamide.
β-blockers	Decreased hypotensive effects of β-blockers.
Diuretics	Decreased diuretic effects with renal or cardiovascular disease.
Heparin	Increased bleeding risk with heparin.
Hypoglycemic agents	Increased effects of hypoglycemic agents.
Methotrexate	Decreased methotrexate clearance; increased risk of bone marrow toxicity.
NSAIDs	Avoid NSAIDs.
Phenytoin	Decreased levels of phenytoin.
Uricosuric agents	Antagonizes uricosuric agents.
Valproic acid	May increase levels of valproic acid.
Warfarin	Increased bleeding risk with warfarin.

Aspirin/Calcium Carbonate/Magnesium Carbonate/Magnesium Oxide (Bufferin, Bufferin Extra Strength)

ACE inhibitors	Diminished hypotensive and hyponatremic effects of ACE inhibitors.
Acetazolamide	May increase levels of acetazolamide.
β-blockers	Decreased hypotensive effects of β-blockers.
Diuretics	Decreased diuretic effects with renal or cardiovascular disease.
Heparin	Increased bleeding risk with heparin.
Hypoglycemic agents	Increased effects of hypoglycemic agents.
Methotrexate	Decreased methotrexate clearance; increased risk of bone marrow toxicity.
NSAIDs	Avoid NSAIDs.
Phenytoin	Decreased levels of phenytoin.
Uricosuric agents	Antagonizes uricosuric agents.
Valproic acid	May increase levels of valproic acid.

Table 3.2: DRUG INTERACTIONS FOR ANALGESICS (cont.)

SALICYLATES & COMBINATIONS (cont.)

Aspirin/Calcium Carbonate/Magnesium Carbonate/Magnesium Oxide (Bufferin, Bufferin Extra Strength)

Warfarin	Increased bleeding risk with warfarin.

Aspirin/Citric Acid/Sodium Bicarbonate (Alka-Seltzer, Alka Seltzer Extra Strength)

ACE inhibitors	Diminished hypotensive and hyponatremic effects of ACE inhibitors.
Acetazolamide	May increase levels of acetazolamide.
β-blockers	Decreased hypotensive effects of β-blockers.
Diuretics	Decreased diuretic effects with renal or cardiovascular disease.
Heparin	Increased bleeding risk with heparin.
Hypoglycemic agents	Increased effects of hypoglycemic agents.
Methotrexate	Decreased methotrexate clearance; increased risk of bone marrow toxicity.
NSAIDs	Avoid NSAIDs.
Phenytoin	Decreased levels of phenytoin.
Uricosuric agents	Antagonizes uricosuric agents.
Valproic acid	May increase levels of valproic acid.
Warfarin	Increased bleeding risk with warfarin.

Aspirin/Diphenhydramine Citrate (Alka-Seltzer PM, Bayer PM Extra Strength)

ACE inhibitors	Diminished hypotensive and hyponatremic effects of ACE inhibitors.
Acetazolamide	May increase levels of acetazolamide.
Alcohol	Increased drowsiness with alcohol.
β-blockers	Decreased hypotensive effects of β-blockers.
Diuretics	Decreased diuretic effects with renal or cardiovascular disease.
Heparin	Increased bleeding risk with heparin.
Hypoglycemic agents	Increased effects of hypoglycemic agents.
Methotrexate	Decreased methotrexate clearance; increased risk of bone marrow toxicity.
NSAIDs	Avoid NSAIDs.
Phenytoin	Decreased levels of phenytoin.
Sedatives	Increased drowsiness with sedatives.
Tranquilizers	Increased drowsiness with tranquilizers.
Uricosuric agents	Antagonizes uricosuric agents.
Valproic acid	May increase levels of valproic acid.
Warfarin	Increased bleeding risk with warfarin.

SALICYLATES & COMBINATIONS *(cont.)*

Choline Magnesium Trisalicylate

Acidifying agents	Urine acidification decreases salicylate clearance.
Antacid	Rise in urine pH (with chronic antacid use) increases salicylate clearance.
Anticoagulants	May potentiate anticoagulants.
Carbonic anhydrase inhibitors	May potentiate carbonic anhydrase inhibitors.
Corticosteroids	Corticosteroids decrease salicylate levels.
Insulin	May potentiate insulin.
Methotrexate	May potentiate methotrexate.
Phenytoin	May potentiate phenytoin.
Sulfonylureas	May potentiate sulfonylureas.
Uricosuric agents	Salicylates may decrease effects of uricosuric agents.
Valproic acid	May potentiate valproic acid.

Diphenhydramine Hydrochloride/Magnesium Salicylate (Doan's PM)

Alcohol	Increased drowsiness with alcohol.
Sedatives	Increased drowsiness with sedatives.
Tranquilizers	Increased drowsiness with tranquilizers.
Varicella virus vaccine	Enhanced risk of developing Reye's syndrome.

Magnesium Salicylate (Doan's Regular, Doan's Extra Strength)

Alcohol	Increased drowsiness with alcohol.
Sedatives	Increased drowsiness with sedatives.
Tranquilizers	Increased drowsiness with tranquilizers.
Varicella virus vaccine	Enhanced risk of developing Reye's syndrome.

Salsalate (Salflex)

Agents that increase urinary pH	Decreased effects with agents that increase urinary pH.
Anticoagulants	Potential bleeding may occur with anticoagulants.
Corticosteroids	Competes for protein binding with corticosteroids.
Food	Food slows absorption.
Methotrexate	Competes for protein binding with methotrexate.
Naproxen	Competes for protein binding with naproxen.
Penicillin	Competes for protein binding with penicillin.

SALICYLATES & COMBINATIONS *(cont.)*

Salsalate (Salflex)

Phenytoin	Competes for protein binding with phenytoin.
Salicylates	Avoid other salicylates.
Sulfinpyrazone	Competes for protein binding with sulfinpyrazone.
Sulfonylureas	Potentiates sulfonylureas.
Thiopental	Competes for protein binding with thiopental.
Thyroxine	Competes for protein binding with thyroxine.
Triiodothyronine	Competes for protein binding with triiodothyronine.
Uricosuric agents	Antagonizes uricosuric agents.
Urinary acidifiers	Potentiated by urinary acidifiers.
Warfarin	Competes for protein binding with warfarin.

TRAMADOL

Acetaminophen/Tramadol Hydrochloride (Ultracet)

Alcohol	Avoid alcohol.
APAP	Avoid other APAP-containing products.
Carbamazepine	May need dose adjustment with carbamazepine.
CNS depressants	Caution and reduce dose with CNS depressants (eg, alcohol, opioids, anesthetics, phenothiazines, tranquilizers, sedatives, hypnotics).
CYP2D6 inhibitors	CYP2D6 inhibitors (eg, fluoxetine, paroxetine, amitriptyline) may potentiate tramadol.
Digoxin	Possible digoxin toxicity.
Drugs that lower seizure threshold	May potentiate seizure risk with drugs that lower seizure threshold.
MAOIs	May potentiate seizure risk with MAOIs.
Naloxone	May potentiate seizure risk with naloxone (with overdose).
Neuroleptics	May potentiate seizure risk with neuroleptics.
Opioids	May potentiate seizure risk with opioids.
Quinidine	Caution with quinidine.
SSRIs	May potentiate seizure risk with SSRIs.
Tricyclics	May potentiate seizure risk with tricyclics (eg, cyclobenzaprine, promethazine).
Warfarin	Possible altered warfarin effects.

Tramadol Hydrochloride (Ultram)

Carbamazepine	May need dose adjustment with carbamazepine.

TRAMADOL *(cont.)*

Tramadol Hydrochloride (Ultram)

CNS depressants	Caution and reduce dose with CNS depressants (eg, alcohol, opioids, anesthetics, phenothiazines, tranquilizers, sedatives, hypnotics).
CYP2D6 inhibitors	CYP2D6 inhibitors (eg, fluoxetine, paroxetine, amitriptyline) may potentiate tramadol.
Digoxin	Possible digoxin toxicity.
Drugs that lower seizure threshold	May potentiate seizure risk with drugs that lower seizure threshold.
MAOIs	May potentiate seizure risk with MAOIs.
Naloxone	May potentiate seizure risk with naloxone (with overdose).
Neuroleptics	May potentiate seizure risk with neuroleptics.
Opioids	May potentiate seizure risk with opioids.
Quinidine	Caution with quinidine.
SSRIs	May potentiate seizure risk with SSRIs.
Tricyclics	May potentiate seizure risk with tricyclics (eg, cyclobenzaprine, promethazine).
Warfarin	Possible altered warfarin effects.

Chapter 4

Hemostatics, Astringents, Gingival Displacement Products and Antiseptics

Kenneth H. Burrell, D.D.S., S.M.

Hemostatics

An understanding of hemostasis, the identification of patients with excessive bleeding tendencies, and interventions to stop abnormal bleeding is essential to the provision of safe and appropriate dental care.

Hemostasis can be divided arbitrarily into four phases: a vascular phase and a platelet phase, also referred to as "primary hemostasis"; and a coagulation phase and a fibrinolytic phase, also referred to as "secondary hemostasis."

Defects in any phase of normal hemostasis have characteristic signs and symptoms. Most commonly, dentists performing surgery will be faced with patients who have defects of the platelet and coagulation phases.

People with quantitative or qualitative platelet disorders usually have superficial signs such as petechiae and ecchymosis on the mucosa and skin. Furthermore, patients may report spontaneous gingival bleeding, epistaxis, prolonged postextraction bleeding or prolonged bleeding after minor trauma. Spontaneous clinical hemorrhage may be present when the platelet count drops below 15,000-20,000/mm³. (For normal laboratory values, see Appendix H.)

The clinical value of a bleeding time for dental procedures is controversial. However, significant prolonged bleeding times beyond 15-20 minutes may suggest significant hemorrhage after dental surgery.

Causes of defects of primary hemostasis include congenital as well as acquired disorders. The most common inherited bleeding disorder in the United States is von Willebrand's disease. This disorder is characterized by various degrees of deficiency and qualitative defects of the von Willebrand factor, which is needed primarily for platelet adhesion in high shear areas. In severe cases of von Willebrand's disease, spontaneous bleeding may occur. However, mild cases may be associated with prolonged bleeding only after major trauma. Common acquired dysfunctions of primary hemostasis include idiopathic thrombocytopenia purpura, liver disease and drug-induced platelet disorders. Also, both acute and chronic leukemia are associated with thrombocytopenia. Some medications are used intentionally to decrease platelet functions in patients with disorders such as coronary artery disease.

Disorders of secondary hemostasis include hemophilia, vitamin K deficiency and liver disease. Hemophilia is usually classified according to the specific factor deficiency, such as hemophilia A for factor VIII deficiency and hemophilia B for factor IX deficiency. Patients with hemophilia lack the ability to form fibrin and have bleeding episodes particularly within stress-bearing joints (deep-seated bleeding). This can cause destruction of these joints.

General dentistry can be performed in patients with > 50% factor activity, but 100% activity is recommended for surgical procedures. In a 60-kg patient with hemophilia A, a 100% plasma level equals 6,000 units of factor VIII.

Vitamin K deficiency causes decreased activation of factors II, VII, IX and X, resulting in a defective coagulation cascade and consequent decreased fibrin production. Virtually all coagulation factors are produced in the liver, and vitamin K is stored in the liver. Thus, liver disease may result in increased bleeding tendencies. Medications such as warfarin, an anticoagulant that impairs the action of vitamin K, are used to prevent thrombosis in patients with such disorders as atrial fibrillation, deep venous thrombosis, ischemic cardiovascular disease and stroke.

A thorough medical history, examination and laboratory evaluation will identify most patients who have increased bleeding tendencies. Included in the patient assessment should be questions addressing whether the patient has relatives with bleeding problems, has experienced prolonged bleeding after trauma, or takes medications or has diseases associated with increased bleeding tendencies. Examination should focus on signs of bruising, jaundice, hyperplastic gingival tissue, spontaneous gingival bleeding and hemarthrosis. Screening tests for impaired hemostasis include platelet count and bleeding time for primary hemostasis, as well as prothrombin time, international normalization ratio, activated partial thromboplastin time and thrombin time for secondary hemostasis. (See Appendix H for normal values.)

Dental treatment of patients with impaired hemostasis may warrant the use of local and/or systemic measures. The use of the appropriate technique or agent depends on the patient's underlying condition and specific hemostatic impairment.

A new category of products called fibrin sealants, such as Crosseal and Tisseel, has been developed to promote hemostasis in liver, lung, splenic and cardiothoracic surgery where conventional methods of hemostasis are not practical. Although research has been conducted using these products in oral surgery, they have not yet been approved for this purpose by the FDA. Fibrin sealants are not exclusively used in patients with bleeding and clotting disorders, since research is showing they promote more rapid postsurgical healing with reduced swelling and ecchymosis. Research may also show these products to be useful in sinus lifts and bone grafting.

Accepted Indications

If blood flow is profuse, mechanical aids such as a compress, hemostatic forceps, a modeling compound splint or hemostatic ligatures can be used. Mechanical obliteration with cryosurgery, electrocauterization and laser can also be used. Although these thermal methods are effective, they may be associated with impaired healing. A third kind of mechanically aided hemostasis is the use of chemical glues, such as n-butyl cyanoacrylate and bone wax. These compounds have a mechanical effect without directly affecting the coagulation process.

For slow blood flow and oozing, a combination of hemostatics can be used. The three kinds of hemostatics to be noted here are absorbable hemostatic agents, agents that modify blood coagulation and vasoconstrictors. Vasoconstrictors act by constricting or closing blood vessels. They are used to a limited extent to control capillary bleeding. Vasoconstrictors are described in detail in Chapter 1. See Table 4.1 for a comparison of various hemostatics useful in dentistry.

Absorbable Gelatin Sponge

The absorbable gelatin sponge consists of a tough, porous matrix prepared from purified pork skin gelatin, granules and water that is indicated as a hemostatic device for control of capillary, venous or arteriolar bleeding when pressure, ligature or other conventional procedures are either ineffective or impractical. It can be used in extraction sites and is absorbed in 4-6 weeks.

Oxidized Cellulose

Oxidized cellulose is a chemically modified form of surgical gauze or cotton that is used to control moderate bleeding by forming an artificial clot when suturing or ligation is impractical and ineffective. Because it is friable, oxidized cellulose is difficult to place and retain in extraction sockets, but can be used as a sutured implant or temporary packing. The cotton or gauze can be removed before dissolution is complete by irrigation with saline or a mildly alkaline solution.

Absorption of oxidized cellulose ordinarily occurs between the second and seventh day after implantation of material, but complete absorption of large amounts of blood-soaked material may take 6 weeks or longer.

Oxidized Regenerated Cellulose

Oxidized regenerated cellulose is prepared from alpha-cellulose by reaction with alkali to form viscose, which is then spun into filaments and oxidized. This process results in greater chemical purity and uniformity of physical structure than oxidized cellulose. It is a sterile, absorbable, knitted fabric that is strong enough to be sutured or cut. It has less tendency to stick to instruments and gloves and is less friable than oxidized cellulose.

Oxidized regenerated cellulose is used to control capillary, venous and small arterial hemorrhage when ligature, pressure, or other conventional methods of control are impractical or ineffective. The product can be used as a surface dressing because it does not retard epithelialization. It is bactericidal against numerous gram-negative and gram-positive microorganisms, both aerobic and anaerobic. It can be placed over extraction sites.

Microfibrillar Collagen Hemostat

Microfibrillar collagen hemostat is a hemostatically active agent prepared from bovine deep flexor tendon (Achilles tendon) as a water-soluble, partial-acid salt of natural collagen. It reduces bleeding from surgical sites such as those involving cancellous bone and gingival graft donor sites. It should not be left in infected or contaminated spaces because it may prolong or promote infection and delay healing.

Collagen Hemostat

Collagen hemostat is absorbable and composed of purified and lyophilized bovine dermal collagen. Used as an adjunct to hemostasis, collagen absorbable hemostat can be sutured into place. It reduces bleeding when ligation and other conventional methods are ineffective or impractical. Excess material should be removed before the wound is closed.

Aminocaproic Acid

Aminocaproic acid, or ε-aminocaproic acid, is used in patients with excessive bleeding due to underlying conditions such as systemic hyper-fibrinolysis and coagulopathies stemming from promyelocytic leukemia. This medication is seldom used for elective oral surgery procedures, but rather during emergency situations in combination with transfusion of fresh frozen blood and fibrinogen.

Desmopressin Acetate

Desmopressin acetate is used primarily to reduce spontaneous bleeding in patients with von Willebrand's disease and in patients with mild-to-moderate hemophilia A (factor VIII levels above 5%). It also is used prophylactically during procedures to reduce the incidence of bleeding, as well as after procedures to achieve better hemostasis in these patient populations.

Tranexamic Acid

Tranexamic acid is used primarily to reduce the amount of factor replacement necessary after dental extractions in hemophiliac patients. It is indicated for only 2-8 days during and after the dental procedure. It also is used for other patient populations with impaired secondary hemostasis, including patients who are receiving anticoagulation therapy.

Vitamin K

Vitamin K therapy is required when hypoprothrombinemia results from inadequately available vitamins K_1 and K_2. This occurs when there is decreased synthesis by intestinal bacteria, inadequate absorption from the intestinal tract or increased requirement by the liver for normal synthesis of prothrombin.

Vitamin K, in its various forms, is an essential component of blood coagulation. Vitamins K_1, K_2 or menadione (vitamin K_3) are required for the activation of the functional forms of six coagulation proteins: prothrombin; factors VII, IX and X; and proteins C and S.

Phytonadione (vitamin K_1)

Phytonadione—known as vitamin K_1—is used for
- anticoagulant-induced prothrombin deficiency;
- prophylaxis and therapy of hemorrhagic disease of the newborn;
- hypoprothrombinemia resulting from oral antibacterial therapy;
- hypoprothrombinemia secondary to factors limiting absorption or synthesis of vitamin K such as obstructive jaundice, biliary fistula, sprue, ulcerative colitis, celiac

disease, intestinal resection, cystic fibrosis of the pancreas and regional enteritis;
- other drug-induced hypoprothrombinemia such as that which results from salicylate use.

Menadione (vitamin K_3)

Menadione is a synthetic form of vitamin K, which is sometimes referred to as vitamin K_3.

Menadiol sodium diphosphate (vitamin K_4)

Menadiol sodium diphosphate is effective as a hemostatic agent only when bleeding results from prothrombin deficiency.

Thrombin

Thrombin is useful as a topical local hemostatic agent when blood is oozing from accessible capillaries or venules. In certain kinds of hemorrhage, it can be used to wet pledgets of absorbable gelatin sponge and placed on bleeding tissue or in extraction sockets with or without sutures. It is particularly useful whenever blood is flowing from accessible capillaries and small venules.

General Dosing Information

Table 4.1 lists general dosing information for specific hemostatics.

Dosage Adjustments

The actual dose for each patient must be individualized according to factors such as his or her size, age and physical status. Reduced doses of vitamin K may be indicated for patients who are taking anticoagulants as opposed to those who have malabsorption problems. The other hemostatic agents should be used as needed.

Special Dental Considerations

Cross-Sensitivity

Patients may experience delayed healing using the gelatin, cellulose and collagen hemostatics. This is more often observed when the surgical site is infected.

Patient Monitoring: Aspects to Watch

Patients receiving vitamin K, especially parenterally, may experience allergic reactions such as rash, urticaria and anaphylaxis.

Adverse Effects and Precautions

The incidence of adverse reactions to hemostatic agents is relatively low. Many reactions are temporary. Idiosyncratic and allergic reactions account for a small minority of adverse responses. See Table 4.1.

Pharmacology

Absorbable Gelatin Sponge

The absorbable gelatin sponge promotes the disruption of platelets and acts as a framework for fibrin, probably because of its physical effect rather than the result of its alteration of the blood clotting mechanism. It can be placed in dry form or may be moistened with sterile saline or thrombin solution and used in extraction sites.

Oxidized Cellulose

Oxidized cellulose is a chemically modified form of surgical gauze or cotton. Its hemostatic action depends on the formation of an artificial clot by cellulosic acid, which has a marked affinity for hemoglobin.

Oxidized Regenerated Cellulose

Oxidized regenerated cellulose probably serves as a hemostatic by providing a physical effect rather than altering the normal physiological clotting mechanism.

Microfibrillar Collagen Hemostat

This hemostatic agent is used topically to trigger the adhesiveness of platelets and stimulate the release phenomenon to produce aggregation of platelets leading to their disintegration and to release coagulation factors that, together with plasma factors, enable fibrin to form. The physical structure of microfibrillar collagen hemostat adds strength to the clot.

Collagen Hemostat

When collagen comes into contact with blood, platelets aggregate and release coagulation factors, which together with plasma factors, cause the formation of fibrin and a clot.

Aminocaproic Acid

Aminocaproic acid is an antifibrinolytic agent that slows or stops fibrinolysis by inhibiting the action of plasminogen. Consequently, it delays the breakdown of the hemostatic plug. This medication is administered both intravenously and orally in the form of tablets and syrup. Concurrent use of other hemostatic agents in patients with significant bleeding tendencies is recommended.

Desmopressin Acetate

Desamino-*D*-arginine vasopressin is a synthetic analogue of the natural pituitary hormone 1-8-D-arginine vasopressin. This medication increases plasma levels of von Willebrand factor-VIII complex and factor VIII levels. It is administered 30 minutes before the dental appointment. It facilitates outpatient care for patients with hemophilia, but should always be used in conjunction with other hemostatic agents.

Tranexamic Acid

Tranexamic acid is an antifibrinolytic hemostatic agent that acts by decreasing conversion of plasminogen to plasmin. At much higher doses, it acts as a noncompetitive inhibitor of plasmin. It is indicated for prophylaxis and treatment of patients with hemophilia, to prevent or reduce hemorrhage during and after tooth extraction. Unlabeled uses include topical use as a mouthwash, along with systemic therapy to reduce bleeding after oral surgery. It is contraindicated for use in patients receiving anticoagulant therapy. This medication is administered both intravenously and orally.

Vitamin K

Two forms of naturally occurring vitamin K have been isolated and prepared synthetically. The naturally occurring forms are designated vitamins K_1 and K_2. Vitamin K_1 is present in most vegetables, particularly in their green leaves. Vitamin K_2 is produced by intestinal bacteria. Menadione has vitamin K activity and is derived from a breakdown of the vitamin K molecule by intestinal bacteria and is sometimes referred to as vitamin K_3. Menadiol sodium diphosphate, or vitamin K_4, is a water-soluble derivative that is converted to menadione in the liver.

Hypoprothrombinemia may result from inadequately available vitamins K_1 and K_2 because of decreased synthesis by intestinal bacteria, inadequate absorption from the intestinal tract or increased requirement by the liver for normal synthesis of prothrombin. Liver dysfunction may also decrease the production of prothrombin, but the hypoprothrombinemia from hepatic cell injury may not respond to the administration of vitamin K as many coagulation proteins are produced in hepatocytes.

Insufficient vitamin K in ingested foods becomes significant only when the synthesis of the vitamin by intestinal bacteria is markedly reduced by the oral administration of antibacterial agents. Biliary obstructions or intestinal disorders may result in an inadequate rate of absorption of vitamin K.

Phytonadione (vitamin K_1)
Vitamin K_1 is required for the production of the functional forms of six coagulation proteins: prothrombin, factors VII, IX and X and proteins C and S.

Menadione (vitamin K_3)
Although it is readily absorbed from the intestine, menadione must be converted to vitamin K_2 by the liver. Therefore, it requires a normal flow of bile into the intestine or the concomitant administration of bile salts.

Menadiol sodium diphosphate (vitamin K_4)
Vitamin K_4, because of its water solubility, is absorbed from the intestinal tract even in the absence of bile salts.

Thrombin

Thrombin is a sterile protein substance that is an essential component of blood coagulation. It activates fibrinogen to form fibrin.

Patient Advice
- Let the patient know that a hemostatic has been used, what kind of hemostatic it is and why it was used.
- Advise the patient to let you know if bleeding continues from the surgical site.

Astringents

Astringents cause contraction of tissues. They accomplish this by constricting small blood vessels, extracting water from tissue or precipitating protein.

Accepted Indications
Dentists can apply astringents to gingival tissues before taking impressions, placing Class V or root-surface restorations. They can be used alone or in combination with retraction cords. Aluminum and iron salts are the compounds used as astringents in dentistry.

Aluminum Chloride
Aluminum chloride causes contraction or shrinking of tissue, making it useful in

retracting gingival tissue. It also reduces secretions and minor hemorrhage.

Aluminum Potassium Sulfate

Aluminum potassium sulfate, or alum, is not widely used even though it is relatively innocuous, because its tissue retraction and hemostatic properties are limited.

Aluminum Sulfate

Aluminum sulfate, as with other aluminum salts, serves as an effective astringent for gingival retraction and hemostatic action.

Ferric Sulfate

Ferric sulfate is an effective and safe astringent and hemostatic for use in gingival retraction. It also can be used in vital pulpotomies.

General Dosing Information

Table 4.1 lists general dosing and administration information for specific astringents.

Adverse Effects

The incidence of adverse reactions to astringents is relatively low. Most reactions are temporary. The adverse effects listed in Table 4.1 apply to all major types of astringents.

Pharmacology

The ability of any astringent to contract or shrink mucous membrane or skin tissue is related to its mode of action involving protein precipitation and water absorption.

Gingival Displacement Products

Gingival displacement products can be used alone or in combination with astringents or vasoconstrictors. They are usually made of cotton and are woven in various ways to suit the practitioner's preferences. These cotton cords are available in a variety of diameters to accommodate the variation in gingival sulcus width and depth. Gingival displacement pastes are also available. One uses kaolin as the vehicle and contains 6.5% aluminum chloride; the other is made of a polymer call PVS that expands into the sulcus as it sets.

The cords can be impregnated with astringents or vasoconstrictors either by the manufacturer or at chairside. Aluminum chloride, aluminum sulfate and ferric sulfate are used as the astringents, while racemic epinephrine is used as the vasoconstrictor.

Epinephrine cord is contraindicated in patients with a history of cardiovascular diseases and dysrhythmias, diabetes and hyperthyroidism and in those taking rauwolfias and ganglionic blocking agents. Caution is advised in patients taking monoamine oxidase inhibitors.

Some practitioners and educators believe that epinephrine-containing displacement cord and solutions should not be used in dentistry. However, plasma epinephrine concentration increased significantly only after 60 minutes in a study of healthy subjects without a history of high blood pressure. In spite of the elevated plasma epinephrine levels, the subjects' heart rates, mean arterial pressures and pulse pressure were not significantly different when the same subjects were exposed to a potassium aluminum sulfate (alum) impregnated cord. The gingival tissues of the subjects were intact, however. Therefore, the patient's medical history, oral health, type of procedure to be done, amount and length of displacement cord, and exposure of the vascular bed should be considered before deciding to use epinephrine-containing retraction cords. Table 4.1 provides gingival displacement cord information, including adverse effects, precautions and contraindications of a variety of commercially available displacement cords.

Accepted Indications

Gingival displacement cord is used for all kinds of gingival displacement before taking impressions or placing restorations.

General Dosing Information

Dosage Adjustments

The actual maximum dose for each patient must be individualized depending on factors such as oral health and sensitivity.

Adverse Effects and Precautions

The incidence of adverse reactions to gingival displacement cords and paste is relatively low. Most reactions are temporary, but gingival tissue destruction may permanently alter gingival architecture, especially after vigorous cord placement.

Pharmacology

Gingival displacement products work mechanically to widen the gingival sulcus. With the addition of astringents or vasoconstrictors, the gingival tissue is retracted further. The astringents act by constricting blood vessels, extracting water from tissue or precipitating proteins.

Suggested Readings

Anderson KW, Baker SR. Advances in facial rejuvenation surgery. Otolaryngol Head Neck Surg 2003;11(4):256–60.

Colman RW, Hirsch J, Marder VJ, Salzman EW, eds. Hemostatics and thrombosis: Basic principles and clinical practice. 4th ed. Philadelphia: Lippincott Williams & Wilkins; 2000.

Donovan TE, Chee WWL. Current concepts in gingival displacement. Dent Clin N Am 2004;48:433–44.

Fat and water soluble vitamins: vitamin K. In: Drug facts and comparisons. St Louis: Facts and Comparisons; 2000:12–13.

Garfunkel AA, Galili D, Findler M, Lubliner J. Bleeding tendency: a practical approach to dentistry. Compend Contin Educ Dent 1999;20:836–52.

Rossman JA, Rees TD. The use of hemostatic agents in dentistry. Postgrad Dent 1996;3:3–12.

Wahl MJ. Myths of dental surgery in patients receiving anticoagulant therapy. JADA 2000;131:77–81.

Antiseptics

An antiseptic is a broad-spectrum antimicrobial chemical solution that is applied topically to body surfaces to reduce the microbial flora in preparation for surgery or at an injection site. The antimicrobial activity of antiseptics usually is weaker than that of disinfectants and sterilants because less harsh, or weaker, chemicals usually must be applied to body surfaces to avoid irritating the tissues. However, the antimicrobial activity of antiseptics can be lethal to the microbes on the body surfaces. The specific activity depends on the nature of the antiseptic chemical and the microbes involved. In dentistry, antiseptics are grouped into three classes: handwashing agents, skin and mucosal antiseptics, and root canal and cavity preparations (see Table 4.2 for usage information).

Table 4.1: USAGE INFORMATION FOR HEMOSTATICS, ASTRINGENTS, AND GINGIVAL DISPLACEMENT PRODUCTS

NAME	FORM/ STRENGTH	DOSAGE	WARNINGS/PRECAUTIONS & CONTRAINDICATIONS	ADVERSE EFFECTS
HEMOSTATICS				
LOCAL AGENTS THAT MODIFY BLOOD COAGULATION				
Absorbable Gelatin Sponge (Gelfoam)	**Dental Packing Blocks:** 20 × 20 × 7 mm; **Pow:** 1g	Absorbable gelatin sponge may be cut; may be applied to bleeding surfaces to cover area.	**W/P:** Should not be overpacked in extraction sites or surgical defects because it may expand to impinge on neighboring structures.	May form a nidus for infection or abscess formation.
Collagen, Bovine/ Glycosamino- glycans (CollaCote★, CollaPlug, Col- laTape★, Integra Bilayer Matrix Wound Dressing, Integra Dermal Regeneration Template)	**CollaCote, Col- laPlug, CollaTape:** 1 × 3, ¾ × 1½, 3/8 × ¾ in	Use as directed.	**W/P:** Do not use on infected or contaminated wounds. Although these dressings will promote hemostasis, they are not intended for use in treating systemic coagulation disorders. **P/N:** Safety during pregnancy unknown.	NA
Collagen Hemostat (Instat)	**Pads:** 1 × 2, 3 × 4 in	Should be applied directly to bleeding surface with pressure; is more effective when applied dry, or may be moistened with sterile saline or thrombin solution; may be left in place as necessary; is absorbed 8-10 w after placement.	**W/P:** Incidence of pain has been reported to increase when this material is placed in extraction sockets. Allergic reactions can occur in patients with known sensitivity to bovine material.	Should not be used in mucous membrane closure because it may interfere with healing due to mechanical interposition. Should not be left in infected or contaminated space because of possible delay in healing and increased likelihood of abscess formation. Should not be used in patients with a known sensitivity to bovine material. Should not be overpacked because collagen absorbable hemostat absorbs water and can expand to impinge on neighboring structures. Should not be used in cases where point of hemorrhage is submerged, because collagen must be in direct contact with bleeding site to achieve desired effect.
Microfibrillar Collagen Hemostat (Avitene, Instat MCH)	**Avitene Flour:** ½-, 1-, 5-g syringes; **Avitene Sheets:** 35 × 35, 70 × 35, 70 × 70 mm; **Instat MCH:** Coherent fibers packaged in 0.5- and 1.0-g containers	Is applied topically and adheres firmly to bleeding surfaces.	**W/P:** Is not intended to treat systemic coagulation disorders. Placement in extraction sites has been reported to increase pain. Should not be left in infected or contaminated spaces because of possible adhesion formation, allergic reaction, foreign body reaction. Interferes with wound margins.	May potentiate abscess formation, hematoma and wound dehiscence.
Oxidized Cellulose (Oxycel)	**Pad:** 3 × 3 in; **Pledget:** 2 × 1 × 1 in; **Strip:** 18 × 2, 5 × ½, 36 × ½ in	Hemostatic effect is greater when material is applied dry as opposed to moistened with water or saline.	**W/P:** Extremely friable and difficult to place. Should not be used at fracture sites because it interferes with bone regeneration. Should not be used as a surface dressing except for the immediate control of hemorrhage, as cellulosic acid inhibits epithelialization. Should not be used in combination with thrombin because the hemostatic action of either alone is greater than that of the combination.	May lead to a foreign-body reaction.

★ indicates a product bearing the ADA Seal of Acceptance.   NA = Not available.

Table 4.1: USAGE INFORMATION FOR HEMOSTATICS, ASTRINGENTS, AND GINGIVAL DISPLACEMENT PRODUCTS (cont.)

NAME	FORM/ STRENGTH	DOSAGE	WARNINGS/PRECAUTIONS & CONTRAINDICATIONS	ADVERSE EFFECTS
HEMOSTATICS (cont.)				
Oxidized Regenerated Cellulose (Surgicel Absorbable Hemostat★, Surgicel Nu-Knit Absorbable Hemostat)	**Surgicel sheets:** 2 × 14, 4 × 8, 2 × 3, ½ × 2 in; **Surgicel Nu-Knit sheets:** 1 × 1, 3 × 4, 6 × 9 in	Can be laid over extraction socket for control of bleeding; minimal amounts of the material should be placed on bleeding site; may be held firmly against tissue.	**W/P:** Placement in extraction sites may delay healing; it should not be placed in fracture sites because it may interfere with callus formation and may cause cyst formation. Encapsulation of fluid and foreign bodies possible.	NA
SYSTEMIC AGENTS THAT MODIFY BLOOD COAGULATION				
Aminocaproic Acid (Amicar)	**Inj:** 250mg/mL; **Syr:** 1.25g/5mL; **Tab:** 500mg*, 1000mg*	**Adults: IV:** 16-20mL (4-5g) in 250mL diluent during 1st hr, then 4mL/hr (1g) in 50mL of diluent. **PO:** 5g during 1st hr, then 5mL (syr) or 1g (tabs) per hr. Continue therapy for 8 hrs or until bleeding is controlled.	**W/P:** Avoid in hematuria of upper urinary tract origin due to risk of intrarenal obstruction from glomerular capillary thrombosis or clots in renal pelvis and ureters. Skeletal muscle weakness with necrosis of muscle fibers reported after prolonged therapy. Consider cardiac muscle damage with skeletal myopathy. Avoid rapid IV infusion. Thrombophlebitis may occur. Contains benzyl alcohol; do not administer to neonates due to risk of fatal gasping syndrome. Do not administer without a definite diagnosis of hyperfibrinolysis. **Contra:** Active intravascular clotting process, disseminated intravascular coagulation without concomitant heparin. **P/N:** Category C, caution in nursing.	Edema, headache, anaphylactoid reactions, injection site reactions, pain, bradycardia, hypotension, abdominal pain, diarrhea, nausea, vomiting, agranulocytosis, increased CPK, confusion, dyspnea, pruritus, tinnitus.
Anti-Inhibitor Coagulation Complex (Autoplex T, Feiba-VH)	**Sol:** 1 IU	**Adults/Pediatrics: Autoplex T:** 25 to 100 units/kg, depending on severity of hemorrhage; repeat after 6 hours if no hemostatic improvement. **Feiba-VH:** 50 to 100 units/kg.	**W/P:** Made from human plasma. May contain infectious agents, such as viruses, that can cause disease. The risk that such products will transmit an infectious agent has been reduced by screening plasma donors for prior exposure to certain viruses, by testing for the presence of certain current virus infections, and by in-activating and/or removing certain viruses. Despite these measures, such products can still potentially transmit disease. Because this product is made from human blood, it may carry a risk of transmit-ting infectious agents, eg, viruses and theoretically, the Creutzfeldt-Jakob disease (CJD) agent. ALL infections thought by a physician possibly to have been transmit-ted by this product should be reported by the physician or other healthcare provider to the U.S. distributor. **Contra:** Bleeding episodes resulting from coagulation factor deficiencies, eg, disseminated intravasular coagulation, fibrinolysis, normal coagula-tion mechanism. **P/N:** Category C, caution in nursing.	Tachycardia, hypotension, chest pain, nausea, dizzi-ness, headache, fever.
Desmopressin Acetate (DDAVP)	**Inj:** 4µg/mL; **Nasal Spray:** 10µg/inh [5mL]; **Tab:** 0.1mg*, 0.2mg*; **Rhinal Tube:** 0.01% [2.5mL]	**Adults: Hemophilia A and von Willebrand Disease:** 0.3µg/kg IV. Add 50mL diluent. Give 30 minutes preoperatively. **Pediatrics: Hemophilia A and von Willebrand Disease: >3 months: (Inj)** 0.3µg/kg IV. Add 50mL diluent if 10kg; add 10mL diluent	**W/P:** Mucosal changes with nasal forms may occur; discontinue until resolved. Decrease fluid intake in pediatrics and el-derly to decrease risk of water intoxication and hyponatremia; monitor osmolality. Caution with coronary artery insufficiency, hypertensive cardiovascular disease, fluid and electrolyte imbalance (eg, cystic fibrosis). Anaphylaxis reported with	**Inj:** Headache, nausea, abdominal cramps, vulval pain, injection site reac-tions, facial flushing, BP changes. **Spray:** Headache, dizziness, rhinitis, nausea, nasal congestion, sore throat, cough, respiratory infection, epistaxis.

*Scored.   ★indicates a product bearing the ADA Seal of Acceptance.   NA = Not available.

NAME	FORM/ STRENGTH	DOSAGE	WARNINGS/PRECAUTIONS & CONTRAINDICATIONS	ADVERSE EFFECTS
Desmopressin Acetate *(cont.)*		if >10kg. Give 30 minutes preoperatively.	IV use. Caution with IV use if history of thrombus formation. For diabetes insipidus, dosage must be adjusted according to diurnal pattern of response; estimate response by adequate duration of sleep and adequate, not excessive, water turnover. **P/N:** Category B, caution in nursing.	**Tab:** Nausea, flushing, abdominal cramps, headache, increased SGOT, water intoxication, hyponatremia.
Epinephrine (Epidri, Orostat, Racellet, Racemistat)	**Sol:** 25% (Racemistat); **Pellet:** 8% (Epidri);**Cotton pellet** (racemic epinephrine): 0.90-1.40mg/pellet #2; 0.42-0.68mg/pellet #3 (Racellet)	Use as directed.	NA	NA
Phytonadione (Mephyton, Vitamin K, Vitamin K₁)	**Tab:** 5mg* (Mephyton); **Inj:**1mg/0.5mL, 10 mg/mL (Vitamin K)	***Adults*: Anticoagulant-Induced Prothrombin Deficiency: Initial:** 2.5-10mg up to 25mg (rarely 50mg). May repeat if PT is still elevated 12-48 hrs after initial dose. **Hypoprothrombinemia Due to Other Causes:** 2.5-25mg or more (rarely up to 50mg). Give bile salts when endogenous bile supply to GIT is deficient.	**W/P:** Does not produce an immediate coagulant effect. Maintain lowest possible dose to prevent original thromboembolic events. Avoid repeated large doses with hepatic disease. Failure to respond may indicate a congenital coagulation defect or a condition unresponsive to vitamin K. Avoid large doses in liver disease. Monitor PT regularly. **P/N:**Category C, caution in nursing.	Severe hypersensitivity reactions (anaphylactoid reactions, death), flushing, peculiar taste sensations, dizziness, rapid and weak pulse, profuse sweating, hypotension, dyspnea, cyanosis.
Tranexamic Acid (Cyklokapron)	**Sol:** 100 mg/mL in 10-mL vials; **Tab:** 500 mg	***Adult/Ped*:** Immediately before surgery, 10mg/kg IV; after surgery, 25mg/kg orally tid or qid for 2-8 days.	**W/P:** Dose should be reduced for patients with renal impairment. Contraindicated in patients with acquired defective color vision and subarachnoid hemorrhage. **P/N:** Category B.	Giddiness, nausea, vomiting, diarrhea, blurred vision; hypotension with IV dose.
Vitamin K₃ or Menadione	**Powder**	***Adults*:** 2-10mg/day, 4-7 days before surgery.	**W/P:** Requires normal flow of bile or administration of bile salts. Patient undergoing prothrombin reduction therapy should not receive vitamin K preparations except under physician supervision.	Adverse reactions are similar to those produced by phytonadione, but incidence is low.
Vitamin K₄ or Menadiol Sodium Diphosphate	**Inj:** 5, 10, 37.5mg/ mL; **Tab:** 5mg	**Injection:** 5-10mg q day, 4-7 days. **Oral:** 5mg q day, 4-7 days.	**W/P:** Before administering drug, determine if patient is receiving anticoagulant therapy; a patient undergoing prothrombin reduction therapy should not receive vitamin K preparations except under physician supervision. If patient is taking anticoagulants, this agent may decrease their effectiveness.	Adverse reactions are similar to those produced by phytonadione, but incidence is low.

THROMBIN (TOPICAL AGENT)

NAME	FORM/ STRENGTH	DOSAGE	WARNINGS/PRECAUTIONS & CONTRAINDICATIONS	ADVERSE EFFECTS
Thrombin (Thrombin-JMI, Thrombinar, Thrombogen, Thrombostat)	**Pow:** 1,000, 5,000, 10,000, 20,000 units; 50,000 units (Thrombinar only); **Pow (with isotonic saline diluent):** 5,000-, 10,000- and 20,000-unit containers with 5-, 10-, and 20-mL of isotonic saline; **Thrombostat:** Also contains 0.02mg/mL phemerol as a preservative	**Profuse Bleeding (Sol):** 1,000-2,000 units/mL. For bleeding from skin or mucosa—solution: 100 units/mL.	**W/P:** Thrombin must not be injected into blood vessels because it might cause serious or even fatal embolism from extensive intravascular thrombosis; instead, should be applied to surface of bleeding tissue as solution or powder. **P/N:** Category C.	Allergic reactions can occur in patients with known sensitivity to bovine material.

Table 4.1: USAGE INFORMATION FOR HEMOSTATICS, ASTRINGENTS, AND GINGIVAL DISPLACEMENT PRODUCTS (cont.)

NAME	FORM/ STRENGTH	DOSAGE	WARNINGS/PRECAUTIONS & CONTRAINDICATIONS	ADVERSE EFFECTS
ASTRINGENTS				
Aluminum Chloride (Gingi-Aid, FS Hemostatic, Hemodent★, Hemodettes, Hemogin-L, Styptin, Ultradent)	**Gel:** 20% (Hemodettes); **Sol:** 20% (Hemodent, Styptin), 25% (Gingi-Aid, FS Hemostatic, Ultradent); **Oint:** 25% (Hemogin-L); **Retraction cords:** Average concentration of 0.915, 3.5mg/in	**Adults:** Apply product directly to tissues using a cotton pledget or apply to gingival retraction cords.	None of significance to dentistry.	Concentrated solutions of aluminum chloride are acidic and may have an irritating and even caustic effect on tissues.
Aluminum Potassium Sulfate	**Pow:** 100%, various concentrations, all available and prepared by chemical supply houses	**Adults:** Any concentration, including 100% powder, can be used.	None of significance to dentistry.	May have an irritating effect.
Aluminum Sulfate (Gel-Cord, Rastringent, Rastringent II)	**Cotton pellet:** 2.20-2.80mg/pellet (Rastringent); **Gel:** In unit-dose cartridge; **Impregnated retraction cord:** Average concentration of 0.48, 0.85, 1.45mg/in; **Topical solution:** 25%	**Adults:** Apply product directly to tissues using a cotton pledget or apply to gingival retraction cords.	None of significance to dentistry.	May have an irritating and even caustic effect.
Ferric Chloride (Viscostat Wintermint)	NA	**Adults:** Apply product directly to tissues using a cotton pledget or apply to gingival retraction cords.	NA	NA
Ferric Subsulfate (Astringyn)	NA	**Adults:** Apply product directly to tissues using a cotton pledget or apply to gingival retraction cords.	NA	NA
Ferric Sulfate (Astringedent★, Hemodent-FS, Stasis, Visco-Stat)	**Sol:** 13.3% (Astringedent), 15.5 (Hemodent-FS), 20% (ViscoStat—for use in infuser kit), 21% (Stasis)	**Adults:** Apply product directly to tissues using a cotton pledget or apply to gingival retraction cords.	None of significance to dentistry.	Compound may cause tissue irritation to a greater degree than aluminum compounds.
Ferric Sulfate/Ferric Subsulfate (Astringedent X)	**Sol:** 25%	**Adults:** Apply product directly to tissues using a cotton pledget or apply to gingival retraction cords.	NA	NA
GINGIVAL DISPLACEMENT PRODUCTS†				
Retraction cord, plain (Gingi-Plain, Gingi-Plain Z-Twist, Hemodent, Retrax, Sil-Trax Plain, Ultrapak)	**Gingi-Plain Firm Cord:** #1 (thin); #2 (medium); #3 (thick); **Gingi-Plain Z-Twist Braided Cord:** #00 (very thin); #1 (thin); #2 (medium); #3 (thick); **Hemodent:** #9 (medium thin); #3 (medium heavy);	Use as directed.	None of significance to dentistry.	None of significance to dentistry.

†A number of retraction cords are available with racemic epinephrine in concentrations ranging from 0.3-1.45mg/in and varying concentration of zinc phenylsulfonate.   ★indicates a product bearing the ADA Seal of Acceptance.   NA = Not available.

NAME	FORM/ STRENGTH	DOSAGE	WARNINGS/PRECAUTIONS & CONTRAINDICATIONS	ADVERSE EFFECTS
Retraction cord, plain *(cont.)*	**Retrax Twisted Cord:** #7 (thin); #8 (small); #9 (medium); #10 (large) **Sil-Trax Plain Braided Cord:** #7 (thin); #8 (small); #9 (medium); #10 (large); **Ultrapak:** Ultrapak #000 (ultra thin); #00 (very thin); #0 (thin); #1 (medium); #2 (thick); #3 (ultra thick)			
Retraction cord with aluminum chloride (Hemodent★, Retreat)	**Hemodent:** #9 (medium thin); #3 (medium heavy), 0.915 mg/in; **Retreat:** #1 (thin); #2 (medium); #3 (thick)	Use as directed.	**Contra:** History of allergy.	May cause irritation or tissue destruction.
Retraction paste, plain (Magic FoamCord)	PVS	Use as directed.	None of significance to dentistry.	None of significance to dentistry.
Retraction paste with aluminum chloride (Expa-syl)	6.5% aluminum chloride	Use as directed.	**Contra:** History of allergy.	May cause irritation or tissue destruction.
Retraction cord with aluminum sulfate (Gingi-Aid Z-Twist, Pascord, R-Cord, Sil-Trax AS)	**Gingi-Aid Z-Twist Braided Cord:** #00 (very thin); #1 (thin); #2 (medium); #3 (thick); 0.5 mg/in; **Pascord Twisted Cord:** #7 (thin), 0.48 mg/in; #8 (small), 0.48 mg/in; #9 (medium), 0.85 mg/in; #10 (large), 1.45 mg/in; **R-Cord:** Braided cord with or without epinephrine; **Sil-Trax AS Braided Cord:** #7 (thin), 0.48 mg/in; #8 (small), 0.48 mg/in; #9 (medium), 0.85 mg/in; #10 (large), 1.45 mg/in	Use as directed.	None of significance to dentistry.	May have an irritating and even caustic effect.
Retraction cord with aluminum potassium sulfate (GingiBraid, GingiKnit, Gingi-Tract, Sulpak, Sultan Ultra, UniBraid)	**GingiBraid:** 0 (fine); 1 (small); 2 (medium); 3 (large); also available plain; **GingiKnit:** 000 (very fine); 00 (fine); 0 (small); 1 (medium); 2 (large); 3 (extra large); **Gingi-Tract:** Thin, medium, thick;	Use as directed.	None of significance to dentistry.	May have an irritating effect.

Table 4.1: USAGE INFORMATION FOR HEMOSTATICS, ASTRINGENTS, AND GINGIVAL DISPLACEMENT PRODUCTS *(cont.)*

NAME	FORM/ STRENGTH	DOSAGE	WARNINGS/PRECAUTIONS & CONTRAINDICATIONS	ADVERSE EFFECTS
GINGIVAL DISPLACEMENT PRODUCTS† *(cont.)*				
Retraction cord with aluminum potassium sulfate *(cont.)*	**Sulpak:** Braided cord in thin, medium, large; **Sultan:** Braided cord in thin, medium, large; available with either aluminum potassium sulfate or racemic epinephrine; **UniBraid:** 0 (fine); 1 (small); 2 (medium); 3 (large); also available plain			
Retraction cord with epinephrine (Gingi-Pak)	#1 (thin); #2 (medium); #3 (thick); 0.5 mg/in	Use as directed.	**W/P:** Patient's medical history and oral health, type of procedure to be done, amount and length of retraction, and exposure of the vascular bed should be considered before epinephrine-containing retraction cords are used. **Contra:** Patients with a history of cardiovascular diseases, diabetes, hyperthyroidism, hypertension or arteriosclerosis and patients taking tricyclic antidepressants, monoamine oxidase inhibitors, rauwolfias, or ganglionic blocking agents.	May cause irritation or tissue destruction.
Retraction cord with racemic epinephrine (R-Cord, Racord, Sil-Trax EPI, Sultan)	**Racord Twisted Cord:** #7 (thin), 0.50 mg/in.; #8 (small), 0.50 mg/in.; #9 (medium), 0.85 mg/in.; #10 (large), 1.15 mg/in; **Sil-Trax EPI Braided Cord:** #7 (thin), 0.50 mg/in; #8 (small), 0.50 mg/in; #9 (medium), 0.85 mg/in; #10 (large), 1.15 mg/in; **Sultan:** 0.108-0.48 mg/in	Use as directed.	**W/P:** Patient's medical history and oral health, type of procedure to be done, amount and length of retraction, and exposure of the vascular bed should be considered before epinephrine-containing retraction cords are used. **Contra:** Patients with a history of cardiovascular diseases, diabetes, hyperthyroidism, hypertension or arteriosclerosis and patients taking tricyclic antidepressants, monoamine oxidase inhibitors, rauwolfias, or ganglionic blocking agents.	May cause irritation or tissue destruction.

†A number of retraction cords are available with racemic epinephrine in concentrations ranging from 0.3-1.45mg/in and varying concentration of zinc phenylsulfonate   ★ indicates a product bearing the ADA Seal of Acceptance.   NA = Not available.

Table 4.2: USAGE INFORMATION FOR TOPICAL ANTISEPTICS, ROOT CANAL MEDICATIONS, AND PERIODONTAL DRESSINGS

NAME	FORM/STRENGTH	WARNINGS/PRECAUTIONS, CONTRAINDICATIONS & ADVERSE EFFECTS	ACTIONS/ USES
HANDWASHING AGENTS			
Chlorhexidine Gluconate, 4% (BrianCare Antimicrobial Skin Cleanser, Dencide Antimicrobial Solution, Dial Surgical Hand Scrub, Dyna-Hex 4% Antimicrobial Skin Cleanser, Endure 400 Scrub-Stat 4, Excell Antimicrobial Skin Cleanser, Hibiclens Antiseptic Antimicrobial Skin Cleanser, Maxiclens, MetriCare Surgical Hand Scrub, Novoclens Topical Solution)	**Sol:** 4% chlorhexidine gluconate; 4% isopropyl alcohol	**W/P:** Use only for topical application on the hands. Chlorhexidine is nontoxic on the skin but may cause damage if placed directly into the eye or ear. It has been reported to cause deafness when instilled in the middle ear through perforated eardrums. **A/E:** Irritation, sensitization, and generalized allergic reactions have been reported with chlorhexidine-containing products, especially in the genital area.	Very effective against gram-positive bacteria, moderately effective against gram-negative bacteria, bacteriostatic only against mycobacteria. According to laboratory studies, can eliminate infectivity of lipophilic viruses such as HIV, influenza and herpes simplex but is not very effective against hydrophilic viruses such as poliovirus and some enteric viruses.
Chlorhexidine Gluconate, 2% (Chlorostat Antimicrobial Skin Cleanser, Dyna-Hex 2% Antimicrobial Skin Cleanser, Endure 420)	**Sol:** 2% chlorhexidine gluconate; 4% isopropyl alcohol	**W/P:** Use only for topical application on the hands. Chlorhexidine is nontoxic on the skin but may cause damage if placed directly into the eye or ear. It has been reported to cause deafness when instilled in the middle ear through perforated eardrums. **A/E:** Irritation, sensitization, and generalized allergic reactions have been reported with chlorhexidine-containing products, especially in the genital area.	Not as effective as the 4% solution but has similar spectrum of activity.
Chlorhexidine Gluconate, 0.75% (Perfect Care)	**Sol:** 0.75% chlorhexidine gluconate	**W/P:** Use only for topical application on the hands. Chlorhexidine is nontoxic on the skin but may cause damage if placed directly into the eye or ear. It has been reported to cause deafness when instilled in the middle ear through perforated eardrums. **A/E:** Irritation, sensitization, and generalized allergic reactions have been reported with chlorhexidine-containing products, especially in the genital area.	Not as effective as the 4% solution; best for nonsurgical routine handwashing.
Chlorhexidine Gluconate Solution, 0.5% (Hibistat Germicidal Hand Rinse)	**Sol:** 0.5% chlorhexidine gluconate; 70% isopropyl alcohol (4oz, 8oz bottles); **Hand Wipe Towelette:** 5mL solution, 50 per box	**W/P:** Use only for topical application on the hands. Chlorhexidine is nontoxic on the skin but may cause damage if placed directly into the eye or ear. It has been reported to cause deafness when instilled in the middle ear through perforated eardrums. **A/E:** Irritation, sensitization, and generalized allergic reactions have been reported with chlorhexidine-containing products, especially in the genital area.	Not as effective as the 4% solution; best for nonsurgical routine handwashing.
Iodophors (Betadine Surgical Scrub, Povidex Surgical Scrub)	**Sol:** 0.75% (available iodine)	**W/P:** Can cause skin irritation; rinse off after handwashing. **Contra:** Do not use iodophors on infants due to risk of iodine-induced hyperthyroidism. **A/E:** Irritation, allergic reaction.	Very effective against gram-positive bacteria and moderately effective against gram-negative bacteria, the tubercle bacillus, fungi and many viruses.
Para-chloro-*meta*-xylenol **(PCMX) (chloroxylenol)** (DermAseptic, DisAseptic, Lurosep Antimicrobial Lotion Soap, OmniCare 7, VioNex, VioNex with with Nonoxynol-9)	**PCMX:** 0.5% (Lurosep Antimicrobial Lotion Soap, OmniCare 7, VioNex); 3% (DermAseptic); 4% (DisAseptic); PCMX 0.5% with Nonoxynol-9 (VioNex with Nonoxynol-9)	**A/E:** Irritation, allergic reaction.	Although some studies have shown chlorhexidine and iodophors to be more active than PCMX against skin flora, PCMX is a fairly broad-spectrum antimicrobial agent that is moderately effective against gram-positive bacteria and somewhat effective against gram-negative bacteria, the tubercle bacillus and some fungi and viruses.

★ indicates a product bearing the ADA Seal of Acceptance. The products listed here might not include all of those that are available. Also, the listing of a product does not denote its superiority to any other product that is either listed or not listed, nor does it guarantee its availability or quality.

Table 4.2: USAGE INFORMATION FOR TOPICAL ANTISEPTICS, ROOT CANAL MEDICATIONS, AND PERIODONTAL DRESSINGS *(cont.)*

NAME	FORM/STRENGTH	WARNINGS/PRECAUTIONS, CONTRAINDICATIONS & ADVERSE EFFECTS	ACTIONS/ USES
HANDWASHING AGENTS *(cont.)*			
Triclosan or Irgasan (Bacti-Stat, Cetaphil Antibacterial Cleansing, Dial Liquid Antimicrobial Soap, Lysol I.C. Antimicrobial Soap, Oilatum-AD Cleansing Lotion, pHisoderm Antibacterial Cleanser, Prevacare Antimicrobial Handwash, SaniSept, Septisol Solution)	**Soap, Sol, Lotion:** 0.2% (Dial Liquid Antimicrobial Soap); 0.3% (Bacti-Stat, Lysol I.C. Antimicrobial Soap, SaniSept); 1% (Prevacare); 0.25% irgasan (Septisol Solution)	**A/E:** Irritation, allergic reaction.	Moderately effective against gram-positive bacteria and most gram-negative bacteria, but it may be less effective against *Pseudomonas aeruginosa;* somewhat effective against the tubercle bacillus; level of its effectiveness against viruses is unknown.
SKIN AND MUCOSAL ANTISEPTICS			
Chlorhexidine gluconate, subgingival delivery (PerioChip)	**Biodegradable chip:** 2.5mg	**W/P:** Use has not been studied in acutely abscessed periodontal pockets and is not recommended. Rarely, infectious events including abscesses and cellulitis have been reported with adjunctive use of the chip post scaling and root planing. Patient management should include consideration of potentially contributing medical disorders (eg, cancer, diabetes, and immunocompromised status). Patients should avoid dental floss at insertion site for 10 days after placement; all other oral hygiene may be continued as usual. Although sensitivity is normal the first week after placement, patients should promptly report pain, swelling or other problems that occur. Use in pediatric patients has not been studied. **Contra:** Hypersensitivity to chlorhexidine. **P/N:** Category C; safety in nursing unknown. **A/E:** Toothache (including dental, gingival or mouth pain; tenderness; aching; throbbing; soreness; discomfort; and sensitivity), upper respiratory tract infection, headache.	Subgingival delivery of chlorhexidine in a biodegradable hydrolyzed gelatin matrix; FDA-approved as an adjunct to periodontal therapy. Chip maintains antimicrobial concentration in periodontal pocket for at least 7 days. Clinical studies have not demonstrated staining or severe adverse effects using this agent in a local delivery system.
Ethanol/Isopropyl Alcohol (Alco-gel, Epi-Clenz, Gel-stat, Isagel, Rubbing Alcohol, BD Alcohol, Lacrosse Isopropyl Alcohol)	**Liq:** 70% ethyl alcohol; 70% isopropyl alcohol	**W/P:** For external use only; produces serious gastric disturbances if taken internally. Flammable; keep away from fire or flame. **Contra:** Do not use in eyes or on mucous membranes, irritated skin, deep wounds, puncture wounds, or serious burns. **A/E:** Defatting of skin and enhanced exposure of bacteria in hair follicles; painful stinging and burning when applied directly to mucosa and wounds.	Very effective; gives rapid protection against most vegetative gram-positive and gram-negative bacteria; has good activity against the tubercle bacillus, most fungi and many viruses.
Iodophors (Betadine Solution, Sana Prep Solution)	**Sol:** 0.75% (Sana Prep), 1% (Betadine) (available iodine)	**Contra:** Do not use iodophors on infants due to risk of iodine-induced hyperthyroidism. **A/E:** Irritation, allergic reaction.	May be applied to oral mucosa to reduce bacteremias during treatment of patients who are at increased risk of developing endocarditis (as indicated by American Heart Association) or who may be immunocompromised and have a neutropenia; antiseptic mouthrinses containing chlorhexidine or phenolic compounds also may be used in these instances (see Chapter 9); aqueous iodine preparations or a tincture of iodine (iodine in alcohol) also may be used for skin antisepsis.

★ indicates a product bearing the ADA Seal of Acceptance. The products listed here might not include all of those that are available. Also, the listing of a product does not denote its superiority to any other product that is either listed or not listed, nor does it guarantee its availability or quality.

NAME	FORM/STRENGTH	WARNINGS/PRECAUTIONS, CONTRAINDICATIONS & ADVERSE EFFECTS	ACTIONS/ USES

ROOT CANAL MEDICATIONS AND PERIODONTAL DRESSINGS

ALDEHYDES

Formocresol (Buckley's Formo Cresol★, Formo Cresol★)	**Liq: (Buckley's)** 35% cresol, 19% formaldehyde, 17.5% glycerine, 28.5% water; **(Formo)** 48.5% cresol, 48.5% formaldehyde, 3% glycerine	**W/P:** Minimize soft-tissue contact. Combined action of cresol, a protein-coagulating phenolic compound, and formaldehyde, an alkylating agent, make formocresol extremely cytotoxic and capable of causing widespread necrosis of vital tissue in the mouth or elsewhere.	Vital pulp therapy in primary teeth.

INTRACANAL MEDICATIONS

Calcium hydroxide (Ca[OH]$_2$) (Generic calcium hydroxide powder★, Pulpdent Temp-Canal★)	**Pow: (generic)** Calcium hydroxide, USP; **Sol: (Pulpdent)** Calcium hydroxide in aqueous methylcellulose	**W/P:** Minimize soft-tissue contact.	Used to create an environment for healing pulpal and periapical tissues, to produce antimicrobial effects, to aid in elimination of apical seepage, to induce formation of calcified tissue, and to prevent inflammatory resorption after trauma.

IRRIGANTS

Ethylenediaminetetra-acetic acid (EDTA) (Generic EDTA, EDTAC, File-EZE, RC Prep★, REDTA)	**Sol: (generic)** 17% in aqueous solution, pH 8.0; **(EDTA)** EDTA with Centrimide; **(File-EZE)** EDTA in an aqueous solution; **(RC)** Urea peroxide 10%, EDTA 15% in a special water soluble base; **(REDTA)** EDTA 17% in an aqueous solution, pH of 8.0	**W/P:** Minimize soft-tissue contact.	In combination with sodium hypochlorite, EDTA removes smear layer; alone, aids in removal of calcified tissue by chelating metal ions.
Hydrogen Peroxide 3% (H$_2$O$_2$)	Generic aqueous solution	**W/P:** Minimize soft-tissue contact. Should be used carefully to avoid emphysema of adjacent soft tissue. **A/E:** Irritation, tooth sensitivity, allergic reaction.	Oxidizing power of hydrogen peroxide kills certain anaerobic bacteria in cultures; in contact with tissues, its germicidal power is very limited because it is readily decomposed by organic matter and antimicrobial effect lasts only as long as oxygen is being released; can be used to cleanse and treat infected pulp canals.
Sodium hypochlorite (NaOCl) (Clorox, Hypogen)	5.25% sodium hypochlorite	**W/P:** Minimize soft-tissue contact. Sodium hypochlorite is caustic and not suitable for application to wounds or areas of infection in soft tissues. **A/E:** Irritation, allergic reaction.	Has a solvent action on pulp tissue and organic debris, is used for irrigation of root canals, and is useful for cleaning dentures; aqueous solutions of 2.5% and 5% sodium hypochlorite are reported to be equally effective in dissolving pulpal debris when used as root canal irrigants.

MISCELLANEOUS PREPARATIONS

Zinc oxide (COE-Pak Periodontal Paste★; COE-Pak Automix Periodontal Paste★; COE-Pak Hard and Fast Set Periodontal Paste★; Pulpdent PerioCare Periodontal Dressing★; Perio-Putty; Zinc Oxide, USP★; Zone Periodontal Pak)	**(COE-Pak) Paste 1:** 45% zinc oxide, 37% magnesium oxide, 11% peanut oil, 6% mineral oil, 1% chloroxylenol, chlorothymol and coumarin, 0.02% Toluidine-Red pigment; **Paste 2:** 43% polymerized rosin, 24% coconut fatty acid, 10% ethyl alcohol, 9% petroleum jelly, 4% gum elemi, 4% lanolin,	**W/P:** Minimize soft-tissue contact.	Periodontal dressing; Perio-Putty also has skin lubricant.

Table 4.2: USAGE INFORMATION FOR TOPICAL ANTISEPTICS, ROOT CANAL MEDICATIONS, AND PERIODONTAL DRESSINGS *(cont.)*

NAME	FORM/STRENGTH	WARNINGS/PRECAUTIONS, CONTRAINDICATIONS & ADVERSE EFFECTS	ACTIONS/ USES
ROOT CANAL MEDICATIONS AND PERIODONTAL DRESSINGS *(cont.)*			
Zinc oxide *(cont.)*	3% ethyl cellulose, 1.5% chlorothy-mol, 1% carnauba, 0.2% zinc acetate, 0.1% spearmint oil; **(PerioCare)** **Paste:** 38.5% magnesium oxide, 29.8% vegetable oils, 19.2% zinc oxide, 12.5% calcium hydroxide, 0.2% coloring; **Gel:** 63.2% resins, 29.8% fatty acids, 3.5% ethyl cellulose, 3.5% lanolin; **(Perio-Putty)** **Base:** 3.1% polyvinylpyrrolidone-iodine complex, 9% polymer, 5% benzocaine, 82.9% fillers; **Catalyst:** 19.9% zinc oxide, 10.3% magnesium oxide, 12.3% mineral and vegetable oils, 58% inert fillers; **Skin Lubricant:** 95% silicone oils, 5% inert fillers; **(Zinc) Pow:** Zinc oxide; **(Zone) Base:** 3.1% polyvinylpyrrolidone-iodine complex, 38.3% rosin, 2% chlorobutanol, 10% mineral oil, 9.3% isopropyl myristate, 37.3% propylene glycol monoisostearate		
Zinc Oxide-Eugenol (Kirkland Periodontal Pak, Peridres)	**(Kirkland) Pow:** 40% zinc oxide, 40% rosin, 20% tannic acid; **Liq:** 46.5% eugenol, 46.5% peanut oil, 7.5% rosin; **(Peridres) Pow:** 49% rosin, 46% zinc oxide, 3% tannic acid, 3% kaolin; **Liq:** 98% eugenol, 2% thymol	**W/P:** Minimize soft-tissue contact.	Periodontal dressing.
PHENOLIC COMPOUNDS			
Parachlorophenol (PCP) (Cresanol Root Canal Dressing, M.C.P. Root Canal Dressing★, Parachlorophenol Liquefied)	**(Cresanol, M.C.P.) Liq:** 25% parachlorophenol, 25% metacresyl acetate, 50% camphor; **(para-chlorophenol liquefied) Liq:** 98% parachlorophenol, 2% glycerin	**W/P:** Minimize soft-tissue contact. Phenolic compounds can destroy tissue cells by binding cell membrane lipids and proteins.	Intracanal medicament.
Parachlorophenol, Camphor-ated (CPC), USP★	**Liq:** 35% parachlorophenol and 65% camphor	**W/P:** Minimize soft-tissue contact. Phenolic compounds can destroy tissue cells by binding cell membrane lipids and proteins.	Intracanal medicament.
Eugenol, USP★	**Liq:** 100% eugenol	**W/P:** Minimize soft-tissue contact. Phenolic compounds can destroy tissue cells by binding cell membrane lipids and proteins.	Anodyne/oral tissues, teeth.

★ indicates a product bearing the ADA Seal of Acceptance. The products listed here might not include all of those that are available. Also, the listing of a product does not denote its superiority to any other product that is either listed or not listed, nor does it guarantee its availability or quality.

Chapter 5

Glucocorticoids

Lida Radfar, D.D.S., M.S.; Martha Somerman, D.D.S., Ph.D.

Glucocorticoids are hormones secreted by the adrenal gland in response to ultradian and circadian rhythms and to stress. The major effects of glucocorticoids can broadly be defined as influencing the metabolism of carbohydrates, protein and fat metabolism, as well as water and electrolyte balance. Consequently, glucocorticoids are involved in the deposition of glucose as glycogen and the conversion of glycogen and protein into glucose when needed; the stimulation of protein loss from specific organs; the redistribution of fatty tissue in facial, abdominal and shoulder regions; and alterations of the filtration rate of specific electrolytes that cause water retention.

Glucocorticoids mainly regulate the metabolic pathways, while mineralcorticoids are involved with electrolyte and water balance. The secretion of glucocorticoids from the adrenal glands is controlled by hormones, such as corticotropin-releasing factor, produced by the hypothalamus, and adrenocorticotropic hormone (ACTH), produced by the anterior pituitary gland. This pathway is often referred to as the hypothalamic-pituitary-adrenal (HPA) axis. Glucocorticoid secretion from the adrenal glands is regulated by a negative feedback mechanism; that is, the adrenal glands will diminish glucocorticoid secretion when excess plasma levels of steroids are present. However, the glands cannot distinguish between endogenously and exogenously supplied glucocorticoids. Consequently, administration of supraphysiological levels of exogenous glucocorticoids for long periods may result in secondary adrenal insufficiency.

Glucocorticoids are, among other things, essential for a person's ability to adapt to stressful situations. Adrenal insufficiency or dysfunction, therefore, may predispose a person to inadequate physiological response to stress. Severe adrenal suppression and accompanied diminished stress response may have clinical significance after 7-10 days of steroid administration. In stressful situations, cardiovascular collapse may ensue and, if not treated appropriately, can result in a high degree of morbidity and even death. This type of response is rare in patients with adrenal insufficiency owing to exogenous glucocorticoids, but may be a concern for patients with Addison's disease. Dentists need to be able to assess the level of patients' adrenal suppression and provide patients with glucocorticoid replacement therapy when necessary.

Assessment of adrenal suppression. Many factors play a role in assessing the diminished output of glucocorticoids from the adrenal glands in patients who are prescribed glucocorticoids. These factors include, but are not limited to, the type of glucocorticoids the patient is prescribed, the route of administration, the dosing schedule, the duration of taking the steroids, concomitant systemic disorders and drug interactions.

Each type and formulation of glucocorticoids has been assigned a specific level of potency that is compared to the potency of hydrocortisone (Table 5.1). Thus, prednisone is four times more potent than hydrocortisone, while betamethasone is 25 times more potent. The more potent the drug, the higher the risk of causing adrenal suppression. The risk of experiencing adverse effects from glucocorticoid administration usually increases with duration of therapy and frequency of administration. Adrenal suppression occurs rapidly and may be present for up to 2 years, even after as little as 2 weeks of glucocorticoid therapy. However, although the adrenal function is suppressed, the stress response returns after approximately 11-14 days. For the purpose of not causing stress-related adverse events, the return of the stress response is of the essence.

Except for the high-potency topical glucocorticoids, topically applied glucocorticoids—including those used intraorally—have not been associated with adrenal suppression. However, aerosol and systemically administered glucocorticoids have been associated with adrenal suppression and diminished stress response in patients. For patients receiving chronic glucocorticoid therapy, alternate-day therapy is used to reduce potential side effects.

Accepted Indications

Glucocorticoids are used to induce immune suppression in patients with a variety of conditions. Patients who have undergone organ transplantations, for example, often are prescribed high doses of glucocorticoids to prevent organ rejection. Although other conditions such as autoimmune diseases, respiratory diseases, dermatologic diseases and some hematologic disorders also require long-term glucocorticoid therapy, there is usually no need for such high doses as used with transplant patients.

Glucocorticoids are also used in dental settings. Various oral conditions such as lichen planus, aphthous ulcers, benign mucous membrane pemphigoid, pemphigus, postherpetic neuralgia, and temporomandibular joint disorders benefit from glucocorticoid therapy. Furthermore, glucocorticoids also are used to reduce swelling after major oral-maxillofacial surgical procedures.

General Dosing Information

Table 5.1 provides dosage and prescribing information for systemic glucocorticoids (separated into low-, intermediate- and high-potency categories); topical glucocorticoids (separated into low-, intermediate-, high- and very high-potency categories); and inhaled glucocorticoids.

When administering glucocorticoids, dentists may use topical formulations, intralesional and intra-articular injections or systemic forms. Topical agents are the ones most commonly used by dentists and, if employed for less than 1 month, usually will not cause significant detrimental effects. However, very high-potency topical glucocorticoids used to treat oral lesions can cause adrenal suppression and should not be used for more than 2 weeks without a thorough medical evaluation of the patient. Creams, ointments and gels all can be used intraorally and are applied to lesions 2-4 times daily. Gels adhere fairly well to the oral mucosa and are applied directly to lesions. To increase penetration and time in contact with lesions, gel formulations also can be placed inside a mouthguard covering the affected area. Ointments usually are mixed with equal amounts of Orabase, a compound that adheres to the oral mucosa, and is placed directly on lesions. Ointments also can be placed inside mouthguards. Although creams can be used for oral lesions, these formulations are not commonly used for this purpose. Dexamethasone elixir and prednisolone syrup are the oral rinses commonly used for topical purposes. The patient is instructed to rinse for 30 seconds with these medications, and then to expectorate them, 2-4 times daily.

Intralesional injections commonly are used only intermittently; when used for soft-tissue pathologies, they have not been associated with systemic complications. Triamcinolone hexacetonide is the most frequently used medication for this purpose.

Intra-articular injections, also predominantly performed with triamcinolone hexacetonide, should be performed only in 3-week intervals to diminish bone pathology.

Systemic glucocorticoid therapy is used in the short term before, during and after oral surgery to reduce postoperative edema. Oral lesions associated with very high morbidity sometimes are treated with systemic glucocorticoid therapy. High doses of prednisone, up to 60-80 mg per day for 7-10 days, can be used for treatment of lichen planus, major aphthous ulcerations, oral pemphigoid and oral pemphigus. Treatment beyond 2 weeks should be coordinated with the patient's physician.

Maximum Recommended Doses

The maximum recommended doses for systemic glucocorticoid formulations per procedure or appointment are 5-20 mg of prednisone for a maintenance dose and 5-60 mg for continuous or alternate-day therapy, but doses depend on the patient's condition. Dosing schedules and maximum doses are based on the assumption that the dentist has determined (through taking a health history and interviewing) that the patient is in general good health and is not taking any medications that can interact with the glucocorticoid agent. The main concerns are patients with hyperglycemic conditions and patients who cannot tolerate immunosuppressive therapy. The potential harmful effects of these medications always must be carefully weighed against the benefit.

Dosage Adjustments

The actual maximum dose for each patient must be individualized depending on his or her size, age and physical status; other drugs he or she may be taking; and duration of existing glucocorticoid therapy (long-term use considerations). Reduced maximum doses may be indicated for pediatric and geriatric patients, patients with serious illness or disability, and patients with medical conditions or who are taking drugs that alter responses to glucocorticoids.

Special Dental Considerations

The effect of glucocorticoids can be divided arbitrarily into two categories that have significance for dentists:

- Dental patients taking glucocorticoids may need modifications and alterations of routine dental therapy, for purposes such as reducing patients' stress response and glucocorticoid replacement.
- Glucocorticoid users may exhibit intra-oral manifestations.

Modifications of routine dental therapy. Is there a need for antibiotic coverage? There are no definitive data regarding the need for patients taking glucocorticoids to receive antibiotic prophylaxis before undergoing dental therapy. However, it is prudent for dental providers to consider antibiotic prophylaxis in patients taking a combined dose of more than 700 mg of prednisone. No antibiotic prophylaxis is recommended if a patient takes less than 10 mg of prednisone per day. Dentists may choose to use the same protocol for antibiotic prophylaxis as that put forth by the American Heart Association for prevention of subacute bacterial endocarditis (see Appendix D). However, the efficacy of this protocol for patients taking glucocorticoids has not been established.

There are two situations in which dentists need to provide patients with extra glucocorticoids. First, patients with dysfunctional adrenal glands may not be able to produce enough glucocorticoids to respond to the stress associated with dental therapy. The most common condition associated with primary adrenal destruction is Addison's disease, an autoimmune destruction of the adrenal glands. Patients with inadequately functioning adrenal glands will need prophylactic glucocorticoid therapy before undergoing dental procedures. Second, patients who have been taking glucocorticoids for a long period may have iatrogenic adrenal suppression and will need glucocorticoid replacement therapy before undergoing dental procedures.

As the stress response returns within 11-14 days after cessation of glucocorticoid therapy, patients do not need replacement therapy after a 2-4 weeks period of not having taken glucocorticoids. Furthermore, patients being switched from daily therapy to alternate-day therapy can be treated without glucocorticoid replacement therapy on the nonglucocorticoid day. As a rule, patients needing replacement therapy should receive the equivalent of up to 300 mg of hydrocortisone or 60-75 mg of prednisone the morning of a dental appointment.

The amount of glucocorticoid replacement should be gauged according to the anticipated level of stress. Accordingly, depending on the patient's level of fear and anxiety, oral examinations generally require no replacement therapy, while any procedure requiring local anesthetics warrants additional glucocorticoid coverage.

Oral health care providers should follow this protocol for the management of patients who are receiving glucocorticoid therapy:

- Schedule elective procedures in the morning.
- Use mild sedatives for apprehensive patients.
- Use glucocorticoid replacement therapy when indicated.
- Always use long-acting local anesthetics.
- Monitor blood pressure during the procedure.
- Use medications to alleviate postoperative pain.

As a rule, replacement therapy is indicated for patients who presently are taking more than 30 mg of hydrocortisone equivalent of glucocorticoids for more than 2 weeks. It also is indicated for patients seeking dental care within the first 2-4 weeks after having stopped glucocorticoid therapy subsequent to having taken at least 30 mg of hydrocortisone equivalent of glucocorticoids for more than 2 weeks.

Intraoral manifestations. Of all the intraoral manifestations caused by glucocorticoids, the most common is oral candidiasis. It has been estimated that up to 75% of people using inhalers that contain glucocorticoids may develop intraoral candidiasis (Table 5.1). These inhalers are used mainly by patients with asthma, but they also can be prescribed for patients with allergies and other respiratory conditions. To diminish the occurrence of candidiasis, dentists should properly instruct patients in the use of spacer devices and to rinse their mouths with water after using the inhalers. Resolution of intraoral candidiasis can be accomplished effectively with antifungal troches, lozenges or oral solutions (see Chapter 7).

Long-term systemic administration of glucocorticoids may impair wound healing. This may be the result of the catabolic effect and the reduced inflammatory response induced by these compounds.

The anti-inflammatory property of glucocorticoids may mask a chronic infection. Glucocorticoids will prevent accumulation of neutrophils and monocytes at sites of inflammation (impaired chemotaxis) and further suppress the phagocytic abilities of cells. Thus, the classic clinical inflammatory response may be greatly blunted.

Intraoral dryness has also been reported in patients taking glucocorticoids, both systemically and in the form of inhalers. An increased caries rate can be anticipated, and patients should be instructed about improved oral hygiene procedures and use of topical fluorides, as well as in-office fluoride therapy.

Drug Interactions of Dental Interest
Table 5.2 lists drug interactions with glucocorticoids and related problems of potential clinical significance in dentistry.

Laboratory Value Alterations

- Low serum cortisol levels, < 5-10 µg/dL in a specimen obtained between 8 and 10 a.m., and increased serum ACTH, 200-1,600 µg/dL, are diagnostic for adrenal insufficiency. Dentists may want to request a complete blood count, as neutropenia and lymphocytosis may be present.

Special Patients

Pregnant and nursing women

All systemic glucocorticoid preparations are classified in pregnancy risk category C and may cause birth defects such as cleft lip and palate. Consequently, glucocorticoid administration during pregnancy and during breast feeding should be avoided.

Pediatric, geriatric and other special patients

Administration of as little as 5 mg of prednisone may cause growth retardation in children. However, if glucocorticoid therapy ceases before the epiphyses close, catch-up growth may take place.

Pediatric patients may have a greater susceptibility to topical glucocorticoid–induced adrenal suppression than adults have, because children have thinner skin and their ratio of skin surface area to body weight is larger than that of adults. Topical glucocorticoids should be used with caution in children.

Geriatric patients exhibit a propensity to develop hypertension, as well as osteoporosis, while receiving glucocorticoid therapy. Glucocorticoid dosage also needs to be adjusted in younger and older patients to minimize damage to kidney and liver functions.

Patient Monitoring: Aspects to Watch

- Symptoms of blood dyscrasias (such as infection, bleeding and poor healing): for patients with these symptoms, the dentist should request a medical consultation for blood studies and postpone dental treatment until normal values are re-established
- Vital signs, at every appointment: necessary to monitor possible cardiovascular side effects
- Salivary flow: as a factor in caries, periodontal disease and candidiasis
- Dose and duration of glucocorticoid therapy: to assess stress tolerance and risk of immunosuppression
- Need for medical consultation: to assess disease control and patient's stress tolerance

Adverse Effects and Precautions

The multitude of potential side effects of systemic glucocorticoids necessitates complete disclosure of the risks to patients (see Table 5.1). Withdrawal of glucocorticoids after patients are treated for more than 10 consecutive days should be accomplished gradually to diminish side effects. Patients taking daily doses of 60 mg of prednisone should reduce their daily intake by 10 mg every day before completely stopping therapy. Too-quick withdrawal of glucocorticoid therapy may result in flare-up of the underlying condition or even adrenal crisis. If it is necessary that a patient continue to receive glucocorticoid therapy for longer than 2 weeks, a consultation with a physician is appropriate.

Severe hepatic disease may prevent prednisone metabolism; when treating such patients, the dentist may have to administer the active form of the medication, prednisolone, to achieve a clinical effect. Furthermore, patients with severe liver disease may not be able to take glucocorticoids with acetaminophen, as acetaminophen toxicity may ensue.

Concurrent administration of other medications such as barbiturates, phenytoin and rifampin may double the clearance of prednisolone. Interactions also may occur with other medications and need to be considered when prescribing glucocorticoids (see Table 5.2).

The most common adverse signs of glucocorticoid therapy include changes in skin (such as acne, ecchymosis, thinning, violaceous abdominal striae), weight gain, truncal obesity, "buffalo hump" (adipose tissue accumulation on the back of the neck), thin extremities, decreased muscle mass and "moon face." These features appear in 13% of patients after as little as 60 days of glucocorticoid use and in up to 50% of patients treated for 5-8 years. Patients with these signs need to be encouraged to keep a low-fat, low-calorie diet and to exercise.

Skeletal fractures may occur in 11-20% of patients treated with daily doses of 7.5-10 mg of prednisone for more than 1 year. The major underlying cause of these osteoporotic changes may be decreased osteoblastic activity and maturation. The most rapid loss of trabecular bone loss occurs within the first 2 months of high-dose glucocorticoid therapy, with an average of 5% bone mass loss within the first year. It is prudent to give calcium and vitamin D supplements and hormone replacements and to initiate weight-bearing exercise programs for patients receiving long-term glucocorticoid therapy. Another complication, more commonly found with patients taking long-term glucocorticoids, is osteonecrosis, which specifically affects the hip joint.

Patients taking a total dose of more than 1,000 mg of prednisone are more predisposed than patients taking lesser doses to develop peptic ulcers. This side effect is aggravated in patients already taking other potentially ulcerogenic medications. Administration of an H_2-antagonist may be beneficial as a prophylactic measure to reduce the incidence of peptic ulcerations.

Glucocorticoids initially may induce a psychological state of well-being, which subsequently may become a state of glucocorticoid-induced depression when the glucocorticoids are withdrawn.

Increased incidence of accelerated atherosclerosis has been noted in patients with systemic lupus erythematosus or rheumatoid arthritis who are treated with long-term glucocorticoids. Furthermore, patients with pre-existing hypertension may experience a worsening of their hypertensive control when treated with glucocorticoids.

Glucocorticoid-induced glucose intolerance is not associated with serious complications, but caution should be heeded when treating diabetic patients.

Progression of carcinoma of the breast and Kaposi's sarcoma has been reported in patients receiving glucocorticoid therapy. Although renewed development of Kaposi's sarcoma may occur, this lesion usually disappears after cessation of glucocorticoid therapy.

Pharmacology

Mechanism of action/effect. The effectiveness of glucocorticoid hormones is based on their ability to bind to cytosolic receptors in target tissues and subsequently enter the nucleus, where the glucocorticoid-receptor complex interacts with nuclear chromatin. This results in a cascade of events including the expression of hormone-specific ribonucleic acids, or RNAs, which in turn increases synthesis of specific proteins that mediate distinct physiological functions. The glucocorticoid cortisol is a normal circulating hormone secreted by the adrenal gland that functions in regulating normal metabolism and providing resistance to stress. In addition, at high levels whether the result of disease or drug intake glucocorticoids can have one or more physiological effects. These include:

- altering levels of blood cells in the plasma (that is, decreasing eosinophils, basophils, monocytes and lymphocytes and increasing levels of hemoglobin, erythrocytes and neutrophils), which decreases circulating levels of cells involved in fighting off infections and results in increased susceptibility to infections;

- reducing the inflammatory response as a result of a decrease in lymphocytes as well as altering lymphocytes' ability to inhibit the enzyme phospholipase A2, which is required for production of prostaglandins and leukotrienes;

- suppressing the HPA axis, thus inhibiting further synthesis of glucocorticoids.

Therefore, patients taking glucocorticoids warrant special attention as discussed in the introduction to this chapter.

Absorption. Systemically, most glucocorticoids are rapidly and readily absorbed from the GI tract because of their lipophilic character. Also, absorption occurs via synovial and conjunctival spaces.

Topically, absorption through the skin is very slow. However, chronic use in a nasal spray (for seasonal rhinitis, for example) can lead to pulmonary epithelial atrophy. Furthermore, excessive or prolonged use of topical glucocorticoids can result in sufficient absorption to cause systemic effects.

Both cortisone and prednisone contain a keto group at position II that must be hydroxylated in the liver to become activated. Thus, these drugs should be avoided in patients with abnormal liver function. Also, topical application of position II ketocorticoids is ineffective as a result of inactivity of this form of the glucocorticoid.

Distribution. In general, circulating cortisol is bound to plasma proteins: about 80-90% bound to transcortin—a cortisol-binding globulin with high affinity—while about 5-10% binds loosely to albumin. About 3-10% remains in the free (bioactive) form. Transcortin can bind to most synthetic glucocorticoids as well. However, some glucocorticoids, such as dexamethasone, do not bind to transcortin and, thus, are almost 100% in free form.

Biotransformation. Inactivation occurs primarily in the liver and also in the kidney, mostly to inactive metabolites. However, cortisone and prednisone are activated only after being metabolized to hydrocortisone and prednisolone, respectively. Fluorinated glucocorticoids are metabolized more slowly than the other members of this group.

Elimination. About 30% of inactive metabolite is metabolized further and then excreted in the urine.

Patient Advice

- Emphasize the importance of good oral hygiene to prevent soft-tissue inflammation.
- Caution the patient to prevent injury when using oral hygiene aids; he or she should use a soft toothbrush and have the dentist or hygienist evaluate his or her brushing and flossing techniques.
- Suggest the use of daily home fluoride preparations if chronic xerostomia occurs.
- Suggest the use of sugarless gum, frequent sips of water or artificial saliva substitutes if chronic xerostomia occurs.
- Caution against using mouthrinses with high alcohol content, as they have drying effects on the oral mucosa.
- The patient should use a topical glucocorticoid after brushing and eating and at bedtime for optimal effect.
- Use of topical glucocorticoids on oral herpetic ulcerations is contraindicated.
- The patient should apply the agent with a cotton-tipped applicator by pressing, not rubbing, the paste on the lesion.
- When a topical glucocorticoid is used to treat oral lesions, a tissue response should be noted within 7-14 days. If not, the patient should return for oral evaluation. If glucocorticoids are used chronically, the patient should return for frequent recall visits.

- If irritation, infection or sensitization occurs at site, the patient should discontinue use and return for evaluation.
- The patient should avoid exposing the affected area to sunlight; burns may occur.
- Topical glucocorticoids are for external use only.
- The patient should prevent the topical glucocorticoid from coming in contact with his or her eyes.
- The patient should not bandage or wrap the affected area unless directed to do so.
- The patient should report adverse reactions.
- The patient should avoid taking anything by mouth for 30 or 60 minutes after topical use in the mouth (as a mouthrinse or an ointment, respectively).

Suggested Readings

Barnes PJ. Molecular mechanisms and cellular effects of glucocorticosteroids. Immunol Allergy Clin North Am 2005;25:451-68.

Effect of corticosteroids for fetal maturation on perinatal outcomes. NIH Consensus Statement 1994;12(2):1-24.

Lester RS, Knowles SR, Shear NH. The risks of systemic corticosteroid use. Dermatol Clin 1998;16(2):277-86.

Miller CS, Little JW, Falace DA. Supplemental corticosteroids for dental patients with adrenal insufficiency: reconsideration of the problem. JADA 2001;132:1570-9.

Siegel MA, Silverman Jr. S, Sollecito TP, eds. Clinician's guide to treatment of common oral conditions. 5th ed. Baltimore: American Academy of Oral Medicine; 2001.

Table 5.1: PRESCRIBING INFORMATION FOR GLUCOCORTICOIDS

NAME	FORM/ STRENGTH	DOSAGE	WARNINGS/PRECAUTIONS & CONTRAINDICATIONS	ADVERSE EFFECTS†
INHALED GLUCOCORTICOIDS (Bronchial)				
Beclomethasone Dipropionate (Qvar)	**MDI:** 40mcg/inh, 80mcg/inh [7.3g]	***Adults:*** **Previous Bronchodilator Only:** 40-80mcg bid. **Max:** 320mcg bid. **Previous Inhaled Cortico-steroid Therapy:** 40-160mcg bid. **Max:** 320mcg bid. **Maint With Oral Corticosteroids:** May attempt gradual reduction of oral dose after 1 week on inhaled therapy. ***Pediatrics:*** **Adolescents: Previous Bronchodilator Only:** 40-80mcg bid. **Max:** 320mcg bid. **Previous Inhaled Corticosteroid Therapy:** 40-160mcg bid. **Max:** 320mcg bid. **5-11 yrs: Previous Bronchodilator Only or Inhaled Corticosteroid Therapy:** 40mcg bid. Max: 80mcg bid. **≥5 yrs: Maint With Oral Corticosteroids:** May attempt gradual reduction of oral dose after 1 week on inhaled therapy.	**W/P:** Deaths due to adrenal insuf-ficiency have occurred with transfer from systemic corticosteroids to inhaled corticosteroids. Resume oral corticosteroids during stress or severe asthma attack. Risk of adrenal insufficiency and withdrawal symptoms when replacing systemic corticoste-roids. May unmask allergic conditions previously suppressed by systemic steroid therapy. Caution with TB, ocular herpes simplex, or untreated systemic bacterial, fungal, parasitic or viral infec-tions. May suppress growth in children. Exposure to chickenpox or measles requires prophylaxis treatment. Not for rapid relief of bronchospasm. **Contra:** Status asthmaticus, acute asthmatic attacks. **P/N:** Category C, not for use in nursing.	Headache, **pharyngi-tis**, upper respiratory tract infection, rhinitis, increased asthma symptoms, sinusitis.
Budesonide (Pulmicort Respules, Pulmi-cort Turbuhaler)	**Powder, Inhalation:** (Turbuhaler) 200mcg/inh; **Sus, Inhalation:** (Respules) 0.25mg/2mL; 0.5mg/2mL [2mL, 30s]	***Adults:*** **(Turbuhaler) Previous Bronchodilator Only: Initial:** 200-400mcg bid. **Max:** 400mcg bid. **Previous Inhaled Corticosteroid: Initial:** 200-400mcg bid [mild-to-moderate asthma patients may use 200-400mcg qd]. **Max:** 800mcg bid. **Previous Oral Corticosteroid: Initial:** 400-800mcg bid. **Max:** 800mcg bid. Gradually reduce PO corticosteroid after 1 week of budesonide. ***Pediatrics:*** **(Turbuhaler) ≥6 yrs: Previous Bronchodilator Only/Inhaled Corticosteroid: Initial:** 200mcg bid. Mild-to-moderate asthma patients previously controlled on inhaled steroids may use 200-400mcg qd. **Max:** 400mcg bid. Oral Corticosteroid: **Max:** 400mcg bid. **(Respules) 1-8 yrs: Previous Bronchodilator Only: Initial:** 0.5mg qd or 0.25mg bid. Administer via jet nebulizer. **Max:** 0.5mg/day. **Previous Inhaled Corticosteroid:** 0.5mg qd or 0.25mg bid. **Max:** 1mg/day. **Previous Oral Corticosteroid:** 1mg qd or 0.5mg bid. **Max:** 1mg/day. Gradually reduce PO corticosteroid after 1 week of budesonide.	**W/P:** Deaths due to adrenal insuf-ficiency have occurred with transfer from systemic corticosteroids to inhaled corti-costeroids. Resume oral corticosteroids during stress or severe asthma attack. Transferring from oral to inhalation therapy may unmask allergic conditions (eg, rhinitis, conjunctivitis, eczema). Ob-serve for adrenal insufficiency, systemic corticosteroid withdrawal effects, and growth suppression (children). More susceptible to infections. Not for acute bronchospasm. Discontinue if bron-chospasm occurs after dosing. Caution with tuberculosis of the respiratory tract; untreated systemic fungal, bacterial, viral or parasitic infections; or ocular herpes simplex. *Candida* infection of the mouth and pharynx reported. **Contra:** Primary treatment of status asthmaticus or other acute asthma attacks. **P/N:** (Respules) Category B, caution in nursing; (Turbu-haler) Category B, not for use in nursing.	**Pharyngitis**, headache, fever, sinusitis, pain, bronchospasm, bronchitis, respiratory infection, monoliasis.
Flunisolide (Aerobid, Aerobid-M)	**MDI:** 0.25mg/inh [7g]	***Adults:*** **Initial:** 2 inh bid. **Max:** 4 inh bid. Rinse mouth after use. ***Pediatrics:*** **6-15 yrs:** 2 inh bid. Rinse mouth after use.	**W/P:** Deaths due to adrenal insuf-ficiency have occurred with transfer from systemic corticosteroids to inhaled corticosteroids. Resume oral corticosteroids during stress or severe asthma attack. Observe for adrenal insufficiency, systemic corticosteroid withdrawal effects, and growth suppression (children). More susceptible to infections. Not for acute bronchospasm. Discontinue if bron-chospasm occurs after dosing. Caution with tuberculosis of the respiratory tract; untreated systemic fungal, bacterial, viral or parasitic infections;	Upper respiratory infection, diarrhea, stomach upset, cold symptoms, nasal congestion, headache, nausea, vomiting, **sore throat, unpleasant taste.**

* Scored.   † Bold entries denote special dental considerations.

Table 5.1: PRESCRIBING INFORMATION FOR GLUCOCORTICOIDS *(cont.)*

NAME	FORM/ STRENGTH	DOSAGE	WARNINGS/PRECAUTIONS & CONTRAINDICATIONS	ADVERSE EFFECTS†
INHALED GLUCOCORTICOIDS (Bronchial) *(cont.)*				
Flunisolide *(cont.)*			or ocular herpes simplex. *Candida* infection of the mouth and pharynx reported. **Contra:** Primary treatment of status asthmaticus or other acute asthma attacks. **P/N:** Category C, caution with nursing.	
Fluticasone Propionate (Flovent, Flovent HFA, Flovent Rotadisk)	**MDI:** 44mcg/inh [7.9g, 13g], 110mcg/inh [7.9g, 13g], 220mcg/inh [7.9g, 13g]; **(HFA)** 44mcg/inh [10.6g], 110mcg/inh [12g], 220mcg/inh [12g]; **Rotadisk:** 50mcg/dose, 100mcg/dose, 250mcg/dose [15 x 4 blisters]	*Adults:* **(MDI, HFA MDI) Previous Bronchodilator Only: Initial:** 88mcg bid. Max: 440mcg bid. **Previous Inhaled Corticosteroids: Initial:** 88-220mcg bid. Max: 440mcg bid. **Previous Oral Corticosteroids: Initial/Max:** 880mcg bid. **(Rotadisk) Previous Bronchodilator Only: Initial:** 100mcg bid. **Max:** 500mcg bid. **Previous Inhaled Corticosteroids: Initial:** 100-250mcg bid. **Max:** 500mcg bid. **Previous Oral Corticosteroids: (Rotadisk) Initial/Max:** 1000mcg bid. Reduce PO prednisone no faster than 2.5mg/day weekly, beginning at least 1 week after starting fluticasone. Rinse mouth after use. *Pediatrics:* **≥12 yrs: (MDI, HFA MDI) Previous Bronchodilator Only: Initial:** 88mcg bid. **Max:** 440mcg bid. **Previous Inhaled Corticosteroids: Initial:** 88-220mcg bid. **Max:** 440 mcg bid. **Previous Oral Corticosteroids: Initial/Max:** 880mcg bid. **(Rotadisk) Previous Bronchodilator Only: Initial:** 100mcg bid. **Max:** 500mcg bid. **Previous Inhaled Corticosteroids: Initial:** 100-250mcg bid. **Max:** 500mcg bid. **Previous Oral Corticosteroids: (Rotadisk) Initial/Max:** 1000mcg bid. **4-11 yrs: (Rotadisk) Previous Bronchodilator Only/Inhaled Corticosteroids: Initial:** 50mcg bid. **Max:** 100mcg bid. Reduce PO prednisone no faster than 2.5mg/day weekly, beginning at least 1 week after starting fluticasone. Rinse mouth after use.	**W/P:** Deaths due to adrenal insufficiency have occurred with transfer from systemic corticosteroids to inhaled corticosteroids. Resume oral corticosteroids during stress or severe asthma attack. Wean slowly from systemic corticosteroid therapy. Observe for adrenal insufficiency, systemic corticosteroid withdrawal effects, hypercorticism, adrenal suppression (including adrenal crisis), reduction in growth velocity (children and adolescents). May increase susceptibility to infections. Not for acute bronchospasm. Discontinue if bronchospasm occurs after dosing. Caution with tuberculosis of the respiratory tract; untreated systemic fungal, bacterial, viral or parasitic infections; or ocular herpes simplex. *Candida* infection of the mouth and pharynx reported. Glaucoma, increased IOP and cataracts reported. **Contra:** Primary treatment of status asthmaticus or other acute asthma attacks. **P/N:** Category C, caution in nursing.	**Pharyngitis,** nasal congestion, sinusitis, rhinitis, dysphonia, **oral candidiasis,** upper respiratory infection, influenza, headache, nasal discharge, allergic rhinitis, fever, osteoporosis, paradoxical bronchospasm, pneumonia.
Mometasone Furoate (Asmanex Twisthaler)	**Twisthaler:** 220mcg/inh	*Adults:* **Previous Therapy with Bronchodilators Alone or Inhaled Corticosteroids: Initial:** 220mcg qpm. **Max:** 440mcg qpm or 220mcg bid. **Previous Therapy with Oral Corticosteroids: Initial:** 440mcg bid. **Max:** 880mcg/day. Titrate to lowest effective dose once asthma stability is achieved. *Pediatrics:* **≥12 yrs: Previous Therapy with Bronchodilators Alone or Inhaled Corticosteroids: Initial:** 220mcg qpm. **Max:** 440mcg qpm or	**W/P:** Deaths due to adrenal insufficiency have occurred with transfer from systemic corticosteroids to inhaled corticosteroids. Wean slowly from systemic corticosteroid therapy. Resume oral corticosteroids during stress or severe asthma attack. May unmask allergic conditions previously suppressed by systemic corticosteroid therapy. May increase susceptibility to infections. Not for rapid relief of bronchospasm or other acute episodes of asthma. Discontinue if bronchospasm occurs after dosing. Observe for systemic corticosteroid withdrawal effects, hypercorticism, reduced bone mineral density, and adrenal suppression; reduce dose slowly if needed. Decreased growth velocity may occur in pediatric patients. Candida infections in	Headache, allergic rhinitis, **pharyngitis,** upper respiratory tract infection, sinusitis, **oral candidiasis,** dysmenorrhea, musculoskeletal pain, back pain, dyspepsia, myalgia, abdominal pain, nausea.

* Scored.   † Bold entries denote special dental considerations.

NAME	FORM/ STRENGTH	DOSAGE	WARNINGS/PRECAUTIONS & CONTRAINDICATIONS	ADVERSE EFFECTS†
Mometasone Furoate *(cont.)*			the mouth and pharynx reported. Caution with active or quiescent TB infection of the respiratory tract; untreated systemic fungal, bacterial, viral, or parasitic infections; or ocular herpes simplex. Glaucoma, increased IOP, and cataracts reported. **Contra:** Primary treatment of status asthmaticus or other acute episodes of asthma where intensive measures are required. **P/N:** Category C, caution in nursing.	
Triamcinolone Acetonide (Azmacort)	**MDI:** 100mcg/ inh [20g]	*Adults:* 2 inh tid-qid or 4 inh bid. **Severe Asthma: Initial:** 12-16 inh/day. **Max:** 16 inh/day. **Rinse mouth after use.** *Pediatrics:* >12 yrs: 2 inh tid-qid or 4 inh bid. **Severe Asthma: Initial:** 12-16 inh/day. **Max:** 16 inh/day. 6-12 yrs: 1-2 inh tid-qid or 2-4 inh bid. **Max:** 12 inh/day. Rinse mouth after use.	**W/P:** Deaths due to adrenal insufficiency have occurred with transfer from systemic corticosteroids to inhaled corticosteroids. Resume oral corticosteroids during stress or severe asthma attack. Observe for adrenal insufficiency, systemic corticosteroid withdrawal effects, hypercorticism and growth suppression (children). More susceptible to infections. Not for acute bronchospasm. Discontinue if bronchospasm occurs after dosing. Caution with tuberculosis of the respiratory tract; untreated systemic fungal, bacterial, viral or parasitic infections; or ocular herpes simplex. *Candida* infection of the mouth and pharynx reported. **Contra:** Primary treatment of status asthmaticus or other acute asthma attacks. **P/N:** Category C, caution in nursing.	**Pharyngitis,** sinusitis, headache, flu syndrome.

INHALED GLUCOCORTICOIDS (Nasal)

NAME	FORM/ STRENGTH	DOSAGE	WARNINGS/PRECAUTIONS & CONTRAINDICATIONS	ADVERSE EFFECTS†
Beclomethasone Dipropionate Monohydrate (Beconase AQ)	**Aerosol:** (Beconase) 0.042mg/ inh [6.7g, 16.8g]; **Spray:** (Beconase AQ) 0.042mg/inh [25g]	*Adults:* **(Inhaler):** 1 spray per nostril bid-qid. **(Spray)** 1-2 sprays per nostril bid. *Pediatrics:* **(Inhaler)** ≥12 yrs: 1 spray per nostril bid-qid. **6-12 yrs:** 1 spray per nostril tid. **(Spray)** ≥6 yrs: 1-2 sprays per nostril bid.	**W/P:** Risk of adrenal insufficiency and withdrawal symptoms when replacing systemic corticosteroids with a topical corticosteroid. Caution with active or quiescent TB, ocular herpes simplex, or untreated bacterial, fungal and systemic viral infections. Avoid with recent nasal trauma, surgery or septum ulcers. Risk for more severe/fatal course of infections (eg, chickenpox, measles) and for *Candida* infection of the nose and pharynx. Potential for growth velocity reduction in pediatrics. **P/N:** Category C, caution in nursing.	**Nasopharyngeal irritation,** sneezing, headache, nausea, lightheadedness, **irritated/dry nose and throat, unpleasant taste/smell.**
Budesonide (Rhinocort Aqua)	**Spray:** 32mcg/ inh [8.6g]	*Adults:* 1 spray per nostril qd. **Max:** 4 sprays/nostril/day. *Pediatrics:* ≥6 yrs: 1 spray per nostril qd. **Max: 6-12 yrs:** 2 sprays/nostril/day. >12 yrs: 4 sprays/nostril/day.	**W/P:** Risk of adrenal insufficiency and withdrawal symptoms when replacing systemic corticosteroids with a topical corticosteroid. Caution with active or quiescent TB, ocular herpes simplex, or untreated bacterial, fungal and systemic viral infections. Avoid with recent nasal trauma, surgery or septum ulcers. Risk for more severe/fatal course of infections (eg, chickenpox, measles) and for Candida infection of the nose and pharynx. Potential for growth velocity reduction in pediatrics. **P/N:** Category B, caution in nursing.	Nasal irritation, **pharyngitis,** cough, epistaxis.

Table 5.1: PRESCRIBING INFORMATION FOR GLUCOCORTICOIDS *(cont.)*

NAME	FORM/ STRENGTH	DOSAGE	WARNINGS/PRECAUTIONS & CONTRAINDICATIONS	ADVERSE EFFECTS†
INHALED GLUCOCORTICOIDS (Nasal) *(cont.)*				
Flunisolide (Nasarel)	**Spray:** 0.029mg/ inh [25mL]	***Adults:* Initial:** 2 sprays per nostril bid. **Titrate:** May increase to 2 sprays per nostril tid. **Max:** 8 sprays per nostril/day. ***Pediatrics:* 6-14 yrs: Initial:** 1 spray per nostril tid or 2 sprays per nostril bid. **Max:** 4 sprays per nostril/day.	**W/P:** Risk of adrenal insufficiency and withdrawal symptoms when replacing systemic corticosteroids with a topical corticosteroid. Caution with active or quiescent TB, ocular herpes simplex, or untreated bacterial, fungal and systemic viral infections. Avoid with recent nasal trauma, surgery or septum ulcers. Risk for more severe/fatal course of infections (eg, chickenpox, measles) and for *Candida* infection of the nose and pharynx. Potential for growth velocity reduction in pediatrics. **Contra:** Untreated localized infection of the nasal mucosa. **P/N:** Category C, caution in nursing.	**Aftertaste**, nasal burning/stinging, cough, epistaxis, nasal dryness.
Fluticasone Propionate (Flonase)	**Spray:** 0.05mg/ inh [16g]	***Adults:* Initial:** 2 sprays per nostril qd or 1 spray per nostril bid. **Maint:** 1 spray per nostril qd. May dose as 2 sprays per nostril qd as needed for seasonal allergic rhinitis. ***Pediatrics:*** **≥4 yrs: Initial:** 1 spray per nostril qd. If inadequate response, may increase to 2 sprays per nostril. **Maint:** 1 spray per nostril qd. **Max:** 2 sprays per nostril/day. **≥12 yrs:** May dose as 2 sprays per nostril qd as needed for seasonal allergic rhinitis.	**W/P:** Risk of adrenal insufficiency and withdrawal symptoms when replacing systemic corticosteroids with a topical corticosteroid. Caution with active or quiescent TB, ocular herpes simplex, or untreated bacterial, fungal and systemic viral infections. Avoid with recent nasal trauma, surgery or septum ulcers. Risk for more severe/fatal course of infections (eg, chickenpox, measles); avoid exposure in patients who have not had disease or been properly immunized. *Candida* infection of nose and pharynx reported (rare). Potential for growth velocity reduction in pediatrics. Excessive use may cause signs of hypercorticism or HPA suppression. **P/N:** Category C, caution with nursing.	Headache, **pharyngitis**, epistaxis, nasal burning/irritation, asthma symptoms, nausea/vomiting, cough.
Mometasone Furoate Monohydrate (Nasonex)	**Spray:** 0.05mg/ inh [17g]	***Adults:* Allergic Rhinitis: Treatment/ Prophylaxis:** 2 sprays per nostril qd. For prophylaxis, start 2-4 weeks before allergy season. **Nasal Polyps:** 2 sprays per nostril bid. ***Pediatrics:*** **≥12 yrs: Treatment/Prophylaxis:** 2 sprays per nostril qd. For prophylaxis, start 2-4 weeks before allergy season. **2-11 yrs: Treatment:** 1 spray per nostril qd.	**W/P:** Risk of adrenal insufficiency and withdrawal symptoms when replacing systemic corticosteroids with a topical corticosteroid. Caution with active or quiescent TB, ocular herpes simplex, or untreated bacterial, fungal and systemic viral infections. Avoid with recent nasal trauma, surgery or septum ulcers. Risk for more severe/fatal course of infections (eg, chickenpox, measles) and for *Candida* infection of the nose and pharynx. Potential for growth velocity reduction in pediatrics. **P/N:** Category C, caution with nursing.	Headache, viral infection, **pharyngitis**, epistaxis, cough, upper respiratory tract infection, dysmenorrhea, myalgia, sinusitis.
Triamcinolone Acetonide (Nasacort AQ)	**AQ Spray:** 55mcg/inh [16.5g]; **HFA Aerosol:** 55mcg/ inh [9.3g]	***Adults:* (AQ Spray) Initial/Max:** 2 sprays per nostril qd. May reduce dose with improvement to 1 spray per nostril qd. **(HFA Aerosol) Initial:** 2 sprays per nostril qd. **Max:** 4 sprays per nostril qd. ***Pediatrics:*** **6-12 yrs: (AQ Spray) Initial:** 1 spray per nostril qd. **Max:** 2 sprays per nostril qd. **≥12 yrs: Initial/Max:** 2 sprays per nostril qd. May reduce dose with improvement to 1 spray per nostril qd. **(HFA Aerosol) ≥6 yrs:** 2 sprays per nostril qd.	**W/P:** Risk of adrenal insufficiency and withdrawal symptoms when replacing systemic corticosteroid with a topical corticosteroid. Caution with active or quiescent TB, ocular herpes simplex, or untreated bacterial, fungal and systemic viral infections. Avoid with recent nasal trauma, surgery or septum ulcers. Risk for more severe/fatal course of infections (eg, chickenpox, measles) and for Candida infection of the nose and pharynx. Potential for growth velocity reduction in pediatrics. **P/N:** Category C, caution in nursing.	**Pharyngitis**, epistaxis, infection, otitis media, headache, sneezing, rhinitis, nasal irritation, cough, sinusitis, vomiting.

* Scored.   † Bold entries denote special dental considerations.

NAME	FORM/ STRENGTH	DOSAGE	WARNINGS/PRECAUTIONS & CONTRAINDICATIONS	ADVERSE EFFECTS[†]

SYSTEMIC GLUCOCORTICOIDS (Low Potency)

CORTISONE ACETATE

NAME	FORM/ STRENGTH	DOSAGE	WARNINGS/PRECAUTIONS & CONTRAINDICATIONS	ADVERSE EFFECTS[†]
Hydrocortisone (Cortef)	**Sus:** (Hydrocortisone Cypionate) 10mg/5mL [120mL]; **Tab:** (Hydrocortisone) 5mg, 10mg, 20mg	**Adults: Initial:** 20-240mg/day depending on disease. Adjust until a satisfactory response. **Maint:** Decrease in small amounts to lowest effective dose. **Pediatrics: Initial:** 20-240mg/day depending on disease. Adjust until a satisfactory response. **Maint:** After favorable response, decrease in small amounts to lowest effective dose.	**W/P:** May need to increase dose before, during, and after stressful situations. May mask signs of infections. Avoid abrupt withdrawal. Prolonged use may produce glaucoma, optic nerve damage, secondary ocular infections. Increases BP, salt/water retention, potassium excretion. More severe/fatal course of infections reported with chickenpox, measles. Caution with TB, hypothyroidism, cirrhosis, ocular herpes simplex, HTN, diverticulitis, fresh intestinal anastomosis, ulcerative colitis, osteoporosis, myasthenia gravis, renal insufficiency, peptic ulcer disease. Growth and development of children on prolonged therapy should be monitored. Monitor for psychic disturbances. Kaposi's sarcoma reported. **Contra:** Systemic fungal infections. **P/N:** Safety in pregnancy and nursing not known.	Fluid and electrolyte disturbances, HTN, osteoporosis, muscle weakness, cushingoid state, menstrual irregularities, nervousness, insomnia, impaired wound healing, ulcerative esophagitis, excessive sweating, increases intracranial pressure, carbohydrate intolerance, glaucoma, cataracts.
Hydrocortisone Sodium Succinate (Solu-Cortef)	**Inj:** 100mg, 250mg, 500mg, 1g	**Adults: Initial:** 100-500mg IV/IM, depending on condition severity. May repeat dose at 2, 4, or 6 hrs based on clinical response. High dose therapy usually not >48-72 hrs; may use antacids prophylactically. **Pediatrics:** Use lower adult doses. Determine dose by severity of condition and response. Dose should not be <25mg/day.	**W/P:** May need to increase dose before, during, and after stressful situations. May mask signs of infection or cause new infections. Prolonged use may produce glaucoma, optic nerve damage, secondary ocular infections. Increases BP, salt/water retention, potassium and calcium excretion. More severe/fatal course of infections reported with chickenpox, measles. Enhanced effect with hypothyroidism or cirrhosis. Caution with Strongyloides, latent TB, ocular herpes simplex, HTN, diverticulitis, fresh intestinal anastomoses, ulcerative colitis, osteoporosis, myasthenia gravis, renal insufficiency, peptic ulcer disease. Kaposi's sarcoma reported. Monitor for psychic disturbances. Acute myopathy with high doses. Avoid abrupt withdrawal. Monitor growth and development of children on prolonged therapy. Hypernatremia may occur with high dose therapy >48-72 hrs. **Contra:** Premature infants, systemic fungal infections. **P/N:** Safety in pregnancy and nursing not known.	Fluid and electrolyte disturbances, HTN, osteoporosis, muscle weakness, cushingoid state, menstrual irregularities, vertigo, headache, impaired wound healing, DM, ulcerative esophagitis, peptic ulcer, pancreatitis, increased sweating, increases intracranial pressure, carbohydrate intolerance, glaucoma, cataracts.

SYSTEMIC GLUCOCORTICOIDS (Intermediate Potency)

NAME	FORM/ STRENGTH	DOSAGE	WARNINGS/PRECAUTIONS & CONTRAINDICATIONS	ADVERSE EFFECTS[†]
Methylprednisolone Sodium Succinate (Solu-Medrol)	**Inj:** 40mg, 125mg, 500mg, 1g, 2g	**Adults: Usual: Initial:** 10-40mg IV over several minutes. May repeat IV/IM dose at intervals based on clinical response. **High-Dose Therapy:** 30mg/kg IV over at least 30 minutes, may repeat q4-6h for 48 hrs. High dose therapy usually not >48-72 hrs. Give antacids prophylactically. **Pediatrics:** Use lower adult doses. Determine dose by severity of condition and response. Dose should not be <0.5mg/kg q24h.	**W/P:** May need to increase dose before, during, and after stressful situations. May mask signs of infection or cause new infections. Prolonged use may produce cataracts, glaucoma, secondary ocular infections. Increases BP, salt/water retention, calcium/potassium excretion. More severe/fatal course of infections reported with chickenpox, measles. Caution with latent TB, hypothyroidism, cirrhosis, ocular herpes simplex, HTN,	Fluid and electrolyte disturbances, HTN, osteoporosis,

Table 5.1: PRESCRIBING INFORMATION FOR GLUCOCORTICOIDS *(cont.)*

NAME	FORM/ STRENGTH	DOSAGE	WARNINGS/PRECAUTIONS & CONTRAINDICATIONS	ADVERSE EFFECTS†
SYSTEMIC GLUCOCORTICOIDS (Intermediate Potency) *(cont.)*				
Methylpredniso-lone Sodium Succinate *(cont.)*			diverticulitis, fresh intestinal anastomoses, ulcerative colitis, osteoporosis, myasthenia gravis, renal insufficiency, peptic ulcer disease. Kaposi's sarcoma reported. Growth and development of children on prolonged therapy should be monitored. Monitor for psychic disturbances. Avoid abrupt withdrawal. Reports of cardiac arrhythmias, circulatory collapse, cardiac arrest following rapid administration of large IV doses. Effectiveness not established for the treatment of sepsis syndrome and septic shock. Bradycardia reported with high doses. **Contra:** Premature infants (due to benzyl alcohol diluent) and systemic fungal infections. **P/N:** Safety in pregnancy and nursing not known.	muscle weakness, cushingoid state, menstrual irregularities, insomnia, impaired wound healing, DM, ulcerative esophagitis, excessive sweating, increases intracranial pressure, carbohydrate intolerance, glaucoma, cataracts, nausea.
Methylpredniso-lone (Medrol)	**Tab:** 2mg*, 4mg*, 8mg*, 16mg*, 32mg*; (Dose-Pak) 4mg* [21]	***Adults:*** **Initial:** 4-48mg/day depending on disease and response. **Maint:** Decrease dose by small amounts to lowest effective dose. ***Pediatrics:*** **Initial:** 4-48mg/day depending on disease and response.	**W/P:** May need to increase dose before, during, and after stressful situations. May mask signs of infection or cause new infections. Prolonged use may produce glaucoma, optic nerve damage, secondary ocular infections. Increases BP, salt/water retention, potassium excretion. More severe/fatal course of infections reported with chickenpox, measles. Caution with Strongyloides, latent TB, hypothyroidism, cirrhosis, ocular herpes simplex, HTN, diverticulitis, fresh intestinal anastomoses, ulcerative colitis, osteoporosis, myasthenia gravis, renal insufficiency, peptic ulcer disease. Kaposi's sarcoma reported. Growth and development of children on prolonged therapy should be monitored. Monitor for psychic disturbances. Avoid abrupt withdrawal. The 24mg tabs contain tartrazine; caution with tartrazine sensitivity. **Contra:** Systemic fungal infections. **P/N:** Safety in pregnancy and nursing not known.	Fluid and electrolyte disturbances, HTN, osteoporosis, muscle weakness, cushingoid state, menstrual irregularities, nervousness, insomnia, impaired wound healing, DM, ulcerative esophagitis, excessive sweating, increases intracranial pressure, carbohydrate intolerance, glaucoma, cataracts, weight gain, nausea, malaise.
Methylpredniso-lone Acetate (Depo-Medrol)	**Inj:** 20mg/mL, 40mg/mL, 80mg/mL	***Adults:*** 10-80mg. ***Pediatrics:*** Use lower adult doses. Determine dose by severity of condition and response.	**W/P:** Dermal and subdermal atrophy reported; do not exceed recommended doses. May need to increase dose before, during, and after stressful situations. May mask signs of infection or cause new infections. Prolonged use may produce cataracts, glaucoma, secondary ocular infections. Increases BP, salt/water retention, potassium and calcium excretion. More severe/fatal course of infections reported with chickenpox, measles. Caution with Strongyloides, latent TB, hypothyroidism, cirrhosis, ocular herpes simplex, HTN, diverticulitis, fresh intestinal anastomoses, ulcerative colitis, osteoporosis, myasthenia gravis, renal insufficiency, peptic ulcer disease. Kaposi's sarcoma reported. Growth and development of children on prolonged therapy should be monitored. Monitor for psychic disturbances. Avoid abrupt	Fluid and electrolyte disturbances, HTN, osteoporosis, muscle weakness, cushingoid state, menstrual irregularities, impaired wound healing, DM, ulcerative esophagitis, excessive sweating,

* Scored.   † Bold entries denote special dental considerations.

NAME	FORM/ STRENGTH	DOSAGE	WARNINGS/PRECAUTIONS & CONTRAINDICATIONS	ADVERSE EFFECTS†
Methylpredniso- lone Acetate *(cont.)*			withdrawal. Do not use intra-articu- larly, intrabursally, or for intratendinous administration in acute infection. Avoid injection into unstable and previously infected joints. Monitor urinalysis, blood sugar, BP, weight, chest x-ray, and upper GI x-ray (if ulcer history) regularly during prolonged therapy. **Contra:** Intrathecal administration, systemic fungal infec- tions. **P/N:** Safety in pregnancy and nursing not known.	increases intracranial pressure, carbohy- drate intolerance, glaucoma,cataracts, urticaria, subcutane- ous/cutaneous atrophy.
Prednisolone (Prelone)	**Syr:** 5mg/5mL [120mL], 15mg/5mL [240mL, 480mL]	***Adults:* Initial:** 5-60mg/day depend- ing on disease and response. **Maint:** Decrease dose by small amounts to lowest effective dose. ***Pediatrics:*** **Initial:** 5-60mg/day depending on disease and response. **Maint:** Decrease dose by small amounts to lowest effective dose.	**W/P:** Adjust dose during stress or change in thyroid status. May mask signs of infection or cause new infec- tions. Prolonged use may produce glaucoma, optic nerve damage, second- ary ocular infections. Increases BP, salt/ water retention, potassium excretion. Avoid exposure to chickenpox, measles. Caution with latent TB, hypothyroidism, cirrhosis, ocular herpes simplex, HTN, diverticulitis, fresh intestinal anasto- mosis, ulcerative colitis, osteoporosis, myasthenia gravis, renal insufficiency, peptic ulcer disease. Growth and development of children on prolonged therapy should be monitored. Monitor for psychic disturbances. Avoid abrupt withdrawal. **Contra:** Systemic fungal infections. **P/N:** Safety in pregnancy and nursing not known.	Fluid and electrolyte disturbances, osteoporosis, muscle weakness, cushingoid state, menstrual irregularities, nervous- ness, insomnia, impaired wound healing, excessive sweating, carbohydrate intolerance, glaucoma, cataracts, weight gain, nausea, malaise.
Prednisolone Acetate	**Sol:** 5mg/mL, 5mg/5mL; **Tab:** 1mg, 2.5mg*, 5mg*, 10mg*, 20mg*, 50mg*	***Adults:* Initial:** 5-60mg/day depend- ing on disease and response. **Maint:** Decrease dose by small amounts to lowest effective dose. ***Pediatrics:*** **Initial:** 5-60mg/day depending on disease and response. **Maint:** Decrease dose by small amounts to lowest effective dose.	**W/P:** May need to increase dose before, during, and after stressful situations. May mask signs of infection or cause new infections. Prolonged use may produce glaucoma, optic nerve damage, secondary ocular infections. Increases BP, salt/water retention, potassium excretion. More severe/fatal course of infections reported with chickenpox, measles. Caution with latent TB, hypothyroidism, cirrhosis, ocular herpes simplex, HTN, diverticulitis, fresh intestinal anastomosis, ulcerative colitis, osteoporosis, myasthenia gravis, renal insufficiency, peptic ulcer disease. Growth and development of children on prolonged therapy should be monitored. Monitor for psychic disturbances. Avoid abrupt withdrawal. **Contra:** Systemic fungal infections. **P/N:** Safety in pregnancy and nursing not known.	Fluid and electrolyte disturbances, HTN, osteoporosis, muscle weakness, cushingoid state, menstrual irreg- ularities, nervousness, insomnia, impaired wound healing, DM, ulcerative esophagitis, excessive sweating, increases intracranial pressure, carbohydrate intolerance, glaucoma, cataracts, weight gain, nausea, malaise.
Prednisolone Sodium Phosphate (Pediapred)	**Sol:** 5mg/5mL [120mL]	***Adults:* Initial:** 5-60mg/day depend- ing on disease and response. **Maint:** Decrease dose by small amounts to lowest effective dose. ***Pediatrics:*** **Initial:** 0.14-2mg/kg/day given tid-qid.	**W/P:** May produce reversible HPA axis suppression. Adjust dose during stress or change in thyroid status. May mask signs of infection or cause new infec- tions. May activate latent amebiasis. Avoid with cerebral malaria. Avoid exposure to chickenpox or measles. Not for treatment of optic neuritis or active ocular herpes simplex. May cause eleva- tion of BP or IOP, cataracts, glaucoma,	Edema, fluid/elec- trolyte disturbances, osteoporosis, muscle weakness, pancreatitis, peptic ulcer, impaired wound healing, increased intracranial pressure, cushingoid state, hirsutism, menstrual

Table 5.1: PRESCRIBING INFORMATION FOR GLUCOCORTICOIDS *(cont.)*

NAME	FORM/ STRENGTH	DOSAGE	WARNINGS/PRECAUTIONS & CONTRAINDICATIONS	ADVERSE EFFECTS†
SYSTEMIC GLUCOCORTICOIDS (Intermediate Potency) *(cont.)*				
Prednisolone Sodium Phosphate *(cont.)*			optic nerve damage, Kaposi's sarcoma, psychic derangements, salt/water retention, increased excretion of potassium and/or calcium, osteoporosis, growth suppression in children, secondary ocular infections. Caution with Strongyloides, CHF, diverticulitis, HTN, renal insufficiency, fresh intestinal anastomoses, active or latent peptic ulcer, ulcerative colitis. Enhanced effect in hypothyroidism or cirrhosis. Avoid abrupt withdrawal. Use with caution in elderly, increased risk of corticosteroid-induced side effects; start at low end of dosing range; monitor bone mineral density. **Contra:** Systemic fungal infections. **P/N:** Category C, caution in nursing.	irregularities, growth suppression in children, glaucoma, nausea, weight gain.
Triamcinolone Acetonide (Kenalog-10, Kenalog-40)	**Inj:** 10mg/mL, 40mg/mL	*Adults:*10-80mg/day. *Pediatrics:* ≥6 yrs: **Arthritis: Initial:** 2.5-15mg intra-articular, intrabursal, or tendon-sheath injections.	**W/P:** Caution with cirrhois, diverticulitis, hypothyroidism, hypertension, myasthenia gravis, ocular herpes simplex, osteoporosis, peptic ulcer, psychotic tendencies, renal insufficiency, ulcerative colitis, untreated systemic infections. **P/N:** Category C, caution with nursing.	Osteoporosis, depression, euphoria, hypercortisolism.
Triamcinolone Hexacetonide (Aristospan)	**Inj:** 5mg/mL, 20mg/mL	*Adults:* Usual: 2-48mg/day. *Pediatrics:* **Initial:** 0.11-1.6mg/ kg/day in 3 or 4 divided doses (3.2-48mg/m²bsa/day).	**W/P:** Caution with cirrhois, diverticulitis, hypothyroidism, hypertension, myasthenia gravis, ocular herpes simplex, osteoporosis, peptic ulcer, psychotic tendencies, renal insufficiency, ulcerative colitis, untreated systemic infections. **P/N:** Category C, caution with nursing.	Osteoporosis, depression, euphoria, hypercortisolism.
SYSTEMIC GLUCOCORTICOIDS (High Potency)				
Betamethasone (Celestone)	**Syrup:** 0.6mg/5mL [118mL]	*Adults:* **Initial:** 0.6-7.2mg/day depending on disease. Maintain until sufficient response. **Maint:** Decrease dose by small amounts to lowest effective dose. Discontinue gradually. *Pediatrics:* **Initial:** 0.6-7.2mg/day depending on disease. Maintain until sufficient response. **Maint:** Decrease dose by small amounts to lowest effective dose. Discontinue gradually.	**W/P:** May need to increase dose before, during, and after stressful situations. May mask signs of infection or cause new infections. Prolonged use may produce posterior subcapsular cataracts, glaucoma, optic nerve damage, secondary ocular infections. Increases BP, salt/water retention, potassium and calcium excretion. More severe/fatal course of infections reported with chickenpox, measles. Caution with threadworm infestation, latent TB, hypothyroidism, cirrhosis, ocular herpes simplex, HTN, diverticulitis, fresh intestinal anastomosis, ulcerative colitis, osteoporosis, myasthenia gravis, renal insufficiency, peptic ulcer disease. Growth and development of children on prolonged therapy should be monitored. Monitor for psychic disturbances. Avoid abrupt withdrawal. **Contra:** Systemic fungal infections. **P/N:** Safety in pregnancy and nursing not known.	Sodium retention, fluid retention, potassium loss, muscle weakness, myopathy, peptic ulcer, impaired wound healing, thin fragile skin, convulsions, menstrual irregularities, cataracts.
Dexamethasone	**Inj:** (Dexamethasone Sodium Phosphate) 4mg/ mL, 10mg/mL; **Sol:** (Dexamethasone)	*Adults:* Individualize for disease and patient response. Withdraw gradually. **(Tab) Initial:** 0.75-9mg/day PO. **Maint:** Decrease in small amounts to lowest effective dose. **(Inj) Usual:** 0.2-9mg. **Maint:** Decrease in small	**W/P:** Increase dose before, during, and after stressful situations. Avoid abrupt withdrawal. May mask signs of infection, activate latent amebiasis, elevate BP, cause salt/water retention, increase excretion of potassium and calcium.	Fluid/electrolyte disturbances, muscle weakness, osteoporosis, peptic ulcer, pancreatitis, ulcerative esophagitis, impaired

* Scored. † Bold entries denote special dental considerations.

NAME	FORM/ STRENGTH	DOSAGE	WARNINGS/PRECAUTIONS & CONTRAINDICATIONS	ADVERSE EFFECTS†
Dexamethasone (cont.)	0.5mg/5mL, 1mg/mL; **Tab:** (Dexamethasone) 0.5mg*, 0.75mg*, 1mg*, 1.5mg*, 2mg*, 4mg*, 6mg*	amounts to lowest effective dose. **Pediatrics:** Individualize for disease and patient response. Withdraw gradually. **(Tab) Initial:** 0.75-9mg/day PO. **Maint:** Decrease in small amounts to lowest effective dose.	Prolonged use may produce cataracts, glaucoma, secondary ocular infections. Caution with recent MI, ocular herpes simplex, emotional instability, non-specific ulcerative colitis, diverticulitis, peptic ulcer, renal insufficiency, HTN, osteoporosis, myasthenia gravis, thread-worm infection, active tuberculosis. Enhanced effect with hypothyroidism, cirrhosis. Consider prophylactic therapy if exposed to measles or chickenpox. Risk of glaucoma, cataracts and eye infections. False negative dexamethasone suppression test with indomethacin. **Contra:** Systemic fungal infections. **P/N:** Safety in pregnancy not known, not for use in pregnancy.	wound healing, headache, psychic disturbances, growth suppression (children), glaucoma, hyperglycemia, weight gain, nausea, malaise.

TOPICAL GLUCOCORTICOIDS (Low Potency)

NAME	FORM/ STRENGTH	DOSAGE	WARNINGS/PRECAUTIONS & CONTRAINDICATIONS	ADVERSE EFFECTS†
Alclometasone Dipropionate (Aclovate)	**Cre, Oint:** 0.05% [15g, 45g, 60g]	**Adults:** Apply bid-tid. Reassess if no improvement after 2 weeks. **Pediatrics:** ≥1 yr: Apply bid-tid. Reassess if no improvement after 2 weeks.	**W/P:** May produce reversible HPA axis suppression. Discontinue if irritation occurs. Use appropriate antifungal agent if fungal infection develops. Pediatrics may be more susceptible to systemic toxicity. **P/N:** Category C, caution in nursing.	Stinging, burning, irritation, secondary fungal infection, mucosal atrophy.
Desonide (DesOwen, Tridesilon)	**Cre, Oint:** 0.05% [15g, 60g]; **Lot:** 0.05% [60mL, 120mL]	**Adults:** Apply bid-tid, depending on severity. Reassess if no improvement after 2 weeks.	**W/P:** May produce reversible HPA axis suppression. Discontinue if irritation occurs. Use appropriate antifungal agent if fungal infection develops. Pediatrics may be more susceptible to systemic toxicity. **P/N:** Category C, caution in nursing.	Stinging, burning, irritation, secondary fungal infection, mucosal atrophy.
Hydrocortisone (Cortaid, Cortizone, Hytone, Hytone 1%)	**(Cortaid) Cre:** 1%; **Spray:** 1%. **(Cortizone) Cre:** 1%; **Oint:** 1%; **Spray:** 1%; **(Hytone) Cre:** 2.5% [30g, 60g]; **Lot:** 2.5% [60mL]; **Oint:** 2.5% [30g]; **(Hytone 1%) Lot:** 1% [30mL, 120mL]	**(Cortaid/Cortizone) Adults & Pediatrics:** ≥2 yrs: Apply to affected area tid-qid. **(Hytone) Adults:** Apply bid-qid depending on the severity. **Pediatrics:** Apply bid-qid depending on the severity. **(Hytone 1%) Adults:** Apply up to tid-qid.	**W/P:** May produce reversible HPA axis suppression. Discontinue if irritation occurs. Use appropriate antifungal agent if fungal infection develops. Pediatrics may be more susceptible to systemic toxicity. (Cortaid/Cortizone/Hytone 1%) Avoid eyes. Discontinue use if condition worsens, if symptoms persist for more than 7 days, or if symptoms recur after clearing up. **P/N:** (Hytone) Category C, caution in nursing. (Cortaid/Cortizone/Hytone 1%) Safety in pregnancy and nursing is not known.	Stinging, burning, irritation, secondary fungal infection, mucosal atrophy.

TOPICAL GLUCOCORTICOIDS (Medium Potency)

NAME	FORM/ STRENGTH	DOSAGE	WARNINGS/PRECAUTIONS & CONTRAINDICATIONS	ADVERSE EFFECTS†
Betamethasone Valerate (Luxiq)	**Foam:** 0.12% [50g, 100g]	**Adults:** Gently massage into affected area bid (am and pm) until foam disappears. Reassess if no improvement after 2 weeks.	**W/P:** May produce reversible HPA axis suppression. Discontinue if irritation occurs. Use appropriate antifungal agent if fungal infection develops. Pediatrics may be more susceptible to systemic toxicity. **P/N:** Category C, caution in nursing.	Stinging, burning, irritation, secondary fungal infection, mucosal atrophy.
Clocortolone Pivalate (Cloderm)	**Cre:** 0.1% [15g, 45g, 90g]	**Adults:** Apply tid. Use with occlusive dressing for management of psoriasis or recalcitrant conditions. **Pediatrics:** Apply tid. Use with occlusive dressing for management of psoriasis or recalcitrant conditions.	**W/P:** May produce reversible HPA axis suppression. Discontinue if irritation occurs. Use appropriate antifungal agent if fungal infection develops. Pediatrics may be more susceptible to systemic toxicity. **P/N:** Category C, caution in nursing.	Stinging, burning, irritation, secondary fungal infection, mucosal atrophy.

Table 5.1: PRESCRIBING INFORMATION FOR GLUCOCORTICOIDS *(cont.)*

NAME	FORM/ STRENGTH	DOSAGE	WARNINGS/PRECAUTIONS & CONTRAINDICATIONS	ADVERSE EFFECTS[†]
TOPICAL GLUCOCORTICOIDS (Medium Potency) *(cont.)*				
Desoximetasone (Topicort-LP)	**Cre:** (LP) 0.05% [15g, 60g], 0.25% [15g, 60g]; **Gel:** 0.05% [15g, 60g]; **Oint:** 0.25% [15g, 60g]	**Adults:** Apply bid. **Pediatrics:** (Cre, Gel) Apply bid. ≥10 yrs: (Oint) Apply bid.	**W/P:** May produce reversible HPA axis suppression. Discontinue if irritation occurs. Use appropriate antifungal agent if fungal infection develops. Pediatrics may be more susceptible to systemic toxicity. **P/N:** Category C, caution in nursing.	Stinging, burning, irritation, secondary fungal infection, mucosal atrophy.
Fluocinolone Acetonide (Derma-Smoothe/ FS, Synalar)	**(Derma-Smoothe/ FS) Oil:** 0.01% [120mL]; **(Synalar) Cre, Oint:** 0.025% [15g, 60g]; **Sol:** 0.01% [20mL, 60mL]	**Adults:** (Derma-Smoothe/FS) Apply tid. **Pediatrics:** ≥2 yrs: Moisten skin and apply bid up to 4 weeks. **(Synalar)** **Adults:** Apply bid-qid. **Pediatrics:** Apply bid-qid.	**W/P:** May produce reversible HPA axis suppression. Discontinue if irritation occurs. Use appropriate antifungal agent if fungal infection develops. Pediatrics may be more susceptible to systemic toxicity. **P/N:** Category C, caution in nursing.	Stinging, burning, irritation, secondary fungal infection, mucosal atrophy.
Flurandrenolide (Cordran, Cordran SP)	**Cre (SP):** 0.05% [15g, 30g, 60g]; **Lot:** 0.05% [15mL, 60mL]; **Tape:** 4mcg/cm²	**Adults:** (Cre, Lot) Apply qd-qid depending on severity. For moist lesions, apply cream bid-tid. Apply lotion bid-tid. **Pediatrics:** (Cre, Lot) Apply qd-qid depending on severity. For moist lesions, apply cream bid-tid. Apply lotion bid-tid.	**W/P:** May produce reversible HPA axis suppression. Discontinue if irritation occurs. Use appropriate antifungal agent if fungal infection develops. Pediatrics may be more susceptible to systemic toxicity. **P/N:** Category C, caution in nursing.	Stinging, burning, irritation, secondary fungal infection, mucosal atrophy.
Fluticasone Propionate (Cutivate)	**Cre:** 0.05% [15g, 30g, 60g]; **Oint:** 0.005% [15g, 30g, 60g]	**Adults:** (Cream) Atopic Dermatitis: Apply qd-bid. **Pediatrics:** ≥3 months: (Cre) Atopic Dermatitis: Apply qd-bid.	**W/P:** May produce reversible HPA axis suppression. Discontinue if irritation occurs. Use appropriate antifungal agent if fungal infection develops. Pediatrics may be more susceptible to systemic toxicity. **P/N:** Category C, caution in nursing.	Stinging, burning, irritation, secondary fungal infection, mucosal atrophy.
Halcinonide (Halog)	**(Halog) Cre, Oint:** 0.1% [15g, 30g, 60g, 240g]; **Sol:** 0.1% [20mL, 60mL]; **(Halog-E) Cre:** 0.1% in a hydrophilic vanishing cream [30g, 60g]	**Adults:** (Cre, Oint, Sol) Apply bid-tid. (Cre in hydrophilic base) Apply qd-tid. **Pediatrics:** Limit to least amount compatible with an effective therapeutic regimen.	**W/P:** May produce reversible HPA axis suppression. Discontinue if irritation occurs. Use appropriate antifungal agent if fungal infection develops. Pediatrics may be more susceptible to systemic toxicity. **P/N:** Category C, caution in nursing.	Stinging, burning, irritation, secondary fungal infection, mucosal atrophy.
Hydrocortisone Butyrate (Locoid, Locoid Lipocream)	**Cre, Oint:** 0.1% [15g, 45g]; **Sol:** 0.1% [20mL, 60mL]	**Adults:** (Cre, Oint) Apply bid-tid. (Sol) Apply bid-tid. **Pediatrics:** (Cre, Oint) Apply bid-tid. (Sol) Apply bid-tid.	**W/P:** May produce reversible HPA axis suppression. Discontinue if irritation occurs. Use appropriate antifungal agent if fungal infection develops. Pediatrics may be more susceptible to systemic toxicity. **P/N:** Category C, caution in nursing.	Stinging, burning, irritation, secondary fungal infection, mucosal atrophy.
Hydrocortisone Probutate (Pandel)	**Cre:** 0.1% [15g, 45g, 80g]	**Adults:** Apply qd-bid depending on severity of condition.	**W/P:** May produce reversible HPA axis suppression. Discontinue if irritation occurs. Use appropriate antifungal agent if fungal infection develops. Pediatrics may be more susceptible to systemic toxicity. **P/N:** Category C, caution in nursing.	Stinging, burning, irritation, secondary fungal infection, mucosal atrophy.
Hydrocortisone Valerate (Westcort)	**Cre, Oint:** 0.2% [15g, 45g, 60g]	**Adults:** Apply bid-tid. **Pediatrics:** Apply bid-tid.	**W/P:** May produce reversible HPA axis suppression. Discontinue if irritation occurs. Use appropriate antifungal agent if fungal infection develops. Pediatrics may be more susceptible to systemic toxicity. **P/N:** Category C, caution in nursing.	Stinging, burning, irritation, secondary fungal infection, mucosal atrophy.
Mometasone Furoate (Elocon)	**Cre, Oint:** 0.1% [15g, 45g]; **Lot:** 0.1% [30mL, 60mL]	**Adults:** (Cream, Oint) Apply qd. (Lotion) Apply a few drops qd. Reassess if no improvement within 2 weeks. **Pediatrics:** (Cream, Oint) ≥2 yrs: Apply qd for up to 3 weeks if needed. Reassess if no improvement within 2 weeks.	**W/P:** May produce reversible HPA axis suppression. Discontinue if irritation occurs. Use appropriate antifungal agent if fungal infection develops. Pediatrics may be more susceptible to systemic toxicity. **P/N:** Category C, caution (cream, ointment) or not for use (lotion) in nursing.	Stinging, burning, irritation, secondary fungal infection, mucosal atrophy.

* Scored.   † Bold entries denote special dental considerations.

NAME	FORM/ STRENGTH	DOSAGE	WARNINGS/PRECAUTIONS & CONTRAINDICATIONS	ADVERSE EFFECTS†
Prednicarbate (Dermatop E)	Cre, Oint: 0.1% [15g, 60g]	Adults: (Cream, Oint) Apply bid. Pediatrics: ≥1 yr: (Cream) Apply bid. Max: 3 weeks of therapy. ≥10 yrs: (Oint) Apply bid.	W/P: May produce reversible HPA axis suppression. Discontinue if irritation occurs. Use appropriate antifungal agent if fungal infection develops. Pediatrics may be more susceptible to systemic toxicity. P/N: Category C, caution in nursing.	Stinging, burning, irritation, secondary fungal infection, mucosal atrophy.
Triamcinolone Acetonide (Aristocort-A, Kenalog)	(Aristocort-A) Cre: 0.025% [15g, 60g], 0.1% [15g, 60g], 0.5% [15g]; Oint: 0.1% [15g, 60g]; (Kenalog) Cre: 0.1% [15g, 60g, 80g], 0.5% [20g]; Lot: 0.025%, 0.1% [60mL]; Oint: 0.1% [15g, 60g]; Spray: 0.147mg/g [63g]	Adults: (Aristocort-A) (Cre, Oint) Apply tid-qid. (Kenalog) (Cre, Lot, Oint) Apply 0.025% bid-qid. Apply 0.1% or 0.5% bid-tid. (Spray) Apply tid-qid.	W/P: May produce reversible HPA axis suppression. Discontinue if irritation occurs. Use appropriate antifungal agent if fungal infection develops. Pediatrics may be more susceptible to systemic toxicity. P/N: Category C, caution in nursing.	Stinging, burning, irritation, secondary fungal infection, mucosal atrophy.

TOPICAL GLUCOCORTICOIDS (High Potency)

NAME	FORM/ STRENGTH	DOSAGE	WARNINGS/PRECAUTIONS & CONTRAINDICATIONS	ADVERSE EFFECTS†
Amcinonide (Cyclocort)	Cre, Oint: 0.1% [15g, 30g, 60g]; Lot: 0.1% [20mL, 60mL]	Adults: Apply bid-tid depending on severity. Pediatrics: Apply bid-tid depending on severity.	W/P: May produce reversible HPA axis suppression. Discontinue if irritation occurs. Use appropriate antifungal agent if fungal infection develops. Pediatrics may be more susceptible to systemic toxicity. P/N: Category C, not for use in nursing.	Stinging, burning, irritation, secondary fungal infection, mucosal atrophy.
Betamethasone Dipropionate, Augmented (Diprolene, Diprolene AF)	Cre (AF), Gel, Oint: 0.05% [15g, 50g]; Lot: 0.05% [30mL, 60mL]	Adults: (Gel, Lot) Apply qd-bid for no more than 2 weeks. Limit to (Gel) 50g/week, (Lot) 50mL/week. (Cre, Oint) Apply qd-bid, up to 45g/week. Pediatrics: ≥13 yrs: (Cre) Apply qd-bid for no more than 2 weeks. Limit to 45g/week. ≥12 yrs: (Gel, Lot) Apply qd-bid for no more than 2 weeks. Limit to (Gel) 50g/week, (Lot) 50mL/week. (Oint) Apply qd-bid, up to 45g/week.	W/P: May produce reversible HPA axis suppression. Discontinue if irritation occurs. Use appropriate antifungal agent if fungal infection develops. Pediatrics may be more susceptible to systemic toxicity. P/N: Category C, (Cre, Lot) not for use in nursing; (Gel, Oint) caution in nursing.	Stinging, burning, irritation, secondary fungal infection, mucosal atrophy.
Desoximetasone (Topicort)	Cre: (LP) 0.05% [15g, 60g], 0.25% [15g, 60g]; Gel: 0.05% [15g, 60g]; Oint: 0.25% [15g, 60g]	Adults: Apply bid. Pediatrics: (Cre, Gel) Apply bid. ≥10 yrs: (Oint) Apply bid.	W/P: May produce reversible HPA axis suppression. Discontinue if irritation occurs. Use appropriate antifungal agent if fungal infection develops. Pediatrics may be more susceptible to systemic toxicity. P/N: Category C, caution in nursing.	Stinging, burning, irritation, secondary fungal infection, mucosal atrophy.
Fluocinonide (Lidex, Lidex-E, Vanos)	(Lidex) Cre, Gel, Oint: 0.05% [15g, 30g, 60g]; Sol: 0.05% [60mL]; (Lidex-E) Cre: 0.05% [15g, 30g, 60g]; (Vanos) Cre: 0.1% [30mg, 60mg]	(Lidex, Lidex-E) Adults: Apply bid-qid. Pediatrics: Apply bid-qid. (Vanos) Adults: Apply thin layer to affected area qd-bid. Max: 60g/week. Do not exceed 2 weeks.	W/P: May produce reversible HPA axis suppression. Discontinue if irritation occurs. Use appropriate antifungal agent if fungal infection develops. Pediatrics may be more susceptible to systemic toxicity. P/N: Category C, caution in nursing.	Stinging, burning, irritation, secondary fungal infection, mucosal atrophy.

TOPICAL GLUCOCORTICOIDS (Very High Potency)

NAME	FORM/ STRENGTH	DOSAGE	WARNINGS/PRECAUTIONS & CONTRAINDICATIONS	ADVERSE EFFECTS†
Betamethasone Dipropionate, Augmented (Diprolene, Diprolene AF)	Cre (AF), Gel, Oint: 0.05% [15g, 50g]; Lot: 0.05% [30mL, 60mL]	Adults: (Gel, Lot) Apply qd-bid for no more than 2 weeks. Limit to (Gel) 50g/week, (Lot) 50mL/week. (Cre, Oint) Apply qd-bid, up to 45g/week. Pediatrics: ≥13 yrs: (Cre) Apply qd-bid for no more than 2 weeks. Limit to 45g/week. ≥12 yrs: (Gel, Lot) Apply qd-bid for no more than 2 weeks. Limit to (Gel) 50g/week, (Lot) 50mL/week. (Oint) Apply qd-bid, up to 45g/week.	W/P: May produce reversible HPA axis suppression. Discontinue if irritation occurs. Use appropriate antifungal agent if fungal infection develops. Pediatrics may be more susceptible to systemic toxicity. P/N: Category C, (Cre, Lot) not for use in nursing; (Gel, Oint) caution in nursing.	Stinging, burning, irritation, secondary fungal infection, mucosal atrophy.

Table 5.1: PRESCRIBING INFORMATION FOR GLUCOCORTICOIDS *(cont.)*

NAME	FORM/ STRENGTH	DOSAGE	WARNINGS/PRECAUTIONS & CONTRAINDICATIONS	ADVERSE EFFECTS†
TOPICAL GLUCOCORTICOIDS (Very High Potency) *(cont.)*				
Clobetasol Propionate (Clobex, Olux, Temovate, Temovate E)	**(Clobex) Lot:** 0.05% [30mL, 59mL]; **Shampoo:** 0.05% [118mL]; **Spray:** 0.05% [2oz]; **(Olux) Foam:** 0.05% [50g, 100g]; **(Temovate) Cre, Oint:** 0.05% [15g, 30g, 45g, 60g]; **Gel:** 0.05% [15g, 30g, 60g]; **Sol:** 0.05% [25mL]; **(Temovate-E) Cre:** 0.05% [15g, 30g, 60g]	**(Clobex)** *Adults:* ≥18 yrs: **(Lot)** Apply bid for up to 2 consecutive weeks. **(Spray)** Spray on affected area(s) **Max:** 50g/week or 50ml/week. bid. Rub in gently and completely. Reassess after 2 weeks; may repeat for additional 2 weeks. Limit treatment to 4 weeks. **Max:** 50g/week. **(Olux)** *Adults:* Apply to affected area bid (am and pm). No more than 1.5 capfuls/application. Limit to 2 consecutive weeks. **Max:** 50g/week. *Pediatrics:* ≥12 yrs: Apply to affected area bid (am and pm). No more than 1.5 capfuls/application. Limit to 2 consecutive weeks. **Max:** 50g/week. **(Temovate)** *Adults:* Apply bid. **Max:** 50g/week or 50mL/week.	**W/P:** May produce reversible HPA axis suppression. Discontinue if irritation occurs. Use appropriate antifungal agent if fungal infection develops. Pediatrics may be more susceptible to systemic toxicity. **P/N:** Category C, caution in nursing.	Stinging, burning, irritation, secondary fungal infection, mucosal atrophy.
Diflorasone Diacetate (Psorcon, Psorcon-E)	**Cre, Oint:** 0.05% [15g, 30g, 60g]	*Adults:* Apply qd-tid **(Psorcon Oint/ Psorcon E Cream)** or qd-qid **(Psorcon E Oint)** or bid **(Psorcon Cream)** depending on the severity.	**W/P:** May produce reversible HPA axis suppression. Discontinue if irritation occurs. Use appropriate antifungal agent if fungal infection develops. Pediatrics may be more susceptible to systemic toxicity. **P/N:** Category C, caution in nursing.	Stinging, burning, irritation, secondary fungal infection, mucosal atrophy.
Halobetasol Propionate (Ultravate)	**Cre, Oint:** 0.05% [15g, 50g]	*Adults:* Apply qd-bid. Rub in gently. Limit treatment to 2 weeks. **Max:** 50g/week. *Pediatrics:* ≥12 yrs: Apply qd-bid. Rub in gently. Limit treatment to 2 weeks. **Max:** 50g/week.	**W/P:** May produce reversible HPA axis suppression. Discontinue if irritation occurs. Use appropriate antifungal agent if fungal infection develops. Pediatrics may be more susceptible to systemic toxicity. **P/N:** Category C, caution in nursing.	Stinging, burning, irritation, secondary fungal infection, mucosal atrophy.

* Scored.   † Bold entries denote special dental considerations.

Table 5.2: DRUG INTERACTIONS FOR GLUCOCORTICOIDS

INHALED GLUCOCORTICOIDS

Beclomethasone Diproionate Monohydrate (Beconase AQ)

Corticosteroids	Concomitant systemic corticosteroids increases risk of hypercorticism and/or HPA axis suppression.

Budesonide (Pulmicort Respules, Pulmicort Turbuhaler, Rhinocort Aqua)

Cimetidine	(Respules) Slight decrease in clearance and increase in oral bioavailabilty with cimetidine. Cimetidine increase plasma levels.
Corticosteroids	Concomitant systemic corticosteroids increases risk of hypercorticism and/or HPA axis suppression.
CYP3A4 inhibitors	CYP3A4 inhibitors (eg, itraconazole, clarithromycin, erythromycin) may inhibit metabolism and increase systemic exposure.
Ketoconazole, oral	Oral ketoconazole increases plasma levels.

Flunisolide (Aerobid, Aerobid-M, Nasarel)

Corticosteroids	Concomitant systemic corticosteroids increases risk of hypercorticism and/or HPA axis suppression.

Fluticasone Propionate (Flonase, Flovent HFA)

Corticosteroids, inhaled	Concomitant inhaled corticosteroids increases risk of hypercorticism and/or HPA axis suppression.
CYP3A4 inhibitors	Caution with other potent CYP3A4 inhibitors, may increase serum fluticasone levels.
Ketoconazole	Caution with ketoconazole, may increase serum fluticasone levels.
Ritonavir	Increased levels with ritonavir; avoid use.

Mometasone Furoate (Asmanex Twisthaler)

Ketoconazole	Ketoconazole may increase plasma levels.

Triamcinolone Acetonide (Azmacort, Nasacort AQ)

Prednisone	Caution with prednisone.

SYSTEMIC GLUCOCORTICOIDS (Low Potency)

Hydrocortisone (Cortef)

Anticoagulants, oral	Effects on oral anticoagulants are variable; monitor PT.
ASA, high dose	Increases clearance of chronic high dose ASA; caution with hypoprothrombinemia.
Hepatic enzyme inducers	Reduced efficacy and increased clearance with hepatic enzyme inducers (eg, phenobarbital, phenytoin, and rifampin).
Hypoglycemic, oral	Increased oral hypoglycemic requirements in DM.
Insulin	Increased insulin requirements in DM.
Ketoconazole	Decreased clearance with ketoconazole.

Table 5.2: DRUG INTERACTIONS FOR GLUCOCORTICOIDS *(cont.)*

SYSTEMIC GLUCOCORTICOIDS (Low Potency) *(cont.)*

Hydrocortisone (Cortef)

Troleandomycin	Decreased clearance with troleandomycin.
Vaccines, killed or inactivated	Possible decreased vaccine response with killed or inactivated vaccines with immunosuppressive doses.
Vaccines, live	Avoid live vaccines with immunosuppressive doses.

Hydrocortisone Sodium Succinate (Solu-Cortef)

Anticoagulants, oral	Effects on oral anticoagulants are variable; monitor PT/INR.
ASA, high dose	Increases clearance of chronic high dose ASA; caution with hypoprothrombinemia.
Hepatic enzyme inducers	Reduced efficacy and increased clearance with hepatic enzyme inducers (eg, phenobarbital, phenytoin, and rifampin).
Hypoglycemic, oral	Increased oral hypoglycemic requirements in DM.
Insulin	Increased insulin requirements in DM.
Ketoconazole	Decreased clearance with ketoconazole.
Troleandomycin	Decreased clearance with troleandomycin.
Vaccines, killed or inactivated	Possible decreased vaccine response with killed or inactivated vaccines with immunosuppressive doses.
Vaccines, live	Avoid live vaccines with immunosuppressive doses.

SYSTEMIC GLUCOCORTICOIDS (Intermediate Potency)

Methylprednisolone Sodium Succinate (Solu-Medrol)

Anticoagulants, oral	Effects on oral anticoagulants are variable; monitor PT/INR.
ASA, high dose	Increases clearance of chronic high dose ASA. Caution with ASA in hypoprothrombinemia.
Cyclosporine	Mutual inhibition of metabolism with cyclosporine; convulsions reported.
Hepatic enzyme inducers	Reduced efficacy with hepatic enzyme inducers (eg, phenobarbital, phenytoin, and rifampin).
Hypoglycemic, oral	Increased oral hypoglycemic requirements in DM.
Insulin	Increased insulin requirements in DM.
Ketoconazole	Decreased clearance with ketoconazole.
Troleandomycin	Decreased clearance with troleandomycin.
Vaccines, killed or inactivated	Possible decreased vaccine response with killed or inactivated vaccines with immunosuppressive doses.
Vaccines, live	Avoid live vaccines with immunosuppressive doses.

SYSTEMIC GLUCOCORTICOIDS (Intermediate Potency) *(cont.)*

Methylprednisolone (Medrol)

Anticoagulants, oral	Effects on oral anticoagulants are variable; monitor PT.
ASA, high dose	Increases clearance of chronic high dose ASA. Caution with ASA in hypoprothrombinemia.
Cyclosporine	Mutual inhibition of metabolism with cyclosporine; convulsions reported.
Hepatic enzyme inducers	Reduced efficacy with hepatic enzyme inducers (eg, phenobarbital, phenytoin, and rifampin).
Hypoglycemic, oral	Increased oral hypoglycemic requirements in DM.
Insulin	Increased insulin requirements in DM.
Ketoconazole	Potentiated by ketoconazole.
Troleandomycin	Potentiated by troleandomycin.
Vaccines, killed or inactivated	Possible decreased vaccine response with killed or inactivated vaccines with immunosuppressive doses.
Vaccines, live	Avoid live vaccines with immunosuppressive doses.

Methylprednisolone Acetate (Depo-Medrol)

Anticoagulants, oral	Effects on oral anticoagulants are variable; monitor PT.
ASA, high dose	Increases clearance of chronic high dose ASA. Caution with ASA in hypoprothrombinemia.
Cyclosporine	Mutual inhibition of metabolism with cyclosporine; convulsions reported.
Hepatic enzyme inducers	Reduced efficacy with hepatic enzyme inducers (eg, phenobarbital, phenytoin, and rifampin).
Hypoglycemic, oral	Increased oral hypoglycemic requirements in DM.
Insulin	Increased insulin requirements in DM.
Ketoconazole	Potentiated by ketoconazole.
Solutions	Do not dilute or mix with other solutions.
Troleandomycin	Potentiated by troleandomycin.
Vaccines, killed or inactivated	Possible decreased vaccine response with killed or inactivated vaccines with immunosuppressive doses.
Vaccines, live	Avoid live vaccines with immunosuppressive doses.

Prednisolone (Prelone)

ASA	Avoid ASA with hypoprothrombinemia.
Antidiabetic agents	May increase blood glucose; adjust antidiabetic agents.
Smallpox vaccination	Avoid smallpox vaccination with immunosuppressive doses.

Table 5.2: DRUG INTERACTIONS FOR GLUCOCORTICOIDS *(cont.)*

SYSTEMIC GLUCOCORTICOIDS (Intermediate Potency) *(cont.)*

Prednisolone (Prelone)

Vaccines, killed or inactivated	Possible decreased vaccine response with killed or inactivated vaccines with immunosuppressive doses.
Vaccines, live	Avoid live vaccines with immunosuppressive doses.

Prednisolone Acetate

Anticoagulants, oral	Variable effect on oral anticoagulants.
ASA	Increases clearance of high dose ASA; caution in hypoprothrombinemia.
Hepatic enzyme inducers	Increased clearance with hepatic enzyme inducers.
Hypoglycemic, oral	Increased oral hypoglycemic requirements in DM.
Insulin	Increased insulin requirements in DM.
Ketoconazole	Decreased metabolism with ketoconazole.
Smallpox vaccination	Avoid smallpox vaccine with immunosuppressive doses.
Troleandomycin	Decreased metabolism with troleandomycin.
Vaccines, killed or inactivated	Possible decreased vaccine response with killed or inactivated vaccines with immunosuppressive doses.
Vaccines, live	Avoid live vaccines with immunosuppressive doses.

Prednisolone Sodium Phosphate (Pediapred)

Anticholinesterase agents	May produce severe weakness in myasthenia gravis patients on anticholinesterase agents.
Antidiabetic agents	May increase blood glucose; adjust antidiabetic agents.
ASA	Increased risk of GI side effects with ASA.
Barbiturates	Enhanced metabolism with barbiturates.
Cyclosporine	Use with cyclosporine may increase activity of both drugs; convulsions reported with concomitant use.
Ephedrine	Enhanced metabolism with ephedrine.
Estrogens	Decreased metabolism with estrogens.
Ketoconazole	Decreased metabolism with ketoconazole.
Neuromuscular drugs	High doses or concurrent neuromuscular drugs may cause acute myopathy.
NSAIDs	Increased risk of GI side effects with other NSAIDs.
Phenytoin	Enhanced metabolism with phenytoin.

SYSTEMIC GLUCOCORTICOIDS (Intermediate Potency) *(cont.)*

Prednisolone Sodium Phosphate (Pediapred)

Potassium-depleting agents	Enhanced possibility of hypokalemia when given with potassium-depleting agents.
Rifampin	Enhanced metabolism with rifampin.
Salicylates	May increase clearance of salicylates.
Skin tests	May suppress reactions to skin tests.
Vaccines, killed or inactivated	Possible diminished response with killed or inactivated vaccines.
Vaccines, live	Avoid live vaccines with immunosuppressive doses.
Warfarin	May inhibit response to warfarin.

Triamcinolone Acetonide (Kenalog-10, Kenalog-40)

Alcuronium	Decreased alcuronium effectiveness; prolonged muscle weakness and myopathy.
Aldesleukin	Reduced antitumor effectiveness.
Amphotericin B Liposome	Increased risk of hypokalemia.
Aspirin	Increased risk of gastrointestinal ulceration and subtherapeutic aspirin serum concentrations.
Atracurium	Decreased atracurium effectiveness; prolonged muscle weakness and myopathy.
Cisatracurium	Decreased cisatracurium effectiveness; prolonged muscle weakness and myopathy.
Doxacurium	Decreased doxacurium effectiveness; prolonged muscle weakness and myopathy.
Echinacea	Decreased effectiveness of corticosteroids.
Flumequine	Increased risk for tendon rupture.
Fluoroquinolones	Increased risk for tendon rupture
Fosphenytoin	Decreased triamcinolone effectiveness.
Gallamine	Decreased gallamine effectiveness; prolonged muscle weakness and myopathy.
Hexafluorenium	Decreased hexafluorenium bromide effectiveness; prolonged muscle weakness and myopathy.
Hydrochlorothiazide	Hypokalemia and subsequent cardiac arrhythmias.
Itraconazole	Increased corticosteroid plasma concentrations and an increased risk of corticosteroid side effects (myopathy, glucose intolerance, Cushing's syndrome).
Licorice	Increased risk of corticosteroid adverse effects.
Ma Huang	Decreased effectiveness of corticosteroids.

Table 5.2: DRUG INTERACTIONS FOR GLUCOCORTICOIDS *(cont.)*

SYSTEMIC GLUCOCORTICOIDS (Intermediate Potency) *(cont.)*

Triamcinolone Acetonide (Kenalog-10, Kenalog-40)

Metocurine	Decreased metocurine effectiveness; prolonged muscle weakness and myopathy.
Mivacurium	Decreased mivacurium effectiveness; prolonged muscle weakness and myopathy.
Pancuronium	Decreased pancuronium effectiveness; prolonged muscle weakness and myopathy.
Phenobarbital	Decreased corticosteroid effectiveness.
Phenytoin	Decreased triamcinolone effectiveness.
Pipecuronium	Decreased pipecuronium effectiveness; prolonged muscle weakness and myopathy.
Primidone	Decreased triamcinolone effectiveness.
Quetiapine	Decreased serum quetiapine concentrations.
Rifampin	Decreased triamcinolone effectiveness.
Rocuronium	Decreased rocuronium effectiveness; prolonged muscle weakness and myopathy.
Saiboku-To	Enhanced and prolonged effect of corticosteroids.
Tretinoin	Decreased efficacy of tretinoin.
Tuberculin	Decreased reactivity to tuberculin.
Tubocurarine	Decreased tubocurarine effectiveness; prolonged muscle weakness and myopathy.
Vaccines	Inadequate immunological response to the vaccine.
Vecuronium	Decreased vecuronium effectiveness; prolonged muscle weakness and myopathy.

Triamcinolone Diacetate (Aristocort, Aristocort-Forte)

Alcuronium	Decreased alcuronium effectiveness; prolonged muscle weakness and myopathy.
Aldesleukin	Reduced antitumor effectiveness.
Amphotericin B Liposome	Increased risk of hypokalemia.
Aspirin	Increased risk of gastrointestinal ulceration and subtherapeutic aspirin serum concentrations.
Atracurium	Decreased atracurium effectiveness; prolonged muscle weakness and myopathy.
Cisatracurium	Decreased cisatracurium effectiveness; prolonged muscle weakness and myopathy.
Doxacurium	Decreased doxacurium effectiveness; prolonged muscle weakness and myopathy.
Echinacea	Decreased effectiveness of corticosteroids.
Flumequine	Increased risk for tendon rupture.
Fluoroquinolones	Increased risk for tendon rupture.
Fosphenytoin	Decreased triamcinolone effectiveness.
Gallamine	Decreased gallamine effectiveness; prolonged muscle weakness and myopathy.

SYSTEMIC GLUCOCORTICOIDS (Intermediate Potency) *(cont.)*

Triamcinolone Diacetate (Aristocort, Aristocort-Forte)

Hexafluorenium	Decreased hexafluorenium bromide effectiveness; prolonged muscle weakness and myopathy.
Hydrochlorothiazide	Hypokalemia and subsequent cardiac arrhythmias.
Itraconazole	Increased corticosteroid plasma concentrations and an increased risk of corticosteroid side effects (myopathy, glucose intolerance, Cushing's syndrome).
Licorice	Increased risk of corticosteroid adverse effects.
Ma Huang	Decreased effectiveness of corticosteroids.
Metocurine	Decreased metocurine effectiveness; prolonged muscle weakness and myopathy.
Mivacurium	Decreased mivacurium effectiveness; prolonged muscle weakness and myopathy.
Pancuronium	Decreased pancuronium effectiveness; prolonged muscle weakness and myopathy.
Phenobarbital	Decreased corticosteroid effectiveness.
Phenytoin	Decreased triamcinolone effectiveness.
Pipecuronium	Decreased pipecuronium effectiveness; prolonged muscle weakness and myopathy.
Primidone	Decreased triamcinolone effectiveness.
Quetiapine	Decreased serum quetiapine concentrations.
Rifampin	Decreased triamcinolone effectiveness.
Rocuronium	Decreased rocuronium effectiveness; prolonged muscle weakness and myopathy.
Saiboku-To	Enhanced and prolonged effect of corticosteroids.
Tretinoin	Decreased efficacy of tretinoin.
Tuberculin	Decreased reactivity to tuberculin.
Tubocurarine	Decreased tubocurarine effectiveness; prolonged muscle weakness and myopathy.
Vaccines	Inadequate immunological response to the vaccine.
Vecuronium	Decreased vecuronium effectiveness; prolonged muscle weakness and myopathy.

Triamcinolone Hexacetonide (Aristospan)

Alcuronium	Decreased alcuronium effectiveness; prolonged muscle weakness and myopathy.
Aldesleukin	Reduced antitumor effectiveness.
Amphotericin B Liposome	Increased risk of hypokalemia.
Aspirin	Increased risk of gastrointestinal ulceration and subtherapeutic aspirin serum concentrations.
Atracurium	Decreased atracurium effectiveness; prolonged muscle weakness and myopathy.

Table 5.2: DRUG INTERACTIONS FOR GLUCOCORTICOIDS *(cont.)*

SYSTEMIC GLUCOCORTICOIDS (Intermediate Potency) *(cont.)*

Triamcinolone Hexacetonide (Aristospan)

Cisatracurium	Decreased cisatracurium effectiveness; prolonged muscle weakness and myopathy.
Doxacurium	Decreased doxacurium effectiveness; prolonged muscle weakness and myopathy.
Echinacea	Decreased effectiveness of corticosteroids.
Flumequine	Increased risk for tendon rupture.
Fluoroquinolones	Increased risk for tendon rupture.
Fosphenytoin	Decreased triamcinolone effectiveness.
Gallamine	Decreased gallamine effectiveness; prolonged muscle weakness and myopathy.
Hexafluorenium	Decreased hexafluorenium bromide effectiveness; prolonged muscle weakness and myopathy.
Hydrochlorothia-zide	Hypokalemia and subsequent cardiac arrhythmias.
Itraconazole	Increased corticosteroid plasma concentrations and an increased risk of corticosteroid side effects (myopathy, glucose intolerance, Cushing's syndrome).
Licorice	Increased risk of corticosteroid adverse effects.
Ma Huang	Decreased effectiveness of corticosteroids.
Metocurine	Decreased metocurine effectiveness; prolonged muscle weakness and myopathy.
Mivacurium	Decreased mivacurium effectiveness; prolonged muscle weakness and myopathy.
Pancuronium	Decreased pancuronium effectiveness; prolonged muscle weakness and myopathy.
Phenobarbital	Decreased corticosteroid effectiveness.
Phenytoin	Decreased triamcinolone effectiveness.
Pipecuronium	Decreased pipecuronium effectiveness; prolonged muscle weakness and myopathy.
Primidone	Decreased triamcinolone effectiveness.
Quetiapine	Decreased serum quetiapine concentrations.
Rifampin	Decreased triamcinolone effectiveness.
Rocuronium	Decreased rocuronium effectiveness; prolonged muscle weakness and myopathy.
Saiboku-To	Enhanced and prolonged effect of corticosteroids.
Tretinoin	Decreased efficacy of tretinoin.
Tuberculin	Decreased reactivity to tuberculin.
Tubocurarine	Decreased tubocurarine effectiveness; prolonged muscle weakness and myopathy.
Vaccines	Inadequate immunological response to the vaccine.
Vecuronium	Decreased vecuronium effectiveness; prolonged muscle weakness and myopathy.

SYSTEMIC GLUCOCORTICOIDS (High Potency)

Betamethasone (Celestone)

ASA	Caution with ASA in hypoprothrombinemia.
Hypoglycemic agents, oral	Increased requirements of oral hypoglycemic agents.
Immunization procedures	Avoid smallpox vaccines and other immunization procedures at high doses.
Immunosuppressives	Increased susceptibility to infections with immunosuppressives.
Insulin	Increased requirements of insulin.
Smallpox vaccines	Avoid smallpox vaccines at high doses.

Dexamethasone

ASA	Caution with ASA.
Coumarins	Antagonizes or potentiates coumarins.
CYP3A4 inducers	Inducers of CYP3A4 (eg, phenytoin, phenobarbital, carbamazepine, rifampin) enhance clearance; increase steroid dose.
CYP3A4 inhibitors	Inhibitors of CYP3A4 (ketoconazole, macrolides) may increase plasma levels.
CYP3A4 metabolizers	Increased clearance of drugs metabolized by CYP3A4 (eg, indinavir, erythromycin).
Ephedrine	Ephedrine enhance clearance; increase steroid dose.
Ketoconazole	Ketoconazole may inhibit adrenal corticosteroid synthesis and cause adrenal insufficiency during corticosteroid withdrawal.
Metabolism-affecting drugs	Drugs that affect metabolism may interfere with dexamethasone suppression tests.
Phenytoin	May increase or decrease phenytoin levels.
Potassium-depleting diuretics	Hypokalemia with potassium-depleting diuretics.
Virus vaccines, live	Live virus vaccines are contraindicated with immunosuppressive doses.

Chapter 6

Antibiotics

Clay Walker, Ph.D.; Luciana Machion, D.D.S., Ph.D.

The term "antibiotic" initially was used to refer to any compound produced by a microorganism that inhibited another microorganism. Through common usage, this definition has evolved to include any natural, semisynthetic or, in some cases, totally manmade antimicrobial agent that inhibits bacterial growth. An antibiotic can be classified as either bactericidal or bacteriostatic. Bactericidal drugs, such as penicillins, directly kill an infecting organism; bacteriostatic drugs, such as tetracyclines and erythromycin, inhibit the proliferation of bacteria by interfering with an essential metabolic process, resulting in the elimination of bacteria by the host's immune defense system.

Antibiotics are used commonly in dentistry for both therapeutic and preventive measures involving oral bacterial infections. Oral infections can occur for a number of reasons and primarily involve pulpal and periodontal tissues. Secondary infections of the soft tissues pose special therapeutic challenges. Regardless of the oral infection being treated, monitoring the course of the infection with observation of the patient between 24 and 72 hours is recommended to ensure efficacy of the drug selected. Although culturing oral infections is not always possible or necessary, consideration of this procedure followed by antibiotic sensitivity testing should be included in the treatment of patients who do not respond to the antibiotic used initially.

Before undertaking the therapeutic use of any antibiotic, the clinician should determine an established need for antibiotic therapy, take a careful history to determine if the patient has experienced any previous adverse reactions or developed a sensitivity to a specific antibiotic, determine which antibiotic is or is most likely to be effective against a bacterium or bacteria, and ensure that he or she has a thorough knowledge of the side effects and drug interactions.

Penicillin is still the drug of choice for treatment of infections in and around the oral cavity. In patients allergic to penicillin, erythromycin or clindamycin may be an appropriate alternative. Finally, if there is no response to penicillin V, then amoxicillin with clavulanic acid may be a good alternative in patients not allergic to penicillin, as the spectrum of sensitivity is altered. In general, there is no advantage in selecting a bactericidal rather than a bacteriostatic antibiotic for the treatment of healthy people. However, if the patient is immunocompromised either by concurrent treatment (such as cancer chemotherapy or drugs associated with a bone-marrow transplant) or by a preexisting disease (such as HIV infection), a bactericidal antibiotic would be indicated.

Prophylactic Use of Antibiotics

Prophylactic use of antibiotics is recommended before the performance of invasive dental procedures on patients who are at risk of developing bacterial endocarditis (Appendix D) and late prosthetic joint infections (those occurring 6 or more months after placement of the prosthesis) (Appendix E). Injudicious use of antibiotics can have dire consequences, and the clinician must carefully consider, and discuss with the patient, the advantages and disadvantages of prescribing an antibiotic (Appendix F).

Antibiotics and Oral Contraceptives

With regard to possible drug interactions with antibiotics, and the common use of oral steroid contraceptives, it is important to recognize a recent American Dental Association report. Dental practitioners have been advised to discuss a possible reduction in efficacy of oral steroid contraceptives during antibiotic therapy with all women of child-bearing age. Furthermore, these patients should be advised to use additional forms of contraception during short-term antibiotic use. The American Medical Association also concluded that women should be informed of the possible interaction, as an interaction could not be completely discounted and could not be predicted. It is the opinion of the ADA Council of Scientific Affairs that, considering the possible consequences of an unwanted pregnancy, when prescribing antibiotics to a patient using oral contraceptives, the dentist should do the following:

- advise the patient of the potential risk of the antibiotic's reducing the effectiveness of the oral contraceptive;
- recommend that the patient discuss with her physician the use of an additional non-hormonal means of contraception;
- advise the patient to maintain compliance with oral contraceptives when concurrently using antibiotics.

Penicillins and Cephalosporins

Antibiotics belonging to these two classes are referred to as "β-lactam antibiotics" owing to the presence of the β-lactam ring common to all drugs in these classes. These drugs are considered bactericidal because they directly result in the death of bacteria by inhibiting specific bacterial enzymes required for the assembly of the bacterial cell wall. Many of the β-lactam antibiotics are rendered inactive by the bacterial production of β-lactamase,

an enzyme that hydrolyzes the β-lactam ring and renders the antibiotic inactive. The bacterial production of β-lactamase is the primary reason that treatment with penicillins or cephalosporins can fail.

The cephalosporins and the closely related cephamycins normally are listed together as a single related group and are similar to the penicillins in structure and action. Although penicillins are usually superior for treating dental-related infections, the cephalosporins/cephamycins are included in this chapter because they are used frequently in medical practice and may be encountered in patients seeking dental treatment. Additionally, they may be indicated in the prevention of infections arising from bacteremias of an oral nidus, as in prophylaxis against late prosthetic joint infections.

Accepted Indications

Table 6.1 lists common indications for penicillins and cephalosporins.

General Dosing and Dosage Adjustments

These are the dosages more frequently recommended for the treatment of dental-related infections (see Table 6.2). Other semisynthetic penicillins (azlocillin, mezlocillin, piperacillin, ticarcillin, and methicillin) as well as most of the cephalosporins/cephamycins (cephalothin, cephapirin, cefazolin, cefamandole, cefoxitin, cefonicid, cefotaxime, ceftizoxime, ceftazidime, and cefoperazone) are available only IM or IV owing to poor oral absorption and instability in the presence of gastric acids. These are generally reserved for the treatment of severe infections and diseases that require hospitalization (see Table 6.2).

Under normal circumstances, penicillins and cephalosporins are rapidly eliminated from the body primarily through the kidneys and, partly, in the bile and by other routes. In the case of patients with reduced renal function, dosages should be adjusted downward relative to creatinine clearance rates in consultation with the patient's physician. In patients undergoing peritoneal dialysis, an alternative antibiotic should be considered because most penicillins and cephalosporins are effectively removed from the bloodstream by hemodialysis.

Special Dental Considerations

Drug Interactions of Dental Interest

Amoxicillin/clavulanic acid should not be coadministered with the antiabuse drug disulfiram. Table 6.3 lists possible interactions between penicillins and cephalosporins and other drugs.

Cross-Sensitivity

Before initiating therapy with any penicillin or cephalosporin, careful inquiry should be made concerning previous hypersensitivity reactions to any penicillin, cephalosporin, or other allergens. Serious and occasionally fatal hypersensitivity (anaphylactoid) reactions have been reported in patients receiving penicillin or cephalosporin therapy. These reactions are more apt to occur in people with a history of penicillin and/or cephalosporin hypersensitivity and/or a history of sensitivity to multiple allergens. Penicillins and cephalosporins should be used with caution in patients who have a history of significant allergies and/or asthma. Because of the similarity in the structure of the penicillins and cephalosporins, patients allergic to one class may manifest cross-reactivity to members of the other class. Cross-reactivity to cephalosporins may occur in as many as 20% of the patients who are allergic to penicillins. Patients with a history or suspected history of hypersensitivity to a penicillin or cephalosporin, if given any antibiotic in this class, should be observed for any difficulty in breathing or other sign of allergic reaction for a minimum of 1 hour before being released.

Special Patients

Pregnant and nursing women

Penicillins and cephalosporins are secreted in human breast milk, and caution should be exercised when a drug from either group is administered to nursing women, as it may lead to sensitization, diarrhea and candidiasis. Clinical experience with the penicillins and cephalosporins during pregnancy has not shown any evidence of adverse effects on the fetus. However, there have been no adequate and well-controlled studies in pregnant women that show conclusively that harmful effects of these drugs on the fetus can be ruled out. Therefore, penicillins and cephalosporins should be used during pregnancy only if clearly needed.

Pharmacology

See Table 6.4 for pharmacologic information on penicillins and cephalosporins.

Patient Advice

- In case of the development of any adverse effect (rash; nausea; vomiting; diarrhea; swelling of lips, tongue or face; fever and so forth), the patient should be advised to stop taking the medication and promptly inform the dentist.
- Encourage compliance with the full course of therapy despite improvement in clinical signs and symptoms of an infection.
- There have been reports of reduced oral contraceptive effectiveness in women taking ampicillin, amoxicillin and penicillin, resulting in unplanned pregnancy. Although the association is weak, advise patients of this information and encourage them to use an alternate or additional method of contraception while taking any of these penicillins.

Macrolides

The macrolide group of antibiotics contains approximately 40 compounds, but only a limited few have clinical use. Erythromycin has generally been the most effective and is widely used as an alternative to penicillins for the treatment and prevention of infections caused by gram-positive microorganisms. Clarithromycin, a semisynthetic macrolide antibiotic, is similar to erythromycin, but has a broader spectrum of activity. Both antibiotics have good activity against most gram-positive bacteria associated with the mouth. Unlike erythromycin, clarithromycin has relatively good activity against a number of gram-negative bacteria.

In recent years, a novel class of antibiotics called the azalides has surfaced. These new macrolide derivatives appear superior to erythromycin and clarithromycin in that they offer better pharmacokinetic properties, excellent tissue distribution, longer therapeutic half-life and activity against many gram-negative and gram-positive bacteria. Of the azalides, azithromycin has received extensive clinical use.

Accepted Indications
Table 6.1 lists common indications for macrolides.

General Dosing and Dosage Adjustments
See Table 6.2 for general dosage and prescribing information. Erythromycin and azithromycin are principally eliminated from the body via the liver. Therefore, dosages and/or the dosage interval should be adjusted when these drugs are administered to a patient with impaired hepatic function. Clarithromycin is eliminated via the liver and kidney and may be administered without dosage adjustment in patients with hepatic impairment and normal renal function. However, in the presence of severe renal impairment with or without coexisting hepatic impairment, decreased dosage or prolonged dosage intervals may be

appropriate. Hepatotoxicity has been associated rarely with all erythromycin salts, but more frequently with erythromycin estolate.

Cross-Sensitivity
Erythromycin, azithromycin or clarithromycin are contraindicated in patients with known hypersensitivity to any of the macrolide antibiotics.

Special Patients
Pregnant and nursing women
Clarithromycin should not be used in pregnant women except in clinical circumstances in which no alternative therapy is appropriate. If pregnancy occurs while taking the drug, the patient should be advised that clarithromycin has demonstrated teratogenicity in animals, but as of yet not in humans. Although no evidence of impaired fertility or harm to the fetus has been found with either erythromycin or azithromycin, these drugs should be used during pregnancy only if needed.

Erythromycin and clarithromycin are secreted in human breast milk and should be used with caution in nursing mothers. As it is not known if azithromycin is secreted in human breast milk, the same cautions should be applied to this drug as well.

Pediatric, geriatric and other special patients
The safety of clarithromycin has not been established for children aged < 12 years, and the safety of azithromycin has not been established for children and youths aged < 16 years.

Dosage adjustment does not appear to be necessary in elderly patients who have normal renal and hepatic function.

Pharmacology
See Table 6.4 for pharmacologic information on macrolides.

Tetracyclines

The tetracyclines, which include tetracycline, doxycycline and minocycline, all have essentially the same broad-spectrum of activity and are frequently indicated in the treatment of gram-positive and gram-negative bacterial infections of the head and neck as well as other regions of the body. They are considered to be bacteriostatic at normal dosages and inhibit bacterial protein synthesis in sensitive bacteria by binding to the 30S ribosomal subunits and preventing the addition of amino acids to the growing peptide chain. At high concentrations, the tetracyclines are bactericidal and may inhibit protein synthesis in mammalian cells. The advantage of using doxycycline or minocycline rather than tetracycline, is that the former two antibiotics are absorbed better after oral administration. This greater absorption results in higher serum levels and a lesser need for frequent dosing. Unfortunately, resistance to one tetracycline often indicates resistance to all tetracyclines.

Accepted Indications

Dental applications include the adjunctive treatment of refractory periodontitis and juvenile periodontitis, dental abscesses, soft tissue abscesses, and as an alternative when penicillins are contraindicated or when β-lactamase-producing microorganisms are involved. Due to bacterial resistance, the tetracyclines are not indicated in the treatment of streptococcal or staphylococcal infections.

Resistance to tetracycline hydrochloride has become so widespread that this drug is rarely used in clinical medicine. However, the drug still appears to be beneficial in the treatment of certain dental infections, including periodontitis that do not respond favorably to conventional periodontal therapy. See Table 6.1 for indications.

Subantimicrobial-Dose Doxycycline

The U.S. Food and Drug Administration has approved the use of a subantimicrobial dose of doxycycline hyclate (20 mg bid, available generically and as the brand Periostat) as an adjunctive to periodontal therapy. Although this drug is classified as an antibiotic, it does not act as one because of its low dose. The major mechanism of action of this drug is the suppression of collagenase, particularly that which is produced by polymorphonuclear leukocytes. As the dose is too low to affect bacteria, resistance to this medication does not seem to develop. The therapeutic objective is to modulate the inflammatory host response, not necessarily kill bacteria. Since a subantimicrobial dose of doxycycline hyclate has no antibacterial properties, it is important that it be used as an adjunct to mechanical therapy. Note: An antibacterial dose of doxycycline hyclate is available in a slow-release tablet (Oracea, 40 mg qd) for treating rosacea.

Treatment with a subantimicrobial dose of doxycycline hyclate, 20 mg q12h, in conjunction with either dental debridment or scaling and root planing, significantly and consistently improved clinical signs of periodontal disease in clinical trials. A subantimicrobial dose of doxycycline hyclate represents the application of the concept of host modulation to the treatment of periodontal disease.

Safety studies showed that use of a subantimicrobial dose of doxycycline hyclate twice daily was well-tolerated for up to 12 months, and that the rates and types of adverse events were not different than those associated with placebos. Furthermore, the dose demonstrated neither an antimicrobial effect on the periodontal microflora nor a shift in normal flora. Lastly, there was no evidence of the development of multiantibiotic resistance.

General Dosing and Dosage Adjustments

See Table 6.2 for dosage and prescribing information.

Because tetracyclines have been shown to depress plasma prothrombin activity, patients receiving anticoagulant therapy may require downward adjustment of the anticoagulant dosage.

If renal impairment exists, the recommended doses for any tetracycline may lead to excessive systemic accumulation of the antibiotic and, possibly, liver toxicity. The antianabolic action of the tetracyclines may cause an increase in blood urea nitrogen. In patients with significant renal insufficiency, this may lead to azotemia, hyperphosphatemia and acidosis. Total dosages of any tetracycline should therefore be decreased in patients with renal impairment by reduction of recommended individual doses and/or by extending the time between doses.

Special Dental Considerations

Special Patients
Pregnant and nursing women
All tetracyclines cross the placenta and form a stable calcium complex in bone-forming tissue. Consequently, use of tetracyclines is not recommended during the last half of pregnancy, as the drugs may cause permanent discoloration of teeth, enamel hypoplasia and inhibition of skeletal growth in the fetus.

Although previous recommendations advised against prescribing tetracycline in nursing mothers, the latest statement of the American Academy of Pediatrics considers tetracycline safe in nursing mothers.

Pediatric, geriatric and other special patients
Tetracycline drugs should not be used in children aged ≤ 8 years because these drugs may cause permanent discoloration of the teeth.

Concurrent, long-term use of tetracyclines with estrogen-containing oral contraceptives may result in reduced contraceptive reliability. Patients should be advised of this information and encouraged to use an alternative or additional method of contraception while taking any tetracycline.

Pharmacology
See Table 6.4 for pharmacologic information on tetracylines.

Locally Delivered Antibiotics

There is evidence that locally delivered, controlled-release antimicrobial agents—such as doxycycline hyclate gel (10%) (Atridox) and minocycline hydrochloride microspheres 1 mg (Arestin)—are effective in the treatment of periodontal pockets. The general benefit of locally delivered, controlled-release antibiotics is the achievement of high site concentrations of antibiotic with low systemic drug levels. Accordingly, one is able to reduce the putative pathogenic bacteria while minimizing the risk of adverse systemic side effects.

Accepted Indications
Clinical studies suggest that subgingival delivery of doxycycline hyclate 10% (Atridox) has a potential periodontal benefit. Doxycycline hyclate gel is injected into a periodontal pocket through a syringe system is intended to deliver an antibacterial concentration for 7-14 days and is biodegradable. The effects of doxycycline hyclate on attachment level gain and probing depth reduction have been shown to be equivalent to those of scaling and root planing alone and also, when used in combination with mechanical instrumentation, it shows better results than instrumentation alone.

Clinical trials suggest that minocycline hydrochloride 1 mg microspheres (Arestin) as an adjunct to scaling and root planing are more effective in reducing pocket depths than scaling and root planing alone. The minocycline hydrochloride microsphere is a bioadhesive, biodegradable polymer in powder form that is injected into the periodontal pocket to maintain a therapeutic drug concentation for 10-14 days.

Reapplication of both of these drugs may be indicated at certain intervals.

Adverse Effects and Precautions

The most common side effect of controlled-release antibiotic agents is localized erythema and rare occurrences of localized candidiasis. The clinician should keep in mind the potential side effects of antibiotics described earlier—such as development of resistant strains or increased growth of opportunistic organisms—when considering prescription of local controlled-release antibiotics for periodontal pocket delivery.

Patient Advice

- Until more evidence becomes available, the clinician would be prudent to advise patients receiving locally delivered antibiotics in the same manner as he or she would those taking the antibiotic in its oral form. Please refer to the section on Patient Advice for each antibiotic.

Clindamycin

Clindamycin is a semisynthetic derivative of lincomycin. Although not structurally related to erythromycin, it shares the same primary mode of action in that it binds to the 50S ribosomal subunits and inhibits bacterial protein synthesis in sensitive organisms (bacteriostatic). At higher concentrations, clindamycin can be bactericidal. Clindamycin is relatively active against gram-positive and gram-negative anaerobic bacteria, including most of those associated with the mouth. Essentially, all gram-negative aerobic bacteria are resistant.

Accepted Indications

Clindamycin is generally reserved for the treatment of serious infections of the respiratory tract, skin and soft tissue, female genital tract, intra-abdominal infections and abscesses, and septicemia involving gram-positive and/or gram-negative anaerobes, streptococci, staphylococci, and mixed infections involving anaerobes and facultative gram-positive bacteria.

However, clindamycin is indicated as a prophylactic antibiotic for dental patients at risk of developing bacterial endocarditis and who are allergic to penicillin and unable to take oral medications. Additionally, clindamycin is effective as adjunctive treatment of chronic and acute osteomyelitis caused by staphylococcus and is an alternative to penicillin V potassium and erythromycin for treatment of orofacial infections. See Table 6.1.

General Dosing and Dosage Adjustments

See Table 6.2 for dosage and prescribing information. In patients with severe renal and/or hepatic impairment, clindamycin should be administered only for very severe infections, with the dosages and dosage intervals adjusted accordingly.

Special Dental Considerations

Drug Interactions of Dental Interest

Table 6.3 lists possible interactions between clindamycin and other drugs.

Cross-Sensitivity

There are no cross-sensitivities reported between clindamycin and any other antibiotic group. However, the 75- and 150-mg capsules of clindamycin hydrochloride contain FD&C Yellow no. 5 (tartrazine), which may cause allergic reactions in some patients with hypersensitivity to aspirin.

Special Patients

Pregnant and nursing women

Clindamycin is secreted in breast milk in sufficient concentrations to cause disturbances of the intestinal flora of infants and should not be administered to nursing mothers unless warranted by clinical circumstances. Jaundice and abnormalities in liver function tests also may occur.

The safety of clindamycin for use during pregnancy has not been established.

Pediatric, geriatric and other special patients
Clindamycin should not be administered to older patients who have an associated severe illness that may render them more susceptible to diarrhea.

The drug should be administered with caution to any patient with a history of gastrointestinal disease, particularly colitis, or to a patient with severe renal disease and/or severe hepatic disease.

Pharmacology
See Table 6.4 for pharmacologic information on clindamycin.

Metronidazole

Metronidazole's primary use is in the bactericidal treatment of obligate anaerobic bacteria associated with the mouth, the intestinal tract and the female genital tract.

As an adjunct to periodontal therapy, metronidazole and amoxicillin are often used in combination at dosages consisted of 250 mg of metronidazole and 250-500 mg of amoxicillin given concurrently at 8-hour intervals (tid) for a period of 7 to 10 days.

Note: The combined use of metronidazole with amoxicillin or amoxicillin/clavulanic acid has not been approved by the U.S. Food and Drug Administration.

Accepted Indications
Metronidazole is generally reserved for the treatment of serious infections of the lower respiratory tract, skin and soft tissue, female genital tract, intra-abdominal infections and abscesses, bones and joints, and bacterial septicemia involving obligate gram-positive anaerobic cocci, gram-negative anaerobic bacilli and *Clostridium* species.

The drug is indicated in the treatment of symptomatic and asymptomatic trichomoniasis in both females and males, amebic dysentery, antibiotic-associated colitis and in pseudomembraneous colitis due to infection by *Clostridium difficile* (see Table 6.1).

Metronidazole has been used with considerable success as an adjunct to the treatment of periodontitis; this probably is related to its high activity against the gram-negative anaerobic bacilli that are often associated with the disease. The concurrent oral administration of metronidazole with amoxicillin has been used with considerable success in the treatment of both juvenile and adult forms of periodontitis and in the treatment of refractory periodontitis that has not responded favorably to other forms of periodontal therapy. It has been reported to be particularly effective in the treatment of Actinobacillus actinomycetemcomitans-associated periodontitis. Additionally, the use of metronidazole and penicillin V for severe mixed odontogenic infections has been a successful adjunct in clinically resolving these infections.

General Dosing and Dosage Adjustments
See Table 6.2 for dosage and prescribing information. Patients with severe hepatic disease or impairment metabolize metronidazole slowly, with a resultant accumulation in the plasma. For such patients, the drug should be given with caution and the dosages adjusted downward from those normally given. However, for patients receiving renal dialysis, adjustment is not necessary because metronidazole is rapidly removed by dialysis.

In elderly patients, the pharmacokinetics of the drug may be altered and monitoring of serum levels may be necessary to adjust the dosage.

Special Dental Considerations

Cross-Sensitivity

Metronidazole is contraindicated in patients with a history of hypersensitivity to metronidazole or any other nitroimidazole derivative.

Special Patients

Pregnant and nursing women

Metronidazole should be used with caution in pregnant women. Animal reproduction studies have failed to demonstrate teratogenic effects on the fetus, and there are no adequate, well-controlled studies in pregnant women. Metronidazole is distributed in breast milk and has been shown in some animal studies to have a carcinogenic effect and possibly adverse effects in infants. Therefore, its use is not recommended in nursing mothers.

Pediatric, geriatric and other special patients

As the pharmacokinetics of metronidazole may be altered in elderly patients, the drug should be given with caution and only when an alternative antibiotic is not available.

Drug serum levels should be watched in elderly patients as well as in patients with severe hepatic disease or impairment to avoid toxicity.

The safety and effectiveness of metronidazole has not been established in children except for the treatment of amebiasis.

Patients with Crohn's disease should not be treated with metronidazole, as the drug may potentiate the tendency for the formation of gastrointestinal and certain extraintestinal cancers.

Pharmacology

See Table 6.4 for pharmacologic information on metronidazole.

Quinolones

The quinolones are a group 1,8-naphthyridine synthetic derivatives that are not chemically related to any other antibacterial agents. These drugs may be divided into the older quinolones, such as nalidixic acid, that have limited antibacterial activity, and the newer fluoroquinolones, which are characterized as having a broad spectrum of activity. Examples of the latter are ciprofloxacin and levofloxacin. Both of these have excellent activity against a wide range of gram-negative and gram-positive bacteria, including many that are resistant to third-generation cephalosporins, broad spectrum semi-synthetic pencillins, and the newer semi-synthetic aminoglycosides. Most anaerobic bacteria, including those of the oral cavity, are resistant to these drugs. Due to their wide spread usage in the treatment of upper respiratory tract and urinary tract infections as well as a host of other bacterial infections, it is very likely that some patients presenting for dental treatment may be taking one of these drugs. Fortunately, neither ciprofloxacin nor levofloxacin are reported to cross-react with most other classes of antibiotics.

Accepted Indications

Both ciprofloxacin and levofloxacin are indicated in the treatment of infections caused by aerobic or facultative gram-negative rods or by *Staphylococcus aureus* (including methacillin-resistant *S. aureus*), *Staphylococcus epidermidis*, *Escherichia coli*, *Streptococcus pyogenes*, or *Enterococcus faecalis* as well as other bacteria involving infections of the sinuses, the respiratory tract, the skin and skin structures, the bones and joints, and the urinary tract. Neither drug is indicated in the treatment of infections caused by obligate anaerobic bacteria. See Table 6.1.

General Dosing and Dosage Adjustments

See Table 6.2 for dosage and prescribing information. In patients who have impaired renal clearance and are not undergoing renal dialysis, dosage intervals should be adjusted based on serum creatinine levels. For patients who are undergoing renal dialysis, dosages of 250-500 mg should be given either qd or should be based on serum creatinine levels.

For patients with changing renal function or for patients with both renal and hepatic insufficiency, adjusted dosages should be based on serum concentrations of ciprofloxacin.

Special Dental Considerations

Cross-Sensitivity
A history of hypersensitivity to ciprofloxacin, levofloxacin, or to any other quinolone is a contraindication to its use.

Special Patients
Pregnant and nursing women
The safety and effectiveness of ciprofloxacin and levofloxacin in pregnant or lactating women has not been established. The drug should be used during pregnancy only if the potential benefit justifies the potential risk to the fetus.

Both drugs are excreted in human milk. Owing to the potential for serious adverse reactions in nursing infants, nursing should be discontinued if it is necessary to administer either ciprofloxacin or levofloxacin to the mother.

Pediatric, geriatric and other special patients
The safety and effectiveness of either ciprofloxacin or levofloxacin in children and adolescents aged < 18 years has not been established.

Patient Monitoring: Aspects to Watch
Serum creatinine levels should be monitored in patients receiving ciprofloxacin who have severe renal impairment.

Owing to the potential for serious adverse reactions, serum levels of theophylline should be monitored closely if it is necessary to administer either drug to patients receiving theophylline.

Adverse Effects and Precautions
The most common side effects are nausea, diarrhea, vomiting, abdominal pain/discomfort, headache, restlessness and rash (see Table 6.2). Each of these has been reported in 1% to 5% of patients receiving quinolones.

Pharmacology
See Table 6.4 for pharmacologic information on quinolones (ciprofloxacin and levofloxacin).

Suggested Readings

American Academy of Pediatrics Committee on Drugs. The transfer of drugs and other chemicals into human milk. Pediatrics 1994;93(1):137-50.

American Dental Association Health Foundation Research Institute, Department of Toxicology. Antibiotic interference with oral contraceptives. JADA 1991;122:79.

American Medical Association Council on Scientific Affairs. Report 8 of the Council on Scientific Affairs (A-00): drug interactions between antibiotics and oral contraceptives. Available at: www.ama-assn.org/ama/pub/article/2036–2927.html. Accessed April 1, 2003.

Consensus reports from the 1996 World Workshop in Periodontics. JADA 1998;29(supplement):1S-69S.

Liu P, Muller M, Derendorf H. Rational dosing of antibiotics: the use of plasma concentrations versus tissue concentrations. Int J Antimicrob Agents 2002;19(4):285-90.

Ramgoolam A, Steele R. Formulations of antibiotics for children in primary care: effects on compliance and efficacy. Paediatr Drugs 2002;4(5):323-33.

United States Pharmacopeial Convention, Inc. Drug information for the health care professional. 18th ed. Rockville, Md.: United States Pharmacopeial Convention, Inc.; 1998.

Walker CB. Antimicrobial agents and chemotherapy. In: Slots J, Taubman M, eds. Contemporary oral microbiology and immunology. St. Louis: Mosby; 1992:242-64.

Walker CB. Selected antimicrobial agents: Mechanisms of action, side effects, and drug interactions. In: Slots J, Rams T, eds. Periodontology 2000. Vol. 10: Systemic and topical antimicrobial therapy in periodontics. Copenhagen: Munksgaard; 1996:12-28.

Table 6.1: ACCEPTED INDICATIONS FOR ANTIBIOTIC USE

NAME	CHARACTERISTICS	COMMON INDICATIONS FOR USE
Clindamycin		
	Active against most gram-positive bacteria, including many staphylococcal and streptococcal species	Treatment of severe infections caused by anaerobic bacteria
	Excellent activity against both gram-positive and gram-negative anaerobic bacteria	Adjunct to treatment of adult refractory periodontitis
		Adjunct to treatment of chronic and acute osteomyelitis caused by staphylococcus
		Alternative to penicillin and erythromycin for treating orofacial infections
		Alternative prophylactic antibiotic for dental patients allergic to penicillin and unable to take oral medication
Macrolides		
Azithromycin	Broad spectrum of activity for both gram-positive and gram-negative bacteria	Indicated in the treatment of patients ≥ age 16 y who have mild-to-moderate infections
	Given once daily	Alternative prophylactic antibiotic for dental patients at risk of bacterial endocarditis and allergic to penicillin
		Alternative to penicillin G and other penicillins for treatment of gram-positive coccoid infections in patients with hypersensitivity to penicillins
Clarithromycin	Active against gram-positive and many gram-negative bacteria	Treatment of mild-to-moderate respiratory infections and uncomplicated skin infections
		Alternative prophylactic antibiotic for dental patients at risk of bacterial endocarditis and allergic to penicillin
		Alternative to penicillin G and other penicillins for treatment of gram-positive coccoid infections in patients with hypersensitivity to penicillins
Erythromycin Base	Active against gram positive bacteria, particularly gram-positive cocci	Treatment of upper and lower respiratory tract, skin and soft tissue infections of mild-to-moderate severity
	Provides only limited activity against gram-negative bacteria	Alternative to penicillin G and other penicillins for treatment of gram-positive coccoid infections in patients with hypersensitivity to penicillins
	Yields irregular and unpredictable serum levels	
	Given during a fasting state	
Erythromycin Ethylsuccinate	Activity same as for erythromycin base	Uses same as for erythromycin base
Erythromycin Stearate	Activity same as for erythromycin base	Uses same as for erythromycin base
	Less subject to gastric acids than erythromycin base	
	Yields more predictable serum levels	
Metronidazole		
	Antibacterial activity against all anaerobic cocci and both gram-negative bacilli and gram-positive spore-forming bacilli	Indicated in treatment of trichomoniasis, amebiasis and giardiasis as well as a variety of infections caused by obligate anaerobic bacteria
	Nonsporulating gram positive bacilli are often resistant as are most facultative bacteria	Indicated in treatment of obligate anaerobic bacterial infections associated with mouth, intestinal tract and female genital tract
		Has been used as adjunct in treatment of periodontitis

Table 6.1: ACCEPTED INDICATIONS FOR ANTIBIOTIC USE *(cont.)*

NAME	CHARACTERISTICS	COMMON INDICATIONS FOR USE
Penicillins and Cephalosporins		
Amoxicillin	Similar to ampicillin but yields higher serum levels	Has same uses as ampicillin
	More rapidly and completely absorbed from stomach than ampicillin	Designed specifically for oral administration
	Penetrates gingival crevicular fluid well but is hydrolyzed rapidly if significant levels of β-lactamases are present	Recommended as a prophylactic antibiotic to prevent bacterial endocarditis and late prosthetic joint infections following invasive dental procedures in at-risk patients
Amoxicillin/Clavulanic Acid	Has same properties as amoxicillin but is resistant to wide range of β-lactamases	Broad-spectrum antibiotic with excellent activity against many β-lactamase producing oral and non-oral bacteria
	Penetrates gingival crevicular fluid well	
	Resistant to most β-lactamases produced by oral bacteria	Recommended as a prophylactic antibiotic to prevent late prosthetic joint infections following invasive dental procedures in at-risk patients
Ampicillin	Provides broad-spectrum activity against both gram-negative and gram-positive bacteria	Broad-spectrum penicillin for use against a variety of bacteria that do not produce β-lactamase (for example, *Escherichia coli*, as well as *Neisseria*, *Haemophilus* and *Proteus* species)
	Stable to stomach acids and readily absorbed from the stomach	For dental patients at risk for bacterial endocarditis and unable to take oral medication, the IM or IV route is recommended
	Susceptible to β-lactamases	
Quinolones (Ciprofloxacin and Levofloxacin)		
	Bactericidal	Indicated in treatment of infections of the lower respiratory tract, skin, bone and joints, and urinary tract and for the treatment of infectious diarrhea
	Broad spectrum of activity against both gram-positive and gram-negative bacteria	As a single agent or in combination with metronidazole in the treatment of periodontitis associated with *Actinobacillus actinomycetemcomitans*
	Inactive against most anaerobic bacteria	
Tetracyclines		
Doxycycline Hyclate	Has the same characteristics as tetracycline except that it is absorbed more completely following oral administration and yields higher serum levels	Adjunctive treatment of adult periodontitis and juvenile periodontitis
		Treatment of acute necrotizing ulcerative gingivitis and dental abscesses
		Alternative to penicillins for treatment of actinomycosis and other oral infections
Minocycline Hydrochloride	Has the same characteristics as tetracycline except that it is absorbed more completely following oral administration and yields higher serum levels	Uses same as for doxycycline (above)
	More lipophilic than doxycycline and provides better tissue penetration	
Tetracycline Hydrochloride	Broad-spectrum antibiotic with activity against gram-positive and gram-negative bacteria, mycoplasmas, rickettsial and chlamydial infections	Uses same as for doxycycline (above)

Table 6.2: PRESCRIBING INFORMATION FOR ANTIBIOTICS

NAME	FORM/ STRENGTH	DOSAGE	WARNINGS/PRECAUTIONS & CONTRAINDICATIONS	ADVERSE EFFECTS†
AMINOCYCLITOL				
Spectinomycin (Trobicin)	**Inj:** 2g	***Adults:*** Administer 2g (5mL) IM into upper outer quandrant of gluteal muscle. Use 4g (10mL) for treatment in geographic areas with prevalent antibiotic resistance. Divide dose between 2 gluteal sites.	**W/P:** Contains benzyl alcohol. May mask or delay symptoms of incubating syphilis. Perform serologic test for syphilis at time of diagnosis and after 3 months. Caution in atopic individuals. Monitor for resistance by N.gonorrhoeae. **P/N:** Category B, caution in nursing.	Injection site soreness, urticaria, dizziness, nausea, chills, fever, and insomnia.
AMINOGLYCOSIDES				
Amikacin Sulfate (Amikin, Amikin Pediatric)	**Sol: (Amikin Pedatric):** 50mg/mL, **(Amikin):** 250mg/mL	***Adults:*** (IM/IV)15mg/kg/day given q8h or q12h. **Max:** 15mg/kg/day. **Heavier Weight** *Patients:* **Max:** 1.5g/day. **Recurrent UnComplicated UTI:** 250mg bid. **Duration:** 7-10 days. Stop therapy if no response after 3-5 days. Reduce dose if suspect renal dysfunction. Discontinue if azotemia increases or if a progressive decrease in urinary output occurs. ***Pediatrics:*** 15mg/kg/day given bid-tid. **Newborns: LD:** 10mg/kg. **MD:** 7.5mg/kg q12h. **Duration:** 7-10 days.	**Potential for ototoxicity and nephrotoxicity. Neuromuscular blockade, respiratory blockade reported. Avoid potent diuretics and other neurotoxic, nephrotoxic, and ototoxic drugs. W/P:** May aggravate muscle weakness; caution with muscular disorders (eg, myasthenia gravis, or parkinsonism). May cause fetal harm in pregnancy. Contains sodium bisulfite, allergic reactions may occur especially in asthmatics. Maintain adequate hydration. Assess kidney function before therapy then daily. **Contra:** History of serious toxic reactions to aminoglycosides. **P/N:** Category D, not for use in nursing.	Ototoxicity, neuromuscular blockage, nephrotoxicity, skin rash, drug fever, headache, paresthesia, tremor, nausea, arthralgia, anemia, and hypotension.
Gentamicin Sulfate (Gentamicin)	**Inj:** 10mg/mL, 40mg/mL	***Adults:*** **IM/IV: Serious Infections:** 3mg/kg/day given q8h. **Life-Threatening Infections:** 5mg/kg/day tid-qid; reduce to 3mg/kg/day as soon as clinically indicated. Treat for 7-10 days; may need longer course in difficult and complicated infections. **Renal Impairment:** Reduced dose given q8h or usual dose given at prolonged intervals based on either CrCl or serum creatinine. **Dialysis:** 1-1.7mg/kg, depending on severity of infection, at end of each dialysis period. **Obese Patients:** Calculate dose based on estimated lean body mass. ***Pediatrics:*** **Children:** 6-7.5mg/kg/day (2-2.5mg/kg given q8h). **Infants and Neonates:** 7.5mg/kg/day (2.5mg/kg given q8h). **Premature and Full-Term Neonates ≤1 week:** 5mg/kg/day (2.5mg/kg given q12h). Treat for 7-10 days; may need longer course in difficult and complicated infections. **Renal Impairment:** Reduced dose given q8h or usual dose given at prolonged intervals based on either CrCl or serum creatinine. **Dialysis:** 2mg/kg at end of each dialysis period. **Obese Patients:** Calculate dose based on estimated lean body mass.	**Risk of toxicity is greater with impaired renal function, high dosage, or prolonged therapy. Monitor serum concentrations closely. Avoid prolonged peak levels >2mcg/mL and trough levels >2mcg/mL. Monitor renal and eight cranial nerve function, urine, BUN, SCr, and CrCl. Obtain serial audiograms. Advanced age and dehydration increase risk of toxicity. Adjust dose or discontinue use with evidence of ototoxicity or nephrotoxicity. May cause fetal harm during pregnancy. Avoid concurrent and/or sequential systemic or topical use of other potentially neurotoxic and/or nephrotoxic drugs, such as cisplatin, cephaloridine, kanamycin, amikacin, neomycin, polymyxin B, colistin, paromomycin, streptomycin, tobramycin, vancomycin, or viomycin. Avoid concurrent use with potent diuretics, such as ethacrynic acid or furosemide. W/P:** Contains metabisulfite. Neuromuscular blockade, respiratory paralysis, ototoxicity, and nephrotoxicity may occur after local irrigation or topical application during surgical procedures. Caution with neuromuscular disorders (eg, myasthenia gravis, or parkinsonism). Caution in elderly; monitor renal function. Keep patients well-hydrated during treatment. May cause fetal harm when administered to pregnant women. **P/N:** Category D, safety not known in nursing.	Nephrotoxicity, neurotoxicity, rash, fever, urticaria, nausea, vomiting, headache, lethargy, confusion, depression, decreased appetite, weight loss, BP changes, blood dyscrasias, and elevated LFTs.

*Scored.   † Bold entries denote special dental considerations.

Table 6.2: PRESCRIBING INFORMATION FOR ANTIBIOTICS (cont.)

NAME	FORM/ STRENGTH	DOSAGE	WARNINGS/PRECAUTIONS & CONTRAINDICATIONS	ADVERSE EFFECTS†
AMINOGLYCOSIDES (cont.)				
Tobramycin (TOBI)	**Sol:** 60mg/mL (300mg/ampule)	**Adults:** Inhale via nebulizer 300mg q12h for 28 days, then stop for 28 days. Resume therapy for next 28 day on/28 day off cycle. **Pediatrics: ≥6 years:** Inhale via nebulizer 300mg q12h for 28 days, then stop for 28 days. Resume therapy for next 28-day-on/28-day-off cycle.	**W/P:** Caution with muscular disorders (eg, myasthenia gravis, or Parkinson's disease), and renal, auditory, vestibular, or neuromuscular dysfunction. May cause hearing loss, bronchospasm. Can cause fetal harm in pregnancy. Discontinue if nephrotoxicity occurs until serum level <2mcg/mL. **P/N:** Category D, not for use in nursing.	Voice alteration, **taste perversion**, and tinnitus.
CARBACEPHEM				
Loracarbef (Lorabid)	**Cap:** 200mg, 400mg; **Sus:** 100mg/5mL, 200mg/5mL [50mL, 100mL]	**Adults: Acute Bronchitis:** 200-400mg q12h for 7 days. **Chronic Bronchitis:** 400mg q12h for 7 days. **Pneumonia:** 400mg q12h for 14 days. **Pharyngitis/Tonsillitis:** 200mg q12h for 10 days. **Sinusitis:** 400mg q12h for 10 days. **Cystitis:** 200mg qd for 7 days. **Pyelonephritis:** 400mg q12h for 14 days. **SSSI:** 200mg q12h for 7 days. **CrCl 10-49mL/min:** Give 50% dose or double interval. **CrCl <10mL/min:** Usual dose every 3-5 days. Take 1hr before or 2hrs after meals. **Pediatrics: ≥13 yrs: Acute Bronchitis:** 200-400mg q12h for 7 days. **ABECB:** 400mg q12h for 7 days. **Pneumonia:** 400mg q12h for 14 days. **Pharyngitis/Tonsillitis:** 200mg q12h for 10 days. **Sinusitis:** 400mg q12h for 10 days. **Cystitis:** 200mg qd for 7 days. **Pyelonephritis:** 400mg q12h for 14 days. **SSSI:** 200mg q12h for 7 days. Take 1hr before or 2hrs after meals. **6 mo-12 yrs: Otitis Media:** (Sus Only) 15mg/kg q12h for 10 days. **Sinusitis:** 15mg/kg q12h for 10 days. **Pharyngitis/Tonsillitis:** 7.5mg q12h for 10 days. **Impetigo:** 7.5mg/kg q12h for 7 days. Take 1hr before or 2hrs after meals.	**W/P:** Determine if history of penicillin, cephalosporin, or other drug allergy. Cross-sensitivity of 10% with penicillin allergy. Caution in renal dysfunction or colitis. May cause superinfection or pseudomembranous colitis. **Contra:** Hypersensitivity to cephalosporins. **P/N:** Category B, caution in nursing.	All patients: Diarrhea, abdominal pain, nausea, vomiting, rash, headache, vaginitis, and vaginal moniliasis. Pediatrics: Anorexia, somnolence, and rhinitis.
CARBAPENEM				
Cilastin Sodium/Imipenem (Primaxin IM)	**Inj:** (Imipenem-Cilastatin) 500mg-500mg, 750mg-750mg	**Adults:** Dose according to imipenem. **Mild to Moderate LRTI/SSSI/Gynecologic Infection:** 500mg or 750mg IM q12h depending on severity. **Intra-Abdominal Infection:** 750mg IM q12h. Continue for at least 2 days after symptoms resolve. **Elderly:** Start at low end of dosing range. Continue for at least 2 days after symptoms resolve; do not treat >14 days. **Max:** 1500mg/day. Avoid if CrCl <20mL/min. **Pediatrics: ≥12 yrs:** Dose according to imipenem. **Mild to Moderate LRTI/SSSI/Gynecologic Infection:** 500mg or 750mg IM q12h depending on severity. **Intra-Abdominal Infection:** 750mg IM q12h. Continue for at least 2 days after symptoms resolve; do not treat >14 days. **Max:** 1500mg/day. Avoid if CrCl <20mL/min.	**W/P:** Serious, fatal hypersensitivity reactions reported. Increased incidence of reactions with previous hypersensitivity to cephalosporins, penicillins, other β-lactams, and other allergens. Pseudomembranous colitis reported. Prolonged use may result in overgrowth of nonsusceptible organisms. Avoid injection into blood vessel. Caution in elderly. CNS adverse events (eg, myoclonic activity, confusion, or seizures) reported most commonly with CNS disorders and renal dysfunction; discontinue if these occur. **Contra:** Severe shock, heart block, or hypersensitivity to local anesthetics of amide type (due to lidocaine diluent). **P/N:** Category C, caution in nursing.	Injection-site pain, nausea, diarrhea, fever, vomiting, rash, hypotension, seizures, dizziness, pruritus, urticaria, and somnolence.

*Scored.   † Bold entries denote special dental considerations.

NAME	FORM/ STRENGTH	DOSAGE	WARNINGS/PRECAUTIONS & CONTRAINDICATIONS	ADVERSE EFFECTS†
Cilastin Sodium/ Imipenem (Primaxin IV)	**Inj:** (Imipe-nem-Cilastatin) 250mg-250mg, 500mg-500mg	**Adults: ≥70kg and CrCl >70mL/min:** Dose based on imipenem component. **Uncomplicated UTI:** 250mg q6h. **Complicated UTI:** 500mg q6h. **Mild Infection:** 250-500mg q6h. **Moderate Infection:** 500mg q6-8h or 1g q8h. **Severe, Life-Threatening Infection:** 500mg-1g q6h or 1g q8h. **Max dose:** 50mg/kg/day or 4g/day, whichever is lower. **Renal Impairment and/or <70kg:** Refer to prescribing information. **CrCl 6-20mL/min:** 125-250mg q12h. **CrCl ≤5mL/min:** Administer hemodialysis within 48hrs of dose.	**W/P:** Serious, fatal hypersensitivity reactions reported. Increased incidence of reactions with previous hypersensitivity to cephalosporins, penicillins, other β-lactams, and other allergens. Pseudomembranous colitis reported. Prolonged use may result in overgrowth of nonsusceptible organisms. CNS adverse events (eg, myoclonic activity, confusion, or seizures) reported most commonly with CNS disorders and renal dysfunction. **P/N:** Category C, caution in nursing.	Phlebitis/thrombophlebitis, nausea, diarrhea, vomiting, rash, fever, hypotension, seizures, dizziness, pruritus, urticaria, and somnolence.
Ertapenem (Invanz)	**Inj:** 1g	**Adults:** 1g IM/IV qd. **Treatment Duration: Intra-Abdominal Infection:** 5-14 days. **SSSI:** 7-14 days. **CAP/UTI:** 10-14 days. **Pelvic Infection:** 3-10 days. May administer IV for up to 14 days and IM for up to 7 days. **CrCl ≤30mL/min:** 500mg IM/IV qd. **HemoDialysis:** Give 150mg IM/IV after dialysis only if 500mg dose was given within 6hrs prior to dialysis.	**W/P:** Anaphylactic reactions reported with β-lactam therapy; increased incidence with sensitivity to multiple allergens. Seizures, CNS adverse experiences, and pseudomembranous colitis reported. Increased risk of seizures with CNS disorders and/or compromised renal function. Use lidocaine HCl as the diluent; avoid dextrose-containing diluents. Monitor renal, hepatic, and hematopoietic functions during prolonged therapy. Do not inject into blood vessel. **Contra:** Hypersensitivity to drugs in same class, anaphylactic reactions to β-lactams, and hypersensitivity to local anesthetics of the amide type (due to lidocaine diluent). **P/N:** Category B, caution in nursing.	Diarrhea, infused vein complication, nausea, headache, vaginitis, edema/swelling, fever, abdominal pain, constipation, altered mental status, headache, insomnia, phlebitis/thrombophlebitis, and vomiting.
Meropenem (Merrem)	**Inj:** 500mg, 1g	**Adults: IV: Intra-Abdominal:** 1g q8h. **CrCl 26-50mL/min:** 1g q12h. **CrCl 10-25mL/min:** 500mg q12h. **CrCl <10mL/min:** 500mg q24h. **SSSI:** 500mg q8h. **CrCl 26-50mL/min:** 500mg q12h. **CrCl 10-25mL/min:** 250mg q12h. **CrCl <10mL/min:** 250mg q24h. **Pediatrics: IV: ≥3 months: >50kg: Intra-Abdominal:** 1g q8h. **Meningitis:** 2g q8h. **SSSI:** 500mg q8h. **≤50kg: Intra-Abdominal:** 20mg/kg q8h. **Max:** 1g q8h. **Meningitis:** 40mg/kg q8h. **Max:** 2g q8h. **SSSI:** 10mg/kg q8h. **Max:** 500mg q8h.	**W/P:** Severe and fatal hypersensitivity reactions reported; increased risk with allergens and/or penicillin sensitivity. Pseudomembranous colitis reported. Seizures and other CNS effects reported particularly with pre-existing CNS disorders, bacterial meningitis, and renal dysfunction. Thrombocytopenia reported with severe renal impairment. Prolonged use may result in superinfection. Use as monotherapy for meningitis caused by penicillin nonsusceptible strains of Streptococcus pneumoniae has not been established. **Contra:** Hypersensitivity to β-lactams. **P/N:** Category B, caution in nursing.	Headache, rash, local reactions, diarrhea, nausea, vomiting, and constipation.

CEPHALOSPORINS

NAME	FORM/ STRENGTH	DOSAGE	WARNINGS/PRECAUTIONS & CONTRAINDICATIONS	ADVERSE EFFECTS†
Cefaclor (Ceclor)	**Cap:** 250mg, 500mg; **Sus:** 125mg/5mL [150mL], 187mg/5mL [100mL], 250mg/5mL [75mL, 150mL], 375mg/5mL [100mL]	**Adults: Usual:** 250mg q8h. **Severe Infections/Pneumonia:** 500mg q8h. Treat β-hemolytic strep for 10 days. **Pediatrics: ≥1 month: Usual:** 20mg/kg/day given q8h. **Otitis Media/Serious Infections:** 40mg/kg/day. **Max:** 1g/day. May administer q12h for otitis media and pharyngitis. Treat β-hemolytic strep for 10 days.	**W/P:** Cross sensitivity to penicillins and other cephalosporins may occur. Pseudomembranous colitis reported. Positive direct Coombs' tests reported. Caution with markedly impaired renal function, history of GI disease. False (+) for urine glucose with Benedict's, Fehling's solution, and Clinitest tablets. **P/N:** Category B, caution in nursing.	Hypersensitivity reactions, diarrhea, eosinophilia, genital pruritus and vaginitis, serum-sickness-like reactions, and superinfection.

Table 6.2: PRESCRIBING INFORMATION FOR ANTIBIOTICS *(cont.)*

NAME	FORM/ STRENGTH	DOSAGE	WARNINGS/PRECAUTIONS & CONTRAINDICATIONS	ADVERSE EFFECTS†
CEPHALOSPORINS *(cont.)*				
Cefadroxil (Duricef)	**Cap:** 500mg; **Sus:** 250mg/5mL [50mL, 100mL], 500mg/5mL [50mL, 75mL, 100mL]; **Tab:** 1g*	***Adults:* Uncomplicated Lower UTI:** 1-2g/day given qd or bid. **Other UTI:** 1gm bid. **SSSI:** 1g qd or 500mg bid. **Group A β-hemolytic Strep Pharyngitis/Tonsillitis:** 1g qd or 500mg bid for 10 days. **CrCl ≤50mL/min: Initial:** 1g. **Maint:** CrCl 25-50mL/min: 500mg q12h; **CrCl 10-25mL/min:** 500mg q24h; **CrCl 0-10mL/min:** 500mg q36h. ***Pediatrics:* UTI/SSSI:** 15mg/kg q12h. **Pharyngitis/Tonsillitis/Impetigo:** 30mg/kg qd or 15mg/kg q12h. Treat β-hemolytic strep infections for at least 10 days.	**W/P:** Caution with markedly impaired renal function, history of GI disease. Cross-sensitivity with cephalosporins and penicillins. False (+) direct Coombs' tests and pseudomembranous colitis reported. **P/N:** Category B, Caution in nursing.	Diarrhea, rash, hypersensitivity reactions, pruritus, hepatic dysfunction, genital moniliasis, vaginitis, fever, and superinfection (prolonged use).
Cefdinir (Omnicef)	**Cap:** 300mg; **Sus:** 125mg/5mL, 250mg/5mL [60mL, 100mL]	***Adults:* (Cap) SSSI/CAP:** 300mg q12h for 10 days. **AECB/Pharyngitis/Tonsillitis:** 300mg q12h for 5-10 days or 600mg q24h for 10 days. **Sinusitis:** 300mg q12h or 600mg q24h for 10 days. **CrCl <30mL/min:** 300mg qd. ***Pediatrics:* (Sus) 6 months-12 years: Otitis Media/Pharyngitis/Tonsillitis:** 7mg/kg q12h for 5-10 days or 14mg/kg q24h for 10 days. **Sinusitis:** 7mg/kg q12h or 14mg/kg q24h for 10 days. **SSSI:** 7mg/kg q12h for 10 days. **(Cap) ≥13 years: CAP/SSSI:** 300mg q12h for 10 days. **AECB/Pharyngitis/Tonsillitis:** 300mg q12h for 5-10 days or 600mg q24h for 10 days. **Sinusitis:** 300mg q12h or 600mg q24h for 10 days. **CrCl <30mL/min/1.73m²:** 7mg/kg qd. **Max:** 300mg qd.	**W/P:** Cross sensitivity to penicillins and other cephalosporins may occur. Pseudomembranous colitis reported. Positive direct Coombs' tests may occur. Caution with renal dysfunction, history of colitis. Suspension contains 2.86g/5mL of sucrose; caution in diabetes. False (+) for urine glucose with Clinitest and Benedict's or Fehling's solution. **P/N:** Category B, Caution in nursing.	Diarrhea, vaginal moniliasis, nausea, headache, abdominal pain, and superinfection (prolonged use).
Cefditoren Pivoxil (Spectracef)	**Tab:** 200mg	***Adults:* ABECB:** 400mg bid for 10 days. **Pharyngitis/Tonsillitis/SSSI:** 200mg bid for 10 days. **CAP:** 400mg bid for 14 days. **CrCl 30-49mL/min:** 200mg bid. **CrCl <30mL/min:** 200mg qd. Take with meals. ***Pediatrics:* ≥12 years: ABECB:** 400mg bid for 10 days. **Pharyngitis/Tonsillitis/SSSI:** 200mg bid for 10 days. **CAP:** 400mg bid for 14 days. **CrCl 30-49mL/min:** 200mg bid. **CrCl <30mL/min:** 200mg qd. Take with meals.	**W/P:** Cross-sensitivity to penicillins and other cephalosporins. Pseudomembranous colitis reported. Not recommended for prolonged antibiotic therapy. Prolonged therapy may cause superinfection. May decrease PT. **Contra:** Milk protein hypersensitivity and carnitine deficiency. **P/N:** Category B, caution in nursing.	Diarrhea, nausea, and vaginal moniliasis.
Cefepime Hydrochloride (Maxipime)	**Inj:** 500mg, 1g, 2g	***Adults:* Moderate-Severe Pneumonia:** 1-2g IV q12h for 10 days. **Febrile Neutropenia Emperic Therapy:** 2g IV q8h for 7 days or until neutropenia resolved. **Mild-Moderate UTI:** 0.5-1g IM/IV q12h for 7-10 days. **Severe UTI/Moderate-Severe SSSI:** 2g IV q12h for 10 days. **Complicated Intra-Abdominal Infections:** 2g IV q12h for 7-10 days. **CrCl ≤60mL/min: Initial:** Same dose as normal renal function. **Maint:** Refer to prescribing information for dose-adjustment. ***Pediatrics:* 2 months-16 years: ≤40kg: UTI/SSSI/Pneumonia:** 50mg/kg IV q12h. **Febrile Neutropenia:** 50mg/kg IV q8h. **Max:** Do not exceed adult dose. **CrCl ≤60mL/min: Initial:** Same dose as normal renal function. **Maint:** Refer to prescribing information for dose-adjustment.	**W/P:** Caution with penicillin sensitivity; cross-hypersensitivity may occur. Pseudomembranous colitis reported. Treatment may result in overgrowth of nonsusceptible organisms. Caution with renal impairment and history of GI disease, especially colitis. Encephalopathy, myoclonus, seizures, and/or renal failure reported. Discontinue if seizure occurs. Associated with a fall in PT; monitor PT with renal or hepatic impairment, poor nutritional state, and protracted course of antimicrobials; give vitamin K as indicated. **P/N:** Category B, caution in nursing.	Local reactions (eg, phlebitis) rash, and diarrhea.

*Scored.   † Bold entries denote special dental considerations.

NAME	FORM/ STRENGTH	DOSAGE	WARNINGS/PRECAUTIONS & CONTRAINDICATIONS	ADVERSE EFFECTS[†]
Cefixime (Suprax)	**Sus:** 100mg/5mL [50mL, 75mL, 100mL]	***Adults:*** Usual: 400mg qd. **Gonorrhea:** 400mg single dose. **CrCl 21-60mL/min/ HemoDialysis:** Give 75% of standard dose. **CrCl <20mL/min/CAPD:** Give 50% of standard dose.	**W/P:** Caution with penicillin or other allergy, GI disease (eg, colitis). Ana-phylactic/anaphylactoid reactions and pseudomembranous colitis reported. May cause false (+) direct Coombs', Benedict's, Fehling's solution, Clinitest. **P/N:** Category B, caution in nursing.	Diarrhea, abdominal pain, nausea, dyspepsia, flatu-lence, and superinfection.
Cefotaxime (Claforan)	**Inj:** 500mg, 1g, 2g, 10g	***Adults:*** **Gonococcal Urethritis/Cervi-citis (males/females):** 500mg single dose IM. **Rectal Gonorrhea:** 0.5g (females) or 1g (males) single dose IM. **Uncomplicated Infections:** 1g IM/IV q12h. **Moderate-Severe Infections:** 1-2g IM/IV q8h. **Septicemia:** 2g IV q6-8h. **Life-Threatening Infections:** 2g IV q4h. **Max:** 12g/day. **Surgical Prophylaxis:** 1g IM/IV 30-90min before surgery. **Cesarean Section:** 1g IV when umbilical cord is clamped, then 1g IV at 6 and 12 hrs after 1st dose. **CrCl <20mL/min/1.73 m²:** Give 50% usual dose. ***Pediatrics:*** ≥50kg: Use adult dose. **Max:** 12g/day. **1 month-12 years and ≤50kg:** 50-180mg/ kg/day IM/IV divided in 4-6 doses. **1-4 weeks:** 50mg/kg IV q8h. **0-1 week:** 50mg/kg IV q12h. **CrCl <20mL/min/1.73 m²:** Give 50% usual dose.	**W/P:** Cross-sensitivity to penicillins and other cephalosporins may occur. Pseudomembranous colitis reported. May result in overgrowth of non-susceptible organisms. Caution with history of GI disease. Reduce dose with renal dysfunction. Granulocyto-penia may occur with long-term use. Monitor blood counts if therapy >10 days. Monitor injection site for tissue inflammation. False positive direct Coombs' tests reported. **P/N:** Category B, caution in nursing.	Injection-site reactions, rash, pruritus, fever, eosinophilia, colitis, and diarrhea.
Cefotetan (Cefotan)	**Inj:** 1g, 1g/50mL, 2g, 2g/50mL, 10g	***Adults:*** Usual: 1-2g IV q6-8h. **Un-complicated Infections:** 1g IV q6-8h. **Moderate-Severe:** 1g IV q4h or 2g IV q6-8h. **Gas Gangrene/Other Infections Requiring Higher Dose:** 2g IV q4h or 3g IV q6h. **Renal Insufficiency: LD:** 1-2g IV. **Maint:** **CrCl 30-50mL/min:** 1-2g IV q8-12h. **CrCl 10-29mL/min:** 1-2g IV q12-24h. **CrCl 5-9mL/min:** 0.5-1g IV q12-24h. **CrCl <5mL/min:** 0.5-1g IV q24-48h. **HemoDialysis: LD:** 1-2g IV after dialysis. **Maint:** See renal insuf-ficiency doses above. **Prophylaxis: Uncontaminated GI Surgery/Hyster-ectomy:** 2g IV 0.5-1hr prior to surgery, then 2g IV q6h after first dose up to 24hrs. **C-Section:** 2g IV single dose after umbilical cord is clamped, or 2g IV after umbilical cord is clamped fol-lowed by 2g IV 4 and 8hrs after initial dose. ***Pediatrics:*** ≥3 months: 80-160mg/kg/day divided into 4-6 equal doses. **Max:** 12g/day. **Prophylaxis: Uncontaminated GI Surgery/Hysterec-tomy:** 30-40mg/kg IV 0.5-1hr prior to surgery, then 30-40mg/kg IV q6h after first dose up to 24hrs.	**W/P:** Possible cross-sensitivity be-tween penicillins and cephalosporins. Pseudomembranous colitis reported. Caution with allergies and GI disease, particularly colitis. Prolonged use may result in overgrowth of nonsusceptible organisms. Monitor renal, hepatic, and hematopoietic functions, especially with prolonged therapy. False positive for urine glucose with Clinitest tablets. **P/N:** Category B, caution in nursing.	Thrombophlebitis, rash, pseudomembranous colitis, pruritus, fever, dyspnea hypotension, diarrhea, blood dyscrasias, elevated LFTs, changes in renal function tests, and exacerbation of myasthenia gravis.
Cefoxitin (Mefoxin)	**Inj:** 1g, 1g/50mL, 2g, 2g/50mL, 10g	***Adults:*** Usual: 1-2g IV q6-8h. **Uncomplicated Infections:** 1g IV q6-8h. **Moderate-Severe:** 1g IV q4h or 2g IV q6-8h. **Gas Gangrene/Other Infections Requiring Higher Dose:** 2g IV q4h or 3g IV q6h. **Renal Insufficiency: LD:** 1-2g IV. **Maint: CrCl 30-50mL/min:** 1-2g IV q8-12h. **CrCl 10-29mL/min:** 1-2g IV q12-24h. **CrCl 5-9mL/min:** 0.5-1g IV q12-24h. **CrCl <5mL/min:** 0.5-1g IV q24-48h. **HemoDialysis: LD:** 1-2g IV after dialysis. **Maint:** See renal insuffiency.	**W/P:** Possible cross-sensitivity be-tween penicillins and cephalosporins. Pseudomembranous colitis reported. Caution with allergies, GI disease, particularly colitis. Prolonged use may result in overgrowth of nonsusceptible organisms. Monitor renal, hepatic, hematopoietic functions, especially with prolonged therapy. False positive for urine glucose with Clinitest tablets. **P/N:** Category B, caution use in nursing.	Thrombophlebitis, rash, pseudomembranous colitis, pruritus, fever, diarrhea, blood dyscrasias, elevated LFTs, changes in renal function tests, and exacerbation of myasthenia gravis.

Table 6.2: PRESCRIBING INFORMATION FOR ANTIBIOTICS (cont.)

NAME	FORM/ STRENGTH	DOSAGE	WARNINGS/PRECAUTIONS & CONTRAINDICATIONS	ADVERSE EFFECTS†
CEPHALOSPORINS (cont.)				
Cefoxitin (cont.)		**Prophylaxis: Uncontaminated GI Surgery/Hysterectomy:** 2g IV 0.5-1 hr prior to surgery, then 2g IV q6h after first dose up to 24hrs. **C-Section:** 2g IV single dose after umbilical cord is clamped, or 2g IV after umbilical cord is clamped followed by 2g IV 4 and 8hrs after initial dose. **Pediatrics: ≥3 months:** 80-160mg/kg/day divided into 4-6 equal doses. **Max:** 12g/day. **Prophylaxis: Uncontaminated GI Surgery/Hysterectomy:** 30-40mg/kg IV 0.5-1 hr prior to surgery, then 30-40mg/kg IV q6h after first dose up to 24hrs.		
Cefpodoxime Proxetil (Vantin)	**Sus:** 50mg/5mL [50mL, 100mL], 100mg/5mL [50mL, 75mL, 100mL]; **Tab:** 100mg, 200mg	**Adults:** Take tabs with food. **Pharyngitis/Tonsillitis:** 100mg q12h for 5-10 days. **CAP:** 200mg q12h for 14 days. **ABECB:** 200mg q12h for 10 days. **Uncomplicated Gonorrhea (men and women)/Rectal Gonococcal Infections (women):** 200mg single dose. **SSSI:** 400mg q12h for 7-14 days. **Sinusitis:** 200mg q12h for 10 days. **UTI:** 100mg q12h for 7 days. **CrCl <30mL/min:** Increase interval to q24h. **HemoDialysis:** Dose 3x weekly after dialysis. **Pediatrics: ≥12 years:** Take tabs with food. **Pharyngitis/Tonsillitis:** 100mg q12h for 5-10 days. **CAP:** 200mg q12h for 14 days. **ABECB:** 200mg q12h for 10 days. **Uncomplicated Gonorrhea (men and women)/Rectal Gonococcal Infections (women):** 200mg single dose. **SSSI:** 400mg q12h for 7-14 days. **Sinusitis:** 200mg q12h for 10 days. **UTI:** 100mg q12h for 7 days. **2 months-11 years: Otitis Media:** 5mg/kg q12h for 5 days. **Max:** 200mg/dose. **Pharyngitis/Tonsillitis:** 5mg/kg q12h for 5-10 days. **Max:** 100mg/dose. **Sinusitis:** 5mg/kg q12h for 10 days. **Max:** 200mg/dose. **CrCl <30mL/min:** Increase interval to q24h. **HemoDialysis:** Dose 3x weekly after dialysis.	**W/P:** Cross-sensitivity to penicillins and other cephalosporins may occur. Pseudomembranous colitis reported. Positive direct Coombs' tests reported. Caution with renal dysfunction. **P/N:** Category B, not for use in nursing.	Diarrhea, nausea, vaginal fungal infections, vulvovaginal infections, abdominal pain, headache, and superinfection.
Cefprozil (Cefzil)	**Sus:** 125mg/5mL, 250mg/5mL [50mL, 75mL, 100mL]; **Tab:** 250mg, 500mg	**Adults: ≥13 yrs: Pharyngitis/Tonsillitis:** 500mg q24h for 10 days. **Acute Sinusitis:** 250-500mg q12h for 10 days. **ABECB/Acute Bronchitis:** 500mg q12h for 10 days. **SSSI:** 250-500mg q12h or 500mg q12h for 10 days. **CrCl <30mL/min:** 50% of standard dose. **Pediatrics: 2-12 years: Pharyngitis/Tonsillitis:** 7.5mg/kg q12h for 10 days. **SSSI:** 20mg/kg q24h for 10 days. **6 months-12 years: Otitis Media:** 15mg/kg q12h for 10 days. **Acute Sinusitis:** 7.5-15mg/kg q12h for 10 days. Do not exceed adult dose. **CrCl >30mL/min:** 50% of standard dose.	**W/P:** Cross-sensitivity with cephalosporins and penicillins. False (+) direct Coombs' tests reported. Pseudomembranous colitis reported. Caution with GI disease, renal impairment, elderly. False (+) for urine glucose with Benedict's, Fehling's solution, and Clinitest tablets. Suspension contains phenylalanine. **P/N:** Category B, caution in nursing.	Diarrhea, nausea, hepatic enzyme elevations, eosinophilia, genital pruritus, genital vaginitis, and superinfection (prolonged use).

*Scored.   † Bold entries denote special dental considerations.

NAME	FORM/ STRENGTH	DOSAGE	WARNINGS/PRECAUTIONS & CONTRAINDICATIONS	ADVERSE EFFECTS†
Ceftazidime (Fortaz, Tazicef)	**Inj:** 500mg, 1g, 1g/50mL, 2g, 2g/50mL, 6g (Fortaz). **Inj:** 1g, 2g, 6g (Tazicef)	***Adults:*** Usual: 1g IM/IV q8-12h. **UnComplicated UTI:** 250mg IM/IV q12h. **Complicated UTI:** 500mg IM/IV q8-12h. **Bone and Joint Infection:** 2g IV q12h. **Uncomplicated Pneumonia/SSSI:** 500mg-1g IM/IV q8h. **Gynecological/Intra-Abdominal/Meningitis/Severe Life-Threatening Infection:** 2g IV q8h. **Lung Infection caused by Pseudomonas in Cystic Fibrosis (normal renal function):** 30-50mg/kg IV q8h. **Max:** 6g/day. **Renal Impairment: CrCl 31-50mL/min:** 1g q12h. **CrCl 16-30mL/min:** 1g q24h. **CrCl 6-15mL/min:** 500mg q24h. **CrCl <5mL/min:** 500mg q48h. For severe infections (6g/day), increase renal impairment dose by 50% or increase dosing interval. Apply reduced dosage recommendations after initial 1g LD is given. **HemoDialysis:** Give 1g before and 1g after each hemodialysis. **Intra-Peritoneal Dialysis/Continuous Ambulatory Peritoneal Dialysis:** Give 1g followed by 500mg q24h, or add to fluid at 250mg/2L. ***Pediatrics:*** **Neonates (0-4 weeks):** 30mg/kg IV q12h. **1 month-12 years:** 30-50mg/kg IV q8h. **Max:** 6g/day. Higher doses for patients with cystic fibrosis or when treating meningitis. **Renal Impairment: CrCl 31-50mL/min:** 1g q12h. **CrCl 16-30mL/min:** 1g q24h. **CrCl 6-15mL/min:** 500mg q24h. **CrCl <5mL/min:** 500mg q48h. For severe infections (6g/day), increase renal impairment dose by 50% or increase dosing interval. Apply reduced dosage recommendations after initial 1g LD is given. **HemoDialysis:** Give 1g before and 1g after each hemodialysis. **Intra-Peritoneal Dialysis/Continuous Ambulatory Peritoneal Dialysis:** Give 1g followed by 500mg q24h, or add to fluid at 250mg/2L.	**W/P:** Monitor renal function; potential for nephrotoxicity. Prolonged use may result in overgrowth of nonsusceptible organisms. Possible cross-sensitivity between penicillins, cephalosporins, and other β-lactam antibiotics. Pseudomembranous colitis reported. Elevated levels with renal insufficiency can lead to seizures, encephalopathy, coma, asterixis, and neuromuscular excitability. Possible decrease in PT; caution with renal or hepatic impairment or poor nutritional state; monitor PT and give vitamin K if needed. Caution with colitis, other GI diseases, and the elderly. Distal necrosis can occur after inadvertent intra-arterial administration. Continue therapy for 2 days after the signs and symptoms of infection have disappeared, but in complicated infections longer therapy may be required. False positive for urine glucose with Benedict's solution, Fehling's solution, and Clinitest tablets. **P/N:** Category B, caution in nursing.	Phlebitis and inflammation at injection site, pruritus, rash, fever, and diarrhea.
Ceftibuten (Cedax)	**Cap:** 400mg; **Sus:** 90mg/5mL [30mL, 60mL, 90mL, 120mL]	***Adults:*** **ABECB/Otitis Media/Pharyngitis/Tonsillitis:** 400mg qd for 10 days. **Max:** 400mg/day. **CrCl 30-49mL/min:** 4.5mg/kg or 200mg qd. **CrCl 5-29mL/min:** 2.25mg/kg or 100mg qd. Take 2hrs before or at least 1hr after a meal. ***Pediatrics:*** **≥6 months: Pharyngitis/Tonsillitis/Otitis Media:** 9mg/kg qd for 10 days. **Max:** 400mg. **ABECB/Otitis Media/Pharyngitis/Tonsillitis:** **≥12 years:** 400mg qd for 10 days. **Max:** 400mg/day. **CrCl 30-49mL/min:** 4.5mg/kg or 200mg qd. **CrCl 5-29mL/min:** 2.25mg/kg or 100mg qd. Take 2hrs before or at least 1hr after a meal.	**W/P:** Pseudomembranous colitis reported. Caution with history of GI disease. Cross-sensitivity with cephalosporins and penicillins. **P/N:** Category B, caution in nursing.	Diarrhea, vomiting, abdominal pain, anorexia, dizziness, dyspepsia, **dry mouth**, dyspnea, dysuria, fatigue, flatulence, loose stools, headache, pruritus, rash, rigors, urticaria, and superinfection (prolonged use).

Table 6.2: PRESCRIBING INFORMATION FOR ANTIBIOTICS *(cont.)*

NAME	FORM/ STRENGTH	DOSAGE	WARNINGS/PRECAUTIONS & CONTRAINDICATIONS	ADVERSE EFFECTS†
CEPHALOSPORINS *(cont.)*				
Ceftizoxime Sodium (Cefizox)	**Inj:** 1g, 2g, 10g	**Adults: UnComplicated UTI:** 500mg q12h IM/IV. **Other Sites:** 1g q8-12h IM/IV. **Severe/Refractory Infections:** 1-2g IM/IV q8-12h. **PID:** 2g IV q8h. **Life-Threatening Infections:** 3-4g IV q8h. **Uncomplicated Gonorrhea:** 1g IM as single dose. **Renal Impairment: LD:** 500mg-1g IM/IV. **Less-Severe Infection: Maint: CrCl 50-79mL/min:** 500mg q8h. **CrCl 5-49mL/min:** 250-500mg q12h. **CrCl 0-4mL/min (Dialysis):** 500mg q48h or 250mg q24h. **Life-Threatening Infection: Maint: CrCl 50-79mL/min:** 0.75-1.5g q8h. **CrCl 5-49mL/min:** 0.5-1g q12h. **CrCl 0-4mL/min (Dialysis):** 0.5-1g q48h or 0.5g q24h. **Pediatrics: ≥6 months:** 50mg/kg IM/IV q6-8h, up to 200mg/kg/day. **Max:** 6g/day for serious infections.	**W/P:** Pseudomembranous colitis reported. Caution with history of GI disease. Cross-sensitivity with cephalosporins and penicillins. Prolonged use may result in overgrowth of super-infection, positive Coombs' test. **P/N:** Category B, caution in nursing.	Rash, pruritus, fever, BUN elevation, injection-site reactions (eg, burning, cellulitis, phlebitis, pain, induration, or tenderness), eosinophilia, thrombocytosis, elevated liver enzymes, and GI effects.
Ceftriaxone (Rocephin)	**Inj:** 250mg, 500mg, 1g, 2g, 10g	**Adults: Usual:** 1-2g/day IV/IM given qd-bid. **Max:** 4g/day. **Gonorrhea:** 250mg IM single dose. **Surgical Prophylaxis:** 1g IV 0.5-2hrs before surgery. **Pediatrics: Skin Infections:** 50-75mg/kg/day IV/IM qd-bid. **Max:** 2g/day. **Otitis Media:** 50mg/kg (up to 1g) IM single dose. **Serious Infections:** 50-75mg/kg/day IM/IV q12h. **Max:** 2g/day. **Meningitis: Initial:** 100mg/kg (up to 4g), then 100mg/kg/day qd-bid for 7-14 days. **Max:** 4g/day.	**W/P:** Cross-sensitivity to penicillins and other cephalosporins may occur. Pseudomembranous colitis reported. May result in overgrowth of nonsusceptible organisms. Altered PT, transient BUN and SCr elevations may occur. Do not exceed 2g/day and monitor blood levels with both hepatic and renal dysfunction. Caution with history of GI disease. Discontinue if develop gallbladder disease. May alter PT; monitor with impaired vitamin K synthesis or low vitamin K stores. Avoid in hyper-bilirubinemic neonates, especially prematures. **P/N:** Category B, caution in nursing.	Injection-site reactions, eosinophilia, thrombocytosis, diarrhea, and SGOT and SGPT elevations.
Cefuroxime Axetil (Ceftin)	**Sus:** 125mg/ 5mL [100mL], 250mg/5mL [50mL, 100mL]; **Tab:** 125mg, 250mg, 500mg	**Adults: (Tab) Pharyngitis/Tonsillitis/Sinusitis:** 250mg bid for 10 days. **ABECB/SSSI:** 250-500mg bid for 10 days. **Acute Bronchitis:** 250-500mg bid for 5-10 days. **UTI:** 125-250mg bid for 7-10 days. **Gonorrhea:** 1000mg single dose. **Lyme Disease:** 500mg bid for 20 days. **Pediatrics: ≥13 years: (Tab) Pharyngitis/Tonsillitis/Sinusitis:** 250mg bid for 10 days. **ABECB/SSSI:** 250-500mg bid for 10 days. **Acute Bronchitis:** 250-500mg bid for 5-10 days. **UTI:** 125-250mg bid for 7-10 days. **Gonorrhea:** 1000mg single dose. **Lyme Disease:** 500mg bid for 20 days. **3 months-12 years: (Sus) Pharyngitis/Tonsillitis:** 10mg/kg bid for 10 days. **Max:** 500mg/day. **Otitis Media/Sinusitis/Impetigo:** 15mg/kg bid for 10 days. **Max:** 1000mg/day. **(Tab-if can swallow whole) Pharyngitis/Tonsillitis:** 125mg bid for 10 days. **Otitis Media/Sinusitis:** 250mg bid for 10 days.	**W/P:** Tablets are not bioequivalent to suspension. Caution with colitis, renal impairment. Cross-sensitivity with cephalosporins and penicillins. Pseudomembranous colitis reported. False (+) for urine glucose with Benedict's, Fehling's solution, and Clinitest tablets. May cause fall in PT; risk in patients stable on anticoagulants, if receiving protracted course of antibiotics, renal/hepatic impairment, or a poor nutritional state; give vitamin K as needed. **P/N:** Category B, not for use in nursing.	All patients: Diarrhea, nausea, vomiting, vaginitis. Pediatrics (suspension): **taste dislike**, superinfection (prolonged use).

*Scored. † Bold entries denote special dental considerations.

NAME	FORM/ STRENGTH	DOSAGE	WARNINGS/PRECAUTIONS & CONTRAINDICATIONS	ADVERSE EFFECTS†
Cefuroxime Sodium (Zinacef)	**Inj:** 750mg, 1.5g, 7.5g, 750mg/50mL, 1.5g/50mL	**Adults:** Usual: 750mg-1.5g q8h, for 5-10 days. **Uncomplicated Pneumonia and UTI/SSSI/Disseminated Gonococcal Infections:** 750mg q8h. **Severe/Complicated Infections:** 1.5g q8h. **Bone and Joint Infections:** 1.5g q8h. **Life-Threatening Infections/Infections With Susceptible Organisms:** 1.5g q6h. **Meningitis: Max:** 3g q8h. **Uncomplicated Gonococcal Infection:** 1.5g IM single dose at two different sites with 1g PO probenecid. **Surgical Prophylaxis:** 1.5g IV 0.5-1 hr before incision, then 750mg IM/IV q8h with prolonged procedure. **Open-Heart Surgery (Perioperative):** 1.5g IV at induction of anesthesia and q12h thereafter for total of 6g. **CrCl 10-20mL/min:** 750mg q12h. **CrCl <10mL/min:** 750mg q24h. **HemoDialysis:** Give further dose at end of dialysis. **Pediatrics: >3 months: Usual:** 50-100 mg/kg/day in divided doses q6-8h. **Severe Infections:** 100mg/kg/day (not to exceed max adult dose). **Bone and Joint Infections:** 150mg/kg/day in divided doses q8h (not to exceed max adult dose). **Meningitis:** 200-240mg/kg/day IV in divided doses q6-8h. **Renal Dysfunction:** Modify dosing frequency consistent with adult recommendations.	**W/P:** Cross-sensitivity to penicillins and other cephalosporins may occur. Pseudomembranous colitis reported. Monitor renal function. May result in overgrowth of nonsusceptible organisms. Caution with history of GI disease, particularly colitis. Hearing loss in pediatics being treated for meningitis. Risk of decreased prothrombin activity with renal or hepatic impairment, poor nutritional state, or protracted course of therapy. False (+) urine glucose with copper reduction tests and false (-) with ferricyanide test. **P/N:** Category B, caution in nursing.	Thrombophlebitis, GI symptoms, decreased Hgb and Hct, and eosinophilia. Transient rise in SGOT, SGPT, alkaline phosphatase, and bilirubin.
Cephalexin (Keflex)	**Cap:** 250mg, 500mg; **Sus:** 125mg/5ml, 250mg/5ml [100ml, 200ml]	**Adults:** Usual: 250mg q6h. **Streptococcal Pharyngitis/SSSI/Uncomplicated Cystitis (>15 years):** 500mg q12h. Treat cystitis for 7-14 days. **Max:** 4g/day. **Pediatrics:** Usual: 25-50mg/kg/day in divided doses. **Streptococcal Pharyngitis (>1 year)/SSSI:** May divide into 2 doses, give q12h. **Otitis Media:** 75-100mg/kg/day given qid.	**W/P:** Caution with markedly impaired renal function, history of GI disease. Cross-sensitivity with cephalosporins and penicillins. Pseudomembranous colitis reported. False (+) direct Coombs' tests reported. False (+) for urine glucose with Benedict's, Fehling's solution, and Clinitest tablets. **P/N:** Category B, caution in nursing.	Diarrhea, allergic reactions, dyspepsia, gastritis, abdominal pain, and superinfection (prolonged use).
Cephalexin (Panixine Disperdose)	**Tab for Oral Sus:** 125mg, 250mg	**Adults: ≥15 yrs:** Usual: 250mg q6h. **Streptococcal Pharyngitis and Skin and Skin-Structure Infections:** 500mg q12h. **Cystitis:** 500mg q12h for min 7-14 days. **Max:** 4g/day. Do not crush, cut, or chew tab. Treat β-hemolytic streptococcal infections for ≥10 days.	**W/P:** Caution with markedly impaired renal function and history of GI disease. Cross-sensitivity with cephalosporins and penicillins. Pseudomembranous colitis reported. False (+) direct Coombs' tests reported. False (+) for urine glucose with Benedict's, Fehling's solution, and Clinitest tablets. **P/N:** Category B, caution in nursing.	Diarrhea, allergic reactions, dyspepsia, gastritis, abdominal pain, rash, urticaria, anal pruritus, monilliasis, vaginitis, dizziness, fatigue, headache, and superinfection (prolonged use).
Cephradine (Velosef)	**Cap:** 250mg, 500mg; **Sus:** 125mg/5ml, 250mg/5ml	**Adults: Infection of Skin or Subcutaneous Tissue:** 250mg qid or 500mg q12hrs. **RTI:** 250mg qid or 500mg qd. **Lobar Pneumonia:** 500mg q6hrs or 1g q12hrs. **UTI Chronic:** up to 1 g q6hrs. **UTI, Serious:** 500mg q6hrs. **UTI Uncomplicated:** 500mg q12hrs. **UTI (Severe):** up to 1g q6hrs. **Pediatrics: Otitis Media:** 25-50mg/kg/day divided q6-12hrs. **Otitis Due to H. influenzae:** 75-100mg/kg/day divided q6-12hrs. **Max:** 4g/day.	**W/P:** Caution with markedly impaired renal function, history of GI disease. Cross-sensitivity with cephalosporins and penicillins. Pseudomembranous colitis reported. False (+) direct Coombs' tests reported. False (+) for urine glucose with Benedict's, Fehling's solution, and Clinitest tablets. **P/N:** Category B, caution in nursing.	Diarrhea, allergic reactions, dyspepsia, gastritis, abdominal pain, rash, urticaria, anal pruritus, monilliasis, vaginitis, dizziness, fatigue, headache, and superinfection (prolonged use).

Table 6.2: PRESCRIBING INFORMATION FOR ANTIBIOTICS *(cont.)*

NAME	FORM/ STRENGTH	DOSAGE	WARNINGS/PRECAUTIONS & CONTRAINDICATIONS	ADVERSE EFFECTS†
CYCLIC LIPOPEPTIDE				
Daptomycin (Cubicin)	**Inj:** 500mg	***Adults:* ≥18 years:** Administer as IV infusion over 30min. 4mg/kg once every 24hrs for 7-14 days. **Renal Impairment: CrCl <30mL/min/Hemodialysis or CAPD:** 4mg/kg once every 48hrs.	**W/P:** Pseudomembranous colitis and neuropathy reported. Monitor CPK levels weekly; discontinue if unexplained signs and symptoms of myopathy occur with CPK elevation >1000 U/L (~5X ULN), or with CPK levels ≥10X ULN. **P/N:** Category B, caution in nursing.	Constipation, nausea, injection-site reactions, headache, diarrhea, insomnia, rash, vomiting, abnormal LFTs, and superinfection.
FLUOROQUINOLONES				
Ciprofloxacin (Cipro IV)	**Inj:** 10mg/mL, 200mg/100mL, 400mg/200mL	***Adults:* ≥18 years: IV: UTI: Mild-Moderate:** 200mg q12h for 7-14 days. **Complicated/Severe:** 400mg q12h for 7-14 days. **LRTI/SSSI: Mild-Moderate:** 400mg q12h for 7-14 days. **Complicated/Severe:** 400mg q8h for 7-14 days. **Bone and Joint: Mild-Moderate:** 400mg q12h for ≥4-6 weeks. **Complicated/Severe:** 400mg q8h for ≥4-6 weeks. Nosocomial **Pneumonia:** 400mg q8h for 10-14 days. **Complicated Intra-Abdominal:** 400mg q12h (w/metronidazole) for 7-14 days. **Acute Sinusitis:** 400mg q12h for 10 days. **Chronic Bacterial Prostatitis:** 400mg q12h for 28 days. **Febrile Neutropenia:** 400mg q8h (w/piperacillin 50mg/kg q4h) for 7-14 days. **Max:** 24g/day. **Inhalational Anthrax:** 400mg q12h for 60 days. Administer over 60min. **CrCl 5-29mL/min:** 200-400mg q18-24h. ***Pediatrics:* <18 yrs: Inhalational Anthrax:** 10mg/kg q12h for 60 days. **Max:** 400mg/dose; 800mg/day. **1-17 years: Complicated UTI/Pyleonephritis:** 6-10mg/kg q8h for 10-21 days. **Max:** 400mg/dose.	**W/P:** Convulsions, increased intracranial pressure, and toxic psychosis reported. Caution with CNS disorders or if predisposed to seizures. Severe, fatal hypersensitivity reactions may occur. Pseudomembranous colitis, achilles, and other tendon ruptures reported. Discontinue at first sign of rash/hypersensitivity or if pain, inflammation, or ruptured tendon occur. May permit overgrowth of clostridia. Maintain hydration; avoid alkaline urine. Avoid excessive sunlight and UV light. Do not give via feeding tube. Monitor renal, hepatic, and hematopoietic function with prolonged use. Dose adjustment with renal dysfunction. **Contra:** Concomitant administration with tizanidine. **P/N:** Category C, not for use in nursing.	Nausea, diarrhea, CNS disturbances, local IV site reactions, hepatic enzyme abnormalities, eosinophilia, headache, restlessness, and rash.
Ciprofloxacin (Cipro)	**Sus:** 250mg/5mL, 500mg/5mL [100mL]; **Tab:** 250mg, 500mg, 750mg	***Adults:* ≥18 years: Acute Sinusitis/Typhoid Fever:** 500mg q12h for 10 days. **LRTI/SSSI: Mild-Moderate:** 500mg q12h for 7-14 days. **Severe/Complicated:** 750mg q12h for 7-14 days. **Cystitis/UTI:** 100-250mg q12h for 3 days. **UTI: Mild-Moderate:** 250mg q12h for 7-14 days. **Severe/Complicated:** 500mg q12h for 7-14 days. **Chronic Bacterial Prostatitis:** 500mg q12h for 28 days. **Intra-Abdominal:** 500mg q12h (w/ metronidazole) for 7-14 days. **Bone and Joint: Mild-Moderate:** 500mg q12h for ≥4-6 weeks. **Severe/Complicated:** 750mg q12h for ≥4-6 weeks. **Infectious Diarrhea:** 500mg q12h for 5-7 days. **Uncomplicated Urethral/Cervical Gonococcal:** 250mg single dose. **Inhalational Anthrax:** 500mg q12h for 60 days. **CrCl 30-50mL/min:** 250-500mg q12h. **CrCl 5-29mL/min:** 250-500mg q18h. **Hemodialysis/Peritoneal Dialysis:** 250-500mg q24h (after dialysis). Administer at least 2hrs before or 6hrs after magnesium or aluminum containing antacids, sucralfate, Videx; (didanosine) chewable/buffered tablets	**W/P:** Convulsions, increased intracranial pressure, and toxic psychosis reported. Caution with CNS disorders or if predisposed to seizures. Severe, fatal hypersensitivity reactions may occur. Pseudomembranous colitis and achilles and other tendon ruptures reported. Discontinue at first sign of rash/hypersensitivity or if pain, inflammation, or ruptured tendon occur. May permit overgrowth of clostridia. Maintain hydration; avoid alkaline urine. Avoid excessive sunlight and UV light. Do not give via feeding tube. Monitor renal, hepatic, and hematopoietic function with prolonged use. Dose adjustment with renal dysfunction. **Contra:** Concomitant administration with tizanidine. **P/N:** Category C, not for use in nursing.	Nausea, dizziness, headache, CNS disturbances, vomiting, diarrhea, rash, and abdominal pain/discomfort.

*Scored. † Bold entries denote special dental considerations.

NAME	FORM/ STRENGTH	DOSAGE	WARNINGS/PRECAUTIONS & CONTRAINDICATIONS	ADVERSE EFFECTS†
Ciprofloxacin (cont.)		or pediatric powder, or other products containing calcium, iron, or zinc. *Pediatrics*: <18 yrs: **Inhalational Anthrax:** 15mg/kg q12h for 60 days. **Max:** 500mg/dose. **1-17 years: Complicated UTI/Pyelonephritis:** 10-20mg/kg q12h for 10-21 days. **Max:** 750mg/dose.		
Ciprofloxacin (Cipro XR)	Tab, ER: 500mg, 1000mg	*Adults*: ≥18 years: **UnComplicated UTI:** 500mg qd for 3 days. **Complicated UTI:** 1000mg qd for 7-14 days. **CrCl <30mL/min:** 500mg qd. **Acute Uncomplicated Pyelonephritis:** 1000mg qd for 7-14 days. **CrCl <30mL/min:** 500mg qd. Take with fluids. Administer at least 2hrs before or 6hrs after magnesium or aluminum containing antacids, sucralfate, Videx; (didanosine) chewable/buffered tablets or pediatric powder, metal cations (eg, iron), or multivitamins with zinc. Avoid concomitant administration with dairy products alone or with calcium-fortified products. Space concomitant calcium intake (>800mg) by at least 2hrs. Do not split, crush, or chew. Swallow tab whole. **Dialysis:** Give after procedure is completed.	**W/P:** Convulsions, increased intracranial pressure, and toxic psychosis reported. Caution with CNS disorders or if predisposed to seizures. Severe, fatal hypersensitivity reactions may occur. Pseudomembranous colitis and achilles and other tendon ruptures reported. Discontinue at first sign of rash/hypersensitivity or if pain, inflammation, or ruptured tendon occur. May permit overgrowth of clostridia. Maintain hydration; avoid alkaline urine. Avoid excessive sunlight and UV light. Do not give via feeding tube. Monitor renal, hepatic, and hematopoietic function with prolonged use. Dose adjustment with renal dysfunction. **Contra:** Concomitant administration with tizanidine. **P/N:** Category C, not for use in nursing.	Nausea and headache.
Gatifloxacin (Tequin)	Inj: 2mg/mL (in 5% dextrose),10mg/mL; Tab: 200mg, 400mg [Teq-Paq, 7 tabs]	*Adults*: ≥18 yrs: **(PO/IV) Complicated UTI/Pyelonephritis/UnComplicated SSSI:** 400mg qd for 7-10 days. **ABECB:** 400mg qd for 5 days. **Sinusitis:** 400mg qd for 10 days. **CAP:** 400mg qd for 7-14 days. **Uncomplicated UTI (cystitis):** 400mg single dose or 200mg qd for 3 days. **Uncomplicated Urethral Gonorrhea (Men)/Endocervical and Rectal Gonorrhea (Women):** 400mg single dose. **CrCl ≥40mL/min:** 400mg qd. **CrCl <40mL/min or Dialysis:** 400mg on day 1, then 200mg qd.	**W/P:** May prolong QTc interval; avoid in patients with QTc-interval prolongation or uncorrected hypokalemia. Caution with proarrhythmic conditions, renal dysfunction, CNS disorders, or conditions that may predispose to seizures. Discontinue at first sign of hypersensitivity (eg, rash). Convulsions, increased intracranial pressure, psychosis, CNS stimulation, and fatal hypersensitivity reactions reported with quinolones. Pseudomembranous colitis reported. Stop therapy if pain, inflammation, or ruptured tendon occurs. May alter glucose levels; monitor closely. Potential for photosensitivity reaction. May cause CNS events (eg, nervousness, agitation, insomnia, anxiety, or nightmares). **P/N:** Category C, caution in nursing.	Nausea, diarrhea, vaginitis, headache, and dizziness.
Gemifloxacin (Factive)	Tab: 320mg	*Adults*: ≥18 years: **ABECB:** 320mg qd for 5 days. **CAP:** 320mg qd for 7 days. **Renal Impairment: CrCl ≤40mL/min or Dialysis:** 160mg qd. Take with fluids.	**W/P:** May prolong QT interval; avoid in patients with a history of prolonged QTc interval or uncontrolled electrolyte disorders. Caution with proarrhythmic conditions or epilepsy or if predisposed to convulsions. Discontinue at first sign of hypersensitivity (eg, rash). CNS effects, photosensitivity reactions, and hypersensitivity reactions (some fatal) reported; discontinue if any of these occur. Pseudomembranous colitis and Achilles and other tendon rupture reported. Stop therapy if rash, pain, inflammation, or ruptured tendon occurs. Avoid excessive sunlight and UV light. Maintain hydration. **P/N:** Category C, not for use in nursing.	Diarrhea, rash, and nausea.

NAME	FORM/ STRENGTH	DOSAGE	WARNINGS/PRECAUTIONS & CONTRAINDICATIONS	ADVERSE EFFECTS†
FLUOROQUINOLONES *(cont.)*				
Levofloxacin (Levaquin)	**Inj:** 5mg/mL, 25mg/mL; **Sol:** 25mg/mL; **Tab:** 250mg, 500mg, 750mg [Leva-pak, 5⁵]	***Adults:*** **≥18 years: IV/PO: ABECB:** 500mg qd for 7 days. **CAP:** 500mg qd for 7-14 days or 750mg qd for 5 days. **Sinusitis:** 500mg qd for 10-14 days or 750mg qd for 5 days. **CBP:** 500mg qd for 28 days. **UnComplicated SSSI:** 500mg qd for 7-10 days. **Complicated SSSI/Nosocomial Pneumonia:** 750mg qd for 7-14 days. **Inhalational Anthrax:** 500mg qd for 60 days. **Complicated SSSI/Nosocomial Pneumonia/CAP/Sinusitis: CrCl 20-49mL/min:** 750mg, then 750mg q48h. **CrCl 10-19mL/min/Hemodialysis/CAPD:** 750mg, then 500mg q48h. **ABECB/CAP/Sinusitis/Uncomplicated SSSI/CBP/Inhalational Anthrax: CrCl 20-49mL/min:** 500mg, then 250mg q24h. **CrCl 10-19mL/min/Hemodialysis/CAPD:** 500mg, then 250mg q48h. **Complicated UTI/Acute Pyelonephritis:** 250mg qd for 10 days. **CrCl 10-19mL/min:** 250mg, then 250mg q48h. **UnComplicated UTI:** 250mg qd for 3 days. Take oral solution 1hr before or 2hrs after eating.	**W/P:** Only administer injection via IV infusion over a period of not less than 60 or 90min, depending on dosage. Convulsions, toxic psychoses, increased ICP, and CNS stimulation reported; Discontinue if any of these occur. Caution with CNS disorders that may predispose to seizures/lower seizure threshold (eg, epilepsy, renal insufficiency, or drug therapy). Hyper- or hypoglycemia with insulin or oral hypoglycemics. Moderate to severe phototoxicity can occur. Serious/fatal hypersensitivity reactions; discontinue at first sign of rash. Pseudomembranous colitis and torsade de pointes (rare) have been reported. May permit overgrowth of clostridia. Caution in renal insufficiency. Stop therapy if pain, inflammation, or ruptured tendon occurs. **P/N:** Category C, not for use in nursing.	Nausea, diarrhea, headache, insomnia, and constipation.
Lomefloxacin (Maxaquin)	**Tab:** 400mg*	***Adults:*** **≥18 years: ABECB:** 400mg qd for 10 days. **Uncomplicated Cystitis:** 400mg qd for 3 days (E.coli) or 10 days (*K. pneumoniae, P. mirabilis,* or *S. saprophyticus*). **Complicated UTI:** 400mg qd for 14 days. **Hemodialysis/ CrCl >10 to <40mL/min: LD:** 400mg. **Maint:** 200mg qd. **Preoperative Prevention: TRPB:** 400mg single dose 1-6hrs before procedure. **TUSP:** 400mg single dose 2-6hrs before procedure.	**W/P:** Moderate to severe phototoxicity, convulsions, pseudomembranous colitis, and serious fatal hypersensitivity reactions reported. Avoid in pregnancy and nursing. Not for empiric treatment of *P. bacteremia* or ABECB caused by *S. pneumoniae.* Caution with CNS disorder or those predisposed to seizures. Adjust dose in renal impairment. Discontinue if pain, inflammation, or tendon rupture occurs. Increased risk of tendon rupture in patients receiving concomitant corticosteriods. Maintain adequate hydration. Rare cases of sensory or sensorimotor axonal polyneuropathy have been reported; discontinue if symptoms of neuropathy occur. **P/N:** Category C, not for use in nursing.	Headache, nausea, photosensitivity, dizziness, diarrhea, and abdominal pain.
Moxifloxacin (Avelox)	**Inj:** 400mg/ 250mL; **Tab:** 400mg [ABC Pack, 5 tabs]	***Adults:*** **≥18 yrs: Sinusitis:** 400mg PO/ IV q24h for 10 days. **ABECB:** 400mg PO/IV q24h for 5 days. **SSSI:** 400mg PO/IV q24h for 7 days. **cSSSI:** 400mg PO/IV q24h for 7-21 days. **cIAI:** 400mg IV q24h for 5-14 days. **CAP:** 400mg PO/IV q24h for 7-14 days.	**W/P:** Avoid in pregnancy, nursing, and patients <18 years. QT prolongation may be dose or infusion rate dependent; do not exceed recommended dose. Avoid with known QT interval prolongation or uncorrected hypokalemia. Caution with ongoing proarrhythmic conditions (eg, significant bradycardia or acute MI). Pseudomembranous colitis reported. Caution with CNS disorders (eg, severe cerebral arteriosclerosis or epilepsy). Discontinue if convulsions, CNS effects, hypersensitivity reaction, or tendon rupture occurs. **P/N:** Category C, not for use in nursing.	Nausea, diarrhea, and dizziness.

*Scored.   † Bold entries denote special dental considerations.

NAME	FORM/ STRENGTH	DOSAGE	WARNINGS/PRECAUTIONS & CONTRAINDICATIONS	ADVERSE EFFECTS†
Norfloxacin (Noroxin)	Tab: 400mg	*Adults:* ≥18 years: **Uncomplicated UTI Due to *E. coli, K. pneumonia, P. mirabilis:*** 400mg q12h for 3 days. **Uncomplicated UTI Due To Other Organisms:** 400mg q12h for 7-10 days. **Complicated UTI:** 400mg q12h for 10-21 days. **CrCl ≤30mL/min:** 400mg qd. **Uncomplicated Gonorrhea:** 800mg single dose. **Acute/Chronic Prostatitis:** 400mg q12h for 28 days. Take 1hr before or 2hrs after meals or milk/dairy products.	**W/P:** Pseudomembranous colitis, convulsions, phototoxicity, and ruptures of the shoulder, hand, and Achilles tendons reported. Avoid in pregnancy and nursing mothers. Convulsions reported. Caution with renal dysfunction. Discontinue if CNS stimulation, increase in intracranial pressure, or toxic psychoses occurs. Not effective for treatment of syphilis. May exacerbate myasthenia gravis. Hemolytic reactions reported with G6P deficiency. **Contra:** History of tendinitis or tendon rupture associated with the use of quinolones. **P/N:** Category C, not for use in nursing.	Dizziness, nausea, headache, abdominal pain, and asthenia.
Ofloxacin (Floxin)	Tab: 200mg, 300mg, 400mg	*Adults:* ≥18 years: **ABECB/CAP/SSSI:** 400mg q12h for 10 days. **Cervicitis/Urethritis:** 300mg q12h for 7 days. **Gonorrhea:** 400mg single dose. **PID:** 400mg q12h for 10-14 days. **Uncomplicated Cystitis:** 200mg q12h for 3 days (*E. coli* or *K. pneumoniae*) or 7 days (other pathogens). **Complicated UTI:** 200mg q12h for 10 days. **Prostatitis:** (*E. coli*) 300mg q12h for 6 weeks. **CrCl 20-50mL/min:** Dose q24h. **CrCl <20mL/min:** After regular initial dose, give 50% of normal dose q24h. **Severe Hepatic Impairment: Max:** 400mg/day.	**W/P:** Convulsions, increased intracranial pressure, toxic psychosis, and CNS stimulation reported; discontinue if this occurs. Serious, fatal hypersensitivity reactions reported. Pseudomembranous colitis and ruptures of shoulder, hand, and Achilles tendon reported. Not shown to be effective for syphilis. Safety and efficacy unknown in patients <18 years old, pregnancy, and nursing. Maintain adequate hydration. Caution with renal or hepatic dysfunction, risk for seizures, and CNS disorder with predisposition to seizures. Avoid excessive sunlight. Monitor blood and renal and hepatic function with prolonged therapy. **P/N:** Category C, not for use in nursing.	Nausea, insomnia, headache, dizziness, diarrhea, vomiting, external genital pruritus in women, and vaginitis.

GLYCOPEPTIDE

NAME	FORM/ STRENGTH	DOSAGE	WARNINGS/PRECAUTIONS & CONTRAINDICATIONS	ADVERSE EFFECTS†
Vancomycin (Vancocin)	Inj: 500mg/100mL, 1g/200mL	*Adults:* **Usual:** 500mg IV q6h or 1g IV q12h. **Mild to Moderate Renal Impairment: Initial:** 15mg/kg/day. **Maint:** 1.9mg/kg/day. Administer 10mg/min or over at least 60min, whichever is longer. **Renal Dysfunction: Initial:** 15mg/kg. Dose is about 15x the GFR in mL/min (refer to table in labeling). **Elderly:** Require greater dose reduction. **Functionally Anephric: Initial:** 15mg/kg, then 1.9mg/kg/24hrs. **Marked Renal Dysfunction:** 250-1000mg every several days. **Anuria:** 1000mg every 7-10 days. *Pediatrics:* **Usual:** 10mg/kg IV q6h. **Infants/Neonates: Initial:** 15mg/kg, then 10mg/kg q12h for neonates in the 1st week of life and q8h thereafter until 1 month. Administer over at least 60min. **Renal Dysfunction: Initial:** 15mg/kg. Dose is about 15x the GFR in mL/min (refer to table in labeling). **Premature Infants:** Require greater dose reduction.	**W/P:** Only for colitis treatment; not systemically absorbed. Rapid bolus may cause hypotension, cardiac arrest (rare). Administer in a dilute solution over at least 60min. Ototoxicity and pseudomembranous colitis reported. Adjust dose in renal dysfunction. Prolonged use may result in the overgrowth of nonsusceptible organisms. Monitor renal and auditory function. Reversible neutropenia reported; monitor leukocyte count periodically. Intrathecal safety has not been assessed. **Contra:** Known allergy to corn or corn products because the solution contains dextrose. **P/N:** Category C, not for use in nursing.	Infusion-related events, hypotension, wheezing, pruritus, pain, chest and head muscle spasm, dyspnea, urticaria, nephrotoxicity, pseudomembranous colitis, ototoxicity, neutropenia, and phlebitis.

Table 6.2: PRESCRIBING INFORMATION FOR ANTIBIOTICS *(cont.)*

NAME	FORM/ STRENGTH	DOSAGE	WARNINGS/PRECAUTIONS & CONTRAINDICATIONS	ADVERSE EFFECTS†
LINCOSAMIDES				
Clindamycin (Cleocin)	**Cap:** (HCl) 75mg, 150mg, 300mg; **Inj:** (Phosphate) 150mg/mL, 300mg/50mL, 600mg/50mL, 900mg/50mL; **Sus:** (HCl) 75mg/5mL [100g]	***Adults:*** **Serious Infection:** 150-300mg PO q6h or 600-1200mg/day IM/IV given bid-qid. **More Severe Infection:** 300-450mg PO q6h or 1200-2700mg/ day IM/IV given bid-qid. **Life-Threatening Infections:** Up to 4800mg/day IV. **Max:** 600mg per IM injection. Take oral form with full glass of water. Treat β-hemolytic strep for at least 10 days. ***Pediatrics:*** **Birth-16 years: Serious Infection:** 8-16mg/kg/day PO. **More Severe Infection:** 16-20mg/kg/day PO. **1 month-16 years:** 20-40mg/kg/day IM/IV given tid-qid; use higher dose for more severe infection. **<1 month:** 15-20mg/kg/day IM/IV given tid-qid. Take oral form with full glass of water. Treat β-hemolytic strep for at least 10 days.	**Pseudomembranous colitis reported; may range in severity from mild to life threatening. W/P:** Discontinue if diarrhea occurs. May permit overgrowth of clostridia. Not for treatment of meningitis. Caution with atopic patients, GI disease (eg, colitis), hepatic disease, and the elderly. Monitor blood and hepatic and renal function with long-term use. Do not give injection undiluted as a bolus. The 75mg and 100mg capsules contain tartrazine. **P/N:** Category B, not for use in nursing.	Abdominal pain, pseudomembranous colitis, esophagitis, nausea, vomiting, diarrhea, hypersensitivity reactions, **metallic taste**. Injection: jaundice, blood dyscrasias, pruritus, vaginitis, and superinfection (prolonged use).
Lincomycin (Linocin)	**Inj:** 300mg/mL	***Adults:*** **IM: Serious Infection:** 600mg q24h. **More Severe Infection:** 600mg q12h or more often. **IV:** Dose depends on severity. **Serious Infection:** 600mg-1g q8-12h. **More Severe Infection:** Increase dose. Infuse over ≥1hr. **Life-Threatening Situation:** Up to 8g/day has been given. **Max:** 8g/day. **Severe Renal Dysfunction:** 25-30% of normal dose. ***Pediatrics:*** **>1 month: IM: Serious Infection:** 10mg/kg q24h. **More Severe Infection:** 10mg/kg q12h or more often. **IV:** 10-20mg/kg/day, depending on severity, infused in divided doses as described for adults. **Severe Renal Dysfunction:** 25-30% of normal dose.	**Diarrhea, colitis, and pseudomembranous colitis reported; may begin up to several weeks after discontinuation. Reserve for serious infections where less toxic antimicrobials are inappropriate. W/P:** May be inadequate for meningitis treatment. Contains benzyl alcohol. Monitor elderly for change in bowel frequency. Caution with severe renal/hepatic dysfunction or history of GI disease (eg, colitis), asthma, or significant allergies. Superinfections may occur. Perform periodic CBC, LFTs, and renal function tests with prolonged therapy. Do not administer undiluted as IV bolus. Cardiopulmonary arrest and hypotension with too rapid IV administration. **P/N:** Category C, not for use in nursing.	Glossitis, stomatitis, nausea, vomiting, diarrhea, colitis, pruritus, blood dyscrasias, hypersensitivity reactions, rash, urticaria, vaginitis, tinnitus, and vertigo.
OXAXOLIDINONE				
Linezolid (Zyvox)	**Inj:** 2mg/mL; **Sus:** 100mg/ 5mL [150mL]; **Tab:** 600mg	***Adults:*** **VRE:** 600mg IV/PO q12h for 14-28 days. **Nosocomial Pneumonia/ Complicated SSSI/CAP:** 600mg IV/PO q12h for 10-14 days. **UnComplicated SSSI:** 400mg PO q12h for 10-14 days. ***Pediatrics:*** **VRE:** Treat for 14-28 days. **≥12 years:** 600mg IV/PO q12h. **Birth-11 years:** 10mg/kg IV/PO q8h. **Nosocomial Pneumonia/Complicated SSSI/CAP:** Treat for 10-14 days. **≥12 years:** 600mg IV/PO q12h. **Birth-11years:** 10mg/kg IV/PO q8h. **UnComplicated SSSI:** Treat for 10-14 days. **≥12 years:** 600mg PO q12h. **5-11 years:** 10mg/kg PO q12h. **<5 yrs:** 10mg/kg PO q8h.	**W/P:** Myelosuppression including anemia, thrombocytopenia, pancytopenia, and leukopenia reported; monitor CBC weekly. Superinfection and pseudomembranous colitis may occur. May permit overgrowth of clostridia. Oral suspension contains phenylalanine. Peripheral and optic neuropathy have been reported. **P/N:** Category C, caution in nursing.	Diarrhea, headache, nausea, and vomiting.
KETOLIDE				
Telithromycin (Ketek)	**Tab:** 300mg [20ˢ], 400mg [60ˢ, Ketek Pak, 10ˢ]	***Adults:*** **ABECB/Sinusitis:** 800mg qd for 5 days. **CAP:** 800mg qd for 7-10 days. **Severe Renal Impairment (CrCl <30mL/min):** 600mg qd. **HemoDialysis:** Give after dialysis session on dialysis	**W/P:** Pseudomembranous colitis, visual disturbances, and hepatic dysfunction reported; avoid with congenital prolongation, ongoing proarrhythmic conditions	Diarrhea, nausea, headache, dizziness, and vomiting.

*Scored.   † Bold entries denote special dental considerations.

NAME	FORM/ STRENGTH	DOSAGE	WARNINGS/PRECAUTIONS & CONTRAINDICATIONS	ADVERSE EFFECTS†
Telithromycin (cont.)		days. **Severe Renal Impairment (CrCl <30mL/min) with Hepatic Impairment:** 400mg qd.	(eg, uncorrected hypokalemia or hypomagnesemia), or significant bradycardia. May exacerbate myasthenia gravis; avoid use. Caution with history of hepatiti or jaundice associated with prior use. **Contra:** Hypersensitivity to macrolide antibiotics, concomitant cisapride, or pimozide. **P/N:** Category C, caution in nursing.	

MACROLIDES

NAME	FORM/ STRENGTH	DOSAGE	WARNINGS/PRECAUTIONS & CONTRAINDICATIONS	ADVERSE EFFECTS†
Azithromycin (Zithromax, Zithromax Tri-Pak, Zithromax Z-pak)	**Inj:** 500mg; **Sus:** 100mg/ 5mL [15mL], 200mg/5mL [15mL, 22.5mL, 30mL], 1g/pkt [3s, 10s]; **Tab:** 250mg [Z-PAK, 6 tabs], 500mg [TRI-PAK, 3 tabs], 600mg	*Adults:* (PO) COPD/CAP/Pharyngitis/ **Tonsillitis (second-line therapy)/ SSSI:** ≥16 years: 500mg on day 1, then 250mg qd on days 2-5. **COPD:** 500mg qd for 3 days. **ABS:** 500mg qd for 3 days. **Genital Ulcer Disease and Non-Gonococcal Urethritis/Cervicitis:** 1g single dose. **Urethritis/Cervicitis due to N. Gonorrhea:** 2g single dose. **MAC Prophylaxis:** 1200mg once weekly. **MAC Treatment:** 600mg qd with ethambutol 15mg/kg/day. **(IV) ≥16 years: CAP:** 500mg qd for at least 2 days, then 500mg PO to complete 7-10-day course. **PID:** 500mg qd for 1-2 days, then 250mg PO to complete 7-day course. *Pediatrics:* (Sus) **Otitis Media: ≥6 months:** 30mg/kg single dose; 10mg/kg qd for 3 days; or 10mg/kg qd on day 1, then 5mg/kg qd on days 2-5. **ABS: ≥6 months:** 10mg/ kg qd for 3 days. **CAP: ≥6 months:** 10mg/kg qd on day 1, then 5mg/kg qd on days 2-5. **(Sus, Tab) Pharyngitis/Tonsillitis: ≥2 years:** 12mg/kg qd for 5 days. 1g suspension is not for pediatric use.	**W/P:** Monitor theophylline, terfenadine, cyclosporine, hexobarbital, phenytoin, and warfarin. May increase digoxin and carbamazepine levels. Potentiates triazolam. Aluminum- and magnesium-containing antacids reduce oral levels. Acute ergot toxicity may occur with ergotamine or dihydroergotamine. Monitor for azithromycin side effects (eg, liver enzyme abnormalities or hearing impairment) with nelfinavir. **P/N:** Category B, caution in nursing.	Diarrhea/loose stools, nausea, and abdominal pain.
Clarithromycin (Biaxin, Biaxin XL)	**Sus:** 125mg/5mL, 250mg/5mL [50mL, 100mL]; **Tab:** 250mg, 500mg	*Adults:* Biaxin: **Pharyngitis/Tonsillitis:** 250mg q12h for 10 days. **Sinusitis:** 500mg q12h for 14 days. **ABECB:** 250-500mg q12h for 7-14 days. **SSSI/CAP:** 250mg q12h for 7-14 days. **MAC Prophylaxis/Treatment:** 500mg bid. **H. pylori: Triple Therapy:** 500mg + amoxicillin 1g + omeprazole 20mg, all q12h for 10 days; or 500mg + amoxicillin 1g + lansoprazole 30mg, all q12h for 10-14 days. Give additional omeprazole 20mg qd for 18 days with active ulcer. **Dual Therapy:** 500mg q8h + omeprazole 40mg qd for 14 days (give additional omeprazole 20mg qd for 14 days with active ulcer); or 500mg q8h or q12h + ranitidine bismuth citrate 400mg q12h for 14 days (give additional ranitidine bismuth citrate 400mg bid for 14 days with active ulcer). Avoid Biaxin and ranitidine bismuth citrate combination with CrCl <25mL/min. **Biaxin XL: Sinusitis:** 1000mg qd for 14 days. **ABECB/CAP:** 1000mg qd for 7 days. **CrCl <30mL/min:** Give 50% dose or double interval. Take with food.	**W/P:** Avoid in pregnancy. Pseudomembranous colitis reported. Adjust dose with severe renal impairment. **Contra:** Concomitant cisapride, pimozide, terfenadine, or other macrolide antibiotics. **P/N:** Category C, caution in nursing	Diarrhea, nausea, abnormal taste, dyspepsia, abdominal pain, headache, vomiting, and rash.

Table 6.2: PRESCRIBING INFORMATION FOR ANTIBIOTICS *(cont.)*

NAME	FORM/ STRENGTH	DOSAGE	WARNINGS/PRECAUTIONS & CONTRAINDICATIONS	ADVERSE EFFECTS†
MACROLIDES *(cont.)*				
Dirithromycin (Dynabac)	**Tab, Delayed Release:** 250mg [D5-Pak, 10 tabs]	*Adults:* **ABECB:** 500mg qd for 5-7 days. **Acute Bronchitis:** 500mg qd for 7 days. **Pharyngitis/Tonsillitis:** 500mg qd for 10 days. **CAP:** 500mg qd for 14 days. **SSSI:** 500mg qd for 5-7 days. Take with food or within 1hr of having eaten. Do not cut, chew, or crush tabs. *Pediatrics:* ≥**12 years: ABECB:** 500mg qd for 5-7 days. **Acute Bronchitis:** 500mg qd for 7 days. **Pharyngitis/Tonsillitis:** 500mg qd for 10 days. **CAP:** 500mg qd for 14 days. **SSSI:** 500mg qd for 5-7 days. Take with food or within 1hr of having eaten. Do not cut, chew, or crush tabs.	**W/P:** Avoid with known, suspected, or potential bacteremias. Pseudomembranous colitis reported. Caution with severe hepatic insufficiency. **P/N:** Category C, caution in nursing.	Abdominal pain, headache, nausea, vomiting, diarrhea, and dyspepsia.
Erythromycin (ERYC, Erythrocin)	**Cap, Delayed Release:** 250mg (ERYC); **Tab:** 250mg, 500mg (Erythrocin); **Cap, Delayed Release:** 250mg (Erythromycin)	*Adults:* **Usual:** 250mg q6h or 500mg q12h. **Max:** 4g/day. Treat strep infections for 10 days. **Chlamydial Urogenital Infection During Pregnancy:** 500mg qid for at least 7 days or 250mg qid for 14 days. **Urethral/Endocervical/Rectal Chlamydial Infections:** 500mg qid for 7 days. **Primary Syphilis:** 30-40g in divided doses for 10-15 days. **Acute PID:** 500mg (erythromycin lactobionate) IV q6h for 3 days, then 250mg PO q6h for 7 days. **Streptococcal Infection Long-Term Prophylaxis of Rheumatic Fever:** 250mg bid. **Intestinal Amebiasis:** 250mg qid for 10-14 days. **Pertussis:** 40-50mg/kg/day in divided doses for 5-14 days. **Legionnaires' Disease:** 1-4g/day in divided doses. **Bacterial Endocarditis Prophylaxis:** 1g 1hr before procedure, then 500mg 6hrs later. *Pediatrics:* **Usual:** 30-50mg/kg/day in divided doses without food. **Max:** 4g/day. **Severe Infections:** Double dose up to 4g/day. Treat strep infections for 10 days. **Intestinal Amebiasis:** 30-50mg/kg/day in divided doses for 10-14 days. **Bacterial Endocarditis Prophylaxis:** 20mg/kg 1hr before procedure, then 10mg/kg 6hrs later.	**W/P:** Pseudomembranous colitis and hepatic dysfunction reported. **Contra:** Concomitant terfenadine or cisapride. **P/N:** Category B, caution in nursing.	Nausea, vomiting, abdominal pain, diarrhea, anorexia, abnormal LFTs, allergic reaction, and superinfection (prolonged use).
Erythromycin (EryPed)	**Sus:** 100mg/ 2.5mL [50mL], 200mg/5mL, 400mg/5mL [5mL, 100mL, 200mL]; **Tab, Chewable:** 200mg*	*Adults:* **Usual:** 1600mg/day given q6h, q8h, or q12h. **Max:** 4g/day. Treat strep infections for 10 days. **Streptococcal Infection Prophylaxis with Rheumatic Heart Disease:** 400mg bid. **Urethritis** (*C. trachomatis* or *U. urealyticum*): 800mg tid for 7 days. **Primary Syphilis:** 48-64g in divided doses over 10-15 days. **Intestinal Amebiasis:** 400mg qid for 10-14 days. **Pertussis:** 40-50mg/ kg/day in divided doses for 5-14 days. **Legionnaires' Disease:** 1.6-4g/day in divided doses. *Pediatrics:* **Usual:** 30-50mg/kg/day in divided doses q6h, q8h, or q12h. Double dose for more severe infections. Treat strep infections for 10 days. **Intestinal Amebiasis:** 30-50mg/kg/day in divided doses for 10-14 days. **Pertussis:** 40-50mg/kg/ day in divided doses for 5-14 days.	**W/P:** Pseudomembranous colitis and hepatic dysfunction reported. **Contra:** Concomitant terfenadine or cisapride. **P/N:** Category B, caution in nursing.	Nausea, vomiting, abdominal pain, diarrhea, anorexia, hepatic dysfunction, abnormal LFTs, allergic reactions, and superinfection (prolonged use).

*Scored.   † Bold entries denote special dental considerations.

NAME	FORM/ STRENGTH	DOSAGE	WARNINGS/PRECAUTIONS & CONTRAINDICATIONS	ADVERSE EFFECTS†
MONOBACTAM				
Azactam (Aztreonam)	**Inj:** 500mg, 1g, 2g, 1g/50mL, 2g/50mL	***Adults:* UTI:** 500mg-1g IM/IV q8-12h. **Moderately Severe Systemic Infections:** 1-2g IM/IV q8-12h. **Severe Systemic/Life-Threatening *P. aeruginosa:*** 2g IV q6-8h. **Max:** 8g/day. **CrCl 10-30mL/min: Initial: LD:** 1 or 2g. **Maint:** 50% of usual dose. **CrCl <10mL/min: Initial: LD:** 500mg, 1g or 2g. **Maint:** 25% of initial dose at usual intervals. **Serious/Life-Threatening Infections:** In addition to maintenance dose, give 1/8 initial dose after each hemodialysis session. IV route is recommended for single dose >1g or for bacterial septicemia, localized parenchymal abscess (eg, intra-abdominal abscess), peritonitis, or other severe systemic or life-threatening infections. Continue for at least 48hrs after patient is asymptomatic or bacterial eradication. ***Pediatrics:* 9 months-16 years: Mild-Moderate Infections:** 30mg/kg IV q8h. **Moderate-Severe Infections:** 30mg/kg IV q6-8h. **Max:** 120mg/kg/day. IV route is recommended for single dose >1g or for bacterial septicemia, localized parenchymal abscess (eg, intra-abdominal abscess), peritonitis, or other severe systemic or life-threatening infections. Continue for at least 48hrs after patient is asymptomatic or evidence of bacterial eradication.	**W/P:** Caution with hypersensitivity to other β-lactams or allergens. Pseudomembranous colitis reported. May promote overgrowth of nonsusceptible organisms. Monitor with renal or hepatic impairment. Toxic epidermal necrolysis reported (rarely) in bone marrow transplant with multiple risk factors including sepsis. **P/N:** Category B, not for use in nursing.	Diarrhea, nausea, vomiting, rash, abdominal cramps, vaginal candidiasis, discomfort/swelling at injection site, and hypersensitivity reaction.
NITROIMIDAZOLE				
Metronidazole (Flagyl)	**CAP:** 375mg; **Tab:** 250mg, 500mg	***Adults:* Trichomoniasis (Female and Male Sex Partner):** (Cap/Tab) 375mg bid or 250mg tid for 7 days. **One-day Therapy:** (Tab) 2gm as single or divided doses. If repeat course needed, reconfirm diagnosis and allow 4-6 weeks between courses. **Abscess:** 500mg or 750mg tid for 5-10 days. **Dysentery:** 750mg tid for 5-10 days. **Anaerobic Bacterial Infection:** Usually IV therapy initially if serious, 7.5mg/kg q6h for 7-10 days or longer. **Max:** 4g/24hrs. **Elderly:** Adjust dose based on serum levels. **Hepatic Disease:** Give lower dose cautiously; monitor levels. ***Pediatrics:* Amebiasis:** 35-50mg/kg/24hrs given tid for 10 days.	**W/P:** Seizures and peripheral neuropathy reported. Discontinue if abnormal neurological signs occur. Caution with severe hepatic impairment, blood dyscrasias, or CNS diseases. Monitor leukocytes before and after therapy. **Contra:** Treatment during 1st trimester of pregnancy. **P/N:** Category B, not for use in nursing.	Seizures, peripheral neuropathy, nausea, vomiting, headache, anorexia, urticaria, rash, **metallic taste**, dysuria, vaginal candidiasis, vaginitis, dizziness, and leukopenia.
Metronidazole (Flagyl IV)	**Inj:** 500mg; 500mg (RTU)	***Adults:* LD:** 15mg/kg IV. **Maint:** 6hrs later, 7.5mg/kg IV q6h for 7-10 days or more. **Max:** 4g/24hrs.	**W/P:** Seizures and peripheral neuropathy reported. Discontinue if abnormal neurological signs occur. Caution with severe hepatic impairment, blood dyscrasias, or CNS disease. Monitor leukocytes before and after therapy. Metronidazole IV is effective in *B. fragilis* infections resistant to clindamycin, chloramphenicol, and penicillin. **P/N:** Category B, not for use in nursing.	Convulsive seizures, peripheral neuropathy, nausea, vomiting, headache, leukopenia, rash, vaginal candidiasis, and thrombophlebitis.

Table 6.2: PRESCRIBING INFORMATION FOR ANTIBIOTICS *(cont.)*

NAME	FORM/ STRENGTH	DOSAGE	WARNINGS/PRECAUTIONS & CONTRAINDICATIONS	ADVERSE EFFECTS†
NITROIMIDAZOLE *(cont.)*				
Metronidazole (Flagyl ER)	**Tab, Extended Release:** 750mg	***Adults:*** 750mg qd for 7 days; take 1hr before or 2hrs after meals. **Elderly:** Adjust dose based on serum levels. **Hepatic Disease:** Give lower dose cautiously; monitor levels.	**W/P:** Seizures and peripheral neuropathy reported. Discontinue if abnormal neurological signs occur. Caution with severe hepatic impairment, blood dyscrasias, or CNS diseases. Monitor leukocytes before and after therapy. **Contra:** Treatment during 1st trimester of pregnancy. **P/N:** Category B, not for use in nursing.	Headache, vaginitis, nausea, **metallic taste**, dizziness, seizures, peripheral neuropathy, vomiting, leukopenia, urticaria, rash, dysuria, and vaginal candidiasis.
PENICILLINS				
Amoxicillin (Amoxil, Amoxil Pediatric, Trimox)	**(Amoxil) Cap:** 250mg, 500mg; **Sus:** 50mg/mL [15mL, 30mL], 125mg/5mL [80mL, 100mL, 150mL], 200mg/5mL [5mL, 50mL, 75mL, 100mL], 250mg/5mL [80mL, 100mL, 150mL], 400mg/5mL [5mL, 50mL, 75mL, 100mL]; **Tab:** 500mg, 875mg; **Tab, Chewable:** 200mg, 400mg; **(Trimox) CAP:** 250mg, 500mg; **Sus:** 125mg/5mL, 250mg/5mL [80mL, 100mL, 150mL]	***Adults:* Ear/Nose/Throat/SSSI/GU:** (Mild/Moderate) 500mg q12h or 250mg q8h. (Severe) 875mg q12h or 500mg q8h. **LRTI:** 875mg q12h or 500mg q8h. Gonorrhea 3g as single dose. ***H. pylori:*** (Dual Therapy) 1g + 30mg lansoprazole, both tid x 14 days. (Triple Therapy) 1g + 30mg lansoprazole + 500mg clarithromycin, all q12h x 14 days. **CrCl 10-30mL/min:** 250-500mg q12h. **>10mL/min:** 250-500mg q24h. **HemoDialysis:** 250-500mg or 250mg q24h, additional dose during and at the end. ***Pediatrics:* Neonates: ≤12 weeks:** Max: 30mg/kg/day divided q12h. **>3 months: Ear/Nose/ Throat/SSSI/GU: (Mild/Moderate):** 25mg/kg/day given q12h or 20mg/kg/day given q8h. **(Severe):** 45mg/kg/day given q12h or 40mg/kg/day given q8h. **LRTI:** 45mg/kg/day given q12h or 40mg/kg/day given q8h. **Gonorrhea:** (Prepubertal) 50mg/kg with 25mg/kg probenecid as single dose. (Not for <2yrs). **>40kg:** Dose as adult.	**W/P:** Monitor renal, hepatic, and blood with prolonged use. 200mg, 400mg chewable tabs contain phenylalanine. **P/N:** Category B, caution in nursing.	Nausea, vomiting, diarrhea, pseudomembranous colitis, hypersensitivity reactions, blood dyscrasias, and superinfection (prolonged use).
Amoxicillin (Dispermox)	**Tab, Dispersible:** 200mg, 400mg, 600mg	***Adults:*ENT/SSSI/GU: (Mild/Moderate):** 500mg q12h or 250mg q8h. **(Severe):** 875mg q12h or 500mg q8h. **LRTI:** 875mg q12h or 500mg q8h. **Gonorrhea:** 3g as single oral dose. Do not chew or swallow dispersible tabs. ***Pediatrics:* Neonates: ≤12 weeks:** Max: 30mg/kg/day divided q12h. **>3 months: ENT/SSSI/GU: (Mild/Moderate):** 25mg/kg/day given q12h or 20mg/kg/day given q8h. **(Severe):** 45mg/kg/day given q12h or 40 mg/ kg/day given q8h. **LRTI:** 45mg/kg/day given q12h or 40mg/kg/day given q8h. **Gonorrhea:** (Prepubertal) 50mg/kg with 25mg/kg probenecid as single dose (regimen not for use if <2 yrs). **>40kg:** Dose as adult. Do not chew or swallow dispersible tabs.	**W/P:** Monitor renal, hepatic, and blood with prolonged use. Dispersible tabs contain phenylalanine. **P/N:** Category B, caution in nursing	Nausea, vomiting, diarrhea, pseudomembranous colitis, hypersensitivity reactions, blood dyscrasias, and superinfection (prolonged use).
Amoxicillin/ Clavulanate (Augmentin)	**(Augmentin) Sus:** 125-31.25mg/5mL [75mL, 100mL,	***Adults:*** (Dose based on amoxicillin) 500mg q12h or 250mg q8h. **Severe Infections/RTI:** 875mg q12h or 500mg q8h. May use 125mg/5mL or	**W/P:** Pseudomembranous colitis reported. Possibility of superinfection. Caution with hepatic dysfunction. Monitor renal, hepatic, and hematopoietic	Diarrhea/loose stools, nausea, skin rashes, urticaria, vomiting, and vaginitis.

*Scored.   † Bold entries denote special dental considerations.

NAME	FORM/ STRENGTH	DOSAGE	WARNINGS/PRECAUTIONS & CONTRAINDICATIONS	ADVERSE EFFECTS†
Amoxicillin/ Clavulanate *(cont.)*	150mL] 200-28.5mg/5mL [50mL, 75mL, 100mL], 250-62.5mg/5mL [75mL, 100mL, 150mL], 400-57mg/5mL [50mL, 75mL, 100mL]; **Tab:** 250-125mg, 500-125mg, 875-125mg*; **Tab, Chewable:** 125-31.25mg, 200-28.5mg, 250-62.5mg, 400-57mg; **(Augmentin ES-600): Sus:** 600mg-42.9mg/ 5mL [50mL, 75mL, 100mL, 150mL]	250mg/5mL sus in place of 500mg tab and 200mg/5mL sus or 400mg/5mL sus in place of 875mg tab. **CrCl <30mL/min:** Do not give 875mg tab. **CrCl 10-30mL/min:** 250-500mg q12h. **CrCl <10mL/min:** 250-500mg q24h. **HemoDialysis:** 250-500mg q24h, give additional dose during and at the end of dialysis. *Pediatrics:* **(Augmentin): Dose based on amoxicillin) ≥40kg:** Use adult dose. **≥12 weeks: Sinusitis/ OM/LRTI/Severe Infections:** (Sus/Tab, Chewable) 45mg/kg/day given q12h or 40mg/kg/day given q8h. **Less Severe Infections:** 25mg/kg/day given q12h or 20mg/kg/day given q8h. **<12 weeks:** 15mg/kg q12h (use 125mg/5mL sus). **(Augmentin ES-600):** Dose based on amoxicillin. **3 months-12 years: <40kg:** 45mg/kg q12h for 10 days.	functions with prolonged use. Avoid with mononucleosis. Fatal hypersensitivity reactions reported. Take with food to reduce GI upset. Chewable tabs and suspension contain phenylalanine. The 250mg tab and chewable tab are not interchangeable due to unequal clavulanic acid amounts. Only use 250mg tab in pediatrics ≥40kg. False (+) for urine glucose with Clinitest and Benedict's or Fehling's solution.**Contra:** History of penicillin allergy or amoxicillin-clavulanate associated cholestatic jaundice/hepatic dysfunction. **P/N:** Category B, caution in nursing.	
Amoxicillin/ Clavulanate (Augmentin XR)	**Tab, ER:** (Amoxicillin-Clavulanate) 1000mg-62.5mg	*Adults:* **Sinusitis:** 2 tabs q12h for 10 days. **CAP:** 2 tabs q12h for 7-10 days. Take at the start of a meal.	**W/P:** Pseudomembranous colitis reported. Possibility of superinfection. Caution with hepatic dysfunction. Monitor renal, hepatic, and hematopoietic functions with prolonged use. Avoid with mononucleosis. Fatal hypersensitivity reactions reported. Take with food to reduce GI upset. Chewable tabs and suspension contain phenylalanine. The 250mg tab and chewable tab are not interchangeable due to unequal clavulanic acid amounts. Only use 250mg tab in pediatrics ≥40kg. False (+) for urine glucose with Clinitest and Benedict's or Fehling's solution. **Contra:** History of penicillin allergy or amoxicillin-clavulanate associated cholestatic jaundice/hepatic dysfunction, severe renal impairment (CrCl >30mL/min), or hemodialysis. **P/N:** Category B, caution in nursing.	Diarrhea, nausea, genital moniliasis, abdominal pain, and vaginal mycosis.
Ampicillin Sodium (Principen)	**Inj:** 125mg, 250mg, 500mg, 1g, 2g, 10g	*Adults:* **IM/IV: Respiratory Tract: ≥40kg:** 250-500mg q8h. **<40kg:** 25-50mg/kg/day given q6-8h. **GI/GU caused by** *N. gonorrhoeae* **(females): ≥40kg:** 500mg q6h. **<40kg:** 50mg/kg/ day given q6-8h. **Urethritis caused by** *N. gonorrhoeae* **(males):** 500mg q8-12h for 2 doses; may retreat if needed. **Bacterial Meningitis:** 150-200mg/ kg/day given q3-4h. **Septicemia:** 150-200mg/kg/day IV for 3 days, continue with IM q3-4h. Treat for minimum of 10 days and 48-72hrs after being asymptomatic. *Pediatrics:* **Bacterial Meningitis:** 150-200mg/kg/day given q3-4h. **Septicemia:** 150-200mg/kg/day IV given q3-4h for 3 days, continue with IM q3-4h. Treat for minimum of 10 days and 48-72hrs after being asymptomatic.	**W/P:** Caution with renal impairment. Cross-sensitivity with other β-lactams. May cause skin rash, especially in mononucleosis; avoid use. Pseudomembranous colitis reported. May result in overgrowth of nonsusceptible organisms. **P/N:** Category B, caution in nursing.	Headache, nausea, vomiting, oral and vaginal candidiasis, diarrhea, urticaria, allergic reactions, anaphylaxis, serum sickness-like reactions, and exfoliative dermatitis.

Table 6.2: PRESCRIBING INFORMATION FOR ANTIBIOTICS *(cont.)*

NAME	FORM/ STRENGTH	DOSAGE	WARNINGS/PRECAUTIONS & CONTRAINDICATIONS	ADVERSE EFFECTS†
PENICILLINS *(cont.)*				
Ampicillin Sodium/Sulbactam (Unasyn)	**Inj:** (Ampicillin-Sulbactam) 1g-0.5g, 2g-1g, 10g-5g	**Adults:**1.5-3g (ampicillin-,sulbactam) IM/IV q6h. **Max:** 4g/day sulbactam. **Renal Impairment: CrCl ≥30mL/min:** 1.5-3g q6-8h. **CrCl 15-29mL/min:** 1.5-3g q12h. **CrCl 5-14mL/min:** 1.5-3g q24h. **Pediatrics:** ≥1 yr: SSSI: 1.5-3g (ampicillin-sulbactam) IM/IV q6h. **Max:** 4g/day sulbactam.	**W/P:** Serious, fatal hypersensitivity reactions reported. Pseudomembranous colitis reported. Increased risk of skin rash with mononucleosis, use alternate agent. **P/N:** Category B, caution in nursing.	Injection-site pain, thrombophlebitis, diarrhea, rash, nausea, vomiting, malaise, headache, chest pain, flatulence, dysuria, edema, erythema, chills, epistaxis.
Dicloxacillin (Dynapen)	**CAP:** 250mg, 500mg; **Sus:** 62.5mg/5mL [100mL]	**Adults: Mild-Moderate Infection:** 125mg q6h. **Severe Infection:** 250mg q6h for at least 14 days. **Pediatrics: <40kg: Mild-Moderate Infection:** 12.5mg/kg/day in divided doses q6h. **Severe Infection:** 25mg/kg/day in divided doses q6h for at least 14 days.	**W/P:** Serious, fatal hypersensitivity reactions reported. Caution with history of allergy and/or asthma. Monitor renal, hepatic, and hematopoietic function with prolonged use. Not for use as initial therapy with serious, life-threatening infections, or with nausea, vomiting, gastric dilation, cardiospasm, or intestinal hypermotility. **P/N:** Category B, caution in nursing	Allergic reactions, nausea, vomiting, diarrhea, stomatitis, **black or hairy tongue,** and superinfection (prolonged use).
Nafcillin Sodium	**Inj:** 1g/50 mL, **Pow:** 1g, 2g, 10g, 200g	**Adults: Bacterial infectious disease, Susceptible:** 0.5-1 g IV every 4-6hrs, depending on type and severity of infection. **Bacterial infectious disease, Susceptible:** 0.5 g IM every 4-6hrs, depending on type and severity of infection. **Endocarditis (Severe):** 1-2 g IV every 4hrs. **Pediatrics: Bacterial infectious disease, Susceptible:** neonates 1 week and younger, 40 mg/kg/day IV/IM divided every 8-12hrs; neonates 1-4 weeks, 60 mg/kg/day IV/IM divided every 8-12hrs, depending on type and severity of infection. **Bacterial infectious disease, Susceptible:** 50-200 mg/kg/day IV/IM divided every 4-6hrs, maximum 12 g/day, depending on type and severity of infection.	**W/P:** Serious hypersensitivity reactions reported; increased risk with sensitivity to multiple allergens. Cross-sensitivity to cephalosporins. Monitor renal, hepatic, and hematopoietic functions with prolonged use. Discontinue if bleeding manifestations occur; increased risk with renal failure. Prolonged use may cause superinfections. May experience neuromuscular excitability or convulsions with higher than recommended doses. Contains 1.85mEq/g sodium; caution with salt restriction. Monitor electrolytes periodically with low potassium levels. May mask symptoms of syphilis. Increased incidence of rash and fever in cystic fibrosis. ADD-Vantage vial is not for IM use. Continue treatment for at least 48-72hrs after patient becomes asymptomatic. **Contra:** Hypersensitivity to cephalosporins. **P/N:** Category B, caution in nursing.	Rash, pruritus, diarrhea, nausea, vomiting, phlebitis, injection-site reaction, pain, and inflammation.
Oxacillin Sodium	**Inj:** 1g/50 mL, 2g/50 mL; **Pow:** 1g, 2g, 10g	**Adults: Bacterial infectious disease, penicillinase-producing staphylococcal infections:** 0.5-1g PO every 4-6hrs. **Bacterial infectious disease, penicillinase-producing staphylococcal infections:** 250mg-2g IV/IM every 4-6hrs; maximum 12g/day. **Endocarditis:** 2g IV every 4hrs for 4-6 weeks. **Infection of skin and/or SC tissue:** 0.5-1g PO every 4-6hrs. **Infection of skin and/or subcutaneous tissue:** 250mg-2g IV/IM every 4-6hrs; maximum 12g/day. **RTI:** 250 mg-2g IV/IM every 4-6hrs; maximum 12g/day. **Septicemia:** 250mg-2g IV/IM every 4-6hrs; maximum 12g/day. **Pediatrics: Bacterial infectious disease, penicillinase-producing staphylococcal infections:** Infants and children under 40kg, 50-100mg/kg/day PO/IV/IM divided every 4-6hrs; children over 40kg, use adult dosing; maximum 12g/day. Bacterial infectious disease, Penicillinase-producing staphylococcal	**W/P:** Serious hypersensitivity reactions reported; increased risk with sensitivity to multiple allergens. Cross-sensitivity to cephalosporins. Monitor renal, hepatic, and hematopoietic functions with prolonged use. Discontinue if bleeding manifestations occur; increased risk with renal failure. Prolonged use may cause superinfections. May experience neuromuscular excitability or convulsions with higher-than-recommended doses. Contains 1.85mEq/g sodium; caution with salt restriction. Monitor electrolytes periodically with low potassium levels. May mask symptoms of syphilis. Increased incidence of rash and fever in cystic fibrosis. ADD-Vantage vial is not for IM use. Continue treatment for at least 48-72hrs after patient becomes asymptomatic. **Contra:** Hypersensitivity to cephalosporins. **P/N:** Category B, caution in nursing.	Rash, pruritus, diarrhea, nausea, vomiting, phlebitis, injection-site reaction, pain, and inflammation.

*Scored.   † Bold entries denote special dental considerations.

NAME	FORM/STRENGTH	DOSAGE	WARNINGS/PRECAUTIONS & CONTRAINDICATIONS	ADVERSE EFFECTS†
Oxacillin Sodium *(cont.)*		**infections:** neonates 7 days and younger, 50-75mg/kg/day IV/IM divided every 8-12hrs. **Bacterial infectious disease, penicillinase-producing staphylococcal infections:** Neonates over 7 days, 75-100mg/kg/day IV/IM divided every 6-8hrs.		
Penicillin V Potassium (Veetids)	**Sus:** 125mg/5mL, 250mg/5mL [100mL, 200mL]; **Tab:** 250mg, 500mg	***Adults:*** Usual: Streptococcal Infections (Scarlet fever, Erysipelas, Upper Respiratory Tract): 125-250mg q6-8h for 10 days. **Pneumococcal Infections (Otitis media, Respiratory Tract):** 250-500mg q6h until afebrile for at least 2 days. **Staphylococcus Infections (Skin/Soft Tissue):** 250-500mg q6-8h. **Fusospirochetosis Infections (Oropharynx):** 250-500mg q6-8h. **Rheumatic Fever/Chorea Prevention:** 125-250mg bid. ***Pediatrics:* ≥12 years:** Usual: Streptococcal Infections (Scarlet fever, Erysipelas, and Upper Respiratory Tract): 125-250mg q6-8h for 10 days. **Pneumococcal Infections (Otitis media, Respiratory Tract):** 250-500mg q6h until afebrile for at least 2 days. **Staphylococcus Infections (Skin/Soft Tissue):** 250-500mg q6-8h. **Fusospirochetosis Infections (Oropharynx):** 250-500mg q6-8h. **Rheumatic Fever/Chorea Prevention:** 125-250mg bid.	**W/P:** Not for severe pneumonia, empyema, bacteremia, pericarditis, meningitis, and arthritis during the acute stage. Serious and fatal anaphylactic reactions reported. Pseudomembranous colitis reported. Oral administration may not be effective with severe illnesses, nausea, vomiting, gastric dilation, cardiospasm, and intestinal hypermobility. Cross-sensitivity with cephalosporins. Caution with asthma and allergies. **P/N:** Category B, caution in nursing	Nausea, vomiting, epigastric distress, diarrhea, hypersensitivity reactions, **black or hairy tongue,** anaphylaxis, and superinfection (prolonged use).
Penicillin G Potassium (Pfizerpen)	**Inj:** 1MU, 5MU, 20MU	***Adults:*** Anthrax/Gonorrheal Endocarditis/Severe Infections (Streptococci, Pneumococci, Staphylococci): Minimum of 5MU/day. **Syphilis:** Administer in hospital. Determine dose and duration based on age and weight. **Meningococcic Meningitis:** 1-2MU IM q2h or 20-30MU/day continuous IV. **Actinomycosis:** 1-6MU/day for cervicofacial cases; 10-20MU/day for thoracic and abdominal disease. **Clostridial Infections:** 20MU/day (adjunct to antitoxin). **Fusospirochetal Severe Infections:** 5-10MU/day for oropharynx, lower respiratory tract, and genital-area infection. **Rat-bite Fever:** 12-15MU/day for 3-4 weeks. **Listeria Endocarditis:** 15-20MU/day for 4 weeks. **Pasteurella Bacteremia/Meningitis:** 4-6MU/day for 2 weeks. **Erysipeloid Endocarditis:** 2-20MU/day for 4-6 weeks. **Gram Negative Bacillary Bacteremia:** 20-80MU/day. **Diphtheria (carrier state):** 0.3-0.4MU/day in divided doses for 10-12 days. **Endocarditis Prophylaxis:** 1MU IM mixed with 0.6MU procaine penicillin G 0.5-1hr before procedure. **Renal/Cardiac/Vascular Dysfunction:** Consider dose reduction. For streptococcal infection, treat for min 10 days. ***Pediatrics:*** Listeria Infections: Neonates: 0.5-1MU/day. **Congenital Syphilis:** Administer in hospital. Determine dose and duration based on age and weight. **Endocarditis Prophylaxis:** 30,000U/kg IM mixed with 0.6MU procaine penicillin G 0.5-1hr before procedure. For streptococcal infection, treat for min 10 days.	**W/P:** Serious and fatal anaphylactic reactions reported; increased risk with hypersensitivity to penicillins, cephalosporins, and other allergens. Avoid IV, intra-arterial administration, or injection into/near major peripheral nerves or blood vessels; may cause severe neurovascular damage. Take culture after therapy completion to determine streptococci eradication. Caution with history of significant allergies or asthma. May result in overgrowth of nonsusceptible organisms. Evaluate renal, hepatic, and hematopoietic systems with prolonged therapy. Administer slowly to avoid electrolyte imbalance from potassium or sodium content; monitor electrolytes and consider dose reductions with renal, cardiac, or vascular dysfunction. Caution in newborns; evaluate organ system function frequently. **P/N:** Category B, caution in nursing.	Skin rash (eg, maculopapular eruption, or exfoliative dermatitis), urticaria, chills, fever, edema, arthralgia, prostration, anaphylaxis, arrhythmias, cardiac arrest, and Jarisch-Herxheimer reaction.

Table 6.2: PRESCRIBING INFORMATION FOR ANTIBIOTICS *(cont.)*

NAME	FORM/STRENGTH	DOSAGE	WARNINGS/PRECAUTIONS & CONTRAINDICATIONS	ADVERSE EFFECTS[†]
PENICILLINS *(cont.)*				
Piperacillin Sodium (Pipracil)	**Inj:** 2g, 3g, 4g	***Adults:*** Usual: 3-4g IM/IV q4-6h. **Max:** 24g/day; **IM:** 2g/site. **Serious Infections:** 200-300mg/kg/day IV divided q4-6h. **Complicated UTI:** 125-200mg/kg/day IV divided q6-8h. **Uncomplicated UTI/Community Acquired Pneumonia:** 100-125mg/kg/day IM/IV divided q6-12h. **Uncomplicated Gonorrhea:** 2g IM single dose with 1g PO probenecid 30min before injection. **Surgical Prophylaxis:** 2g IV 20-30min just prior to anesthesia. **C-Section:** 2g IV after cord is clamped. (See labeling for follow-up dosing). **Renal Impairment: Uncomplicated/Complicated UTI: CrCl <20mL/min:** 3g q12h. **Complicated UTI: CrCl 20-40mL/min:** 3g q8h. **Serious Infection: CrCl 20-40mL/min:** 4g q8h. **CrCl <20mL/min:** 4g q12h. **HemoDialysis:** Give 1g additional dose after each dialysis. **Max:** 2g q8h. Usual treatment is for 7-10 days; treat gynecologic infections for 3-10 days; treat Group A β-hemolytic strep infections for at least 10 days. ***Pediatrics:*** **≥12 years:** Usual: 3-4g IM/IV q4-6h. **Max:** 24g/day; **IM:** 2g/site. **Serious Infections:** 200-300mg/kg/day IV divided q4-6h. **Complicated UTI:** 125-200mg/kg/day IV divided q6-8h. **Uncomplicated UTI/Community-Acquired Pneumonia:** 100-125mg/kg/day IM/IV divided q6-12h. **Uncomplicated Gonorrhea:** 2g IM single dose with 1g PO probenecid 30min before injection. **Surgical Prophylaxis:** 2g IV 20-30min just prior to anesthesia. **C-Section:** 2g IV after cord is clamped. (See labeling for follow-up dosing). **Renal Impairment: Uncomplicated/Complicated UTI: CrCl <20mL/min:** 3g q12h. **Complicated UTI: CrCl 20-40mL/min:** 3g q8h. **Serious Infection: CrCl 20-40mL/min:** 4g q8h. **CrCl <20mL/min:** 4g q12h. **HemoDialysis:** Give 1g additional dose after each dialysis. **Max:** 2g q8h. Usual treatment is for 7-10 days; treat gynecologic infections for 3-10 days; treat Group A β-hemolytic strep infections for at least 10 days.	**W/P:** Serious hypersensitivity reactions reported; increased risk with sensitivity to multiple allergens. Cross sensitivity to cephalosporins. Monitor renal, hepatic, and hematopoietic functions with prolonged use. Discontinue if bleeding manifestations occur; increased risk with renal failure. Prolonged use may cause superinfections. May experience neuromuscular excitability or convulsions with higher than recommended doses. Contains 1.85mEq/g sodium; caution with salt restriction. Monitor electrolytes periodically with low potassium levels. May mask symptoms of syphilis. Increased incidence of rash and fever in cystic fibrosis. ADD-Vantage vial is not for IM use. Continue treatment for at least 48-72hrs after patient becomes asymptomatic. **Contra:** Hypersensitivity to cephalosporins. **P/N:** Category B, caution in nursing.	Thrombophlebitis, erythema and pain at injection site, diarrhea, headache, dizziness, anaphylaxis, rash, and superinfections.
Piperacillin Sodium/ Tazobactam (Zosyn)	**Inj:** (Piperacillin-Tazobactam) 40mg-5mg/mL, 60mg-7.5mg/mL, 2g-0.25g, 3g-0.375g, 4g-0.5g, 4g-0.5g/100mL, 36g-4.5g	***Adults:*** Usual: 3.375g q6h for 7-10 days. **Nosocomial Pneumonia:** 4.5g q6h for 7-14 days plus aminoglycoside. **CrCl 20-40mL/min:** 2.25g q6h. **CrCl <20mL/min:** 2.25g q8h. **HemoDialysis: Max:** 2.25g q12h. Give 1 additional 0.75g dose after each dialysis period.	**W/P:** Serious, fatal hypersensitivity reactions may occur with penicillin allergy. Pseudomembranous colitis reported. Discontinue if bleeding manifestations occur. May experience neuromuscular excitability or convulsions with higher doses. Contains 2.35mEq/g Na; caution with restricted salt intake. Increased incidence of rash and fever in cystic fibrosis. Monitor electrolyte periodically with low K⁺ reserves. **Contra:** Hypersensitivity to cephalosporins. **P/N:** Category B, caution in nursing.	Rash, pruritus, diarrhea, nausea, vomiting, phlebitis, injection site reaction, pain, and inflammation.

*Scored.   † Bold entries denote special dental considerations.

NAME	FORM/ STRENGTH	DOSAGE	WARNINGS/PRECAUTIONS & CONTRAINDICATIONS	ADVERSE EFFECTS†
Ticarcillin/ Clavulanate Potassium (Timentin)	**Inj:** (Ticarcillin-Clavulanate) 3g-100mg, 3g-100mg/100mL, 30g-1g	*Adults:* ≥60kg: **UTI/Systemic Infection:** 3g-100mg (3.1g vial) IV q4-6h. **Gynecologic Infections: Moderate:** 200mg/kg/day ticarcillin IV given q6h. **Severe:** 300mg/kg/day ticarcillin IV given q4h. **<60kg: Usual:** 200-300mg/kg/day ticarcillin IV given q4-6h. **UTI:** 3g-200mg (3.2g vial) q8h. **Renal Impairment (based on ticarcillin): CrCl 60-30mL/min:** 2g IV q4h. **CrCl 30-10mL/min:** 2g IV q8h. **CrCl <10mL/min:** 2g IV q12h (2g IV q24h with hepatic dysfunction). **Peritoneal Dialysis:** 3.1g IV q12h. **HemoDialysis:** 2g IV q12h, and 3.1g after each dialysis. Apply reduced dosage after initial 3.1g LD is given. *Pediatrics:* ≥3 months: ≥60kg: **Mild to Moderate:** 3g-100mg (3.1g vial) IV q6h. **Severe:** 3g-100mg (3.1g vial) IV q4h. **<60 kg: Mild to Moderate:** 50mg/kg ticarcillin IV q6h. **Severe:** 50mg/kg ticarcillin IV q4h. **Renal Impairment (based on ticarcillin): CrCl 60-30mL/min:** 2g IV q4h. **CrCl 30-10mL/min:** 2g IV q8h. **CrCl <10mL/min:** 2g IV q12h (2g IV q24h with hepatic dysfunction). **Peritoneal Dialysis:** 3.1g IV q12h. **HemoDialysis:** 2g IV q12h, and 3.1g after each dialysis. Apply reduced dosage after initial 3.1g LD is given.	**W/P:** Prolonged use may result in overgrowth of nonsusceptible organisms. Caution with penicillin, cephalosporin, and other allergen sensitivities. Pseudomembranous colitis reported. Risk of convulsions with high doses especially with renal impairment. Monitor renal, hepatic, hematopoietic functions, and serum K+ with prolonged therapy. Caution with fluid and electrolyte imbalance; hypokalemia reported. Clotting time, platelet aggregation, and PT abnormalities may occur especially with renal impairment; discontinue therapy. Continue therapy for at least 2 days after signs/symptoms disappear. **P/N:** Category B, caution in nursing.	Hypersensitivity reactions, headache, giddiness, **taste/smell disturbances**, stomatitis, flatulence, nausea, vomiting, diarrhea, hematologic disturbances, hepatic/renal function tests abnormalities, and local reactions.

POLYPEPTIDE

NAME	FORM/ STRENGTH	DOSAGE	WARNINGS/PRECAUTIONS & CONTRAINDICATIONS	ADVERSE EFFECTS†
Colistimethate (Coly-Mycin)	**Inj:** 150mg	*Adults:* **Usual:** 2.5-5mg/kg/day IV/IM in 2-4 divided doses. **Max:** 5mg/kg/day. **SCr 1.3-1.5mg/dL:** 2.5-3.8mg/kg/day IV/IM in 2 divided doses. **SCr 1.6-2.5mg/dL:** 2.5mg/kg/day IV/IM in 1-2 divided doses. **SCr 2.6-4mg/dL:** 1.5mg/kg/day IV/IM q36h. **Obesity:** Base dose on IBW. *Pediatrics:* **Usual:** 2.5-5mg/kg/day IV/IM in 2-4 divided doses. **Max:** 5mg/kg/day. **SCr 1.3-1.5mg/dL:** 2.5-3.8mg/kg/day IV/IM in 2 divided doses. **SCr 1.6-2.5mg/dL:** 2.5mg/kg/day IV/IM in 1-2 divided doses. **SCr 2.6-4mg/dL:** 1.5mg/kg/day IV/IM q36h. **Obesity:** Base dose on IBW.	**W/P:** Transient neurological disturbances may occur; dose reduction may alleviate symptoms. Respiratory arrest reported after IM administration. Increased risk of apnea and neuromuscular blockade with renal impairment. Reversible dose-dependent nephrotoxicity reported. Pseudomembranous colitis reported. May permit overgrowth of clostridia. Use extreme caution with renal impairment; discontinue with further impairment. **P/N:** Category C, caution in nursing.	GI upset, **tingling of extremities and tongue**, **slurred speech**, dizziness, vertigo, paresthesia, itching, urticaria, rash, fever, increased BUN and creatinine, decreased creatinine clearance, respiratory distress, apnea, nephrotoxicity, and decreased urine output.

STREPTOGRAMIN

NAME	FORM/ STRENGTH	DOSAGE	WARNINGS/PRECAUTIONS & CONTRAINDICATIONS	ADVERSE EFFECTS†
Dalfopristin/ Quinupristin (Synercid)	**Inj:** (Dalfopristin-Quinupristin) 350mg-150mg per 500mg vial	*Adults:* **VREF:** 7.5mg/kg IV q8h. Duration depends on site and severity of infection. **Complicated SSSI:** 7.5mg/kg IV q12h for at least 7 days. **Hepatic Cirrhosis (Child Pugh A or B):** May need dose reduction. *Pediatrics:* ≥6 yrs: **VREF:** 7.5mg/kg IV q8h. Duration depends on site and severity of infection. **Complicated SSSI:** 7.5mg/kg IV q12h for at least 7 days. **Hepatic Cirrhosis (Child Pugh A or B):** May need dose reduction.	**W/P:** Pseudomembranous colitis reported. Flush vein with 5% dextrose after infusion to minimize venous irritation. Arthralgia, myalgia, and bilirubin elevation reported. **P/N:** Category B, caution in nursing.	Infusion site reactions (inflammation, pain, edema), nausea, diarrhea, and rash.

Table 6.2: PRESCRIBING INFORMATION FOR ANTIBIOTICS (cont.)

NAME	FORM/STRENGTH	DOSAGE	WARNINGS/PRECAUTIONS & CONTRAINDICATIONS	ADVERSE EFFECTS†
SULFONAMIDES				
Sulfamethoxazole/Trimethoprim (Bactrim)	(Sulfamethoxazole [SMX]-Trimethoprim [TMP]) Tab: 400mg-80mg*; Tab, DS: 800mg-160mg*	***Adults:*** **UTI:** 800mg SMX-160mg TMP q12h for 10-14 days. **Shigellosis:** 800mg SMX-160mg TMP q12h for 5 days. **AECB:** 800mg SMX-160mg TMP q12h for 14 days. **PCP Treatment:** 15-20mg/kg TMP and 75-100mg/kg SMX per 24hrs given q6h for 14-21 days. **PCP Prophylaxis:** 800mg SMX-160mg TMP qd. **Traveler's Diarrhea:** 800mg SMX-160mg TMP q12h for 5 days. **CrCl: 15-30mL/min:** 50% usual dose. **CrCl: <15mL/min:** Not recommended. ***Pediatrics:*** **≥2 months: UTI/Otitis Media:** 4mg/kg TMP and 20mg/kg SMX q12h for 10 days. **Shigellosis:** 8mg/kg TMP and 40mg/kg SMX per 24hrs given q12h for 5 days. **PCP Treatment:** 15-20mg/kg TMP and 75-100mg/kg SMX per 24hrs given q6h for 14-21 days. **PCP Prophylaxis:** 150mg/m²/day TMP with 750mg/m²/day SMX given bid, on 3 consecutive days/week. **Max:** 320mg TMP/1600mg SMX/day. **CrCl: 15-30mL/min:** 50% usual dose. **CrCl: <15mL/min:** Not recommended.	**W/P:** Fatal hypersensitivity reactions (eg, Stevens-Johnson syndrome, toxic epidermal necrolysis, fulminant hepatic necrosis, agranulocytosis, or aplastic anemia) may occur. Pseudomembranous colitis, cough, SOB, and pulmonary infiltrates reported. Avoid with group A β-hemolytic streptococcal infections. Caution with hepatic/renal impairment, elderly, folate deficiency (eg, chronic alcoholics, anticonvulsants, malabsorption, malnutrition), bronchial asthma, and other allergies). In G6PD deficiency, hemolysis may occur. Increased incidence of adverse events with AIDS. Ensure adequate fluid intake and urinary output. Caution with porphyria or thyroid dysfunction. **Contra:** Megaloblastic anemia due to folate deficiency, pregnancy, nursing, infants <2 months, marked hepatic damage, or severe renal insufficiency if cannot monitor renal status. **P/N:** Category C, contraindicated in nursing.	Nausea, vomiting, anorexia, rash, and urticaria.
Sulfamethoxazole/Trimethoprim (Septra)	(Sulfamethoxazole [SMX]-Trimethoprim [TMP]) Inj: (Septra) 80mg-16mg/mL; Sus: (Sulfatrim Pediatric, Septra) 200mg-40mg/5mL [100mL, 473mL]; Tab: (Septra) 400mg-80mg*; Tab, DS: (Septra) 800mg-160mg*	***Adults:*** **(Sus, Tab) UTI:** 800mg-160mg PO q12h for 10-14 days. **Shigellosis/Traveler's Diarrhea:** 800mg-160mg PO q12h for 5 days. **AECB:** 800mg-160mg PO q12h for 14 days. **PCP Treatment: 15-20mg/kg TMP and 75-100mg/kg SMX per 24hrs given PO q6h for 14-21 days PCP Prophylaxis:** 800mg-160mg PO qd. **(Inj) Severe UTI:** 8-10mg/kg TMP IV given in divided doses q6, 8 or 12h for up to 14 days. **PCP Treatment:** 15-20mg/kg TMP IV given in divided doses q6-8h for up to 14 days. **Shigellosis:** 8-10mg/kg TMP IV given in divided doses q6, 8 or 12h for 5 days. **(Inj, Sus, Tab) Renal Impairment: CrCl 15-30mL/min:** 50% usual dose. **CrCl <15mL/min:** Not recommended. ***Pediatrics:*** **(Sus, Tab) ≥2 months: UTI/Otitis Media:** 4mg/kg TMP and 20mg/kg SMX q12h for 10 days. **Shigellosis/Traveler's Diarrhea:** 4mg/kg TMP and 20mg/kg SMX q12h for 5 days. **PCP Treatment:** 15-20mg/kg TMP and 75-100mg/kg SMX/24hrs given q6h for 14-21 days. **PCP Prophylaxis:** 150mg/m²/day TMP and 750mg/m²/day SMX PO given bid, on 3 consecutive days per week. **Max:** 320mg TMP and 1600mg SMX per day. **(Inj) Severe UTI:** 8-10mg/kg TMP IV given in divided doses q6, 8 or 12h for up to 14 days. **PCP Treatment:** 15-20mg/kg TMP IV given in divided doses q6-8h for up to 14 days. **Shigellosis:** 8-10mg/kg TMP IV given in divided doses q6, 8 or 12h for 5 days. **(Inj, Sus, Tab) Renal Impairment: CrCl 15-30mL/min:** 50% usual dose. **CrCl <15mL/min:** Not recommended.	**W/P:** Fatal hypersensitivity reactions (eg, Stevens-Johnson syndrome, toxic epidermal necrolysis, fulminant hepatic necrosis, agranulocytosis, or aplastic anemia) may occur. Pseudomembranous colitis, cough, SOB, and pulmonary infiltrates reported. Avoid with group A β-hemolytic streptococcal infections. Caution with hepatic/renal impairment, elderly, folate deficiency (eg, chronic alcoholics, anticonvulsants, malabsorption, or malnutrition), bronchial asthma, and other allergies). In G6PD deficiency, hemolysis may occur. Increased incidence of adverse events in AIDS patients. Maintain adequate fluid intake. **Contra:** Megaloblastic anemia due to folate deficiency, pregnancy at term, nursing, infants <2 months old **P/N:** Category C, contraindicated in nursing.	Anorexia, nausea, vomiting, rash, urticaria, cholestatic jaundice, agranulocytosis, anemia, hyperkalemia, renal failure, interstitial nephritis, hyponatremia, convulsions, arthralgia, myalgia, and weakness.

*Scored. † Bold entries denote special dental considerations.

NAME	FORM/ STRENGTH	DOSAGE	WARNINGS/PRECAUTIONS & CONTRAINDICATIONS	ADVERSE EFFECTS†
TETRACYCLINE DERIVATIVES				
Demeclocycline (Declomycin)	**Tab:** 150mg, 300mg	**Adults: Usual:** 150mg qid or 300mg bid. **Gonorrhea: Initial:** 600mg, then 300mg q12h for 4 days. **Gonorrhea:** 600mg followed by 300mg q12h for 4 days to a total of 3g. **Renal/Hepatic Impairment:** Reduce dose and/or extend dose intervals. Continue therapy for at least 24-48hrs after symptoms subside. Treat strep infections for at least 10 days. Take at least 1hr before or 2hrs after meals with plenty of fluids. **Pediatrics: >8 yrs: Usual:** 3-6mg/lb/day given bid-qid. **Gonorrhea:** 600mg followed by 300mg q12h for 4 days to a total of 3g. **Renal/Hepatic Impairment:** Reduce dose and/or extend dose intervals. Continue therapy for at least 24-48hrs after symptoms subside. Treat strep infections for at least 10 days. Take at least 1hr before or 2hrs after meals with plenty of fluids.	**W/P:** May cause fetal harm during pregnancy. Use during tooth development (last half of pregnancy, infancy, <8yrs), or long-term use, or repeated short-term use may cause permanent discoloration of the teeth. Pseudotumor cerebri (adults), bulging fontanels (infants) reported. Caution with renal or hepatic impairment. Long-term use may cause reversible, nephrogenic diabetes insipidus syndrome. May result in overgrowth of nonsusceptible organisms; discontinue if superinfection develops. CNS symptoms may occur; caution when operating machinery. May decrease bone growth in premature infants. Monitor hematopoietic, renal, and hepatic function with long-term use. Discontinue at first evidence of skin erythema after sun/UV light exposure. **Contra:** Hypersensitivity to any of the tetracyclines. **P/N:** Category D, not for use in nursing.	GI problems, rash, esophageal ulceration, hypersensitivity reactions, dizziness, headache, tinnitus, blood dyscrasias, photosensitivity reactions, enamel hypoplasia, and elevated BUN.
Doxycycline (Aridox, Monodox)	**Cap:** 50mg, 100mg	**Adults: Usual:** 100mg q12h or 50mg q6h for 1 day, then 100mg/day. **Severe Infection:** 100mg q12h. **Uncomplicated Gonococcal Infections (except anorectal infections in men):** 100mg bid for 7 days or 300mg stat, then repeat in 1hr. **Acute Epididymo-Orchitis caused by _N. gonorrhoeae_ or _C. trachomatis_:** 100mg bid for at least 10 days. **Primary/Secondary Syphilis:** 300mg/day in divided dose for at least 10 days. **Uncomplicated Urethral/Endocervical/Rectal Infection caused by _C. trachomatis_:** 100mg bid for at least 7 days. **Nongonococcal Urethritis caused by _C. trachomatis_ and _U. urealyticum_:** 100mg bid for at least 7 days. Take with full glass of water. Take with food if GI upset occurs. **Pediatrics: >8 yrs: ≤100 lbs:** 2mg/lb divided in 2 doses for 1 day, then 1mg/lb daily in single or 2 divided doses. **Severe Infection:** May use up to 2mg/lb/day. **>100 lbs:** 100mg q12h or 50mg q6h for 1 day, then 100mg/day. **Severe Infection:** 100mg q12h. Take with a full glass of water. Take with food if GI upset occurs.	**W/P:** Avoid direct sunlight or UV light. May cause permanent tooth discoloration during tooth development (last half of pregnancy and children <8 years). Monitor renal/hepatic function and blood with long-term therapy. May increase BUN. Photosensitivity and pseudotumor cerebri reported. Discontinue if superinfection occurs. Bulging fontanels in infants and intracranial HTN in adults reported. **Contra:** Hypersensitivity to any of the tetracyclines. **P/N:** Category D, not for use in nursing.	GI effects, photosensitivity, rash, blood dyscrasias, and hypersensitivity reactions.
Doxycycline (Doryx)	**CAP:** 75mg, 100mg	**Adults: Usual:** 100mg q12h on 1st day, followed by 100mg qd. **Severe Infections/Chronic UTI:** 100mg q12h. **Uncomplicated Gonococcal Infections (Men, except anorectal infections):** 100mg bid for 7 days, or 300mg followed in 1hr by another 300mg dose. **Acute Epididymo-Orchitis:** 100mg bid for at least 10 days. **Primary/Secondary Syphilis:** 300mg/day in divided doses for at least 10 days. **Nongonococcal Urethritis, Uncomplicated Urethral/Endocervical/Rectal**	**W/P:** May cause fetal harm during pregnancy. Use during tooth development (last half of pregnancy, infancy, <8yrs) may cause permanent discoloration of the teeth or enamel hypoplasia. Photosensitivity, increased BUN, or superinfection may occur. Monitor hematopoietic, renal, and hepatic values periodically with long-term therapy. Bulging fontanels in infants and benign intracranial HTN in adults reported. May decrease bone growth in premature infants. **Contra:** Hypersensitivity	Anorexia, nausea, vomiting, diarrhea, dysphagia, enterocolitis, rash, exfoliative dermatitis, renal toxicity, hypersensitivity reactions, and blood dyscrasias.

Table 6.2: PRESCRIBING INFORMATION FOR ANTIBIOTICS *(cont.)*

NAME	FORM/ STRENGTH	DOSAGE	WARNINGS/PRECAUTIONS & CONTRAINDICATIONS	ADVERSE EFFECTS†
TETRACYCLINE DERIVATIVES *(cont.)*				
Doxycycline *(cont.)*		**Infection:** 100mg bid for at least 7 days. **Inhalational Anthrax (post-exposure):** 100mg bid for 60 days. Treat Strep infections for 10 days. *Pediatrics:* **>8 yrs: >100lbs:** 100mg q12h on 1st day, followed by 100mg qd. **Severe Infections/Chronic UTI:** 100mg q12h. **≤100lbs:** 2mg/lb given bid on day 1, followed by 1mg/lb given qd-bid thereafter. **Severe Infections:** Up to 2mg/lb. **Inhalational Anthrax (Post-Exposure): <100lbs:** 1mg/lb bid for 60 days. **≥100lbs:** 100mg bid for 60 days.	to any of the tetracyclines. **P/N:** Category D, not for use in nursing.	
Doxycycline (Atridox★, Periostat★, Vibramycin, Vibra-tabs)	**Cap:** (Doxycycline Hyclate) 50mg, 100mg; **Cap (low dose‡):** (Doxycycline Hyclate [Periostat]) 20mg; **Gel syringe§:** (Doxycycline Hyclate 10% [Atridox]) 50mg in a 500-mg blended formulation; **Syr:** (Doxycycline Calcium) 50mg/5mL; **Sus:** (Doxycycline Monohydrate) 25mg/5mL [60mL]; **Tab:** (Vibra-Tabs) 100mg	*Adults:* (Atridox) Single injection of gel into periodontal pocket; repeat at 4 mo. One dose delivers local antibacterial concentrations for 7-14 days. **Max:** 1 injection per pocket every 7 days. **(Periostat) Usual:** 20mg q12h. **Max:** Same as usual dose. Give 1 hr before or 2 hr after meal. **(Vibramycin, Vibra-tabs) Usual:** 100mg q12h on day 1, then 100mg qd or 50mg q12h. **Severe Infection:** 100mg q12h. Treat for 10 days with strep infection. **Uncomplicated Gonococcal Infection (Except Anorectal in Men):** 100mg bid for 7 days or 300mg followed by 300mg in 1hr. **Uncomplicated Urethral/Endocervical/Rectal Infection and Nongonococcal Urethritis:** 100mg bid for 7 days. **Syphilis:** 100mg bid for 2 weeks. **Syphilis for >1 yr:** 100mg bid for 4 weeks. **Acute Epididymo-orchitis:** 100mg bid for at least 10 days. **Inhalation Anthrax (Post-Exposure):** 100mg bid for 60 days. **Malaria Prophylaxis:** 100mg qd. Begin 1-2 days before travel and continue for 4 weeks after leaving malarious area. *Pediatrics:* **(Vibramycin, Vibra-tabs) >8 yrs: ≥100 lbs:** 1mg/lb bid on day 1, then 1mg/lb qd or 0.5mg/lb bid. **Severe Infections: Maint:** 2mg/lb. **>100lbs: Usual:** 100mg q12h on day 1, then 100mg qd or 50mg q12h. **Severe Infection:** 100mg q12h. Treat for 10 days with strep infection. **Inhalation Anthrax (Post-Exposure): <100lbs:** 1mg/lb bid for 60 days. **≥100lbs:** 100mg bid for 60 days. **Malaria Prophylaxis:** 2mg/kg qd. **Max:** 100mg/day. Begin 1-2 days before travel and continue for 4 weeks after leaving malarious area.	**W/P:** May cause fetal harm with pregnancy. Permanent tooth discoloration during tooth development (last half of pregnancy and children <8 yrs) reported. May increase BUN. Photosensitivity, enamel hypoplasia reported. Superinfection with prolonged use. Syrup contains sodium metabisulfite. Bulging fontanels in infants and benign intracranial HTN in adults reported. Monitor renal/hepatic and hematopoietic function with long-term use. Take adequate fluids with caps or tabs to reduce esophageal irritation. Take with food or milk if GI irritation occurs. (Atridox) Use with caution in patients with history or predisposition to oral candidiasis. Mechanical oral hygiene procedures (ie, tooth brushing, flossing) should be avoided on treated areas for 7 days. May result in overgrowth of nonsusceptible organisms; effects of prolonged treatment (> 6 mo) have not been studied. Atridox has not been tested in the following: pregnant women, patients with severe periodontal defects, immunocompromised patients; or for use in regeneration of alveolar bone. **Contra:** Hypersensitivity to any of the tetracyclines. **P/N:** Category D, not for use in nursing.	GI effects, photosensitivity, increased BUN, hypersensitivity reactions, and blood dyscrasias. (Atridox) Cold- and flu-like symptoms; **gum discomfort, pain, or soreness;** headache; **pressure sensitivity of tooth; toothache.**
Minocycline (Arestin, Dynacin, Minocin)	**Cap:** 50mg, 75mg, 100mg; **Tab:** 50mg, 75mg, 100mg (Dynacin); **Cap:** 50mg, 100mg (Minocin); **Cartridge:** 1mg (Arestin)	*Adults:* (Arestin) Single injection of one unit dosage into periodontal pocket, 5mm or deeper, after scaling and root planing. One dose delivers antibacterial concentrations for 10-14 days. **Max:** 1 injection per pocket every 3 mo. **(Dynacin, Minocin) Usual:** 200mg initially, then 100mg q12h; alternative is 100-200mg initially, then 50mg qid.	**W/P:** May cause fetal harm during pregnancy. Use during tooth development (last half of pregnancy, infancy, <8yrs) may cause permanent discoloration of the teeth or enamel hypoplasia; avoid use during this period. Renal toxicity, hepatotoxicity, photosensitivity, increased BUN, superinfection, or pseudotumor cerebri may occur;	Anorexia, nausea, vomiting, diarrhea, dysphagia, enterocolitis, pancreatitis, increased LFTs, hepatitis, liver failure, renal toxicity, rash, exfoliative dermatitis, Stevens-Johnson syndrome, skin and mucous membrane pigmentation,

*Scored.   † Bold entries denote special dental considerations.   ‡ At this dose, not antibacterial, but modulates the inflammatory host response.   § Locally delivered sustained-release system.   ★ indicates a drug bearing the ADA Seal of Acceptance.

NAME	FORM/ STRENGTH	DOSAGE	WARNINGS/PRECAUTIONS & CONTRAINDICATIONS	ADVERSE EFFECTS[†]
Minocycline (cont.)		**Uncomplicated Gonococcal Infection (Men, other than urethritis and anorectal infections):** 200mg initially, then 100mg q12h for min 4 days. **Uncomplicated Gonococcal Urethritis (Men):** 100mg q12h for 5 days. **Syphilis:** Administer usual dose for 10-15 days. **Meningococcal Carrier State:** 100mg q12h for 5 days. *Mycobacterium marinum:* 100mg q12h for 6-8 weeks. **Uncomplicated urethral, endocervical, or rectal infection:** 100mg q12h for at least 7 days. **Renal Dysfunction:** Reduce dose and/or extend dose intervals. *Pediatrics:* **(Dynacin, Minocin) >8 yrs:** 4mg/kg initially followed by 2mg/kg q12h. Take with plenty of fluids.	perform hematopoietic, renal, and hepatic monitoring. May impair mental/physical abilities. Use alternate form of contraception other than oral contraceptives. May decrease bone growth in premature infants. (Arestin) Use with caution in patients with history or predisposition to oral candidiasis. May result in overgrowth of nonsusceptible organisms; effects of prolonged treatment (> 6 mo) have not been studied. Use has not been studied in acutely abscessed periodontal pockets and is not recommended. Arestin has not been tested in pregnant women or immunocompromised patients; or for use in regeneration of alveolar bone. Advise patients of the following: avoid hard, crunchy, or sticky foods for 1 wk after treatment; wait 12 hrs after treatment before brushing teeth; postpone use of interproximal cleaning devices for 10 days after treatment; do not touch treated areas. Although sensitivity is normal the first week after treatment, patients should promptly report pain, swelling or other problems that occur. **Contra:** Hypersensitivity to any of the tetracyclines. **P/N:** Category D, not for use in nursing.	blood dyscrasias, headache, **tooth discoloration**. (Arestin) **Bleeding gums**; chills; **dental pain; fever, pain, redness, and swelling in the mouth; problems with teeth; redness or swelling of gums; toothache.**
Tetracycline (Sumycin)	**Sus:** 125mg/5mL; **Tab:** 250mg, 500mg	*Adults:* **Mild-Moderate:** 250mg qid or 500mg bid. **Severe:** 500mg qid. Continue for 24-48hrs after symptoms subside (minimum 10 days with Group A β-hemolytic streptococci). **Severe Acne: Initial:** 1g/day in divided doses. **Maint:** After improvement, 125-500mg/day. **Brucellosis:** 500mg qid for 3 weeks plus streptomycin 1g IM bid for 1 week, then qd for 1 week. **Syphilis:** 30-40g equally divided over 10-15 days. **Gonorrhea:** 500mg q6h for 7 days. **Chlamydia:** 500mg qid for at least 7 days. **Renal Dysfunction:** Reduce dose or extend dose interval. *Pediatrics:* **>8 yrs: Usual:** 25-50mg/kg divided bid-qid. Continue for 24-48hrs after symptoms subside (minimum 10 days with Group A β-hemolytic streptococci). **Severe Acne: Initial:** 1g/day in divided doses. **Maint:** After improvement, 125-500mg/day. **Renal Dysfunction:** Reduce dose or extend dose interval.	**W/P:** May cause fetal harm with pregnancy, permanent tooth discoloration during tooth development (last half of pregnancy and children <8 yrs). May increase BUN. Photosensitivity and enamel hypoplasia reported. Superinfection with prolonged use. Suspension contains sodium metabisulfite. Bulging fontanels in infants and benign intracranial HTN in adults reported. Monitor renal/hepatic and hematopoietic function with long-term use. Caution with history of asthma, hay fever, urticaria, and allergy. **P/N:** Category D, not for use in nursing	GI effects, photosensitivity, increased BUN, hypersensitivity reactions, blood dyscrasias, dizziness, and headache.

Table 6.3: DRUG INTERACTIONS FOR ANTIBIOTICS

AMINOGLYCOSIDES

Amikacin Sulfate (Amikin, Amikin Pediatric)

Aminoglycosides	Crossed allergenicity with aminoglycosides.
Anesthetics	Increased risk of neuromuscular blockade and respiratory paralysis with anesthetics.
β-lactams	Significant mutual inactivation may occur with β-lactams.
Cephalosporins	Increased nephrotoxicity with cephalosporins.
Diuretics	Avoid diuretics and other nephrotoxic agents.
Neuromuscular blockers	Increased risk of neuromuscular blockade and respiratory paralysis with neuromuscular blockers.
Neurotoxic drugs	Avoid use.
Ototoxic drugs	Avoid use.

Gentamicin Sulfate (Gentamicin)

Cephalosporins	Increased nephrotoxicity with cephalosporins.
Neuromuscular blockers	Increased risk of neuromuscular blockade and respiratory paralysis with neuromuscular blockers.

Tobramycin (TOBI)

Aminoglycosides	Hearing loss reported with previous or concomitant aminoglycosides.
Diuretics	Avoid diuretics and other nephrotoxic agents.
Neurotoxic drugs	Avoid use.
Ototoxic drugs	Avoid use.

CARBACEPHEM

Loracarbef (Lorabid)

Diuretics	Use with caution.
Probenecid	Potentiated by probenecid.

CARBAPENEM

Cilastin Sodium/Imipenem (Primaxin IM)

Antibiotics	Do not mix physically with other antibiotics; may give concomitantly with other antibiotics.
Probenecid	Avoid use.

Cilastin Sodium/Imipenem (Primaxin IV)

Antibiotics	Do not mix physically with other antibiotics; may give concomitantly with other antibiotics.
Ganciclovir	Seizures reported with ganciclovir; avoid concomitant use.
Probenecid	Avoid use.

Ertapenem (Invanz)

Probenecid	Decreased clearance with probenecid.

CARBAPENEM (cont.)

Meropenem (Merrem)

Probenecid	Probenecid inhibits renal excretion; avoid concomitant use.
Valproic acid	May reduce valproic acid levels.

CEPHALOSPORINS

Cefaclor (Ceclor)

Probenecid	Renal excretion inhibited by probenecid.
Warfarin	May potentiate warfarin and other anticoagulants; monitor PT/INR.

Cefdinir (Omnicef)

Antacids (aluminum- or magnesium-containing drugs)	Reduced absorption with antacids; separate doses by 2hrs.
Iron-fortified foods	Reduced absorption with iron-fortified drugs; separate doses by 2hrs.
Iron supplements	Reduced absorption with iron supplements; separate doses by 2hrs; reddish stools reported.
Probenecid	Inhibits renal secretion.

Cefditoren Pivoxil (Spectracef)

Antacids	Avoid use.
H_2-receptor antagonists	May reduce absorption.
Probenecid	Increased plasma levels with probenecid.

Cefepime Hydrochloride (Maxipime)

Aminoglycosides	Increased risk of nephrotoxicity and ototoxicity with aminoglycosides.
Diuretics	Risk of nephrotoxicity with diuretics.

Cefixime (Suprax)

Anticoagulants	Increased PT with anticoagulants.
Carbamazepine	May increase carbamazepine levels.

Cefotaxime (Claforan)

Aminoglycosides	Increased risk of nephrotoxicity with aminoglycosides.

Cefotetan (Cefotan)

Alcohol	Possible disulfiram-like reaction within 72hrs with alcohol.
Aminoglycosides	Increased risk of nephrotoxicity; monitor renal function with aminoglycosides.

Cefoxitin (Mefoxin)

Aminoglycosides	Increased risk of nephrotoxicity with aminoglycosides.

Table 6.3: DRUG INTERACTIONS FOR ANTIBIOTICS *(cont.)*

CEPHALOSPORINS *(cont.)*

Cefpodoxime Proxetil (Vantin)

Antacids	Decreased plasma levels and absorption with antacids.
Anticholinergics	Delayed peak plasma levels with anticholinergics.
H_2-blockers	Decreased plasma levels and absorption with H_2-blockers.
Nephrotoxic agents	Closely monitor renal function with nephrotoxic agents.
Probenecid	Inhibits renal excretion.

Cefprozil (Cefzil)

Aminoglycosides	Increased risk of nephrotoxicity with aminoglycosides.
Diuretics	Caution with agents causing adverse effects on renal function.

Ceftazidime (Fortaz, Tazicef)

β-lactams	May decrease effect of β-lactams.
Cephalosporins	Increased nephrotoxicity with cephalosporins.
Chloramphenicol	Avoid use.
Diuretics	Increased nephrotoxicity with diuretics.

Ceftizoxime Sodium (Cefizox)

Aminoglycosides	Increased risk of nephrotoxicity with aminoglycosides.

Ceftriaxone (Rocephin)

Diuretics	Caution with agents causing adverse effects on renal function.
Drugs that lower gastric acidity	Lower bioavailability when used with such drugs.
Probenecid	Increases plasma levels.

Cefuroxime Sodium (Zinacef)

Aminoglycosides	Possible nephrotoxicity with concomitant use.
Anticoagulants	May decrease prothrombin activity; use with caution.
Diuretics	Caution with agents causing adverse effects on renal function.

Cephalexin (Keflex)

Probenecid	Inhibits excretion.

Cephalexin (Panixine Disperdose)

Probenecid	Inhibits excretion.

CYCLIC LIPOPEPTIDE

Daptomycin (Cubicin)

Statins	Consider temporarily suspending statins.

CYCLIC LIPOPEPTIDE *(cont.)*

Daptomycin (Cubicin)

Tobramycin	Use tobramycin with caution; may affect levels.
Warfarin	Monitor PT/INR for first several days with warfarin.

FLUOROQUINOLONES

Ciprofloxacin (Cipro IV)

Anticoagulants	Enhances anticoagulant effects.
Caffeine	Increases caffeine levels and prolongs effects.
Cyclosporine	Transient serum creatinine elevations with cyclosporine.
Drugs that lower seizure threshold	Use with caution.
Glyburide	Severe hypoglycemia (rare) with glyburide.
Phenytoin	Altered serum levels of phenytoin.
Probenecid	Potentiated by probenecid.
Theophylline	Increases theophylline levels and prolongs effects.

Ciprofloxacin (Cipro)

Antacids (aluminum- or magnesium-containing drugs)	Space doses at least 2 hrs before or 6hrs after administration with antacids.
Anticoagulants	Enhances anticoagulant effects.
Caffeine	Increases caffeine levels and prolongs effects.
Calcium	Decreased serum and urine levels with calcium; space doses at least 2hrs before or 6hrs after administration.
Cyclosporine	Transient serum creatinine elevations with cyclosporine.
Didanosine	Space doses at least 2 hrs before or 6hrs after administration with didanosine.
Drugs that lower seizure threshold	Use with caution.
Glyburide	Severe hypoglycemia (rare) with glyburide.
Iron	Decreased serum and urine levels with iron; space doses at least 2hrs before or 6hrs after administration.
Phenytoin	Altered serum levels of phenytoin.
Probenecid	Potentiated by probenecid.
Sucralfate	Space doses at least 2 hrs before or 6 hrs after administration with sucralfate.
Theophylline	Increases theophylline levels and prolongs effects; fatal reactions have occurred.
Zinc	Space doses at least 2 hrs before or 6 hrs after administration with zinc.

Table 6.3: DRUG INTERACTIONS FOR ANTIBIOTICS (cont.)

FLUOROQUINOLONES (cont.)

Gemifoxacin (Factive)

Amiodarone	Avoid Class III antiarrhytmics such as amiodarone.
Antacids (aluminum- or magnesium- containing drugs)	Space doses at least 2hrs before or 6hrs after administration with antacids.
Antipsychotics	Caution with drugs that prolong the QTc interval, such as antipsychotics.
Didanosine	Space doses at least 2hrs before or 6hrs after administration with didanosine.
Erythromycin	Caution with drugs that prolong the QTc interval, such as erythromycin.
Iron	Decreased serum and urine levels with iron; space doses at least 2hrs before or 6hrs after administration.
Probenecid	Potentiated by probenecid.
Procainamide	Avoid Class IA antiarrhytmics such as procainamide.
Quinidine	Avoid Class IA antiarrhytmics such as quinidine.
Sotalol	Avoid Class III antiarrhytmics such as sotalol.
Sucralfate	Space doses at least 2hrs before or 6hrs after administration with sucralfate.
Tricyclic antidepressants	Caution with drugs that prolong the QTc interval, such as TCAs.
Zinc	Space doses at least 2hrs before or 6hrs after administration with zinc.

Levofloxacin (Levaquin)

Antacids (aluminum- or magnesium- containing drugs)	Space doses at least 2hrs before or 6hrs after administration.
Didanosine	Space doses at least 2hrs before or 6hrs after administration; didanosine may decrease levels.
NSAIDs	May increase seizure risk and CNS stimulation.
Theophyline	Monitor theophylline levels.
Warfarin	Increases PT; monitor closely.

Lomefloxacin (Maxaquin)

Antacids (aluminum- or magnesium- containing drugs)	Space doses at least 2hrs before or 6hrs after administration.
Cimetidine	May increase effects.
Cyclosporine	May enhance cyclosporine.

FLUOROQUINOLONES *(cont.)*

Lomefloxacin (Maxaquin)

Didanosine	Space doses at least 2hrs before or 6hrs after administration with didanosine; may decrease levels.
Probenecid	Slows renal elimination.
Sucralfate	Space doses at least 2hrs before or 6hrs after administration with sucralfate.
Warfarin	May enhance warfarin effects.

Moxifloxacin (Avelox)

Amiodarone	Avoid Class III antiarrhytmics such as amiodarone.
Antacids (aluminum- or magnesium-containing drugs)	Decreased bioavailability; space doses at least 4hrs before or 8hrs after administration.
Antipsychotics	Caution with drugs that prolong the QTc interval, such as antipsychotics.
Cisapride	Caution with drugs that prolong the QTc interval, such as cisapride.
Corticosteroids	Concomitant use may increase risk of tendon rupture in elderly.
Didanosine	Decreased bioavailability; space doses at least 4hrs before or 2hrs after administration.
Erythromycin	Caution with drugs that prolong QTc interval.
Iron	Decreased bioavailability; space doses at least 4hrs before or 8hrs after administration.
NSAIDs	May increase seizure risk and CNS stimulation.
Procainamide	Avoid Class IA antiarrhytmics such as procainamide.
Sotalol	Avoid Class III antiarrhytmics such as sotalol.
Sucralfate	Decreased bioavailability; space doses at least 4hrs before or 8hrs after administration.
TCAs	Caution with drugs that prolong the QTc interval
Quinidine	Avoid Class IA antiarrhytmics.
Warfarin	Monitor PT.
Zinc	Decreased bioavailability; space doses at least 4hrs before or 8hrs after administration.

Norfloxacin (Noroxin)

Antacids	May interfere with absorption; space dose by 2hrs.
Caffeine	May reduce clearance of caffeine.
Cyclosporine	May increase cyclosporine levels.
Didanosine	May interfere with absorption; space dose by 2hrs.
Iron	May interfere with absorption; space dose by 2 hrs.
Nitrofurantoin	Antagonized effects with nitrofurantoin.
Probenecid	Diminished urinary excretion with probenecid.

Table 6.3: DRUG INTERACTIONS FOR ANTIBIOTICS *(cont.)*

FLUOROQUINOLONES *(cont.)*

Norfloxacin (Noroxin)

Theophylline	Increases theophylline levels and prolongs effects; fatal reactions have occurred.
Warfarin	May enhance effects of warfarin.
Zinc	May interfere with absorption; space dose by 2 hrs.

Ofloxacin (Floxin)

Antacids	May interfere with absorption; space dose by 2 hrs.
CYP450	May increase half life of drugs metabolized by CYP450.
Didanosine	May interfere with absorption; space dose by 2 hrs.
Hypoglycemics	May potentiate oral hypoglycemics; discontinue if hypoglycemia occurs.
Insulin	May potentiate insulin; discontinue if hypoglycemia occurs.
NSAIDs	May increase seizure risk and CNS stimulation.
Sucralfate	May interfere with absorption; space dose by 2 hrs.
Theophylline	May potentiate theophylline.
Warfarin	May potentiate warfarin.
Zinc	May interfere with absorption; space dose by 2 hrs.

GLYCOPEPTIDE

Vancomycin (Vancocin)

Anesthetics	Increase in infusion-related events (erythema, flushing, anaphylactoid reactions).
Nephrotoxic agents	Carefully monitor with use.
Neurotoxic drugs	Carefully monitor with use.

LINCOSAMIDES

Clindamycin (Cleocin)

Erythromycin	Antagonism may occur with erythromycin.
Neuromuscular blockers	May potentiate neuromuscular blockers.

Lincomycin (Lincocin)

Erythromycin	Antagonism may occur with erythromycin.
Kaolin-pectin	Kaolin-pectin inhibits oral lincomycin.
Neuromuscular blockers	May potentiate neuromuscular blockers.

OXAXOLIDINONE

Linezolid (Zyvox)

Adrenergic agents	Potential interaction with adrenergic agents.
Dopamine	Use with caution.
Dopaminergic agents	May enhance pressor response to dopaminergic agents.
Epinephrine	Use with caution.
Phenylpropanol-amine	Use with caution.
Pseudoephedrine	Use with caution.
Serotonergic agents	Potential interaction; serotonin syndrome may occur.
Sympathomimet-ics	May enhance pressor response to sympathomimetics.
Tyramine-containing foods	Avoid large quantities.
Vasopressors	May enhance pressor response to vasopressors.

KETOLIDE

Telithromycin (Ketek)

Anticoagulants	May potentiate effects of anticoagulants.
Atorvastatin	Avoid use.
Cisapride	Avoid use.
Ergot alkaloid derivatives	Avoid use.
Lovastatin	Avoid use.
CYP3A4 Inducers	Decreased effects with CYP3A4 inducers.
CYP450	Increases levels of drugs metabolized by CYP450 system.
Digoxin	Monitor use.
Dofetilide	Avoid Class III antiarrhythimcs such as dofetilide.
Itraconazole	Increased levels with concomitant use.
Ketoconazole	Increased levels with concomitant use.
Midazolam	Monitor use.
Pimozide	Avoid use.

Table 6.3: DRUG INTERACTIONS FOR ANTIBIOTICS (cont.)

KETOLIDE (cont.)

Telithromycin (Ketek)

Procainamide	Avoid Class 1A antiarrhythmics such as procainaminde.
Quinidine	Avoid Class IA antiarrhythmics.
Rifampin	Avoid use.
Simvastatin	Avoid use.
Sotalol	Decreases levels of sotalol.
Theophylline	Space dosing by 1hr to reduce GI effects.

MACROLIDES

Azithromycin (Zithromax, Zithromax Tri-Pak, Zithromax Z-pak)

Antacids	May reduce oral levels of magnesium- or aluminum-containing antacids.
Carbamazepine	May increase carbamazepine levels.
Cyclosporine	Monitor use.
Digoxin	May increase digoxin levels.
Dihydroergota-mine	Acute ergot toxicity may occur.
Ergotamine	Acute ergot toxicity may occur.
Hexobarbital	Monitor use.
Nelfinavir	Monitor for azithrymycin side effects (liver enzyme abnormalities, hearing impairment).
Phenytoin	Monitor use.
Terfenadine	Monitor use.
Theophylline	Monitor use.
Triazolam	Potentiates triazolam.
Warfarin	Monitor use.

Clarithromycin (Biaxin, Biaxin XL)

Anticoagulant	Potentiates anticoagulant effects.
Astemizole	Avoid use.
Bismuth citrate	Avoid use if CrCl < 25mL/min or history of porphyria.
Carbmazepine	Increases serum levels of carbamazepine.
CYP450	Increases serum levels of drugs metabolized by CYP450.
Digoxin	Increases serum levels of digoxin.
Dihydroergota-mine	Acute ergot toxicity reported.
Ergotamine	Acute ergot toxicity reported.

MACROLIDES *(cont.)*

Clarithromycin (Biaxin, Biaxin XL)

Fluconazole	Increased levels with fluconazole.
HMG-CoA reductase inhibitors	Increases serum levels of HMG-CoA reductase inhibitors.
Omeprazole	Increases serum levels of omeprazole.
Ranitidine	Avoid use if CrCl < 25mL/min or history of porphyria.
Ritonavir	Avoid use if CrCl < 60 mL/min.
Theophylline	Increases serum levels of theophylline.
Triazolam	Decreased clearance of triazolam.
Zidovudine	Decreases zidovudine plasma levels.

Dirithromycin (Dynabac)

Alfentanil	Use with caution.
Antacids	Increased absorption with antacids.
Anticoagulants	Increased effects of anticoagulants.
Astemizole	Use with caution.
Bromocriptine	Use with caution.
Carbamazepine	Use with caution.
Cyclosporine	Monitor use.
Digoxin	Increases serum levels of digoxin.
Dihydroergotamine	Acute ergot toxicity reported.
Disopyramide	Use with caution.
Ergotamine	Acute ergot toxicity reported.
H_2-receptor antagonists	Increased absorption with H_2-receptor antagonists.
Lovastatin	Use with caution.
Phenytoin	Use with caution.
Theophylline	Possible dosage adjustment needed.
Triazolam	Decresed clearance of triazolam.
Valproate	Use with caution.

Erythromycin (ERYC, Erythrocin)

Anticoagulants	Increased effects of anticoagulants.
Cisapride	Avoid use.
CYP450	Increases serum levels of drugs metabolized by CYP450.

Table 6.3: DRUG INTERACTIONS FOR ANTIBIOTICS *(cont.)*

MACROLIDES *(cont.)*

Erythromycin (ERYC, Erythrocin)

Digoxin	Increases serum levels of digoxin.
Dihydroergota-mine	Acute ergot toxicity reported.
Ergotamine	Acute ergot toxicity reported.
Terfenadine	Avoid use.
Theophylline	Increases serum levels of theophylline.
Triazolam	Potentiates triazolam.

Erythromycin (EryPed)

Anticoagulants	Increased effects of anticoagulants.
Astemizole	Avoid use.
CYP450	Increases serum levels of drugs metabolized by CYP450.
Cisapride	Avoid use.
Digoxin	Increases serum levels of digoxin.
Dihydroergota-mine	Acute ergot toxicity reported.
Ergotamine	Acute ergot toxicity reported.
Lovastatin	Rhabdomyolysis reported with lovastatin.
Midazolam	Increases effects of midazolam.
Pimozide	Avoid use.
Sildenafil	May potentiate sildenafil.
Terfenadine	Avoid use.
Theophylline	Increases serum levels of theophylline.
Triazolam	Potentiates triazolam.

MONOBACTAM

Azactam (Aztreonam)

Aminoglycosides	Monitor renal function; increased risk of nephrotoxicity and ototoxicity.
Radiaton therapy	Toxic epidermal necrolysis reported (rarely) in bone marrow transplant.

NITROIMIDAZOLE

Metronidazole (Flagyl, Flagyl IV, Flagyl ER)

Alcohol	Avoid alcohol during and for 3 days after use.
Cimetidine	Potentiated by cimetidine.

NITROIMIDAZOLE *(cont.)*

Metronidazole (Flagyl, Flagyl IV, Flagyl ER)

Disulfiram	Avoid within 2 weeks of disulfiram use; increased possibility of psychotic reactions.
Lithium	Increased lithium levels.
Phenobarbital	Increased elimination with phenobarbital.
Phenytoin	Increased elimination with phenytoin; may impair phenytoin clearance.
Warfarin	Potentiates anticoagulant effects of warfarin; monitor PT.

PENICILLINS

Amoxicillin (Amoxil, Amoxil Pediatric, Trimox)

Chloramphenicol	May interfere with bactericidal effects.
Macrolides	May interfere with bactericidal effects.
Probenecid	Increased levels with probenecid.
Sulfonamides	May interfere with bactericidal effects.
Tetracycline	May interfere with bactericidal effects.

Amoxicillin (Dispermox)

Chloramphenicol	May interfere with bactericidal effects.
Macrolides	May interfere with bactericidal effects.
Probenecid	Increased levels with probenecid.
Sulfonamides	May interfere with bactericidal effects.
Tetracycline	May interfere with bactericidal effects.

Amoxicillin/Clavulanate (Augmentin, Augmentin XR)

Allopurinol	May increase incidence of rash.
Anticoagulants	May increase PT with anticoagulant therapy.
Disulfiram	Increased risk of side effects.
Oral contraceptives	May reduce effects of oral contraceptives.
Probenecid	Increased levels with probenecid.

Ampicillin Sodium (Principen)

Allopurinol	May increase incidence of rash.
Bacteriostatic antibiotics	May interfere with bactercidal activity.
Oral contraceptives	May reduce effects of oral contraceptives.
Probenecid	Increased levels with probenecid.

Table 6.3: DRUG INTERACTIONS FOR ANTIBIOTICS *(cont.)*

PENICILLINS *(cont.)*

Ampicillin Sodium/Sulbactam (Unasyn)

Allopurinol	May increase incidence of rash.
Aminoglycosides	Do not reconstitute with aminoglycosides; may inactivate aminoglycosides.
Probenecid	Increased levels with probenecid.

Dicloxacillin (Dynapen)

Probenecid	Potentiated by probenecid.
Tetracycline	Tetracycline may antagonize the bactercidal effects.

Penicillin G Potassium (Pfizerpen)

Bacteriostatic antibiotics	May diminish effects of penicillin.
Probenecid	Prolonged levels with probenecid.

Piperacillin Sodium (Pipracil)

Aminoglycosides	Do not mix with aminoglycoside in a syringe or infusion bottle; may cause inactivation of aminoglycoside.
Cytotoxic therapy	Increased risk of hypokalemia.
Diuretics	Increased risk of hypokalemia.
Methotrexate	May reduce methotrexate clearance.
Vecuronium	May prolong neuromuscular blockade of nondepolarizing muscle relaxants.

Piperacillin Sodium/Tazobactam (Zosyn)

Aminoglycosides	Do not mix with aminoglycoside in a syringe or infusion bottle; may cause inactivation of aminoglycoside.
Cytotoxic therapy	Increased risk of hypokalemia.
Diuretics	Increased risk of hypokalemia.
Methotrexate	May reduce methotrexate clearance.
Vecuronium	May prolong neuromuscular blockade of non-depolarizing muscle relaxants.

Ticarcillin/Clavulanate Potassium (Timentin)

Aminoglycosides	May inactivate aminoglycosides if mixed together in parenteral solution.
Probenecid	Increased serum levels and prolonged half-life with probenecid.

POLYPEPTIDE

Colistimethate (Coly-Mycin)

Aminoglycosides	Avoid use.
Decamethonium	Extreme caution with curariform muscle relaxants; may potentiate neuromuscular-blocking effect.

POLYPEPTIDE *(cont.)*

Colistimethate (Coly-Mycin)

Gallamine	Extreme caution with curariform muscle relaxants; may potentiate neuromuscular-blocking effects.
Polymyxin	Avoid use.
Sodium cephalothin	May enhance neurotoxicity.
Sodium citrate	Extreme caution with curariform muscle relaxants; may potentiate neuromuscular-blocking effects.
Succinylcholine	Extreme caution with curariform muscle relaxants; may potentiate neuromuscular-blocking effects.
Tubocurarine	Extreme caution with curariform muscle relaxants; may potentiate neuromuscular-blocking effects.

STREPTOGRAMIN

Dalfopristin/Quinupristin (Synercid)

Cyclosporine	Monitor cyclosporine levels.
CYP3A4 drugs	Significant inhibition of CYP3A4 drugs; use with caution. Avoid drugs metabolized by CYP3A4 that prolong the QTc interval.
Digoxin	May inhibit digoxin.

SULFONAMIDES

Sulfamethoxazole/Trimethoprim (Bactrim)

Amantadine	Single case of delirium with amantadine.
Cyclosporine	Marked but reversible nephrotoxicity reported.
Digoxin	Increased plasma levels of digoxin (especially in elderly).
Diuretics	May increase risk of thrombocytopenia with purpura in elderly patients.
Hypoglycemics (oral)	Increased effects of oral hypoglycemics.
Indomethacin	Increased levels with indomethacin.
Methotrexate	Increased plasma levels of methotrexate.
Phenytoin	Increased effects of phenytoin.
Pyrimethamine	May develop megaloblastic anemia.
Tricyclic antidepressants	May decrease effects of TCAs.
Warfarin	Use with caution; may prolong PT.

Table 6.3: DRUG INTERACTIONS FOR ANTIBIOTICS (cont.)

SULFONAMIDES (cont.)

Sulfamethoxazole/Trimethoprim (Septra)

Diuretics	May increase risk of thrombocytopenia with purpura in elderly patients.
Methotrexate	Increased plasma levels of methotrexate.
Phenytoin	Increased effects of phenytoin.
Warfarin	Use with caution; may prolong PT.

TETRACYCLINE DERIVATIVES

Demeclocycline (Declomycin)

Anticoagulants	Decreases PT; may need to decrease the dose of anticoagulants.
Antacids (aluminum-, calcium-, and magnesium-containing products)	Decreased absorption with antacids.
Dairy products	Interfere with absorption.
Iron	Decreased absorption with iron-containing products.
Methoxyflurane	Fatal renal toxicity reported.
Oral contraceptives	May decrease efficacy of oral contraceptives; use alternate method of birth control.
Penicillin	May interfere with bactericidal action of penicillin; avoid concomitant use.

Doxycycline (Aridox, Monodox)

Anticoagulants	Decreases PT; may need to decrease anticoagulant dose.
Antacids (aluminum-, calcium-, and magnesium-containing products)	Decreased absorption with antacids.
Barbituates	Decreases half-life of doxycycline.
Carbamazepine	Decreases half-life of doxycycline.
Dairy products	Take 1hr before or 2hrs after dairy products.
Methoxyflurane	Fatal renal toxicity reported.
Oral contraceptives	May decrease efficacy of oral contraceptives; use alternate method of birth control.
Penicillin	May interfere with bactericidal action of penicillin; avoid concomitant use.
Phenytoin	Decreaes half-life of doxycycline.

TETRACYCLINE DERIVATIVES *(cont.)*

Doxycycline (Doryx, Vibramycin, Vibra-tabs)

Anticoagulants	Decreases PT; may need to decrease anticoagulant dose.
Antacids (aluminum-, calcium-, and magnesium-containing products)	Decreased absorption with antacids.
Iron	Decreased absorption with iron-containing products.
Penicillin	May interfere with bactericidal action of penicillin; avoid concomitant use.

Minocycline (Arestin, Dynacin, Minocin)

Antacids (aluminum-, calcium-, and magnesium-containing products)	Decreased absorption with antacids.
Anticoagulants	Decreases PT; May need to decrease the dose of anticoagulants.
Ergotamine	Risk of ergotism with ergot alkaloids.
Hepatoxic drugs	Use with caution.
Iron	Decreased absorption with iron-containing products.
Isotretinoin	Avoid isotretinoin shortly before, during, and after therapy.
Methoxyflurane	Fatal renal toxicity reported.
Oral contraceptives	May decrease efficacy of oral contraceptives; use alternate method of birth control.
Penicillin	May interfere with bactericidal action of penicillin; avoid concomitant use.

Tetracycline (Sumycin)

Antacids (aluminum-, calcium-, and magnesium-containing products)	Decreased absorption with antacids.
Anticoagulants	Decreases PT; may need to decrease anticoagulant dose.
Methoxyflurane	Fatal renal toxicity reported.
Penicillin	May interfere with bactericidal action of penicillin; avoid concomitant use.

Table 6.4: PHARMACOLOGIC PROPERTIES OF ANTIBIOTICS

DRUG	ACTION	ABSORPTION	DISTRIBUTION	EXCRETION
Clindamycin				
	Bacteriostatic: inhibits bacterial protein synthesis. At higher concentrations, clindamycin can be bactericidal.	Nearly completely absorbed from the stomach after oral administration; absorption is not appreciably influenced by the presence of food.	The drug is widely distributed to many fluids and tissues, including bone. It crosses the placental barrier and enters the fetal circulation.	The drug is excreted in the urine and the feces. Antimicrobial activity may persist in the colonic contents for up to 1 week after therapy.
Macrolides				
	Inhibit bacterial protein synthesis by binding reversibly to the 50S ribosomal subunits of sensitive bacteria.	Food in stomach delays drug's ultimate absorption. Clarithromycin and azithromycin are better absorbed than erythromycin and yield higher serum levels.	Diffuse readily into intracellular fluids, and antibacterial activity can be achieved at essentially all body sites with the exception of the brain and cerebrospinal fluid.	Erythromycin and azithromycin are mainly eliminated via the liver. Clarithromycin is eliminated via the liver and kidneys.
Metronidazole				
	Bactericidal: inhibits DNA synthesis; it also modifies cell-mediated immunity, thereby normalizing excessive immune reactions.	Usually completely and promptly absorbed after oral administration and achieves therapeutic levels in the serum about 1 hour after the first dosage.	Penetrates well into body tissues and fluids, including vaginal secretions, saliva, breast milk and cerebrospinal fluid; passes the placental barrier and enters fetal circulation.	The liver accounts for more than 50% of the drug's systemic clearance. However, unchanged metronidazole and its metabolites are excreted in various proportions in the urine.
Penicillins and Cephalosporins				
	Bactericidal: inhibit specific bacterial enzymes required for the assembly of the bacterial cell wall.	Excellent absorption; more predictable blood levels can be obtained if given on an empty stomach.	Widely distributed throughout the body, including the saliva and gingival crevicular fluid; crosses the placenta.	Rapidly eliminated from plasma by the kidneys.
Quinolones (Ciprofloxacin and Levofloxacin)				
	Bactericidal: inhibit DNA synthesis.	Rapidly absorbed from the stomach after oral administration; maximum serum concentrations are obtained 1-2 hours after oral administration.	Present in antibacterial concentrations in saliva, nasal and bronchial secretions, sputum, breast milk, skin blister fluid, lymph, peritoneal fluid and prostatic secretions.	In patients with reduced renal function, drug half-life is slightly prolonged and dosage adjustments may be required.
Tetracyclines				
	Bacteriostatic: inhibit bacterial protein synthesis. Bactericidal at high concentrations; may inhibit protein synthesis in mammalian cells.	Doxycycline and minocycline possess greater absorption than tetracycline. Absorption is greater in the fasting state.	Tetracyclines penetrate soft tissues, the CNS and the brain, cross the placenta and enter fetal circulation and amniotic fluid. High concentrations are also present in breast milk.	Excretion is via the urine and feces. Renal clearance of minocycline is lower than tetracycline. Doxycycline does not accumulate significantly in the blood of patients with renal failure.

Chapter 7

Antifungal and Antiviral Agents

Brian C. Muzyka, D.M.D., M.S., M.B.A.;
Martha Somerman, D.D.S., Ph.D.

Antifungal Agents

The most common oral fungal infection is caused by *Candida* species. Oral *Candida* infections may have four clinical presentations. Pseudomembranous candidiasis (thrush) appears as white or yellow plaque on mucosal surfaces that may be wiped away easily. Erythematous (atrophic) candidiasis appears as red patches on any mucosal surface. When found on the tongue, it may cause depapillation. Hyperplastic (chronic) candidiasis is similar to the pseudomembranous variant, but the plaques cannot readily be removed. Angular chelitis (perleche), the last variant of oral *Candida* infection, is a mixed *Candida* and bacterial infection. Angular chelitis appears as red radiating fissures from the corners of the mouth and is often accompanied by a pseudomembranous covering.

Candida infections may be diagnosed empirically or through oral cultures or cytological smears. As *Candida* is a normal constituent of the oral cavity, care should be used to interpret findings of oral *Candida* species.

Pharmacological treatment for oral fungal infections is limited to three classes of antifungal agents: azoles, polyenes and echinocandins. The azole group is further subdivided into imidazole and triazole groups. Echinocandins are a newer class of antifungals that inhibit synthesis of β (1-3)-d-glucan, an integral part of fungal cell walls. β (1-3)-d-glucan is not found in mammalian cells and, therefore, limited adverse effects have been reported.

Table 7.1 provides dosage and prescribing information on antifungal drugs.

Accepted Indications
Superficial oral fungal infections are most commonly treated with topical antifungal agents. These agents are available in several forms such as rinses, troches and creams. Cutaneous fungal infections are most often treated with topical agents such as creams and ointments. Systemic fungal infections with an oral presentation are treated with systemic medications.

Drug Categories
Azole antifungal agents
These drugs are divided into the following subgroups:
- Imidazoles: clotrimazole, miconazole and ketoconazole;
- Triazoles: fluconazole and itraconazole. Many of the azoles are used to treat oropharyngeal candidiasis. They are also used for other fungal infections, such as aspergillosis, blastomycosis, chromomycosis, coccidioidomycosis, cryptococcosis and histoplasmosis.

Polyene antifungal agents
Polyenes are amphotericin B and nystatin. Polyenes are used for local treatment of fungal infections of the mouth caused by

Candida albicans and other *Candida* species. Intravenous formulations of amphotericin B are used for treatment of severe systemic fungal infections.

The pharmokinetics of the different formulations of amphotericin can differ substantially. In general, usual dosages of amphotericin B cholesteryl sulfate complexes (ABCD), amphotericin B lipid complexes (ABLC) and liposomal amphotericin B (L-AmB) are tolerated better than the conventional formulation of amphotericin B.

ABCD is labeled for treatment of invasive aspergillosis in people who are nonresponsive to amphotericin and in people who are unable to tolerate amphotericin secondary to renal impairment or toxicity. It also is being investigated for treatment of other invasive fungal infections, including *Candida*.

ABLC is labeled for the use of invasive fungal infections in people who are intolerant of or refractory to treatment with conventional amphotericin B.

L-AmB is labeled for the use of cryptococcalmeningitis in people with HIV infection and in empiric therapy of presumed fungal infections in people with neutropenia who have fevers.

Echinocandins

Echinocandins sometimes are referred to as glucan synthesis inhibitors because they inhibit synthesis of β (1-3)-d-glucan, an integral component of the yeast cell wall. At present, echinocandins are used for the treatment of nonresponsive or refractory aspergillosis, esophageal candidasis and candidemia.

General Dosing Information

General dosing information is provided in Table 7.1. The selection of agent and dosage depends on the extent of the oral fungal infection. Topical forms of treatment are recommended for superficial infections in patients who are immunocompetent, and systemic medications are recommended for

deep fungal infections or for the treatment of patients who are immunocompromised.

Special Dental Considerations

General Considerations

- The oral mucosa should be examined for signs of fungal infection such as white plaque, erythematous areas, ulcerations, nodules or granulomas.
- Laboratory confirmation should be considered for deep fungal or superficial fungal disease in patients who are immunocompromised.
- Removable dental prosthetics and oral appliances should be disinfected with a 1:1 solution of hydrogen peroxide and water during the treatment period for superficial disease.
- Toothbrushes, denture brushes and other oral hygiene devices that may be contaminated with fungal organisms should be replaced.
- Systemic formulations of antifungal medications should be considered for use with dentate patients who have poor oral hygiene or a high Caries Index, as the troche formulations have high sugar content.
- Topical solutions, topical creams or systemic treatment should be considered for use with patients with xerostomia who may have difficulty using troches.

Drug Interactions of Dental Interest

Table 7.2 lists interactions of potential concern to clinicians administering antifungal drugs.

Azoles

- Absorption of itraconazole and ketoconazole can be affected by concomitant use of antacids. If concomitant administration of sulcralfate or of drugs that affect gastric acidity is necessary, it is recommended that these drugs should be given at least 2 hours after or 1 hour before ketoconazole or itraconazole administration.

- Other drug classes that may affect absorption of itraconazole and fluconazole include anticholinergics, antispasmodics, antimuscarinics, H_2-histamine receptor agonists, omeprazole and sulcralfate.
- Increased anticoagulant effects may occur in patients who are taking antifungal agents in conjunction with coumadin. Anticoagulation levels should be closely monitored and anticoagulation medication dosage adjusted accordingly.
- Concomitant use of antihistamines such as terfenadine and astemizole—neither of which is available in the United States any longer—with itraconazole and ketoconazole has led to cardiac dysrhythmias and is contraindicated.
- Concomitant use of cisapride (no longer available in the United States) and ketoconazole is contraindicated and has resulted in serious cardiovascular effects.
- Concomitant use of ketoconazole and rifampin has resulted in decreased serum concentrations of ketoconazole. These drugs should not be administered concomitantly.
- Concomitant use of ketoconazole with cyclosporine or phenytoin may increase plasma levels of cyclosporine and phenytoin. Patients taking these drugs should be monitored closely.
- Concomitant administration of ketoconazole and the steroid drugs methylprednisolone or prednisolone may result in increased plasma levels of the steroids.
- Concomitant use of alcohol and antifungal drugs may increase liver damage. Patients should be counseled not to drink alcohol while taking antifungal medications. Additionally, a disulfiram-type reaction (such as flushing, rash, peripheral edema, nausea or headache) has occurred in patients ingesting alcohol while receiving ketoconazole therapy.
- Concomitant use of ketoconazole and the benzodiazepines midazolam or triazolam may result in increased plasma concentration of the benzodiazepine agents. Because of the potentiated hypnotic and sedative effects, these agents should not be used concomitantly with ketoconazole.
- Itraconazole and ketoconazole may increase serum digoxin levels; therefore, digoxin levels should be closely monitored when administered with itraconazole or ketoconazole.

Polyenes
- Nephrotoxic effects of certain drugs (such as aminoglycosides, capreomycin, cisplatin, colistin, cyclosporine, methoxyflurane, pentamidine, polymixin B and vancomycin) may be additive with the concurrent or sequential use of IV amphotericin B and should be avoided. Intensive monitoring of renal function is recommended if amphotericin B is used in conjunction with any nephrotoxic agent.
- Serum potassium concentrations should be monitored closely in patients receiving any amphotericin B formulation concomitantly with a cardiac glycoside or skeletal muscle relaxant.
- Corticosteroids may enhance potassium depletion caused by amphotericin B and should not be used concomitantly.

Echinocandins
Clinicians should be cautious when using echinocandins in people with hepatic impairment. Dosage reduction may be required for those with moderate hepatic impairment.

Concomitant use of caspofungin acetate with cyclosporine is not recommended secondary to elevated hepatic transaminase levels unless the benefit of using the drug outweighs the risk.

Limited data suggest that coadministration of drug clearance–inducers, inducer/inhibitors, or both with caspofungin acetate may result in reduced doses of caspofungin acetate. These inducer and inducer/inhibitors include efavirenz, nelfinavir, nevaripine, phenytoin, rifampin, dexamethasone or carbamazepine. Increase in dosage of caspofungin acetate to 70 mg should be considered in nonresponsive patients who are coadministered one or more of the inducer or inducer/inhibitor agents.

Concomitant use of micafungin sodium with nifedipine may cause increase nifedipine levels. Use of micafungin sodium with sirolimus may increase sirolimus levels.

Special Patients

Pregnant and nursing women

Most antifungal drugs are classified in pregnancy risk category B or C. Caution should be taken in prescribing these agents to pregnant women. As some antifungal agents may enter breast milk, the clinician should use caution in prescribing these agents to women who are nursing.

Pediatric, geriatric and other special patients

Many antifungal agents can alter kidney and liver function, which may be severely damaging to older and younger patients. Therefore, dentists may need to adjust doses of antifungal agents accordingly.

Adverse Effects and Precautions

Table 7.1 lists adverse effects and precautions related to antifungal agents.

Pharmacology

The azole antifungal agents interfere with cytochrome P-450 activity, which is necessary for the demethylation of 14-α methylsterol to ergosterol. Ergosterol is the major sterol associated with fungal cell membranes. This interference in ergosterol causes changes in the cell membrane permeability and allows fungal cell elements to escape from the cell.

The polyenes inhibit fungal growth by binding with sterol in the fungal cell wall to interfere with cell membrane permeability, resulting in cell lysis.

The class of echinocandins inhibits the synthesis of β (1-3)-d-glucan, an integral part of fungal cell walls. This class at present is limited to caspofungin acetate and micafungin sodium, and they do not inhibit the enzymes in the cytochrome P-450 system.

Patient Advice

The following advice can be given to all patients diagnosed with oral fungal infections.

- Long-term therapy may be indicated to clear the infection and prevent relapse.
- Patients should take the medication as prescribed and should complete the course of the medication.
- Patients should not use commercial alcohol-based mouthrinses during treatment unless they are prescribed by the dentist.
- Removable oral appliances and dental prosthetics should be treated daily with a 1:1 disinfection solution of hydrogen peroxide and water during the treatment period for superficial disease.
- Oral hygiene devices (such as toothbrushes and denture brushes) that may be contaminated should be replaced.

Antiviral Agents

Viruses are among the simplest and smallest forms of life and must use a living host to replicate. Human viral infections have a wide spectrum of presentation, from subclinical infection to lethal infection. Viruses that affect the oral cavity, however, usually are self-limiting and heal spontaneously in a host with an intact immune system. Oral viral infections encountered in dental practice are usually limited to Coxsackie-type viruses (such as herpangina, acute lymphonodular pharyngitis and hand-foot-and-mouth disease); treatment for herpangina and acute lymphonodular pharyngitis is usually supportive. Other viral infections include herpes-type viruses (herpes labialis, chicken pox and shingles) and human papilloma viruses (HPV). Viral diseases that affect the delivery of dental care include all forms of viral hepatitis and human immunodeficiency virus (HIV) disease. As a description of these disease processes would be lengthy, the reader may learn more about these diseases by reviewing the suggested readings.

Coxsackie virus infection. Coxsackie viruses are a group of RNA viruses responsible for herpangina, acute lymphonodular pharyngitis and hand-foot-and-mouth disease. Herpangina occurs in epidemics with symptoms a bit milder than those of herpetic infections.

Herpes virus infection. Clinical signs of herpes-type viruses often are preceded by a prodromal period in which a sharp burning or shooting pain occurs along the affected nerve distribution. Vesicles appear and rupture, leaving a raw ulcerated hemorrhagic surface that is quite painful. Multiple intraoral lesions may interfere with the ability to maintain an adequate nutritional status, and supportive therapy will be required. Diagnosis of herpetic infections can be difficult, and a cytological smear or biopsy of the affected site may be necessary to rule out other disease processes such as aphthous ulcerations, pemphigus, pemphigoid or lichen planus.

Recurrent herpes labialis is estimated to affect up to 40% of the U.S. population annually. Treatment for herpes labialis has usually been relegated to formulations that contain an anesthetic and/or a moistening agent.

One agent used in the treatment of recurrent herpes labialis is docosanol. Docosanol is reported to reduce herpes labialis symptoms and reduces healing time by 0.72 days.

Valacyclovir, an acyclovir analogue, also is used in the treatment of herpes labialis.

In a study where the majority of patients initiated treatment within 2 hours of onset of symptoms, the mean duration of herpes labialis episodes were about 1 day shorter in subjects treated with 2 g twice daily for 1 day.

Oral herpetic infections usually are self-limiting, and treatment consists mainly of nutritional support and pain palliation. Patients with compromised immune function are at increased risk of reactivation of viral disease, and often the reactivated disease will be more involved and more difficult to control. Patients with HIV may develop severe HSV infections that affect the oral cavity. These infections can be life-threatening, and appropriate diagnosis and treatment are crucial. Acyclovir and acyclovir analogues are most commonly used for the treatment of HSV infection in this population.

Aphthous ulcers. Quite often, recurrent aphthous ulcers are misdiagnosed as herpes. Recurrent aphthous ulcers (RAUs) are characterized by periodic ulcerations confined to the oral mucosa. No single etiologic agent has been implicated for RAUs; however, many theories have been put forward, suggesting multifactorial causes including stress, vitamin deficiency, diet, hormonal changes, allergies, trauma and immune dysfunction.

Minor aphthous ulcers (ulcers less than 1 cm in diameter) usually are found on the less keratinized tissues in the oral cavity such as the buccal mucosa, the floor of the mouth and the ventral surface of the tongue. In certain susceptible individuals the use of dentifrices formulated without sodium lauryl sulfate may decrease the incidence of aphthous ulcers.

A prescription drug, amlexanox (Aphthasol), is approved for the treatment of aphthous ulcerations. Amlexanox is a potent inhibitor of the formation and release of inflammatory mediators from mast cells. A number of nonprescription products also are available for treatment of aphthous ulcers and other oral ulcerative conditions. Peroxide gel (Peroxyl Gel) is a hydrogen peroxide-based gel used to debride ulcerations in an effort to promote healing. Other agents exert their major effect by providing a protective coating over the ulcer to decrease pain and promote healing. These agents include Orabase Soothe and Seal, a liquid formulation of 2-octyl cyanoacrylate that forms a protective barrier that can last up to 6 hours. Another agent, Gelclair, is an adherent oral gel that forms a film over the affected areas. A glycyrrhetinic acid and sodium hyaluronate preparation (Rincinol PRN) has a similar action in that it forms a barrier over the ulcer.

Human papilloma virus (HPV). Presently, 17 different subtypes of HPV have been isolated from oral mucosa. HPV lesions in the oral cavity may present as verrucous, hyperplastic or papillomatous growths that are asymptomatic. Various modalities of treatment for HPV have been employed with limited success. These treatments include excision, laser ablation, cryotherapy, application of keratinolytic agents and injection of antiviral agents.

Conditions treated with interferon alfa (Intron A, Roferon-A, Peg Intron). The interferons are a group of naturally occurring biologic response modifiers. These agents have antiviral properties and they also have some antiproliferative, immune enhancing, and differentiating effects. There are three main types of interferons: alpha and beta interferons (type 1), and gamma interferon (type 2), which is different in structure and function from both the alpha and beta interferons.

Accepted Indications

Because of substantial toxicity and side effects, antiviral agents usually are reserved for immunocompromised patients with mucocutaneous HSV-associated lesions. Studies in immunocompetent patients have shown little clinical benefit of using topical acyclovir in treatment of herpes labialis. Application of penciclovir to herpes labialis lesions decreased the duration of pain, viral shedding and time required for healing. The clinical benefit of penciclovir is modest, however; on average, it shortens the duration of pain and viral shedding by less than one day.

General Dosing Information

Dosage and prescribing information for antiviral agents and aphthous ulcer medications can be found in Table 7.1.

Special Dental Considerations

Drug Interactions of Dental Interest

Table 7.2 presents information regarding drug interactions with antiviral agents.

- Systemic acyclovir, ganciclovir and valacyclovir are nephrotoxic and should be used with caution in patients who have renal disease or in patients who are receiving other nephrotoxic medications.
- Concomitant administration of acyclovir and probenecid may delay the urinary excretion and renal clearance of acyclovir. Probenecid also may interfere with the renal clearance and urinary excretion of ganciclovir.
- Concomitant use of acyclovir and zidovudine (AZT) may increase CNS symptoms such as drowsiness or lethargy; therefore, patients should be monitored closely.
- Famciclovir and valacyclovir are eliminated by the kidneys. Its dosage should be adjusted accordingly for patients with renal impairment.
- Foscarnet has a high toxic profile and should be used with care, especially in patients with a history of renal impairment.

Adjunctive Therapy

For relief of pain associated with viral lesions and aphthous ulcers, typical anesthetic agents bring temporary relief. Lidocaine viscous, 2%, can be of value. Diphenhydramine elixir, an antihistamine containing 12.5 mg of diphenhydramine per mL, also can be used for its topical anesthetic properties. Lidocaine viscous sometimes is mixed with equal parts of antacids and diphenhydramine elixir to improve adherence to the oral mucosa.

If patients are experiencing difficulty in eating, liquid dietary supplements may be recommended.

Adverse Effects and Precautions

Table 7.1 lists adverse effects, precautions and contraindications associated with antiviral agents.

Pharmacology

Viral resistance to antiviral agents has become an increasing problem. Drug resistance has many causes and, depending on the specific drug, can have many mechanisms. With acyclovir, it is believed that resistant herpes simplex viruses have developed because of alterations in either the viral thymidine kinase or the viral DNA polymerase. Viral thymidine kinase starts the process through which acyclovir is transformed to its active derivative, acyclovir triphosphate. This process does not occur in uninfected cells to any great extent, and because acyclovir is taken up selectively by infected cells, the concentration of acyclovir triphosphate in infected cells is 40-100 times greater than in uninfected cells. Clinically, acyclovir-resistant HSV infections are seen in patients whose immunodeficiency is increasing. Other antiviral medications, such as foscarnet, must be used to treat such acyclovir-resistant patients.

Interferons bind to specific cell receptors, activating the synthesis of different proteins including 2'-5' oligoadenylate synthetase and protein-kinase. This interaction causes an interference with viral replication, assembly and release. Included is a change in cellular glycosylation that produces a glycoprotein-deficient virus that shows lower infectivity. Interferons also exert their actions by immune modulation, thereby increasing the lytic effects of cytotoxic T lymphocytes.

Effects of IFN-a can include fever, myalgias, lethargy, headaches (flu-like syndrome), central nervous system dysfunction, gastrointestinal disturbances and bone marrow suppression.

Currently, IFN-a has FDA approval for the treatment of hairy cell leukemia, Kaposi's sarcoma (HHV-8), condylomata acuminata (HPV), chronic HBV or HCV infection, and melanoma after wide local excision. Recently approved peg-interferon has proven more effective than standard interferon therapy for HCV infection.

Patient Advice

- Topical acyclovir and penciclovir should be applied using a finger cot or some type of protective covering.
- Patients who have oral viral disease should avoid using mouthrinses with a high alcohol content.
- Patients who have oral viral disease should dispose of toothbrushes used during periods of infection.
- Amlexanox paste should be applied using a finger cot. If a protective finger covering is not used, the hands should be washed immediately after applying the medication.

Suggested Readings

Hairston BR, Bruce AJ, Rogers III RS. Viral diseases of the oral mucosa. Dermatol Clin 2003;21:17-32.

Lalla RV, Peterson DE. Oral mucositis. Dent Clin N Am 2005;49:167-84.

Letsinger JA, McCarty MA, Jorizzo JL. Complex aphthosis: a large case series with evaluation algorithm and therapeutic ladder from topicals to thalidomide. J Am Acad Dermatol 2005;52(3 pt 1):500-8.

Muzyka BC. Oral fungal infections. Dent Clin N Am 2005;49:49-65.

Pallasch TJ. Antifungal and antiviral chemotherapy. Periodontology 2000. 2002;28:240-55.

Patton LL. HIV disease. Dent Clin N Am 2003;47:467-92.

Preiser W, Doerr HW, Vogel JU. Virology and epidemiology of oral herpesvirus infections. Med Microbiol Immunol 2003;192(3):133-6.

Scully C, Felix DH. Oral medicine — Update for the dental practitioner. Aphthous and other common ulcers. Br Dent J 2005;199:259-64.

Stoopler ET, Greenberg MS. Update on herpesvirus infections. Dent Clin N Am 2003;47:517-32.

Table 7.1: PRESCRIBING INFORMATION FOR ANTIFUNGAL AND ANTIVIRAL AGENTS

NAME	FORM/ STRENGTH	DOSAGE	WARNINGS/PRECAUTIONS & CONTRAINDICATIONS	ADVERSE EFFECTS†
ANTIFUNGAL AGENTS, SYSTEMIC				
Amphotericin B Cholesteryl Sulfate Complex (Amphotec)	Inj: 50mg, 100mg	*Adults:* Test Dose: Infuse small amount over 15-30 minutes. *Treatment:* 3-4mg/kg/day IV at 1mg/kg/hr. *Pediatrics:* Test Dose: Infuse small amount over 15-30 minutes. *Treatment:* 3-4mg/kg/day IV at 1mg/kg/hr.	W/P: Anaphylaxis may occur. Discontinue if severe respiratory distress occurs. Acute reactions (eg, fever, shaking chills, hypotension, nausea, tachypnea) 1-3 hrs after start infusion. Monitor renal/hepatic function, electrolytes, CBC, PT during therapy. P/N: Category B, not for use in nursing.	Chills, fever, headache, hypotension, tachycardia, HTN, nausea, vomiting, thrombocytopenia, increased creatinine, hypokalemia, dyspnea, hypoxia.
Amphotericin B lipid Complex (Abelcet)	Inj: 5mg/mL	*Adults:* 5mg/kg IV at 2.5mg/kg/h. *Pediatrics:* 5mg/kg IV at 2.5mg/kg/h.	W/P: Anaphylaxis reported. Discontinue if respiratory distress occurs. Monitor SCr, LFTs, serum electrolytes, CBC during therapy. P/N: Category B, not for use in nursing.	Chills, fever, increased SCr, multiple organ failure, nausea, hypotension, respiratory failure, vomiting, dyspnea, sepsis, diarrhea, headache, heart arrest, HTN, hypokalemia, infection, kidney failure, pain, thrombocytopenia.
Amphotericin B Liposome (Ambisome)	Inj: 50mg	*Adults:* Empiric Therapy: 3mg/kg/day IV. Systemic Infections (Aspergillus, Candida, Cryptococcus): 3-5mg/kg/day IV. Cryptococcal Meningitis in HIV: 6mg/kg/ day IV. Visceral Leishmaniasis: Immunocompetent: 3mg/kg/day IV on days 1-5, 14, 21. May repeat course if needed. Immunocompromised: 4mg/kg/day IV on days 1-5, 10, 17, 24, 31, 38. *Pediatrics:* 1 month-16 yrs: Empirical Therapy: 3mg/kg/day IV. Systemic Infections (Aspergillus, Candida, Cryptococcus): 3-5mg/kg/day IV. Cryptococcal Meningitis in HIV: 6mg/kg/day IV. Visceral Leishmaniasis: Immunocompetent: 3mg/kg/day IV on days 1-5, 14, 21. May repeat course if needed. Immunocompromised: 4mg/kg/day IV on days 1-5, 10, 17, 24, 31, 38.	W/P: If anaphylaxis occurs, discontinue all further infusions. Significantly less toxic than amphotericin B deoxycholate. Monitor renal, hepatic, hematopoietic function and electrolytes (especially K$^+$, Mg^{++}). P/N: Category B, not for use in nursing.	Chills, asthenia, back pain, pain, infection, chest pain, HTN, hypotension, tachycardia, GI hemorrhage, diarrhea, nausea, vomiting, hyperglycemia, hypokalemia, dyspnea.
Caspofungin Acetate (Cancidas)	Inj: 50mg, 70mg	*Adults:* Invasive Aspergillosis: LD: 70mg IV on Day 1. Maint: 50mg IV qd. Empirical Therapy: LD: 70mg IV on Day 1. Maint: 50mg IV qd. If 50mg is well tolerated but does not provide adequate clinical response, daily dose can be increased to 70mg. Fungal infections should be treated for a minimum of 14 days. Continue treatment 7 days after neutropenia and clinical symptoms are resolved. Esophageal Candidiasis: 50mg IV qd. Consider suppressive therapy in HIV patients. Candidemia/Candida Infections: LD: 70mg IV on Day 1. Maint: 50mg IV qd. Moderate Hepatic Insufficiency: LD: 70mg IV on Day 1. Maint: 35mg IV qd. Concomitant Rifampin: 70mg IV qd. Concomitant Nevirapine/ Efavirenz/Carbamazepine/Dexamethasone/Phenytoin: May need to increase dose to 70mg IV qd. Base duration of treatment on severity of disease, clinical response, microbiological response, and recovery from immunosuppression.	P/N: Category C, caution in nursing.	Fever, infused vein complications, nausea, vomiting, flushing, rash, facial edema.

*Scored.   †Bold entries denote special dental considerations.

Table 7.1: PRESCRIBING INFORMATION FOR ANTIFUNGAL AND ANTIVIRAL AGENTS (cont.)

NAME	FORM/ STRENGTH	DOSAGE	WARNINGS/PRECAUTIONS & CONTRAINDICATIONS	ADVERSE EFFECTS†
ANTIFUNGAL AGENTS, SYSTEMIC (cont.)				
Clotrimazole (Mycelex Troche)	**Loz/Troche:** 10mg [70 loz, 140 loz]	***Adults:* Treatment:** Slowly dissolve 1 troche in mouth 5 times/day for 14 days. **Prophylaxis:** Slowly dissolve 1 troche in mouth tid for duration of chemotherapy or until steroids are reduced. ***Pediatrics:*** ≥3 yrs: **Treatment:** Slowly dissolve 1 troche in mouth 5 times/day for 14 days.	**W/P:** Not for systemic mycoses. May cause abnormal LFTs; monitor hepatic function. Only use in patients mentally and physically able to dissolve the troche. Confirm diagnosis by KOH smear and/or culture. **P/N:** Category C, safety in nursing is not known.	Abnormal LFTs, nausea, vomiting, **unpleasant mouth sensations**, pruritus.
Fluconazole (Diflucan)	**Inj:** 200mg/100mL, 400mg/200mL; **Sus:** 50mg/5mL, 200mg/5mL [35mL]; **Tab:** 50mg, 100mg, 150mg, 200mg	***Adults:* Vaginal Candidiasis:** 150mg PO single dose. **IV/PO: Oropharyngeal Candidiasis:** 200mg 1st day then 100mg qd for minimum 2 weeks. **Esophageal Candidiasis:** 200mg 1st day then 100mg qd for minimum 3 weeks then treat 2 weeks following resolution of symptoms. **Max:** 400mg/day. **Systemic Infections:** 400mg/day. **UTI/Peritonitis:** 50-200mg/day. **Cryptococcal Meningitis:** 400mg 1st day then 200mg qd for 10-12 weeks after negative CSF culture. **Suppression of relapse in AIDS:** 200mg/day. **Prophylaxis in BMT:** 400mg/day. **CrCl <50mL/min: Initial:** LD 50-400mg. **Maint:** Give 50% of recommended dose. ***Pediatrics:* IV/PO: Oropharyngeal Candidiasis:** 6mg/kg 1st day then 3mg/kg/day for minimum of 2 weeks. **Esophageal Candidiasis:** 6mg/kg 1st day then 3mg/kg/day for minimum 3 weeks and 2 weeks following resolution of symptoms. **Max:** 12mg/kg/day. **Systemic Infections:** 6-12mg/kg/day. **Cryptococcal Meningitis:** 12mg/kg 1st day then 6mg/kg/day for 10-12 weeks after negative CSF culture. **Suppression of relapse in AIDS:** 6mg/kg/day. **CrCl <50mL/min: Initial:** 50-400mg. **Maint:** Give 50% of recommended dose.	**W/P:** Monitor LFTs. Discontinue if hepatic dysfunction develops or exfoliative skin disorder progresses. Anaphylaxis reported. **Contra:** Coadministration with cisapride or terfenadine (with multiple diflucan doses of ≥400mg). Caution if hypersensitive to other azoles. **P/N:** Category C, not for use in nursing.	Headache, nausea, abdominal pain, diarrhea, skin rash, vomiting.
Flucytosine (Ancobon)	**Cap:** 250mg, 500mg	***Adults:*** 50-150mg/kg/day given q6h. **Renal Impairment:** Reduce initial dose. Take a few caps over 15 minutes to reduce nausea/vomiting.	**Extreme caution with renal dysfunction. Monitor hematologic, renal, and hepatic status closely. W/P:** Caution with renal dysfunction and bone marrow depression. Bone marrow depression can be irreversible and fatal. **P/N:** Category C, not for use in nursing.	Myocardial toxicity, chest pain, dyspnea, rash, pruritus, urticaria, photosensitivity, nausea, vomiting, jaundice, renal failure, pyrexia, crystalluria, anemia, leukopenia, eosinophilia, thrombocytopenia, ataxia, hearing loss, neuropathy.
Griseofulvin, Microcrystalline (Grifulvin V)	**Sus:** 125mg/5mL [120mL]; **Tab:** 500mg	***Adults:* Tinea Capitis:** 500mg qd for 4-6 weeks. **Tinea Corporis:** 500mg qd for 2-4 weeks. **Tinea Pedis:** 1g qd for 4-8 weeks. **Tinea Cruris:** 500mg qd. **Tinea Unguium:** 1g qd for at least 4 months (fingernail) or at least 6 months (toenails). ***Pediatrics: Usual:*** 5mg/lb/day. 30-50lb: 125-250mg qd. **>50lb:** 250-500mg qd. **Tinea Capitis:** Treat for 4-6 weeks. **Tinea Corporis:** Treat for 2-4 weeks. **Tinea Pedis:** Treat for 4-8 weeks. **Tinea Unguium:** Treat for at least 4 months (fingernail) or at least 6 months (toenails).	**W/P:** Confirm diagnosis. Not for prophylactic use. Monitor renal, hepatic, and hematopoietic functions periodically with prolonged therapy. Cross-sensitivity with penicillin may exist. Photosensitivity reported. Discontinue if granulocytopenia occurs. **Contra:** Porphyria, hepatocellular failure, pregnancy. **P/N:** Not for use in pregnancy and in nursing.	Rash, urticaria, **oral thrush**, nausea, vomiting, epigastric distress, diarrhea, headache, dizziness, insomnia, mental confusion.
Itraconazole (Sporanox)	**Cap:** 100mg; **Inj:** 10mg/mL;	***Adults:* (Cap)** Take with full meal. If patient has achlorhydria or is also taking	**Contraindicated with cisapride, pimozide, quinidine, or dofetilide.**	Nausea, diarrhea, vomiting, abdominal pain,

*Scored.   †Bold entries denote special dental considerations.

NAME	FORM/ STRENGTH	DOSAGE	WARNINGS/PRECAUTIONS & CONTRAINDICATIONS	ADVERSE EFFECTS†
Itraconazole *(cont.)*	**Sol:** 10mg/mL [150mL]	gastric acid suppressors give with a cola beverage. **Toenail Onchomycosis:** 200mg qd for 12 weeks. **Fingernail Onchomycosis:** 200mg bid for 1 week, then skip for 3 weeks, then 200mg bid for 1 week. **Blastomycosis/Histoplasmosis:** 200mg qd. May increase by 100mg increments if no improvement. **Max:** 400mg/day. Give bid if dose <200mg/day. **Aspergillosis:** 200-400mg/day. **Life-Threatening Infections: LD:** 200mg tid for 1st 3 days. Continue for at least 3 months. **(IV)** Give by IV infusion over 1 hour. Blastomycosis/Histoplasmosis/Aspergillosis: 200mg bid for 4 doses, then 200mg qd, up to 14 days. Continue with caps for at least 3 months. Treat for at least 3 months. **ETFN/Life-Threatening Infections:** 200mg IV bid for 4 doses, then 200mg qd for up to 14 days. Continue with solution 200mg PO bid, up to 28 days. **(Sol)** Oropharyngeal Candidiasis: 200mg/day for 1-2 weeks. **Refractory to Fluconazole:** 100mg bid (response in 2-4 weeks, may relapse shortly after discontinuation). **Esophageal Candidiasis:** 100-200mg/day for at least 3 weeks. Continue for 2 weeks after symptoms resolve. Take on empty stomach. Swish 10mL at a time for several seconds, then swallow.	**Serious cardiovascular events (eg, QT prolongation, torsade de pointes, ventricular tachycardia, cardiac arrest, and/or sudden death) reported with cisapride, pimozide, quinidine and other CYP3A4 inhibitors. Do not use caps for onychomycosis with ventricular dysfunction. W/P:** Rare cases of hepatotoxicity reported. Monitor LFTs; discontinue if hepatic dysfunction develops. Avoid with liver disease. Discontinue if neuropathy or CHF occurs. Solution and capsules are not interchangeable. Consider alternative therapy if unresponsive in patients with cystic fibrosis. Avoid with ventricular dysfunction. Caution with ischemic/valvular disease, pulmonary disease, renal failure, other edematous disorders. Avoid injection if CrCl <30mL/min. **Contra:** (Cap, Inj, Sol) Concomitant cisapride, oral midazolam, pimozide, quinidine, dofetilide, triazolam, and HMG CoA-reductase inhibitors metabolized by CYP3A4 (eg, lovastatin, simvastatin). (Cap) Treatment of onychomycosis if pregnant or contemplating pregnancy, ventricular dysfunction (eg, CHF). **P/N:** Category C, not for use in nursing.	fever, cough, rash, increased sweating, headache, hypokalemia.
Ketoconazole	**Tab:** 200mg*	*Adults:* **Initial:** 200mg qd. **Max:** 400mg qd. *Pediatrics:* >2 yrs: 3.3-6.6mg/kg/day.	**Risk of fatal hepatotoxicity. Concomitant terfenadine, astemizole and cisapride are contraindicated due to serious cardiovascular adverse events. W/P:** Hepatotoxicity reported. Monitor LFTs prior to therapy and periodically thereafter. Serum testosterone levels may be lowered. Hypersensitivity reactions reported. Tablets require acidity for dissolution. Not for use in children unless benefit outweighs risk. **Contra:** Concomitant terfenadine, astemizole, cisapride or triazolam. **P/N:** Category C, not for use in nursing.	Nausea, vomiting, abdominal pain, pruritus.
Micafungin Sodium (Mycamine)	**Inj:** 50mg	*Adults:* **Esophageal Candidiasis:** 150mg/day IV infusion over 1 hour (usual range 10-30 days). *Candida* **Infection Prophylaxis in HSCT:** 50mg/day IV infusion over 1 hour (usual range 6-51 days). Do not mix or co-infuse with other drugs.	**W/P:** Report of serious hypersensitivity (eg, anaphylaxis, anaphylactoid, shock). Liver function test abnormalities, monitor for evidence of worsening. Reports of significant renal dysfunction, acute renal failure, and elevations in BUN and creatinine. Reports of acute intravascular hemolysis and hemoglobinuria. May precipitate when mixed or co-infused with other drugs. **P/N:** Category C, caution in nursing.	Hyperbilirubinemia, leukopenia, headache, rash, phlebitis, nausea.
Nystatin (Mycostatin)	**Loz: (Pastille)** 200,000U [30 loz]; **Sus:** 100,000U/mL [60mL, 480mL]; **Tab:** 500,000U	*Adults:* **Oral Candidiasis: (Loz)** 200,000-400,000U 4-5 times/day. **Max:** 14 days. Dissolve slowly in mouth. **(Sus)** 4-6mL qid. Retain in mouth as long as possible before swallowing. **GI Candidiasis: (Tab)** 500,000-1,000,000U tid. *Pediatrics:* **Oral Candidiasis: (Loz)** 200,000-400,000U	**W/P:** Not for systemic mycoses. Discontinue if irritation/hypersensitivity occurs. Confirm diagnosis with KOH smear and/or cultures if symptoms persist after course of therapy. Continue at least 48 hrs after clinical response. **P/N:** Category C, caution in nursing.	Diarrhea, nausea, vomiting, GI distress, rash, urticaria, Stevens-Johnson syndrome, oral irritation.

Table 7.1: PRESCRIBING INFORMATION FOR ANTIFUNGAL AND ANTIVIRAL AGENTS *(cont.)*

NAME	FORM/ STRENGTH	DOSAGE	WARNINGS/PRECAUTIONS & CONTRAINDICATIONS	ADVERSE EFFECTS†
ANTIFUNGAL AGENTS, SYSTEMIC *(cont.)*				
Nystatin *(cont.)*		4-5 times/day. **Max:** 14 days. Dissolve slowly in mouth. **(Sus)** 4-6mL qid. **Infants:** 2mL qid. Retain in mouth as long as possible before swallowing.		
Terbinafine Hydrochloride (Lamisil)	**Tab:** 250mg	**Adults:** Fingernail: 250mg qd for 6 weeks. **Toenail:** 250mg qd for 12 weeks.	**W/P:** Liver disease and serious skin reactions reported; stop therapy if these develop. Avoid with liver disease or renal impairment (CrCl ≤50 mL/min). Check serum transaminases before therapy. Monitor CBC if immunocompromised and taking terbinafine >6 weeks. Stop therapy if neutrophil count ≤1,000 cells/mm³. Changes in ocular lens and retina reported (unknown significance). **P/N:** Category B, not for use in nursing.	Headache, diarrhea, dyspepsia, rash, liver enzyme abnormalities.
Voriconazole (Vfend)	**Inj:** 200mg; **Sus:** 40mg/mL [100mL]; **Tab:** 50mg, 200mg	**Adults:** Invasive Aspergillosis: **(Inj)** LD: 6mg/kg IV q12h x 2 doses. **Maint:** 4mg/kg IV q12h. Switch to PO when appropriate. **(PO) Maint:** >40kg: 200mg q12h; 300mg q12h if inadequate response. <40kg: 100mg q12h; 150mg q12h if inadequate response. **Esophageal Candidiasis: (PO)** >40kg: 200mg q12h. <40kg: 100mg q12h. Treat for minimum of 14 days and at least 7 days following resolution of symptoms. **Candidemia Nonneutropenic Patients/Deep Tissue Candida Infections: (Inj)** LD: 6mg/kg IV q12h x 2 doses. **Maint:** 3-4mg/kg IV q12h or 200mg PO q12h. **Intolerant: (Inj/PO) Maint:** IV: 3mg/kg q12h. **PO:** Reduce by 50mg steps to minimum of 200mg q12h for >40kg or 100mg q12h for <40kg. **Concomitant Phenytoin: Maint:** IV: 5mg/kg q12h. **PO:** >40kg: 400mg q12h. <40kg: 200mg q12h. **Mild to Moderate Hepatic Cirrhosis: Maint:** 1/2 of maint dose. **CrCl <50mL/min:** Use PO. Take PO 1 hr before or 1 hr after a meal. Base duration on severity of underlying disease, recovery from immunosuppression, and clinical response.	**W/P:** Monitor visual function with treatment >28 days. Hepatic reactions (clinical hepatitis, cholestasis, fulminant hepatic failure) reported; monitor LFTs at initiation and during therapy. Discontinue if liver dysfunction occurs. Tabs contain lactose; avoid with galactose intolerance, Lapp lactase deficiency, or glucose-galactose malabsorption. Anaphylactoid-type reactions reported with injection. Avoid strong, direct sunlight. Monitor renal function. May prolong QT interval; caution with proarrhythmic conditions. Correct electrolyte disturbances before starting therapy. **Contra:** Concomitant terfenadine, astemizole, cisapride, pimozide, quinidine, sirolimus, rifampin, carbamazepine, long-acting barbiturates, ritonavir, efavirenz, rifabutin, ergot alkaloids. **P/N:** Category D, not for use in nursing.	Visual disturbances, fever, rash, headache, nausea, vomiting, diarrhea, sepsis, peripheral edema, abdominal pain, respiratory disorder, increased LFTs.
ANTIFUNGAL AGENTS, TOPICAL				
Butenafine Hydrochloride (Mentax)	**Cre:** 1% [15g, 30g]	**Adults:** T.pedis: Apply bid for 7 days or qd for 4 weeks. **T.corporis/ t.cruris/t.versicolor:** Apply qd for 2 weeks. **Pediatrics:** ≥12 yrs: T.pedis: Apply bid for 7 days or qd for 4 weeks. **T.corporis/t.cruris/t.versicolor:** Apply qd for 2 weeks.	**W/P:** Avoid eyes, nose, mouth, and other mucous membranes. Discontinue if irritation or sensitivity develops. Confirm diagnosis. Caution if sensitive to other allylamine antifungals. **P/N:** Category B, caution in nursing.	Burning, stinging, itching, contact dermatitis, irritation, erythema, worsening of condition.
Ciclopirox (Loprox, Loprox TS)	**Cre:** 0.77% [15g, 30g, 90g]; **Gel:** 0.77% [30g, 45g, 100g]; **Shampoo:** 1%	**Adults: (Cre/Gel/Sus)** Massage affected and surrounding areas bid (am and pm) up to 4 weeks. **(Shampoo)** Apply about 5mL (up to 10mL for long hair) to wet scalp. Lather and rinse off after 3 minutes. Repeat twice	**Contra:** Avoid eyes, mucous membranes, occlusive wrappings or dressings. Discontinue if sensitization or chemical irritation occurs. **P/N:** Pregnancy B, caution in nursing.	Contact dermatitis, pruritus, burning.

*Scored.   †Bold entries denote special dental considerations.

NAME	FORM/ STRENGTH	DOSAGE	WARNINGS/PRECAUTIONS & CONTRAINDICATIONS	ADVERSE EFFECTS†
Ciclopirox *(cont.)*	[120mL]; **Sus: (Loprox TS)** 0.77% [30mL, 60mL]	weekly for 4 weeks, at least 3 days apart. *Pediatrics:* ≥10 yrs: (Cre/Sus) Massage affected and surrounding areas bid (am and pm) up to 4 weeks. Gel or Shampoo not recommended in pediatrics <16 yrs.		
Clotrimazole (Lotrimin)	**Cre:** 1% [15g, 30g, 45g]; **Lot:** 1% [30mL]; **Sol:** 1% [10mL, 30mL]	*Adults:* Apply bid (am and pm). Re-evaluate if no improvement after 4 weeks. *Pediatrics:* Apply bid (am and pm). Re-evaluate if no improvement after 4 weeks.	**W/P:** Discontinue if irritation or sensitivity occurs. Not for opthalmic use. **P/N:** Category B, caution in nursing.	Erythema, stinging, blistering, peeling, edema, pruritus, urticaria, burning, irritation.
Clotrimazole w/ betamethasone dipropionate (Lotrisone)	(Betamethasone-Clotrimazole) **Cre:** 0.05-1% [15g, 45g]; **Lot:** 0.05-1% [30mL]	*Adults:* ≥17 yrs: Massage sufficient amount bid (am and pm) to area for 2 weeks for T.cruris and T.corporis and 4 weeks for T.pedis. Discontinue if condition persists after 2 weeks for T.cruris and T.corporis, and after 4 weeks for T.pedis.	**W/P:** May produce reversible HPA axis suppression, Cushing's syndrome, hyperglycemia, and glucosuria. Discontinue if irritation develops. Pediatrics may be more susceptible to systemic toxicity. Not for use with occlusive dressing. **P/N:** Category C, caution in nursing.	Paresthesia, rash, edema, secondary infection.
Econazole Nitrate (Spectazole)	**Cre:** 1% [15g, 30g, 85g]	*Adults:* T.cruris/t.corporis/t.versicolor: Apply qd for 2 weeks. T.pedis: Apply qd for 4 weeks. **Cutaneous candidiasis:** Apply bid for 2 weeks.	**W/P:** Avoid eyes. **P/N:** Category C, caution with nursing.	Burning, itching, stinging, erythema.
Ketoconazole (Nizoral, Nizoral AD)	**Shampoo:** 2% [120mL]; **Shampoo:** 1% [4 oz, 7 oz]	**(Nizoral)** *Adults:* Apply to damp skin and lather. Rinse with water after 5 minutes. One application should be sufficient. **(Nizoral AD)** *Adults:* Wet hair and lather. Rinse thoroughly and repeat. Apply every 3-4 days up to 8 weeks if needed. *Pediatrics:* ≥12 yrs: Wet hair. Apply and lather. Rinse thoroughly and repeat. Apply every 3-4 days up to 8 weeks if needed.	**W/P:** Shampoo may remove curl from permanently waved hair. Avoid eyes. Discontinue if rash appears, or if condition worsens or does not improve in 2-4 weeks. **P/N: (Nizoral)** Category C, caution in nursing. **(Nizoral AD)** Use in pregnancy and nursing not known.	Abnormal hair texture, scalp pustules, mild skin dryness, pruritus, increase in normal hair loss, oily or dry scalp and hair.
Miconazole Nitrate (Desenex, Lotrimin AF, Micatin, Monistat-Derm, Neosporin AF)	**Cre:** 2%; **Lot:** 2%; **Powder:** 2%; **Spray:** 2%	*Adults:* Cleanse skin with soap and water and dry thoroughly. Apply to affected area am and pm. **Athlete's Foot and Ringworm:** Treat for 4 weeks. **Jock Itch:** Treat for 2 weeks. *Pediatrics:* ≥2 yrs: Cleanse skin with soap and water and dry thoroughly. Apply to affected area am and pm. **Athlete's Foot and Ringworm:** Treat for 4 weeks. **Jock Itch:** Treat for 2 weeks.	**W/P:** Discontinue if irritation occurs or no improvement in 4 weeks (T.pedis or T. corporis) or 2 weeks (T. cruris). Avoid eye contact. Not effective on scalp or nails. **P/N:** Safety in pregnancy and nursing not known.	
Naftifine Hydrochloride (Naftin)	**Cre:** 1% [15g, 30g, 60g]; **Gel:** 1% [20g, 40g, 60g]	*Adults:* Massage into affected and surrounding areas **(Cream)** qd or **(Gel)** bid (am and pm). Wash hands after use. Re-evaluate if no improvement after 4 weeks.	**W/P:** Stop therapy if irritation develops. Avoid eyes, nose, and mucous membranes. **P/N:** Category B, caution in nursing.	Burning/stinging, rash, erythema, itching, dryness, skin tenderness.
Nystatin (Mycostatin)	**Cre:** 100,000U/g [30g]; **Powder, Topical:** 100,000U/g [15g]	*Adults:* **(Cre)** Apply to affected area bid until healing is complete. **(Powder)** Apply to lesions bid-tid until healing is complete. For fungal infections of the feet, dust powder on feet and in shoes also. *Pediatrics:* **Neonates and Older: (Cre)** Apply to affected area bid until healing is complete. **(Powder)** Apply to lesions bid-tid until healing is complete. For fungal infections of the feet, dust powder on feet and in shoes also.	**W/P:** Discontinue if irritation or sensitization occurs. Confirm diagnosis. Not for systemic, oral, intravaginal, or ophthalmic use. For fungal infections of the feet, dust powder on feet as well as in all footwear. Moist lesions are best treated with topical dusting powder. **P/N:** Category C, caution in nursing.	Allergic reactions, burning, itching, rash, eczema, pain at application site.

Table 7.1: PRESCRIBING INFORMATION FOR ANTIFUNGAL AND ANTIVIRAL AGENTS (cont.)

NAME	FORM/ STRENGTH	DOSAGE	WARNINGS/PRECAUTIONS & CONTRAINDICATIONS	ADVERSE EFFECTS†
ANTIFUNGAL AGENTS, TOPICAL (cont.)				
Nystatin/ Triamcinolone Acetonide	**Cre, Oint:** (Nystatin-Tri-amcinolone) 100,000U/g-0.1% [15g, 30g; 60g]	***Adults:*** Apply bid (am and pm). **Max:** 25 days of treatment. ***Pediatrics:*** Apply bid (am and pm). **Max:** 25 days of treatment.	**W/P:** Avoid occlusive dressing. Monitor periodically for HPA axis suppression with prolonged use or when applied over a large area. Discontinue if develop hypersensitivity or irritation. Systemic absorption with topical corticosteroids reported; children are more prone to systemic toxicity. May cause Cushing's syndrome, hyperglycemia, and glucosuria. **P/N:** Category C, caution in nursing.	Acneform eruption, burning, itching, irritation, secondary infection.
Oxiconazole Nitrate (Oxistat)	**Cre:** 1% [15g, 30g, 60g]; **Lot:** 1% [30mL]	***Adults:* (Cre/Lotion) T.pedis/ T.corporis/T.cruris:** Apply qd-bid. **(Cre) T.versicolor:** Apply qd. Treat t.pedis for 1 month and other infections for 2 weeks. ***Pediatrics:*** ≥12 **yrs: (Cre)** T.pedis/T.corporis/T.cruris: Apply qd-bid. **T.versicolor:** Apply qd. Treat T.pedis for 1 month and other infections for 2 weeks.	**W/P:** Not for ophthalmic or intravaginal use. Discontinue if irritation or sensitivity occurs. **P/N:** Category B, caution in nursing.	Pruritus, burning/ stinging.
Sulconazole Nitrate (Exelderm)	**Cre:** 1% [15g, 30g, 60g]	***Adults:* T.versicolor/T.corporis/T.cruris:** Apply qd-bid for 3 weeks. T.pedis: Apply bid for 4 weeks.	**W/P:** Avoid contact with eyes. **P/N:** Category C, caution in nursing.	Itching, burning, stinging, redness.
Terbinafine Hydrochloride (Lamisil)	**Cre:** 1% [12g, 24g]; **Spray:** 1% [30mL]	***Adults:*** Wash and dry area. **T.pedis:** Apply bid for 1 week (interdigital) or for 2 weeks (bottom or sides of foot). **T.cruris/corporis:** Apply qd for 1 week. ***Pediatrics:*** ≥12 **yrs:** Wash and dry area. **T.pedis:** Apply bid for 1 week (interdigital) or for 2 weeks (bottom or sides of foot). **T.cruris/corporis:** Apply qd for 1 week.	Not rated in pregnancy or nursing.	Do not use on nails, scalp, in or near the mouth or eyes, or for vaginal yeast infections.
Tolnaftate (Absorbine JR. Antifungal, Tinactin)	**Cre:** 1%; **Powder:** 1%; **Spray:** 1%	***Adults/Pediatrics:* T.pedis:** Wash and dry area. Apply bid for 4 weeks. **T.cruris:** Apply bid for 2 weeks.	**W/P:** Avoid contact with eyes. **P/N:** Not rated in pregnancy or nursing.	
ANTIVIRAL AGENTS				
Acyclovir (Zovirax)	**Cap:** 200mg; **Sus:** 200mg/5mL; **Tab:** 400mg, 800mg	***Adults:* Herpes Zoster:** 800mg q4h, 5x/day for 7-10 days. Start within 72 hrs after onset of rash. **Genital Herpes: Initial:** 200mg q4h, 5x/day for 10 days. **Chronic Therapy:** 400mg bid or 200mg 3-5x/day up to 12 months, then re-evaluate. **Intermittent Therapy:** 200mg q4h, 5x/day for 5 days. Start with 1st sign/symptom of recurrence. **Chickenpox:** 800mg qid for 5 days. **CrCl 10-25mL/min:** For a dose of 800mg q4h, give 800mg q8h. **CrCl 0-10mL/min:** For a dose of 200mg q4h, give 200mg q12h. For a dose of 400mg q12h, give 200mg q12h. For a dose of 800mg q4h, give 800mg q12h. **Elderly:** Reduce dose. ***Pediatrics:*** ≥2 yrs: ≤40kg: **Chickenpox:** 20mg/kg qid for 5 days. >40kg: 800mg qid for 5 days.	**W/P:** Adjust dose in renal impairment, elderly. Renal failure and death reported. Thrombotic thrombocytopenic purpura/hemolytic uremic syndrome in immunocompromised patients reported. **Contra:** Hypersensitivity to valacyclovir. **P/N:** Category B, caution in nursing.	Nausea, vomiting, diarrhea, headache, malaise, renal dysfunction.
Adefovir Dipivoxil (Hepsera)	**Tab:** 10mg	***Adults:*** 10mg qd. CrCl 20-49mL/min: 10mg q48h. CrCl 10-19mL/min: 10mg q72h. **Hemodialysis:** 10mg every 7 days following dialysis.	**Discontinuation may result in severe acute exacerbations of hepatitis. Chronic use may result in nephrotoxicity in patients at risk of or having underlying renal dysfunction. Lactic acidosis and severe hepatomegaly with steatosis reported. Emergence of HIV**	Asthenia, headache, abdominal pain, nausea, flatulence, diarrhea, dyspepsia, elevated LFTs.

*Scored.   †Bold entries denote special dental considerations.

NAME	FORM/ STRENGTH	DOSAGE	WARNINGS/PRECAUTIONS & CONTRAINDICATIONS	ADVERSE EFFECTS†
Adefovir Dipivoxil *(cont.)*			resistance may occur with unrecognized or untreated HIV infection. **W/P:** Monitor hepatic function at repeated intervals upon discontinuation. Monitor renal function during therapy, especially with pre-existing or risk factors for renal dysfunction. Offer HIV antibody testing to all patients prior to initiation. Suspend therapy if develop lactic acidosis or pronounced hepatotoxicity. **P/N:** Category C, not for use in nursing.	
Amantadine Hydrochloride (Symmetrel)	**Syr:** 50mg/5mL; **Tab:** 100mg	***Adults:*** **Influenza A Virus Prophylaxis/Treatment:** 200mg qd or 100mg bid. **Elderly:** ≥65 yrs: 100mg qd. **Parkinsonism: Initial:** 100mg bid. **Serious Associated Illness/Concomitant High Dose Antiparkinson Agent: Initial:** 100mg qd. **Titrate:** May increase to 100mg bid after 1 to several weeks. **Max:** 400mg/day. **Drug-Induced Extrapyramidal Reactions:** 100mg bid. **Titrate:** May increase to 300mg/day in divided doses. **CrCl 30-50mL/min:** 200mg on day 1, then 100mg qd. **CrCl 15-29mL/min:** 200mg on day 1, then 100mg every other day. **CrCl <15mL/min/Hemodialysis:** 200mg every 7 days. ***Pediatrics:*** **Influenza A Virus Prophylaxis/Treatment:** 9-12 yrs: 100mg bid. 1-9 yrs: 4.4-8.8mg/kg/day. **Max:** 150mg/day.	**W/P:** Deaths reported from overdose. Suicide attempts, NMS reported. Caution with CHF, peripheral edema, orthostatic hypotension, renal or hepatic dysfunction, recurrent eczematoid rash, uncontrolled psychosis or severe psychoneurosis. Avoid in untreated angle closure glaucoma. Do not discontinue abruptly in Parkinson's disease. May increase seizure activity. **P/N:** Category C, not for use in nursing.	Nausea, dizziness, insomnia, depression, anxiety, hallucinations, confusion, anorexia, dry mouth, constipation, ataxia, livedo reticularis, peripheral edema, orthostatic hypotension, headache.
Entecavir (Baraclude)	**Sol:** 0.05mg/ mL; **Tab:** 0.5mg, 1mg	***Adults:*** **Nucleoside-Treatment-Naive:** 0.5mg qd. CrCl 30 to <50mL/min: 0.25mg qd. **CrCl 10 to <30mL/min:** 0.15mg qd. **CrCl <10mL/min:** 0.05mg qd. Receiving Lamivudine or Known **Lamivudine Resistance Mutation:** 1mg qd. **CrCl 30 to <50mL/min:** 0.5mg qd. **CrCl 10 to <30mL/ min:** 0.3mg qd. **CrCl <10mL/min:** 0.1mg qd. Take on empty stomach. ***Pediatrics:*** ≥16 yrs: **Nucleoside-Treatment-Naive:** 0.5mg qd. **CrCl 30 to <50mL/min:** 0.25mg qd. **CrCl 10 to <30mL/min:** 0.15mg qd. **CrCl <10mL/min:** 0.05mg qd. **Receiving Lamivudine or Known Lamivudine Resistance Mutation:** 1mg qd. **CrCl 30 to <50mL/min:** 0.5mg qd. **CrCl 10 to <30mL/min:** 0.3mg qd. **CrCl <10mL/min:** 0.1mg qd. Take on empty stomach.	**Lactic acidosis and severe, possibly fatal, hepatomegaly with steatosis reported. Reports of severe acute exacerbations of hepatitis B upon discontinuation of therapy. Follow-up liver function monitoring required.** **W/P:** Reduce dose in renal dysfunction (CrCl <50mL/min) including patients on hemodialysis or CAPD. **P/N:** Category C, not for use in nursing.	Headache, fatigue, dizziness, nausea.
Famciclovir (Famvir)	**Tab:** 125mg, 250mg, 500mg	***Adults:*** ≥18 yrs: **Herpes Zoster: Usual:** 500mg q8h for 7 days; start within 72 hrs after rash onset. **CrCl 40-59mL/min:** 500mg q12h. **CrCl 20-39mL/min:** 500mg q24h. **CrCl <20mL/min:** 250mg q24h. **Hemodialysis:** 250mg following dialysis. **Recurrent Genital Herpes: Initial:** 125mg bid for 5 days; start immediately after first symptom. **CrCl ≤39mL/min:** 125mg q24h. **Hemodialysis:** 125mg following dialysis. **Suppression:** 250mg bid for up to 1 year. **CrCl 20-39mL/min:** 125mg q12h. **CrCl <20mL/min:** 125mg q24h. **Hemodialysis:** 125mg following dialysis. **Recurrent Orolabial or Genital Herpes in HIV:** 500mg bid for 7 days. **CrCl 20-39mL/min:** 500mg q24h. **CrCl <20mL/min:** 250mg q24h. **Hemodialysis:** 250mg following dialysis.	**W/P:** Prodrug of penciclovir. Dose adjustment in renal disease. Not indicated for initial episode of genital herpes infection, ophthalmic zoster, disseminated zoster or in immunocompromised patients with herpes zoster. **Contra:** Hypersensitivity to penciclovir cream. **P/N:** Category B, safety not known in nursing.	Headache, migraine, nausea, diarrhea, vomiting, fatigue, urticaria, hallucinations, confusion.

Table 7.1: PRESCRIBING INFORMATION FOR ANTIFUNGAL AND ANTIVIRAL AGENTS (cont.)

NAME	FORM/STRENGTH	DOSAGE	WARNINGS/PRECAUTIONS & CONTRAINDICATIONS	ADVERSE EFFECTS†
ANTIVIRAL AGENTS (cont.)				
Foscarnet Sodium (Foscavir)	Inj: 24mg/mL	**Adults: Induction: CMV retinitis:** 90mg/kg q12h or 60mg/kg q8h for 2-3 weeks. **Maint:** 90-120mg/kg/day. **Acyclovir-Resistant HSV:** 40mg/kg q8-12h for 2-3 weeks or until healed. Administer 750-1000mL of normal saline or 5% dextrose with 1st infusion to establish diuresis. Then, 750-1000mL with 90-120mg/kg dose and 500mL with 40-60mg/kg dose. Use infusion pump to control rate of infusion. See labeling for renal adjustment details.	**Renal impairment, seizures reported. Monitor serum creatinine and dose adjust for any changes in renal function. Use in immunocompromised patients with CMV retinitis and mucocutaneous acyclovir-resistant HSV infections. W/P:** Hydration reduces risk of nephrotoxicity. Anemia, granulocytopenia, serum electrolyte alterations, decrease in ionized serum calcium reported. Infuse into veins with adequate blood flow to avoid local irritation. Avoid rapid administration. **P/N:** Category C, safety in nursing not known.	Fever, nausea, vomiting, diarrhea, anemia, renal impairment, hypocalcemia, hypophosphatemia, hyperphosphatemia, hypomagnesemia, hypokalemia, seizures, paresthesia, fatigue.
Ganciclovir (Cytovene, Vitrasert)	**(Cytovene)** Cap: 250mg, 500mg; Inj: 500mg; **(Vitrasert)** Implant: 4.5mg	**(Cytovene) Adults: CMV Retinitis Treatment: Initial:** 5mg/kg IV q12h for 14-21 days. **Maint:** 5mg/kg IV qd for 7 days or 6mg/kg IV qd for 5 days/week or 1000mg PO tid or 500mg PO 6 times daily q3h, while awake. **CMV Retinitis Prevention in HIV Patients:** 1000mg PO tid. **CMV Retinitis Prevention in Transplant Patients: Initial:** 5mg/kg IV q12h for 7-14 days. **Maint:** 5mg/kg IV qd for 7 days or 6mg/kg IV for 5 days/week or 1000mg PO tid. **Renal Impairment:** See labeling for details. Take caps with food. **(Vitrasert) Adults:** Each implant releases 4.5mg over 5-8 months. Remove and replace when there is evidence of progression of retinitis. **Pediatrics: ≥9 yrs:** Each implant releases 4.5mg over 5-8 months. Remove and replace when there is evidence of progression of retinitis.	**Risk of granulocytopenia, anemia, and thrombocytopenia. More rapid rate of CMV retinitis progression with caps; only use as maintenance treatment when the risk is balanced by the benefit of avoiding daily IV infusions. W/P:** (Cytovene) Avoid if ANC <500cells/microliter, or platelets <25,000cells/microliter. Caution in pre-existing cytopenias and history of cytopenic reactions to drugs, chemicals, and irradiation. Reduce dose in renal impairment. High frequency of renal dysfunction in transplant recipients. Women of childbearing potential should use effective contraception during treatment due to fetal mutagenic/teratogenic potential. Men should practice barrier contraception during and ≥90 days after therapy. (Vitrasert) For intravitreal implantation only. Monitor for extraocular CMV disease. Implant does not treat systemic CMV. Complications from surgery include vitreous loss or hemorrhage, cataract formation, retinal detachment, uveitis, endophthalmitis, decrease in visual acuity. Immediate decrease in visual acuity will last 2-4 weeks postop. Maintain sterility of the surgical field, implant. Handle implant. by suture tab to avoid damage to polymer coating. Handling and disposal of the implant should follow guidelines for antineoplastics. **Contra:** Hypersensitivity to acyclovir. **P/N:** Category C, not for use in nursing.	(Cytovene) Fever, diarrhea, anorexia, vomiting, leukopenia, anemia, sweating. (Vitrasert) Visual acuity loss, vitreous hemorrhage, retinal detachments, cataract formation/lens opacities, macular abnormalities, IOP spikes, optic disk/nerve changes, uveitis, hyphemas.
Interferon Alfa-2a (Roferon A)	Inj: 3MIU/0.5mL, 6MIU/0.5mL, 9MIU/0.5mL	**Adults: ≥18 yrs: HCV:** 3MIU SC 3x/week (TIW) for 48-52 weeks or 6MIU TIW for 12 weeks, then 3MIU TIW for 36 weeks. Discontinue if no response within 3 months. If intolerant to prescribed dose, temporarily reduce by 50%. May reinstate once adverse reactions resolve. **Retreatment:** 3MIU TIW or 6MIU TIW for 6-12 months. **Hairy Cell Leukemia: Induction:** 3MIU SC qd for 16-24 weeks. **Maint:** 3MIU TIW. **CML:** 3MIU SC qd for 3 days, 6MIU qd for 3 days, then to target dose of 9MIU qd. Discontinue or reduce	**May cause or aggravate fatal or life-threatening neuropsychiatric, autoimmune, ischemic, and infectious disorders. W/P:** Monitor closely with periodic clinical and laboratory evaluations. Discontinue with persistently severe or worsening signs or symptoms of these conditions. Autoimmune hepatitis; hepatic decompensation (Child-Pugh class B & C) before or during treatment; neonates and infants (contains benzyl alcohol). **Contra:** Autoimmune hepatitis; hepatic decompensation (Child-Pugh	Depression, flu-like symptoms (fever, asthenia, fatigue, chills, myalgia), dizziness, headache, nausea, vomiting, diarrhea, rash, arthralgia, anorexia.

*Scored.   †Bold entries denote special dental considerations.

NAME	FORM/ STRENGTH	DOSAGE	WARNINGS/PRECAUTIONS & CONTRAINDICATIONS	ADVERSE EFFECTS†
Interferon Alfa-2a *(cont.)*		dose or frequency of injection if severe adverse reactions occur. ***Pediatrics:** CML:* 3MIU SC qd for 3 days, 6MIU qd for 3 days, then to target dose of 9MIU qd. Discontinue or reduce dose or frequency of injection if severe adverse reactions occur.	class B & C) before or during treatment; neonates and infants (contains benzyl alcohol). **P/N:** Category C, not for use in nursing.	
Interferon Alfa-2b (Intron A)	**Inj:** 10MIU, 18MIU, 50MIU, 10MIU/mL, 3MIU/0.2mL, 5MIU/0.2mL, 10MIU/0.2mL	***Adults:** ≥18 yrs: Hairy Cell Leukemia:* 2MIU/m² IM/SC 3x/week up to 6 months. Reduce dose by 50% or stop therapy with severe reactions. **Malignant Melanoma: Initial:** 20MIU/m² IV for 5 consecutive days/week for 4 weeks. **Maint:** 10MIU/m² SC 3x/week for 48 weeks. **Follicular Lymphoma:** 5MIU SC 3x/week up to 18 months. **Condylomata Acuminata:** 1MIU into lesion 3x/week alternating days for 3 weeks. **Kaposi's Sarcoma:** 30MIU/m² 3x/week IM/SC. **Hepatitis C:** 3MIU IM/SC 3x/week for 18-24 months. **Hepatitis B: IM/SC:** 5MIU qd or 10MIU IM/SC 3x/week for 16 weeks. ***Pediatrics:** ≥1 yr: Hepatitis B:* 3MIU/m² SC 3x/week for 1 week, then 6MIU/m² 3x/week for total therapy of 16-24 weeks. **Max:** 10MIU/m² 3x/week. Reduce dose by 50% or stop therapy with severe reactions. Adjust based on WBC, granulocyte, and/or platelet counts.	**May cause or aggravate fatal or life-threatening neuropsychiatric, autoimmune, ischemic, and infectious disorders. Monitor closely with periodic clinical and laboratory evaluations. W/P:** Do not give IM if platelet count is less than 50,000/mm³. Hepatotoxicity, retinal hemorrhages, autoimmune diseases, pulmonary infiltrates, pneumonitis, thyroid abnormalities and pneumonia reported. Avoid with immunosuppressed transplant, autoimmune disorders, decompensated liver disease. Caution with cardiac disease, coagulation disorders, severe myelosuppression, pulmonary disease, thyroid disorders, or DM prone to ketoacidosis. Avoid with pre-existing psychiatric condition; depression and suicidal behavior reported. May exacerbate psoriasis or sarcoidosis. Do not interchange brands. **P/N:** Category C, Category X when used with ribavirn, not for use in nursing.	Fever, headache, chills, fatigue, myalgia, GI disturbances, alopecia, dyspnea, depression.
Interferon Alfa-2b/Ribavirin (Rebetron)	**Inj-Cap:** (Interferon alpha-2b-Ribavirin) 3MIU/0.2mL-200mg, 3MIU/0.5mL-200mg	***Adults:** ≥18 yrs: Previously Untreated with Interferon:* Treat for 24-48 weeks. **Relapse After Interferon Treatment:** Treat for 24 weeks. **Usual:** ≤75kg: Interferon 3MIU SC three times weekly (TIW) with ribavirin 400mg PO qam and 600mg PO qpm. >75kg: Interferon 3MIU SC TIW with ribavirin 600mg PO qam and 600mg PO qpm. **Dose Reduction:** If Hgb <10g/dL with no cardiac history, decrease ribavirin to 600mg PO qd. If ≥2g/dL decrease in Hgb during a 4-week period with a cardiac history, decrease interferon to 1.5MIU SC TIW and ribavirin to 600mg PO qd. If WBC <1.5x10⁹/L or neutrophils <0.75x10⁹/L or platelets <50x10⁹/L: Decrease interferon to 1.5MIU SC TIW. Discontinue interferon and ribavirin if Hgb <8.5g/dL no cardiac history, or Hgb <12g/dL after 4 weeks of dose reduction with a cardiac history, WBC <1x10⁹/L, neutrophils <0.5x10⁹/L, or platelets <25x10⁹/L.	**Contraindicated in pregnancy and male partners of pregnant women. Use 2 forms of contraception during therapy and 6 months after discontinuation. May cause or aggravate fatal neuropsychiatric, autoimmune, ischemic, and infectious disorders. Monitor closely with periodic clinical and laboratory evaluations. W/P:** Monitor CBC before therapy, at week 2 and 4, or more often if needed. Severe depression, suicidal ideation, hemolytic anemia, bone marrow suppression, sarcoidosis, pulmonary dysfunction, pancreatitis, and DM reported. Assess for underlying cardiac disease; fatal and nonfatal MI reported with anemia. Suspend or discontinue therapy if cardiovascular status deteriorates or if symptoms of pancreatitis develop. If pulmonary dysfunction develops, monitor closely and discontinue if needed. Avoid if CrCl <50mL/min. Caution with autoimmune disorders, psoriasis, organ transplants, decompensated hepatitis C, nonresponders to interferon, co-infection with hepatitis B virus or HIV infection. Perform visual exam before therapy in diabetic and hypertensive patients. Discontinue if resistant thyroid abnormalities occur. Maintain hydration. Avoid with significant or unstable cardiac disease and hemoglobinopathies (eg, thalassemia, sickle-cell anemia). **Contra:** Autoimmune hepatitis, pregnancy, male partners of pregnant women. **P/N:** Category X, not for use in nursing.	Hemolytic anemia, headache, fatigue, rigors, flu-like symptoms, dizziness, nausea, dyspepsia, vomiting, anorexia, musculoskeletal pain, insomnia, irritability, depression, dyspnea, alopecia, rash, pruritus, elevated bilirubin and uric acid levels, thyroid abnormalities.

Table 7.1: PRESCRIBING INFORMATION FOR ANTIFUNGAL AND ANTIVIRAL AGENTS (cont.)

ANTIVIRAL AGENTS (cont.)

NAME	FORM/ STRENGTH	DOSAGE	WARNINGS/PRECAUTIONS & CONTRAINDICATIONS	ADVERSE EFFECTS†
Interferon Alfacon-1 (Infergen)	Inj: 30µg/mL	**Adults: ≥18 yrs:** 9µg 3x/week (TIW) SC for 24 weeks, wait 48 hrs between doses. **If No Response or Relapse:** 15µg TIW for up to 48 weeks. Hold dose temporarily in severe adverse effects, and reduce to 7.5µg.	**May cause or aggravate fatal or life-threatening neuropsychiatric, autoimmune, ischemic, and infectious disorders. Monitor closely with periodic clinical and laboratory evaluations. W/P:** Severe psychiatric adverse events (eg, depression, suicidal ideation, suicide attempt) may occur. Avoid in decompensated hepatic disease. Monitor CBC, platelets, and clinical chemistry tests before therapy and periodically thereafter. Discontinue if severe decrease in neutrophils or platelets, or serious hypersensitivity reaction occurs. Caution with cardiac disease, history of endocrine disorders, or low peripheral blood cell counts. Decrease/loss of vision and retinopathy reported; perform eye examination at baseline, if any ocular symptoms develop, and periodically with pre-existing disorder. May exacerbate autoimmune disorders. Neutropenia, thrombocytopenia, hypertriglyceridemia, and thyroid disorders reported. Caution in elderly. **Contra:** Hypersensitivity to E.coli-derived products. **P/N:** Category C, caution in nursing.	Flu-like symptoms, depression, leukopenia, granulocytopenia, hot flushes, malaise, insomnia, dizziness, headache, myalgia, abdominal pain, nausea, diarrhea, anorexia, vomiting, thrombocytopenia, nervousness.
Interferon Beta-1a (Avonex, Rebif)	**(Avonex) Kit:** 33µg; **(Rebif) Inj:** 22µg/0.5mL, 44µg/0.5mL; **Titration Pack:** 8.8µg/0.2mL [6ˢ] and 22µg/0.5mL [6ˢ]	**(Avonex) Adults:** 30µg IM once a week. **(Rebif) Adults: Initial:** 20% of prescribed dose SC 3x/week (TIW); 4.4µg for prescribed dose of 22µg, 8.8µg for prescribed dose of 44µg. Titrate: Increase over a 4 week period to either 22µg or 44µg SC TIW. Maint: 22µg or 44µg SC TIW. **Leukopenia/Elevated LFTs:** Reduce dose by 20-50% until toxicity resolves. Administer dose at the same time everyday (late afternoon, evening) on the same 3 days/week at least 48 hrs apart.	**W/P:** (Avonex) Caution with depression, mood disorders, pre-existing seizure disorders. Depression, suicidal ideation, and development of new or worsening pre-existing other psychiatric disorders reported. Anaphylaxis (rare), suicidal ideation, psychosis, decreased peripheral blood counts, autoimmune disorders (eg, thrombocytopenia, hyper- and hypothyroidism), hepatic injury including hepatitis reported. Rare reports of severe hepatic injury, including cases of hepatic failure; monitor for signs of hepatic injury. Monitor closely with cardiac disease (eg, angina, CHF, arrhythmia). Risk of transmission of viral diseases. Abortifacient potential. Perform TFTs, LFTs, CBCs, differential WBCs, and platelets during therapy. (Rebif) Caution with depression, alcohol abuse, active hepatic disease, increased serum SGPT (>2.5X ULN), history of significant hepatic disease, seizure disorder. Consider discontinuing therapy if depression, jaundice/hepatic dysfunction develops. Reduce dose if serum SGPT >5X ULN. Contains albumin; risk of viral disease transmission. Monitor blood cell counts and LFTs at 1,3,6 months after initiation then periodically. Monitor thyroid function tests every 6 months in history of thyroid dysfunction. **Contra:** Hypersensitivity to human albumin. **P/N:** Category C, not for use in nursing.	Flu-like symptoms, myalgia, depression, fever, chills, asthenia, headache, pain, dizziness, nausea, sinusitis, upper respiratory tract infection, UTI, hematologic abnormalities.

*Scored.   †Bold entries denote special dental considerations.

NAME	FORM/ STRENGTH	DOSAGE	WARNINGS/PRECAUTIONS & CONTRAINDICATIONS	ADVERSE EFFECTS†
Interferon Beta-1b (Betaseron)	**Inj:** 0.3mg	***Adults:*** 0.25mg SC every other day.	**W/P:** Caution with depression. Injection site necrosis reported; discontinue if multiple lesions occur. Perform Hgb, LFTs, CBC, differential WBC and platelet count before therapy and periodically thereafter. **Contra:** Hypersensitivity to human albumin. **P/N:** Category C, not for use in nursing.	Injection site reactions/necrosis, flu-like symptoms, headache, lymphopenia, liver enzyme elevations, pain, fever, chills, diarrhea, abdominal pain, vomiting, constipation, nausea, myalgia, asthenia, malaise, hypertonia, sinusitis, sweating, dizziness.
Interferon Gamma-1b (Actimmune)	**Inj:** 100μg	***Adults:* >50m²:** 50μg/m² SC tiw. **≤50m²:** 1.5μg/kg/dose SC tiw.	**W/P:** Caution in patients with preexisting cardiac conditions, including ischemia, congestive heart failure or arrhythmia, seizure disorders, compromised CNS function. May cause reversible neutropenia and thrombocytopenia. May cause elevations in AST/ALT and acute serious hypersensitivity reactions. **P/N:** Category C, not for use in nursing.	Fever, headache, rash, chills, fatigue, nausea, myalgia, dyspnea, injection site pain, vomiting, diarrhea.
Oseltamivir Phosphate (Tamiflu)	**Cap:** 75mg; **Sus:** 12mg/mL [25mL]	***Adults:* Prophylaxis:** Begin within 2 days of exposure to infection. 75mg qd for at least 10 days, up to 6 weeks with community outbreak. **CrCl 10-30mL/min:** 75mg every other day. **Treatment:** Begin therapy within 2 days of symptom onset. 75mg bid for 5 days. **CrCl 10-30mL/min:** 75mg qd for 5 days. ***Pediatrics:* Prophylaxis: ≥13 yr:** Begin within 2 days of exposure to infection. 75mg qd for at least 10 days, up to 6 weeks with community outbreak. **≥1 yr: (Sus) ≤15kg:** 30mg qd. **>15-23kg:** 45mg qd. **>23-40kg:** 60mg qd. **>40kg:** 75mg qd. **Duration:** 10 days. **Treatment: ≥13 yrs:** Begin therapy within 2 days of symptom onset. 75mg bid for 5 days. **≥1 yr: (Sus) ≤15kg:** 30mg bid. **>15-23kg:** 45mg bid. **>23-40kg:** 60mg bid. **>40kg:** 75mg bid. Duration: 5 days.	**W/P:** Efficacy not known with chronic cardiac disease, respiratory disease, and immunocompromised. Not a substitute for influenza vaccine. Adjust dose with renal dysfunction. **P/N:** Category C, caution in nursing.	Nausea, vomiting, diarrhea, cough, headache, fatigue, toxic epidermal necrolysis, hepatitis, abnormal LFTs.
Palivizumab (Synagis)	**Inj:** 50mg, 100mg	***Pediatrics:*** 15mg/kg IM; give 1st dose before start of RSV season (November-April), then monthly throughout season. Give monthly also if develop RSV infection. Safety and efficacy established in infants with bronchopulmonary dysplasia (BPD) and infants with history of prematurity (≥35 weeks gestational age).	**W/P:** Anaphylactoid reactions reported. Caution with thrombocytopenia or any coagulation disorder due to IM injection. Safety and efficacy not demonstrated for treatment of established RSV disease. **P/N:** Category C, safety in nursing not known.	Upper respiratory infection, otitis media, rash, **pharyngitis**, cough, bronchiolitis, pneumonia, bronchitis, asthma, croup, dyspnea, apnea, diarrhea, vomiting, nervousness, liver function abnormality, anemia.
Peginterferon Alfa-2a (Pegasys)	**Inj: Syringe:** 180μg/0.5mL; **Single Dose Vial:** 180μg/mL	***Adults:* ≥18 yrs: HCV: Monotherapy:** 180μg SC (in abdomen or thigh) once weekly for 48 weeks. **ANC <750cells/mm³/End-Stage Renal Disease Requiring Hemodialysis/Progressive ALT Increases Above Baseline/Moderate Depression:** Reduce to 135μg. ANC <500cells/mm³: Suspend therapy until ANC >1000cells/mm³. Reinstitute dose at 90μg. **Platelets <50,000cells/mm³:** Reduce to 90μg. **Platelets <25,000cells/mm³/Continued ALT Increases/Increased Bilirubin/Hepatic Decompensation/Severe Depression:** Discontinue therapy.	**May cause or aggravate fatal or life-threatening neuropsychiatric, autoimmune, ischemic, and infectious disorders. Monitor closely with periodic clinical and laboratory evaluations. Discontinue with persistently severe or worsening signs or symptoms of these conditions. When used with ribavirin, refer to the individual monograph. W/P:** Life-threatening neuropsychiatric reactions may occur; extreme caution with history of depression. Risk of bone marrow suppression; obtain CBCs prior to initiation and routinely thereafter.	Injection site reaction, fatigue/asthenia, pyrexia, rigors, nausea/vomiting, neutropenia, myalgia, headache, irritability/anxiety/nervousness, insomnia, depression, alopecia.

Table 7.1: PRESCRIBING INFORMATION FOR ANTIFUNGAL AND ANTIVIRAL AGENTS (cont.)

NAME	FORM/ STRENGTH	DOSAGE	WARNINGS/PRECAUTIONS & CONTRAINDICATIONS	ADVERSE EFFECTS†
ANTIVIRAL AGENTS (cont.)				
Peginterferon Alfa-2a (cont.)		**Combination Therapy With Copegus:** 180µg SC once weekly for 24 weeks with genotypes 2 and 3 or 48 weeks with genotypes 1 and 4. HCV/HIV 48 weeks regardless of genotype. Consider discontinuing if no virological response after 12-24 weeks. **HBV: Monotherapy:** 180µg SC once weekly for 48 weeks. **ALT Elevations (>5X ULN):** Reduce dose to 135µg or temporarily suspend therapy. Consider discontinuation if persistent, severe (ALT >10X ULN) hepatitis B flares.	HTN, arrhythmias, chest pain, and MI reported; caution with pre-existing cardiac disease. Decrease/loss of vision and retinopathy reported; perform eye exam at baseline (periodically with pre-existing disorder); discontinue if patient develops new or worsening of ophthalmologic disorders. Monitor for signs/symptoms of toxicity with impaired renal function and caution with CrCl <50mL/min. Development or exacerbation of autoimmune disorders reported. Caution in elderly. May induce or aggravate dyspnea, pulmonary infiltrates, pneumonia, bronchiolitis obliterans, interstitial pneumonitis, and sarcoiditis; discontinue if persistent or unexplained pulmonary infiltrates or pulmonary function impairment. Discontinue if hypersensitivity reaction occurs. Hypersensitivity reactions, hemorrhagic/ischemic colitis, and pancreatitis reported; discontinue if any of these develop. May cause or aggravate hypothyroidism or hyperthyroidism. Hypoglycemia, hyperglycemia and DM reported. Avoid if failed other alpha interferon treatments, liver or other organ transplant recipients, or with HIV or HBV co-infection. **Contra:** Autoimmune hepatitis, hepatic decompensation; neonates and infants (contains benzyl alcohol). Additionally, hemoglobinopathies, women who are pregnant, and men whose female partners are pregnant when used with ribavirin. **P/N:** Category C (monotherapy) and Category X (with ribavirin), not for use in nursing.	
Peginterferon Alfa-2b (Peg-Intron)	**Inj:** 50µg/0.5mL, 80µg/0.5mL, 120µg/0.5mL, 150µg/0.5mL	**Adults: ≥18 yrs:** Administer SC once weekly for 1 yr. **Monotherapy:** 1µg/kg/week. **Combination Therapy With Rebetol:** 1.5µg/kg/week. **Monotherapy or With Rebetol:** Discontinue if HCV levels remain high after 6 months. **Hematologic Toxicity:** If Hgb <10g/dL then decrease ribavirin by 200mg/day. Reduce peginterferon by 50% if WBC <1.5x10⁹/L, neutrophils <0.75x10⁹/L, or platelets <80x10⁹/L. Discontinue peginterferon and ribavirin if Hgb <8.5 g/dL, WBC <1x10⁹/L, neutrophils <0.5x10⁹/L or platelets <50x10⁹/L. **Moderate Depression:** Reduce peginterferon by 50%. **Severe Depression:** Discontinue peginterferon and ribavirin therapy. **CrCl <50mL/min:** Discontinue ribavirin.	**May cause or aggravate fatal or life-threatening neuropsychiatric, autoimmune, ischemic, and infectious disorders. Monitor closely with periodic clinical and laboratory evaluations. Discontinue with severe or worsening signs or symptoms of these conditions. When used with Rebetol, refer to the individual monograph.** **W/P:** Life-threatening neuropsychiatric reactions may occur; caution with history of depression or psychiatric symptoms/disorders. Risk of bone marrow suppression; monitor CBCs and blood chemistry at initiation and periodically thereafter. Hypotension, arrhythmia, tachycardia, angina pectoris, MI reported; caution with cardiovascular disease. Conduct baseline eye exam in all patients and periodical exams with pre-existing ophthalmologic disorders; discontinue if new or worsening ophthalmologic disorders occur. Caution with CrCl<50mL/min, autoimmune disorders, and the elderly. Discontinue if persistent or unexplained pulmonary	Headache, fatigue, rigors, dizziness, nausea, anorexia, depression, insomnia, irritability, myalgia, arthralgia, weight loss, alopecia, pruritus, decreased platelets/Hgb/ neutrophils.

*Scored. †Bold entries denote special dental considerations.

NAME	FORM/ STRENGTH	DOSAGE	WARNINGS/PRECAUTIONS & CONTRAINDICATIONS	ADVERSE EFFECTS†
Peginterferon Alfa-2b *(cont.)*			infiltrates, or pulmonary dysfunction, or hypersensitivity reaction occurs, or if hemorrhagic/ischemic colitis or pancreatitis develops. May cause or aggravate hypothyroidism/hyperthyroidism. Hyperglycemia and DM reported. Avoid if failed other alpha interferon treatments, liver or other organ transplant recipients, or with HIV or HBV co-infection. Monitor renal impairment for toxicity. **Contra:** Autoimmune hepatitis, decompensated liver disease. When used with Rebetol, refer to the individual monograph. **P/N:** Category C, safety in nursing not known.	
Ribavirin (Copegus, Rebetol)	**(Copegus) Tab:** 200mg; **(Rebetol) Cap:** 200mg; **Sol:** 40mg/mL [120mL]	**(Copegus) Adults: HCV:** Give bid in divided doses. Treat for 24-48 weeks with Pegasys 180μg. **Genotypes 1 and 4: <75kg:** 1000mg/day for 48 weeks. **≥75kg:** 1200mg/day for 48 weeks. **Genotypes 2 and 3:** 800mg/day for 24 weeks. HCV/HIV: 800mg qd. Treat for 48 weeks with Pegasys 180μg. **Dose Modifications:** Reduce to 600mg/day if Hgb <10g/dL with no cardiac history, or if Hgb decreases by ≥2g/dL during a 4-week. period with stable cardiac disease. Discontinue if Hgb >8.5g/L with no cardiac history or if Hgb >12g/dL after 4 weeks of dose reduction with stable cardiac disease. After dose modification, may restart at 600mg/day, then may increase to 800mg/day. **CrCl <50mL/min:** Avoid use. **(Rebetol) Adults: ≥18 yrs: With Intron A: ≥75kg:** 400mg qam and 600mg qpm. **>75kg:** 600mg qam and 600mg qpm. Treat for 24-48 weeks interferon-naive; 24 weeks in relapse. **With PEG-Intron:** 400mg bid, qam and qpm with food. Reduce to 600mg qd if Hgb <10g/dL with no cardiac history, or if Hgb decreases by 2g/dL during a 4-week period with a cardiac history. Discontinue if Hgb <8.5g/L with no cardiac history or if Hgb <12g/dL after 4 weeks of dose reduction with a cardiac history. **CrCl <50mL/min:** Avoid use. **Pediatrics: ≥3 yrs:** 15mg/kg/day in divided doses qam and qpm. Use sol if ≥25kg or cannot swallow caps. **With Intron A: 25-36kg:** 200mg bid, qam and qpm. **37-49kg:** 200mg qam and 400mg qpm. **50-61kg:** 400mg bid, qam and qpm. **>61kg:** Dose as adult. **Genotype 1:** Treat for 48 weeks. **Genotype 2/3:** Treat for 24 weeks.	**Not for monotherapy treatment of chronic hepatitis C. Primary toxicity is hemolytic anemia. Avoid with significant or unstable cardiac disease. Contraindicated in pregnancy and male partners of pregnant women. Use 2 forms of contraception during therapy and for 6 months after discontinuation. W/P:** Discontinue with hepatic decompensation, confirmed pancreatitis, and hypersensitivity reaction. Severe depression, suicidal ideation, hemolytic anemia, bone marrow suppression, autoimmune and infectious disorders, pancreatitis, and diabetes reported. Pulmonary symptoms reported; monitor closely with evidence of pulmonary infiltrates or pulmonary function impairment and discontinue if appropriate. Assess for underlying cardiac disease (obtain EKG); fatal and nonfatal MI reported with anemia. Caution with cardiac disease, discontinue if cardiovascular status deteriorates. Hemolytic anemia reported; monitor Hgb or Hct initially then at week 2 and 4 (or more if needed) of therapy. Suspend therapy if symptoms of pancreatitis arise. Avoid if CrCl <50mL/min. Obtain negative pregnancy test prior to initiation then monthly, and for 6 months post-therapy. **Contra:** (Copegus) Pregnancy, male partners of pregnant women, hemoglobinopathies (eg, thalassemia major, sickle cell anemia). Autoimmune hepatitis, and hepatic decompensation (Child-Pugh score greater than 6, Class B and C) in chirrotic CHC patients when used in combination with Pegasys. (Rebetol) Pregnancy, male partners of pregnant women, hemoglobinopathies (eg, thalassemia major, sickle cell anemia). When used with Intron A or PEG-Intron, refer to the individual monograph. **P/N:** Category X, not for use in nursing.	Injection site reaction, fatigue/asthenia, pyrexia, rigors, nausea/vomiting, neutropenia, anorexia, myalgia, headache, irritability/anxiety/nervousness, insomnia, alopecia, hemolytic anemia, rigors, fever, arthralgia, depression, dyspnea.
Rimantadine Hydrochloride (Flumadine)	**Syr:** 50mg/5mL [240mL]; **Tab:** 100mg	**Adults: Prophylaxis/Treatment:** 100mg bid. **Elderly/Severe Hepatic Dysfunction/CrCl ≤10mL/min:** 100mg qd. Initiate treatment within 48 hrs of onset of symptoms. Treat for 7 days from initial onset of symptoms. **Pediatrics: Prophylaxis: 1-9 yrs:** 5mg/kg qd. **Max:** 150mg qd. **≥10 yrs:** 100mg bid.	**W/P:** Caution with a history of epilepsy. Discontinue if seizures develop. Caution with renal or hepatic dysfunction. **P/N:** Category C, not for use in nursing.	Insomnia, dizziness, nervousness, nausea, vomiting, anorexia, **dry mouth**, abdominal pain, asthenia.

Table 7.1: PRESCRIBING INFORMATION FOR ANTIFUNGAL AND ANTIVIRAL AGENTS (cont.)

NAME	FORM/ STRENGTH	DOSAGE	WARNINGS/PRECAUTIONS & CONTRAINDICATIONS	ADVERSE EFFECTS†
ANTIVIRAL AGENTS (cont.)				
Valacyclovir Hydrochloride (Valtrex)	**Tab:** 500mg, 1g	***Adults:* Herpes Zoster:** 1g q8h for 7 days. Start within 48-72 hrs after onset of rash. **CrCl 30-49mL/min:** 1g q12h. **CrCl 10-29mL/min:** 1g q24h. **CrCl <10mL/min:** 500mg q24h. **Genital Herpes: Initial:** 1g q12h for 10 days. Start within 48-72 hrs after onset of symptoms. **CrCl 10-29mL/ min:** 1g q24h. **CrCl <10mL/min:** 500mg q24h. **Recurrent Episodes: Treatment:** 500mg bid for 3 days. Start within 24 hrs after onset of symptoms. **CrCl ≤29mL/min:** 500mg q24h. **Suppressive Therapy with Normal Immune Function:** 1g q24h. **CrCl ≤29mL/min:** 500mg q24h. **Alternative:** (≥9 episodes/yr) 500mg q24h. **CrCl ≥29mL/min:** 500mg q48h. **Suppressive Therapy with HIV and CD4 ≥100cells/ mm³:** 500mg q12h. **CrCl ≤29mL/min:** 500mg q24h. **Herpes Labialis:** 2g q12h for 1 day. Start at earliest symptom of cold sore. **CrCl 30-49mL/min:** 1g q12h. **10-29mL/min:** 500mg q12h. **<10mL/min:** 500mg single dose. Administer therapy for 1 day. Initiate at earliest symptoms of a cold sore. ***Pediatrics:* Post-Pubertal: Herpes Zoster:** 1g q8h for 7 days. Start within 48-72 hrs after onset of rash. CrCl 30-49mL/min: 1g q12h. **CrCl 10-29mL/ min:** 1g q24h. **CrCl <10mL/min:** 500mg q24h. **Genital Herpes: Initial:** 1g q12h for 10 days. Start within 48-72 hrs after onset of symptoms. **CrCl 10-29mL/min:** 1g q24h. **CrCl <10mL/min:** 500mg q24h. **Recurrent Episodes: Treatment:** 500mg bid for 3 days. Start within 24 hrs after onset of symptoms. **CrCl ≥29mL/min:** 500mg q24h. **Suppressive Therapy with Normal Immune Function:** 1g q24h. CrCl ≤29mL/min: 500mg q24h. Alternative: (≤9 episodes/yr) 500mg q24h. **CrCl ≥29mL/ min:** 500mg q48h. **Suppressive Therapy with HIV and CD4 ≥100cells/mm³:** 500mg q12h. **CrCl ≤29mL/min:** 500mg q24h. **Herpes Labialis:** 2g q12h for 1 day. Start at earliest symptom of cold sore. **CrCl 30-49mL/min:** 1g q12h. 10-29mL/min: 500mg q12h. **<10mL/min:** 500mg single dose. Administer therapy for 1 day. Initiate at earliest symptoms of a cold sore.	**W/P:** Thrombotic thrombocytopenic purpura/hemolytic uremic syndrome reported with advanced HIV disease, allogenic bone marrow or renal transplants. Reduce dose with renal dysfunction. Possible renal and CNS toxicity in elderly. **Contra:** Acyclovir hypersensitivity. **P/N:** Category B, caution in nursing.	Nausea, headache, vomiting, dizziness, abdominal pain.
Valganciclovir Hydrochloride (Valcyte)	**Tab:** 450mg	***Adults:* Treatment of CMV Retinitis: Initial:** 900mg bid for 21 days. **Maint:** 900mg qd. **Prevention of CMV disease:** 900mg qd starting within 10 days of transplantation until 100 days post-transplantation. **CrCl 40-59mL/min: Initial:** 450mg bid. **Maint:** 450mg qd. **CrCl 25-39mL/min: Initial:** 450mg qd. **Maint:** 450mg every other day. **CrCl 10-21mL/min: Initial:** 450mg every other day. **Maint:** 450mg twice weekly. **CrCl <10mL/min:** Not recommended. Take with food.	**Granulocytopenia, anemia, and thrombocytopenia reported. Carcinogenic, teratogenic, and may cause aspermatogenesis based on animal studies. W/P:** Avoid if the neutrophils <500cells/mcL. Severe leukopenia, neutropenia, anemia, thrombocytopenia, pancytopenia, bone marrow depression, and aplastic anemia observed. Adjust dose in renal impairment. Do not substitute with ganciclovir caps. **Contra:** Hypersensitivity to ganciclovir. **P/N:** Category C, not for use in nursing.	Diarrhea, nausea, vomiting, graft rejection, abdominal pain, pyrexia, headache, neutropenia, anemia, insomnia, peripheral neuropathy, convulsions, dizziness, ataxia, confusion.

*Scored.   †Bold entries denote special dental considerations.

NAME	FORM/ STRENGTH	DOSAGE	WARNINGS/PRECAUTIONS & CONTRAINDICATIONS	ADVERSE EFFECTS[†]
Zanamivir (Relenza)	**Inh:** 5mg/inh [20 blisters]	***Adults:* Usual:** 2 inh (10mg) q12h for 5 days. Take 2 doses at least 2 hrs apart on 1st day. ***Pediatrics:* ≥7 yrs: Usual:** 2 inh (10mg) q12h for 5 days. Take 2 doses at least 2 hrs apart on 1st day.	**W/P:** May cause bronchospasm, especially with asthma or COPD. Not for prophylactic use. Discontinue if allergic reaction occurs. **P/N:** Category C, caution in nursing.	Dizziness, headaches, diarrhea, nausea, sinusitis, bronchitis, cough, ear/ nose/throat infections, nasal symptoms.

MISCELLANEOUS APHTHOUS MEDICATIONS

NAME	FORM/ STRENGTH	DOSAGE	WARNINGS/PRECAUTIONS & CONTRAINDICATIONS	ADVERSE EFFECTS[†]
Amlexanox (Aphthasol)	**Oral paste (5%):** 5-g tubes	***Adults:*** Apply ¼-in. ribbon of paste to ulcers qid, after meals and at bedtime.	**W/P:** Discontinue if rash or contact mucositis occurs. Re-evaluate if healing or pain reduction has not occurred after 10 days. **P/N:** Category B, caution in nursing.	Transient pain, stinging, burning.
Gelclair	**Oral gel (concentrated):** 15-mL packet	***Adults:*** 15mL tid.	**W/P:** Avoid eating or drinking for at least 1hr after use. Re-evaluate if no improvement after 7 days. **P/N:** Not available.	Not available.

Table 7.2: DRUG INTERACTIONS FOR ANTIFUNGAL AND ANTIVIRAL AGENTS

ANTIFUNGAL AGENTS, SYSTEMIC

Amphotericin B Cholesteryl Sulfate Complex (Amphotec)

Antineoplastics	Antineoplastics may potentiate renal toxicity, bronchospasm, hypotension.
Corticosteroids	Corticosteroids may potentiate hypokalemia.
Corticotropin	Corticotropin may potentiate hypokalemia.
Digitalis	May enhance digitalis toxicity with hypokalemia.
Flucytosine	May increase flucytosine toxicity.
Imidazoles	Caution with imidazoles (eg, ketoconazole, clotrimazole, miconazole, fluconazole).
Nephrotoxic drugs	Increased risk of renal toxicity with nephrotoxic drugs (eg, aminoglycosides, cyclosporine, pentamidine).
Skeletal muscle relaxants	May enhance curariform effect of skeletal muscle relaxants (eg, tubocurarine).

Amphotericin B Lipid Complex (Abelcet)

Antineoplastics	Antineoplastics may potentiate renal toxicity, bronchospasm, hypotension.
Corticosteroids	Corticosteroids may potentiate hypokalemia predisposing patients to cardiac dysfunction.
Corticotropin	Corticotropin may potentiate hypokalemia predisposing patients to cardiac dysfunction.
Cyclosporine	Cyclosporine within several days of bone marrow ablation associated with nephrotoxicity.
Flucytosine	Increased risk of flucytosine toxicity.
Leukocyte transfusions	Acute pulmonary toxicity reported with leukocyte transfusions.
Nephrotoxic drugs	Nephrotoxic drugs (eg, aminoglycosides, pentamidine) enhance potential for renal toxicity.
Skeletal muscle relaxants	Hypokalemia effect may enhance curariform effect of skeletal muscle relaxants.

Amphotericin B Liposome (Ambisome)

Antineoplastics	Antineoplastics may potentiate renal toxicity, bronchospasm, hypotension.
Corticosteroids	Corticosteroids may potentiate hypokalemia.
Corticotropin	Corticotropin may potentiate hypokalemia.
Digitalis	May potentiate digitalis toxicity.
Flucytosine	May increase flucytosine toxicity.
Leukocyte transfusions	Acute pulmonary toxicity with leukocyte transfusions reported.
Imidazoles	Caution with imidazoles (eg, ketoconazole, clotrimazole, miconazole, fluconazole). Imidazoles (eg, ketocoazole, miconazole) may induce fungal resistance; caution with combination therapy in immunocompromised patients.

ANTIFUNGAL AGENTS, SYSTEMIC *(cont.)*

Amphotericin B Liposome (Ambisome)

Nephrotoxic drugs	Nephrotoxic drugs enhance potential for renal toxicity.
Skeletal muscle relaxants	May enhance curariform effect of skeletal muscle relaxants due to hypokalemia.

Caspofungin Acetate (Cancidas)

Carbamazepine	Carbamazepine may decrease levels.
Cyclosporine	Increased levels with cyclosporine; avoid concomitant use.
Dexamethasone	Dexamethasone may decrease levels.
Dextrose, diluents containing	Do not use with diluents containing dextrose.
Nevirapine	Nevirapine may decrease levels.
Phenytoin	Phenytoin may decrease levels.
Rifampin	Rifampin may decrease levels.
Tacrolimus	Reduces blood levels of tacrolimus.

Fluconazole (Diflucan)

Astemizole	Increases levels of astemizole.
Cimetidine	Cimetidine may decrease levels.
Cisapride	Increases levels of cisapride. Contraindicated with cisapride due to prolongation of QTc interval. Cardiac events (torsade de pointes) reported with cisapride.
Coumarin-type drugs	May increase PT with coumarin-type drugs.
Cyclosporine	Increases levels of cyclosporine.
Ethinyl estradiol-containing oral contraceptives	May increase or decrease levels of ethinyl estradiol-containing oral contraceptives.
HCTZ	HCTZ may increase levels.
Hypoglycemics, oral	Severe hypoglycemia with oral hypoglycemics.
Levonorgestrel-containing oral contraceptives	May increase or decrease levels of levonorgestrel-containing oral contraceptives.
Tacrolimus	Nephrotoxicity reported with tacrolimus.
Phenytoin	Increases levels of phenytoin.
Rifabutin	Uveitis reported with rifabutin.
Rifampin	Rifampin enhances metabolism of fluconazole.

Table 7.2: DRUG INTERACTIONS FOR ANTIFUNGAL AND ANTIVIRAL AGENTS (cont.)

ANTIFUNGAL AGENTS, SYSTEMIC (cont.)

Fluconazole (Diflucan)

Terfenadine	Contraindicated with terfenadine due to prolongation of QTc interval.
Theophylline	Increases levels of theophylline.
Zidovudine	Increases levels of zidovudine.

Flucytosine (Ancobon)

Antibiotics (polyene)	Antifungal synergism with polyene antibiotics (eg, amphotericin B).
Cytosine	Antagonized by cytosine.
Glomerular filtration impairing drugs	Drugs that impair glomerular filtration may prolong half-life.

Griseofulvin, Microcrystalline (Grifulvin V)

Anticoagulants, oral	Oral anticoagulants may need adjustment.
Barbiturates	Barbiturates decrease effects.
Contraceptives, oral	Decreases effects of oral contraceptives; may increase incidence of breakthrough bleeding.

Itraconazole (Sporanox)

Alfentanil	Increases levels of alfentanil.
Alprazolam	Increases levels of alprazolam.
Antacids	Decreased absorption of with antacids.
Astemizole	Increases levels of astemizole.
Buspirone	Increases levels of buspirone.
Busulfan	Increases levels of busulfan.
Calcium channel blockers	Additive negative inotropic effects with calcium channel blockers.
Calcium channel blockers (dihydropyridine)	Increases levels of dihydropyridine calcium channel blockers. Edema reported with dihydropyridine calcium channel blockers; adjust dose.
Carbamazepine	Increases levels of carbamazepine.
Cisapride	Increased levels with cisapride; concurrent use is contraindicated.
CYP3A4 inducers	CYP3A4 inducers (eg, carbamazepine, phenobarbital, phenytoin, isoniazid, rifabutin, rifampin, nevirapine) decrease itraconazole levels.
CYP3A4 inhibitors	CYP3A4 inhibitors (eg, erythromycin, clarithromycin, indinavir, ritonavir) may increase itraconazole levels.
Diazepam	Increases levels of diazepam.

ANTIFUNGAL AGENTS, SYSTEMIC *(cont.)*

Itraconazole (Sporanox)

Digoxin	Increases levels of digoxin.
Docetaxel	Increases levels of docetaxel.
Dofetilide	Increased levels with dofetilide; concurrent use is contraindicated.
Gastric secretion suppressors	Decreased absorption of capsules with gastric secretion suppressors.
HMG-CoA-reductase inhibitors	Increased levels with HMG-CoA-reductase inhibitors; concurrent use is contraindicated.
Hypoglycemics, oral	Increases levels of oral hypoglycemics. Severe hypoglycemia with oral hypoglycemics.
Immunosuppres-sants	Increases levels of immunosuppressants.
Methylprednisolone	Increases levels of methylprednisolone.
Midazolam, oral	Increased levels with oral midazolam; concurrent use is contraindicated. Increases levels of oral midazolam.
Pimozide	Increased levels with pimozide; concurrent use is contraindicated.
Protease inhibitors	Increases levels of protease inhibitors.
Quinidine	Increased levels with quinidine; concurrent use is contraindicated.
Rifabutin	Increases levels of rifabutin.
Triazolam	Increased levels with triazolam; concurrent use is contraindicated. Increases levels of triazolam.
Trimetrexate	Increases levels of trimetrexate.
Verapamil	Increases levels of verapamil.
Vinca alkaloids	Increases levels of vinca alkaloids.
Warfarin	Increases levels of warfarin.

Ketoconazole

Antacids	Give antacids 2 hrs after ketoconazole.
Anticholinergics	Give anticholinergics 2 hrs after ketoconazole.
Astemizole	Contraindicated with astemizole due to cardiac adverse effects.
Cisapride	Contraindicated with cisapride due to cardiac adverse effects.
Coumarin-like drugs	May enhance anticoagulant effect of coumarin-like drugs.
Cyclosporine	May alter metabolism of cyclosporine.
CYP3A4, drugs metabolized by	May alter metabolism of drugs metabolized by CYP3A4.
Digoxin	Monitor digoxin.

Table 7.2: DRUG INTERACTIONS FOR ANTIFUNGAL AND ANTIVIRAL AGENTS *(cont.)*

ANTIFUNGAL AGENTS, SYSTEMIC *(cont.)*

Ketoconazole

H₂ blockers	Give H₂ blockers 2 hrs after ketoconazole.
Hypoglycemics, oral	May potentiate oral hypoglycemics.
Isoniazid	Avoid isoniazid.
Methylprednisolone	May alter metabolism of methylprednisolone.
Midazolam	May potentiate midazolam.
Phenytoin	Monitor phenytoin.
Rifampin	Avoid rifampin.
Tacrolimus	May alter metabolism of tacrolimus.
Terfenadine	Contraindicated with terfenadine due to cardiac adverse effects.
Triazolam	May potentiate triazolam.

Micafungin Sodium (Mycamine)

Nifedipine	Monitor for nifedipine toxicity; reduce nifedipine dose if toxicity occurs.
Sirolimus	Monitor for sirolimus toxicity; reduce sirolimus dose if toxicity occurs.

Terbinafine Hydrochloride (Lamisil)

Cimetidine	Clearance increased by cimetidine.
Cyclosporin	Increased clearance of cyclosporine.
CYP2D6 metabolized drugs	May potentiate levels of drugs metabolized by CYP2D6 (eg, TCA's, beta-blockers, SSRI's, MAOIs-type B).
IV caffeine	Decreased clearance of IV caffeine.
Rifampin	Clearance increased by rifampin.

Voriconazole (Vfend)

Astemizole	Avoid with astemizole.
Barbiturates, long acting	Avoid with long-acting barbiturates.
Benzodiazepines	May increase levels; monitor for adverse events and toxicity with benzodiazepines.
Blood products	Do not infuse simultaneously with blood products.
Calcium channel blockers (dihydropyridine)	May increase levels; monitor for adverse events and toxicity with dihydropyridine calcium channel blockers.

ANTIFUNGAL AGENTS, SYSTEMIC *(cont.)*

Voriconazole (Vfend)

Carbamazepine	Avoid with carbamazepine.
Cimetidine	Cimetidine may increase levels.
Cisapride	Avoid with cisapride.
Cyclosporine	May increase levels; monitor cyclosporine (reduce cyclosporine to 1/2 of initial dose).
CYP2C9 inhibitors	May increase levels of CYP2C9 inhibitors.
CYP3A4 inhibitors	May increase levels of CYP3A4 inhibitors.
Drug infusions	Do not infuse into same line or cannula with other drug infusions.
Efavirenz	Avoid with efavirenz.
Electrolyte supplements	Do not infuse simultaneously with electrolyte supplements.
Ergot alkaloids	Avoid with ergot alkaloids.
HIV protease inhibitors	May increase levels; monitor for adverse events and toxicity with HIV protease inhibitors.
HMG-CoA reductase inhibitors	May increase levels; monitor for adverse events and toxicity with HMG-CoA reductase inhibitors.
Hypoglycemics	May increase levels; monitor hypoglycemics.
Methadone	May increase levels of methadone; may prolong QT interval; dose reduction may be needed.
NNRTIs	May increase levels; monitor for adverse events and toxicity with NNRTIs.
Omeprazole	Omeprazole is CYP2C19/3A4 inhibitor; reduce omeprazole by 1/2 if voriconazole ≥40mg.
Parenteral nutrition	Do not infuse into same line or cannula with parenteral nutrition.
Phenytoin	May increase levels; monitor phenytoin. Phenytoin decreases levels.
Pimozide	Avoid with pimozide.
Proton pump inhibitors	Proton pump inhibitors that are CYP2C19 substrates may increase levels.
Quinidine	Avoid with quinidine.
Rifabutin	Avoid with rifabutin.
Rifampin	Avoid with ergot rifampin.
Ritonavir	Avoid with ritonavir.
Sirolimus	Avoid with sirolimus.
Tacrolimus	May increase levels; monitor tacrolimus (reduce tacrolimus to 1/3 of initial dose).
Terfenadine	Avoid with terfenadine.
Vinca alkaloids	May increase levels; monitor for adverse events and toxicity with vinca alkaloids.
Warfarin	May increase levels; monitor warfarin.

Table 7.2: DRUG INTERACTIONS FOR ANTIFUNGAL AND ANTIVIRAL AGENTS (cont.)

ANTIVIRAL AGENTS

Acyclovir (Zovirax)

Probenecid	Probenecid increased levels of IV formulation.
Nephrotoxic agents	Caution with potentially nephrotoxic agents.

Adefovir Dipivoxil (Hepsera)

Active tubular secretion, drugs competing for	Administration with drugs that compete for active tubular secretion may increase serum levels of adefovir or co-administered drugs.
Nephrotoxic drugs	Caution with nephrotoxic drugs (eg, cyclosporine, tacrolimus, aminoglycosides, vancomycin, NSAIDs).
Renal function reducing drugs	Administration with drugs that reduce renal function may increase serum levels of adefovir or co-administered drugs.

Amantadine Hydrochloride (Symmetrel)

Anticholinergic agents	Anticholinergic agents may potentiate the anticholinergic side effects.
CNS stimulants	Caution with CNS stimulants.
Thioridazine	Increased tremor in elderly Parkinson's disease patients with thioridazine.

Entecavir (Baraclude)

Tubular secretion (drugs undergoing)	May increase serum concentrations of entecavir or coadministered drug with drugs that compete for active tubular secretion.
Renal function reducers	May increase serum concentrations of entecavir or coadministered drug with drugs that reduce renal function or compete for active tubular secretion.

Famciclovir (Famvir)

Tubular secretion (drugs undergoing)	Increased plasma levels of penciclovir with drugs significantly eliminated by active renal tubular secretion.
Aldehyde oxidase metabolized drugs	Potential interaction with drugs metabolized by aldehyde oxidase.
Probenecid	Increased plasma levels of penciclovir with probenecid.

Foscarnet Sodium (Foscavir)

Nephrotoxic drugs	Avoid potentially nephrotoxic drugs (eg, aminoglycosides, amphotericin B).
Pentamidine	Possible hypocalcemia with pentamidine.
Plasma calcium affecting drugs	Caution with drugs that affect plasma calcium levels.
Ritonavir	Renal dysfunction reported with ritonavir.
Saquinavir	Renal dysfunction reported with saquinavir.

ANTIVIRAL AGENTS *(cont.)*

Ganciclovir (Cytovene, Vitrasert)

Adriamycin	Extreme caution with adriamycin; potential additive toxicity.
Amphotericin B	Extreme caution with amphotericin B; potential additive toxicity.
Bactrim	Extreme caution with bactrim; potential additive toxicity.
Cyclosporine	Extreme caution with cyclosporine; potential additive toxicity.
Dapsone	Extreme caution with dapsone; potential additive toxicity.
Didanosine	Increased didanosine serum levels.
Flucytosine	Extreme caution with flucytosine; potential additive toxicity.
Imipenem-cilastatin	Avoid imipenem-cilastatin; may precipitate seizures.
Nucleoside analogues	Extreme caution with other nucleoside analogues; potential additive toxicity.
Pentamidine	Extreme caution with pentamidine; potential additive toxicity.
Probenecid	Potentiated by probenecid.
Vinblastine	Extreme caution with vinblastine; potential additive toxicity.
Vincristine	Extreme caution with vincristine; potential additive toxicity.
Zidovudine	Decreased effects with zidovudine; combination may potentiate zidovudine and cause severe neutropenia.

Interferon Alfa-2a (Roferon A)

Anti-diabetic regimens	Anti-diabetic regimens may need adjustments.
Cardiotoxicity	May increase cardiotoxic effects of other drugs.
CYP450 metabolizing agents	Caution with agents that are metabolized by CYP450.
Hematotoxicity	May increase hematotoxic effects of other drugs.
Interleukin-2	Use with interleukin-2 may increase risk of renal failure.
Myelosuppressive agents	Caution with agents that cause myelosuppression.
Neurotoxicity	May increase neurotoxic effects of other drugs.
Theophylline	May reduce theophylline clearance.
Zidovudine	Synergistic myelosuppression with zidovudine.

Interferon Alfa-2b (Intron A)

Antidiabetics	Antidiabetics may need adjustments.
Myelosuppressive agents	Caution with myelosuppressive agents (eg, zidovudine).

Table 7.2: DRUG INTERACTIONS FOR ANTIFUNGAL AND ANTIVIRAL AGENTS *(cont.)*

ANTIVIRAL AGENTS *(cont.)*

Interferon Alfa-2b (Intron A)

Ribavirin	Increased risk of hemolytic anemia when coadministered with ribavirin.
Theophylline	Increases theophylline levels by 100%.
Thyroid agents	Thyroid agents may need adjustments.

Interferon Alfa-2b/Ribavirin (Rebetron)

Antacids	Reduced absorption with antacids.
Myelosuppressives	Caution with myelosuppressives.
Nucleoside analogues	Caution with coadministration of ribavirin with nucleoside analogues; may cause lactic acidosis. Only coadminister if benefit outweighs risks.

Interferon Alfacon-1 (Infergen)

CYP450 metabolizing agents	Caution with agents that are metabolized by CYP450.
Myelosuppressive agents	Caution with agents that cause myelosuppression.

Interferon Beta-1a (Avonex, Rebif)

Hepatic toxic drugs	Caution with other drugs associated with hepatic injury.
Myelosuppressive agents	Monitor with myelosuppressive agents.

Interferon Beta-1b (Betaseron)

Antipyrine	May inhibit antipyrine elimination.

Interferon Gamma-1b (Actimmune)

Myelosuppressive agents	Monitor with myelosuppressive agents.

Palivizumab (Synagis)

CYP1A2	May inhibit CYP1A2.
NRTIs	Hepatic decompensation can occur with concomitant use of NRTIs and peginterferon alpha-2a/ribavirin.
Peginterferon alpha-2a/ribavirin	Hepatic decompensation can occur with concomitant use of NRTIs and peginterferon alpha-2a/ribavirin.
Theophylline	May increase theophylline AUC; monitor theophylline serum levels.

Peginterferon Alfa-2a (Pegasys)

CYP1A2	May inhibit CYP1A2.
NRTIs	Hepatic decompensation can occur with concomitant use of NRTIs and peginterferon alpha-2a/ribavirin.

ANTIVIRAL AGENTS *(cont.)*

Peginterferon Alfa-2a (Pegasys)

Peginterferon alpha-2a/ribavirin	Hepatic decompensation can occur with concomitant use of NRTIs and peginterferon alpha-2a/ribavirin.
Theophylline	May increase theophylline AUC; monitor theophylline serum levels.

Peginterferon Alfa-2b (Peg-Intron)

Methadone	May increase AUC of methadone, resulting in an increased narcotic effect.
Ribavirin	Hemolytic anemia reported with ribavirin.

Ribavirin (Copegus, Rebetrol)

Didanosine	Avoid concomitant use with didanosine.
NRTIs	Hepatic decompensation can occur with concomitant use of NRTIs and Pegasys/Copegus.
Pegasys	Hepatic decompensation can occur with concomitant use of NRTIs and Pegasys/Copegus.
Stavudine	Avoid concomitant use with stavudine.
Zidovudine	Avoid concomitant use with zidovudine.

Rimantadine Hydrochloride (Flumadine)

APAP	APAP may decrease levels of rimantadine.
ASA	ASA may decrease levels of rimantadine.
Cimetidine	May be potentiated by cimetidine.

Valacyclovir Hydrochloride (Valtrex)

Nephrotoxic drugs	Renal and CNS toxicity with nephrotoxic drugs.

Valganciclovir Hydrochloride (Valcyte)

Didanosine	Increased risk of didanosine toxicity.
Irradiation	Caution with irradiation.
Mofetil	Increased levels of metabolites of both drugs with mycophenolate mofetil.
Myelosuppressive drugs	Caution with myelosuppressive drugs.
Probenecid	Monitor for toxicity with probenecid.
Zidovudine	Greater risk for neutropenia and anemia with zidovudine.

Zanamivir (Relenza)

Inhaled bronchodilator	Use inhaled bronchodilator before zanamivir.

Chapter 8

Agents Affecting Salivation

John A. Yagiela, D.D.S., Ph.D.

Anticholinergic Drugs

Saliva plays a vital role in protecting the health of soft and hard tissues of the mouth and in such functions as taste, mastication and deglutition. Excessive salivation, however, can complicate the performance of dental procedures such as the taking of impressions and the placement of restorations. If chronic, hypersalivation can cause psychosocial problems and both local and systemic disorders.

A number of anticholinergic drugs—otherwise referred to as cholinergic antagonists, antimuscarinic agents or parasympatholytics—are effective antisialogogues and are used by dentists and physicians for treating inappropriate salivary secretions and for reducing normal salivation to facilitate the performance of intraoral procedures. Because none of these agents is selective in action, they all have a tendency to produce side effects, and this must be considered before proceeding with antisialogogue therapy. The anticholinergic drugs included in this chapter are limited to agents that have been approved for use to control salivation or that are used in dentistry for that purpose.

Accepted Indications

The control of salivation for dental procedures is a generally recognized but not officially accepted indication for these drugs. Atropine, glycopyrrolate, propantheline and scopolamine are the most commonly used agents. These drugs also have several medical indications. For example, parenteral atropine has been approved for these uses:

- the control of bradycardia and first-degree heart block associated with excessive vagal activity or administration of succinylcholine;
- to inhibit salivation and respiratory tract secretions during general anesthesia;
- to minimize the muscarinic side effects of cholinesterase inhibitors used to reverse the action of neuromuscular blocking drugs.

Parenteral glycopyrrolate has been approved for the same purposes, except for the prophylaxis of succinylcholine-induced bradydysrhythmias. It also is indicated before general anesthesia to reduce secretion of gastric acid and to minimize the danger of pulmonary aspiration. Parenteral scopolamine has been approved for the control of secretions during general anesthesia and as a preanesthetic sedative and anesthetic adjunct in conjunction with opioid analgesics.

Anticholinergic drugs also have been approved for the management of peptic ulcers and various gastrointestinal, biliary and genitourinary disorders. For most drugs and conditions, these indications are considered obsolete. Transdermal scopolamine remains a useful agent for the prophylaxis and treatment of motion sickness. Selected anticholinergic drugs also are used to treat parkinsonism and as mydriatics and cycloplegics in ophthalmology. Atropine and hyoscyamine (the active isomer of atropine) are recognized antidotes for the muscarinic toxicity of mushrooms, parasympathomimetic agonists and anticholinesterase drugs, insecticides and nerve gases.

Atropine usually is the anticholinergic of choice for most uses in dentistry. Oral dosage forms of atropine are not widely available in neighborhood pharmacies, however, so the dentist should be familiar with the use of other antisialogogues. By parenteral injection, glycopyrrolate is excellent for the control of salivation; scopolamine is a suitable parenteral choice when its sedative, amnestic and antiemetic effects are desired.

General Dosing Information

Low doses of the anticholinergic drugs described in this chapter for blocking excessive salivary secretion, properly adjusted for route of administration, are relatively selective in effect. Larger doses, such as those required to treat vagally induced bradydysrhythmias, uniformly produce side effects, including pronounced dryness of the mouth. General dosing guidelines for the control of salivation provided in Table 8.1.

To control salivation when performing restorative dentistry, the dentist should time drug administration so that the peak effect occurs when a dry operative field is most needed. Thus, atropine, hyoscyamine or scopolamine tablets should be given to the patient 60-90 minutes before the taking of impressions or placement of composite restorations. The analogous interval for oral glycopyrrolate or propantheline is 45-75 minutes.

Maximum Recommended Doses

Maximum recommended doses have not been established for single administrations of anticholinergics beyond the usual doses indicated in Table 8.1.

Dosage Adjustments

Within the recommended range, the dose of an anticholinergic drug may be adjusted according to need. For control of salivation, a low dose may be adequate when only moderation of salivation is required, whereas a larger dose may be necessary if secretions are preventing the successful accomplishment of a procedure, such as an impression. Reduced doses should be considered for infants, geriatric patients and those with medical conditions that alter their responses to anticholinergic drugs.

Special Dental Considerations

Drug Interactions of Dental Interest

Drug interactions and related problems involving anticholinergic antisialogogues listed in Table 8.2 are potentially of clinical significance in dentistry.

Laboratory Value Alterations

- Gastric acid secretion tests are impaired by anticholinergic drugs because they decrease stimulation of gastric acids.
- Radionuclide gastric emptying tests are impaired by anticholinergic drugs because of delayed gastric emptying.
- Phenolsulfonphthalein excretion tests are impaired by atropine because the two agents compete for the same transport mechanism.
- Serum uric acid is decreased in patients with hyperuricemia or gout who are receiving glycopyrrolate.

Cross-Sensitivity

A person with a sensitivity to any belladonna alkaloid may also have a sensitivity to atropine or scopolamine.

Special Patients

Pregnant and nursing women
Atropine, hyoscyamine and scopolamine cross the placenta. Although there is no evidence of teratogenic effects, intravenous atropine can cause tachycardia in the fetus, and parenteral scopolamine given during labor may adversely affect the neonate by

depressing the CNS and reducing vitamin K-dependent clotting factors. Glycopyrrolate and propantheline are quaternary ammonium compounds, and it is unlikely that they reach the fetal circulation in large amounts.

All anticholinergic drugs may inhibit lactation. In addition, atropine and scopolamine are distributed into breast milk. Although single doses to control salivation have not been associated with any health problem, it may be advisable for nursing mothers to collect sufficient milk to cover the 8-hour period after taking an anticholinergic drug.

Pediatric, geriatric and other special patients

Pediatric patients. Infants and small children are especially sensitive to the toxic effects of anticholinergic drugs, even when the dose is corrected for body size. Because of their high metabolic rate, children generate relatively large amounts of heat and must dissipate that heat in a warm environment by sweating. Blockade of acetylcholinemediated perspiration by these agents can quickly lead to grossly elevated temperatures. Flushing of the skin is an important early visual cue that steps must be taken to improve heat loss. Young children may also be especially sensitive to the CNS effects of atropine and scopolamine.

Geriatric patients. Geriatric patients are particularly susceptible to the parasympatholytic effects of anticholinergic drugs on visceral smooth muscle. Although single doses, as used in dentistry for control of salivation, are generally well tolerated by elderly people, large doses of atropine and scopolamine have been associated with excessive depressant and excitatory CNS reactions. Repeated doses can cause constipation and, especially in men, urinary retention. Xerostomia and associated increased dental caries and fungal infections are dental concerns linked to chronic use of these drugs in elderly patients. In addition, patients aged > 40 years are at increased risk of an acute attack of previously undiagnosed angle-closure glaucoma.

Patients with medical problems. Patients with certain medical problems are especially susceptible to the adverse effects of anticholinergic drugs. These include patients with obstructive or paralytic gastrointestinal and urinary tract disorders, cardiac disease and angle-closure glaucoma. Specific recommendations regarding these patients are listed in Table 8.1.

Patient Monitoring: Aspects to Watch

• Cardiovascular status (arterial blood pressure, heart rate, electrocardiogram) with parenteral anticholinergic drugs.

Adverse Effects and Precautions

The adverse effects of the anticholinergic drugs are the predictable consequences of the inhibition of various physiological actions of acetylcholine. Single oral doses of agents used to control salivation are usually well tolerated, but large parenteral doses invariably induce a host of side effects. Although these effects may be unpleasant, they are virtually never life-threatening except in small children and medically compromised patients. The adverse effects, precautions and contraindications listed in Table 8.1 apply to all routes of administration.

Pharmacology

Anticholinergic drugs competitively block the effects of acetylcholine and cholinergic drugs at muscarinic receptor sites. Muscarinic receptors mediate tissue responses to parasympathetic nervous system stimulation and cholinergic-induced sweating and vasodilation. Tertiary amines, such as atropine and especially scopolamine, may produce CNS effects because of their ability to cross the blood-brain barrier. Quaternary amines, such as glycopyrrolate and propantheline, are largely excluded from the brain and do not act directly on the CNS. The existence of muscarinic receptor subtypes (designated M_1 through M_5) also accounts for some of the differences in peripheral effects among the anticholinergic drugs because of different relative affinities of the drugs for these subtypes. It has been determined that the M_3 receptor supports serous salivary gland secretion and the M_2 receptor is responsible for parasympathomimetic cardiac effects. In tissues where acetylcholine release at muscarinic receptors is chronically active, anticholinergic drugs will exert pronounced antimuscarinic effects. If acetylcholine or other cholinergic drugs are absent, anticholinergic drugs will elicit little or no observable effect.

Atropine, hyoscyamine and scopolamine, all naturally occurring belladonna alkaloids, are well absorbed from the gastrointestinal tract; however, absorption is less complete with the synthetic quaternary ammonium drugs. Atropine is partially metabolized in the liver and excreted in the urine as both the parent compound and metabolites. A similar fate presumably occurs with the other anticholinergic agents. Table 8.3 lists the time to effect and duration of effect of anticholinergic drugs used orally for control of salivation.

Patient Advice

- Patients should be aware of the potential common side effects, such as dryness of the mouth, nose and throat; difficulty in swallowing; and inhibition of sweating.
- Parents should be warned of the potential for hyperthermia in small children, especially when the children are overdressed, physically active or in a warm environment.
- Because of the possibility of psychomotor impairment after use of scopolamine, driving or other tasks requiring alertness and coordination should be avoided or performed with added caution, as

appropriate, on the day of treatment. It is also desirable to avoid the use of alcohol or other CNS depressants during this time.

Suggested Readings

Anticholinergics. JADA 2001;132:1021–2.

Dowd FJ. Antimuscarinic drugs. In: Yagiela JA, Dowd FJ, Neidle EA, eds. Pharmacology and therapeutics for dentistry. 5th ed. St. Louis: Mosby; 2004:139-46.

Sherman CR, Sherman BR. Atropine sulfate—a current review of a useful agent for controlling salivation during dental procedures. Gen Dent 1999;47(1):56-60.

Cholinergic Drugs

In contrast to the anticholinergic agents, cholinergic drugs produce effects that mimic those of acetylcholine, the natural ligand for cholinergic receptors. Additional terms used to identify cholinergic drugs include cholinergic agonists, cholinomimetics, parasympathomimetics and muscarinic agonists. The only recognized use for these drugs in dentistry is in the management of xerostomia. Diseases or conditions that cause xerostomia commonly result in opportunistic infection, increased caries and difficulty in speaking and in maintaining normal dietary intake. Although pilocarpine, a naturally occurring cholinergic agonist, has been used as a sialogogue for nearly a century, it was approved for this purpose by the U.S. Food and Drug Administration only in 1994, after being developed under the provisions of the Orphan Drug Act of 1983. Cevimeline, a recently developed cholinergic agonist chemically unrelated to pilocarpine, received approval for clinical use in 2000.

Successful stimulation of salivary secretion by cholinergic drugs requires the presence of intact salivary gland tissue and nerve supply. In the case of radiation therapy, this requirement may be met by residual active tissue in the irradiated field or healthy tissue outside the field.

Accepted Indications

Pilocarpine has been approved for the relief of xerostomia caused by radiation therapy of the head and neck and for the management of xerostomia and keratoconjunctivitis sicca in patients with Sjögren's syndrome. In its topical forms, pilocarpine has also been approved for treating various types of glaucoma and producing pupillary constriction (miosis) after surgery or ocular examination. Cevimeline is approved only for the treatment of xerostomia associated with Sjögren's syndrome.

General Dosing Information

As shown in Table 8.1, the usual adult daily dose of pilocarpine is 5 mg tid, usually 30 minutes before meals. A dose of 10 mg tid may be tried in refractory cases; however, the incidence of dose-related side effects increases at this dosage and, as a general rule, the dentist should use the lowest effective dose that is tolerated by the patient. Cevimeline generally is prescribed as a dose of 30 mg tid. Absorption is best if the drug is taken on an empty stomach. Neither pilocarpine nor cevimeline has been tested in children.

Special Dental Considerations

Drug Interactions of Dental Interest

Table 8.2 lists possible drug interactions and related problems involving cholinergic drugs that are potentially of clinical significance in dentistry.

Cross-Sensitivity

Patients sensitive to other forms of pilocarpine dosage (that is, ophthalmic) should be considered sensitive to oral pilocarpine.

Special Patients

Pregnant and nursing women
There are no data regarding the influence of pilocarpine on reproduction and fetal development. High doses of cevimeline decrease fertility in female rats. Both drugs have been designated as FDA pregnancy category C. It has not been determined if these drugs are distributed into breast milk, and there are no reports of related problems in humans. However, the potential for adverse effects in nursing infants must be considered.

Pediatric, geriatric and other special patients
These cholinergic drugs have not been tested for, nor are they indicated for, use in children. There appears to be no special concern regarding pilocarpine and cevimeline and the geriatric population, although elderly people are more likely to have specific medical problems, such as angle-closure glaucoma, pulmonary disease or cardiovascular disease, that may complicate therapy.

Adverse Effects and Precautions

Most of the adverse effects observed with cholinergic agonists (Table 8.1) are dose-dependent extensions of the drugs' ability to stimulate cholinergic muscarinic receptors. Hypertension may be an important exception to this generalization. Excessive secretions (sweating, bronchial secretions, rhinitis) are the most common side effects associated with oral cholinergic agonists.

Pharmacology

Pilocarpine and cevimeline stimulate muscarinic receptors to elicit most of their effects. Muscarinic receptors are linked to specific G proteins that mediate intracellular signaling in response to drug-receptor binding. For the M_{3943} receptor involved in salivary secretion, stimulation of its G protein causes the intracellular formation of inositol 1,4,5-trisphosphate and diacylglycerol, which promote secretion and smooth muscle contraction. Anomalous hypertensive responses to these drugs may be due to ganglionic or adrenal medullary stimulation. Both drugs, as tertiary amines, gain access to the brain and can produce CNS reactions.

Pilocarpine is readily absorbed from the gastrointestinal tract. Peak drug effects occur within 1 hour and last 3-5 hours. Pilocarpine is partially metabolized, possibly in the plasma or at neuronal synapses, and is then excreted in the urine. Cevimeline is similarly absorbed when taken between meals but is longer lasting. Most of the drug is metabolized in the liver (elimination half-life: 5 hours) before being excreted by the kidneys.

Patient Advice

- Because adverse effects are dose-dependent, patients should be cautioned to take the medication as directed.
- If dizziness, lightheadedness or blurred vision occurs, patients should refrain from driving or other tasks requiring alertness, coordination and visual acuity until the problem is resolved.

Suggested Readings

Chambers MS, Garden AS, Kies MS, Martin JW. Radiation-induced xerostomia in patients with head and neck cancer: pathogenesis, impact on quality of life, and management. Head Neck 2004;26(9):796-807.

Davies AN, Daniels C, Pugh R, Sharma K. A comparison of artificial saliva and pilocarpine in the management of xerostomia in patients with advanced cancer. Palliative Med 1998;12(2):105-11.

Porter SR, Scully C, Hegarty AM. An update of the etiology and management of xerostomia. Oral Surg Oral Med Oral Pathol Oral Radiol Endod 2004(1);97:28-46.

Vivino FB, Al-Hashimi I, Khan Z, et al. Pilocarpine tablets for the treatment of dry mouth and dry eye symptoms in patients with Sjögren syndrome: a randomized, placebo-controlled, fixed-dose, multicenter trial. Arch Intern Med 1999;159(2):174-81.

Saliva Substitutes

When salivary function is absent or minimal, cholinergic drug therapy with pilocarpine or related agents is ineffective. Replacement of missing saliva is a natural therapeutic alternative. Water is most commonly used by patients afflicted with chronic xerostomia because of its unique advantages of availability and low cost. Water is a poor substitute for saliva, however, because it lacks necessary ions, buffering capacity, lubricating mucins and protective proteins. Saliva substitutes, or artificial salivas, are designed to more closely match the chemical and physical characteristics of saliva. These preparations often contain complex mixtures of salts, with cellulose derivatives or animal mucins added to increase viscosity (often to a viscosity greater than that of natural saliva, in an attempt to improve retention within the mouth). Flavoring agents, usually sorbitol or xylitol, generally are added to improve taste, and parabens are sometimes included to inhibit bacterial growth. A general deficiency of artificial salivas is their complete lack of anti-infective proteins, such as secretory immunoglobulin A, histatins, and lysozyme. A saliva substitute in the form of a long-lasting moisturizing gel (oral*balance*; see Table 8.4) contains various ingredients that are claimed to be biologically active, but data supporting their clinical effectiveness are limited.

Accepted Indications

Saliva substitutes are indicated for the symptomatic relief of dry mouth and dry throat in patients with xerostomia.

General Dosing Information

Saliva substitutes are meant to be taken ad libitum throughout the day, usually in the form of sprays, to keep the oral mucosa moist. There are no specific dosing guidelines, nor are there specific recommendations for special patients. Table 8.4 lists, by manufacturer's brand name, the ingredients of some commercially available preparations.

Special Dental Considerations

Patients with severe xerostomia who use a saliva substitute containing sorbitol on a regular basis may be at increased risk of caries associated with a very limited fermentation of sorbitol. A proper professionally designed topical fluoride treatment program undertaken to protect from caries the teeth of the patient with xerostomia should also overcome any problem posed by sorbitol. Use of sugarless chewing gum, some of which may contain a remineralizing agent, and sugarless citrus-flavored lozenges may increase salivary flow. Some patients have claimed benefits from use of Biotène products (oral-*balance*), but there is little information from properly controlled trials to substantiate these claims.

There are no known drug interactions involving saliva substitutes, nor any need for patient monitoring pertaining to these products. Laboratory tests are likewise unaffected.

Cross-Sensitivity

Saliva substitutes containing parabens pose a risk of cross-sensitivity in patients allergic to parabens, para-aminobenzoic acid or its derivatives, such as ester local anesthetics. Some products contain other ingredients that pose additional risks of allergic cross-reactions.

Adverse Effects and Precautions

Aside from the allergic potential of parabens or other components of selected preparations and the possibility of increased caries incidence with sorbitol, there are few potential adverse effects or precautions associated with saliva substitutes. Microbial contamination is a possibility with multiple dose formulations, but this risk is partially offset by the inclusion of paraben preservatives.

Pharmacology

Saliva substitutes are physically active agents. When used regularly, they help minimize the sequelae of xerostomia by keeping the oral mucosa moist and lubricated. Surface abrasion is reduced, and patients are more able to perform the everyday activities of speaking, eating and sleeping. Long-term compliance, however, is a problem with these products because of their perceived inconvenience and relatively high cost.

Because saliva substitutes are quickly swallowed and their activity is of limited duration, they must be administered repeatedly. The components of the ingested solution undoubtedly undergo gastrointestinal absorption; however, there is no information on the pharmacokinetics of the currently available saliva substitutes.

Patient Advice

- Patients should be informed of the necessity of the continual use of saliva substitutes.
- Patients with chronic xerostomia should be educated on the need for regular professional care and for a high degree of compliance with the dental professional's recommendations for minimizing caries and soft-tissue pathology.

Suggested Readings

Alves MB, Motta AC, Messina WC, Migliari DA. Saliva substitute in xerostomic patients with primary Sjogren's syndrome: a single-blind trial. Quintessence Int 2004;35(5):392-6.

Dodds MWJ, Johnson DA, Yeh C-K. Health benefits of saliva: a review. J Dent 2005;33(3):223-33.

Fox PC. Management of dry mouth. Dent Clin North Am 1997;41(4):863-75.

Levine MJ. Development of artificial salivas. Crit Rev Oral Biol Med 1993;4:279-86.

Meyer-Lueckel H, Schulte-Monting J, Kielbassa AM. The effect of commercially available saliva substitutes on predemineralized bovine dentin in vitro. Oral Dis 2002;8(4):192-8.

Table 8.1: PRESCRIBING INFORMATION FOR ANTICHOLINERGIC AND CHOLINERGIC DRUGS

NAME	FORM/ STRENGTH	DOSAGE	WARNINGS/PRECAUTIONS & CONTRAINDICATIONS	ADVERSE EFFECTS†
Atropine Sulfate (Anticholinergic) (Sal-Tropine★, generic)	**Sol, Inj:** Atropine sulfate 0.05mg/ mL, 0.1mg/mL, 0.4mg/mL, 0.5mg/mL,1mg/ mL; **Tab:** Sal-Tropine 0.4mg	**Adults: Sol, Inj: Usual:** 0.4-0.6mg IM/IV/SC. **Range:** 0.3-1.2mg. **Tab: Usual:** 0.4mg. **Range:** 0.4-1.2mg. **Pediatrics: Sol, Inj: Usual:** 0.01mg/ kg up to 0.4mg. **Range:** 0.1mg (newborn) to 0.6mg (>12 yrs). **Tab: Usual:** 0.01mg/kg up to 0.4mg.	**W/P:** Avoid overdose. Increased susceptibility to toxic effects in children. Caution in patients >40 yrs. Conventional doses may precipitate acute angle-closure glaucoma in susceptible patients, convert partial organic pyloric stenosis into complete obstruction, lead to complete urinary retention in patients with prostatic hypertrophy or cause inspissation of bronchial secretions and formation of dangerous viscid plugs in patients with chronic lung disease. **Contra:** Hypersensitivity to atropine or other naturally occurring belladonna alkaloids, angle-closure glaucoma, pyloric stenosis or prostatic hypertrophy except in doses used for preanesthetic medication. **P/N:** Category C, safety in nursing not known.	Urinary hesitancy and retention; **dryness of the mouth**, nose, throat, eyes, skin; blurred vision, photophobia; tachycardia; palpitation; anhidrosis; hyperthermia; drowsiness; dizziness; confusion; hallucinations; delirium.
Cevimeline Hydrochloride (Cholinergic) (Evoxac)	**Cap:** 30mg	**Adults:** 30mg tid.	**W/P:** Caution with significant cardiovascular disease, night driving, performing hazardous activities in reduced lighting, nephrolithiasis, cholelithiasis, biliary tract disease, controlled asthma, chronic bronchitis, or COPD requiring pharmacotherapy. Monitor for toxicity and dehydration. Possible dose-related CNS effects. **Contra:** Hypersensitivity to cevimeline, uncontrolled asthma, when miosis is undesirable (eg, acute iritis, narrow-angle glaucoma). **P/N:** Category C, safety in nursing not known.	Excessive sweating, nausea, rhinitis, diarrhea, headache, sinusitis, upper respiratory tract infection, **coughing, pharyngitis**, vomiting, injury, back pain, rash, conjunctivitis, dizziness, bronchitis, arthralgia, fatigue, pain.
Glycopyrrolate (Anticholinergic) (Robinul, Robinul Forte)	**Sol, Inj:** Robinul 0.2mg/mL **Tab:** Robinul 1mg, Robinul Forte 2mg	**Adults: Sol, Inj: Range:** 0.1-0.2 mg. **Maint:** q6-8h up to 0.8mg/day. **Adults and adolescents: Tab: Usual:** 1mg. **Range:** 1-2mg. **Maint:** 1mg bid up to 8mg/day. **Pediatrics: Sol, Inj: Range** 4-10µg/kg up to 0.2 mg. **Maint:** q3-4h up to 0.8 mg/day.	**W/P:** May produce drowsiness and blurred vision; avoid operating machinery. Risk of heat prostration with high environmental temperature. Diarrhea may be early symptom of incomplete intestinal obstruction especially with ileostomy or colostomy. Caution in elderly, autonomic neuropathy, hepatic/renal disease, ulcerative colitis, hyperthyroidism, coronary heart disease, CHF, tachyarrhythmias, tachycardia, HTN, prostatic hypertrophy, hiatal hernia associated with reflux esophagitis. **Contra:** Hypersensitivity to glycopyrrolate, angle-closure glaucoma, obstructive uropathy, GI tract obstruction, paralytic ileus, intestinal atony of elderly or debilitated, unstable cardiovascular status in acute hemorrhage, severe ulcerative colitis, toxic megacolon complicating ulcerative colitis, myasthenia gravis. **P/N:** Category C, caution in nursing.	Blurred vision, **dry mouth,** urinary retention and hesitancy, increased ocular tension, tachycardia, decreased sweating, hyperthermia, **xerostomia, loss of taste**, headache.
Hyoscyamine Sulfate (Anticholinergic) (Anaspaz, Cystospaz-m, Ib-Stat, Levbid, Levsin, Levsinex, Nulev)	**Cap ER:** Cystospaz-m 0.375mg, Levsinex 0.375mg; **Drop:** Levsin 0.125mg/mL; **Elixir:** Levsin 0.125mg/5mL; **Sol, Inj:** Levsin 0.5mg/mL; **Spray:** Ib-Stat 0.125mg/mL; **Tab:** Anaspaz	**Adults and adolescents: Cap ER, Tab ER:** 0.375-0.75mg q12h, or 1 cap/tab may be given q8h. Do not crush or chew. **Drops, Elixer, Spray, Tab, Tab ODT, Tab SL** (may also chew or swallow SL tabs)**: Usual:** 0.125-0.25mg. **Range:** 0.125-0.5mg. **Maint:** q4-6h. **Max:** 1.5mg/day. **Solution, Inj:** 0.25-0.5mg IM/IV/SC. **Maint:** q4h. **Pediatrics: Drops, Elixer: 2.3-3.3kg:** 12.5µg. **3.4-4.4kg:** 15.6µg. **4.5-6.7kg:** 18.8µg. **6.8-9kg:** 25µg. **9.1-13.5kg:** 31.3µg.	**W/P:** Risk of heat prostration with high environmental temperature. Avoid activities requiring mental alertness. Psychosis has been reported. Caution with diarrhea, autonomic neuropathy, hyperthyroidism, coronary heart disease, CHF, dysrhythmias/tachycardia, HTN, renal disease and hiatal hernia associated with reflux esophagitis. **Contra:** Hypersensitivity to hyoscyamine, atropine or other naturally occurring belladonna alkaloids, angle-closure glaucoma, obstructive uropathy, GI tract obstructive	Urinary hesitancy and retention; **dryness of the mouth**, nose, throat, eyes, skin; blurred vision, photophobia; tachycardia; palpitation; anhidrosis; hyperthermia; drowsiness; dizziness; confusion; hallucinations; delirium.

★indicates a drug bearing the ADA Seal of Acceptance.   †Bold entries denote special dental considerations.

NAME	FORM/ STRENGTH	DOSAGE	WARNINGS/PRECAUTIONS & CONTRAINDICATIONS	ADVERSE EFFECTS†
Hyoscyamine Sulfate (Anticholinergic) *(cont.)*	0.125mg, Levsin 0.125mg; **Tab ER:** Levbid 0.375mg, Levsin 0.375mg; **Tab ODT:** Nulev 0.125mg; **Tab SL:** Levsin 0.125mg	**13.6-22.6kg:** 63µg. **22.7-33kg:** 94-125µg. **34-36kg:** 125-187µg. **Tab, Tab ODT, Tab SL: 2 to 12 yrs:** 0.0625-0.125mg. Maint: q4-6h. **Sol, Inj: 2 to 12 yrs:** 5µg/kg IM/IV/SC.	disease, paralytic ileus, intestinal atony of elderly/debilitated, unstable cardiovascular status in acute hemorrhage, severe ulcerative colitis, toxic megacolon, myasthenia gravis. **P/N:** Category C, caution in nursing.	
Pilocarpine Hydrochloride (Cholinergic) (Salagen)	**Tab:** 5mg, 7.5mg	*Adults:* **Cancer Patients: Initial:** 5mg tid. **Usual:** 15-30mg/day. **Max:** 10mg/dose. **Sjögren's Syndrome: Usual:** 5mg qid.	**W/P:** Caution with significant cardiovascular disease, night driving, performing hazardous activities in reduced lighting, cholelithiasis, biliary tract disease, controlled asthma, chronic bronchitis, or COPD requiring pharmacotherapy. Monitor for toxicity and dehydration. May cause renal colic. Possible dose-related CNS effects. **Contra:** Hypersensitivty to pilocarpine, uncontrolled asthma, when miosis is undesirable (eg, acute iritis, narrow-angle glaucoma). **P/N:** Category C, not for use in nursing.	Sweating, nausea, rhinitis, diarrhea, chills, flushing, urinary frequency, dizziness, asthenia, headache, dyspepsia, lacrimation, edema, amblyopia, vomiting, pharyngitis, HTN, bradycardia, tachycardia.
Propantheline Bromide (Anticholinergic) (Pro-Banthine)	**Tab:** 7.5mg, 15mg	*Adults and adolescents:* **Usual:** 15-30mg. **Range:** 7.5-60mg. **Maint:** tid-qid up to 120mg/day.	**W/P:** In presence of a high environmental temperature, heat prostration can occur, diarrhea may be an early symptom of incomplete intestinal obstruction; in this instance, treatment with propantheline would be inappropriate and possibly harmful with heart disease, may increase heart rate, autonomic neuropathy, cardiac tachyarrhythmias, caution when operating motor vehicle or other machinery, congestive heart failure, coronary heart disease, hepatic or renal disease, hiatal hernia associated with reflux esophagitis, hypertension, hyperthyroidism. **Contra:** Hypersensitivity to propantheline or other anticholinergics, angle-closure glaucoma, intestinal atony of elderly or debilitated patients, myasthenia gravis, obstructive disease of gastrointestinal tract, obstructive uropathy, severe ulcerative colitis/ toxic megacolon, unstable cardiovascular adjustment in acute hemorrhage. **P/N:** Category C, caution in nursing.	Diminished sweating, constipation, **xerostomia**, dizziness, drowsiness, confusion, blurred vision, hyperthermia, headache, nausea, vomiting.
Scopolamine Hydrobromide (Anticholinergic) (Scopace, Transderm Scop, generic)	**Patch:** Transderm Scop 0.33mg/24 hrs; **Sol, Inj:** scopolamine hydrobromide 0.4mg/mL; **Tab:** Scopace 0.4mg	*Adults:* **Patch: Motion Sickness:** Apply 1 patch 4 hrs before travel. Replace after 3 days; **Post-OP N/V:** Apply 1 patch the evening before surgery. Keep in place for 24 hrs. Apply patch to a hairless area behind the ear. Do not cut patch in half. **Sol, Inj: Anesthesia: Excessive Salivation:** 0.2-0.6mg IM 30-60 min before induction of anesthesia; **Preoperative Sedation:** 0.32-0.65mg IM/IV/SC; **Vomiting:** 0.6-1mg SC. **Tab: Usual:** 0.4mg. **Range:** 0.4-0.8mg. *Pediatrics:* **Sol, Inj: Anesthesia: Excessive Salivation: 4-7 mo:** 0.1mg IM 45-60 min before anesthesia. **7 mo-3 yrs:** 0.15mg IM 45-60 min before anesthesia. **3-8 yrs:** 0.2mg IM 45-60 min before anesthesia. **8-12 yrs:** 0.3mg IM 45-60 min before anesthesia; **Vomiting:** 6µg/kg/dose SC.	**W/P:** Monitor IOP with open-angle glaucoma. Not for use in children. Caution with pyloric obstruction, urinary bladder neck or intestinal obstruction, elderly. Increased CNS effects with liver or kidney dysfunction. May aggravate seizures or psychosis. Idiosyncratic reactions reported (rare). **Contra:** Angle-closure glaucoma, hypersensitivity to belladonna alkaloids. **P/N:** Category C, caution in nursing.	**Dry mouth,** drowsiness, blurred vision, dilation of pupils, dizziness, disorientation, confusion.

Table 8.2: DRUG INTERACTIONS FOR ANTICHOLINERGIC AND CHOLINERGIC DRUGS

ALL ANTICHOLINERGIC DRUGS

Antacids or absorbent antidiarrheal drugs	May impair absorption of anticholinergic drug. Avoid administration within 2-3 hours.
Antimyasthenics	Muscarinic effects are blocked by anticholinergic drugs, possibly obscuring early signs of an antimyasthenic overdose. Use cautiously.
CNS depressants	Summation of CNS depression with scopolamine; hallucination and behavioral disturbances have been reported with parenteral lorazepam and scopolamine. Use cautiously.
Drugs with anticholinergic side effects	Additive anticholinergic effects. Use cautiously with antiparkinsonism drugs, antipsychotic agents, carbamazepine, digoxin, dronabinol, orphenadrine, procainamide, quinidine, sedative antihistamines, and tricyclic antidepressants.
Haloperidol	Antipsychotic effects of haloperidol may be impaired. Use cautiously.
Ketoconazole	Absorption may be impaired by increased gastric pH. Take ketoconazole at least 2 hours before the anticholinergic drug.
Metoclopramide	Effect of hastening gastric emptying may be blocked. Use cautiously.
Opioid analgesics	Summation of constipating effects. Use cautiously.
Potassium chloride	Delayed absorption may increase gastrointestinal toxicity of potassium chloride. Avoid concurrent use.

ALL CHOLINERGIC DRUGS

β-adrenergic blocking drugs	Summation of drug effects on cardiac automaticity and conduction. Use cautiously.
Drugs with anticholinergic activity	Antagonistic drug effects. Use cautiously when the anticholinergic effect of the interacting drug is not the goal of therapy; consult with a physician to optimize drug treatment. Drugs requiring caution include anticholinergics, antiparkinson drugs, antipsychotic agents, carbamazepine, digoxin, dronabinol, orphenadrine, procainamide, quinidine, sedative antihistamines, and tricyclic antidepressants.
Drugs with cholinergic activity	Summation of drug effects. Use cautiously with cholinergic antiglaucoma drugs, antimyasthenic agents, and bethanechol.
Hepatic enzyme inhibitors	Inhibition of cevimeline metabolism. Use cautiously with azole antifungals, erythromycins, nefazodone, protease inhibitors, and selective serotonin reuptake inhibitors.

Table 8.3: PHARMACOKINETIC PARAMETERS OF ANTICHOLINERGIC DRUGS

DRUG	TIME OF ONSET (MIN)	DURATION OF EFFECT (H)	AMINE STRUCTURE
Atropine	30-60	4-6	Tertiary
Hyoscyamine	30-60	4-6	Tertiary
Scopolamine	30-60	4-6	Tertiary
Glycopyrrolate	30-45	6-8	Quaternary
Propantheline	30-45	6	Quaternary

Table 8.4: SALIVA SUBSTITUTES PRODUCT INFORMATION

BRAND NAME(S)	CONTENT/FORM
Entertainer's Secret	**Solution:** sodium carboxymethylcellulose, dibasic sodium phosphate, potassium chloride, parabens, aloe vera gel, glycerin, flavor, water in 60-mL spray
Moi-Stir, Moi-Stir Swabsticks	**Solution:** sodium carboxymethylcellulose; dibasic sodium phosphate; calcium, magnesium, potassium and sodium chlorides; parabens; sorbitol; water in 4-oz spray and 3-stick packets
MouthKote	**Solution:** Yerba Santa, citric acid, ascorbic acid, sodium benzoate, flavor, sodium saccharin, sorbitol, xylitol, water in 2- and 8-oz spray
Optimoist	**Solution:** hydroxyethylcellulose, acesulfame potassium, calcium phosphate monobasic, citric acid, sodium benzoate, sodium hydroxide, sodium monofluorophosphate in 60- and 355-mL spray
Oralbalance	**Gel:** hydroxyethylcellulose, hydrogenated starch, glycerate polyhydrate, potassium thiocyanate, glucose oxidase, lactoperoxidase, lysozyme, lactoferrin, aloe vera, xylitol in 1.5-oz tubes
Saliva Substitute ★	**Solution:** sodium carboxymethylcellulose, flavor, sorbitol, water in 120-mL squeeze bottles
Salivart ★	**Solution:** sodium carboxymethylcellulose; dibasic potassium phosphate; calcium, magnesium, potassium and sodium chlorides; sorbitol; water; nitrogen propellant in 1- and 2.48-oz spray cans
SalivaSure	**Lozenge:** sodium carboxymethylcellulose, dicalcium phosphate, malic acid, sodium citrate dihydrate, citric acid, silica colloidal, magnesium stearate, stearic acid, sorbitol
Xero-Lube	**Solution:** hydroxyethylcellulose; dibasic and monobasic potassium phosphates; calcium, magnesium and potassium chlorides; sodium fluoride; methylparaben; flavor; xylitol in 6-oz spray

★ indicates a product bearing the ADA Seal of Acceptance.

Chapter 9

Mouthrinses and Dentifrices

Angelo J. Mariotti, D.D.S., Ph.D.; Kenneth H. Burrell, D.D.S., S.M.

Mouthrinses

Mouthrinses are solutions formulated to control or reduce halitosis through topical deoxidization, to act as antibacterial agents to reduce and prevent gingivitis, to interact with saliva and mucosal proteins, or to help prevent caries. The major components of mouthrinses are water, flavoring, humectant, surfactant, alcohol and the active ingredients.

Water is the major vehicle used to solubilize the ingredients. The flavor is designed to make the mouthrinse pleasant to use. The humectant adds substance or "body" to the product and inhibits crystallization around the opening of the container. The surfactant is used to solubilize the flavoring agent and provide foaming action. In addition, the surfactant helps remove oral debris and has some limited antimicrobial properties. If the formulation requires an antimicrobial agent, the surfactant must be compatible with it. Alcohol also helps solubilize some of the ingredients present in the formulation. There has been some concern about the association between mouthrinses containing alcohol and oral cancers, but current findings do not establish a causal relationship.

Active ingredients vary considerably within the product category, but they can be placed into four general groups: antimicrobial agents, fluoride, astringent salts and chlorophyllins.

Antimicrobial agents can be useful in reducing plaque formation, decreasing the severity of gingivitis and controlling halitosis. At this time, chlorhexidine and delmopinol hydrochloride (Decapinol) are the only products that have received FDA approval for efficacy in reducing plaque and gingival inflammation and both will require a prescription for use. Delmopinol hydrochloride is a heterocyclic amino alcohol with both hydrophilic and lipophilic properties. It is a surface active agent which prevents bacteria from adhering to and colonizing tooth surfaces. At the time of publication, only chlorhexidine is available commercially.

Numerous antibacterial agents have been used as subgingival irrigants in patients with gingivitis and periodontitis. In general, both home-applied and professionally applied subgingival antimicrobial agents have been shown to reduce gingivitis; however, subgingival irrigation as an adjunct to conventional periodontal therapy has produced equivocal results. Moreover, subgingival irrigation with antimicrobial agents does not appear to have significantly greater benefits than irrigation with water alone.

Fluoride rinses will reduce carious lesions substantially. However, these agents have little or no effect in reducing supragingival plaque.

Oxygenating compounds with concentrations of 3% or greater of hydrogen peroxide should not be considered for frequent and extended use, as such use can result in damage to oral tissues. In solutions containing carbamide peroxide, one-third of the carbamide peroxide is converted to hydrogen peroxide, which has the potential to damage oral tissue if the dose exceeds 3% hydrogen peroxide. A solution of 10% carbamide peroxide releases approximately 3% hydrogen peroxide when introduced into the mouth.

Some studies have reported plaque reductions in patients using prebrushing rinses, but a large number of studies found no advantage to using prebrushing rinses for the purpose of reducing plaque levels. Thus, the recommendation of prebrushing rinses for increased plaque removal is questionable.

The reasons for halitosis are complex, and dentists recognize that a mouthrinse may treat the symptoms and not the causes of halitosis. Astringent salts present in mouthwashes can interact with salivary and mucosal proteins to control halitosis, and chlorophyllins can serve as topical deodorizers to mask halitosis. However, the effect of using mouthrinses to disguise malodor is transitory. To diagnose and treat the cause of halitosis effectively, the dentist must perform a thorough examination.

Accepted Indications

Mouthrinses are used in dentistry for a variety of reasons: to freshen breath (reduce halitosis), to prevent or control dental caries, to reduce plaque formation on teeth and gingiva, to prevent or reduce gingivitis, to reduce the rate of supragingival calculus accumulation, or to produce a combination of these effects.

Gingivitis

To receive the ADA Seal of Acceptance, a mouthrinse used for the control of gingival inflammation must demonstrate a statistically significant reduction in gingival inflammation that represents a proportionate reduction of at least 15% in favor of the mouthrinse in any one study and an average of 20% reduction in two studies.

Halitosis

Mouthrinses used to mask oral odor pose several problems. Breath odors can result for a myriad of reasons, including poor oral hygiene, oral or systemic disease, types of food eaten and bacterial flora in the alimentary canal and on the tongue. Furthermore, the duration of action of mouthrinses in masking halitosis is quite variable, but these agents generally have a short duration of action because of poor substantivity.

Mouthrinses thought to be useful in the control of halitosis either contain agents that limit the growth of bacteria responsible for common mouth odors or inactivate the malodorous volatile sulfur-containing compounds that are present owing to amino acid degradation. The antimicrobial agents include chlorhexidine, chlorine dioxide, cetylpyridium chloride and oral rinses based on a mixture of the essential oils (such as eucalyptol, menthol, thymol and methyl salicylate). Examples of agents that inhibit odor-causing compounds are zinc salts, ketone, terpene and ionone, a compound found in tomato juice.

At press time, there were no ADA-accepted mouthrinses for the control of halitosis. Although several ADA-accepted mouthrinses can substantiate their claims using criteria that are currently used by the oral care industry, these criteria may not reflect the ADA-established guidelines for evaluating products' effectiveness against oral malodor. Mouthrinses containing chlorine dioxide are available, but there are no adequately controlled clinical trials to determine their efficacy in controlling sulfide-associated odors from bacteria or oral mucosa.

Supragingival Calculus Accumulation (Antitartar)

An antimicrobial mouthrinse containing essential oils and zinc chloride has been shown to reduce the rate of supragingival calculus accumulation. This product has been clinically shown to have plaque-, gingivitis- and calculus-reducing properties.

General Dosing Information

The usual adult dosage (and often the geriatric dosage) for mouthrinses (see Table 9.1) is 10-20 mL for therapeutic rinses; it is not established for cosmetic and prebrushing rinses and so can be dictated by individual choice. For oxygenating agents, dosage regimens are more restrictive in terms of frequency and duration of usage. Duration of rinsing varies by the type of agent used. Safety and efficacy typically have not been established for antigingivitis mouthrinse use by pediatric patients.

Maximum Recommended Doses

Maximum recommended doses for mouthrinses are typically what can be held in the mouth comfortably (10-20mL). The exception is an oxygenating agent of 1.5% hydrogen peroxide (Peroxyl), which is used in 10-mL quantities. Depending on whether the formulations are purchased over the counter (with directions on packaging) or are prescribed (with directions on the label), additional mouthrinse should be taken only after sufficient time has been allowed to prove that the therapeutic effect of the previous dose requires augmentation.

Dosage Adjustments

The actual maximum dose for each patient must be individualized depending on factors such as his or her size, age and physical status; ability to effectively rinse and expectorate; oral health; and sensitivity. Mouthrinses are not often prescribed for young pediatric patients. As patients often swallow some of the product, reduced maximum doses may be indicated for geriatric patients, patients with serious illness or disability and patients with medical conditions who are taking drugs that alter oral responses to mouthrinses.

Special Dental Considerations

Drug Interactions of Dental Interest

Concurrent use of agents that contain either calcium hydroxide or aluminum hydroxide may form a complex with fluoride ions and reduce a rinse's effectiveness in the mouth. Concomitant use of chlorhexidine and stannous fluoride mouthrinses may reduce the efficacy of each agent.

Cross-Sensitivity

Some patients can develop allergic reactions (such as skin rash, hives and facial swelling) to rinses. If this occurs, treatment should be discontinued immediately.

Special Patients

Problems in women who are pregnant or breastfeeding have not been documented with normal daily use of oral rinses containing fluorides.

Patient Monitoring: Aspects to Watch

- Extrinsic staining and increased calculus buildup is possible in some instances (see Table 9.1).
- Caution should be used in prescribing mouthrinses containing alcohol to patients in recovery from alcoholism.
- Rinsing with water or drinking anything after using the mouthrinse should be avoided for at least 30 minutes to prevent clearance of the drug from the mouth and reduction in effectiveness of the mouthrinse.

Adverse Effects and Precautions

The incidence of adverse reactions to mouthrinses is relatively low. Many reactions (burning, taste alterations, tooth staining) are temporary. Idiosyncratic and allergic reactions account for a small minority of adverse responses. The adverse effects listed in Table 9.1 apply to all major types of mouthrinses.

Pharmacology

Chlorhexidine

Chlorhexidine is a bisbiguanide with broad-spectrum antibacterial activity. It is a symmetrical, cationic molecule that binds strongly to hydroxylapatite, the organic pellicle of the tooth, oral mucosa, salivary proteins and bacteria. As a result of the binding of chlorhexidine to oral structures, the drug exhibits substantivity (for example, 30% of the drug is retained after rinsing, with subsequent slow release over time). Chlorhexidine is poorly absorbed from the gastrointestinal tract, and whatever is absorbed is excreted primarily in the feces. Depending on the dose, chlorhexidine can be bacteriostatic or bactericidal. Bacteriostasis results from interference with bacterial cell wall transport systems. Bactericidal concentrations disrupt the cell wall, which leads to leakage of intracellular proteins.

Chlorhexidine can also be administered to subgingival sites in a controlled local delivery system called PerioChip. Subgingival delivery of chlorhexidine in a biodegradable hydrolyzed gelatin matrix maintains an antimicrobial concentration in the periodontal pocket for at least 7 days. Clinical studies have not demonstrated staining or adverse effects using this agent in a local delivery system (see Chapter 4, Table 4.2, for usage information).

Essential Oils

Antibacterial activity is created by a combination of essential oils (eucalyptol [0.092%], thymol [0.062%], methyl salicylate [0.06%] and menthol [0.042%]) in an alcohol-based (21.6-26.9%) vehicle. Essential oils have been implicated in inhibiting bacterial enzymes and reducing pathogenicity of plaque. The substantivity of these agents, also called phenolics, is poor.

Fluorides

Fluoride has been shown to reduce carious lesions dramatically in both children and adults. Fluoride ion is assimilated into the apatite crystal of enamel and stabilizes the crystal, making teeth more resistant to decay. Fluoride also has been shown to help remineralize incipient carious lesions. The germicidal activity of these agents, which include various liquid formulations of stannous fluoride, is negligible.

Oxygenating Agents

Oxygenating agents release oxygen as an active intermediate, loosening debris in inaccessible areas. Oxygenating agents also have been reported to induce damage in bacterial cells by altering membrane permeability. The germicidal activity of these agents is negligible. The substantivity of oxygenating agents is poor.

Prebrushing Rinses

The exact mechanism that prebrushing rinses use to "loosen" plaque is not known and is questionable. However, it has been suggested that surface-active agents (sodium lauryl sulfate and sodium benzoate, for example) make plaque soluble and therefore easier to remove.

Herbal Agents

Some mouthrinses and dentifrices contain a variety of mixtures of herbal agents (such as aloe vera, sodium carrageenan, echinacea, goldenseal, bee propolis and many others). At this time, controlled long-term studies to ascertain the efficacy of these agents in patients are lacking.

Note: Although alcohol can denature bacterial cell walls, it serves as a nontherapeutic vehicle in most mouthrinses.

Patient Advice

* The effectiveness of any mouthrinse is tied to the use of the agent as prescribed by the dentist. This means the proper dose, duration of time in the mouth and frequency of rinsing must be carefully followed. If a patient misses a dose, he or she should apply the mouthrinse as soon as possible; however, doubling the dose will offer no benefit.
* To receive the greatest antiplaque or anticaries benefit, the patient should rinse before retiring to bed.
* After using a mouthrinse, the patient should not rinse with water or drink anything for at least 30 minutes. Immediately drinking or rinsing with water will increase the drug's clearance from the mouth and reduce its effectiveness. Furthermore, changes in taste sensation may occur if the mouth is rinsed with water immediately after mouthrinse use.
* These mouthrinses should be kept out of the reach of young children, as their ingestion of 4 or more ounces of rinses containing alcohol can cause alcohol intoxication.

Dentifrices

Oral hygiene is a critical aspect of all dental therapy. Proper oral hygiene reduces the buildup of dental plaque on tooth surfaces and reduces the incidence of dental caries as well as various types of periodontal diseases. Dentifrices are pastes, gels or powders used to help remove dental plaque by enhancing the mechanical scrubbing and cleaning power of a toothbrush. Dentifrices typically contain abrasives (to remove debris and residual stain), foaming agents or detergents (a preference of consumers), humectants (to prevent loss of water from the preparation), thickening agents or binders (to stabilize dentifrice formulations and prevent separation of liquid and solid phases), flavoring (a preference of consumers) and therapeutic agents (see Table 9.2).

Depending on the dentifrice, the principal outcomes can include reduction of caries incidence by assimilation of the fluoride ion into the apatite crystal of enamel (as a result of sodium fluoride, stannous fluoride or sodium monofluorophospate); reduction of tooth hypersensitivity by blocking the pain caused by fluid exchange between dentinal tubules and pulp (as a result of arginine bicarbonate, calcium carbonate complex, potassium nitrate or stabilized stannous fluoride); cosmetic whitening of teeth (as a result of hydrogen peroxide, papain/sodium citrate, or sodium tripolyphosphate and/or abrasives); reduction of calculus (as a result of pyrophosphates, zinc citrate, chloride, triclosan or stabilized stannous fluoride); and reduction of plaque formation by reducing enzymatic activity of microorganisms and by an antibacterial effect (as a result of triclosan with vinylmethyl-ether maleic acid, zinc citrate, stannous fluoride or a combination of essential oils) (see Table 9.2).

It should be noted that with few exceptions, whitening toothpastes are different from agents that bleach. Bleaching involves free radicals (usually derived from hydrogen peroxide), whereas whitening or stain removal is accomplished by abrasive agents, phosphate compounds or papain/sodium citrate (citroxain) (see Chapter 12).

Most dentifrices marketed to the public can be broadly classified as agents for:
* antitartar activity (reduction of calculus formation)
* caries prevention
* cosmetic effect (tooth whitening)

- gingivitis reduction
- plaque formation reduction
- reduction of tooth sensitivity

Accepted Indications

Dentifrices are used in dentistry for cosmetic purposes and to provide caries prevention, reduce tooth sensitivity, reduce calculus formation, reduce plaque formation, reduce gingivitis or provide a combination of all of these.

General Dosing Information

Depending on the patient's age and the dentifrice used (see Table 9.3), the usual adult dosage is approximately 1.5 mg of fluoride. The dosage for children younger than 6 years is about 0.25 g (a pea-sized amount).

Dosage Adjustments

The actual maximum dose for each patient must be individualized depending on factors such as his or her size, age and physical status; ability to effectively rinse and expectorate; oral health; and sensitivity. Highly fluoridated dentifrices are not often prescribed for pediatric patients, and reduced maximum doses may be indicated for certain patients, such as those with physical or mental disabilities.

Special Dental Considerations

Drug Interactions of Dental Interest

The following drug interactions and related problems involving dentifrices are potentially of clinical significance in dentistry.

Many of the ingredients of dentifrices, as well as products containing stannous fluoride, interact with chlorhexidine and reduce its efficacy. Dentifrice ingredients can also interact with cetylpyridinium chloride. Therefore, these agents should not be used concomitantly but, rather, used at least 30 minutes apart. Use of a chlorhexidine rinse followed immediately by a fluoride dentifrice may reduce the efficacy of each agent.

Cross-Sensitivity

Some patients can develop allergic reactions (skin rash, hives, desquamation) to dentifrices and should discontinue use of the product immediately.

Special Patients

Patients with physical or mental disabilities may have difficulty clearing dentifrices from the mouth. These patients should receive additional help from caretakers.

Patient Monitoring: Aspects to Watch

See Table 9.3.

Adverse Effects and Precautions

The incidence of adverse reactions to dentifrices is relatively low. Many reactions (burning or taste alterations) are temporary. Idiosyncratic and allergic reactions account for a small minority of adverse responses.

The adverse effects listed in Table 9.3 apply to all major types of dentifrices. Some patients cannot use tartar-control products because of the development of dentinal hypersensitivity or soft tissue irritation. For information on desensitizing agents, see Chapter 11. A small percentage of patients have an adverse reaction to sodium lauryl sulfates, a detergent that is added to some toothpastes. In such instances, switching to a dentifrice without sodium lauryl sulfate (such as Rembrandt or Sensodyne Gel) may be beneficial. Chlorhexidine and cetylpyridinium chloride have been reported to produce an extrinsic stain on teeth with the incidence being higher for chlorhexidine than for cetylpyridinium chloride.

Pharmacology

Antitartar Formulas

The precise mechanism of supragingival calculus formation is not known. However, it is assumed that most calculus-reducing formulas reduce crystal growth on tooth surfaces. One way in which they accomplish this is the chelation of cations by the dentifrices' active ingredient.

Cosmetic Formulas

Whitening of teeth can occur by two mechanisms. One method is mechanical, in which an abrasive is used to remove debris and surface stains from the tooth. The other method involves the use of phosphate compounds such as sodium tripolyphosphate and sodium hexametaphosphate that break down pigments that accumulate on or in tooth enamel. Sodium bicarbonate acts as both a mild abrasive and an agent for dissolving stain pigments.

Fluoride Formulas

Fluoride has been shown to reduce carious lesions dramatically in both children and adults. Fluoride ion is assimilated into the apatite crystal of enamel and stabilizes the crystal, making it more resistant to decay. Fluoride also has been shown to remineralize carious lesions.

Gingivitis- and Plaque-Reduction Formulas

Triclosan is both a bisphenol and a nonionic germicide that is effective against gram-positive and gram-negative bacteria, and it has been shown to reduce plaque accumulation and decrease the severity of gingivitis. A dentifrice containing stabilized stannous fluoride also has been shown to reduce gingivitis. The mechanism of action is thought to depend on the inhibition of bacterial metabolism and concomitant plaque acid reduction. Dentifrices containing zinc citrate have been reported to prevent the attachment of bacteria to teeth and to be antibacterial. A dentifrice containing a combination of essential oils (eucalyptol 0.738%, menthol 0.340%, methyl salicylate 0.480%, thymol 0.511%) also has been shown to reduce plaque accumulation and gingivitis.

Herbal Agents

Some toothpastes contain a variety of mixtures of herbal agents (such as aloe vera, sodium carrageenan, echinacea, goldenseal and bee propolis). Currently, controlled, long-term studies to ascertain the efficacy of these agents in patients are lacking.

Sensitivity-Reduction Formulas

The mechanisms of action to reduce tooth sensitivity are not well-established. It has been hypothesized that pain sensation in teeth can be reduced by blocking dentin tubule fluid exchange, by depolarizing pulpal nerves or by both means. Currently available sensitive-teeth formulas act via the topical application of agents to root surfaces.

Suggested Readings

Ciancio SG. Chemical agents: plaque control, calculus reduction and treatment of dentinal hypersensitivity. Periodontology 2000 1995;8:75-86.

Davies RM, Ellwood RP, Davies GM. The effectiveness of a toothpaste containing triclosan and polyvinyl-methyl ether maleic acid copolymer in improving plaque control and gingival health: a systematic review. J Clin Periodontol 2004;31:1029-33.

Mariotti A, Hefti A. Drugs for the control of supragingival plaque. In: Stitzel CR, Craig RE, eds. Modern pharmacology. 5th ed. Boston: Little, Brown; 1997:533-40.

Panagakos FS, Volpe AR, Petrone ME, DeVizio W, Davies RM. Advanced oral antibacterial/anti-inflammatory technology: a comprehensive review of the clinical benefits of a triclosan/copolymer/fluoride dentifrice. J Clin Dent 2005;16:S1-S19.

Paraskevas S, van der Weijden GA. A review of the effects of stannous fluoride on gingivitis. J Clin Periodontol 2006;33(1):1-13.

Quirynen M, Zhao H, van Steenberghe D. Review of the treatment strategies for oral malodour. Clin Oral Investig 2002;6:1-10.

Rolla G, Ogaard B, Cruz R de A. Clinical effect and mechanism of cariostatic action of fluoride-containing toothpastes: a review. Int Dent J 1991;41(3):171-4.

Topping G, Assaf A. Strong evidence that daily use of fluoride toothpaste prevents caries. Evid Based Dent 2005;6(2):32.

Table 9.1: USAGE INFORMATION FOR MOUTHRINSES

BRAND NAME/CONTENT	DOSAGE*	WARNINGS/PRECAUTIONS & CONTRAINDICATIONS	ADVERSE EFFECTS
ANESTHETIC MOUTHRINSE			
Chloraseptic Mouthwash: 1.4% phenol, 12.5% alcohol.	**Adults:** 10mL prn (no more often than q 3 h). **Pediatrics:** Not recommended.	NA	NA
ANTITARTAR MOUTHRINSES			
Advanced Listerine Antiseptic with Tartar Protection (Arctic Mint)★: 0.064% thymol, 0.092% eucalyptol, 0.060% methyl salicylate, 0.042% menthol, 0.09% zinc chloride, 21.6% alcohol, miscellaneous ingredients; **Vi-Jon Ice Mint Tartar Control Antiseptic Mouthrinse ★†:** miscellaneous ingredients.	**Adults:** Rinse with 20mL for 30 sec.	NA	NA
CETYLPYRIDINIUM CHLORIDE‡			
Cepacol: 14.5% alcohol, 0.05% cetylpyridinium chloride, miscellaneous ingredients; **Crest Pro-Health Rinse (Clean Mint, Wintergreen) (alcohol-free):** 0.07% cetylpyridinium chloride, miscellaneous ingredients; **Scope Mouthwash and Gargle:** 18.9% alcohol, sodium benzoate, cetylpyridinium chloride, benzoic acid, domiphen bromide, miscellaneous ingredients; **Scope Mouthwash and Gargle with Baking Soda:** 9.9% alcohol, cetylpyridinium chloride, domiphen bromide, miscellaneous ingredients; **Viadent Advanced Care Oral Rinse:** 6.1% SD alcohol 38-B, 0.05% cetylpyridinium chloride, miscellaneous ingredients.	**Adults:** (Crest Pro-Health) 20mL (4 tsp) swished for 30 sec bid. Do not swallow. When used after brushing, rinse mouth with water first. (All other brands) Amount, duration and frequency depend on individual choice. **Pediatrics:** (Crest Pro-Health) < 6yrs: Do not use. ≥ 6yrs to < 12yrs: Supervise use. (All other brands) Not recommended.	**W/P:** Should be used cautiously in young children. **Contra:** Patients with known allergies to ingredients.	NA
CHLORHEXIDINE§			
G-U-M Chlorhexidine Gluconate Oral Rinse, USP (alcohol-free): 0.12% chlorhexidine; **Peridex★:** 0.12% chlorhexidine, 11.6% alcohol; **PerioGard:** 0.12% chlorhexidine, 11.6% alcohol.	**Adults:** 15mL swished for 30 sec and expectorated; use bid. Do not swallow; do not rinse with water immediately after use.	**W/P:** Permanent staining of margins of restorations or composite restorations. Should not be used as sole treatment of gingivitis. **Contra:** Patients with sensitivity to chlorhexidine. **P/N:** Category B.	Allergic reaction (skin rash, hives, swelling of face), alteration of taste, staining of teeth, staining of restorations, discoloration of tongue, increase in calculus formation, parotid duct obstruction, parotitis, desquamation of oral mucosa, irritation to lips or tongue, oral sensitivity.
COSMETIC MOUTHRINSES			
Listerine Whitening Pre-Brush Rinse: 8% alcohol, 2% hydrogen peroxide, miscellaneous agents; **Rembrandt Age Defying Mouthrinse:** 0.05% sodium fluoride wt/vol, 1.5% hydrogen peroxide solution, miscellaneous agents; **Rembrandt Dazzling Fresh Mouthrinse:** methylparaben, sodium citrate, sodium lauryl sulfate, miscellaneous ingredients.	**Adults:** Amount, duration, and frequency of use depend on individual choice. **Pediatrics:** Not recommended.	**W/P:** Should be used cautiously in young children and in people who have low salivary flow due to age or drugs. **Contra:** Patients with allergic reactions, oral ulcerations, and oral desquamative diseases.	NA

★ indicates a product bearing the ADA Seal of Acceptance.
NA = not available.
*Pediatric safety and efficacy have not been established except with fluoride rinses in children 6 years and older.
†Private label manufacturer.
‡Depending on the formulation, products containing cetylpyridinium chloride are used for various purposes, including control of plaque, gingivitis and halitosis.
§Pregnancy risk category B. Pregnancy risk categories have not been established for other products.
¶Although Listerine was the first antiseptic oral rinse formulated, today there are a significant number of generic compounds with similar antibacterial properties. Various mouthrinses that carry the ADA seal are generic versions of Listerine.
**There are a significant number of generic fluoride rinse products that carry the ADA seal.

BRAND NAME/CONTENT	DOSAGE*	WARNINGS/PRECAUTIONS & CONTRAINDICATIONS	ADVERSE EFFECTS
Targon: 15.6% alcohol, PEG-40, hydrogenated castor oil, sodium lauryl sulfate, disodium phosphate, miscellaneous ingredients.	**Adults:** Before brushing, rinse with 20mL for 30 sec.	NA	NA

DELMOPINOL

Decapinol Oral Rinse: classified as medical device; forms a barrier by adhering to tooth surfaces.	**Adults:** 10mL swished for 60 sec and expectorated; use bid after brushing. **Pediatrics < 12yrs:** Not recommended.	**W/P:** Not recommended during pregnancy due to lack of studies.	NA

ESSENTIAL OILS

Listerine Antiseptic¶ (Original ★, Cool Mint ★, FreshBurst ★, Natural Citrus ★, and Vanilla Mint): 0.092% eucalyptol, 0.062% thymol, 0.06% methyl salicylate, 0.042% menthol, and alcohol ranging from 21.6% for the flavored versions and 26.9% for the original version; **Swan (Amber, Blue Mint, Spring Mint) Antiseptic Mouthrinse ★†, Vi-Jon (Regular, Blue Mint, Citrus, Fresh Mint) Antiseptic Mouthrinse ★†:** ingredients equivalent to Listerine.	**Adults:** 20mL swished full strength for 30 sec and expectorated; do not swallow. Use bid or prn. **Pediatrics:** Do not use in children < 12yrs.	**W/P:** Should not be used as sole treatment of gingivitis. **Contra:** Children < 12yrs.	NA

FLUORIDES**

Fluorigard Anti-Cavity Dental Rinse, Phos-Flur Anti-Cavity Fluoride Rinse ★, Pro-DenRx Daily APF Fluoride Rinse ★, Tom's of Maine Natural Anticavity Fluoride Mouthwash ★: 0.02% sodium fluoride; **ACT Anticavity Fluoride Rinse for Kids ★, NaFrinse Acidulated Oral Rinse ★, NaFrinse Neutral/Daily Mouthrinse ★, Oral-B Rinse Therapy Anti-Cavity Treatment, Reach Fluoride Dental Rinse, Swan Anticavity Fluoride Rinse ★†:** 0.05% sodium fluoride; **ACT Anticavity Fluoride Rinse ★:** 0.05% sodium fluoride, 7% alcohol; NaFrinse Mouthrinse Powder, 0.2% ★, **NaFrinse Neutral/Weekly Mouthrinse ★, NaFrinse Unit Dose Mouthrinse Solution ★, Pro-DenRx 0.2% Neutral Sodium Fluoride Rinse ★:** 0.2% sodium fluoride; **PreviDent Dental Rinse ★:** 0.2% sodium fluoride, 6% alcohol; **Dentinbloc Dentin Desensitizer:** 1.09% sodium fluoride, 0.4% stannous fluoride, 0.14% hydrogen fluoride.	**Adults:** 10mL of sodium fluoride swished for 60 sec and expectorated qd; patient should not eat or drink for 30 min after rinsing. **Pediatrics:** < 6yrs: Not recommended. ≥ 6yrs: 10mL of 0.05% sodium fluoride swished for 60 sec and expectorated qd; patient should not eat or drink for 30 min after rinsing.	**W/P:** Chronic systemic overdose may induce fluorosis and changes in bone. **Contra:** Patients with dental fluorosis, fluoride toxicity from systemic ingestion, and severe renal insufficiency.	Ulcerations of oral mucosa, fluorosis, osteosclerosis, diarrhea, bloody vomit, nausea, stomach cramps, black tarry stools, drowsiness, faintness, stomach cramps or pain, unusual excitement if swallowed.

MOUTHRINSES FOR HALITOSIS

Astring-O-Sol (concentrate): SD alcohol 38-B, 75.6% methyl salicylate, miscellaneous ingredients; **Lavoris Crystal Fresh (Original, Peppermint):** alcohol, citric acid, sodium hydroxide, zinc oxide, miscellaneous ingredients; **Lavoris (Mint, Cinnamon):** alcohol, aromatic oils, zinc chloride and/or zinc oxide; **Listermint Mint (alcohol-free):** zinc chloride, sodium benzoate, sodium lauryl sulfate, miscellaneous ingredients; **Oxyfresh Natural Mouthrinse (alcohol-free):** oxygene (contains chlorine dioxide), miscellaneous ingredients; **Platinum:** monofluorophosphate, tetra	**Adults:** Amount, duration and frequency depend on individual choice. **Pediatrics:** Not recommended.	**W/P:** Should be used cautiously in young children. **Contra:** Patients with known allergies to ingredients.	NA

Table 9.1: USAGE INFORMATION FOR MOUTHRINSES *(cont.)*

BRAND NAME/CONTENT	DOSAGE*	WARNINGS/PRECAUTIONS & CONTRAINDICATIONS	ADVERSE EFFECTS
MOUTHRINSES FOR HALITOSIS *(cont.)*			
potassium pyrophosphate, miscellaneous ingredients; **Rembrandt Mouth Refreshing Rinse (alcohol-free):** sodium benzoate, methyl paraben, miscellaneous ingredients; **Retardex Oral Rinse (alcohol free):** ciosysii (contains chlorine dioxide), miscellaneous ingredients; **TherSol Mouthwash:** 6.4% SD alcohol 38B, 6% glycerine, 0.4% ethoxylated tertiary amine, 0.1% capryl/capramidopropyl betaine, miscellaneous ingredients; **Tom's of Maine Natural Mouthwash:** aloe vera, ascorbic acid, menthol, spearmint, witch hazel, miscellaneous ingredients.			
MOUTHRINSE FOR PAIN RELIEF (CANKER AND MOUTH SORES, ETC)			
Rincinol P.R.N. Soothing Oral Rinse: sodium hyaluronate, polyvinylpyrrolidone, glycyrrhetinic acid, aloe vera extract, miscellaneous ingredients.	***Adults/Pediatrics:*** Swish for 60 sec and expectorate; use prn.	NA	NA
OXYGENATING AGENTS			
Gly-Oxide: 10% carbamide peroxide; **Orajel Rinse:** 4% alcohol, 1.5% hydrogen peroxide; **Perimax Hygenic Perio Rinse:** 1.5% hydrogen peroxide; **Peroxyl Mouthrinse:** 1.5% hydrogen peroxide, 6% alcohol.	***Adults:*** Regimens used for rinses containing oxygenating agents will vary depending on formulation: eg, recommendation for Gly-Oxide is that several drops be applied to affected areas, followed by a 2-3 min rinsing; the recommendation for Peroxyl Mouthrinse is that 10mL of it be used, followed by a 60-sec rinsing.	**W/P:** Should not be used for extended periods of time because of possible side effects mentioned at left. **Contra:** Treatment of periodontitis or gingivitis.	Chemical burns of oral mucosa, decalcification of teeth, black hairy tongue.
PREBRUSHING RINSE			
Advanced Formula Plax (Original, Mint Sensation, SoftMint): 8.7% alcohol, tetrasodium pyrophosphate, benzoic acid, sodium lauryl sulfate, sodium benzoate, miscellaneous ingredients.	***Adults:*** Efficacy has not been established for adult or geriatric population.	NA	Negligible effects on plaque make these agents of little use in the treatment of carious lesions or periodontal diseases, including gingivitis.

★indicates a product bearing the ADA Seal of Acceptance.
NA = not available.
*Pediatric safety and efficacy have not been established except with fluoride rinses in children 6 years and older.
†Private label manufacturer.
‡Depending on the formulation, products containing cetylpyridinium chloride are used for various purposes, including control of plaque, gingivitis and halitosis.
§Pregnancy risk category B. Pregnancy risk categories have not been established for other products.
¶Although Listerine was the first antiseptic oral rinse formulated, today there are a significant number of generic compounds with similar antibacterial properties. Various mouthrinses that carry the ADA seal are generic versions of Listerine.
**There are a significant number of generic fluoride rinse products that carry the ADA seal.

Table 9.2: COMPONENTS OF DENTIFRICES

INGREDIENTS	FUNCTION
Abrasives: Calcium carbonate, dehydrated silica gels, hydrated aluminum oxides, magnesium carbonate, phosphate salts, silicates	Remove debris and residual stain, remove surface stains on teeth
Fluoride	Reduces caries
Peroxides, sodium tripolyphosphate, sodium hexametaphosphate, papain/sodium citrate	Remove surface stains on teeth
Potassium nitrate, sodium citrate, strontium chloride	Reduce dentinal sensitivity
Pyrophosphates, triclosan, zinc citrate	Reduce supragingival calculus
Stannous fluoride, triclosan	Reduce gingival inflammation
Detergents: Sodium lauryl sulfate, sodium N-lauryl sarcosinate	Create foaming action and may help increase the solubility of plaque and accretions during brushing
Flavoring agents: Diverse and complex agents that may contain saccharin as a sweetener	Provide taste to dentifrice (consumer preference)
Humectants: Glycerol, propylene glycol, sorbitol	Prevent water loss
Thickening agents or binders: Mineral colloids, natural gums, seaweed colloids, synthetic celluloses	Stabilize formulations

Table 9.3: USAGE INFORMATION FOR DENTIFRICES

NAME/ACTIVE INGREDIENTS	WARNINGS/PRECAUTIONS	ADVERSE EFFECTS
ANTITARTAR*		
Aim Anti-Tartar Gel Formula with Fluoride, Aim Tartar Control Gel Toothpaste: Zinc citrate, 0.76% sodium monofluorophosphate	See manufacturer's labeling for specific brand information.	Development of dentinal hypersensitivity and tissue irritation, but incidence is low.
Aquafresh ALL with Tartar Control Toothpaste★: Tetrapotassium pyrophosphate, tetrasodium pyrophosphate, 0.243% sodium fluoride		
Aquafresh Whitening Tartar Protection Toothpaste★: 0.243% sodium fluoride, sodium tripolyphosphate		
Close-Up Tartar Control Gel: Zinc citrate, 0.76% sodium monofluorophosphate		
Colgate Tartar Control Baking Soda and Peroxide Toothpaste★: Sodium monofluorophosphate, 0.15% w/v fluoride ion		
Colgate Tartar Control Toothpaste★ or Gel★: Tetrasodium pyrophosphate, 0.243% sodium fluoride		
Colgate Tartar Control Plus Whitening Gel★ or Mint Paste★: 0.243% sodium fluoride, 1% tetrasodium pyrophosphate		
Colgate Total Toothpaste★, Colgate Total Clean Mint Toothpaste★, Colgate Total Fresh Stripe Toothpaste★, Colgate Total Mint Stripe Gel★: 0.243% sodium fluoride, 0.30% triclosan		
Colgate Total Advanced Clean Toothpaste★, Colgate Total Advanced Fresh Gel★, Colgate Total 2 in 1 Advanced Fresh Liquid Toothpaste★: 0.243% sodium fluoride, 0.30% triclosan		
Colgate Total Plus Whitening Toothpaste★, Colgate Total Plus Whitening Gel★: 0.243% sodium fluoride, 0.30% triclosan		
Crest Extra Whitening With Tartar Protection★: 0.243% sodium fluoride, 5.045% tetrasodium pyrophosphate		
Crest MultiCare★: 0.243% sodium fluoride, tetrasodium pyrophosphate		
Crest MultiCare Whitening★: 0.243% sodium fluoride, 5.045% tetrasodium pyrophosphate		
Crest Pro-Health Toothpaste (Clean Cinnamon, Clean Mint)★: 0.454% stannous fluoride (active ingredient), sodium hexametaphosphate (tartar reduction and stain inhibition ingredient)		
Crest Tartar Protection Fluoride Gel★ or Toothpaste★: 0.243% sodium fluoride, tetrapotassium pyrophosphate, disodium pyrophosphate, tetrasodium pyrophosphate		
Dr. Fresh Complete Fluoride Toothpaste (MFP)★: 0.24% W/W sodium fluoride		
Listerine Essential Care Tartar Control Powerful Mint Gel: 0.76% sodium monofluorophosphate, 0.738% eucalyptol, 0.340% menthol, 0.480% methyl salicylates, 0.511% thymol, zinc citrate trihydrate, miscellaneous ingredients		
Pepsodent Tartar Control Toothpaste: Ingredients not available.		
Prevent Tartar Prevention Toothpaste with Fluoride: 0.76% monofluorophosphate, zinc chloride		
Viadent Advanced Care Toothpaste: 2% zinc citrate, 0.8% sodium monofluorophosphate		

★indicates a product bearing the ADA Seal of Acceptance.
*These dentifrices also possess caries-preventive properties.
†Fluoride from sodium fluoride, sodium monofluorophosphate or stannous fluoride.
‡Private label manufacturer.
§All these dentifrices also possess caries-preventive properties except for Protect Desensitizing Solution.
¶In sensitivity-reduction dentifrices, fluoride is the active agent only for caries prevention; the exception is stannous fluoride, which has both caries-preventive and sensitivity-reducing properties.

NAME/ACTIVE INGREDIENTS	WARNINGS/PRECAUTIONS	ADVERSE EFFECTS
CARIES PREVENTION (Active Ingredient: Fluoride†)		
Aim Cavity Protection Gel Toothpaste Aquafresh Extra Fresh Toothpaste Aquafresh Fluoride Protection Toothpaste Aquafresh for Kids Toothpaste★ Aquafresh Kids Bubblemint Toothpaste Aquafresh Triple Protection Toothpaste★ Arm & Hammer Advance Care Toothpaste★ Arm & Hammer Complete Care Toothpaste★ Arm & Hammer Dental Care Toothpaste★ Arm & Hammer Dental Care Advanced Cleaning Mint Toothpaste w/ Baking Soda★ Arm & Hammer Enamel Care Toothpaste★ Arm & Hammer Peroxide Care Toothpaste★ Biotene Toothpaste Close-Up Anticavity Gel Toothpaste Close-Up Freshening Gel Toothpaste Colgate Advanced Freshness Toothpaste Colgate 2-in-1 Advanced Fresh Liquid Toothpaste★ Colgate 2-in-1 Kids Toothpaste★ Colgate Cavity Protection Gel with Baking Soda★ Colgate Cavity Protection Great Regular Flavor Fluoride Toothpaste★ Colgate Cavity Protection Toothpaste with Baking Soda★ Colgate Cavity Protection Winterfresh Gel★ Colgate Fresh Confidence Toothpaste Colgate for Kids Toothpaste★ Colgate Junior Toothpaste★ Colgate Tartar Control Plus Whitening Gel★ or Mint Paste★ Colgart Tartar Control Toothpaste★ or Gel★ Colgate Total Toothpaste★ Colgate Total 2 in 1 Advanced Fresh Liquid Toothpaste★ Colgate Total Advanced Clean Toothpaste★ Colgate Total Advanced Fresh Toothpaste Gel★ Colgate Total Clean Mint Toothpaste★ Colgate Total Fresh Stripe Toothpaste★ or Mint Stripe Gel★ Colgate Total Toothpaste★ Colgate Total Advanced Freshness Toothpaste★ Colgate Total Plus Whitening Liquid Toothpaste★ Colgate Total Plus Whitening Toothpaste★ or Gel★ Cool Wave Fresh Mint Gel Fluoride Anticavity Toothpaste★ Crest Advanced Cleaning Toothpaste Crest Cavity Protection Cool Mint Gel★ Crest Cavity Protection Icy Mint★ Crest Cavity Protection Toothpaste★ Crest Intelliclean Toothpaste Crest Kids SparkleFun Cavity Protection Gel★ Crest MultiCare Toothpaste★ Crest Multicare Whitening Toothpaste★ Crest Pro-Health Toothpaste (Clean Cinnamon, Clean Mint)★ Crest Rejuvenating Effects Toothpaste Crest Sensitivity Protection Mild Mint Paste★ DTI Toothpaste and Gel (Bubble Gum, Mint)★‡ Dr. Fresh Complete Care Toothpaste★ Dr. Fresh Fluoride Toothpaste★ Enamel Care Toothpaste Equate Cavity Protection Toothpaste★ Gleem Sodium Fluoride Anticavity Toothpaste Goofy Grape Natural Anticavity Fluoride Toothpaste/Liquid Gel for Children★ Mentadent Cavity Fighting Toothpaste★ Mentadent Fluoride Toothpaste w/Baking Soda &Peroxide★ Orajel Sensitive Pain Relieving Toothpaste for Adults★ OraLine Fluoride Toothpaste★	Tell caregivers of pediatric patients to make sure a pea-sized amount is used on toothbrush to minimize amount of fluoride ingested. **Usual adult dosage:** 1.5mg; **pediatrics < 6 yrs:** ~0.25g (pea-sized amount). See manufacturer's labeling for specific brand information.	Fluorosis.

Table 9.3: USAGE INFORMATION FOR DENTIFRICES *(cont.)*

NAME/ACTIVE INGREDIENTS	WARNINGS/PRECAUTIONS	ADVERSE EFFECTS
CARIES PREVENTION (Active Ingredient: Fluoride[†]) *(cont.)*		
OraLine Kids Bubblegum Toothpaste★ OraLine Secure Clear Fluoride Mint Toothpaste★ Pepsodent Original Toothpaste with Cavity Protection Pepsodent Baking Soda Toothpaste Plak Smacker Dinosaur Fluoride Gel Toothpaste(Bubblegum)★ Plak Smacker Great White Shark Fluoride Toothpaste(Cool Berry)★ Quality Choice Mint Flavor Toothpaste★ Rembrandt Whitening Toothpaste★ Shane Fluoride Toothpaste★ Sheffield Fluoride Toothpaste★Original, Bubble Gum, Mint)★‡ Stages Toothpaste Suave Cavity Protection Clean Mint Toothpaste Tom's of Maine Natural Baking Soda Toothpaste(Gingermint, Peppermint)★ Tom's of Maine Natural Fluoride Toothpaste for Children★ Tom's of Maine Natural Fluoride Toothpaste(Wintermint)★ Tom's of Maine Natural Toothpaste (Cinnamint, Fennel,Spearmint)★ Topol Whitening Anticavity Toothpaste Ultra Brite Advanced Whitening Fluoride Toothpaste Ultra Fresh Fluoride Toothpaste★ Unique Fluoride Toothpaste★ Viadent Advanced Care Toothpaste Zooth Children's Toothpaste★		
COSMETIC*		
Aim Whitening Gel Toothpaste with Baking Soda: 0.8% sodium monofluorophosphate **Aquafresh Multi-Action Whitening Toothpaste:** 0.243% sodium fluoride, sodium tripolyphosphate **Aquafresh Whitening Advanced Freshness:** 0.243% sodium fluoride, sodium tripolyphosphate **Aquafresh Whitening Toothpaste★:** 0.243% sodium fluoride, 10% sodium tripolyphosphate **Caffree Anti-Stain Fluoride Toothpaste:** Fluoride **Close-Up Whitening Gel Toothpaste:** Ingredients not available. **Colgate Baking Soda & Peroxide Whitening Toothpaste:** 0.15% W/V fluoride ion, sodium monofluorophosphate **Colgate Luminous Fluoride Toothpaste★:** 0.243% sodium fluoride, tetrasodium pyrophosphate **Colgate Platinum Tooth Whitener Toothpaste:** 2% tetrasodium phosphate, 10% aluminum oxide, 0.76% sodium monofluorophosphate **Colgate Simply White Toothpaste:** 0.24% sodium fluoride 0.24% (0.13% W/V fluoride ion) **Colgate Sparkling White Toothpaste:** 0.24% sodium fluoride 0.24% (0.13% W/V fluoride ion) **Colgate Total Advanced Clean Toothpaste★, Colgate Total 2-in-1 Advanced Fresh Liquid Toothpaste★:** 0.243% sodium fluoride, 0.30% triclosan **Colgate Total Plus Whitening Gel★, Liquid Toothpaste★ or Toothpaste★:** 0.243% sodium fluoride, 0.30% triclosan **Crest Baking Soda Whitening Tartar Protection Toothpaste:** 0.243% sodium fluoride	Not all discolorations of enamel (for example, enamel mottling, tetracycline staining, aging-extrinsic enamel) are responsive to extrinsic bleaching via dentifrices. See manufacturer's labeling for specific brand information.	Burning sensation, drying out of mucous membranes, taste alteration, gingival abrasion, enamel erosion.

★indicates a product bearing the ADA Seal of Acceptance.
*These dentifrices also possess caries-preventive properties.
†Fluoride from sodium fluoride, sodium monofluorophosphate or stannous fluoride.
‡Private label manufacturer.
§All these dentifrices also possess caries-preventive properties except for Protect Desensitizing Solution.
¶In sensitivity-reduction dentifrices, fluoride is the active agent only for caries prevention; the exception is stannous fluoride, which has both caries-preventive and sensitivity-reducing properties.

NAME/ACTIVE INGREDIENTS	WARNINGS/PRECAUTIONS	ADVERSE EFFECTS
COSMETIC* *(cont.)*		
Crest Dual Action Whitening Toothpaste: 0.243% sodium fluoride, 0.15% W/V fluoride ion		
Crest Extra Whitening With Tartar Protection★: 0.243% sodium fluoride, 5.045% tetrasodium pyrophosphate		
Crest MultiCare Whitening★: 0.243% sodium fluoride, 5.045% tetrasodium pyrophosphate		
Crest Pro-Health Toothpaste (Clean Cinnamon, Clean Mint)★: 0.454% stannous fluoride (active ingredient), sodium hexametaphosphate (tartar reduction and stain inhibition ingredient)		
Crest Rejuvenating Effects Toothpaste: 0.243% sodium fluoride, silica		
Crest Vivid White Toothpaste: 0.243% sodium fluoride, 0.15% W/V fluoride ion		
Crest Whitening Expressions Toothpaste & Liquid Gel, Crest Whitening Plus Scope: 0.243% sodium fluoride, 0.15% W/V fluoride ion		
Mentadent Advanced Whitening Toothpaste, Mentadent Replenishing White Toothpaste: 0.24% sodium fluoride		
Pearl Drops Baking Soda Whitening Toothpaste: Fluoride		
Pearl Drops Extra Strength Whitening Toothpaste with Fluoride: Fluoride		
Pearl Drops Whitening Gel: Fluoride		
Pearl Drops Whitening Toothpolish with Fluoride: Fluoride		
Rembrandt Age Defying Toothpaste: 0.76% sodium monofluorophosphate, tribon, papain/sodium citrate (citroxain), dicalcium orthophosphate, 6% carbamide peroxide		
Rembrandt Dazzling White Toothpaste: 0.76% sodium monofluorophosphate, 6% carbamide peroxide, papain/sodium citrate (citroxain)		
Rembrandt Whitening Toothpaste★: 44% dicalcium phosphate dihydrate, 0.76% sodium monofluorophosphate (1,000 ppm), papain/sodium citrate (citroxain)		
Sensiv for Sensitive Teeth: Ingredients not available.		
Sensodyne Extra Whitening: 5% potassium nitrate, 0.243% sodium fluoride, pentasodium triphosphate		
PLAQUE AND/OR GINGIVITIS REDUCTION*		
Colgate Total Toothpaste★, Colgate Total Clean Mint Toothpaste★, Colgate Total Fresh Stripe Toothpaste★, Colgate Total Mint Stripe Gel★: 0.243% sodium fluoride, 0.30% triclosan	See manufacturer's labeling for specific brand information.	Allergic reaction, burning sensation, bitter taste. Products containing stannous fluoride may produce reversible staining of teeth.
Colgate Total Advanced Clean Toothpaste★, Colgate Total Advanced Fresh Gel★, Colgate Total 2 in 1 Advanced Fresh Liquid Toothpaste★: 0.243% sodium fluoride, 0.30% triclosan		
Crest Pro-Health Toothpaste (Clean Cinnamon, Clean Mint)★: 0.454% stannous fluoride (active ingredient), sodium hexametaphosphate (tartar reduction and stain inhibition ingredient)		
Viadent Advanced Care Toothpaste: 2% zinc citrate, 0.8% sodium monofluorophosphate		

Table 9.3: USAGE INFORMATION FOR DENTIFRICES *(cont.)*

NAME/ACTIVE INGREDIENTS	WARNINGS/PRECAUTIONS	ADVERSE EFFECTS
SENSITIVITY REDUCTION§¶		
Aquafresh Sensitive Toothpaste: 5% potassium nitrate, 0.243% sodium fluoride	Differential diagnosis is important to rule out other reasons for sensitivity—for example, cracked tooth or caries. Toothpastes containing 5% potassium nitrate are not recommended for children < 12 yrs. See manufacturer's labeling for specific brand information.	Allergic reactions (most products contain parabens, to which some patients may be allergic).
Butler Maximum Strength Sensitive Toothpaste: 5% potassium nitrate, 0.22% sodium fluoride		
Colgate Sensitive Maximum Strength: 5% potassium nitrate, 0.454% stannous fluoride		
Colgate Sensitive Plus Whitening Toothpaste: 5% potassium nitrate; 0.24% sodium fluoride (0.14% W/V fluoride ion)		
Crest Pro-Health Toothpaste (Clean Cinnamon, Clean Mint)★: 0.454% stannous fluoride (active ingredient), sodium hexametaphosphate (tartar reduction and stain inhibition ingredient)		
Crest Sensitivity Protection Soothing Whitening Mint Paste★: 5% potassium nitrate, 0.243% sodium fluoride		
Dr. Fresh T-Sensitive Toothpaste, Dr. Fresh T-Sensitive Tartar Control Toothpaste		
Orajel Sensitive Pain-Relieving Toothpaste for Adults★: 5% potassium nitrate, 1.15% sodium monofluorophosphate		
Oral-B Sensitive with Fluoride Paste: 5% potassium nitrate, sodium fluoride (0.14% w/v fluoride ion)		
Protect Sensitive Teeth Gel Toothpaste: 5% potassium nitrate, 0.243% sodium fluoride		
Protect Desensitizing Solution (with activating swabs): hydroxypropyl cellulose, potassium fluoride, polyethyleneglycol dimethacrylate and other methacrylates		
Rembrandt Whitening Toothpaste for Sensitive Teeth: 5% potassium nitrate, 0.76% sodium monofluorophosphate, sodium citrate		
Sensodyne Baking Soda, Sensodyne Cool Gel, Sensodyne Fresh Impact: 5% potassium nitrate, 0.243 % sodium fluoride		
Sensodyne Original, Sensodyne Fresh Mint: 5% potassium nitrate, sodium fluoride (0.13% w/v fluoride ion)		
Sensodyne Extra Whitening: 5% potassium nitrate, 0.243% sodium fluoride, pentasodium triphosphate		
Sensodyne Tartar Control Plus Whitening: 5% potassium nitrate, sodium fluoride (0.145% w/v fluoride ion), tetrasodium pyrophosphate		
Sensodyne Toothpaste for Sensitive Teeth, Tartar Control Plus Whitening: 5% potassium nitrate, sodium fluoride (0.145% w/v fluoride ion), tetrasodium pyrophosphate		

★indicates a product bearing the ADA Seal of Acceptance.
*These dentifrices also possess caries-preventive properties.
†Fluoride from sodium fluoride, sodium monofluorophosphate or stannous fluoride.
‡Private label manufacturer.
§All these dentifrices also possess caries-preventive properties except for Protect Desensitizing Solution.
¶In sensitivity-reduction dentifrices, fluoride is the active agent only for caries prevention; the exception is stannous fluoride, which has both caries-preventive and sensitivity-reducing properties.

Chapter 10

Fluorides

Kenneth H. Burrell, D.D.S., S.M.

With today's array of available fluoride products, it is not surprising that confusion abounds concerning their proper use. Factors that should be taken into account when considering a fluoride regimen are the age of the patient, the patient's caries risk and other caries-producing factors.

Age of the patient. Patients less than 6 years are at risk of developing enamel fluorosis from excessive amounts of fluoride in the water supply, inappropriate and injudicious use of fluoride supplements and regular, inadvertent ingestion of fluoride-containing over-the-counter products such as toothpaste. Ingestion of fluoride in food products also contributes to a child's total daily fluoride intake.

Improper use of fluoride supplements by itself can cause fluorosis. Patients should follow instructions on the labels of over-the-counter fluoride-containing products so that they can avoid unintended fluoride ingestion.

The patient's caries risk. According to the Centers for Disease Control and Prevention, "populations believed to be at increased risk for dental caries are those with low socioeconomic status or low levels of parental education, those who do not seek regular dental care, and those without dental insurance or access to dental services. Individual factors that possibly increase risk include active dental caries; a history of high caries experience in older siblings or caregivers; root surfaces exposed by gingival recession; high levels of infection with cariogenic bacteria; impaired ability to maintain oral hygiene; malformed enamel or dentin; reduced salivary flow because of medications, radiation treatment,

or disease; low salivary buffering capacity (i.e., decreased ability of saliva to neutralize acids); and the wearing of space maintainers, orthodontic appliances, or dental prostheses. Risk can increase if any of these factors are combined with dietary practices conducive to dental caries (i.e., frequent consumption of refined carbohydrates). Risk decreases with adequate exposure to fluoride." Patients without caries or with a low risk of caries may require nothing more than the 0.7 to 1.2 parts per million fluoride in the municipal water supply or, if at increased risk, an appropriate fluoride-supplement dosage schedule, along with the daily use of a fluoride-containing dentifrice. Patients with moderate risk may require the additional use of a 0.05% sodium fluoride over-the-counter mouthrinse or a 0.4% stannous fluoride gel, preferably at times other than when brushing with a fluoride toothpaste. Patients with an increased risk of caries may also require the daily use of neutral or acidulated 1.1% sodium fluoride gel and annual or semiannual applications of higher concentration fluoride gels, solutions or varnishes.

Other caries-producing factors. A patient's existing fluoride regimen is an important part of his or her dental history, but, of course, it is not the only consideration when trying to determine risk of caries. The patient's oral hygiene regimen, diet and medical history, and whether pit and fissure sealants have been placed on newly erupted teeth must also be taken into account. Twice-daily brushing and once-daily interdental cleaning, usually with floss, should be adequate for patients with low caries risk, provided these procedures are done properly and thoroughly. A well-balanced diet with a minimum amount of snacking also should reduce the risks of dental caries. Important events in a patient's medical history can change that regimen, however. Diminished salivary flow, or xerostomia, can be caused by medications, head and neck irradiation for cancer treatments and some diseases, such as Sjögren's syndrome. Xerostomia can increase the caries risk dramatically so that a patient's diet, oral hygiene and fluoride use may require modification after its onset.

Clinical judgment is important for successful treatment. Correct diagnosis as a result of careful history-taking, meticulous examination and competent interpretation of diagnostic tests can increase the likelihood of successful prevention or treatment outcome.

Fluoridated Water and Fluoride Supplements

Accepted Indications

Fluoride in community and school water supplies is responsible to a great degree for the fact that most people in the United States have a low risk of experiencing dental caries. When fluoride levels in drinking water are below 0.6 ppm and when children from 6 months to 16 years are considered to be at increased risk of experiencing dental caries, a fluoride supplement should be prescribed (see Table 10.1). An analysis of the home drinking water may not be adequate, however. The patient's parents or guardians may need to be questioned about the child's usual source of drinking water. For example, daycare centers may have fluoridated drinking water that is at levels adequate to preclude prescribing a fluoride supplement.

General Dosing Information

The recommended concentration of fluoride in fluoridated water supply systems that offers the maximum reduction in dental caries with the minimal amount of enamel mottling or fluorosis varies with the annual average of maximum daily air temperature (people living in warmer climates tend to drink more water than those in cooler climates). It may range from 0.7 ppm in Houston, Texas, to 1.2 ppm in Duluth, Minnesota.

The fluoride level in drinking water is a major factor in determining the dosage for fluoride supplements that are used for children between the ages of 6 months and 16 years. Many bottled waters do not contain optimal amounts of fluoride. Table 10.1 shows the recommended fluoride supplement dosage schedule.

Systemic dosing of fluoride supplements is typically prescribed in the form of either drops, tablets or swish-and-swallow solutions.

General dosage forms include tablets and lozenges available in 0.25 mg, 0.50 mg and 1 mg. Fluoride drops are available in various concentrations, which affects the number of drops per dose. Thus, it is important to specify the concentration of the drops prescribed. A combination fluoride supplement/mouthrinse is also available, with each 5 mL (one teaspoonful) containing 1 mg of fluoride from 2.20 mg of sodium fluoride and orthophosphoric acid.

Prenatal fluoride. The efficacy of prenatal dietary fluoride supplements in preventing dental caries has been well-established in animal studies. However, well-designed clinical studies to demonstrate the safety and efficacy of prenatal fluoride in preventing caries in human subjects still are lacking. Therefore, no definitive recommendations regarding the use of prenatal fluoride can be made. Furthermore, prenatal dietary fluoride supplements will not affect the permanent dentition because permanent teeth do not begin to develop in utero.

Maximum Recommended Doses

No more than 120 mg of fluoride should be dispensed per household at one time. One tablet of the prescribed dose should be taken per day with water or juice. Taking fluoride supplements with milk and other dairy products is not recommended because they can combine with the calcium to become poorly absorbed calcium fluoride. The tablet strength is determined by the concentration of fluoride in the patient's source of drinking water and the age of the child. Tables 10.1 and 10.2 show the maximum recommended dose: 1 mg per day.

Dosage Adjustments

The actual maximum dose for each patient must be individualized depending on the patient's weight, age, physical status and other dietary sources of fluoride intake. Reduced doses may be indicated for patients based on changes in their water supply's fluoride content, which may result from relocation or any adverse side effects experienced.

Special Dental Considerations

Drug Interactions of Dental Interest

Calcium-containing products and food interfere with the absorption of systemic fluoride.

Cross-Sensitivity

Allergic rash and other idiosyncratic reactions have rarely been reported. Gastric distress, headache and weakness have been reported in cases of excessive ingestion.

Special Patients

Fluoride supplements are not recommended for patients other than children with high caries risk who live in areas with fluoride levels such as those described in Table 10.1.

Patient Monitoring: Aspects to Watch

Fluoride supplements can cause fluorosis in children living in areas where drinking water contains fluoride levels at or above 0.6 ppm (Table 10.1).

Adverse Effects and Precautions

No adverse reactions or undesirable side effects have been reported when fluoride supplements have been taken as directed. Excessive use may result in dental fluorosis, especially in areas where the fluoride level in drinking water is high. Therefore, fluoride supplements are not recommended where the water content of fluoride is at or above 0.6 ppm.

In children, acute ingestion of 10-20 mg of sodium fluoride can cause excessive salivation and gastrointestinal disturbances. Ingestion of 500 mg can be fatal. Oral or intravenous fluids containing calcium, or both, may be indicated.

Precautions. If the fluoride level is unknown, the drinking water must be tested for fluoride content before supplements are prescribed. For testing information, ask the local or state health department or dental school. Determining a proper dosage schedule can be a complex task if a patient has exposure to a number of different water supplies. Once a proper schedule is established, however, the effectiveness of the schedule requires the patient's long-term compliance.

Contraindications. The fluoride dosage schedule was designed to take into account the widespread use of fluorides that can contribute to the increased frequency and severity of fluorosis. Fluoride supplements are contraindicated for children drinking water with fluoride concentrations at or above 0.6 ppm.

Pharmacology

Mechanism of action/effect. After early studies showed that fluoride reduced the solubility of powdered enamel and dentin, investigators began trying to determine how fluoride works to reduce dental caries. However, the mechanism or mechanisms of action are still incompletely understood. Nevertheless, fluoride is thought to work topically. It has been speculated that a combination of actions work to reduce the severity and frequency of dental caries, which is the result of excessive demineralization in the demineralization-remineralization process. This excessive demineralization occurs after repeated acid attacks that result when bacterial plaque metabolizes sugars ingested during meals and snacks. Clinical manifestations of dental caries become evident when demineralization predominates over time and upsets the demineralization-remineralization equilibrium. Fluoride reduces the demineralization of enamel and dentin by reducing the acid production of bacterial plaque and decreasing the solubility of apatite crystals. When fluoride is exposed to apatite crystals, it readily becomes incorporated to reduce the dissolution of apatite during acid attacks. The presence of fluoride, therefore, inhibits demineralization and helps to maintain the equilibrium between demineralization and remineralization during acid attacks.

Absorption. Fluoride is absorbed in the gastrointestinal tract, 90% of it in the stomach. Calcium, iron or magnesium ions may delay absorption.

Distribution. After absorption, 50% of fluoride is deposited in bones and teeth in healthy young adults, 80% in children. Bones and teeth account for 99% of the fluoride taken up by the body.

Elimination. The major route of excretion is the kidneys. Fluoride is also excreted by the sweat glands, the tear glands, the gastrointestinal tract and in breast milk.

Patient Advice

- Patients and their parents or guardians should be advised to take systemic fluorides as directed.
- Patients or their parents or guardians should notify the prescriber when their water supply has changed as the result of a move or a change in schools or by the addition of fluoride to the water supply.

- These products should be kept from children's reach; they are often formulated to have a pleasant taste and children therefore are more likely to consume them if they are easily accessible.

Topically Applied Fluorides

Accepted Indications

Topically applied preparations are used in the prevention and treatment of dental caries. Concentrations of 1,500 ppm or below are sold as over-the-counter preparations for the prevention of dental caries. Preparations that are prescribed for topical home use generally consist of higher concentrations of fluoride and are indicated for both treatment and prevention. Patients who are either at high risk of developing dental caries or who experience high caries rates are candidates for daily use of these products. However, high-concentration preparations that are usually applied annually in children are applied to prevent caries.

Some kinds of fluoride compounds at certain concentrations can be used to reduce dentinal hypersensitivity. Sodium fluoride (151,000 ppm fluoride ion), in equal amounts of kaolin and glycerin, has been shown to be effective for this purpose when professionally applied and burnished into affected areas using orangewood sticks. A water-free 0.4% (1,000 ppm fluoride ion) stannous fluoride gel has also been demonstrated to reduce dentinal hypersensitivity when patients use it daily at home. A dentifrice containing 0.454% stannous fluoride and 5% potassium nitrate also has been shown to reduce dentin hypersensitivity.

Further, a stabilized 0.454% stannous fluoride toothpaste has been shown to reduce plaque activity, gingivitis and dentinal hypersensitivity.

General Dosing Information

Topical dosing is typically provided in the form of liquid solutions, gels, foams, varnishes, pastes, rinses and dentifrices. Concentrations can vary depending on oral health and sensitivity, the particular indication involved, region of treatment, response to previous or existing concentrations and doses of fluoride as well as individual patient characteristics such as age, weight, physical status, and ability to effectively rinse and expectorate. See Table 10.3.

Doses of topically applied solutions, gels, foams and varnishes are typically applied with a cotton swab, a toothbrush, a carrier or as a rinse. To control the dosing of high fluoride concentrations so that excessive amounts of fluoride are not in the mouth and to control salivary contamination, cotton rolls, a saliva ejector or high vacuum suction can be used. Because varnishes are applied to adhere to teeth for prolonged periods, all residual fluoride is swallowed. Between 0.3 and 0.5 mL of varnish is used per patient so that about 5-11 mg is ingested. This amount is consistent with ingestion calculations for other professionally applied fluoride preparations.

With fluoride dentifrices, brushing more than twice a day may be required, but this depends on the patient's caries risk. A 0.4% stannous fluoride gel might be considered as an alternative to brushing with a dentifrice, however. In this way, the patient can receive the benefit of the same fluoride exposure as with the dentifrice without a dentifrice's cleansing properties, which may not be necessary.

Maximum Recommended Doses

The maximum recommended doses for topical fluoride formulations per procedure or appointment are listed in Table 10.4.

Dosage Adjustments

The actual maximum dose for each patient can be individualized depending on the patient's age and physical status, ability to effectively rinse and expectorate, and oral health and sensitivity.

Special Dental Considerations

Cross-Sensitivity

Although allergies to fluoride probably do not exist, patients may be allergic to some of the ingredients in the various formulations. Some of the 1.23% acidulated phosphate fluoride solutions and gels and some dentifrices contain tartrazines used as color additives. They can cause allergic reactions, especially in patients with hypersensitivity to aspirin.

Adverse Effects and Precautions

Excessive ingestion of fluoride products can produce acute and chronic effects. Ingestion of quantities of fluoride as low as 1 mg per day have been shown to produce mild fluorosis in a small percentage of the population if the ingestion takes place during tooth crown development. The severity and frequency of fluorosis can increase in a population if the recommended dose is exceeded and if the quantity of daily fluoride ingestion increases. Chronic fluoride toxicity, or skeletal fluorosis, may occur after years of daily ingestion of 20-80 mg of fluoride; however, such heavy doses are far in excess of the average intake in the United States. There is no evidence that skeletal changes are produced by ingestion of therapeutic doses of fluoride, however.

Accidental ingestion of fluoride, > 120 mg in the form of fluoride supplements and mouthrinses or > 260 mg in a toothpaste, can cause gastrointestinal disturbances such as excessive salivation, nausea, vomiting, abdominal pain and diarrhea. Central nervous system disturbances that have been observed include irritability, paresthesia, tetany and convulsions. Respiratory and cardiac failure have also been observed. See Table 10.3.

Therefore, as a precautionary measure, no large quantities of fluoride-containing products should be stored in the home. The American Dental Association recommends that no more than 120 mg should be prescribed at one time in the form of monthrinses and supplements and no individual toothpaste tube should contain more than 260 mg of fluoride. Toothpaste may contain the greater quantity of fluoride because dentifrice humectants and detergents induce vomiting.

Laboratory studies have shown that low-pH topical fluoride preparations react with glass and quartz filler particles in resin-based composites and dental ceramics (porcelains). Although this reaction is not noticeable after one application, the cumulative effect of several applications may compromise the esthetic appearance of these kinds of restorations. Therefore, it is prudent to consider using nonacidic fluoride preparations with patients who have extensive ceramic and composite restorations when daily applications are required.

Pharmacology
See the discussion earlier in this chapter.

Patient Advice
Although the gel form of 2% neutral sodium fluoride may be more easily applied, clinical evidence of its effectiveness has not been demonstrated. The original application schedule was 4 times per year and was for children at the specific ages of 3, 7, 10, and 13 years. Currently the caries-inhibiting properties of this solution are considered to be equivalent to the APF gels and solutions, which contain a higher concentration of fluoride (12,300 ppm).

Suggested Readings

American Dental Association Council on Scientific Affairs. Professionally applied topical fluoride: evidence-based clinical recommendations. JADA 2006;137(8):1151-59.

Centers for Disease Control and Prevention, National Center for Chronic Disease Prevention and Health Promotion, Division of Oral Health. Recommendations for using fluoride to prevent and control dental caries in the United States. MMWR Recomm Rep 2001 Aug 17;50(RR-14):1-42.

Levy SM. Review of fluoride exposures and ingestion. Community Dent Oral Epidemiol 1994;22(3):173-80.

Newbrun E. Current regulations and recommendations concerning water fluoridation, fluoride supplements, and topical fluoride agents. J Dent Res 1992;71(5):1255-65.

Ripa LW. A critique of topical fluoride methods (dentifrices, mouthrinses, operator-, and self-applied gels) in an era of decreased caries and increased fluorosis prevalence. J Public Health Dent 1991;51(1):23-41.

Ripa LW. Review of the anticaries effectiveness of professionally applied and self-applied topical fluoride gels. J Public Health Dent 1989;49(5):297-309.

Twetman S, Axelsson S, Dahlgren H, et al. Caries-preventive effect of fluoride toothpaste: a systematic review. Acta Odontol Scand 2003 Dec;61(6):347-55.

Twetman S, Petersson L, Axelsson S, et al. Caries-preventive effect of sodium fluoride mouthrinses: a systematic review of controlled clinical trials. Acta Odontol Scand 2004 Aug;62(4):223-30.

Warren DP, Chan JT. Topical fluorides: efficacy, administration, and safety. J Acad Gen Dent 1997;45(2):134-40, 142.

Whitford GM, Allmann DW, Shaked AR. Topical fluoride: effects on physiologic and biochemical process. J Dent Res 1987;66(5):1072-8.

Table 10.1: DOSAGE FOR SYSTEMIC FLUORIDE SUPPLEMENTS*

AGE	FLUORIDE ION LEVEL IN DRINKING WATER (PPM)†		
	< 0.3	0.3-0.6	>0.6
Birth-6 mo	None	None	None
6 mo-3 yrs	0.25 mg/day‡	None	None
3-6 yrs	0.50 mg/day	0.25 mg/day	None
6-16 yrs	1.0 mg/day	0.50 mg/day	None

*Recommended dosage schedule of the American Dental Association, the American Academy of Pediatric Dentistry and the American Academy of Pediatrics.
†1.0 ppm = 1mg/liter.
‡2.2mg sodium fluoride contains 1mg fluoride ion.

Table 10.2: PRESCRIBING INFORMATION FOR FLUORIDE SUPPLEMENTS

NAME/STRENGTH	FORM/BRAND(S)	CHILD DOSAGE[†]	MAX CHILD DOSAGE
Sodium fluoride, drops—2mg/mL fluoride	**Drops:** Luride★, Pediaflor	½ dropperful = 0.25mg 1 dropperful = 0.5mg 2 droppersful = 1mg	Prescribe no more than 200 mL per household.
Sodium fluoride, drops—flouride	**Drops:** Karidium	2 drops = 0.25mg 4 drops = 0.5mg 8 drops = 1mg	Prescribe no more than 30 mL per household.
Sodium fluoride, drops—2.5mg/mL flouride	**Drops:** Fluor-A-Day★	2 drops = 0.25mg 4 drops = 0.5mg 8 drops = 1mg	Prescribe no more than 30 mL per household.
Sodium fluoride, drops—5mg/mL flouride	**Drops:** Fluoritab★, Flura-Drops	1 drop = 0.25mg 2 drops = 0.5mg 4 drops = 1mg	Prescribe no more than 23 mL per household.
Sodium fluoride, rinse—0.2mg/mL fluoride	**Rinses:** Phos-Flur★	1mg fluoride/teaspoonful (0.2mg fluoride/mL) swished for 1 min then swallowed	Prescribe no more than 500mL per household.
Sodium fluoride, tablets and lozenges—0.25mg fluoride	**Tablets:** Fluor-A-Day★, Fluoritab★, Luride Lozi-Tabs★ **Lozenges:** Fluor-A-Day★	1 tablet or lozenge per day taken with water or juice and dissolved in mouth or chewed	Prescribe no more than 480 tablets or lozenges per household.
Sodium fluoride, tablets and lozenges—0.5mg fluoride	**Tablets:** Fluor-A-Day★, Fluoritab★, Luride Lozi-Tabs★ **Lozenges:** Fluor-A-Day★, Fluorodex Pharmaflur 1.1	1 tablet or lozenge per day taken with water or juice and dissolved in mouth or chewed	Prescribe no more than 240 tablets or lozenges per household.
Sodium fluoride, tablets and lozenges—1mg fluoride	**Tablets:** Fluor-A-Day★, Fluoritab★, Flura-Loz, Luride Lozi-Tabs★ **Lozenges:** Fluor-A-Day★, Pharmaflur, Pharmaflur df	1 tablet or lozenge per day taken with water or juice and dissolved in mouth or chewed	Prescribe no more than 120 tablets or lozenges per household.

★indicates a product bearing the ADA Seal of Acceptance.
[†]These supplements are for children only. There is no dose for adult or geriatric patients.

Table 10.3: PRESCRIBING INFORMATION FOR TOPICAL FLUORIDES

NAME	DOSAGE†	WARNINGS/PRECAUTIONS & CONTRAINDICATIONS	ADVERSE EFFECTS
PROFESSIONALLY APPLIED FLUORIDE PRODUCTS			
Acidulated phosphate fluoride solutions, gels and foams (1.23% fluoride ion, 12,300 ppm fluoride ion) (AllSolutions APF Foam or Gel, Butler APF Fluoride Foam or Gel, Laclede, Oral-B Minute Foam, Care-4, Fluorident, FluoroCare Time Saver, Oral-B Minute Gel, Perfect Choice, Pro-DenRx, Puff Fluoride Foam, Topex 00:60 Second Fluoride Foam, Gel or Rinse)	**Adults:** 5mL (approximately one-third of a tray) of solution or gel with 12,300 ppm fluoride ion per fluoride carrier; apply for 4 min once/y or more frequently as needed. **Max:** 10mL.	**W/P:** Some preparations may contain tartrazines (FDC Yellow No. 5), which are used as color additives; tartrazine can cause allergic reactions, including bronchial asthma. Allergic response is rare, but is frequently observed in patients who also experience hypersensitivity to aspirin. **Contra:** Patients allergic to tartrazine.	(CNS) Inadvertent ingestion can produce headaches and weakness; more severe instances of excessive ingestion can cause CNS problems such as irritability, paresthesia, tetany, convulsions, respiratory failure and cardiac failure; fluoride has direct toxic action on nerve tissue. (GI) Excessive salivation, nausea, vomiting. Hema: Excessive amounts of fluoride can also cause electrolyte disturbances leading to hypocalcemia and hyperkalemia; hypoglycemia is a result of failure of enzyme systems. (Musc) Fluoride has a direct toxic action on muscle and nerve tissue.
2% neutral sodium fluoride solutions, gels or foams (0.90% fluoride ion, 9,050 fluoride ion) (AllSolutions Fluoride Foam or Rinse; Butler Neutral Fluoride Foam, Gel or Rinse; FluoroCare Neutral; Neutra-Foam; Oral-B Neutrafoam; Pro-DenRx Gel or Rinse; Topex Neutral pH)	**Adults:** 5mL (approximately one-third of a tray) of solution, gel or foam with 9,050 ppm fluoride ion per fluoride carrier; apply once/y or more frequently as needed. **Max:** 10mL.	**W/P:** Not to be used with other professionally applied topical fluoride preparations.	(CV) Excessive amounts of fluoride can produce cardiac failure. (CNS) Excessive amounts of fluoride can produce irritability, paresthesia, tetany, convulsions; fluoride has direct toxic action on nerve tissue. (GI) Excessive amounts of fluoride can produce GI disturbances such as excess salivation, nausea, abdominal pain, vomiting and diarrhea. Hema: Excessive amounts of fluoride can cause electrolyte disturbances leading to hypocalcemia and hyperkalemia. Hypoglycemia is a result of enzyme systems failure. (Musc) Fluoride has direct toxic action on muscle tissue. (Resp) Excessive amounts of fluoride can produce respiratory failure.
Fluoride-containing varnishes, 5% sodium fluoride (2.26% fluoride ion, 22,600 ppm fluoride ion) (AllSolutions Varnish, CavityShield, Duraflor, Duraphat, Fluor Protector, Varnish America)	**Adults:** 0.3-0.5mL of varnish containing 22,600 ppm fluoride ion after dental prophylaxis. **Max:** 0.5mL.	**W/P:** Not to be used in conjunction with other high-concentration topical fluoride solutions when varnish is applied to all tooth surfaces; use of some formulations can result in a temporary yellow discoloration of teeth, which patient can brush away 2-6 h after fluoride application.	(CNS) Inadvertent ingestion can produce headaches and weakness; more severe instances of excessive ingestion can cause CNS problems such as irritability, paresthesia, tetany, convulsions, respiratory failure and cardiac failure; fluoride has direct toxic action on nerve tissue. (Hema) Excessive amounts of fluoride can also cause electrolyte disturbances leading to hypocalcemia and hyperkalemia; hypoglycemia is a result of failure of enzyme systems. (Musc) Fluoride has a direct toxic action on muscle and nerve tissue.
Fluoride prophylaxis pastes (0.40% - 2% fluoride ion, 4,000-20,000 ppm fluoride) (Butler Fluoride Prophylaxis Paste, Butler NuCare Prophy Paste with Novamin, Glitter, Masnasil, Post Prophy, Prophy Gems, Radent, Teledyne Waterpik Prophylaxis Paste, Topex, Unipro Prophy Paste, Zircon F, Ziroxide)	**Adults:** Use amount sufficient to polish the teeth (4,000-20,000 ppm fluoride ion). **Max:** Use no more than the amount required to polish the teeth.	**W/P:** Should be thoroughly rinsed from mouth on completion of prophylaxis.	(Oral) Excessive polishing may remove more fluoride from the enamel surface than fluoride prophylaxis paste can replace.

★indicates a product bearing the ADA Seal of Acceptance.   NA = not available.   †Geriatric dosage is same as adult dosage.

Table 10.3: PRESCRIBING INFORMATION FOR TOPICAL FLUORIDES (cont.)

NAME	DOSAGE†	WARNINGS/PRECAUTIONS & CONTRAINDICATIONS	ADVERSE EFFECTS
PRESCRIPTION FLUORIDES			
1.1% neutral or acidulated sodium fluoride gel or dentifrice (0.50% fluoride ion, 5,000ppm fluoride ion) (Cavarest, ControlRx, EtheDent, Karigel-N★, Luride Lozi-Tabs★, Oral-B Neutracare, NeutraGard Advanced Gel, PreviDent Gel, PreviDent 5000 Booster, PreviDent 5000 Plus, Pro-DenRx 1.1% Plus, Theraflur-N★)	***Adults:*** 4-8 drops on inner surface of each custom-made tray per day (5,000 ppm fluoride ion). **Max:** Maximum amount pre-scribed is one 24-mL plastic squeeze bottle; maximum adult dose is 16 drops/day.	**W/P:** Repeated use of acidulated fluoride has been shown to etch glass filler particles in composite restorations and porcelain crowns, facings and laminates. As with all fluoride products, children < age 6yrs should be supervised to prevent their swallowing the product, which can lead to fluorosis, nausea and vomiting.	(Oral) Patients with mucositis may report irritation to the acidulated preparation.
0.2% neutral sodium fluoride rinses (0.09% fluoride ion, 905 ppm fluoride ion solution) (CaviRinse, NaFrinse★, Oral-B Fluorinse, PreviDent Dental Rinse★)	***Adults:*** Recommended for use by children (905 ppm fluoride ion solution): 10mL (2mg fluoride); swish for 1 min, then spit out the solu-tion; use once/day.	**Contra:** Should not be used in children < age 6 yrs because they cannot rinse without significant swallowing and this product is not for systemic use. Should not be swallowed by children of any age and should be kept from their reach.	(General) Allergic reaction could result from flavoring agent. (GI) Nausea and vomiting may result from inadvertent swallowing. (Oral) Irritation of oral tissues, especially in children with mucositis, may result from alcohol that might be part of the formulation.
0.044% sodium fluoride and acidulated phosphate fluoride rinses (0.02% fluoride ion) (OrthoWash, Phos-Flur★)	***Adults:*** 10mL once daily after brushing (200 ppm fluoride ion solution).	NA	NA
OVER-THE-COUNTER FLUORIDES			
Fluoride-containing dentifrices (0.10- 0.15% fluoride ion, 1,000-1,500 ppm fluoride ion)‡	***Adults:*** Amount sufficient to cover toothbrush bristles: ≈1g per day (1,000-1,500 ppm fluoride ion). **Max:** Twice a day or more as recommended.	**W/P:** To prevent fluorosis, supervise children < age 6yrs so that swal-lowing does not occur. Accidental ingestion of a single dose, which contains 1-2mg of fluoride ion, is not harmful. Intentional ingestion of large amounts of fluoride toothpaste can cause gastric irritation, nausea and vomiting. No single container should exceed 260mg of fluoride ion (it is thought that quantity of fluoride in dentifrice can exceed the 120-mg limit ADA has established for other fluoride containing products because dentifrices contain humectants and detergents that induce vomiting).	(General) Allergic reactions thought to be caused by flavoring agents in some formulations (mintflavored products have been reported to cause these reac-tions; however, as a variety of flavoring agents is available, patient should be advised to change to another flavor until a suitable product is found).
0.4% stannous fluoride gels (0.10% fluoride ion, 1,000 ppm fluoride ion) (Alpha-Dent★, Easy-Gel, Florentine II, Gel-Kam★, Gel- Kam Oral Rinse, Gel-Tin★, Kids Choice★, Omnii Gel★, Omnii Just for Kids★, Oral-B Stop, Perfect Choice★, Periocheck Oral Med★, PerioMed, Plak Smacker★, Pro-DenRx, Schein Home Care, Super-Dent★, Tandem Perio Rinse, Topex Take Home Care)	***Adults:*** Amount sufficient to cover toothbrush bristles: ≈1g per day (1,000 ppm fluoride ion). **Max:** Once a day or more as recommended.	**W/P:** Children < age 6yrs should be supervised to prevent swallowing and fluorosis; accidental ingestion of a single dose (1- to 2-mg ribbon of gel) is not harmful. Intentional ingestion of large amounts of gel can cause gastric irritation, nausea and vomiting. No single container should exceed 120mg of fluoride.	(General) Allergic reactions thought to be caused by flavoring agents in some formulations (mintflavored products have been reported to cause these reactions; however, as a variety of flavoring agents is available, patient should be advised to change to another flavor until a suitable product is found). Reversible black stain may occur in pits and fissures and along cervical aspect of a tooth or teeth.

★indicates a product bearing the ADA Seal of Acceptance.
NA = not available.
†Geriatric dosage is same as adult dosage.
‡See Table 9.3 in Chapter 9 for a list of products.

NAME	DOSAGE†	WARNINGS/PRECAUTIONS & CONTRAINDICATIONS	ADVERSE EFFECTS
0.05% sodium fluoride rinses (0.02% fluoride ion) (ACT Anticavity Fluoride Rinse★, ACT Anticavity Fluoride Rinse for Kids★, Fluorigard, NaFrinse Acidulated Oral Rinse★, NaFrinse Neutral/Daily Mouthrinse★, REACH ACT Restoring★)	***Adults:*** 10mL of solution with 230 ppm fluoride ion. **Max:** Rinse for 1 min, once daily.	**W/P:** Children aged < 6 yrs generally should not use this product because of their inability to rinse without swallowing; otherwise, accidental ingestion of a single dose is not harmful. Intentional ingestion of several doses can cause gastric irritation, nausea and vomiting. Some of these products contain alcohol to promote solubility of flavoring agents; these products should be kept out of children's reach and in childproof caps/packaging.	(General) Allergic reactions thought to be caused by flavoring agents in some formulations (mintflavored products have been reported to cause these reactions; however, as a variety of flavoring agents is available, patient should be advised to change to another flavor until a suitable product is found).

Table 10.4: MAXIMUM RECOMMENDED FLUORIDE DOSES PER APPOINTMENT

FORM	MAXIMUM DOSE
1.23% acidulated phosphate fluoride solution, gel or foam	10mL
5% sodium fluoride-containing varnish	0.3-0.5mL
Fluoride toothpaste for children < 6 yrs	Pea-sized amount (0.25g)
1.1% neutral and acidulated sodium fluoride gel drops	0.2-0.4mL
2% neutral sodium fluoride	10mL
0.05% sodium fluoride mouthrinse for children > 6 yrs*	10mL

*Mouthrinses are not recommended for children <6 yrs.

Chapter 11

Desensitizing Agents

Martha Somerman, D.D.S., Ph.D.

Dentin hypersensitivity is characterized by a sharp pain produced in response to mild stimuli that usually disappears with removal of the stimulus. Root sensitivity is a significant problem for many patients and may be a result of, or associated with, scaling and root planing, periodontal surgery, gingival recession, toothbrush abrasion, attrition, erosion, trauma or chronic periodontal disease. It is important to rule out active pathology (for example, root fracture or root surface decay) before providing treatment for root sensitivity. In many situations, root sensitivity decreases with time, but when it does not, it results in extreme discomfort or an inability to eat or drink certain foods, inability to function outdoors in cold weather and, at times, poor oral hygiene that can result in periodontal-related problems. Unfortunately, ideal OTC and professional desensitizing agents with predictable outcomes have not been developed.

Desensitizing agents can be separated into two types: agents applied to the tooth by a practitioner and agents that are for home use. Table 11.1 provides information about currently available products for use in the clinical setting. A major concern with products for home use is the abrasiveness of the paste; however, all ADA-accepted toothpastes have safe levels of abrasive materials.

In-Office Products

Accepted Indications
In-office desensitizing agents are used to provide relief from thermal and tactile sensitivity on exposed root surfaces when pathological causes for pain have been ruled out. Agents containing fluoride also provide an anticaries function. Differential diagnoses for dentinal hypersensitivity are listed in Table 11.2.

Some of the desensitizing agents may be applied in conjunction with iontophoresis, which is the electrical transport of positively or negatively charged drugs across surface tissues. One of the uses of iontophoresis in dentistry is in the treatment of dentinal hypersensitivity with fluoride. Usually a 1% sodium fluoride solution is employed. Results are variable, and the time and cost of the treatment may limit patients' acceptance of it. Nd:YAG and CO_2 lasers also have been used for treating root sensitivity; however, results are not conclusive, and long-term effects on pulp have not been investigated.

General Usage Information

Usage and Administration for Adults and Children
See Table 11.1 for information on usage and administration. As with any agent, if pain persists or worsens, the situation should be re-evaluated. Overuse can be detrimental to tooth structure. Therefore, continued sensitivity, after ruling out other symptoms, can be treated by changing the product versus increasing the dose. Use of increased amounts, beyond those shown in Table 11.1, has not been reported to be effective in decreasing sensitivity.

Special Dental Considerations
- Fluorides interact with calcium-containing products—for example, to form calcium fluoride, which is poorly absorbed.

- Also, certain agents—for example, chlorhexidine—may decrease fluoride's ability to bind to root surfaces. Thus, after using fluoride agents, the patient should not rinse or eat for 1 hour.
- Because products with calcium sodium phosphosilicates do not contain fluoride, individuals may require additional agents/rinses with fluoride for caries control; fluoride products should be used at least 1 hour after the sensitivity treatment.
- Some agents are acidic and thus may cause sensitivity in patients with mucositis.
- Some acidic compounds—for example, oxalate—may cause dulling of porcelain ceramics and decreased effectiveness of bonding cements. Therefore, surfaces treated with oxalate should be pumiced before a bonding agent is used.

Special Patients

Pregnant and nursing women

There is no evidence that desensitizing agents are harmful to pregnant women or during breast feeding. While a minimal amount does cross the placental barrier if these agents are ingested and traces also are found in breast milk, no contraindications are reported when these agents are used as recommended.

Pediatric, geriatric and other special patients

In children, ingestion of high levels of fluoride will cause fluorosis of teeth and osseous changes. In older patients, there is no evidence suggesting a need to modify existing procedures.

Patient Monitoring: Aspects to Watch

- Persistent or increased pain: may require re-evaluation of differential diagnosis as well as consideration of alternative agents, therapies or both.

Adverse Effects and Precautions

Fluorides

Fluoride preparations should be kept out of reach of children. On rare occasions, adverse reactions to fluorides, including skin rash, GI upset and headaches, may be noted. Such reactions are reversible upon discontinuing use. Fluoride should not be swallowed.

Patients with gingival sensitivity may be sensitive to the acidity of certain fluoride solutions.

Acidic fluoride solutions may cause dulling of porcelain and ceramic restorations.

Oxalates

Acids may decrease the effectiveness of bonding cements; thus, teeth treated with oxalates should be pumiced before application of bonding agents.

Varnishes, Sealants and Bonding Agents

Copal-based products, such as Zarosen, cannot be used with bonding agents. No other adverse effects or precautions have been reported.

Pharmacology

The general principle guiding the development of desensitizing agents is that the number of dental tubules exposed to the mouth correlates with sensitivity; thus, many of the agents are designed to occlude tubules. The most popular theory, the "hydrodynamic theory," is that sensitivity in this situation results from the movement of fluid through the exposed tubules, which results in activation of the nerves within the pulp, subsequently registered as pain. A strategy used to decrease sensitivity, based on the hydrodynamic theory, includes the development of agents that can depolarize nerves directly.

Another theory of dentin hypersensitivity is that of the "dentinal receptor mechanism," which proposes that odontoblasts play a more receptive role; however, agents that induce pain normally fail to evoke pain when applied to exposed dentin. Yet a third theory is that certain polypeptides present within the pulp can modulate nerve impulses within the pulp. Thus, therapies have been directed at agents or procedures or both that can depolarize nerves directly.

Patient Advice

- Patients should be aware that, in general, several factors must be carefully considered in treatment of tooth sensitivity: severity of the problem, physical findings and past treatment. Proper diagnosis is required before initiation of treatment, whether in office or at home.
- Patients must realize that use of a desensitizing agent may not prove effective over a short time (for example, less than 2 weeks).

Home Use Products

Accepted Indications

Desensitizing toothpaste agents are used to provide relief from thermal and tactile sensitivity on exposed root surfaces when pathological causes for pain have been ruled out. In addition, many of these toothpastes contain fluoride to prevent caries.

General Usage Information

Usage and Administration

See Table 11.3 for general usage information on desensitizing toothpastes.

Special Dental Considerations

Following are special dental considerations for home use desensitizing agents, which are the same as or very similar to those for in-office products listed earlier in this chapter.

Drug Interactions of Dental Interest

- There is some suggestion of interaction of fluorides with calcium-containing products—for example, formation of calcium fluoride, which is poorly absorbed.

- Certain agents—for example, chlorhexidine—may decrease fluoride's ability to bind to the root surface. Thus, after using fluoride agents, the patient should not use any rinses or eat for 1 hour.
- Some agents are acidic and thus may cause sensitivity in patients with mucositis.
- Some acidic compounds—for example, oxalate—may cause dulling of porcelain ceramics and decreased effectiveness of bonding cements. Therefore, pumicing the root surface before use of some desensitizing agents is recommended.

Special Patients

There is no evidence that desensitizing agents are harmful to pregnant women or during breast feeding. In children, high levels of fluoride will cause fluorosis of teeth and osseous changes. In older patients, no alteration of dose is required.

Patient Monitoring: Aspects to Watch

- Persistent or increased pain may require re-evaluation of differential diagnosis and consideration of alternative agents, therapies or both.

Adverse Effects and Precautions

No adverse effects are reported beyond those related to high-dose fluoride. Precautions include the underlying possibility of an undiagnosed serious dental problem that may need prompt dental care. Products should not be used for more than 4 weeks unless recommended by the dentist. Keep out of reach of children. All patients, and especially those with severe dental erosion, should brush properly and lightly with any dentifrice to avoid further removal of tooth structure.

Pharmacology

The general principle guiding development of desensitizing agents, including toothpastes, is that the number of dental tubules exposed to the mouth correlates with sensitivity; thus, most agents are designed to occlude tubules. The most popular theory is that sensitivity in this situation is due to the movement of fluid through the exposed tubules, which results in activation of the nerves within the pulp and subsequently is registered as pain.

Patient Advice

* Patients should be aware that, in general, several factors must be carefully considered in treatment of tooth sensitivity: severity of the problem, physical findings and past treatment. Proper diagnosis is required before initiation of treatment, whether in office or at home.
* Patients must realize that use of a desensitizing agent will not prove effective over a short time unless the product is used for at least 2 weeks.

Suggested Reading

Gaffar A. Treating hypersensitivity with fluoride varnishes. Compend Contin Educ Dent 1998;19(11):1088-4.

Hilton TJ, Summitt JB. Pulpal considerations. In: Robbins JW, Schwartz RS, Summitt JB, eds. Fundamentals of operative dentistry: a contemporary approach. Chicago: Quintessence Publishing; 2001:91-113.

Jacobsen PL, Bruce G. Clinical dentin hypersensitivity: understanding the causes and prescribing a treatment. J Contemp Pract 2001;2(1):1-12.

Lier BB, Rosing CK, Aass AM, Gjermo P. Treatment of dentin hypersensitivity by Nd:YAG laser. J Clin Periodontol 2002;29:501-6.

MacCarthy D. Dentine hypersensitivity: a review of the literature. J Ir Dent Assoc 2004;50(1):36-41.

Markowitz K. Tooth sensitivity: mechanisms and management. Compendium 1993;14(8):1032-4.

Schiff T, Dos Santos M, Laffi S, et al. Efficacy of a dentifrice containing 5% potassium nitrate and 1500 PPM sodium monofluorophosphate in a precipitated calcium carbonate base on dentinal hypersensitivity. J Clin Dent 1998;9(1):22-5.

West NX, Addy M, Jackson RJ, Ridge DB. Dentine hypersensitivity and the placebo response: a comparison of the effect of strontium acetate, potassium nitrate and fluoride toothpastes. J Clin Periodontol 1997;24(4):209-15.

Zhang C, Matsumoto K, Kimura Y, et al. Effects of CO_2 laser in treatment of cervical dentinal hypersensitivity. J Endod 1998;24(9):595-7.

Zhang Y, Agee K, Pashley DH, Pashley EL. The effects of Pain-Free Desensitizer on dentine permeability and tubule occlusion over time, in vitro. J Clin Periodontol 1998;25(11):884-91.

Table 11.1: USAGE INFORMATION FOR IN-OFFICE DESENSITIZING PRODUCTS

NAME	FORM/CONTENT	USAGE AND ADMINISTRATION	WARNINGS/PRECAUTIONS & CONTRAINDICATIONS
BONDING AGENTS*			
Methacrylate Polymer (All-Bond DS Desensitizer, MicroPrime, Confi-Dental, Gluma Desensitizer)	NA	**Adults:** Apply chairside according to manufactuer's recommendations.	**P/N:** Effects on pregnancy and nursing are unknown.
Polyethylene Glycol Dimethacrylate and Glutaraldehyde (Systemp Densensitizer)	**Liq:** 35% polyethylene glycol dimethacrylate, 5% glutaraldehyde	**Adults:** Apply chairside according to manufactuer's recommendations.	**P/N:** Effects on pregnancy and nursing are unknown.
DESENSITIZING AGENTS†			
Aluminum Oxalate (Dentin Conditioners)	**Liquid**	**Adults:** Dry dentins surface; dispense 10-12 drops into plastic dappen dish; apply saturated cotton pellets to sensitive area for 1 full minute; use light pressure and do not burnish; have patients expectorate after application; to overcome pain threshold, sequential 1-minute treatments may be required. Do not apply with wooden stick.	**W/P:** For chairside treatment of dentinal hypersensitivity, acidic reagents remove smear layer and demineralize root surface (and may also leave crystals of calcium oxalate on the root surfaces), which may decrease effectiveness of bond cements and adhesives' interaction with the root surface; therefore, surfaces treated with an oxalate should be pumiced before a bonding agents is used. **P/N:** Effects on pregnancy and nursing are unknown.
Calcium Sodium Phosphosilicates (Butler NuCare Prophylaxis Paste with NovaMin, Butler NuCare Tooth Root Conditioner with NovaMin)	**Paste:** 1.23% fluoride ion, 48% NovaMin	**Adults:**	
Chlorhexidine/HEMA (HemaSeal & Cide)	**Liquid**	**Adults:** Use as directed.	**P/N:** Effects on pregnancy and nursing are unknown.
Fluoride Ion (Butler APF Fluoride Foam, Butler Neutral Fluoride Foam, Butler APF Fluoride Gel, Butler Neutral Fluoride Rinse)	**Foam:** 1.23% (Butler APF Fluoride Foam), 0.9% (Butler Neutral Fluoride Foam); **Gel:** 1.23% (Butler APF Fluoride Gel), 0.9% (Butler Neutral Fluoride Gel); **Rinse:** 0.9% (Butler Neutral Fluoride Rinse)	**Adults:** Use as directed.	NA
Potassium Oxalate (SuperSeal)	**Liq:** 5mL bottle	**Adults:** Dry dentins surface; dispense 10-12 drops into plastic dappen dish; apply saturated cotton pellets to sensitive area for 1 full minute; use light pressure and do not burnish; have patients expectorate after application; to overcome pain threshold, sequential 1 minute treatments may be required. Do not apply with wooden stick.	**W/P:** For chairside treatment of dentinal hypersensitivity, acidic reagents remove smear layer and demineralize root surface (and may also leave crystals of calcium oxalate on the root surfaces), which may decrease effectiveness of bond cements and adhesives' interaction with the root surface; therefore, surfaces treated with an oxalate should be pumiced before a bonding agents is used. **P/N:** Effects on pregnancy and nursing are unknown.

★indicates a product bearing the ADA Seal of Acceptance.
NA = Not available.
*Mode of action: seals dentinal tubules and reduces fluid shifting.
†Mode of action: has been shown to form particles that block dentinal tubules, thereby providing temporary relief from pain.
‡Mode of action: NuCare Prophy Paste occludes tubules; NuCare Root Conditioner seals tubules. Rincinol P.R.N. forms a protective barrier. Protect Desensitizing Solution removes smear layer to expose tubules; calcium and protein plugs form deep in tubules, assisted by varnish.
§Mode of action: appears to close dentinal tubules, protect pulp, and reduce sensitivity to temperature extremes; compatible with all restorative materials, dental cements, and cavity liners.
¶Mode of action: occludes dentinal tubules.

Table 11.1: USAGE INFORMATION FOR IN-OFFICE DESENSITIZING PRODUCTS *(cont.)*

NAME	FORM/CONTENT	USAGE AND ADMINISTRATION	WARNINGS/PRECAUTIONS & CONTRAINDICATIONS
DESENSITIZING AGENTS† *(cont.)*			
Potassium Mono-Oxalate (Protect)	**Liq:** 2.70%	***Adults:*** Dry dentins surface; dispense 10-12 drops into plastic dappen dish; apply saturated cotton pellets to sensitive area for 1 full minute; use light pressure and do not burnish; have patients expectorate after application; to overcome pain threshold, sequential 1 minute treatments may be required. Do not apply with wooden stick.	**W/P:** For chairside treatment of dentinal hypersensitivity, acidic reagents remove smear layer and demineralize root surface (and may also leave crystals of calcium oxalate on the root surfaces), which may decrease effectiveness of bond cements and adhesives' interaction with the root surface; therefore, surfaces treated with an oxalate should be pumiced before a bonding agents is used. **P/N:** Effects on pregnancy and nursing are unknown.
Potassium Nitrate (Den-Mat Desensitize)	**Kit**	***Adults:*** Use as directed.	**W/P:** Do not exceed recommended dose. **Contra:** Do not use in areas where water fluoride content is greater than 0.6 ppm; some brands of tablets contain too much fluoride for certain age groups or for use in areas of higher water fluoride content. If pain persists more than 4 weeks, patients should be re-evaluated to determine cause of sensitivity. **P/N:** Effects on pregnancy and nursing are unknown.
Potassium Nitrate (Professional Tooth Desensitizing Gel)	**Gel**	***Adults:*** Use as directed.	**W/P:** Do not exceed recommended dose. **Contra:** Do not use in areas where water fluoride content is greater than 0.6 ppm; some brands of tablets contain too much fluoride for certain age groups or for use in areas of higher water fluoride content. If pain persists more than 4 weeks, patients should be re-evaluated to determine cause of sensitivity. **P/N:** Effects on pregnancy and nursing are unknown.
Potassium Nitrate, Fluoride (UltraEZ)	**Gel**	***Adults:*** Use as directed.	**W/P:** Do not exceed recommended dose. **Contra:** Do not use in areas where water fluoride content is greater than 0.6 ppm; some brands of tablets contain too much fluoride for certain age groups or for use in areas of higher water fluoride content. If pain persists more than 4 weeks, patients should be re-evaluated to determine cause of sensitivity. **P/N:** Effects on pregnancy and nursing are unknown.
Potassium Nitrate, Triclosan (Triclosan)	**Paste:** 5% potassium nitrate, 0.3% triclosan	***Adults:*** Apply at least a 1-inch strip of toothpaste onto a soft bristle toothbrush. Brush teeth thoroughly for at least 1 minute twice a day or as recommended.	**W/P:** Do not exceed recommended dose. **Contra:** Do not use in areas where water fluoride content is greater than 0.6 ppm; some brands of tablets contain too much fluoride for certain age groups or for use in areas of higher water fluoride content. If pain persists more than 4 weeks, patients should be re-evaluated to determine cause of sensitivity. **P/N:** Effects on pregnancy and nursing are unknown.
Sodium Fluoride (Crayola Kids Fluoride Anticavity Toothpaste)	**Paste:** 0.239%	***Pediatrics:*** Use as directed.	**W/P:** Do not exceed recommended dose. **Contra:** Do not use in areas where water fluoride content is greater than 0.6 ppm; some brands of tablets contain too much fluoride for certain age groups or for use in areas of higher water fluoride content. If pain persists more than 4 weeks, patients should be re-evaluated to determine cause of sensitivity. **P/N:** Effects on pregnancy and nursing are unknown.

★ indicates a product bearing the ADA Seal of Acceptance.
NA = Not available.
*Mode of action: seals dentinal tubules and reduces fluid shifting.
†Mode of action: has been shown to form particles that block dentinal tubules, thereby providing temporary relief from pain.
‡Mode of action: NuCare Prophy Paste occludes tubules; NuCare Root Conditioner seals tubules. Rincinol P.R.N. forms a protective barrier. Protect Desensitizing Solution removes smear layer to expose tubules; calcium and protein plugs form deep in tubules, assisted by varnish.
§Mode of action: appears to close dentinal tubules, protect pulp, and reduce sensitivity to temperature extremes; compatible with all restorative materials, dental cements, and cavity liners.
¶Mode of action: occludes dentinal tubules.

NAME	FORM/CONTENT	USAGE AND ADMINISTRATION	WARNINGS/PRECAUTIONS & CONTRAINDICATIONS
Sodium Fluoride, Neutral (NiteWhite NSF)	**Liquid**	***Adults:*** Apply in a tray and wear as directed for 5 min/day.	**W/P:** Caution in use of fluorides as desensititizing agents in children owing to possibility of fluorosis. **P/N:** Effects on pregnancy and nursing are unknown.
Sodium Fluoride (Sultan Sodium Fluoride Paste★)	**Paste:** 33.50%	***Adults:*** Burnish onto sensitive area using an orangewood stick for 1 minute; followed by rinsing; to overcome pain threshold, sequential 1 minute treatments may be required.	**W/P:** Do not exceed recommended dose. **Contra:** Do not use in areas where water fluoride content is greater than 0.6 ppm; some brands of tablets contain too much fluoride for certain age groups or for use in areas of higher water fluoride content. If pain persists more than 4 weeks, patients should be re-evaluated to determine cause of sensitivity. **P/N:** Effects on pregnancy and nursing are unknown.
Sodium Fluoride, Potassium Nitrate (Aquafresh Sensitive Teeth, Arm & Hammer Dentacare, Crest Sensitivity Protection, Sensodyne Cool Gel, Sensodyne Tartar Control, Protect Sensitive Teeth, Sensodyne w/Fluoride Tartar Control, Sensodyne w/Fluoride/Baking Soda, Butler Maximum Strength Sensitive Toothpaste)	**Paste:** 5% potassium nitrate	***Adults:*** Apply at least a 1-inch strip of toothpaste onto a soft bristle toothbrush. Brush teeth thoroughly for at least 1 minute twice a day or as recommended.	**W/P:** Do not exceed recommended dose. **Contra:** Do not use in areas where water fluoride content is greater than 0.6 ppm; some brands of tablets contain too much fluoride for certain age groups or for use in areas of higher water fluoride content. If pain persists more than 4 weeks, patients should be re-evaluated to determine cause of sensitivity. **P/N:** Effects on pregnancy and nursing are unknown.
Sodium Fluoride, Stannous Fluoride (Gel-Kam Dentin Block★)	**Gel**	***Adults:*** Dry dentin surface; dispense 10-12 drops into plastic dappen dish; apply saturated cotton pellets to sensitive area for 1 full minute; use light pressure and do not burnish; have patients expectorate after application; to overcome pain threshold, sequential 1-minute treatments may be required. Do not apply with wooden stick.	**W/P:** Caution in use of fluorides as desensititizing agents in children owing to possibility of fluorosis. **P/N:** Effects on pregnancy and nursing are unknown.
Sodium Fluorescein (Plak-Check)	**Sol:** 0.75%	***Adults:*** Use as directed.	NA
Sodium Monofluorophosphate, Potassium Nitrate (Oral-B Sensitive, Den-Mat Sensitive, Rembrandt Whitening Sensitive, Sensodyne Fresh Mint, Sensodyne Original, Sensodyne w/Fluoride)	**Paste:** 5% potassium nitrate	***Adults:*** Apply at least a 1-inch strip of toothpaste onto a soft bristle toothbrush. Brush teeth thoroughly for at least 1 minute twice a day or as recommended.	**W/P:** Do not exceed recommended dose. **Contra:** Do not use in areas where water fluoride content is greater than 0.6 ppm; some brands of tablets contain too much fluoride for certain age groups or for use in areas of higher water fluoride content. If pain persists more than 4 weeks, patients should be re-evaluated to determine cause of sensitivity. **P/N:** Effects on pregnancy and nursing are unknown.
Stannous Fluoride (Stani-Max Pro)	**Liq:** 3.28%	***Adults:*** Dilute 1:1 with water, preferably distilled water to provide a 1.64% SnF_2 rinse. Use in office irrigation or rinse. Recommended rinse after scaling and root planning.	**W/P:** Caution in use of fluorides as desensititizing agents in children owing to possibility of fluorosis. **P/N:** Effects on pregnancy and nursing are unknown.

Table 11.1: USAGE INFORMATION FOR IN-OFFICE DESENSITIZING PRODUCTS *(cont.)*

NAME	FORM/CONTENT	USAGE AND ADMINISTRATION	WARNINGS/PRECAUTIONS & CONTRAINDICATIONS
DESENSITIZING AGENTS† *(cont.)*			
Stannous Fluoride, Potassium Nitrate (Colgate Sensitive Maximum Strength, Colgate Sensitive Maximum Strength plus Whitening)	**Paste:** 5% potassium nitrate	***Adults:*** Apply at least a 1-inch strip of toothpaste onto a soft bristle toothbrush. Brush teeth thoroughly for at least 1 minute twice a day or as recommended.	**W/P:** Do not exceed recommended dose. **Contra:** Do not use in areas where water fluoride content is greater than 0.6 ppm; some brands of tablets contain too much fluoride for certain age groups or for use in areas of higher water fluoride content. If pain persists more than 4 weeks, patients should be re-evaluated to determine cause of sensitivity. **P/N:** Effects on pregnancy and nursing are unknown.
Stannous Fluoride, Sodium Fluoride, Hydrogen Fluoride (Gel-Kam★, ProDentx Comfort Desensitizer, Dentiblock Dentin Desensitizer, ProDentx Office Fluorides)	**Paste:** 0.4% stannous fluoride, 1.09% sodium fluoride, 0.14% hydrogen fluoride	***Adults:*** Dry dentins surface; dispense 10-12 drops into plastic dappen dish; apply saturated cotton pellets to sensitive area for 1 full minute; use light pressure and do not burnish; have patients expectorate after application; to overcome pain threshold, sequential 1 minute treatments may be required.	**W/P:** Caution in use of fluorides as desensititizing agents in children owing to possibility of fluorosis. **P/N:** Effects on pregnancy and nursing are unknown.
Strontium Chloride (Thermodent Toothpaste)	**Paste:** 10%	***Adults:*** Apply at least a 1-inch strip of toothpaste onto a soft bristle toothbrush. Brush teeth thoroughly for at least 1 minute twice a day or as recommended. Do not apply with wooden stick.	**W/P:** Do not exceed recommended dose. **Contra:** Do not use in areas where water fluoride content is greater than 0.6 ppm; some brands of tablets contain too much fluoride for certain age groups or for use in areas of higher water fluoride content. If pain persists more than 4 weeks, patients should be re-evaluated to determine cause of sensitivity. **P/N:** Effects on pregnancy and nursing are unknown.
Strontium Chloride, Sodium Fluoride (Health-Dent Desensitizer, Hema-Glu Desensitizer)	**Liq:** 3.9% strontium chloride, 0.42% sodium fluoride	***Adults:*** Dry dentins surface; dispense 10-12 drops into plastic dappen dish; apply saturated cotton pellets to sensitive area for 1 full minute; use light pressure and do not burnish; have patients expectorate after application; to overcome pain threshold, sequential 1 minute treatements may be required.	**W/P:** Caution in use of fluorides as desensititizing agents in children owing to possibility of fluorosis. **P/N:** Effects on pregnancy and nursing are unknown.
DEVICES‡			
Calcium Sodium Phosphosilicates (Butler NuCare Prophylaxis Paste with NovaMin, Butler NuCare Tooth Root Conditioner with NovaMin)	**NuCare Prophy Paste:** 1.23% fluoride ion, 48% NovaMin; prophy cups: 2 grits (stain removing, gentle); 3 flavors (bubble gum, mint, raspberry cream); **NuCare Root Conditioner:** 2 syringes; **Powder:** NovaMin, 2µ average particle size; **Liquid:** 1% NovaMin in sterile water	***Adults:*** **NuCare Prophy Paste:** Use as directed. **NuCare Root Conditioner:** In-office 2-phase product as a root conditioner including 2 subgingival syringes connected and mixed for 15 sec then expressed from syringe around the gingival margins of sensitive areas.	NA

★indicates a product bearing the ADA Seal of Acceptance.
NA = Not available.
*Mode of action: seals dentinal tubules and reduces fluid shifting.
†Mode of action: has been shown to form particles that block dentinal tubules, thereby providing temporary relief from pain.
‡Mode of action: NuCare Prophy Paste occludes tubules; NuCare Root Conditioner seals tubules. Rincinol P.R.N. forms a protective barrier. Protect Desensitizing Solution removes smear layer to expose tubules; calcium and protein plugs form deep in tubules, assisted by varnish.
§Mode of action: appears to close dentinal tubules, protect pulp, and reduce sensitivity to temperature extremes; compatible with all restorative materials, dental cements, and cavity liners.
¶Mode of action: occludes dentinal tubules.

NAME	FORM/CONTENT	USAGE AND ADMINISTRATION	WARNINGS/PRECAUTIONS & CONTRAINDICATIONS
Hydroxypropyl Cellulose, Potassium Fluoride, Polyethyleneglycol Dimethacrylate and other methacrylates (Protect Desensitizing Solution)	**Kit:** Bottle (4g), 45 applicator sticks, mixing pad	***Adults:*** Dry tooth and apply liquid with applicator provided. Do not apply with wooden stick.	NA
Sodium Hyaluronate, Polyvinylpyrrolidone, Glycyrrhetinic Acid, Aloe Vera Extract (Rincinol P.R.N. Soothing Oral Rinse)	**Packet:** Each single-dose packet contains bio-adherent mucosal coating	***Adults/Pediatrics ≥ 6 yrs:*** Use as directed.	NA

SEALANTS[§]

Barrier Dental Sealant, Pain-Free Desensitizer (active ingredients not available)	NA	***Adults:*** Apply chairside according to manufacturer's recommendations.	**P/N:** Effects on pregnancy and nursing are unknown.

VARNISHES[¶]

Sodium Fluoride (Duraflor, Duraphate, Fluor Protector, Fluocal solution)	**Tubes:** 50mg/mL, 10mL	***Adults:*** Apply chairside according to manufacturer's recommendations.	**W/P:** Not to be used with other professional applied topical fluoride preparations. **P/N:** Effects on pregnancy and nursing are unknown.
Strontium Chloride, Copal Resin (Zarosen)	**Liq:** 0.145% strontium chloride, 6.9% copal resin	***Adults:*** Apply topically to dentin, enamel or cementum with cotton or brush; wipe dry with cotton roll or gauze pad; do not dry with air syringe.	**W/P:** Not to be used with other professional applied topical fluoride preparations. **P/N:** Effects on pregnancy and nursing are unknown.

Table 11.2: DIFFERENTIAL DIAGNOSES FOR DENTINAL HYPERSENSITIVITY

PATHOLOGY	SIGNS AND SYMPTOMS	CLINICAL EVALUATION
Chipped tooth	Thermal sensitivity, pain from abrasion	Visual examination
Cracked tooth	Pain from pressure (biting)	Percussion, biting, application of dye to disclose fracture
Dental caries	Thermal sensitivity (cold), pain from pressure	Radiographic or clinical examination
Dentin hypersensitivity	Sharp, sudden, short pain; thermal sensitivity; pain from abrasion	Osmotic solution, thermal testing, mechanical abrasion, normal electrical pulp test
Fractured restoration	Thermal sensitivity, pain from pressure	Visual examination, biting on plastic or wood sticks
Postoperative sensitivity	Thermal sensitivity with moderate short pain	History of recent operative work
Trauma from occlusion	Thermal sensitivity, pain from pressure, mobility, wear facets, short pain	Occlusal equilibration

Table 11.3: USAGE INFORMATION FOR DESENSITIZING TOOTHPASTES

NAME	FORM/CONTENT	USAGE AND ADMINISTRATION	FEATURE/USES
Calcium sodium phosphosilicates (Oravive [5% NovaMin], Soothe Rx [7.5% NovaMin])	**Oravive:** 4 oz tube; 0.5 oz travel-size unit (5 pack); **Soothe Rx: Kit:** 1.5 oz tube w/ 24 unit dose packets, 0.05 oz each	**Adults/Pediatrics (Oravive):** Apply toothpaste onto soft-bristle toothbrush; brush teeth thoroughly for at least 1 min bid (morning and evening) or as recommended by a dentist or physician; make sure to brush all sensitive areas of the teeth. Do not use mouthrinses, eat or drink for at least 30 min after brushing. **Adults (Soothe Rx):** Use bid for 2 weeks then once per week thereafter. **Pediatrics (Soothe Rx):** Not recommended.	Calcium sodium phosphosilicates decrease dentinal hypersensitivity through tubule occlusion; if pain persists more than 4 weeks, patient should be re-evaluated to determine cause of sensitivity.
Sodium fluoride, 5% potassium nitrate (Aquafresh Sensitive Teeth, Arm & Hammer Dentacare, Butler Maximum Strength Sensitive Toothpaste, Crest Sensitivity Protection★, Desensitize Plus, Oral-B Sensitive, Protect Sensitive Teeth, Sensodyne Cool Gel, Sensodyne Tartar Control)	**Tube:** 1, 3, 4, 4.5 or 6 oz	**Adults:** Apply toothpaste onto soft-bristle toothbrush; brush teeth thoroughly for at least 1 min bid (morning and evening) or as recommended by a dentist or physician; make sure to brush all sensitive areas of the teeth. **Pediatrics:** <**12 yrs:** Dentist or physician should be consulted before children use this product. <**6 yrs:** Children should be supervised when using this product; keep out of reach of children.	Fluoride products are used for prevention of cavities, and potassium nitrate is considered to decrease dentinal hypersensitivity through nerve inhibition; if pain persists more than 4 weeks, patient should be re-evaluated to determine cause of sensitivity.
Sodium monofluorophosphate, 5% potassium nitrate (Den-Mat Sensitive, Orajel Sensitive Pain-Relieving Toothpaste★, Rembrandt Whitening Sensitive, Sensodyne Fresh Mint, Sensodyne Original)	**Tube:** 0.8, 1, 3, 4, or 6 oz	**Adults:** Apply toothpaste onto soft-bristle toothbrush; brush teeth thoroughly for at least 1 min bid (morning and evening) or as recommended by a dentist or physician; make sure to brush all sensitive areas of the teeth. **Pediatrics:** <**12 yrs:** Dentist or physician should be consulted before children use this product. <**6 yrs:** Children should be supervised when using this product; keep out of reach of children.	Fluoride products are used for prevention of cavities, and potassium nitrate is considered to decrease dentinal hypersensitivity through nerve inhibition; if pain persists more than 4 weeks, patient should be re-evaluated to determine cause of sensitivity.
Stannous fluoride, 5% potassium nitrate (Colgate Sensitive Maximum Strength)	**Tube:** 3.2 oz	**Adults:** Apply toothpaste onto soft-bristle toothbrush; brush teeth thoroughly for at least 1 min bid (morning and evening) or as recommended by a dentist or physician; make sure to brush all sensitive areas of the teeth. **Pediatrics:** <**12 yrs:** Dentist or physician should be consulted before children use this product. <**6 yrs:** Children should be supervised when using this product; keep out of reach of children.	Fluoride products are used for prevention of cavities, and potassium nitrate is considered to decrease dentinal hypersensitivity through nerve inhibition; if pain persists more than 4 weeks, patient should be re-evaluated to determine cause of sensitivity.
Stannous fluoride, 5% potassium nitrate, titanium dioxide-coated mica (Colgate Sensitive Maximum Strength Plus Whitening)	**Tube:** 3.2 oz	**Adults:** Apply toothpaste onto soft-bristle toothbrush; brush teeth thoroughly for at least 1 min bid (morning and evening) or as recommended by a dentist or physician; make sure to brush all sensitive areas of the teeth. **Pediatrics:** Recommended for ≥12 yrs.	Fluoride products are used for prevention of cavities, and potassium nitrate is considered to decrease dentinal hypersensitivity through nerve inhibition; if pain persists more than 4 weeks, patient should be re-evaluated to determine cause of sensitivity.
Stannous fluoride, sodium hexametaphosphate (Crest Pro-Health Toothpaste, Clean Cinnamon or Clean Mint★)	**Tube:** 0.85 oz, 4.2 oz	**Adults:** Apply toothpaste onto soft-bristle toothbrush; brush teeth thoroughly for at least 1 min bid (morning and evening) or as recommended by a dentist or physician; make sure to brush all sensitive areas of the teeth. **Pediatrics:** <**12 yrs:** Dentist or physician should be consulted before children use this product. <**6 yrs:** Children should be supervised when using this product; keep out of reach of children.	Fluoride products are used for prevention of cavities, and potassium nitrate is considered to decrease dentinal hypersensitivity through nerve inhibition; if pain persists more than 4 weeks, patient should be re-evaluated to determine cause of sensitivity.

★indicates a product bearing the ADA Seal of Acceptance.

Chapter 12

Bleaching Agents

B. Ellen Byrne, R.Ph., D.D.S., Ph.D.; Frederick McIntyre, D.D.S., M.S.

Tooth bleaching agents can be classified as to whether they are used for external or internal bleaching and whether the procedure is performed in the office by a dentist or at home by a patient. For tooth bleaching, hydrogen peroxide (H_2O_2) is used alone at levels of 15% to 35% or at 10% to 44% levels in a stable gel of carbamide peroxide (urea peroxide) that breaks down to form hydrogen peroxide (3.35% hydrogen peroxide from 10% carbamide peroxide), urea, ammonia and carbon dioxide.

The terms "whitening" and "bleaching," unfortunately, have been used interchangeably. While the mechanism is not completely understood, bleaching involves free radicals and breakdown of pigment, while whitening is accomplished by abrasive agents in the dentifrice (see Chapter 9).

Internal bleaching. Internal bleaching produces reliable results when used to eliminate intrinsic stains in dentin caused by blood breakdown products or endodontics or for stains in receded pulp chambers. However, bleaching should be confined to the dentin; bleaching the cementum, which provides an attachment for the periodontal ligament, has been associated with external root resorption. External root resorption below the gingival attachment is associated with internal bleaching on nonvital teeth that have sustained trauma, poorly sealed canal spaces or heating during the bleaching procedure. It is felt that the bleaching agent diffuses through the dentinal tubules and initiates an inflammatory resorptive response in the cervical area. Unfortunately, external cervical resorption is not seen for approximately 5 to 6 years after internal bleaching. The use of heat is not essential and should be avoided whenever possible.

Internal bleaching is always performed in the dental office. There are two common approaches to internal bleaching: the "office bleach" (a one-time application) and the "walking bleach" (sealed inside the tooth for 2 to 3 days). The office bleaching agent is a mixture of 30% to 35% hydrogen peroxide and perborate, to which heat has been applied by the use of a hot instrument, such as a ball burnisher or an electric heat-producing instrument, for 2 to 5 minutes to accelerate the bleaching process. However, heat also has been associated with external root resorption and should not be used. Walking bleach seals the hydrogen peroxide and perborate mixture inside the tooth for 2 to 3 days. The sodium perborate, a stable white powder that is soluble in water, decomposes into sodium metaborate and hydrogen peroxide, thus releasing nascent oxygen. The sodium perborate, which is mixed with the hydrogen peroxide, also releases oxygen. This combination is thought to be synergistic and very effective in bleaching. There is evidence that sodium perborate may be safer alone than in combination with 30% to 35% hydrogen peroxide. Since sodium perborate is slower-acting than the combination, it requires a longer therapeutic period when used alone. This technique is called "walking bleach" because the bleaching process actually occurs between dental appointments, during which time the bleaching agents are sealed in the pulp chamber.

External bleaching. External bleaching is indicated for teeth that are discolored from aging, fluorosis or staining due to the effects of tetracycline. External bleaching can be applied by the dentist or staff or can be applied by the patient in home-use bleaching. When dentist-administered and home-use bleaching are used together, it is called "dual or combination bleaching."

Dentist-applied external bleaching can be accomplished with periodically repeated use of an office-bleaching agent. Dentist-applied bleaching procedures can be divided into two types:

- Power bleaching with high concentrations of hydrogen peroxide (30% to 40%)
- Assisted bleaching with high concentrations of carbamide peroxide (35% to 44%)

The power bleaching systems are gels that either are premixed or can be prepared chair-side by the mixing of liquid bleach with powder. These products are caustic and, thus, can cause significant soft-tissue injury. The safest, most reliable gingival protection is a properly placed, sealed rubber dam. Assisted bleaches can be used to boost a home-bleaching program or as an easier, low-cost, in-office bleaching method. Because carbamide peroxide is not as strong as hydrogen peroxide, it cannot yield the same results as hydrogen peroxide. Even though these assisted bleaches are not as caustic as high concentrations of hydrogen peroxide, they do have the capability to irritate the gingiva.

An etching gel containing phosphoric acid that is applied to selected dark areas increases the penetration of the bleach. Light is used to produce heat, which accelerates the bleaching process. The light/heat source can be a visible curing light, overhead operatory light, light-emitting diode (LED), plasma arc or argon laser. Externally bleached teeth may need touch-up treatment every 6 months or 1 year. Severely stained teeth may require more frequent retreatment (see Table 12.1).

Home bleaching, supervised by the dentist, is done by the patient at home using a custom-made plastic carrier that holds the bleach against the patient's teeth. After the desired result is achieved, overnight use on a periodic basis (1 to 4 times per month) or daily use of a whitening dentifrice can maintain the lightening that has been achieved.

These products vary in their viscosity, flavor and packing. Most of the home-use bleaches are supplied with material for bleaching trays. In addition, these products contain various concentrations of carbamide peroxide, hydrogen peroxide or both. The concentrations of carbamide peroxide range from 10% to 22%; the hydrogen peroxide concentrations range from 4.5% to 9.5%. Bleaching agents are available for the patient to purchase over the counter. The product may contain hydrogen peroxide or carbamide peroxide. The delivery system varies with the product. Currently, hydrogen peroxide is available impregnated into a thin, flexible, textured strip made of polyethylene, or incorporated into mouthrinses. Carbamide peroxide is available as a gel to be used in bleaching trays. Fluoride, potassium nitrate or both have been added to some products to reduce tooth sensitivity. The majority of side effects involving tooth sensitivity resolve within 24 to 48 hours after use of the product is discontinued.

External bleaching is seldom permanent, lasting approximately 6 months to 2 years after which teeth gradually return to their original color. Usually, the younger the patient, the longer the bleaching will last. The more difficult it is to bleach a tooth, the more likely it is to discolor again. Bluish-gray stains seem to reappear more quickly than yellow stains. Because reoccurrence of staining is unpredictable, promises about longevity should not be made. Internal bleaching usually lasts longer than external bleaching.

The patient must understand that the bleaching agent will not lighten resin-based composite restorations as much as it will natural tooth structure. While there is evidence that resin-based composites will bleach, the results may not match those achieved in natural tooth structure. Patients should be informed that existing restorations will need to be replaced. There is in vitro evidence supporting the fact that bonding of resin-based composites to etched enamel after vital bleaching procedures results in a decreased bond strength. However, within hours to days, the bond strength returns to that achieved with nonbleached enamel. Restoration replacement should be delayed for about 48 hours to allow for return of bond strength and color rebound after bleaching.

Accepted Indications

Types and causes of tooth discoloration and response to bleaching are provided in Table 12.1. Information on in-office bleaching techniques, dentist-supervised home bleaching and over-the-counter home bleaching agents is provided in Table 12.2. Brown, blue-gray and gray stains are usually caused by caries, porphyria, fluorosis, dentinogenesis imperfecta and erythroblastosis fetalis. They need microabrasion and restorative care and should not be bleached.

General Usage Information

Maximum Recommended Amounts

Average treatment time is generally 2 to 6 weeks. More difficult cases require extended treatment and may result in teeth that look chalky. In some patients, stains relapse when treatment is discontinued.

Usage Adjustments
Adults
When having bleaching done at the dental office, some patients, especially those with severe erosion, abrasion or recession, may find the combination of heat and peroxide uncomfortable. These patients are not good candidates for office bleaching. For at-home bleaching, the recommended wearing time varies greatly; the wearing times are determined by the clinical study designs and vary considerably between products. The daily dosage is between one-half hour and 10 hours for one or two treatments per day.

Special Dental Considerations

Drug Interactions of Dental Interest
Possible interactions with bleaching agents are provided in Table 12.3.

Special Patients
Pregnant and nursing women
The long-term effects of using in-office or home bleaching agents on the teeth of pregnant women have not been studied; therefore, women who are pregnant or who have a reasonable expectation that they could become pregnant should not undergo treatment. Pregnancy risk category has not been determined.

Pediatric, geriatric and other special patients
Bleaching agents have been used on the permanent teeth of children aged 10 to 14 years.

Patient Monitoring: Aspects to Watch
Long-term use can alter normal oral flora and contribute to lingual papillary hypertrophy (hairy tongue) and *Candida albicans*.

Adverse Effects and Precautions
See Table 12.4 for adverse effects, precautions and contraindications for in-office and home use of bleaching agents.

Pharmacology
The mechanism of tooth bleaching is not fully understood; however, it is felt that the

unstable peroxide breaks down to highly unstable free radicals. These free radicals chemically break larger pigmented organic molecules in the enamel matrix into smaller less pigmented constituents. Higher concentrations, such as 30% or higher, of hydrogen peroxide remove the enamel matrix, thereby creating microscopic voids that scatter light and increase the appearance of whiteness until remineralization occurs and the color partly relapses. When the morphology of unbleached teeth is compared to that of teeth that have been treated with lower concentrations of peroxide, such as carbamide peroxide 10%, the latter seem not to be affected; therefore, different bleaching materials and concentrations may have different modes of action.

The addition of carbopol, a carboxypolymethylene polymer, prolongs the release of hydrogen peroxide from carbamide peroxide. Carbopol, a water-soluble resin used in many household products such as shampoo and toothpaste, is used as a thickening agent. It does not break down, nor does it increase the breakdown of the bleaching agent. The carbopol binds to the peroxide and triples or quadruples the active release time of peroxide. Products without carbopol are more fluid and bleach more slowly due to the reduced activity time and greater loss of bleach from the tray. See the ADA's statement on the safety of home-use tooth whitening products on the next page.

Patient Advice

The following advice pertains to patients who are using home bleaching agents:

- The more treatments per day, the faster the bleaching; however, this concentrated use of bleaching agents can also increase sensitivity.
- The bleaching agent should be tightly capped and refrigerated.
- The patient should not wear the appliance while eating.
- Users should discontinue treatment with the bleaching agent if the teeth, gums or bite become uncomfortable.
- The dentist should check the patient's mouth every 1 to 6 weeks to ensure that no damage has been done to the teeth, gums or dental restorations.
- Use of a whitening dentifrice after treatment may extend the whitening effect of the treatment.

Suggested Readings

Albers HF. Lightening natural teeth. ADEPT Report 1991;2(1):1-24.

Dishman MV, Covey DA, Baughan LW. The effect of peroxide bleaching on composite to enamel bond strength. Dent Materials 1994;9(1):33-6.

Harrington GW, Natkin F. External resorption associated with bleaching of pulpless teeth. J Endod 1979;5:344-8.

Haywood VB, Leonard RH, Nelson CF, Brunson WD. Effectiveness, side effects and long-term status of nightguard vital bleaching. JADA 1994;125(9):1219-26.

Heithersay GS. Invasive cervical resorption: an analysis of potential predisposing factors. Quintessence Int 1999;30(2):83-95.

Jorgensen MG, Carroll WB. Incidence of tooth sensitivity after home whitening treatment. JADA 2002;133:1076-82.

Monaghan P, Trowbridge T, Lautenschlager E. Composite resin color change after vital tooth bleaching. J Prosthet Dent 1992;67:778-81.

Reality: The information source for esthetic dentistry. Houston: Reality Publishing Co.; 1999, 2000, 2001, 2005.

For more than a decade, the ADA Council on Scientific Affairs has monitored the development and the increasing numbers of whitening oral hygiene products. As the market for these products grew, the association recognized a need for uniform definitions when discussing whiteners.

For example, "whitening" is any process that will make teeth appear whiter. This can be achieved in two ways. A product can bleach the tooth, which means that it actually changes the natural tooth color. Bleaching products contain peroxide(s) that help remove deep (intrinsic) and surface (extrinsic) stains. By contrast, nonbleaching whitening products contain agents that work by physical or chemical action to help remove surface stains only.

Whitening products may be administered or dispensed by dentists or purchased over-the-counter (OTC) and can be categorized into two major groups:

- peroxide-containing whiteners or bleaching agents; and
- whitening toothpastes (dentifrices).

Peroxide-Containing Whiteners or Bleaching Agents

Dentist-dispensed and OTC home-use products

The dentist-dispensed products usually contain 10% carbamide peroxide (equivalent to about 3% hydrogen peroxide), which is the most commonly used active ingredient in home-use tooth bleaching products. All of the products in this category that bear the ADA Seal of Acceptance contain 10% carbamide peroxide; however, participation in the program is not limited to products of this concentration. Although bleaching agents are available OTC, only those dispensed through the dental office are considered for the Seal ADA because professional consultation is important to the procedure's safety and effectiveness.

In a water-based solution, carbamide peroxide breaks down into hydrogen peroxide and urea, with hydrogen peroxide being the active bleaching agent. Other ingredients of peroxide-containing tooth whiteners may include glycerin, carbopol, sodium hydroxide and flavoring agents.

Accumulated clinical data on neutral pH 10% carbamide peroxide continue to support both the safety and effectiveness of this kind of tooth-whitening agent. The most commonly observed side effects to hydrogen or carbamide peroxide are tooth sensitivity and occasional irritation of the soft tissues in the mouth (oral mucosa), particularly the gums. Tooth sensitivity often occurs during early stages of bleaching treatment. Tissue irritation, in most cases, results from an ill-fitting tray rather than the tooth-bleaching agents. Both of these conditions usually are temporary and stop after the treatment.

Professionally applied bleach whiteners

There are many professionally applied tooth whitening bleach products. These products use hydrogen peroxide in concentrations ranging from 15% to 35% and are sometimes used together with a light or laser, which reportedly accelerates the whitening process. Prior to application of professional products, gum tissues are isolated either with a rubber dam or a protective gel. Whereas home-use products are intended for use over a 2- to 4-week period, the professional procedure is usually completed in about one hour. Currently, all of the professionally applied whiteners that have the ADA Seal contain 35% hydrogen peroxide, although this concentration is not a requirement of the program.

As with the 10% home-use carbamide peroxide bleach products, the most commonly observed side effects of professionally applied hydrogen peroxide products are temporary tooth sensitivity and occasional irritation of oral tissues. On rare occasions, irreversible tooth damage has been reported.

The ADA advises patients to consult with their dentists to determine the most appropriate treatment. This is especially important for patients with many fillings, crowns, and extremely dark stains. A thorough oral examination, performed by a licensed dentist, is essential to determine if bleaching is an appropriate course of treatment. The dentist then supervises the use of bleaching agents within the context of a comprehensive, appropriately sequenced treatment plan.

Whitening Toothpastes

Whitening toothpastes (dentifrices) in the ADA Seal of Acceptance program contain polishing or chemical agents to improve tooth appearance by removing surface stains through gentle polishing, chemical chelation, or some other nonbleaching action. Several whitening toothpastes that are available OTC have received the ADA Seal of Acceptance [Editor 's note: Interested readers may visit http://www.ada.org/ada/seal/adaseal_productlist.pdf and search for "whitening"].

Table 12.1: TYPES OF TOOTH DISCOLORATION

COLOR OF STAIN/ETIOLOGY	EASE OR DIFFICULTY OF BLEACHING
White	
Fluorosis	Degree of difficulty depends on extent of fluorosis.
Blue-gray	
Dentinogenesis imperfecta, erythroblastosis fetalis, tetracycline	Deeply stained blue-gray discolorations, especially those associated with tetracycline, are more difficult to treat than yellow stains.
Gray	
Silver oxide from root canal sealers	Dark stains from root canal sealers seldom bleachable, should be treated restoratively.
Yellow	
Fluorosis, physiological changes due to aging, obliteration of the pulp chamber	Mild uniform yellow discoloration associated with aging or mild uniform fluorosis is easiest to treat.
Brown	
Fluorosis, caries, porphyria, tetracycline, dentinogenesis imperfecta	Stains that are deeper in color are more difficult to treat.
Black	
Mercury stain (amalgam), caries, fluorosis	Very dark or black stains from silver-containing root canal sealers or from mercury are seldom bleachable; should be treated restoratively.
Pink	
Internal resorption	Bleaching is not indicated; treatment consists of endodontics and calcium hydroxide treatment.

Table 12.2: USAGE INFORMATION FOR BLEACHING AGENTS

GENERIC NAME	BRAND NAME(S)
PROFESSIONALLY APPLIED AGENTS–INTERNAL[†]	
Hydrogen peroxide 35%	Opalescence Endo; Superoxol★ (with sodium perborate)
PROFESSIONALLY APPLIED AGENTS–EXTERNAL	
Assisted Bleaches	
Carbamide peroxide 30%	VivaStyle 30%
Carbamide peroxide 35%	Opalescence Quick; Pola Zing; Quick Start; White Speed (35% equivalent; 18% hydrogen peroxide and 22% carbamide peroxide)
Carbamide peroxide 44%	Generic
Power Bleaches	
Hydrogen peroxide 15%	BriteSmile Whitening
Hydrogen peroxide 22%	Contrast AM
Hydrogen peroxide 25-27%	GC TiON Whitening In Office Kit, 25%; Niveous 27%; Zoom Whitening Kit, 25%
Hydrogen peroxide 30-35%	ArcBrite, 30%; Hi Lite, 35%; Illuminé, 30%; Kreativ PowerGel, 35%; Laser Smile, 35%; Luma Arch Bleaching System, 35%; Opalescence Xtra, 35%; Pola Office Kit, 35%; Rembrandt Lightening Plus, 35%; Rembrandt One-Hour, 35%; Virtuoso Lightening, 32%
Hydrogen peroxide 38%	Opalescence Xtra Boost
Miscellaneous	
Chlorine dioxide (strength not available)	GentleBright Single Patient Kit
DENTIST-DISPENSED HOME BLEACHING AGENTS	
Carbamide Peroxide	
Carbamide peroxide 6%	VivaStyle Paint On Varnish (6% when applied; concentration is five times higher once dried)
Carbamide peroxide 10%	Colgate Platinum Daytime Professional Whitening System★; Colgate Platinum Overnight Professional Whitening System; Natural Elegance; Nite White Classic★; Patterson Brand Toothwhitening; Rembrandt Lighten
Carbamide peroxide 10% and 15%	Nupro White Gold
Carbamide peroxide 10%, 15% and 20%	Contrast P.M.; Opalescence (10%)★; Opalescence F; Opalescence PF
Carbamide peroxide 10%, 15% and 22%	Rembrandt Bleaching Gel Plus
Carbamide peroxide 10% and 16%	VivaStyle
Carbamide peroxide 10%, 16% and 22%	Nite White Excel 3; Nite White Excel 3NSF; Nite White Excel 3Z
Carbamide peroxide 10% and 22%	Gel White; Zaris
Carbamide peroxide 11%, 13%, 16% and 21%	Perfecta Trio
Carbamide peroxide 12%, 16%, 22% and 30%	Rembrandt Xtra Comfort
Carbamide peroxide 15% and 20%, with 0.11% fluoride ion	Opalescence F
Carbamide peroxide 10%, 15% and 20%, with 0.11% fluoride ion and 3% potassium nitrate	Opalescence PF

GENERIC NAME	BRAND NAME(S)

DENTIST-DISPENSED HOME BLEACHING AGENTS *(cont.)*
Hydrogen Peroxide

Hydrogen peroxide 3%, 7.5% and 9.5%	Poladay
Hydrogen peroxide 4% and 6%	Zoom! Take-Home
Hydrogen peroxide 4.5%	Perfecta 3/15 Extra Strength
Hydrogen peroxide 6%	Nite White Excel 3 Turbo
Hydrogen peroxide 7.5% and 9.5%	Day White Excel 3
Hydrogen peroxide 9%	trèswhite
Hydrogen peroxide 14%	Crest Whitestrips Supreme

OVER-THE-COUNTER HOME BLEACHING AGENTS
Carbamide Peroxide

Carbamide peroxide 9%	Power Brush Whitening Gel; Rembrandt Dazzling White Toothpaste; Rembrandt Plus Gel and Toothpaste
Carbamide peroxide 10%	Natural White Extreme Sensitive Toothpaste
Carbamide peroxide (strength not available)	Rembrandt 2 Hour White Kit

Hydrogen Peroxide

Hydrogen peroxide 0.75%	Mentadent Tooth Whitening System
Hydrogen peroxide 1.5%	Age Defying Whitening Mouthrinse; Rembrandt Plus Peroxide Whitening Rinse
Hydrogen peroxide 2%	Listerine Whitening Pre-Brush Rinse
Hydrogen peroxide 2.5% and 2.7%	Rembrandt 3-in-1; Rembrandt Whitening Wand
Hydrogen peroxide 3%	Age Defying Whitening Toothpaste; Natural White 5-Minute Kit; Natural White Pro; Rapid White
Hydrogen peroxide 4%	Quick White Portable Whitening System
Hydrogen peroxide 6.5% and 10%	Crest Whitestrips; Crest Whitestrips Premium
Hydrogen peroxide 6% (as 30% PVP-hydrogen peroxide)	Natural White 3-in-3
Hydrogen peroxide 6.3%	Colgate Simply White Clear Whitening Gel
Hydrogen peroxide 8.7%	Colgate Simply White Night Clear Whitening Gel
Hydrogen peroxide (strength not available)	Rembrandt Whitening Pen; Rembrandt Whitening Strips

★indicates a product bearing the ADA Seal of Acceptance.
†Indications: Yellow or black stains from endodontics or tetracycline; intrinsic stains when teeth have darkened from blood breakdown products; or in receded pulp chambers. Usual adult dosage: Sealed into pulp chamber for up to 7 days.

Table 12.3: POSSIBLE INTERACTIONS WITH BLEACHING AGENTS

Beverages	
Coffee and tea	May compromise treatment results. Advise patients to avoid these beverages.
Heavy use of alcohol	May possibly result in additive carcinogenicity because peroxides have mutagenic potential and may boost the effects of known carcinogens. Advise patients to avoid drinking excessive amounts of alcohol.
Wine, whiskey and liqueurs	May compromise treatment results. Advise patients to avoid these beverages.
Tobacco	
Heavy use of tobacco	May compromise treatment results; may possibly result in additive carcinogenicity because peroxides have mutagenic potential and may boost the effects of known carcinogens. Advise patients to avoid tobacco products.

Table 12.4: PRECAUTIONS AND ADVERSE EFFECTS FOR BLEACHING AGENTS

PRECAUTIONS	ADVERSE EFFECTS
General	
Patients should not smoke or use other potential carcinogens during treatment.	Prolonged use of 30% or higher H_2O_2 can destroy cells, and for cells that are not destroyed, prolonged use may potentiate the carcinogenic effects of carcinogens.
Oral	
Patients with root sensitivity may not want to have treatment because it can aggravate sensitivity. In cases of tissue burns (see adverse effects at right), rinse affected area for 1-5 min.	Owing to the acidic nature of some of these products, patients can experience transient dentin sensitivity, especially in patients with gingival recession. High concentrations of H_2O_2 used in office bleaching may produce what appear to be tissue burns—white areas on the gingiva that are caused by oxygen gas bubbles and are not true burns, although discomfort can feel like a burn.

Chapter 13

Drugs for Medical Emergencies in the Dental Office

Richard E. Hall, D.D.S., M.D., Ph.D., F.A.C.S.; Stanley F. Malamed, D.D.S.

Medical emergencies can and do occur in dental offices. Surveys have demonstrated that it is likely that at least one potentially life-threatening emergency situation will develop during a dentist's practice lifetime.

Each professional staff member in every dental office should be trained to recognize and manage any emergency situation that might arise.

Although certain categories of emergency drugs are suggested for the dental office emergency kit, it must be emphasized that administering emergency drugs will always be secondary to providing basic life support during an emergency. Indeed, during all emergency situations, health care professionals should strictly adhere to the P,A,B,C,D emergency management protocol:

P = position;
A = airway;
B = breathing;
C = circulation;
D = definitive treatment (which might include administration of drugs).

Because dentists' levels of training in emergency management can vary significantly, it is impossible to recommend any one list of emergency drugs or any one proprietary emergency drug kit that meets the needs and abilities of all dentists. For this reason, dentists should develop their own emergency drug and equipment kits, based on their level of expertise in managing emergencies.

Although no state dental boards have established specific recommendations as to which emergency drugs and equipment a dentist must have available, state boards of dental examiners do mandate that certain drugs and items of emergency equipment be available in offices where dentists employ intramuscular or intravenous parenteral sedation or general anesthesia and, increasingly, where oral conscious sedation is administered to pediatric patients. Specialty groups, such as the American Dental Society of Anesthesiology, the American Association of Oral and Maxillofacial Surgeons and the Academy of Pediatric Dentistry, have instituted guidelines for the use of sedation and general anesthesia, which dictate the emergency drugs that must be readily available. The following drug categories are mandated by many state boards of dental examiners for doctors who have been permitted to use oral conscious sedation in pediatric patients, parenteral conscious sedation, deep sedation or general anesthesia:

- vasoconstrictor;
- corticosteroid;
- bronchodilator;
- muscle relaxant;
- opioid antagonist;
- benzodiazepine antagonist;
- antihistamine (histamine blocker);
- anticholinergic;
- cardiac medications: epinephrine, antidysrhythmic, vasodilator;
- antihypertensive.

Dentists should not include in the emergency kit any drug or item of emergency equipment they are not trained to use. For example, dentists who are not well-trained in tracheal intubation should not include a laryngoscope and endotracheal tubes in their emergency kits; likewise, dentists who are not proficient in venipuncture should not have an anticonvulsant drug, such as diazepam, in their kits because anticonvulsant drugs must be administered intravenously. Also, dentists should not use anticonvulsants if they are unable to ventilate a patient who is unconscious and apneic, as is likely to occur when anticonvulsant drugs are administered to terminate a seizure.

Table 13.1 lists four levels of drugs and medical equipment that can help the dentist design an emergency kit that will be suitable for the level of emergency preparedness of his or her dental office:

- Level 1 drugs are those deemed most important or critical;
- Level 2 drugs are less critical but can be included in the emergency drug kits of dentists trained to use them;
- Level 3 drugs are those employed for advanced cardiac life support;
- Level 4 includes antidotal drugs that are used to reverse the clinical actions of previously administered medications.

Accepted Indications

Table 13.2 describes the emergency clinical indications for injectable and noninjectable drugs.

General Dosing Information

Table 13.2 provides dosing information for injectable and noninjectable drugs.

Special Dental Considerations

Drug Interactions of Dental Interest

Table 13.3 lists the possible interactions of injectable and noninjectable emergency drugs with other drugs.

Adverse Effects and Precautions

Table 13.2 lists the adverse effects and precautions related to injectable and noninjectable emergency drugs with other drugs.

Pharmacology

Injectable Drugs

Level 1 (Basic, critical drugs)

Epinephrine (1:1,000): Epinephrine, a sympathomimetic drug, acts on both α- and β-adrenergic receptors. It is the most potent α-adrenergic receptor agonist available. Clinical actions of benefit during anaphylaxis include increased systemic vascular resistance, increased arterial blood pressure, increased coronary and cerebral blood flow and bronchodilation.

Histamine blockers (diphenhydramine and chlorpheniramine): Histamine blockers appear to compete with histamine for cell-receptor sites on effector cells. These drugs also have anticholinergic and sedative properties.

Level 2 (Noncritical drugs)

Anticonvulsant (diazepam): Diazepam, a central nervous system (CNS) depressant that acts on parts of the limbic system, thalamus and hypothalamus, provides anticonvulsant effects.

Analgesic (morphine sulfate): Morphine exerts its primary effects on the CNS and organs containing smooth muscle. Pharmacological effects include analgesia, drowsiness, euphoria (mood alteration), reduction in body temperature (at low doses), dose-related respiratory depression, interference with adrenocortical response to stress (at high doses) and reduction of peripheral resistance with little or no effect on the cardiac index.

Antihypoglycemic (glucagon, dextrose 50%): Glucagon, which causes an increase in blood glucose concentration, is used to treat hypoglycemia. It is effective in small doses, and no evidence of toxicity has been reported with its use. Glucagon acts only on liver glycogen by converting it to glucose. Intravenous administration of 50% dextrose also can be used to manage hypoglycemia.

Anti-inflammatory adrenal corticosteroid (hydrocortisone sodium succinate): Hydrocortisone sodium succinate has the same metabolic and anti-inflammatory actions as hydrocortisone. After intravenous administration of hydrocortisone sodium succinate, demonstrable effects are evident within 1 hour and persist for a variable period. The preparation also may be administered IM.

Antihypertensive, antianginal, β-adrenergic blocking agents (esmolol, labetalol): Esmolol is a $β_1$ (cardioselective) adrenergic receptor blocking agent with rapid onset, a very short duration of action and no significant membrane-stabilizing or intrinsic sympathomimetic (partial agonist) activities at therapeutic doses. Esmolol inhibits $β_1$ receptors located chiefly in cardiac muscle. At higher doses, it can inhibit $β_2$ receptors located chiefly in the bronchial and vascular musculature. Clinical actions include a decrease in heart rate, an increase in sinus cycle length, prolongation of sinus node recovery time, prolongation of the A-H interval during normal sinus rhythm and during atrial pacing, and an increase in the antegrade Wenckebach cycle length.

Labetalol combines both selective competitive $α_1$-adrenergic blocking and nonselective competitive β-adrenergic blocking activity. Blood pressure is lowered more when the patient is in the standing rather than in the supine position, and symptoms of postural hypotension can occur. During IV dosing, the patient should not be permitted to move to an erect position unmonitored until ability to do so has been established. Labetalol is metabolized primarily through conjugation to glucuronide metabolites.

Anticholinergic, antidysrhythmic (atropine): Though commonly classified as an anticholinergic drug, atropine is more precisely an antimuscarinic agent. Atropine-induced parasympathetic inhibition can be preceded by a transient phase of stimulation. This is most notable in the heart, where small doses often first slow the rate before the more characteristic tachycardia develops owing to inhibition of vagal control. Compared with scopolamine, atropine's actions on the heart, intestine and bronchial smooth muscle are more potent and longer-lasting. Also unlike scopolamine, atropine, in clinical doses, does not depress the CNS, but may stimulate the medulla and higher cerebral centers.

Adequate doses of atropine abolish various types of reflex vagal cardiac slowing, or asystole. It also prevents or eliminates bradycardia (asystole produced by injection of choline esters, anticholinesterase agents or other parasympathomimetic drugs) and cardiac arrest produced by vagal stimulation. Atropine can also lessen the degree of partial heart block when vagal activity is an etiologic factor.

Systemic doses can raise systolic and diastolic pressures slightly and can produce significant postural hypotension. Such doses also slightly increase cardiac output and decrease central venous pressure. Occasionally, therapeutic doses dilate cutaneous blood vessels, particularly in the blush area, producing atropine flush, and can cause atropine fever owing to suppression of sweat gland activity in infants and small children.

Atropine disappears from the blood rapidly after administration and is metabolized primarily by enzymatic hydrolysis in the liver.

Level 3 (Advanced Cardiac Life-Support Drugs)

Endogenous catecholamine (epinephrine [1:10,000]): Epinephrine is an endogenous catecholamine with both α- and β-adrenergic activity. Clinical actions of benefit during cardiac arrest include increased systemic vascular resistance, increased arterial blood pressure, increased heart rate, increased coronary and cerebral blood flow, increased myocardial contraction and increased myocardial oxygen requirements, and increased automaticity.

Anticholinergic, antidysrhythmic (atropine): See description under Level 2.

Antidysrhythmic (lidocaine): Lidocaine suppresses ventricular dysrhythmias primarily by decreasing automaticity, by reducing the slope of Phase 4 diastolic depolarization. Its local anesthetic properties also may help to depress ventricular ectopy after acute myocardial infarction. During acute myocardial ischemia, the threshold for the induction of ventricular fibrillation is reduced. Some studies have shown that lidocaine elevates the fibrillation threshold; therefore, elevation of the fibrillation threshold correlates closely with blood levels of lidocaine.

Lidocaine usually does not affect myocardial contractility, arterial blood pressure, atrial dysrhythmogenesis or intraventricular conduction. It can, on occasion, facilitate atrioventricular conduction.

Antidysrhythmic (procainamide): Procainamide effectively suppresses ventricular ectopy and may be effective when lidocaine has not achieved suppression of life-threatening ventricular dysrhythmias. Procainamide suppresses Phase 4 diastolic depolarization, reducing the automaticity of ectopic pacemakers. Procainamide also slows intraventricular conduction.

Antidysrhythmic (verapamil): Verapamil is a calcium ion influx inhibitor (slow-channel blocker or calcium-ion inhibitor) that exerts its pharmacological effects by modulating the influx of ionic calcium across the cell membrane of the arterial smooth muscle as well as in conductile and contractile myocardial cells.

Alkalinyzing agent (sodium bicarbonate): Intravenous sodium bicarbonate therapy increases plasma bicarbonate, buffers excess hydrogen ion concentration, raises blood pH and reverses the clinical manifestations of acidosis. Administration of sodium bicarbonate does not facilitate ventricular defibrillation or survival in patients who have had a cardiac arrest.

Calcium salt (calcium chloride): Calcium ions increase the force of myocardial contraction. Calcium's positive inotropic effects are modulated by its action on systemic vascular resistance. Calcium can either increase or decrease systemic vascular resistance.

Level 4 (Antidotal Drugs)

Opioid antagonist (naloxone): Naloxone prevents or reverses the actions of opioids, including respiratory depression, sedation and hypotension. It also can reverse the psychotomimetic and dysphoric effects of agonist-antagonists such as pentazocine.

As a "pure" opioid antagonist, naloxone does not produce respiratory depression, psychotomimetic effects or pupillary constriction. In the absence of opioids or agonistic effects of other opioid antagonists, naloxone exhibits essentially no pharmacological activity.

Naloxone is a competitive antagonist for opioid receptor sites. The onset of action after IV administration is apparent within 2 minutes, with an only slightly slower onset after subcutaneous or IM administration. Duration depends on the route of administration; IM administration produces a more prolonged effect than IV administration. The need for repeated doses of naloxone depends on the dose, route of administration and the type of opioid being antagonized.

Naloxone is rapidly distributed in the body and is metabolized in the liver.

Benzodiazepine antagonist (flumazenil): Flumazenil, which antagonizes the actions of benzodiazepines on the CNS, competitively inhibits the activity at the benzodiazepine recognition site on the GABA/benzodiazepine receptor complex. Flumazenil has little or no agonist activity in humans. Flumazenil does not antagonize the CNS effects of drugs affecting GABA-ergic neurons by means other than the benzodiazepine receptor (that is, ethanol, barbiturates or general anesthetics) and does not reverse the effects of opioids.

Flumazenil antagonizes sedation, impairment of recall and psychomotor impairment produced by benzodiazepines in healthy human volunteers. The duration and degree of reversal of benzodiazepine effects are related to the dose and plasma concentration of flumazenil as well as that of the sedating benzodiazepine. Onset of reversal is usually evident within 1 to 2 minutes after IV injection. An 80% response is reached within 3 minutes, with peak effect noted at 6 to 10 minutes.

Noninjectable Drugs

Level 1 (Basic, critical drugs)

Vasodilators (nitroglycerin): The primary action of the vasodilator nitroglycerin is to relax vascular smooth muscle. Although venous effects predominate, nitroglycerin produces, in a dose-related manner, dilation of both venous and arterial beds. It decreases venous return to the heart and reduces systemic vascular resistance and arterial pressure. These effects lead to a decrease in myocardial oxygen consumption, resulting in a more favorable supply-demand ratio and the cessation of anginal discomfort.

Bronchodilator (albuterol): Compared with isoproterenol, albuterol has a preferential effect on β_2-adrenergic receptors. β_2-adrenergic receptors are the predominant receptors in bronchial smooth muscle. Data indicate that β-adrenergic receptors also exist in the human heart in a concentration from approximately 10% to 50%. The action of albuterol is attributable, at least in part, to stimulation through β-adrenergic receptors of ATP to cyclic-AMP. Increased cyclic-AMP levels are associated with bronchial smooth muscle relaxation and the inhibition of the

release of mediators of immediate hypersensitivity from cells, especially mast cells.

Albuterol has a greater effect on the respiratory tract, in the form of bronchial smooth muscle relaxation, while producing fewer cardiovascular (CV) side effects than most bronchodilators at comparable doses. However, in some patients, albuterol, like other bronchodilators, can produce significant CV effects, such as increased pulse rate, blood pressure, symptoms such as palpitation and tremor, and/or electrocardiographic changes.

Antihypoglycemics (orange juice, regular [not diet] soft drinks): Antihypoglycemics are rapidly absorbed sources of glucose for the management of hypoglycemia.

Fibrinolytic (aspirin): Aspirin, in a dose of 81-325 mg, is recommended in the prehospital phase of out-of-hospital myocardial infarction. Its fibrinolytic properties may help in the reperfusion of ischemic myocardium.

Level 2 (Noncritical drugs)

Respiratory stimulant (aromatic ammonia, spirits of ammonia): Ammonia, which is a noxious-smelling vapor, acts by irritating the mucous membrane of the upper respiratory tract, thereby stimulating the respiratory and vasomotor centers of the medulla. This, in turn, increases respiration and blood pressure.

Histamine blocker (for oral administration): Diphenhydramine (50-mg capsules) is recommended for postoperative management of mild allergy (itching, hives, rash).

Suggested Readings

Fast TB, Martin MD, Ellis TM. Emergency preparedness: a survey of dental practitioners. JADA 1986;112:499-501.

Malamed SF. Managing medical emergencies. JADA 1993;124:40-53.

Office anesthesia evaluation manual. 4th ed. Rosemont, Ill.: American Association of Oral and Maxillofacial Surgeons; 1991.

Table 13.1: DRUGS AND EQUIPMENT FOR DENTAL OFFICE EMERGENCIES

INJECTABLE DRUGS	NONINJECTABLE DRUGS	EQUIPMENT
Level 1 (basic, critical drugs)		
Endogenous catecholamine: Epinephrine (1:1,000) **Histamine blocker:** Diphenhydramine, chlorpheniramine	**Oxygen** **Vasodilator:** Nitroglycerin **Bronchodilator:** Albuterol **Antihypoglycemic:** Orange juice, regular (not diet) soft drinks **Fibrinolytic:** Aspirin (chewable)	**Oxygen delivery system** including positive-pressure/demand valve, bag, valve, mask device, pocket mask; **high-volume suction and aspirator tips or tonsillar suction; syringes; tourniquets; Magill intubation; forceps**
Level 2 (noncritical drugs)		
Analgesic: Morphine sulfate **Anticonvulsant:** Diazepam **Antihypertensive:** Antianginal, β-adrenergic blocking agents such as esmolol, labetalol **Antihypoglycemic:** Glucagon HCl, 50% dextrose **Glucocorticoid:** Hydrocortisone sodium succinate	**Anticholinergic:** Atropine **Respiratory stimulant:** Aromatic ammonia, spirits of ammonia **Histamine blocker:** Diphenhydramine (oral administration)	**Airway equipment:** Oropharyngeal or nasopharyngeal airways, or both; laryngoscope and endotracheal tubes **Equipment for intravenous infusion:** Infusion solution such as 5% dextrose and water (D5W); intravenous tubing; catheters, winged infusion sets, or both **Cricothyrotomy device**
Level 3 (advanced cardiac life-support drugs)		
Alkalinizing agent: Sodium bicarbonate **Analgesic:** Morphine sulfate **Antidysrhythmic:** Lidocaine **Antidysrhythmic:** Procainamide **Antidysrhythmic:** Verapamil **Anticholinergic, antidysrhythmic:** Atropine **Calcium salt:** Calcium chloride **Endogenous catecholamine:** Epinephrine (1:10,000, for IV administration)		
Level 4 (antidotal drugs)		
Benzodiazepine antagonist: Flumazenil **Opioid antagonist:** Naloxone		

Table 13.2: PRESCRIBING INFORMATION FOR EMERGENCY DRUGS

NAME	FORM/ STRENGTH	DOSAGE	WARNINGS/PRECAUTIONS, CONTRAINDICATIONS & ADVERSE EFFECTS	INDICATIONS
ANALGESIC				
Morphine Sulfate (Duramorph, Roxanol, Infumorph)	**Sol:** 10mg/5mL, 20mg/5mL [100mL, 500mL]; **Tab:** 15mg*, 30mg*	*Adults:* **(Sol)** 10-20mg q4h. **(Tab)** 15-30mg q4h.	**W/P:** May cause tolerance or psychological/physical dependence; avoid abrupt withdrawal. Caution with head injury, increased intracranial pressure, acute asthma attack, chronic COPD or cor pulmonale, decreased respiratory reserve, pre-existing respiratory depression, hypoxia, hypercapnia, elderly, debilitated, severe hepatic/renal impairment, hypothyroidism, Addison's disease, prostatic hypertrophy, or urethral stricture. May cause severe hypotension. May obscure diagnosis or clinical course with abdominal conditions. May impair mental/physical abilities. **Contra:** Respiratory insufficiency or depression, severe CNS depression, attack of bronchial asthma; heart failure secondary to chronic lung disease, cardiac arrhythmias, increased intracranial or cerebrospinal pressure, head injuries; brain tumor, acute alcoholism, delirium tremens, convulsive disorders, after biliary tract surgery, suspected surgical abdomen, surgical anastomosis, or concomitantly with MAOIs or within 14 days of such treatment. **P/N:** Category C, caution in nursing. **A/E:** Respiratory depression, lightheadedness, dizziness, sedation, nausea, vomiting, and sweating.	To manage pain that is not responsive to nonopioid analgesics; for treatment of pain and anxiety associated with acute myocardial infarction.
ANTICHOLINERGIC				
Atropine Sulfate (Sal-Tropine★, generic)	**Inj:** 0.05mg/mL, 0.1mg/mL, 0.4mg/ mL, 0.5mg/mL, 1mg/mL	*Adults:* **Usual:** 0.5mg IM/IV/SC. **Range:** 0.4-0.6mg. If used as an antisialagogue, **inject IM** prior to anesthesia induction. **Bradyarrhythmias:** 0.4-1mg every 1-2 hrs prn. **Max:** 2mg/dose. May be used as an **antidote for cardiovascular collapse resulting from injudicious administration of choline ester.** When cardiac arrest has occurred, external cardiac massage or other method of resuscitation is required to distribute the drug after IV injection. **Anticholinesterase Poisoning From Insecticide Poisoning:** 2-3mg IV. Repeat until signs of atropine intoxication appear. **Mushroom Poisoning:** Administer sufficient doses to control parasympathomimetic signs before coma and cardiovascular collapse supervene. *Pediatrics:* **Range:** 0.1mg (newborn) to 0.6mg (>12 years). Inject SC 30 min before surgery. **Bradyarrhythmias: Range:** 0.01-0.03mg/kg IV.	**W/P:** Avoid overdose in IV administration. Increased susceptibility to toxic effects in children. Caution in patients >40 years. Conventional doses may precipitate glaucoma in susceptible patients, convert partial organic pyloric stenosis into complete obstruction, lead to complete urinary retention in patients with prostatic hypertrophy, or cause inspissation of bronchial secretions and formation of dangerous viscid plugs in patients with chronic lung disease. **Contra:** Glaucoma, pyloric stenosis, or prostatic hypertrophy except in doses used for preanesthetic medication. **P/N:** Category C, safety in nursing not known. **A/E:** Dry mouth, blurred vision, photophobia, tachycardia, and anhidrosis.	As an antisialagogue for preanesthetic medication; to restore cardiac rate and arterial pressure when vagal stimulation causes a sudden decrease in pulse rate and cardiac action; to lessen the degree of atrioventricular heart block when increased vagal tone is a major factor in conduction defect (as in some cases due to digitalis); to overcome severe bradycardia and syncope owing to hyperactive carotid sinus reflex.

★indicates a product bearing the ADA Seal of Acceptance.
*Scored.

Table 13.2: PRESCRIBING INFORMATION FOR EMERGENCY DRUGS (cont.)

NAME	FORM/ STRENGTH	DOSAGE	WARNINGS/PRECAUTIONS, CONTRAINDICATIONS & ADVERSE EFFECTS	INDICATIONS
ANTICONVULSANTS				
Diazepam (Valium)	**Tab:** 2mg*, 5mg*, 10mg*; **Inj:** 5mg/mL	***Adults:*Tab: Anxiety:** 2-10mg bid-qid. **Alcohol Withdrawal:** 10mg tid-qid for 24 hrs. **Maint:** 5mg tid-qid prn. **Skeletal Muscle Spasm:** 2-10mg tid-qid. **Seizure Disorders:** 2-10mg tid-qid. **Elderly/Debilitated:** 2-2.5mg qd-bid initially. ***Pediatrics:*** **≥6 months**: 1-2.5mg tid-qid initially; may increase gradually as needed and tolerated. ***Adults:* Inj: Anxiety (moderate):** 2-5mg IM/IV, may repeat in 3-4 hrs. **Anxiety (severe):** 5-10mg IM/IV, may repeat in 3-4 hrs. **Alcohol Withdrawal (acute):** 10mg IM/IV, then 5-10mg in 3-4 hrs if needed. **Endoscopic Procedures: Usual:** ≤10mg IV (up to 20mg) or 5-10mg IM 30 min prior to procedure. **Muscle Spasm:** 5-10mg IM/IV, then 5-10mg in 3-4 hrs if needed. **Status Epilepticus/Severe Seizures: Initial:** 5-10mg IV. **Maint:** May repeat at 10- to 15-minute intervals. **Max:** 30mg. **Preoperative:** 10mg IM. **Cardioversion:** 5-15mg IV, 5-10 min prior to procedure. **Elderly/Debilitated:** Usual: 2-5mg. ***Pediatrics:* Tetanus:** 30 days-5 years: 1-2mg IM/IV (slowly), may repeat every 3-4 hrs prn. ≥5 years: 5-10mg IM/IV, may repeat every 3-4 hrs. **Status Epilepticus/Severe Seizures:** 30 days-5 years: 0.2-0.5mg IV (slowly) every 2-5 min up to 5mg. ≥5 years: 1mg IV (slowly) every 2-5 min up to 10mg, may repeat in 2-4 hrs.	**W/P:** Monitor blood counts and LFTs in long-term use. Neutropenia and jaundice reported. Increase in grand mal seizures reported. Avoid abrupt withdrawal. Caution with kidney or hepatic dysfunction. Inject slowly and avoid small veins with IV. Do not mix or dilute with other products in syringe or infusion flask. Extreme caution in elderly, severely ill, and those with limited pulmonary reserve. Avoid if in shock, coma, or acute alcohol intoxication with depressed vital signs. May impair mental/physical abilities. **Contra:** Acute narrow angle glaucoma, untreated open-angle glaucoma, and pediatrics <6 months. **P/N:** Not for use during pregnancy, safety in nursing not known. **A/E:** Drowsiness, fatigue, ataxia, paradoxical reactions, minor EEG changes, and phlebitis (injection site).	A useful adjunct in treating status epi-lepticus and severe recurrent convulsive seizures.
Midazolam Hydrochloride	**Inj:** 1mg/mL, 5mg/mL; **Syrup:** 2mg/mL [118mL]	***Adults:* IV: Sedation/Anxiolysis/Amnesia Induction: <60 years: Initial:** 1-2.5mg IV over 2 min. **Max:** 5mg. **Titrate:** In small increments at 2-min intervals if needed. Concomitant Narcotics/Other CNS Depressants: Reduce by 30%.**≥60 years/ Debilitated/Chronically Ill: Initial:** 1-1.5mg IV over 2 min. **Max:** 3.5mg. **Titrate:** In small increments at 2-min intervals if needed. Concomitant Narcotics/Other CNS Depressants. Reduce by 50%. **Maint:** 25% of sedation dose by slow titration. **IM: Preoperative Sedation/Anxiolysis/ Amnesia: <60 years:** 0.07-0.08mg/kg IM up to 1 hrs before surgery. **≥60 years/Debilitated:** 1-3mg IM.	**Associated with respiratory depression and respiratory arrest especially when used for sedation in noncritical care settings. Do not administer by rapid injection to neonates. Continuous monitoring required. W/P:** Agitation, involuntary movements, hyperactivity, and combativeness reported. Caution with CHF, chronic renal failure, pulmonary disease, uncompensated acute illnesses (eg, severe fluid or electrolyte disturbances), elderly, or debilitated. Avoid use with shock or coma, or in acute alcohol intoxication with depression of vital signs. Contains benzyl alcohol. **Contra:** Acute narrow-angle glaucoma, untreated open-angle glaucoma, and intrathecal or epidural use. **P/N:** Category D, caution in nursing. **A/E:** Decreased tidal volume and/or respiratory rate, BP/HR variations, apnea, hypotension, pain and local injection-site	A useful adjunct in treating status epi-lepticus and severe recurrent convulsive seizures.

*Scored.

NAME	FORM/ STRENGTH	DOSAGE	WARNINGS/PRECAUTIONS, CONTRAINDICATIONS & ADVERSE EFFECTS	INDICATIONS
Midazolam Hydrochloride *(cont.)*		**Anesthesia Induction: Unpremedicated: <55 years: Initially:** 0.3-0.35mg/kg IV over 20-30 sec . May give additional doses of 25% of initial dose to complete induction. **≥55 years: Initial:** 0.3mg/kg IV. **Debilitated: Initial:** 0.15-0.25mg/kg IV. **Premedicated: <55 years: Initial:** 0.25mg/kg IV over 20-30 sec. **≥55 years: Initial:** 0.2mg/kg IV. **Debilitated:** 0.15mg/kg IV. **Maintenance Sedation: LD:** 0.01-0.05mg/kg IV. May repeat dose at 10-15 min intervals until adequate sedation. **Maint:** 0.02-0.1mg/kg/hr. **Titrate** to desired level of sedation using 25-50% adjustments. Infusion rate should be decreased 10-25% every few hours to find minimum effective infusion rate. ***Pediatrics:*** **Sedation/Anxiolysis/Amnesia Induction: IV: <6 months:** Limited information; titrate with small increments and monitor. 6 months-5 years: **Initial:** 0.05-0.1mg/kg IV over 2-3 min, up to 0.6mg/kg if needed. **Max:** 6mg. **6-12 years: Initial:** 0.025-0.05mg/kg IV over 2-3 min, up to 0.4mg/kg if needed. **Max:** 10mg. 12-16 years: 1-2:5mg IV over 2 min. **Titrate:** In small increments at 2-min intervals if needed. **Max:** 10mg. **IM:** 0.1-0.15mg/kg IM, up to 0.5mg/kg if needed. **Max:** 10mg. **Sedation: LD:** 0.05-0.2mg/kg IV infusion over 2-3 min. **Maint:** 0.06-0.12mg/kg/hr IV infusion. May adjust dose by 25%. **Sedation in Critical Care: Neonatal Dose: <32 weeks: Initial:** 0.03mg/kg/hr IV infusion. >32 weeks: **Initial:** 0.06mg/kg/hr IV infusion. Adjust to lowest effective dose. **(Syrup)** ***Pediatrics:*** 0.25-1mg/kg single dose. **Max:** 20mg.	reactions, hiccups, nausea, vomiting, and desaturation. Emesis, nausea, agitation, hypoxia, laryngospasm, bradycardia, prolonged sedation, and rash.	

ANTIDYSRHYTHMICS

NAME	FORM/ STRENGTH	DOSAGE	WARNINGS/PRECAUTIONS, CONTRAINDICATIONS & ADVERSE EFFECTS	INDICATIONS
Lidocaine Hydrochloride (Xylocaine, Lidocaine)	**Inj:** 0.5%, 1%, 2%; (MPF) 0.5%, 1%, 1.5%, 2%; **Sol:** 2% [100mL, 450mL]	***Adults:*** Dosage varies depending on procedure, depth and duration of anesthesia, degree of muscular relaxation, and patient physical condition. **Max:** 4.5mg/kg or total dose of 300mg.**Epidural/Caudal Anesthesia: Max:** Intervals not less than 90 min. **Paracervical Block: Max:** 200mg/90 min. **Regional Anesthesia: IV: Max:** 4mg/kg. **Children/Elderly/Debilitated/Cardiac**	**W/P:** Acidosis, cardiac arrest, and death reported from delay in toxicity management. Local anesthetic solutions containing antimicrobial preservatives should not be used for epidural or spinal anesthesia. Use lowest effective dose. During epidural anesthesia, administer initial test dose and monitor for CNS and CV toxicity as well as for signs of unintended intrathecal administration. Reduce dose with debilitated, elderly, acutely ill, and pediatrics Extreme caution when using	For the acute management of ventricular dysrhythmias such as those occurring in relation to acute myocardial infarction; drug of choice for suppression of ventricular tachycardia and ventricular fibrillation, as well as ventricular premature

Table 13.2: PRESCRIBING INFORMATION FOR EMERGENCY DRUGS *(cont.)*

NAME	FORM/ STRENGTH	DOSAGE	WARNINGS/PRECAUTIONS, CONTRAINDICATIONS & ADVERSE EFFECTS	INDICATIONS
ANTIDYSRHYTHMICS *(cont.)*				
Lidocaine Hydrochloride *(cont.)*		**or Liver Disease**: Reduce dose. *Pediatrics*: >3 years: **Max**: 1.5-2mg/lb. **Regional Anesthesia: IV: Max**: 3mg/kg. **(Sol)** *Adults*: **Irritated/ Inflamed Mucous Membranes**: Usual: 15mL undiluted. (Mouth) Swish and spit out. (Pharynx) Gargle and may swallow. Do not administer in less than 3-hr intervals. **Max**: 8 doses/24 hrs; (Single Dose) 4.5mg/kg or total of 300mg. *Pediatrics*: >3 years: **Max**: Determine by age and weight. **Infants <3 years**: Apply 1.25mL with cotton-tipped applicator to immediate area. Do not administer in less than 3-hr intervals. **Max**: 8 doses/24 hrs.	lumbar and caudal epidural anesthesia with existing neurological disease, spinal deformities, septicemia, and severe HTN. Monitor CV and respiratory vital signs and state of consciousness after each injection. Caution with hepatic disease and CVD. Monitor circulation and respiration with injections into head and neck area. Excessive dosage or too frequent administration may result in high plasma levels and serious adverse effects requiring resuscitative measures. **P/N**: Category B, caution in nursing. **A/E**: Lightheadedness, nervousness, euphoria, confusion, dizziness, drowsiness, tinnitus, blurred vision, vomiting, heat/cold sensations, twitching, tremors, convulsions, respiratory depression, bradycardia, hypotension, urticaria, edema, and anaphylactoid reactions.	complexes in critically ill patients.
Procainamide Hydrochloride	**Tab, Extended Release**: 500mg, 1000mg	*Adults*: Initial: 25mg/kg q12h. **>50 years or Renal/Hepatic/Cardiac Insufficiency**: Reduce dose or increase intervals. Swallow tab whole.	**W/P**: Monitor for QRS widening or QT prolongation. Should cardioconvert or digitalize before use with A-Fib/Flutter. Caution with AV conduction disturbances and 1st-degree heart block; reduce dose. Caution with myasthenia gravis; adjust dose of anticholinesterases. Caution in digitalis intoxication, pre-existing marrow failure, cytopenia, CHF, ischemic heart disease, or cardiomyopathy. May induce lupoid syndrome. Reserve for life-threatening ventricular arrhythmias. Fatal blood dyscrasias reported; obtain CBC, WBC, differential, and platelets weekly for 1st 3 months, then periodically. **Contra**: Complete heart block, 2nd-degree AV block, SLE, or torsade de pointes. **P/N**: Category C, not for use in nursing. **A/E**: GI disturbances, lupus-like symptoms, elevated LFTs, bitter taste, angioneurotic edema, flushing, psychosis, dizziness, depression, urticaria, pruritus, rash, and agranulocytosis.	Useful in suppressing premature ventricular complexes and recurrent ventricular tachycardia that cannot be controlled by lidocaine; rarely used to treat ventricular fibrillation because it takes so long to reach adequate blood levels even after intravenous administration; can also be used to convert supraventricular dysrhythmias.
Verapamil Hydrochloride **(Calan)**	**Tab**: 40mg, 80mg*, 120mg*	*Adults*: **HTN**: **Initial**: 80mg tid. **Usual**: 360-480mg/day. **Elderly/Small Stature**: **Initial**: 40mg tid. **Angina**: Usual: 80-120mg tid. **Elderly/Small Stature**: **Initial**: 40mg tid. **Titrate**: Increase daily or weekly. **A-Fib (Digitalized)**: Usual: 240-320mg/day given tid-qid. **PSVT Prophylaxis (Non-Digitalized)**: 240-480mg/day given tid-qid. **Max**: 480mg/day. **Severe Hepatic Dysfunction**: Give 30% of normal dose.	**W/P**: Avoid with moderate to severe cardiac failure, and ventricular dysfunction if taking a β-blocker. May cause hypotension, AV block, transient bradycardia, or PR interval prolongation. Monitor LFTs periodically; hepatocellular injury reported. Caution with hypertrophic cardiomyopathy or renal or hepatic dysfunction. Decrease dose with decreased neuromuscular transmission. **P/N**: Category C, not for use in nursing. **A/E**: Constipation, dizziness, nausea, hypotension, headache, edema, CHF, fatigue, elevated liver enzymes, dyspnea, bradycardia, AV block, rash, and flushing.	For management of paroxysmal supraventricular tachycardia that does not require cardioversion.
ANTIHYPOGLYCEMIC				
Dextrose 50%	**Glass ampules**: 50mL	*Adults*: IV: 20-50mL at a rate of 10mL/min; most patients regain consciousness rapidly (5-10 min);	**W/P**: Use in caution in patients with renal dysfuntion, diabetes mellitus or carbohydrate intolerance; when highly	For the management of severe hypoglycemic reactions.

*Scored.

NAME	FORM/ STRENGTH	DOSAGE	WARNINGS/PRECAUTIONS, CONTRAINDICATIONS & ADVERSE EFFECTS	INDICATIONS
Dextrose 50% *(cont.)*		additional 50mL may be needed in some patients; supplementary carbohydrates should be given as soon as possible. Is generally well-tolerated. *Pediatrics:* 0.5-1g/kg/dose; D50W is diluted 1:1, producing D25W to avoid hypertonicity. Supplementary carbohydrates should be given as soon as possible, especially to children or adolescent patients.	concentrated dextrose infusion is abruptly withdrawn, administer 5% or 10% dextrose to avoid reactive hypoglycemia. **Contra:** Allergy to corn or corn products. Do not use concentrated solutions of dextrose in patients with: anuria, diabetic coma and hyperglycemia, intracranial or intraspinal hemorrhage, delirium tremens in dehydrated patients, glucose-galactose malabsorption syndrome. **P/N:** Category C, safety in nursing not known. **A/E:** Injection-site reaction, hyperglycemia, aluminum toxicity in patients with renal dysfunction, fluid and electrolyte disturbances (eg, hypokalemia, hypomagnesemia, hypophosphatemia), glycosuria.	Patients with type I diabetes do not have as great a response to blood glucose levels as do stable type II diabetes patients.
Glucagon Hyrochloride (Glucagen)	**Inj:** 1mg	*Adults:* **Severe Hypoglycemia:** 1mg (1U) SC/IM/IV. May give another dose after 15 min if patient does not respond, but IV glucose would be a better alternative. Use immediately after reconstitution; discard unused portion. **Diagnostic Aid: Stomach/ Duodenum/Small Bowel:** 0.5mg (0.5U) IV or 2mg (2U) IM before procedure. Colon: 2mg (2U) IM 10 min before procedure. *Pediatrics:* **Severe Hypoglycemia: ≥20kg:** 1mg (1U) SC/IM/IV. **<20kg:** 0.5mg (0.5U) or 20-30µg/kg. May give another dose after 15 min if patient does not respond, but IV glucose would be a better alternative. Use immediately after reconstitution; discard unused portion.	**W/P:** Caution with history suggestive of insulinoma and/or pheochromocytoma. Glucagon can cause pheochromocytoma tumor to release catecholamines, which may result in a sudden and marked increase in BP. Effective in treating hypoglycemia only if sufficient liver glycogen is present. Glucagon is not effective in states of starvation, adrenal insufficiency, or chronic hypoglycemia; use glucose to treat instead. **Contra:** Pheochromocytoma. **P/N:** Category B, caution in nursing. **A/E:** Nausea, vomiting, allergic reactions, urticaria, respiratory distress, and hypotension.	For the management of severe hypoglycemic reactions. Patients with type I diabetes do not have as great a response to blood glucose levels as do stable type II diabetes patients.
Orange Juice, Nondiet Soft Drinks	**Liquid**	*Adults/Pediatrics:* Orange juice or regular (not diet) soda is administered in 4-oz increments every 5-10 min until patient has returned to normal level of consciousness.	**W/P:** Should not be given to patients who are unconscious or unable to swallow due to risk of choking and aspiration.	For hypoglycemia in the conscious patient.

ANTI-INFLAMMATORY CORTICOSTEROID

NAME	FORM/ STRENGTH	DOSAGE	WARNINGS/PRECAUTIONS, CONTRAINDICATIONS & ADVERSE EFFECTS	INDICATIONS
Hydrocortisone Sodium Succinate (Solu-Cortef)	**Inj:** 100mg, 250mg, 500mg, 1g	*Adults:* **Initial:** 100-500mg IV/IM, depending on condition severity. May repeat dose at 2, 4, or 6 hrs based on clinical response. High dose therapy usually not more than 48-72 hrs; may use antacids prophylactically. *Pediatrics:* Use lower adult doses. Determine dose by severity of condition and response. Dose should not be less than 25mg/day.	**W/P:** May need to increase dose before, during, and after stressful situations. May mask signs of infection or cause new infections. Prolonged use may produce glaucoma, optic nerve damage, or secondary ocular infections. Increases BP, salt/water retention, and potassium and calcium excretion. More severe/fatal course of infections reported with chickenpox and measles. Enhanced effect with hypothyroidism or cirrhosis. Caution with Strongyloides, latent TB, ocular herpes simplex, HTN, diverticulitis, fresh intestinal anastomoses, ulcerative colitis, osteoporosis, myasthenia gravis, renal insufficiency, or peptic ulcer disease. Kaposi's sarcoma reported. Monitor for psychotic disturbances. Acute myopathy with high doses. Avoid abrupt withdrawal. Monitor growth and development of children on prolonged therapy. Hypernatremia may occur with	For treating primary or secondary adrenocortical insufficiency as well as acute adrenocortical insufficiency; also for treatment of shock that proves unresponsive to conventional therapy if adrenocortical insufficiency exists or is suspected; to control severe or incapacitating allergic conditions intractable to adequate trials of conventional treatment in bronchial asthma and drug hypersensitivity reactions.

Table 13.2: PRESCRIBING INFORMATION FOR EMERGENCY DRUGS *(cont.)*

NAME	FORM/ STRENGTH	DOSAGE	WARNINGS/PRECAUTIONS, CONTRAINDICATIONS & ADVERSE EFFECTS	INDICATIONS
ANTI-INFLAMMATORY CORTICOSTEROID *(cont.)*				
Hydrocortisone Sodium Succinate *(cont.)*			high dose therapy >48-72 hrs. **Contra:** Premature infants, systemic fungal infections. **P/N:** Safety in pregnancy and nursing not known. **A/E:** Fluid and electrolyte disturbances, HTN, osteoporosis, muscle weakness, cushingoid state, menstrual irregularities, vertigo, headache, impaired wound healing, DM, ulcerative esophagitis, peptic ulcer, pancreatitis, increased sweating, increases intracranial pressure, carbohydrate intolerance, glaucoma, and cataracts.	
β-ADRENERGIC BLOCKING AGENTS				
Esmolol Hydrochloride (Brevibloc)	**Inj:** 10mg/mL [10mL, 250mL], 20mg/mL [5mL, 100mL], 250mg/mL [10mL]	***Adults:* Supraventricular Tachycardia:** Titrate dose based on ventricular rate. **Load:** 0.5mg/kg over 1 min. **Maint:** 0.05mg/kg/min for next 4 min. May increase by 0.05mg/kg/min at intervals of 4 min or more up to 0.2mg/kg/min. Rapid slowing of ventricular response: Repeat 0.5mg/kg load over 1 min, then 0.1mg/kg/min for 4 min. If needed, another (final) load of 0.5mg/kg over 1 min, then 0.15mg/kg/min for 4 min up to 0.2mg/kg/min. May continue infusions for 24-48 hrs. **Intraoperative/Postoperative Tachycardia and/or HTN: Immediate Control: Initial:** 80mg bolus over 30 sec . **Maint:** 0.15mg/kg/min. May titrate up to 0.3mg/kg/min. **Gradual Control: Initial:** 0.5mg/kg over 1 min. **Maint:** 0.05mg/kg/min for 4 min. Then, if needed, may repeat load and increase to 0.1mg/kg/min.	**W/P:** Hypotension may occur; monitor BP and reduce dose or discontinue if needed. May cause cardiac failure; withdraw at 1st sign of impending cardiac failure. Caution with supraventricular arrhythmias when patient is compromised hemodynamically or is taking other drugs that decrease peripheral resistance, myocardial filling/contractility, and/or electrical-impulse propagation in the myocardium. Not for HTN associated with hypothermia. Caution in bronchospastic diseases; titrate to lowest possible effective dose and terminate immediately in the event of bronchospasm. Caution in diabetics; may mask tachycardia occurring with hypoglycemia. Caution in impaired renal function. Avoid concentrations >10mg/mL and infusions into small veins or through butterfly catheters. Sloughing of skin and necrosis reported with infiltration and extravasation. Use caution when discontinuing infusion in CAD patients. **Contra:** Sinus bradycardia, heart block greater than first degree, cardiogenic shock, or overt heart failure. **P/N:** Category C, caution in nursing. **A/E:** Hypotension, dizziness, diaphoresis, somnolence, confusion, headache, agitation, nausea, and infusion-site reactions.	For treatment of tachycardia and hypertension that occur intraoperatively and postoperatively during surgery or emergence from anesthesia.
Labetalol Hydrochloride (Normodyne, Trandate)	**Inj:** 5mg/mL; **Tab:** 100mg*, 200mg*, 300mg	***Adults:* (Tab) HTN: Initial:** 100mg bid. **Titrate:** 100mg bid every 2-3 days. **Maint:** 200-400mg bid. **Severe HTN:** 1200-2400mg/day given bid-tid. Increments should not exceed 200mg bid for titration. **Elderly: Initial:** 100mg bid. **Titrate:** May increase by 100mg bid. **Maint:** 100-200mg bid. **(Inj) Severe HTN:** Administer in supine position. Repeated IV Infusion: **Initial:** 20mg over 2 min. **Titrate:** Give additional 40-80mg at 10-minute intervals if needed. **Max:** 300mg. **Slow Continuous Infusion:** 200mg at a rate of 2mg/min.	**W/P:** Severe hepatocellular injury reported; caution with hepatic dysfunction. Monitor LFTs periodically; discontinue at 1st sign of hepatic injury. Caution with well-compensated heart failure. Can cause heart failure. Exacerbation of ischemic heart disease with abrupt withdrawal. Caution in nonallergic bronchospasm patients refractory to or intolerant to other antihypertensives. May mask hypoglycemia symptoms. Withdrawal before surgery is controversial. Paradoxical HTN may occur with pheochromocytoma. Death reported during surgery. Avoid injection with low cardiac indices and elevated systemic vascular resistance.	For control of blood pressure in patients with severe hypertension.

*Scored.

NAME	FORM/ STRENGTH	DOSAGE	WARNINGS/PRECAUTIONS, CONTRAINDICATIONS & ADVERSE EFFECTS	INDICATIONS
Labetalol Hydrochloride (cont.)		May adjust dose according to BP. Switch to tabs when BP is stable while in hospital. **Initial:** 200mg, then 200-400mg 6-12 hrs later on Day 1. **Titrate:** May increase at 1-day interval.	**Contra:** Bronchial asthma, obstructive airway disease, overt cardiac failure, >1st-degree heart block, cardiogenic shock, severe bradycardia, or other conditions associated with severe and prolonged hypotension. **P/N:** Category C, caution in nursing. **A/E:** Dizziness, fatigue, nausea, vomiting, dyspepsia, paresthesia, nasal stuffiness, ejaculation failure, impotence, edema, dyspnea, headache, vertigo, postural hypotension, and increased sweating.	

BENZODIAZEPINE ANTAGONIST

NAME	FORM/ STRENGTH	DOSAGE	WARNINGS/PRECAUTIONS, CONTRAINDICATIONS & ADVERSE EFFECTS	INDICATIONS
Flumazenil (Romazicon, generic)	**Inj (Sol):** 0.1mg/mL in 5mL, 10mL multiple-use vials	**For Reversal of Conscious Sedation or in General Anesthesia: IV Only:** Initially, 0.2mg (2mL) administered over 15 sec; if desired level of consciousness has not been obtained after waiting an additional 45 sec, further dose of 0.2mg can be injected and repeated at 60-sec intervals, where necessary, up to additional 4 doses to maximum total dose of 1mg (10mL); dose should be individualized according to patient's response; most patients respond to doses of 0.6-1mg. **Resedation:** Repeated doses can be administered at 20-min intervals, as needed. **Repeat treatment:** No more than 1mg (administered at 0.2mg/min) should be administered at any one time; no more than 3mg should be given in any 1-hr period.	**W/P:** Caution in overdoses involving multiple drug combinations. Risk of seizures, especially with long-term BZD-induced sedation, cyclic antidepressant overdose, concurrent major sedative-hypnotic drug withdrawal, recent therapy with repeated doses of parenteral BZDs, myoclonic jerking or seizure prior to flumazenil administration. Monitor for resedation, respiratory depression, or other residual BZD effects (up to 2hr). Avoid use in the ICU; increased risk of unrecognized BZD dependence. Caution with head injury, alcoholism, and other drug dependencies. Does not reverse respiratory depression/hypoventilation or cardiac depression. May provoke panic attacks with history of panic disorder. Adjust subsequent doses in hepatic dysfunction. Not for use as treatment for BZD dependence or for management of protracted abstinence syndromes. May trigger dose-dependent withdrawal syndromes. **Contra:** Patients given BZDs for life-threatening conditions (eg, control of intracranial pressure or status epilepticus), signs of serious cyclic antidepressant overdose. **P/N:** Category C, caution in nursing. **A/E:** Nausea, vomiting, dizziness, injection site pain, increased sweating, headache, abnormal or blurred vision, agitation.	For complete or partial reversal of sedative effects of benzodiazepines in cases in which general anesthesia has been induced and/or maintained with benzodiazepines or sedation has been produced with benzodiazepines for diagnostic and therapeutic procedures, and for management of an overdose of benzodiazepine.

BRONCHODILATORS

NAME	FORM/ STRENGTH	DOSAGE	WARNINGS/PRECAUTIONS, CONTRAINDICATIONS & ADVERSE EFFECTS	INDICATIONS
Albuterol Sulfate (AccuNeb, Proventil, Proventil HFA, Ventolin HFA)	**(Accuneb) Sol:** 1.25mg/3mL, 0.63mg/3mL [3mL, 25ˢ] **(Proventil/Proventil HFA) Aerosol:** 0.09mg/inh [17g], **(HFA)** 0.09mg/inh [6.7g]; **Sol (neb):** 0.083% [3mL, 25ˢ], 0.5% [20mL]; **Syrup:** 2mg/5mL; **Tab:** 2mg*, 4mg*; **Tab, Extended**	**(AccuNeb)** *Pediatrics:* **2-12 years: Initial:** 0.63mg or 1.25mg tid-qid via nebulizer. **6-12 years with severe asthma or >40kg or 11-12 years: Initial:** 1.25mg tid-qid. **(Proventil/Proventil HFA)** *Adults:* **Bronchospasm: (Aerosol, HFA Aerosol)** 2 inh q4-6h or 1 inh q4h. **(Repetabs) Initial:** 4-8mg q12h. **Max:** 32mg/day. **(Sol)** 2.5mg tid-qid by nebulizer. **(Syrup, Tabs)** 2-4mg tid-qid. **Max:** 32mg/day (8mg qid). **Elderly/Beta-Adrenergic**	**W/P:** (Accuneb) Hypersensitivity reactions reported. Fatalities reported with excessive use. Caution with cardiovascular disorders, especially coronary insufficiency, arrhythmias and HTN. May need concomitant anti-inflammatory agents. Can produce paradoxical bronchospasm. Caution with DM. May cause hypokalemia. (Proventil/Proventil HFA/Ventolin HFA) Discontinue if paradoxical bronchospasm or CV events occur. Avoid excessive use. Caution with coronary insufficiency, arrhythmias, HTN, DM, hyperthyroidism, seizures, and sensitivity to sympathomimetics. Hypersensitivity reactions may occur.	For relief of bronchospasm in patients ≥ 4yr who have reversible obstructive airway disease; for prevention of exercise-induced bronchospasm in patients ≥ 4yr.

Table 13.2: PRESCRIBING INFORMATION FOR EMERGENCY DRUGS *(cont.)*

NAME	FORM/ STRENGTH	DOSAGE	WARNINGS/PRECAUTIONS, CONTRAINDICATIONS & ADVERSE EFFECTS	INDICATIONS
BRONCHODILATORS *(cont.)*				
Albuterol Sulfate *(cont.)*	**Release (Repetabs):** 4mg* **(Ventolin HFA) MDI:** 0.09mg/inh [18g]	**Sensitivity: (Syr, Tabs) Initial:** 2mg tid-qid. **Max: (Tabs)** 8mg tid-qid. **Exercise-Induced Bronchospasm: (Aerosol, HFA Aerosol)** 2 inh 15 min (up to 30 min for HFA) before activity. *Pediatrics:* **Bronchospasm: >14 yrs: (Syr) Initial:** 2-4mg tid-qid. **Max:** 8mg qid. ≥12 yrs: (Aerosol, HFA Aerosol)** 2 inh q4-6h or 1 inh q4h. **(Sol)** 2.5mg tid-qid by nebulizer. **(Tabs) Initial:** 2-4mg tid-qid. **Max:** 8mg qid. **>12 years: (Repetabs) Initial:** 4-8mg q12h. **Max:** 32mg/day. **6-14 years: (Syr) Initial:** 2mg tid-qid. **Max:** 24mg/day. **6-12 years: (Repetabs) Initial:** 4mg q12h. **Max:** 24mg/day. **(Tabs) Initial:** 2mg tid-qid. **Max:** 24mg/day. **2-5 years: (Syr) Initial:** 0.1mg/kg tid (not to exceed 2mg tid). **Titrate:** May increase to 0.2mg/kg/day. **Max:** 4mg tid. ≥4 years: (HFA Aerosol)** 2 inh q4-6h or 1 inh q4h. **Exercise-Induced Bronchospasm:** ≥12 years: (Aerosol)** 2 inh 15 min before activity. ≥4 years: (HFA Aerosol)** 2 inh 15-30 min before activity. **(Ventolin HFA)** *Adults:* **Bronchospasm:** 2 inh q4-6h or 1 inh q4h. **EIB:** 2 inh 15-30 min before activity. *Pediatrics:* ≥4 years: **Bronchospasm:** 2 inh q4-6h or 1 inh q4h. **EIB:** 2 inh 15-30 min before activity.	May cause transient hypokalemia. **P/N:** Category C, not for use in nursing. **A/E:** Asthma exacerbation, otitis media, allergic reaction, gastroenteritis, cold symptoms, throat irritation, viral respiratory infections, upper respiratory inflammation, cough, and musculoskeletal pain.	
ENDOGENOUS CATECHOLAMINE				
Epinephrine (Epipen, Twinject)	**Inj: (Epipen Jr)** 0.5mg/mL, **(Epipen)** 1mg/mL	*Adults:* 0.3mg IM in thigh. May repeat with severe anaphylaxis. *Pediatrics:* 0.15mg or 0.3mg (0.01mg/kg) IM in thigh. May repeat with severe anaphylaxis.	**W/P:** Not for IV use. Contains sulfites. Extreme caution with heart disease. Anginal pain may be induced with coronary insufficiency. Increased risk of adverse reactions with hyperthyroidism, CVD, HTN, DM, elderly, pregnancy, pediatrics <30kg with Epipen and <15kg with Epipen, Jr. **P/N:** Category C, safety in nursing not known. **A/E:** Palpitations, tachycardia, sweating, nausea, vomiting, respiratory difficulty, pallor, dizziness, weakness, tremor, headache, apprehension, and anxiety.	For relief of respiratory distress due to bronchospasm; to provide rapid relief of hypersensitivity reactions from drugs and other allergens, anaphylaxis, or anaphylactic shock.
FIBRINOLYTIC				
Aspirin (Bayer Aspirin Regimen, Bayer Genuine Aspirin, Bayer Extra Strength, Bayer Children's Low Dose Chewable)	**Tab: (Genuine Bayer Aspirin)** 325mg; **Tab: (Bayer Extra Strength)** 500mg; **Tab: (Bayer Aspirin Regimen with Calcium)** 81mg;	*Adults:* **Ischemic Stroke/TIA:** 50-325mg qd. **Suspected Acute MI: Initial:** 160-162.5mg qd as soon as suspect MI. **Maint:** 160-162.5mg qd for 30 days post-infarction, consider further therapy for prevention/recurrent MI.	**W/P:** Increased risk of bleeding with heavy alcohol use (≥3 drinks/day). May inhibit platelet function; can adversely affect inherited (hemophilia) or acquired (hepatic disease, vitamin K deficiency) bleeding disorders. Monitor for bleeding and ulceration. Avoid in	For fibrinolysis in suspected myocardial infarction; administered in prehospital phase of management .

*Scored.

NAME	FORM/ STRENGTH	DOSAGE	WARNINGS/PRECAUTIONS, CONTRAINDICATIONS & ADVERSE EFFECTS	INDICATIONS
Aspirin *(cont.)*	**Tab, Chewable**: (Bayer Aspirin Children's) 81mg; **Tab, Delayed Release**: (Bayer Aspirin Regimen) 81mg, 325mg	**Prevention or Recurrent MI/Unstable Angina/Chronic Stable Angina**: 75-325mg qd. **CABG**: 325mg qd, start 6 hrs post-surgery. Continue for 1 year. **PTCA: Initial**: 325mg, 2 hrs pre-surgery. **Maint**: 160-325mg qd. **Carotid Endarterectomy**: 80mg qd to 650mg bid, start presurgery. **RA: Initial**: 3g qd in divided doses. Increase for anti-inflammatory efficacy to 150-300µg/mL plasma salicylate level. **Spondyloarthropathies**: Up to 4g/day in divided doses. **OA**: Up to 3g/day in divided doses. **Arthritis/SLE Pleurisy: Initial**: 3g/day in divided doses. Increase for anti-inflammatory efficacy to 150-300µg/mL plasma salicylate level. **Pain**: 325-650mg q4-6h. **Max**: 4g/day. *Pediatrics*: **Juvenile RA: Initial**: 90-130mg/kg/day in divided doses. Increase for anti-inflammatory efficacy to 150-300µg/mL plasma salicylate level. **Pain: ≥12 years**: 325-650mg q4-6h. **Max**: 4g/day.	history of active peptic ulcer, severe renal failure, severe hepatic insufficiency, and sodium restricted diets. Associated with elevated LFTs, BUN, and serum creatinine; hyperkalemia; proteinuria; and prolonged bleeding time. Avoid 1 week before and during labor. **Contra**: NSAID allergy, viral infections in children or teenagers, syndrome of asthma, rhinitis, and nasal polyps. **P/N**: Avoid in 3rd trimester of pregnancy and nursing. **A/E**: Fever, hypothermia, dysrhythmias, hypotension, agitation, cerebral edema, dehydration, hyperkalemia, dyspepsia, GI bleed, hearing loss, tinnitus, problems in pregnancy.	

HISTAMINE BLOCKERS

NAME	FORM/ STRENGTH	DOSAGE	WARNINGS/PRECAUTIONS, CONTRAINDICATIONS & ADVERSE EFFECTS	INDICATIONS
Chlorpheniramine Maleate (Chlor-Trimeton Allergy, Diabetic Tussin Allergy Relief)	**Syr**: 2mg/5mL; **Tab**: 4mg; **Tab, ER**: 8mg, 12mg	*Adults*: (Tab/Syrup) 4mg q4-6h. (Tab, ER) 8mg q8-12h or 12mg q12h. **Max**: 24mg/day. *Pediatrics*: **≥12 yrs**: (Tab/Syrup) 4mg q4-6h. **Tab, ER**: 8mg q8-12h or 12mg q12h. **Max**: 24mg/day. **6-12 years**: (Tab/Syrup) 2mg q4-6h. **Max**: 12mg/24 hrs.	**W/P**: Avoid with emphysema, chronic bronchitis, glaucoma, and difficulty in urination due to prostate gland enlargement. **P/N**: Safety in pregnancy and nursing not known. **A/E**: Drowsiness and excitability.	For allergic reactions, allergies, anaphylactic reactions, angioedema; mild, uncomplicated skin manifestation of urticaria and angioedema. (Age ≥ 60 yr) More likely to cause dizziness, sedation and hypotension.
Diphenhydramine Hydrochloride (Benadryl, Benadryl Allergy)	**Cap**: 25mg; **Sol**: 12.5mg/5mL; **Tab**: 25mg; **Tab, Chewable**: 12.5mg	*Adults*: 25-50mg q4-6h. **Max**: 300mg/24 hrs. *Pediatrics*: **≥12 years**: 25-50mg q4-6h. **Max**: 300mg/24 hrs. **6-11 years**: 12.5-25mg q4-6h. **Max**: 150mg/24 hrs.	**W/P**: Caution with emphysema, chronic bronchitis, glaucoma, or difficulty in urination due to prostate gland enlargement. May impair mental/physical abilities. **P/N**: Safety in pregnancy and nursing not known. **A/E**: Drowsiness and excitability (especially in children).	For allergic reactions, allergies, anaphylactic reactions, angioedema; mild, uncomplicated skin manifestation of urticaria and angioedema. (Age ≥ 60 yr) More likely to cause dizziness, sedation and hypotension.

OPIOID ANTAGONIST

NAME	FORM/ STRENGTH	DOSAGE	WARNINGS/PRECAUTIONS, CONTRAINDICATIONS & ADVERSE EFFECTS	INDICATIONS
Naloxone Hydrochloride (Narcan)	**Inj**: 0.4mg/mL, 1mg/mL	*Adults*: **Opioid Overdose: Initial**: 0.4-2mg IV every 2-3 min up to 10mg. IM/SC if IV route not available. **Post-op Opioid Depression**: 0.1-0.2mg IV every 2-3 min to desired response.	**W/P**: Caution in patients (including newborns of addicted mothers) with known or suspected opioid physical dependence. May precipitate acute withdrawal syndrome. Have other resuscitative measures available.	For complete or partial reversal of opioid depression (including respiratory depression) induced by opioids,

Table 13.2: PRESCRIBING INFORMATION FOR EMERGENCY DRUGS (cont.)

NAME	FORM/STRENGTH	DOSAGE	WARNINGS/PRECAUTIONS, CONTRAINDICATIONS & ADVERSE EFFECTS	INDICATIONS
OPIOID ANTAGONIST (cont.)				
Naloxone Hydrochloride (cont.)		May repeat in 1- to 2-hr intervals. Supplemental IM doses last longer. **Narcan Challenge Test: IV:** 0.1-0.2mg, observe 30 sec for signs of withdrawal, then 0.6mg, observe for 20 min **SC:** 0.8mg, observe for 20 min. **Pediatrics: Opioid Overdose: Initial:** 0.01mg/kg IV. Inadequate Response: repeat 0.01mg/kg once. IM/SC in divided doses if IV route not available. **Post-op Opioid Depression:** 0.005-0.01mg IV every 2-3 min to desired response. May repeat in 1- to 2-hr intervals. Supplemental IM doses last longer. **Neonates: Opioid-induced Depression:** 0.01mg/kg IV/IM/SC, may repeat every 2-3 min until desired response.	Caution with cardiac, renal, or hepatic disease. Monitor patients satisfactorily responding due to extended opioid duration of action. Abrupt postoperative opioid depression reversal may result in serious adverse effects leading to death. **P/N:** Category B, caution in nursing. **A/E:** Hypotension, hypertension, ventricular tachycardia and fibrillation, dyspnea, pulmonary edema, cardiac arrest, nausea, vomiting, sweating, seizures, body aches, fever, and nervousness.	including natural and synthetic opioids, propoxyphene, methadone and the opioid antagonist analgesics nalbuphine, pentazocine and butorphanol; also indicated for suspected acute opioid overdosage.
VASODILATOR				
Nitroglycerin (Nitrostat, Nitrolingual Spray)	**Sublingual Tab:** 0.15, 0.3, 0.4, 0.6mg **Translingual Spray:** Nitrolingual, 0.4, 0.8mg/dose **Vaporoles:** amyl nitrite (yellow), 0.3mL	**Oral—Sublingual Tab:** One tablet (0.15-0.6mg) should be dissolved under tongue or in buccal pouch at first sign of an acute anginal attack; dose may be repeated every 5 min until relief is obtained; if pain persists after administration of 3 tablets in a 15-min period, a physician should be notified. **Oral—Lingual Aerosol Spray:** At onset of an anginal attack, 1 (0.4-0.8mg) or 2 metered doses should be sprayed onto or under the tongue; no more than 3 metered doses are recommended during a 15-min period; if chest pain persists, prompt medical attention is recommended.	**W/P:** Severe hypotension may occur; caution with severe hepatic or renal disease, volume depletion or hypotension. Vasodilatory effects with phosphodiesterase inhibitors (eg, sildenafil) can result in severe hypotension. May aggravate angina caused by hypertrophic cardiomyopathy. Tolerance to other nitrate forms may decrease effects. Monitor with acute MI or CHF. **Contra:** Hypersensitivity to nitroglycerin or other organic nitrates, hypotension or uncorrected hypovolemia, increased intracranial pressure and inadequate cerebral circulation. **P/N:** Category C, caution in nursing. **A/E:** Headache, tachycardia, nausea, vomiting, apprehension, restlessness, muscle twitching, retrosternal discomfort, palpitations, dizziness and abdominal pain.	For the prophylaxis, treatment and management of patients with angina pectoris.
MISCELLANEOUS				
Aromatic Ammonia, Spirits of Ammonia	**Vaporoles:** 0.3mL	**Inhalation:** Vaporole containing ammonia is crushed between the user's fingers and held beneath patient's nose, thus permitting patient to inhale the ammonia.	**Contra:** Patients with chronic obstructive pulmonary disease or asthma due to risk of bronchospasm resulting from mucous membrane irritation in upper respiratory tract. **A/E:** May induce brochospasm in asthmatics and others with chronic lung disease.	Repiratory stimulants used for respiratory depression not induced by opioid analgesics; vasodepressor syncope.
Calcium Chloride	**Sol:** 10%	**Adults:** IV: 500-1000mg every 10 min as needed. **Pediatrics:** IV: 20mg/kg every 10 min as needed. Use for hypocalcemia, hyperkalemia, or calcium channel blocker toxicity.	**W/P:** Calcium enhances the effect of cardiac glycosides on the heart and may precipitate arrhythmias. Extravasation of calcium chloride may cause necrosis and skin sloughing. **Contra:** Digitalis toxicity, hypercalcemia, blood hypercoagula bility, IM/SC injection, renal failure, and ventricular fibrillation. **P/N:** Category C, safety in nursing not known. **A/E:** Extravasation necrosis, vasodilation, hypotension, bradycardia, arrhythmia, syncope, mania, erythema.	Only for the treatment of acute hyperkalemia, hypocalcemia or calcium channel blocker toxicity.

*Scored.

NAME	FORM/ STRENGTH	DOSAGE	WARNINGS/PRECAUTIONS, CONTRAINDICATIONS & ADVERSE EFFECTS	INDICATIONS
Oxygen	In compressed gas cylinders in a variety of sizes; portability of the oxygen cylinder is a desirable characteristic; a minimum supply for emergency use is one E-cylinder.	*Adults/Pediatrics*: **Inhalation:** Administered at a flow rate, calculated in L/min, that is adequate to alleviate the presenting signs and symptoms.	**Contra:** Not indicated for patients experiencing hyperventilation.	Any emergency situation in which respiratory distress is evident.
Sodium Bicarbonate	**Sol:** 4.2%, 8.4%	*Adults*: **Metabolic Acidosis: Initial:** 1mEq/kg, **Max:** 50-100mEq, adjust based on ABG or laboratory values; do not give more frequently than q 10 min. *Pediatrics*: 1mEq/kg; do not give more frequently than q 10 min.	**W/P:** Can cause hypochoridemia, hypocalcemia, or alkalosis. Use with great caution if patient has electrolyte imbalances (eg, CHF, cirrhosis, edema, corticosteroid use, or renal failure). When administering, avoid extravasation because it can cause tissue necrosis. **P/N:** Category C, safety in nursing not known. **A/E:** Metabolic alkalosis, injection site pain, hypernatremia, edema.	Used as alkalinyzing agent. Because of absence of proven efficacy and numerous adverse effects, for use (if at all) only after application of more definitive and better substantiated interventions: prompt defibrillation, effective chest compression, endotracheal intubation and hyperventilation with 100% oxygen, and use of such drugs as epinephrine and lidocaine (these interventions take 10 min; thereafter, sodium bicarbonate therapy, although not recommended, can be considered in specific clinical circumstances, such as documented pre-existing metabolic acidosis with or without hyperkalemia).

Table 13.3: DRUG INTERACTIONS FOR EMERGENCY DRUGS

Level 1 (basic, critical drugs)

Bronchodilator (albuterol)	Other sympathomimetic aerosol inhalers should not be used concomitantly with albuterol so as to minimize the risk of deleterious CV events. Albuterol should be administered with extreme caution to patients receiving MAO inhibitors or tricyclic antidepressants because the action of albuterol on the CV system can be potentiated. In the case of an emergency, there is no situation in which a drug-to-drug interaction would be of concern.
Fibrinolytic (aspirin)	When used with NSAIDs, aspirin can increase the risk of GI bleeding and ulceration. There are no drug-to-drug interactions of concern. In the case of an emergency, there is no situation in which a drug-to-drug interaction would be of concern.
Histamine blockers (diphenhydramine, chlorpheniramine)	Histamine blockers have additive effects with alcohol and other central nervous system depressants (sedatives, hypnotics and tranquilizers). In the case of an emergency, there is no situation in which a drug-to-drug interaction would be of concern.

Level 2 (noncritical drugs)

Analgesic (morphine)	Depressant effects of morphine are potentiated by either concomitant administration or the presence of other.central nervous system depressants (alcohol, sedatives, histamine-blockers or psychotropic drugs such as MAO inhibitors, phenothiazines, butyrophenones and tricyclic antidepressants). In the case of an emergency, there is no situation in which a drug-to-drug interaction would be of concern.
Anticonvulsant (diazepam, midazolam)	If combined with other psychotropic or anticonvulsant drugs (phenothiazines, opioids, barbiturates, MAO inhibitors and other antidepressants) CNS and respiratory depressant actions of diazepam can be potentiated. In the case of an emergency, there is no situation in which a drug-to-drug interaction would be of concern.

Level 3 (advanced cardiac life-support drugs)

Antidysrhythmic agent, oral (verapamil)	Concomitant therapy with β-adrenergic blockers and verapamil can result in additive negative effects on heart rate, atrioventricular conduction or cardiac contractility or both. Concomitant administration of verapamil with oral antihypertensive agents will usually have an additive effect on lowering blood pressure; patients should be monitored. In the case of an emergency, there is no situation in which a drug-to-drug interaction would be of concern.
Antidysrhythmic agents, injectable (lidocaine, procainamide)	Lidocaine should be used with caution in patients with digitalis toxicity that is accompanied by atrioventricular block; concomitant use of β-blocking agents or cimetidine can reduce hepatic blood flow and thereby reduce lidocaine clearance. When administering procainamide, additive effects can occur if other antidysrhythmic drugs are given concomitantly; dosage reduction may be necessary. In the case of an emergency, there is no situation in which a drug-to-drug interaction would be of concern.

Level 3 (advanced cardiac life-support drugs) *(cont.)*	
Calcium chloride (calcium salt)	Interaction with CNS depressants other than benzodiazepines has not been specifically studied; no deleterious interactions were seen when flumazenil was administered after opioids, inhalational anesthetics, muscle relaxants and muscle relaxant antagonists with sedatives or anesthesia. In the case of an emergency, there is no situation in which a drug-to-drug interaction would be of concern.
Level 4 (antidotal drugs)	
Benzodiazepine antagonist (flumazenil)	Interaction with CNS depressants other than benzodiazepines has not been specifically studied; no deleterious interactions were seen when flumazenil was administered after opioids, inhalational anesthetics, muscle relaxants and muscle relaxant antagonists with sedatives or anesthesia. In the case of an emergency, there is no situation in which a drug-to-drug interaction would be of concern.

Section II.

Drugs Used in Medicine: Treatment and Pharmacological Considerations for Dental Patients Receiving Medical Care

Chapter 14

Cardiovascular Drugs

Steven Ganzberg, D.M.D., M.S.

Cardiovascular disease affects one in six men and one in seven women aged 45-64 years in the United States. The incidence increases to one in three people aged >65 years. A wide array of medications, with considerably different mechanisms of action, are prescribed to treat these disorders. Primary mechanisms involve the renin-angiotensin system mediated via renal mechanisms and nervous system control via adrenergic supply. Not surprisingly, medications to treat hypertension modify these systems or associated receptor systems.

This chapter will discuss the medications used for the following cardiovascular disorders: dysrhythmias, congestive heart failure, angina, hypertension and hypercholesterolemia. The chapter is organized by drug class and provides a brief explanation of each. It should be noted that drugs utilized for erectile dysfunction are included in the antihypertensive drugs section of this chapter because they are vasodilators. (Sildenafil [Viagra] was originally tested as an antihypertensive and did not succeed.)

Special Dental Considerations

Before performing any dental procedure with a patient who has cardiovascular disease, the dentist should evaluate the patient's blood pressure, heart rate and regularity of rhythm. Any change in medication regimen should be reviewed. It is important for patients to take their cardiovascular medications at their usual scheduled time, irrespective of a dental appointment, to minimize the possibility of intraoperative hypertension or tachycardia.

Noncompliance with medication regimens is not uncommon. The dentist should take special precautions to minimize the stress or pain of a dental procedure so that adverse cardiovascular responses are, in turn, minimized.

Many of these drugs can cause orthostatic hypotension. The dentist should have the patient sit up in the dental chair for 1-2 minutes after being in a supine position and monitor the patient when he or she is standing. Use of epinephrine in local anesthetic solutions should be minimized, and extra care should be taken with aspiration to avoid intravascular injection. If local anesthetic solutions containing epinephrine are deemed necessary, it has been recommended that no more than 40 µg of epinephrine (0.04 mg or approximately two 1.8-cubic-centimeter cartridges of local anesthetic with 1:100,000 epinephrine) should be used for successive dental anesthetic injections in patients with cardiovascular disease. Vital sign monitoring may be of value between injections for selected patients with severe disease. Additional injections of local anesthetic with epinephrine can be given after approximately 5-10 minutes if vital signs are satisfactory. The use of gingival retraction cord with epinephrine is absolutely contraindicated in all patients with cardiovascular disease; this cord should be used with extreme caution, if at all, in other patients.

Patients taking some cardiovascular medications may also be taking anticoagulants. Therefore, before dental procedures involving bleeding are performed, consultation with the patient's physician may be indicated to adjust the anticoagulant dose as discussed in Chapter 19, Hematologic Drugs.

Antiarrhythmic Drugs

In cardiac dysrhythmia, some aspect of normal cardiac electrophysiology is disturbed. This may manifest in one or more of the following: the sinoatrial (SA) node, atrioventricular (AV) node, Bundle of His, Purkinje fibers or in cardiac muscle itself. Antidysrhythmic drugs modify aberrant electrophysiological processes to help restore or improve either an unacceptable rate, an unacceptable rhythm, or both. Some antidysrhythmic drugs, such as β-blockers and calcium channel blockers, are also used for the treatment of other cardiovascular diseases, such as hypertension.

See Tables 14.1 and 14.2 for basic information on antidysrhythmic drugs.

Special Dental Considerations

If dental patients have been taking these drugs for long periods and their symptoms are under adequate control, the management of these patients in an outpatient dental setting without continuous cardiac monitoring is generally acceptable. Hypotension may be encountered. Quinidine is used for several dysrhythmias, but commonly for atrial fibrillation. Other Class I and Class III agents are frequently administered either intravenously or orally for severe cardiac dysrhythmias such as ventricular tachycardia. Class II and Class IV agents can be used for either hypertension, dysrhythmia control or angina. The dentist should consider ECG and continual vital-sign monitoring for patients with serious dysrhythmia. In addition, the dentist should follow the recommendations listed under Special Dental Considerations at the beginning of this chapter for all drugs in this category.

Use of large quantities of injected local anesthetics may have additive and possibly detrimental cardiac effects. Use of epinephrine in local anesthetic solutions should be minimized, and extra care should be taken with aspiration to avoid intravascular injection. A stress-reduction protocol is appropriate.

Most Class I and Class III agents may, in rare cases, cause leukopenia, thrombocytopenia or agranulocytosis. Consider medication-induced adverse effects if gingival bleeding or infection occurs. Elective dental treatment should be deferred if hematologic parameters are compromised.

Quinidine and amiodarone can cause bitter or altered taste. Amiodarone can cause facial flushing.

In orofacial pain management, oral analogues of lidocaine, such as mexiletine, have been reported to be of some use in certain neuropathic pain states. The dentist using these drugs as therapeutic agents is presumed to be proficient in prescribing and managing these medications.

Drug Interactions of Dental Interest

The use of local anesthetics with or without vasoconstrictors is described earlier under Special Dental Considerations. There may be additive anticholinergic effects, such as dry mouth and constipation, with anticholinergic drugs and some sedating antihistamines. Additionally, the cardio-accelerating effect of these medications may be undesirable. Barbiturates, especially when chronically administered, may induce hepatic enzymes and decrease the plasma levels of many antidysrhythmics. Neuromuscular blockade during general anesthesia may be prolonged. Phenytoin interactions are covered in Chapter 17, Neurological Drugs, although this agent typically is used as an antidysrhythmic only in acute cases, for digitalis overdose.

Laboratory Value Alterations

- Most Class I and Class III agents may cause leukopenia, thrombocytopenia or agranulocytosis in rare cases. Bleeding times may be affected.

- Quinidine may cause anemia.
- Disopyramide may lower blood glucose levels.

Pharmacology

The antidysrhythmic drugs, classified in four groups from Class I to Class IV, modify the aberrant electrophysiological process to help restore more normal rate and rhythm. The classification of antidysrhythmic drugs is based on the predominant electrophysiological effect of each drug on the various components of the cardiac conduction system in regard to automaticity, refractoriness and responsiveness. Examples of conditions in which these drugs are useful include atrial fibrillation and other atrial dysrhythmias, emergency treatment of ventricular fibrillation, ventricular dysrhythmias (including premature ventricular contractions, or PVCs), ventricular tachycardia and drug-induced dysrhythmias.

Cardiac Glycosides

These drugs are used mainly to treat congestive heart failure and certain cardiac dysrhythmias such as atrial fibrillation. Digoxin is the only commonly used cardiac glycoside in the U.S.

See Tables 14.1 and 14.2 for basic information on cardiac glycosides.

Special Dental Considerations

Increased gag reflex is possible. Bright dental lights may not be tolerated. The patient's anticoagulation status, as well as the patient's need for bacterial endocarditis prophylaxis, should be evaluated. In addition, the dentist should follow the recommendations listed under Special Dental Considerations at the beginning of this chapter for drugs in this category.

Drug Interactions of Dental Interest

Use of epinephrine in local anesthetic solutions should be minimized, and extra care should be taken with aspiration to avoid intravascular injection.

Sudden increases in potassium, such as through rapid IV administration of penicillin G potassium or succinylcholine, may precipitate digitalis-induced dysrhythmia.

Pharmacology

These drugs increase the force of cardiac contraction and decrease heart rate. By these mechanisms, an enlarged heart is allowed to function more efficiently and its size may be reduced. Because of the rate-slowing effects of these drugs, they are also used to treat specific supraventricular tachycardias. The primary mechanisms of action include inhibition of the sodium-potassium adenosinetriphosphatase, or ATPase, pump and increases in the availability of myocardial Ca^{++} ions intracellularly. This drug has a narrow therapeutic index which necessitates frequent plasma level determinations.

Antianginal Agents

Angina pectoris, literally "pain in the chest," usually results from a lack of adequate oxygen (ischemia) for myocardial need secondary to coronary atherosclerosis. There are three types of angina—chronic stable exertional angina, vasospastic (Prinzmetal's) angina and unstable angina. Chronic stable exertional angina usually occurs in patients when increased activity is such that myocardial oxygen requirement exceeds supply. These patients typically carry a sublingual tablet or spray nitroglycerin, which usually aborts attacks. Vasospastic angina usually occurs at rest secondary to coronary vasospasm rather than atherosclerosis. Unstable angina is, as the name implies, new-onset angina or worsening angina in a patient who was previously stable.

No elective dental procedures should be performed for patients with unstable angina until medically stabilized.

Immediate-acting nitrates, long-acting nitrates, β-blockers and calcium channel blockers are used in the management of angina.

See Tables 14.1 and 14.2 for basic information on antianginal drugs.

Special Dental Considerations

Patients with angina who are taking sublingual nitroglycerin on an as-needed basis should have this medication available at all dental appointments. In the event of chest pain during a dental visit, the prompt use of nitroglycerin is indicated. Supplemental oxygen and vital-sign monitoring are appropriate. Nitroglycerin in the dentist's emergency kit should be checked regularly, as its shelf life is generally short. This is especially true of sublingual nitroglycerin tablets after the container has been opened.

In addition, the dentist should follow the recommendations listed under Special Dental Considerations at the beginning of this chapter.

Nitroglycerin may cause flushing of the face, headache and xerostomia.

Drug Interactions of Dental Interest

Use of epinephrine in local anesthetic solutions should be minimized, and extra care should be taken with aspiration to avoid intravascular injection. Opioids may have added hypotensive effects.

Laboratory Value Alterations

- Use of nitrate-based antianginal agents may increase the risk of methemoglobinemia. Pulse oximetry may overestimate oxygen saturation.

Pharmacology

Four types of drugs are used to treat angina. The nitrates, typified by nitroglycerin, are direct-acting vasodilators. The primary effect is reduction in venous and arterial tone (former more than latter) leading to decreased myocardial workload and less so, coronary vasodilation. Long-acting nitrates, such as isosorbide dinitrate, are also somewhat effective; however, tolerance to these agents limits their long-term value. β-blockers, which block adrenergic responses, may be helpful in treating angina by decreasing myocardial rate and workload. Calcium channel blockers cause vasodilation and slow heart rate, thus decreasing anginal attacks. Lastly, antiplatelet and anticoagulation agents, such as aspirin, may be of value in preventing myocardial infarction.

Antihypertensive Agents

Hypertension is common in the American population, affecting 15-20% of people. The risk of hypertension increases dramatically with age. Physiological blood pressure regulation is a complex interrelationship of multiple overlapping systems. Generally, ACE inhibitors or diuretics are considered first-line agents. Other medications—such as β-blockers, calcium channel blockers, α-blockers and direct-acting vasodilators—are then used, alone or in combination, to control blood pressure. Most patients require a multiple medication regimen.

As dental therapeutic agents, many of these drugs are used to treat chronic orofacial pain conditions. β-blockers and calcium channel blockers are used to manage migraine and other neurovascular conditions. Verapamil is used for prevention of cluster headache. β-blockers and α-blockers are used in the management of complex regional pain syndrome (sympathetically maintained pain). Intravenous phentolamine is currently being used as a diagnostic tool to help determine if pain is being influenced by the sympathetic nervous system. Clonidine is used for a variety of painful conditions.

The dentist using these drugs as therapeutic agents is presumed to be proficient in prescribing and managing these medications.

Diuretics

Diuretic drugs generally exert an antihypertensive effect by increasing sodium and water excretion, thus decreasing blood volume. This decrease in blood volume decreases arterial tone and reduces myocardial workload. These drugs are commonly first-line agents and frequently are combined with other antihypertensives.

See Tables 14.1 and 14.2 for basic information on diuretics.

Special Dental Considerations
Potassium-sparing diuretics may rarely cause agranulocytosis and thrombocytopenia. Consider medication-induced adverse effects if gingival bleeding or infection occurs. In addition, some patients taking diuretics may experience xerostomia, which may require special dental care.

In addition, the dentist should follow the recommendations listed under Special Dental Considerations at the beginning of this chapter.

Drug Interactions of Dental Interest
NSAIDs may antagonize natriuresis and the antihypertensive effects of some diuretics.

Diflunisal, specifically, may increase the plasma concentration of hydrochlorothiazide. Excessive use of epinephrine in local anesthetic solutions may antagonize the antihypertensive effects of these agents. All diuretics, except potassium-sparing agents, may enhance neuromuscular blockade during general anesthesia.

Laboratory Value Alterations
* Loop diuretics and thiazide diuretics can increase blood glucose levels.

* Potassium-sparing diuretics may rarely cause agranulocytosis and thrombocytopenia.

Pharmacology
The site of action of these drugs can be any portion of the kidney from the glomerulus to the distal tubule. Modulation of electrolyte and water reabsorption are common mechanisms of action. It should be noted that patients may be taking these drugs for conditions other than essential hypertension such as renal failure, glaucoma or congestive heart failure. A thorough health history review should provide the necessary information.

Adrenergic Blocking Agents

Adrenergic blocking agents include β-blockers, α-blockers, and combined α- and β-blockers. These drugs are used to manage hypertension by decreasing sympathetic nervous system activity.

See Tables 14.1 and 14.2 for basic information on adrenergic blocking agents.

Special Dental Considerations
Rarely, taste changes have been reported. In addition, the dentist should follow the recommendations listed under Special Dental Considerations at the beginning of this chapter.

A rebound hypertensive crisis may occur if patients abruptly stop taking drugs in this category prior to a dental appointment. Dental patients should be instructed to take their medications at the usual time irrespective of the time of their dental appointment.

Drug Interactions of Dental Interest

Vasoconstrictors in local anesthetics
β-*blockers.* Hypertension and bradycardia can occur when epinephrine or levonordefrin in local anesthetic solutions is

administered to patients taking nonselective β-blockers. Vital sign monitoring before and after injection of local anesthetics containing vasoconstrictors is recommended. There is generally minimal interaction of local anesthetic solutions containing epinephrine with cardioselective β-blockers.

α-blockers. Hypotension and tachycardia can rarely occur when commonly used doses of epinephrine in local anesthetic solutions is administered to patients taking α-blockers. Vital sign monitoring before and after injection of local anesthetics containing vasoconstrictors is highly recommended.

Combined α- and β-blockers. There is generally minimal interaction with local anesthetic solutions containing epinephrine or levonordefrin.

For patients taking medications with β-blockade, long-term NSAID use can lead to significant renal compromise and careful monitoring is recommended.

All adrenergic blocking agents

NSAIDs may partially antagonize the antihypertensive effects of these medications. Opioids may potentiate the hypotensive effect of these medications.

β-blockers only

These agents may decrease the clearance of injected local anesthetics from the peripheral circulation. Phenothiazines may increase the plasma concentration of both drugs.

Pharmacology

The peripheral adrenergic autonomic system principally consists of β_1, β_2, α_1 and α_2 receptors. Catecholamines, such as epinephrine and norepinephrine, act as agonists at these receptors, which have numerous physiological effects. In regard to blood pressure control,

- β_1 activity increases force and rate of cardiac contraction, thus causing tachycardia and increase in blood pressure;

- β_2 activity causes vasodilation in skeletal muscles, thus decreasing blood pressure;
- α_1 receptors cause peripheral vasoconstriction, thus causing an increase in blood pressure;
- α_2 activity causes a decrease in the release of norepinephrine, thus decreasing adrenergic tone.

Adrenergic blocking agents work on one or more of these receptors to alter the sympathetic nervous system response.

β-blockers

β-blockers provide blood pressure control by decreasing the force and rate of cardiac contraction. They are also useful in tachydysrhythmias and angina pectoris. β-blockers are either nonselective or cardioselective. The nonselective β-blockers are antagonists at both the β_1 and β_2 receptors. The cardioselective β-blockers are antagonists at predominantly the β_1 receptor. Because of this difference in receptor activity, patients taking β_1 cardioselective agents experience little interaction with epinephrine in local anesthetic solutions.

α-blockers

α-blockers block either the α_1 receptor (making them selective) or both the α_1 and α_2 receptors (making them nonselective). These drugs control blood pressure by decreasing peripheral vascular tone. They are also used to improve urinary flow in prostatic hypertrophy. Since activation of α_2 receptors decreases adrenergic tone, agents that block both α_1 and α_2 receptors may not be desirable in some patients.

Combined α- and β-blockers

Labetalol and carvedilol block both α_1 and β_1/β_2 receptors with more activity at α-receptors than at β-receptors. Labetalol and carvedilol thus possess properties of a nonselective β-blocker and a vasodilator.

Direct-Acting Vasodilators

Vasodilators include hydralazine, minoxidil, diazoxide, nitroglycerin and derivatives, as well as the calcium channel blockers, which are discussed in a separate section below. These drugs work directly on the peripheral vasculature to decrease arterial and/or venous tone. See Tables 14.1 and 14.2 for basic information on direct-acting vasodilators.

Special Dental Considerations

Hydralazine may, rarely, cause agranulocytosis and thrombocytopenia. The dentist should consider medication effects if gingival bleeding or infection occurs. Facial flushing may occur. Excessive facial hair growth may be seen with minoxidil.

In addition, the dentist should follow the recommendations listed under Special Dental Considerations at the beginning of this chapter.

Drug Interactions of Dental Interest

Excessive use of epinephrine in local anesthetic solutions may antagonize the antihypertensive effects of these agents. NSAIDs may partially antagonize the antihypertensive effects of these medications. Opioids may potentiate the hypotensive effect of these medications.

Laboratory Value Alterations

- Erythrocyte concentration, hemoglobin and hematocrit may be artificially decreased due to hemodilution.

Pharmacology

These agents provide hypertension control predominantly by various direct actions on vascular smooth muscle. The mechanism of action is believed to be mediated via nitric oxide, which alters Ca^{++} dependent muscular contractility and thus produces vascular muscle relaxation.

Vasodilators Used for Erectile Dysfunction

Erectile dysfunction is caused by organic, psychogenic or mixed etiologies. Diseases such as diabetes and peripheral vascular disease, as well as postsurgical sequelae such as those following prostatectomy, can cause erectile dysfunction. See Tables 14.1 and 14.2 for basic information on vasodilators used for erectile dysfunction.

Special Dental Considerations

Glossitis, stomatitis, gingivitis and xerostomia have been reported; however, a causal relationship to drug use is unclear.

Drug Interactions of Dental Interest

Erythromycin, ketaconazole and itraconazole may increase plasma levels of erectile dysfunction vasodilators.

Pharmacology

The mechanism of erection of the penis involves release of nitric oxide (NO) in the corpus cavernosum during sexual stimulation. NO activates guanylate cyclase, which increases cGMP levels to produce smooth muscle relaxation and increase blood flow to the corpus cavernosum. Sildenafil inhibits the degradation of cGMP, thus increasing the effects of NO. At recommended doses, sildenafil has no effect in the absence of sexual stimulation.

Calcium Channel Blockers

Calcium channel blockers are commonly prescribed antihypertensive, antianginal and antidysrhythmic agents. See Tables 14.1 and 14.2 for basic information on calcium channel blockers.

Special Dental Considerations

Gingival enlargement can occur with these agents. Meticulous oral hygiene can reduce these effects. If gingival enlargement occurs, the patient's physician should be consulted about changing the medication to a non-calcium channel blocker antihypertensive. Nimodipine may cause thrombocytopenia. Other agents rarely cause blood dyscrasias. Consider medication-induced adverse effects if gingival bleeding or infection occurs.

In addition, the dentist should follow the recommendations listed under Special Dental Considerations at the beginning of this chapter.

Drug Interactions of Dental Interest

Excessive use of epinephrine in local anesthetic solutions may antagonize the antihypertensive effects of these agents. NSAIDs may partially antagonize the antihypertensive effects of these medications. Opioids may potentiate the hypotensive effect of these medications. There is a possible increased hypotensive effect with aspirin.

Pharmacology

These drugs decrease peripheral vascular tone by decreasing calcium influx in vascular smooth muscle. The antidysrhythmic effect is due primarily to decreasing the slow inward Ca^{++} current in the cardiac conduction system. The agents also depress force and rate of cardiac contraction to various degrees. For instance, verapamil and diltiazem control heart rate more effectively than other calcium channel blockers while most other agents act more prominently by direct vasodilation.

Drugs Acting on the Renin-Angiotensin System

These drugs are considered first-line agents in the control of hypertension. By blocking the effects of angiotensin II, a potent vasoconstrictor, these agents decrease high blood pressure in many patients. The angiotensin receptor blockers exert antagonist activity at the receptor on the blood vessel wall while angiotensin-converting enzyme inhibitors block the formation of angiotensin II. See Tables 14.1 and 14.2 for basic information on drugs acting on the renin-angiotensin system.

Special Dental Considerations

These agents may cause neutropenia or agranulocytosis. Consider medication-induced adverse effects if gingival bleeding or infection occurs. Angioneurotic edema may occur on the face, tongue or glottis. Coughing is a common side effect. Loss of taste has been reported, but rarely.

In addition, the dentist should follow the recommendations listed under Special Dental Considerations at the beginning of this chapter.

Drug Interactions of Dental Interest

Excessive use of epinephrine in local anesthetic solutions may antagonize the antihypertensive effects of these agents. NSAIDs may partially antagonize the antihypertensive effects of these medications. Long term NSAID use can lead to significant renal compromise and careful monitoring is recommended. Opioids may potentiate the hypotensive effect of these medications. Potassium-containing medications, such as penicillin G potassium administered IV, may exacerbate medication-induced hyperkalemia.

Laboratory Value Alterations

- Agranulocytosis and neutropenia may occur.

Pharmacology

Under normal conditions, the reninangiotensin system provides for an increase in blood pressure when hypotension occurs.

Renin released from the renal glomerulus leads to the formation of angiotensin I, which is converted to angiotensin II, primarily in the lung. Angiotensin II is a potent vasoconstrictor and also stimulates aldosterone release. The antihypertensive effect of these agents occurs when angiotensin II is blocked, either at the angiotensin II receptor on the blood vessel wall or by decreased formation of angiotensin II itself. This latter effect occurs when angiotensin-converting enzyme (ACE) in the lung is inhibited, thus blocking the metabolism of angiotensin I to angiotensin II. The term "ACE inhibitor" is therefore commonly used with these medications. Renin inhibiting agents are currently being developed.

Centrally Acting Antihypertensive Agents

These drugs act in the central nervous system (CNS) to decrease peripheral sympathetic tone. See Tables 14.1 and 14.2 for basic information on centrally acting antihypertensive agents.

Special Dental Considerations
A rebound hypertensive crisis may occur if patients abruptly stop taking drugs in this category prior to a dental appointment. Dental patients should be instructed to take their medications at the usual time irrespective of the time of their dental appointment.

These drugs may inhibit salivary flow. Parotid pain may occur.

In addition, the dentist should follow the recommendations listed under Special Dental Considerations at the beginning of this chapter.

Drug Interactions of Dental Interest
Excessive use of epinephrine in local anesthetic solutions may antagonize the antihypertensive effects of these agents and produce a serious hypertensive crisis. NSAIDs may partially antagonize the antihypertensive effects of these medications. Opioids may potentiate the hypotensive and sedative effects of these medications. Other oral or IV sedative agents may be potentiated by these agents. There may be a decreased antihypertensive effect with tricyclic antidepressants. Methyldopa may increase the anticoagulant effect of coumarin anticoagulants.

Pharmacology
The mechanism of action of these agents is chiefly via a CNS α_2 agonist action. As the α_2 receptor decreases adrenergic tone, there is a decrease in sympathetic outflow. This causes a decrease in blood pressure and heart rate.

Peripheral Adrenergic Neuron Antagonists

This diverse group of drugs is rarely prescribed today due to numerous undesirable side effects and the availability of other more efficacious agents. See Tables 14.1 and 14.2 for basic information on peripheral adrenergic neuron antagonists.

Special Dental Considerations
These drugs may inhibit salivary flow.

In addition, the dentist should follow the recommendations listed under Special Dental Considerations at the beginning of this chapter.

Drug Interactions of Dental Interest
Peripheral adrenergic neuron antagonists can cause administered epinephrine to have an exaggerated cardiovascular effect. Blood pressure and heart rate should be carefully monitored if local anesthetic solutions containing epinephrine are deemed essential. NSAIDs may partially antagonize the

antihypertensive effects of these medications. Opioids may potentiate the hypotensive and sedative effects of these medications. Other oral or IV sedative agents may be potentiated by these agents. Phenothiazines may exhibit increased extrapyramidal reactions.

Pharmacology

These drugs act principally by depleting norepinephrine and other catecholamines from the adrenergic nerve endings. Therefore, decreases in heart rate, force of cardiac contraction and peripheral vascular resistance result. These drugs can have complex effects when initially administered.

Anticholesterol Drugs

3-hydroxy-3-methylglutaryl coenzyme A (HMG CoA) reductase inhibitors are the primary drugs used to lower cholesterol, predominantly low-density lipoproteins (LDLs), also called "bad cholesterol." Some agents increase HDLs, the "good cholesterol." Colloquially, these drugs are termed "statins." Drugs that lower LDLs and raise HDLs can prevent the formation of, slow the progression of, or decrease already-formed atherosclerotic plaques. This can lead to improved coronary blood flow and a decrease in morbidity and mortality associated with coronary artery disease.

Other agents used to modify triglyceride levels and cholesterol include resins (cholestyramine and colestipol), fibrates (clofibrate, gemfibrozil and fenofibrate), inhibitors of cholesterol absorption (ezetimibe) and niacin.

See Tables 14.1 and 14.2 for dosage and prescribing information on anticholesterol drugs.

Special Dental Considerations

There are no specific dental considerations other than evaluating the overall cardiovascular risk in patients who are hypercholesteremic, as this indicates at least one risk factor for coronary artery disease.

Drug Interactions of Dental Interest

Use of erythromycin with lovastatin has been associated with increased risk of rhabdomyolysis and acute renal failure. Although this has not been reported for other HMG CoA reductase inhibitors, it is recommended that erythromycin not be given to patients taking any agent in this class. It is not clear if other macrolides, such as clarithromycin, also exhibit this interaction.

Laboratory Value Alterations

* Levels of serum transaminase may increase.
* Creatinine kinase levels may increase, although this usually is not associated with myositis or rhabdomyolysis.

Pharmacology

The conversion of HMG CoA to mevalonate is the rate-limiting step in the synthesis of cholesterol, primarily in the liver. The inhibition of cholesterol synthesis by HMG CoA reductase inhibitors, which block this rate-limiting step, leads to upregulation of LDL receptors and a subsequent increase in degradation of LDLs. There also is a decrease in the synthesis of LDLs.

Adverse Effects

Table 14.1 lists adverse effects of cardiovascular medications.

Suggested Readings

Drugs for cardiac arrhythmias. Med Lett Drugs Ther 1991;33(846):55-60.

Follath F. Clinical pharmacology of antiarrhythmic drugs: variability of metabolism and dose requirements. J Cardiovasc Pharmacol 1991;17(Suppl 6):S74-6.

Friedman L, Schron E, Yusuf S. Risk-benefit assessment of antiarrhythmic drugs: an epidemiological perspective. Drug Saf 1991;6:323-31.

Kaplan NM, ed. Clinical hypertension. 6th ed. Baltimore: Williams & Wilkins; 1994.

Laragh JH, Brenner BM, eds. Hypertension: Pathology, diagnosis, and management. New York: Raven Press; 1990.

Muzyka BC, Glick M. The hypertensive dental patient. JADA 1997;128:1109-20.

Nichols C. Dentistry and hypertension. JADA 1997; 128:1557-2.

Veterans Administration Cooperative Study Group on Antihypertensive Agents. Effects of treatment on morbidity in hypertension. JAMA 1967;202:1028-34.

Table 14.1 PRESCRIBING INFORMATION FOR CARDIOVASCULAR DRUGS

NAME	FORM/ STRENGTH	DOSAGE	WARNINGS/PRECAUTIONS & CONTRAINDICATIONS	ADVERSE EFFECTS†
ACE INHIBITORS				
Benazepril Hydrochloride (Lotensin)	**Tab:** 5mg, 10mg, 20mg, 40mg	***Adults:*** If possible, discontinue diuretic 2-3 days prior to therapy. **Initial:** 10mg qd, 5mg with concomitant diuretic. **Maint:** 20-40mg/day given qd-bid. Resume diuretic if BP not controlled. **Max:** 80mg/day. **CrCl <30mL/min: Initial:** 5mg qd. **Max:** 40mg/day.	**ACE inhibitors can cause death/injury to developing fetus during 2nd and 3rd trimesters. Stop therapy if pregnancy detected. W/P:** Discontinue if angioedema, jaundice, or if marked LFT elevation occurs. Risk of hyperkalemia with DM, renal dysfunction. Persistent nonproductive cough reported. Monitor WBCs in renal and collagen vascular disease. Anaphylactoid reactions reported. Fetal/neonatal morbidity and death reported. Monitor for hypotension in high risk patients (eg, surgery/anesthesia, prolonged diuretic therapy, heart failure, volume and/or salt depletion, etc). Caution with CHF, renal dysfunction, and renal artery stenosis. Less effective on BP in blacks and more reports of angioedema than nonblacks. **P/N:** Category C (1st trimester) and D (2nd and 3rd trimesters), safety not known in nursing.	Cough, dizziness, headache, fatigue, somnolence, postural dizziness, nausea.
Captopril (Capoten)	**Tab:** 12.5mg*, 25mg*, 50mg*, 100mg*	***Adults:*** Take 1 hour before meals. **HTN:** If possible, discontinue recent antihypertensive drug for 1 week prior to therapy. **Initial:** 25mg bid-tid. **Titrate:** May increase to 50mg bid-tid after 1-2 weeks. **Usual:** 25-150mg bid-tid. **Max:** 450mg/day. **CHF: Initial:** 25mg tid; 6.25-12.5mg tid with risk of hypotension or salt/volume depletion. **Usual:** 50-100mg tid. **Max:** 450mg/day. **Left Ventricular Dysfunction Post-MI: Initial:** 6.25mg single dose, then 12.5mg tid. **Titrate:** Increase to 25mg tid over next several days, then to 50mg tid over next several weeks. **Usual:** 50mg tid. **Diabetic Nephropathy:** 25mg tid. **Significant Renal Dysfunction:** Decrease initial dose and titrate slowly.	**ACE inhibitors can cause death/injury to developing fetus during 2nd and 3rd trimesters. Stop therapy if pregnancy detected. W/P:** Discontinue if jaundice or marked LFT elevation occurs. Risk of hyperkalemia with DM, renal dysfunction. Persistent nonproductive cough, anaphylactoid reactions, neutropenia with myeloid hypoplasia reported. Fetal/neonatal morbidity and death reported. Monitor for hypotension in high risk patients (surgery/anesthesia, dialysis, heart failure, volume/salt depletion, etc). Caution with CHF, renal dysfunction, renal artery stenosis, collagen vascular disease (especially with renal dysfunction). Monitor WBC before therapy, then every 2 weeks for 3 months, then periodically. Less effective on BP in blacks and more reports of angioedema than nonblacks. **Contra:** History of ACE inhibitor associated angioedema. **N/P:** Category C (1st trimester) and D (2nd and 3rd trimesters), not for use in nursing.	Proteinuria, rash, hypotension, dysgeusia, cough, MI, CHF.
Enalapril Maleate (Vasotec)	**Tab:** 2.5mg*, 5mg*, 10mg, 20mg	***Adults:* HTN:** If possible, discontinue diuretic 2-3 days prior to therapy. **Initial:** 5mg qd, 2.5mg qd with concomitant diuretic. **Usual:** 10-40mg/day given qd or bid. Resume diuretic if BP not controlled. CrCl <30mL/min: **Initial:** 2.5mg/day. **Dialysis:** 2.5mg/day on dialysis days. **Heart Failure: Initial:** 2.5mg/day. **Usual:** 2.5-20mg given bid. **Max:** 40mg/day. **Left Ventricular Dysfunction: Initial:** 2.5mg bid. **Titrate:** Increase to 20mg/day. Hyponatremia or SrCr 1.6mg/dL with **Heart Failure: Initial:** 2.5mg qd. **Titrate:** Increase to 2.5mg bid, then 5mg bid. **Max:** 40mg/day. ***Pediatrics:* HTN:** 1 month-16 yrs: **Initial:** 0.08mg/kg (up to 5mg) qd. **Titrate:** Adjust according to response.	**ACE inhibitors can cause death/injury to developing fetus during 2nd and 3rd trimesters. Stop therapy if pregnancy detected. W/P:** Discontinue if angioedema, jaundice, or if marked LFT elevation occurs. Risk of hyperkalemia with DM, renal dysfunction. Persistent nonproductive cough reported. Monitor WBCs in renal or collagen vascular disease. Anaphylactoid reactions reported. Fetal/neonatal morbidity and death reported. Monitor for hypotension in high risk patients (heart failure, surgery/anesthesia, hyponatremia, high dose diuretic therapy, severe volume and/or salt depletion, etc). Caution with CHF, obstruction to left ventricle outflow tract, renal dysfunction, and renal artery stenosis. Less effective on BP in blacks and more reports of angioedema than nonblacks. **Contra:** History of ACE inhibitor associated angioedema and hereditary or idiopathic angioedema.	Fatigue, orthostatic effects, asthenia, diarrhea, nausea, headache, dizziness, cough, rash, hypotension, vomiting.

*Scored.   †Bold entries denote special dental considerations.

NAME	FORM/STRENGTH	DOSAGE	WARNINGS/PRECAUTIONS & CONTRAINDICATIONS	ADVERSE EFFECTS[†]
Enalapril Maleate *(cont.)*		**Max:** 0.58mg/kg/dose (or 40mg/dose). Avoid if GFR <30mL/min/1.73m². **To prepare 200mL of 1mg/mL Sus:** Add 50mL of Bicitra to polyethylene terephthalate bottle with ten 20mg tabs and shake for at least 2 minutes. Let stand for 60 minutes, then shake again for 1 minute. Add 150mL of Ora-Sweet SF and shake, then refrigerate. Can store up to 30 days.	**P/N:** Category C (1st trimester) and D (2nd and 3rd trimesters), not for use in nursing.	
Fosinopril Sodium (Monopril)	**Tab:** 10mg*, 20mg, 40mg	**Adults:** If possible, discontinue diuretic 2-3 days before therapy. **Initial:** 10mg qd, monitor carefully if cannot discontinue diuretic. **Maint:** 20-40mg/day. Resume diuretic if BP not controlled. **Max:** 80mg/day. **Heart Failure: Initial:** 10mg qd, 5mg with moderate to severe renal failure or vigorous diuresis. **Titrate:** Increase over several weeks. **Maint:** 20-40mg qd. Max: 40mg qd. **Elderly:** Start at low end of dosing range.	**ACE inhibitors can cause death/injury to developing fetus during 2nd and 3rd trimesters. Stop therapy if pregnancy detected. W/P:** Discontinue if angioedema, jaundice, or if marked LFT elevation occurs. Risk of hyperkalemia with DM, renal dysfunction. Persistent nonproductive cough reported. Monitor WBCs in renal and collagen vascular disease. Anaphylactoid reactions reported. Fetal/neonatal morbidity and death reported. Monitor for hypotension in high risk patients (heart failure, volume and/or salt depletion, surgery/anesthesia, etc). Less effective on BP in blacks and more reports of angioedema than nonblacks. Caution with CHF, renal or hepatic dysfunction, renal artery stenosis. May cause false low measurement of serum digoxin level. **Contra:** History of ACE inhibitor associated angioedema. **P/N:** Category C (1st trimester) and D (2nd and 3rd trimesters), not for use in nursing.	Dizziness, cough, hypotension, musculoskeletal pain.
Lisinopril (Zestril, Prinivil)	**Tab:** 2.5mg, 5mg*, 10mg, 20mg, 30mg, 40mg	**Adults: HTN:** If possible, discontinue diuretic 2-3 days prior to therapy. **Initial:** 10mg qd, 5mg qd with diuretic. **Usual:** 20-40mg qd. Resume diuretic if BP not controlled. **Max:** 80mg/day. **CrCl 10-30mL/min: Initial:** 5mg/day. **Max:** 40mg/day. **CrCl <10mL/min: Initial:** 2.5mg/day. **Max:** 40mg/day. **Heart Failure: Initial:** 5mg qd. **Usual:** 5-40mg qd. May increase by 10mg every 2 weeks. **Max:** 40mg/day. **Hyponatremia or CrCl ≤30mL/min: Initial:** 2.5mg qd. **AMI: Initial:** 5mg within 24 hrs, then 5mg after 24 hrs, then 10mg after 48 hrs, then 10mg qd. Use 2.5mg during 1st 3 days with low systolic BP. **Maint:** 10mg qd for 6 weeks, 2.5-5mg with hypotension. Discontinue with prolonged hypotension. **Elderly:** Caution with dose adjustment.	**ACE inhibitors can cause death/injury to developing fetus during 2nd and 3rd trimesters. Stop therapy if pregnancy detected. W/P:** Discontinue if angioedema, jaundice, or if marked LFT elevation occurs. Risk of hyperkalemia with DM, renal dysfunction. Persistent nonproductive cough reported. Monitor WBCs in renal and collagen vascular disease. Anaphylactoid reactions reported. Fetal/neonatal morbidity and death reported. Monitor for hypotension in high risk patients (heart failure with systolic BP <100 mmHg, surgery/anesthesia, hyponatremia, high dose diuretic therapy, severe volume and/or salt depletion, etc). Caution with CHF, renal dysfunction, and renal artery stenosis. Less effective on BP in blacks and more reports of angioedema than nonblacks. **Contra:** History of ACE inhibitor associated angioedema. **P/N:** Category C (1st trimester) and D (2nd and 3rd trimesters), not for use in nursing.	Hypotension, diarrhea, headache, dizziness, hyperkalemia, increase creatinine and nonprotein nitrogen, syncope, chest pain.
Moexipril Hydrochloride (Univasc)	**Tab:** 7.5mg*, 15mg*	**Adults:** If possible, discontinue diuretic 2-3 days prior to therapy. Take 1 hr before meals. **Initial:** 7.5mg qd, 3.75mg with concomitant diuretic therapy. **Maint:** 7.5-30mg/day given qd-bid. Resume diuretic if BP not controlled. **Max:** 60mg/day. **CrCl ≤40mL/min: Initial:** 3.75mg qd. **Max:** 15mg/day.	**ACE inhibitors can cause death/injury to developing fetus during 2nd and 3rd trimesters. Stop therapy if pregnancy detected. W/P:** Discontinue if angioedema, jaundice, or if marked LFT elevation occurs. Intestinal angioedema reported. Risk of hyperkalemia with DM, renal dysfunction. Persistent nonproductive cough reported. Monitor WBCs in renal and collagen vascular	Cough, dizziness, diarrhea, flu syndrome, fatigue, pharyngitis, flushing, rash, myalgia.

Table 14.1 PRESCRIBING INFORMATION FOR CARDIOVASCULAR DRUGS *(cont.)*

NAME	FORM/ STRENGTH	DOSAGE	WARNINGS/PRECAUTIONS & CONTRAINDICATIONS	ADVERSE EFFECTS†
ACE INHIBITORS *(cont.)*				
Moexipril Hydrochloride *(cont.)*			disease. Anaphylactoid reactions reported. Fetal/neonatal morbidity and death reported. Monitor for hypotension in high risk patients (heart failure, surgery/anesthesia, prolonged diuretic therapy, volume and/or salt depletion, etc). Caution with CHF, renal dysfunction, and renal artery stenosis. Less effective on BP in blacks and more reports of angioedema than nonblacks. **P/N:** Category C (1st trimester) and D (2nd and 3rd trimesters), not for use in nursing.	
Perindopril Erbumine (Aceon)	**Tab:** 2mg*, 4mg*, 8mg*	***Adults:* HTN:** If possible, discontinue diuretic 2-3 days prior to therapy. **Initial:** 4mg qd; 2-4mg/day given qd-bid with concomitant diuretic. **Maint:** 4-8mg/day given qd-bid. Resume diuretic if BP not controlled. **Max:** 16mg/day. **Elderly (>65 yrs): Initial:** 4mg/day given qd-bid. **Max (usual):** 8mg/day. **Renal Impairment: CrCl >30mL/min: Initial:** 2mg/day. Max: 8mg/day. **CAD: Initial:** 4mg qd for 2 weeks. **Maint:** 8mg qd. **Elderly (>70 yrs): Initial:** 2mg qd for 1 week. **Titrate:** 4mg qd for Week 2. **Maint:** 8mg qd.	**ACE inhibitors can cause death/injury to developing fetus during 2nd and 3rd trimesters. Stop therapy if pregnancy detected. W/P:** Discontinue if angioedema, jaundice, or if marked LFT elevation occurs. Risk of hyperkalemia with DM, renal dysfunction. Persistent nonproductive cough reported. Monitor WBCs in renal and collagen vascular disease. Anaphylactoid reactions reported. Fetal/neonatal morbidity and death reported. Monitor for hypotension in high risk patients (heart failure, surgery/anesthesia, hyponatremia, prolonged diuretic therapy, or volume and/or salt depletion). Caution with CHF, renal dysfunction, and renal artery stenosis. Less effective on BP in blacks and more reports of angioedema than nonblacks. Avoid if CrCl ≥30mL/min. **Contra:** History of ACE inhibitor associated angioedema. **P/N:** Category C (1st trimester) and D (2nd and 3rd trimesters), caution in nursing.	Cough, headache, asthenia, dizziness, diarrhea, edema, respiratory infection, lower extremity pain.
Quinapril Hydrochloride (Accupril)	**Tab:** 5mg*, 10mg, 20mg, 40mg	***Adults:* HTN:** If possible, discontinue diuretic 2-3 days prior to therapy. **Initial:** 10-20mg qd; 5mg qd with concomitant diuretic. Titrate at intervals of at least 2 weeks. **Usual:** 20-80mg/day given qd-bid. **CrCl >60mL/min: Initial:** 10mg/day. **CrCl 30-60mL/min: Initial:** 5mg/day. **CrCl 10-30mL/min: Initial:** 2.5mg/day. **Heart Failure: Initial:** 5mg bid. Titrate at weekly intervals. **Usual:** 10-20mg bid. **CrCl >30mL/min: Initial:** 5mg/day. **CrCl 10-30mL/min: Initial:** 2.5mg/day.	**ACE inhibitors can cause death/injury to developing fetus during 2nd and 3rd trimesters. Stop therapy if pregnancy detected. W/P:** Discontinue if angioedema, jaundice, or if marked LFT elevation occurs. Risk of hyperkalemia with DM, renal dysfunction. Persistent nonproductive cough reported. Monitor WBCs in renal or collagen vascular disease. Anaphylactoid reactions reported. Fetal/neonatal morbidity and death reported. Monitor for hypotension in high risk patients (heart failure, surgery/anesthesia, hyponatremia, high dose diuretic therapy, recent intensive diuresis, dialysis, or severe volume and/or salt depletion,etc.). Caution with CHF, renal dysfunction, and renal artery stenosis. Less effective on BP in blacks and more reports of angioedema than nonblacks. **Contra:** History of ACE inhibitor associated angioedema. **P/N:** Category C (1st trimester) and D (2nd and 3rd trimesters), not for use in nursing.	Fatigue, headache, dizziness, cough, nausea, vomiting, hypotension, chest pain.

*Scored.   †Bold entries denote special dental considerations.

NAME	FORM/ STRENGTH	DOSAGE	WARNINGS/PRECAUTIONS & CONTRAINDICATIONS	ADVERSE EFFECTS†
Ramipril (Altace)	**Cap:** 1.25mg, 2.5mg, 5mg, 10mg	**Adults: HTN: Initial:** 2.5mg qd. **Maint:** 2.5-20mg/day given qd or bid. Add diuretic if BP not controlled. **CrCl <40mL/min: Initial:** 1.25mg qd. **Titrate/Max:** 5mg/day. **CHF Post-MI: Initial:** 2.5mg bid, 1.25mg bid if hypotensive. **Titrate:** Increase to 5mg bid. **CrCl <40mL/ min: Initial:** 1.25mg qd. **Titrate:** May increase to 1.25mg bid. **Max:** 2.5mg bid. **Reduction in Risk of MI, Stroke, Death (≥55 yrs): Initial:** 2.5mg qd for 1 week. Increase to 5mg qd for the next 3 weeks. **Maint:** 10mg qd. Reduce/discontinue diuretic if possible. **Volume Depletion/Renal Artery Stenosis: Initial:** 1.25 mg qd.	**ACE inhibitors can cause death/injury to developing fetus during 2nd and 3rd trimesters. Stop therapy if pregnancy detected. W/P:** Discontinue if angioedema, jaundice, or if marked LFT elevation occurs. Risk of hyperkalemia with DM, renal dysfunction. Persistent nonproductive cough and anaphylactoid reactions reported. Monitor WBCs in renal and collagen vascular disease. Fetal/neonatal morbidity and death reported. Monitor for hypotension in high risk patients (heart failure, surgery/anesthesia, hyponatremia, high dose diuretic therapy, recent intensive diuresis, dialysis, or severe volume and/or salt depletion, etc). Caution with CHF, renal dysfunction, severe liver cirrhosis and/or ascites, and renal artery stenosis. Less effective on BP in blacks and more reports of angioedema than nonblacks. May reduce RBC, Hgb, WBC or platelets. May cause agranulocytosis, pancytopenia and bone marrow depression. **Contra:** History of ACE inhibitor associated angioedema. **P/N:** Category C (1st trimester) and D (2nd and 3rd trimesters), not for use in nursing.	Hypotension, cough, dizziness, fatigue, angina, impotence, Stevens-Johnson syndrome.
Trandolapril (Mavik)	**Tab:** 1mg*, 2mg, 4mg	**Adults: HTN:** If possible, discontinue diuretic 2-3 days before therapy. **Initial:** 1mg qd in non-black patients; 2mg qd in black patients; 0.5mg with concomitant diuretic. **Titrate:** Adjust at 1 week intervals. **Usual:** 2-4mg qd. Resume diuretic if not controlled. **Max:** 8mg/day. **Post-MI: Initial:** 1mg qd. **Titrate:** Increase to target dose of 4mg qd as tolerated. **CrCl <30mL/min/Hepatic Cirrhosis for HTN or Post-MI: Initial:** 0.5mg qd.	**ACE inhibitors can cause death/injury to developing fetus during 2nd and 3rd trimesters. Stop therapy if pregnancy detected. W/P:** Discontinue if angioedema or jaundice occurs. Risk of hyperkalemia with DM, renal dysfunction. Persistent nonproductive cough reported. Monitor WBCs in renal impairment and/or collagen vascular disease. Anaphylactoid reactions reported. Fetal/neonatal morbidity and death reported. Monitor for hypotension in high risk patients (heart failure, surgery/anesthesia, prolonged diuretic therapy, volume and/or salt depletion, etc). Caution with CHF, renal dysfunction, and renal artery stenosis. More reports of angioedema in blacks than nonblacks. **Contra:** History of ACE inhibitor associated angioedema. **P/N:** Category C (1st trimester) and D (2nd and 3rd trimesters), not for use in nursing.	Cough, dizziness, hypotension, elevated serum uric acid, elevated BUN, elevated creatinine, asthenia, syncope, myalgia, gastritis, hypocalcemia, hyperkalemia, dyspepsia.

ACE INHIBITORS/DIURETICS

Benazepril Hydrochloride/ Hydrochlorothiazide (Lotensin HCT)	**Tab: (Benazepril-HCTZ)** 5mg-6.25mg*, 10mg-12.5mg*, 20mg-12.5mg*, 20mg-25mg*	**Adults: Initial (if not controlled on benazepril monotherapy):** 10mg-12.5mg tab or 20mg-12.5mg tab. **Titrate:** May increase after 2-3 weeks. **Initial (if controlled on 25mg HCTZ/day with hypokalemia):** 5mg-6.25mg tab. **Replacement Therapy:** Substitute combination for titrated components.	**ACE inhibitors can cause death/injury to developing fetus during 2nd and 3rd trimesters. Stop therapy if pregnancy detected. W/P:** Avoid if CrCl ≥30mL/min/ 1.73m². Discontinue if angioedema, jaundice, or if marked LFT elevation occurs. Risk of hyperkalemia with DM, renal dysfunction. May cause persistent nonproductive cough, hypokalemia, hyperuricemia, hypomagnesemia, hypercalcemia, hypophosphatemia.	Cough, dizziness/ postural dizziness, headache, fatigue.

Table 14.1 PRESCRIBING INFORMATION FOR CARDIOVASCULAR DRUGS *(cont.)*

NAME	FORM/ STRENGTH	DOSAGE	WARNINGS/PRECAUTIONS & CONTRAINDICATIONS	ADVERSE EFFECTS†
ACE INHIBITORS/DIURETICS *(cont.)*				
Benazepril Hydrochloride/ Hydrochloro- thiazide *(cont.)*			Monitor WBCs in renal and collagen vascular disease. Anaphylactoid reactions reported. Fetal/neonatal morbidity and death reported. Monitor for hypotension in high risk patients (eg, surgery/anesthesia, prolonged diuretic therapy, heart failure, volume and/or salt depletion, etc). Caution with CHF, renal dysfunction, and renal artery stenosis. More reports of angioedema in blacks than nonblacks. Monitor f-r fluid/electrolyte imbalance. May increase cholesterol and TG levels. May exacerbate/activate SLE. **Contra:** Anuria, su'fonamide hypersensitivity. **P/N:** Category C (1st trimester) and D (2nd and 3rd trimesters), not for use in nursing.	
Captopril/ Hydrochloro- thiazide (Capozide)	**Tab: (Captopril-HCTZ)** 25mg-15mg*, 25mg-25mg*, 50mg-15mg*, 50mg-25mg*	***Adults:*** **Initial:** 25mg-15mg tab qd. **Titrate:** Adjust dose at 6-week intervals. **Max:** 150mg captopril/50mg HCTZ per day. **Replacement Therapy:** Substitute combination for titrated components. **Renal Impairment:** Decrease dose or increase interval. Take 1 hr before meals.	**ACE inhibitors can cause death/injury to developing fetus during 2nd and 3rd trimesters. Stop therapy if pregnancy detected. W/P:** Discontinue if angioedema, jaundice, or if marked LFT elevation occurs. Risk of hyperkalemia with DM, renal dysfunction. Monitor WBCs in renal and collagen vascular disease. Fetal/neonatal morbidity and death reported. Monitor for hypotension in high risk patients (eg, surgery/anesthesia, volume/salt depletion). Caution with renal or hepatic dysfunction. More reports of angioedema in blacks than nonblacks. May exacerbate or activate SLE. Monitor electrolytes. Hypercalcemia, hypomagnesemia, hyperuricemia may occur. With renal impairment, monitor WBCs and differential before therapy, every 2 weeks for 3 months, then periodically. Neutropenia with myeloid hypoplasia, persistent non-productive cough, anaphylactoid reactions, proteinuria reported. **Contra:** History of ACE inhibitor associated angioedema, anuria, sulfonamide hypersensitivity. **P/N:** Category C (1st trimester) and D (2nd and 3rd trimesters), not for use in nursing.	Cough, hypotension, rash, pruritus, fever, arthralgia, eosinophilia, dysgeusia, neutropenia/thrombocytopenia.
Enalapril Maleate/ Hydrochloro- thiazide (Vaseretic)	**Tab: (Enalapril-HCTZ)** 5mg-12.5mg, 10mg-25mg	***Adults:*** **Initial (if not controlled with enalapril/HCTZ monotherapy):** 5mg-12.5mg tab or 10mg-25mg tab qd. **Titrate:** May increase after 2-3 weeks. **Max:** 20mg enalapril/50mg HCTZ per day. **Replacement Therapy:** Substitute combination for titrated components.	**ACE inhibitors can cause death/injury to developing fetus during 2nd and 3rd trimesters. Stop therapy if pregnancy detected. W/P:** Discontinue if angioedema, jaundice, or if marked LFT elevation occurs. Risk of hyperkalemia with DM, renal dysfunction. Persistent nonproductive cough reported. Monitor WBCs in renal and collagen vascular disease. Anaphylactoid reactions reported. Fetal/neonatal morbidity and death reported. Monitor for hypotension in high risk patients (surgery/anesthesia, hyponatremia, severe volume/salt depletion, etc). Caution with CHF, renal or hepatic dysfunction, obstruction to left ventricle outflow tract, elderly, renal artery stenosis. More reports of angioedema in blacks than nonblacks. May exacerbate or activate SLE. Monitor serum electrolytes. Avoid if CrCl $\geq$30mL/min/1.73m^2. May increase	Dizziness, cough, fatigue, orthostatic effects, diarrhea, nausea, muscle cramps, asthenia, impotence.

*Scored. †Bold entries denote special dental considerations.

NAME	FORM/ STRENGTH	DOSAGE	WARNINGS/PRECAUTIONS & CONTRAINDICATIONS	ADVERSE EFFECTS†
Enalapril Maleate/ Hydrochloro- thiazide *(cont.)*			cholesterol, TG, uric acid levels, and blood glucose. **Contra:** History of ACE inhibitor associated angioedema and hereditary or idiopathic angioedema. Anuria, sulfonamide hypersensitivity. **P/N:** Category C (1st trimester) and D (2nd and 3rd trimesters), not for use in nursing.	
Fosinopril Sodium/ Hydrochloro- thiazide (Monopril HCT)	**Tab: (Fosinopril- HCTZ)** 10mg- 12.5mg, 20mg- 12.5mg	*Adults:* Initial (if not controlled with fosinopril/HCTZ monotherapy): 12.5mg-10mg tab or 12.5mg-20mg tab qd.	**ACE inhibitors can cause death/injury to developing fetus during 2nd and 3rd trimesters. Stop therapy if pregnancy detected. W/P:** Discontinue if angioedema, jaundice, or if marked LFT elevation oc- curs. Risk of hyperkalemia with DM, renal dysfunction. Persistent nonproductive cough reported. Monitor WBCs in renal and collagen vascular disease. Anaphylactoid reactions reported. Fetal/neonatal morbidity and death reported. Monitor for hypotension in high risk patients (eg, surgery/anesthesia, volume/salt depletion). Caution with CHF, renal or hepatic dysfunction. More reports of angioedema in blacks than nonblacks. May exacerbate or activate SLE. Monitor electro- lytes. Avoid if CrCl <30mL/min/1.7m². May increase cholesterol, TG. Hypercalcemia, hypomagnesemia, hyperuricemia may occur. **Contra:** Anuria, sulfonamide hypersensitiv- ity. **P/N:** Category C (1st trimester) and D (2nd and 3rd trimesters), not for use in nursing.	Headache, cough, fa- tigue, dizziness, upper respiratory infection, musculoskeletal pain.
Hydrochloro- thiazide/ Lisinopril (Prinzide)	**Tab: (Lisinopril- HCTZ)** 10mg-12.5mg, 20mg-12.5mg, 20mg-25mg	*Adults:* Initial (if not controlled with lisinopril/HCTZ monotherapy): 10mg-12.5mg tab or 20mg-12.5mg tab daily. **Titrate:** May increase after 2-3 weeks. **Initial (if controlled on 25mg HCTZ/day with hypokalemia):** 10mg-12.5mg tab. **Replacement Therapy:** Substitute combination for titrated components.	**ACE inhibitors can cause death/injury to developing fetus during 2nd and 3rd trimesters. Stop therapy if pregnancy detected. W/P:** Discontinue if angioedema, jaundice, or if marked LFT elevation oc- curs. Risk of hyperkalemia with DM, renal dysfunction. Persistent nonproductive cough reported. Monitor WBCs in renal and collagen vascular disease. Anaphylactoid reactions reported. Fetal/neonatal morbidity and death reported. Monitor for hypotension in high risk patients (eg, surgery/anesthesia, volume/salt depletion). Caution with CHF, renal or hepatic dysfunction, obstruction to left ventricle outflow tract, renal artery ste- nosis, elderly. More reports of angioedema in blacks than nonblacks. May exacerbate or activate SLE. Monitor electrolytes. Avoid if CrCl ≥30mL/min/1.73m². May increase cholesterol, TG. Hypercalcemia, hypergly- cemia, hypomagnesemia, hyperuricemia may occur. **Contra:** History of ACE inhibitor associated angioedema and hereditary or idiopathic angioedema. Anuria, sulfonamide hypersensitivity. **P/N:** Category C (1st trimester) and D (2nd and 3rd trimesters), not for use in nursing.	Dizziness, cough, fatigue, orthostatic ef- fects, diarrhea, nausea, muscle cramps, angioedema.
Hydrochloro- thiazide/ Lisinopril (Zestoretic)	**Tab: (Lisino- pril-HCTZ)** 10mg-12.5mg, 20mg-12.5mg, 20mg-25mg	*Adults:* Initial (if not controlled with lisinopril/HCTZ monotherapy): 10mg-12.5mg tab or 20mg-12.5mg tab daily. **Titrate:** May increase after 2-3 weeks. **Initial (if controlled on**	**ACE inhibitors can cause death/injury to developing fetus during 2nd and 3rd trimesters. Stop therapy if pregnancy detected. W/P:** Discontinue if angioedema, jaundice, or if marked LFT elevation occurs.	Dizziness, headache, cough, fatigue, ortho- static effects, diarrhea, nausea, muscle cramps, angioedema.

Table 14.1 PRESCRIBING INFORMATION FOR CARDIOVASCULAR DRUGS (cont.)

NAME	FORM/STRENGTH	DOSAGE	WARNINGS/PRECAUTIONS & CONTRAINDICATIONS	ADVERSE EFFECTS†
ACE INHIBITORS/DIURETICS (cont.)				
Hydrochloro-thiazide/ Lisinopril (cont.)		**25mg HCTZ/day with hypokalemia):** 10mg-12.5mg tab. **Replacement Therapy:** Substitute combination for titrated components.	Risk of hyperkalemia with DM, renal dysfunction. Persistent nonproductive cough reported. Monitor WBCs in renal and collagen vascular disease. Anaphylactoid reactions reported. Fetal/neonatal morbidity and death reported. Monitor for hypotension in high risk patients (eg, surgery/anesthesia, volume/salt depletion). Caution with CHF, renal or hepatic dysfunction. More reports of angioedema in blacks than nonblacks. May exacerbate or activate SLE. Monitor electrolytes. Avoid if CrCl $\geq$30mL/min/1.7m^2. May increase cholesterol, TG. Hypercalce-mia, hypomagnesemia, hyperuricemia may occur. Caution with left ventricle outflow obstruction. **Contra:** History of ACE inhibitor associated angioedema, hereditary or idiopathic angioedema, anuria, sulfonamide hypersensitivity. **P/N:** Category C (1st trimester) and D (2nd and 3rd trimesters), not for use in nursing.	
Hydrochloro-thiazide/ Moexipril Hydrochloride (Uniretic)	**Tab: (Moexipril-HCTZ)** 7.5mg-12.5mg*, 15mg-12.5mg*, 15mg-25mg*	***Adults:*** **Initial (if not controlled on moexipril/HCTZ monotherapy):** Switch to 7.5mg-12.5mg tab, 15mg-12.5mg tab, or 15mg-25mg tab qd. **Titrate:** May increase after 2-3 weeks. **Initial (if controlled on 25mg HCTZ/day with hypokalemia):** 3.75mg-6.25mg (1/2 of 7.5mg-12.5mg tab). If excessive Reduction with 7.5mg-12.5mg tab, may switch to 3.75mg-6.25mg. **Replacement Therapy:** Substitute combination for titrated components. Take 1 hr before meals.	**ACE inhibitors can cause death/injury to developing fetus during 2nd and 3rd trimesters. Stop therapy if pregnancy detected. W/P:** Discontinue if angioedema, jaundice, or if marked LFT elevation occurs. Intestinal angioedema reported. Risk of hyperkalemia with DM, renal dysfunction. Persistent nonproductive cough reported. Monitor WBCs in renal and collagen vascular disease. Anaphylactoid reactions reported. Fetal/neonatal morbidity and death reported. Monitor for hypotension in high risk patients (eg, surgery/anesthesia, volume/salt deple-tion). Caution in elderly, CHF, renal or hepatic dysfunction. More reports of angioedema in blacks than nonblacks. May exacerbate or ac-tivate SLE. Monitor electrolytes. Avoid if CrCl $\geq$40mL/min/1.73m^2. May increase choles-terol, TG. Hypercalcemia, hypomagnesemia, hyperuricemia may occur. **Contra:** History of ACE inhibitor-associated angioedema, anuria, sulfonamide hypersensitivity. **P/N:** Category C (1st trimester) and D (2nd and 3rd trimesters), not for use in nursing.	Cough, dizziness, fatigue.
Hydrochloro-thiazide/ Quinapril Hydrochloride (Accuretic)	**Tab: (Quinapril-HCTZ)** 10mg-12.5mg*, 20mg-12.5mg*, 20mg-25mg*	***Adults:*** **Initial** (if not controlled on quinapril monotherapy): 10mg-12.5mg or 20mg-12.5mg tab qd. **Ti-trate:** May increase after 2-3 weeks. **Initial (if controlled on HCTZ 25mg/day but significant K$^+$ loss):** 10mg-12.5mg or 20mg-12.5mg tab qd. If previously treated with 20mg quinapril and 25mg HCTZ, may switch to 20mg-25mg tab qd.	**ACE inhibitors can cause death/injury to developing fetus during 2nd and 3rd trimesters. Stop therapy if pregnancy detected. W/P:** Discontinue if angioedema, jaundice, or if marked LFT elevation oc-curs. Risk of hyperkalemia with DM, renal dysfunction. Persistent nonproductive cough reported. Monitor WBCs in renal or collagen vascular disease. Anaphylactoid reactions reported. Fetal/neonatal morbidity and death reported. Monitor for hypotension in high risk patients (heart failure, surgery/anesthe-sia, hyponatremia, severe volume/salt deple-tion, etc.). Caution with CHF, renal or hepatic dysfunction, and renal artery stenosis. Less effective on BP in blacks and more reports of angioedema than nonblacks.	Dizziness, headache, cough, myalgia.

*Scored.   †Bold entries denote special dental considerations.

NAME	FORM/ STRENGTH	DOSAGE	WARNINGS/PRECAUTIONS & CONTRAINDICATIONS
Hydrochloro-thiazide/ Quinapril Hydrochloride (cont.)			May exacerbate or activate SLE. Monitor serum electrolytes. Avoid if CrCl $\geq$30mL/min/1.73m^2. May increase cholesterol, TG, and uric acid levels and decrease glucose tolerance. **Contra:** History of ACE inhibitor associated angioedema, anuria, sulfonamide hypersensitivity. **P/N:** Category C (1st trimester) and D (2nd and 3rd trimesters), not for use in nursing.

α_2-ADRENERGIC AGONISTS, CENTRALLY ACTING

NAME	FORM/ STRENGTH	DOSAGE	WARNINGS/PRECAUTIONS & CONTRAINDICATIONS
Clonidine Hydrochloride (Catapres)	**Patch, Extended Release (TTS):** 0.1mg/24hr [12^s], 0.2mg/24hr [12^s], 0.3mg/24hr [4^s], **Tab:** 0.1mg*, 0.2mg*, 0.3mg*	**Adults: (Patch)** Apply to hairless, intact area of upper arm or chest weekly. Taper withdrawal of previous antihypertensive. **Initial:** 0.1mg/24hr patch weekly. **Titrate:** May increase after 1-2 weeks. **Max:** 0.6mg/24hr. **(Tab)** Initial: 0.1mg bid. **Titrate:** May increase by 0.1mg weekly. **Usual:** 0.2-0.6mg/day in divided doses. **Max:** 2.4mg/day. **(Patch, Tab) Renal Impairment:** Adjust according to degree of impairment.	**W/P:** Avoid abrupt discontinuation. Tabs may cause rash if have allergic reaction to patch. Continue tabs to within 4 hrs of surgery resume and as soon as possible thereafter. Do not remove patch for surgery. Caution with severe coronary insufficiency, conduction disturbances, recent MI, cerebrovascular disease or chronic renal failure. Remove patch before defibrillation or cardioversion. **P/N:** Category C, caution in nursing.
Guanfacine Hydrochloride (Tenex)	**Tab:** 1mg, 2mg	**Adults:** 1mg qhs. **Titrate:** May increase to 2mg qhs after 3-4 weeks. **Max:** 3mg/day.	**W/P:** Caution with severe coronary insufficiency, recent MI, cerebrovascular disease, chronic renal or hepatic failure. Avoid abrupt discontinuation. Dose-related drowsiness and sedation. **P/N:** Category B, caution with nursing.
Methyldopa, Methyldopate Hydrochloride	**Tab:** 125mg, 250mg, 500mg; **Inj:** 50mg/mL	**Adults:** Initial: 250mg bid-tid for 48 hrs. Adjust dose at intervals of not less than 2 days. **Maint:** 500mg-2g/day given bid-qid. **Max:** 3g/day. **Concomitant Antihypertensives (other than thiazides): Initial:** Limit to 500mg/day. **Renal Impairment:** May respond to lower doses. **Pediatrics: Initial:** 10mg/kg/day given bid-qid. **Max:** 65mg/kg/day or 3g/day, whichever is less. **(Inj)** 250-500mg IV q6h as needed. **Max:** 1gm q6h. **Elderly/Renal Dysfunction:** May reduce dose. Switch to oral therapy once BP is controlled.	**W/P:** Positive Coombs test, hemolytic anemia, and liver disorders may occur. Fever reported within the 1st 3 weeks of therapy. HTN has recurred after dialysis. Caution with liver disease or dysfunction. Discontinue if develop signs of heart failure, or involuntary choreoathetotic movements. Edema and weight gain reported. Blood count, Coombs test and LFTs prior to therapy and periodically thereafter. **Contra:** Hypersensitivity to sulfites, active hepatic disease, history of methyldopa associated liver disorder, concomitant MAOIs. **P/N:** Category B, caution in nursing.

α-ADRENERIC BLOCKERS

NAME	FORM/ STRENGTH	DOSAGE	WARNINGS/PRECAUTIONS & CONTRAINDICATIONS
Doxazosin Mesylate (Cardura)	**Tab:** 1mg*, 2mg*, 4mg*, 8mg*	**Adults: HTN: Initial:** 1mg qd (am or pm). Monitor BP 2-6 hrs and 24 hrs after 1st dose. **Titrate:** Increase to 2mg qd then upwards as needed. **Max:** 16mg/day. **BPH: Initial:** 1mg qd (am or pm). **Titrate:** May double the dose every 1-2 weeks. **Max:** 8mg/day.	**W/P:** Monitor for orthostatic hypotension and syncope with 1st dose and dose increase. Caution with hepatic dysfunction. Rule out prostate cancer. Priapism (rare), leukopenia/neutropenia reported. **P/N:** Category C, caution with nursing.
Phenoxybenza-mine Hydrochloride (Dibenzyline)	**Cap:** 10mg	**Adults: Initial:** 10mg bid. **Titrate:** Increase every other day to 20-40mg bid-tid, until BP is controlled.	**W/P:** Caution with marked cerebral or coronary arteriosclerosis, or renal damage. May aggravate symptoms of respiratory infections. **Contra:** Conditions where fall in BP may be undesirable. **P/N:** Category C, not for use in nursing.

*Scored

Table 14.1 PRESCRIBING INFORMATION FOR CARDIOVASCULAR DRUGS (cont.)

NAME	FORM/ STRENGTH	DOSAGE	WARNINGS/PRECAUTIONS & CONTRAINDICATIONS	ADVERSE EFFECTS†
-ADRENERIC BLOCKERS (cont.)				
azosin drochloride nipress)	**Cap:** 1mg, 2mg, 5mg	**Adults: Initial:** 1mg bid-tid. **Maint:** 6-15mg/day in divided doses. **Max:** 40mg/day. **Concomitant Diuretic/ Antihypertensive:** Reduce to 1-2mg tid, then retitrate.	**W/P:** Syncope may occur, usually after initial dose or dose increase. Excessive postural hypotensive effects. Avoid driving for 24 hrs after 1st dose or dose increase. Always start on 1mg cap. False (+) for pheochromocytoma. **P/N:** Category C, caution in nursing.	Dizziness, headache, drowsiness, lack of energy, weakness, palpitations, nausea.
azosin rochloride trin)	**Cap:** 1mg, 2mg, 5mg, 10mg	**Adults: HTN: Initial:** 1mg hs, then slowly increase dose. **Usual:** 1-5mg/ day. **Max:** 20mg/day. If response is substantially diminished at 24 hrs, may increase dose or give in 2 divided doses. **BPH: Initial:** 1mg qhs. **Titrate:** Increase stepwise as needed. **Usual:** 10mg/day. May increase to 20mg/day after 4-6 weeks. **Max:** 20mg/day. If discontinue for several days, restart at initial dose.	**W/P:** Monitor for orthostatic hypotension and syncope initially and with dose increase. Rule out prostate cancer. Priapism (rare) reported. Possibility of hemodilution. **P/N:** Category C, caution with nursing.	Asthenia, postural hypotension, headache, dizziness, dyspnea, nasal congestion/rhinitis, somnolence, impotence, blurred vision, palpitations, nausea, peripheral edema, priapism, thrombocytopenia, atrial fibrillation.
GIOTENSIN II RECEPTOR ANTAGONISTS				
desartan xetil cand)	**Tab:** 4mg, 8mg, 16mg, 32mg	**Adults: HTN: Monotherapy without Volume Depletion: Initial:** 16mg qd. Usual: 8-32mg/day given qd-bid. May add diuretic if BP not controlled. **Intravascular Volume Depletion/Moderate Hepatic Impairment:** Lower initial dose. **Heart Failure: Initial:** 4mg qd. **Usual:** 32mg qd. **Titrate:** Double dose q 2 weeks as tolerated.	**Can cause death/injury to developing fetus during 2nd and 3rd trimesters. Stop therapy if pregnancy detected. W/P:** Can cause fetal injury/death. Correct volume or salt depletion before therapy or monitor closely. Changes in renal function may occur; caution with renal artery stenosis, CHF. Risk of hypotension; caution when initiating therapy in heart failure. **P/N:** Category C (1st trimester) and D (2nd and 3rd trimesters), not for use in nursing.	Back pain, dizziness, upper respiratory infection.
sartan ylate ten)	**Tab:** 400mg*, 600mg	**Adults: Initial:** 600mg qd. **Usual:** 400-800mg/day, given qd-bid. **Moderate to Severe Renal Impairment: Max:** 600mg/day.	**Can cause death/injury to developing fetus during 2nd and 3rd trimesters. Stop therapy if pregnancy detected. W/P:** Can cause fetal injury/death. Correct volume or salt depletion before therapy. Changes in renal function may occur; caution with renal artery stenosis, severe CHF. **P/N:** Category C (1st trimester) and D (2nd and 3rd trimesters), not for use in nursing.	Upper respiratory infection, rhinitis, pharyngitis, cough.
artan ro)	**Tab:** 75mg, 150mg, 300mg	**Adults: HTN: Initial:** 150mg qd. **Titrate:** May increase to 300mg qd. May add low dose diuretic. **Salt/Volume Depletion: Initial:** 75mg qd. **Nephropathy: Maint:** 300mg qd. **Pediatrics: HTN: 13-16 yrs: Initial:** 150mg qd. **Titrate:** May increase to 300mg qd. **6-12 yrs: Initial:** 75mg qd. **Titrate:** May increase to 150mg qd.	**Can cause death/injury to developing fetus during 2nd and 3rd trimesters. Stop therapy if pregnancy detected. W/P:** Can cause fetal injury/death. Correct volume or salt depletion before therapy. Changes in renal function may occur; caution with renal artery stenosis, severe CHF. Angioedema reported. **P/N:** Category C (1st trimester) and D (2nd and 3rd trimesters), not for use in nursing.	Diarrhea, dyspepsia/ heartburn, musculoskeletal trauma, fatigue, upper respiratory infection.
an ium r)	**Tab:** 25mg, 50mg, 100mg	**Adults: HTN: Initial:** 50mg qd. Usual: 25-100mg/day given qd-bid. **Intravascular Volume Depletion/Hepatic Impairment: Initial:** 25mg qd. HTN with LVH: **Initial:** 50mg qd. **Nephropathy: Initial:** 50 mg qd. **Titrate:** Increase to 100mg qd based on BP response.	**Can cause death/injury to developing fetus during 2nd and 3rd trimesters. Stop therapy if pregnancy detected. W/P:** Can cause fetal injury/death. Correct volume or salt depletion before therapy. Changes in renal function may occur; caution with renal artery stenosis, severe CHF. Angioedema reported. Consider dose adjustment with hepatic dysfunction. **P/N:** Category C (1st trimester) and D (2nd and 3rd trimesters), not for use in nursing.	Dizziness, cough, upper respiratory infection, diarrhea.

†Bold entries denote special dental considerations.

NAME	FORM/ STRENGTH	DOSAGE	WARNINGS/PRECAUTIONS & CONTRAINDICATIONS	ADVERSE EFFECTS†
Olmesartan Medoxomil (Benicar)	Tab: 5mg, 20mg, 40mg	**Adults: Monotherapy Without Volume Depletion: Initial:** 20mg qd. **Titrate:** May increase to 40mg qd after 2 weeks if needed. May add diuretic if BP not controlled. **Intravascular Volume Depletion (eg, with diuretics, impaired renal function):** Lower initial dose; monitor closely.	**Can cause death/injury to developing fetus during 2nd and 3rd trimesters. Stop therapy if pregnancy detected. W/P:** Can cause fetal injury/death. Symptomatic hypotension may occur in volume- and/or salt-depleted patients; monitor closely. Changes in renal function may occur; caution with severe CHF. Increases in serum creatinine or BUN reported with renal artery stenosis. **P/N:** Category C (1st trimester) and D (2nd and 3rd trimesters), not for use in nursing.	Dizziness, transient hypotension.
Telmisartan (Micardis)	Tab: 20mg, 40mg*, 80mg*	**Adults: Initial:** 40mg qd. **Usual:** 20-80mg/day. May add diuretic if need additional BP reduction after 80mg/day.	**Can cause death/injury to developing fetus during 2nd and 3rd trimesters. Stop therapy if pregnancy detected. W/P:** Can cause fetal injury/death. Correct volume or salt depletion before therapy. Changes in renal function may occur; caution with renal artery stenosis, severe CHF. Closely monitor with biliary obstructive disorders or hepatic dysfunction. **P/N:** Category C (1st trimester) and D (2nd and 3rd trimesters), not for use in nursing.	Upper respiratory infection, back pain, diarrhea.
Valsartan (Diovan)	Tab: 40mg, 80mg, 160mg, 320mg	**Adults: HTN: Monotherapy Without Volume Depletion: Initial:** 80mg or 160mg qd. **Titrate:** Increase to 320mg qd or add diuretic (greater effect than increasing dose >80mg). **Hepatic/Renal Dysfunction:** Caution with dosing. **Heart Failure: Initial:** 40mg bid. **Titrate:** Increase to 80mg or 160mg bid (use highest dose tolerated). **Max:** 320mg/day in divided doses. **Post-MI: Initial:** 20mg bid. **Titrate:** Increase to 40mg bid within 7 days, with subsequent titrations up to 160mg bid. **Renal Dysfunction:** Caution and possible dose reduction and/or discontinuation.	**Can cause death/injury to developing fetus during 2nd and 3rd trimesters. Stop therapy if pregnancy detected. W/P:** Can cause fetal injury/death. Correct volume or salt depletion before therapy. Changes in renal function may occur; caution with renal artery stenosis, severe CHF. Caution with hepatic dysfunction, renal dysfunction, and obstructive biliary disorder. Risk of hypotension; caution when initiating therapy in heart failure or post-MI. **P/N:** Category C (1st trimester) and D (2nd and 3rd trimesters), not for use in nursing.	(HTN) Viral infection, fatigue, abdominal pain, (Heart Failure) dizziness, hypotension, diarrhea.

ANGIOTENSIN II RECEPTOR ANTAGONISTS/DIURETICS

NAME	FORM/ STRENGTH	DOSAGE	WARNINGS/PRECAUTIONS & CONTRAINDICATIONS	ADVERSE EFFECTS†
Candesartan Cilexetil/ Hydrochloro-thiazide (Atacand HCT)	**Tab: (Candesartan-HCTZ)** 16mg-12.5mg, 32mg-12.5mg	**Adults: Initial:** If BP not controlled on HCTZ 25mg/day or controlled but serum potassium decreased;16mg-12.5mg tab qd. If BP not controlled on 32mg candesartan/day, give 32mg-12.5mg qd; may increase to 32mg-25mg qd.	**Can cause death/injury to developing fetus during 2nd and 3rd trimesters. Stop therapy if pregnancy detected. W/P:** Can cause fetal injury/death. Correct volume or salt depletion before therapy. Caution with hepatic or renal dysfunction, renal artery stenosis, severe CHF, history of allergies, and asthma. May exacerbate or activate SLE. Monitor serum electrolytes. Avoid if CrCl ≥30mL/min. Hyperuricemia, hyperglycemia, hypokalemia, hypomagnesemia, hypercalcemia may occur. Enhanced effects in post-sympathectomy patient. May increase cholesterol and triglyceride levels. **Contra:** Anuria, sulfonamide hypersensitivity. **P/N:** Category C (1st trimester) and D (2nd and 3rd trimesters), not for use in nursing.	Upper respiratory infection, back pain, influenza-like symptoms, dizziness, headache.
Eprosartan Mesylate/ Hydrochloro-thiazide (Teveten HCT)	**Tab: (Eprosartan-HCTZ)** 600mg-12.5mg, 600mg-25mg	**Adults: Usual (Not Volume Depleted):** 600mg-12.5mg qd. **Titrate:** May increase to 600mg-25mg qd if needed. **Renal Impairment: Max:** 600mg/day (eprosartan).	**Can cause death/injury to developing fetus during 2nd and 3rd trimesters. Stop therapy if pregnancy detected. W/P:** Hypersensitivity reactions reported. Fetal/neonatal morbidity and death reported.	Dizziness, headache, back pain, fatigue, myalgia, upper respiratory tract infection, sinusitis, viral infection.

Table 14.1 PRESCRIBING INFORMATION FOR CARDIOVASCULAR DRUGS (cont.)

NAME	FORM/ STRENGTH	DOSAGE	WARNINGS/PRECAUTIONS & CONTRAINDICATIONS	ADVERSE EFFECTS†
ANGIOTENSIN II RECEPTOR ANTAGONISTS/DIURETICS (cont.)				
Eprosartan Mesylate/ Hydrochloro- thiazide (cont.)			Monitor for hypotension in volume/salt depletion. Caution with CHF, renal or hepatic dysfunction. May exacerbate or activate SLE. Monitor electrolytes periodically. Hypercal- cemia, hypomagnesemia, hyperuricemia, hyperglycemia may occur. Enhanced effects in post-sympathectomy patient. **Contra:** Anuria, sulfonamide hypersensitivity. **P/N:** Category C (1st trimester) and D (2nd and 3rd trimesters), not for use in nursing.	
Hydrochloro- thiazide/ Irbesartan (Avalide)	**Tab: (Irbesartan-HCTZ)** 150mg-12.5mg, 300mg-12.5mg, 300mg-25mg	**Adults:** Usual: 1 tab qd. **Max:** 300mg irbesartan qd. **Elderly:** Start at low end of dosing range. Avoid with CrCl ≤30mL/min.	**Can cause death/injury to developing fetus during 2nd and 3rd trimesters. Stop therapy if pregnancy detected. W/P:** Can cause fetal injury/death. Correct volume or salt depletion before therapy. Caution with hepatic or renal dysfunction, renal artery stenosis, severe CHF, history of allergies, elderly, and asthma. May exacerbate or activate SLE. Monitor serum electrolytes. Avoid if CrCl ≥30mL/min. Hyperuricemia, hyperglycemia, hypokalemia, hypomagne- semia, hypercalcemia may occur. Enhanced effects in post-sympathectomy patient. May increase cholesterol and triglyceride levels. Caution in elderly. **Contra:** Anuria, sulfon- amide hypersensitivity. **P/N:** Category C (1st trimester) and D (2nd and 3rd trimesters), not for use in nursing.	Dizziness, fatigue, musculoskeletal pain, influenza, edema, nausea, vomiting.
Hydrochloro- thiazide/ Losartan Potassium (Hyzaar)	**Tab: (Losartan-HCTZ)** 50mg-12.5mg, 100mg-25mg	**Adults: HTN:** If BP uncontrolled on losartan monotherapy, HCTZ alone or controlled with HCTZ 25mg/day but hypokalemic: 50mg-12.5mg tab qd. **Titrate/Max:** If uncontrolled after 3 weeks, increase to 2 tabs of 50mg-12.5mg qd or 1 tab of 100mg-25mg qd. **Severe HTN: Initial:** 50mg-12.5mg qd. **Titrate/Max:** If inadequate response after 2-4 weeks, increase to 1 tab of 100mg-25mg qd. **HTN With Left Ventricular Hypertrophy: Initial:** Losartan 50mg qd. If BP reduction inadequate, add HCTZ 12.5mg or substitute losartan/HCTZ 50-12.5. If additional BP reduction is needed, losartan 100mg and HCTZ 12.5mg may be substituted, followed by losartan 100mg and HCTZ 25mg or losartan/HCTZ 100-25.	**Can cause death/injury to developing fetus during 2nd and 3rd trimesters. Discontinue if pregnancy detected.** Can cause fetal injury/death. Correct volume or salt depletion before therapy. Caution with hepatic or renal dysfunction, renal artery stenosis, severe CHF, history of allergies, asthma. May exacerbate or activate SLE. Monitor serum electrolytes. Avoid if CrCl ≥30mL/min. Observe for signs of fluid or electrolyte imbalance. May precipitate hyperuricemia or gout. Enhanced effects in post-sympathectomy patient. May increase cholesterol, TG levels. Angioedema reported. Not recommended with hepatic dysfunction requiring losartan titration. **Contra:** Anuria, sulfonamide hypersensitivity. **P/N:** Category C (1st trimester) and D (2nd and 3rd trimes- ters), not for use in nursing.	Dizziness, upper respiratory infection, back pain, cough.
Hydrochloro- thiazide/ Olmesartan Medoxomil (Benicar HCT)	**Tab: (Olmesartan-HCTZ)** 20mg-12.5mg, 40mg-12.5mg, 40mg-25mg	**Adults: If BP not Controlled with Olmesartan Alone:** Add HCTZ 12.5mg qd. May titrate to 25mg qd if BP uncontrolled after 2-4 weeks. **If BP not Controlled with HCTZ Alone:** Add olmesartan 20mg qd. May titrate to 40mg qd if BP uncontrolled after 2-4 weeks. **Intravascular Vol- ume Depletion (eg, with diuretics, impaired renal function):** Lower initial dose; monitor closely. **Elderly:** Start at lower end of dosing range.	**Can cause death/injury to developing fetus during 2nd and 3rd trimesters. Stop therapy if pregnancy detected. W/P:** Can cause fetal injury/death. Correct volume or salt depletion before therapy or monitor closely. Caution with hepatic or severe renal dysfunction, progressive liver disease, history of allergies or asthma, renal artery stenosis, severe CHF. Avoid if CrCl ≥30mL/min. May exacerbate or activate SLE. Monitor serum electrolytes. Hyperuricemia, hyperglycemia, hypercalcemia,	Dizziness, upper respiratory tract infec- tion, hyperuricemia, nausea.

*Scored.   †Bold entries denote special dental considerations.

NAME	FORM/ STRENGTH	DOSAGE	WARNINGS/PRECAUTIONS & CONTRAINDICATIONS	ADVERSE EFFECTS†
Hydrochloro-thiazide/ Olmesartan Medoxomil *(cont.)*			hypomagnesemia may occur. May increase cholesterol and triglyceride levels. **Contra:** Sulfonamide hypersensitivity. **P/N:** Category C (1st trimester) and D (2nd and 3rd trimesters), not for use in nursing.	
Hydrochloro-thiazide/ Telmisartan (Micardis HCT)	**Tab: (HCTZ-Telmisartan)** 12.5mg-40mg, 12.5mg-80mg, 25mg-80mg	*Adults:* If BP not controlled on 80mg telmisartan, or 25mg HCTZ/day, or controlled on 25mg HCTZ/day but serum K+ decreased, 80mg-12.5mg tab qd. **Titrate/Max:** If uncontrolled after 2-4 weeks, increase to 160mg-25mg. **Biliary Obstruction/Hepatic Dysfunction: Initial:** 40mg-12.5mg tab qd; monitor closely.	**Can cause death/injury to developing fetus during 2nd and 3rd trimesters. Stop therapy if pregnancy detected. W/P:** Can cause fetal injury/death. Correct volume or salt depletion before therapy. Caution with hepatic or renal dysfunction, biliary obstructive disorders, renal artery stenosis, severe CHF, history of allergies, and asthma. May exacerbate or activate SLE. Monitor serum electrolytes. Avoid if CrCl ≥30mL/min. Hyperuricemia, hyperglycemia, hypokalemia, hypomagnesemia, hypercalcemia may occur. Enhanced effects in post-sympathectomy patient. May increase cholesterol and triglyceride levels. **Contra:** Anuria, sulfonamide hypersensitivity. **P/N:** Category C (1st trimester) and D (2nd and 3rd trimesters), not for use in nursing.	Dizziness, fatigue, sinusitis, upper respiratory infection, diarrhea.
Hydrochloro-thiazide/ Valsartan (Diovan HCT)	**Tab: (Valsartan-HCTZ)** 80mg-12.5mg, 160mg-12.5mg, 160mg-25mg	*Adults:* **Initial:** 80mg-12.5mg qd or 160mg-12.5mg qd if BP not controlled on valsartan alone, or 25mg qd HCTZ alone, or controlled on 25mg qd HCTZ but serum K+ decreased. **Titrate/Max:** If uncontrolled after 3-4 weeks, may increase up to 160mg-25mg qd.	**Can cause death/injury to developing fetus during 2nd and 3rd trimesters. Stop therapy if pregnancy detected. W/P:** Can cause fetal injury/death. Correct volume or salt depletion before therapy. Caution with hepatic or renal dysfunction, biliary obstructive disorders, renal artery stenosis, severe CHF, history of allergies, and asthma. May exacerbate or activate SLE. Monitor serum electrolytes. Avoid if CrCl >30mL/min. Hyperuricemia, hyperglycemia, hypokalemia, hypomagnesemia, hypercalcemia may occur. Enhanced effects in post-sympathectomy patient. May increase cholesterol and triglyceride levels. **Contra:** Anuria, sulfonamide hypersensitivity. **P/N:** Category C (1st trimester) and D (2nd and 3rd trimesters), not for use in nursing.	Cough, headache, dizziness, fatigue, viral infection, pharyngitis, diarrhea.

ANTIARRHYTHMICS

NAME	FORM/ STRENGTH	DOSAGE	WARNINGS/PRECAUTIONS & CONTRAINDICATIONS	ADVERSE EFFECTS†
Disopyramide Phosphate (Norpace)	**Cap: (Norpace)** 100mg, 150mg; **Cap, ER: (Norpace CR)** 100mg, 150mg	*Adults:* **Usual:** 400-800mg/day in divided dose. Recommended: 150mg q6h immediate-release (IR) or 300mg q12h extended-release (CR). Adjust dose with anticholinergic effects. **Weight <110lbs/Moderate Hepatic or Renal Insufficiency (CrCl >40mL/min):** 100mg q6h IR or 200mg q12h CR. **Severe Renal Insufficiency (with or without initial 150mg LD):** CrCl 30-40mL/min: 100mg q8h IR. CrCl 30-15mL/min: 100mg q12h IR. **CrCl <15mL/min:** 100mg q24h IR. **Rapid Control of Ventricular Arrhythmia: LD:** 300mg IR (200mg if <110lbs). Follow with maint dose. **Cardiomyopathy/Cardiac Decompensation: Initial:** 100mg q6-8h IR. Adjust gradually. See labeling if no response or toxicity occurs.	**W/P:** Proarrhythmic; reserve for life-threatening ventricular arrhythmias. May cause or worsen CHF and produce hypotension due to negative inotropic properties. Reduce dose if 1st-degree heart block occurs. Avoid with urinary retention, glaucoma, and myasthenia gravis unless adequate overriding measures taken. Atrial flutter/fibrillation; digitalize first. Monitor closely or withdraw if QT prolongation >25% occurs and ectopy continues. Discontinue if QRS widening >25% occurs. Avoid LD with cardiomyopathy or cardiac decompensation. Correct K+ abnormalities before therapy. Reduce dose with renal/hepatic dysfunction; monitor ECG. Avoid CR formulation with CrCl ≥40mL/min. Caution with sick sinus syndrome, Wolff-Parkinson-White syndrome, bundle branch block, in elderly. May significantly lower blood glucose. **Contra:** Cardiogenic	**Dry mouth,** urinary retention/frequency/ urgency, constipation, blurred vision, GI effects, dizziness, fatigue, headache.

Table 14.1 PRESCRIBING INFORMATION FOR CARDIOVASCULAR DRUGS *(cont.)*

NAME	FORM/ STRENGTH	DOSAGE	WARNINGS/PRECAUTIONS & CONTRAINDICATIONS	ADVERSE EFFECTS†
ANTIARRHYTHMICS *(cont.)*				
Disopyramide Phosphate *(cont.)*		**Elderly:** Start at low end of dosing range. **Pediatrics: <1 yr:** 10-30mg/kg/day. **1-4 yrs:** 10-20mg/kg/day. **4-12 yrs:** 10-15mg/kg/day. **12-18 yrs:** 6-15mg/kg/day. Give in equally divided doses q6h. Hospitalize patient during initial therapy. Start dose titration at lower end of range.	shock, 2nd- or 3rd-degree AV block (if no pacemaker present), congenital QT prolongation. **P/N:** Category C, not for use in nursing.	
Flecainide Acetate (Tambocor)	**Tab:** 50mg, 100mg*, 150mg*	**Adults: PSVT/PAF: Initial:** 50mg q12h. **Titrate:** May increase by 50mg bid every 4 days. **Max:** 300mg/day. **Sustained VT: Initial:** 100mg q12h. **Titrate:** May increase by 50mg bid every 4 days. **Max:** 400mg/day. **CrCl ≥35mL/min: Initial:** 100mg qd or 50mg bid. Reduce dose by 50% with amiodarone. **Pediatrics: <6 months: Initial:** 50mg/m²/day given bid-tid. **≥6 months: Initial:** 100mg/m²/day given bid-tid. **Max:** 200mg/m²/day. Reduce dose by 50% with amiodarone.	**W/P:** Avoid with non-life-threatening ventricular arrhythmias. Increased mortality and non-cardiac arrests reported. Ventricular proarrhythmic effects may occur with atrial fibrillation/flutter. May cause or worsen CHF, arrhythmias. Slows cardiac conduction; dose related increases in PR, QRS, and QT intervals reported. Conduction changes may cause sinus pause, sinus arrest, bradycardia, 2nd- or 3rd-degree AV block. Extreme caution with Sick Sinus Syndrome. May increase endocardial pacing thresholds and suppress ventricular escape with pacemakers. Correct hypokalemia or hyperkalemia before therapy. Monitor with significant hepatic impairment. Initiate treatment of sustained VT in the hospital. **Contra:** Right bundle branch block associated with left hemiblock (without a pacemaker), pre-existing 2nd- or 3rd-degree AV block, cardiogenic shock. **P/N:** Category C, safety in nursing unknown.	Arrhythmias, hepatic dysfunction, cardiac arrest, CHF, flushing, anxiety, vomiting, diarrhea, tinnitus.
Ibutilide Fumarate (Corvert)	**Inj:** 0.1mg/mL	**Adults: ≥60kg:** 1mg over 10 minutes. **<60kg:** 0.01mg/kg over 10 minutes. If arrhythmia still present within 10 minutes after the end of the initial infusion, repeat infusion 10 minutes after completion of 1st infusion.	**W/P:** Proarrhythmic; can cause potentially fatal arrhythmias. Administer in setting with continuous ECG monitoring and person able to treat acute ventricular arrhythmia. Adequately anticoagulate if A-Fib >2-3 days. Correct hypokalemia and hypomagnesemia before therapy. Caution in elderly. **P/N:** Category C, not for use in nursing.	Sustained and non-sustained polymorphic ventricular tachycardia, sustained and nonsustained monomorphic ventricular tachycardia, bundle branch and AV block, ventricular and supraventricular extrasystoles, hypotension, bradycardia.
Mexiletine Hydrochloride	**Cap:** 150mg, 200mg, 250mg	**Adults: Initial:** 200mg q8h when rapid control is not essential. **Titrate:** Adjust by 50-100mg, not less than every 2-3 days. **Usual:** 200-300mg q8h. **Max:** 1200mg/day. If control with ≤300mg q8h, then may divide daily dose and give q12h. **Max:** 450mg q12h. **For Rapid Control: LD:** 400mg, then 200mg in 8 hrs. **Transfer from Class I Oral Agents: Initial:** 200mg and titrate as above, 6-12 hrs after last quinidine sulfate or disopyramide dose, 3-6 hrs after last procainamide dose, or 8-12 hrs after last tocainide dose. **Severe Hepatic Disease:** May need lower dose. Take with food or antacid.	**W/P:** Reserve for life-threatening arrhythmias. May treat patients with 2nd- or 3rd-degree AV block with a pacemaker; monitor continuously. Can worsen arrhythmias. Caution with hypotension, severe CHF, seizure disorder, hepatic impairment, sinus node dysfunction, or intraventricular conduction abnormalities. Leukopenia, agranulocytosis, and abnormal LFTs reported. Monitor ECG. **Contra:** Cardiogenic shock, pre-existing 2nd- or 3rd-degree AV block (without a pacemaker). **P/N:** Category C, not for use in nursing.	Coordination difficulties, tremor, GI distress, lightheadedness.
Procainamide Hydrchloride (Procanbid, Pronestyl)	**Tab, ER:** 500mg, 1000mg	**Adults: Initial:** 25mg/kg q12h. **>50 yrs** or **Renal/Hepatic/Cardiac Insufficiency:** Reduce dose or increase intervals. Swallow tab whole.	**Positive ANA titer may develop with prolonged use. W/P:** Monitor for QRS widening or QT prolongation. Should cardioconvert or digitalize before use with A-Fib/Flutter.	GI disturbances, lupus-like symptoms, elevated LFTs, **bitter taste**, angioneurotic

*Scored. †Bold entries denote special dental considerations.

NAME	FORM/ STRENGTH	DOSAGE	WARNINGS/PRECAUTIONS & CONTRAINDICATIONS	ADVERSE EFFECTS†
Procainamide Hydrchloride *(cont.)*			Caution with AV conduction disturbances and 1st-degree heart block; reduce dose. Caution with myasthenia gravis; adjust dose of anticholinesterases. Caution in digitalis intoxication, pre-existing marrow failure, cytopenia, CHF, ischemic heart disease, cardiomyopathy. May induce lupoid syndrome. Reserve for life-threatening ventricular arrhythmias. Fatal blood dyscrasias reported; obtain CBC, WBC, differential, and platelets weekly for 1st 3 months, then periodically. **Contra:** Complete heart block, 2nd-degree AV block, SLE, torsade de pointes. **P/N:** Category C, not for use in nursing.	edema, flushing, psychosis, dizziness, depression, urticaria, pruritus, rash, agranu-locytosis.
Propafenone Hydrochloride (Rythmol, Rythmol SR)	**Tab:** 150mg*, 225mg*, 300mg*. **(Rythmol SR) Cap, ER:** 225mg, 325mg, 425mg	*Adults:* **Initial:** 150mg q8h. **Titrate:** May increase at minimum 3-4 day intervals to 225mg q8h, then to 300mg q8h if needed. **Max:** 900mg/day. **Elderly/Marked Myocardial Damage:** Increase more gradually during initial phase. **Hepatic Dysfunction:** Reduce dose by 20-30%. **(Rythmol SR) Initial:** 225mg q12h. **Titrate:** May increase at minimum 5 day intervals to 325mg q12h, then to 425mg q12h if needed. **Hepatic Impairment/QRS Widening/2nd- or 3rd-degree AV Block:** Reduce dose.	**W/P:** Avoid with non-life-threatening ventricular arrhythmias, bronchospastic disorders. May cause new or worsened arrhythmias. Caution with hepatic or renal dysfunction. Slows AV conduction and causes 1st-degree AV block. Discontinue if CHF worsens. Agranulocytosis, myasthenia gravis exacerbation, positive ANA titers reported. May alter pacing and sensing thresholds of artificial pacemakers. **Contra:** Uncontrolled CHF, cardiogenic shock, bradycardia, marked hypotension, bronchospastic disorders, electrolyte imbalance, and sinoatrial, atrioventricular (AV) and intraventricular disorders of impulse generation and/or conduction (eg, sick sinus node syndrome, AV block) in the absence of an artificial pacemaker. **P/N:** Category C, not for use in nursing.	**Taste disturbances**, nausea, vomiting, constipation, headache, fatigue, blurred vision, blood dyscrasias.
Quinidine Gluconate, Quinidine Sulfate	**Inj:** 80mg/mL, **Tab, ER:** 324mg. **Quinidine Sulfate Tab, ER:** 300mg	*Adults:* **(Inj) Malaria: LD:** 15mg/kg base (24mg/kg gluconate) over 4 hrs. **Maint:** After 8 hrs, 7.5mg/kg (12mg/kg gluconate) IV q8h for 7 days. **Alternate: Initial:** 6.25mg/kg base (10mg/kg gluconate) IV over 1-2 hrs. **Maint:** 12.5µg/kg/min base (20µg/kg/min gluconate) for 72h. Switch to PO therapy when possible. **A-Fib/Flutter and Ventricular Arrhythmia:** 0.25mg/kg/minute. **Max:** 5-10mg/kg. Consider alternate therapy if conversion to sinus rhythm not achieved. **Renal/Hepatic Impairment or CHF:** Reduce dose. **Elderly:** Start at low end of dosing range. *Pediatrics:* **Malaria: LD:** 15mg/kg base (24mg/kg gluconate) over 4 hrs. **Maint:** After 8 hrs, 7.5mg/kg (12mg/kg gluconate) IV q8h for 7 days. **Alternate: Initial:** 6.25mg/kg base (10mg/kg/min gluconate) IV over 1-2 hrs. **Maint:** 12.5µg/kg/min base (20µg/kg/min gluconate) for 72h. Switch to PO therapy when possible. **A-Fib/Flutter Conversion: (Tab) Initial:** 2 tabs q8h. **Titrate:** Increase cautiously if no effect after 3-4 doses. **Alternate Regimen:** 1 tab q8h for 2 days, then 2 tabs q12h for 2 days, then 2 tabs q8h up to 4 days. **A-Fib/Flutter Relapse Reduction:** 1 tab q8-12h.	**W/P:** Increases risk of mortality, especially with structural heart disease. Rapid infusion can cause peripheral vascular collapse and hypotension. May prolong QTc interval. Paradoxical increase in ventricular rate in A-Fib/Flutter. Caution in those at risk of complete AV block without implanted pacemakers, renal/hepatic dysfunction, elderly, and CHF. Physical/pharmacologic maneuvers to terminate paroxysmal supraventricular tachycardia may be ineffective. Exacerbated bradycardia in sick sinus syndrome. **Contra:** Cardiac rhythm dependent upon a junctional or idioventricular pacemaker (absent of functioning pacemaker), thrombocytopenic purpura with previous treatment, patients adversely affected by anticholinergics (eg, myasthenia gravis). **P/N:** Category C, not for use in nursing.	GI distress, lightheadedness, fatigue, palpitations, weakness, visual problems, nausea, vomiting, diarrhea, fever arrhythmia, abnormal ECG, sleep disturbances, rash, headache, cinchonism, hepatotoxicity, autoimmune/inflammatory syndromes.

Table 14.1 PRESCRIBING INFORMATION FOR CARDIOVASCULAR DRUGS (cont.)

NAME	FORM/ STRENGTH	DOSAGE	WARNINGS/PRECAUTIONS & CONTRAINDICATIONS	ADVERSE EFFECTS†
ANTIARRHYTHMICS (cont.)				
Quinidine Gluconate, Quinidine Sulfate (cont.)		**Titrate:** Increase cautiously if needed. **Ventricular Arrhythmia:** Dosing regimens not adequately studied. **Generally similar to A-Fib/Flutter. Renal/Hepatic Impairment or CHF:** Reduce dose. May break tab in half. Do not chew or crush.		
β-BLOCKERS, CARDIOSELECTIVE				
Atenolol (Tenormin)	**Inj:** 0.5mg/mL; **Tab:** 25mg, 50mg*, 100mg	***Adults:* HTN: Initial:** 50mg qd. **Titrate:** May increase after 1-2 weeks. **Max:** 100mg qd. **Angina: Initial:** 50mg qd. **Titrate:** May increase to 100mg after 1 week. **Max:** 200mg qd. **AMI: Initial:** 5mg IV over 5 minutes, repeat 10 minutes later. If tolerated, give 50mg PO 10 minutes after the last IV dose followed by another 50mg PO 12 hrs later. **Maint:** 100mg qd or 50mg bid for 6-9 days. **Renal Impairment/Elderly: HTN: Initial:** 25mg qd. **HTN/Angina/AMI: Max: CrCl 15-35mL/min:** 50mg/day. **CrCl <15mL/min:** 25mg/day. **Hemodialysis:** 25-50mg after each dialysis.	**W/P:** Withdrawal before surgery is not recommended. Caution with bronchospastic disease, conduction abnormalities, left ventricular dysfunction, heart failure controlled by digitalis and/or diuretics, renal or hepatic dysfunction. Can cause heart failure with prolonged use, hyperuricemia, hypercalcemia, hypokalemia, hypophosphatemia. May mask hypoglycemia or hyperthyroidism symptoms. Avoid abrupt discontinuation. Avoid with untreated pheochromocytoma. Possible fetal harm in pregnancy. May aggravate peripheral arterial circulatory disorders. May manifest latent DM. Monitor for fluid or electrolyte imbalance. May develop antinuclear antibodies (ANA). Neonates born to mothers receiving atenolol may be at risk of hypoglycemia and bradycardia. **Contra:** Sinus bradycardia, >1st-degree heart block, cardiogenic shock, overt cardiac failure. **P/N:** Category D, caution in nursing.	Bradycardia, hypotension, dizziness, fatigue, nausea, depression, dyspnea.
Bisoprolol Fumarate (Zebeta)	**Tab:** 5mg*, 10mg	***Adults:* Initial:** 2.5-5mg qd. **Max:** 20mg/day. **Hepatic Dysfunction or CrCl <40mL/min: Initial:** 2.5mg qd; caution with dose titration.	**W/P:** Avoid abrupt withdrawal. May mask hypoglycemia or hyperthyroidism symptoms. Caution with compensated cardiac failure, DM, bronchospastic disease, hepatic/renal impairment, or peripheral vascular disease. May precipitate cardiac failure. **Contra:** Cardiogenic shock, overt cardiac failure, 2nd- or 3rd-degree AV block, marked sinus bradycardia. **P/N:** Category C, caution in nursing.	Diarrhea, upper respiratory infection, fatigue.
Esmolol Hydrochloride (Brevibloc)	**Inj:** 10mg/mL [10mL, 250mL], 20mg/mL [5mL, 100mL], 250mg/ mL [10mL]	***Adults:* Supraventricular Tachycardia:** Titrate dose based on ventricular rate. **Load:** 0.5mg/kg over 1 min. **Maint:** 0.05mg/kg/min for next 4 min. May increase by 0.05mg/kg/min at intervals of 4 min or more up to 0.2mg/kg/min. **Rapid slowing of Ventricular Response:** Repeat 0.5mg/kg load over 1 min, then 0.1mg/kg/min for 4 min. If needed, another (final) load of 0.5mg/kg over 1 min, then 0.15mg/kg/min for 4 min up to 0.2mg/kg/min. May continue infusions for 24-48 hrs. **Intraoperative/ Postoperative Tachycardia and/or HTN: Immediate Control: Initial:** 80mg bolus over 30 sec. **Maint:** 0.15mg/kg/min. May titrate up to 0.3mg/kg/min. **Gradual Control: Initial:** 0.5mg/kg over 1 min. **Maint:** 0.05mg/kg/min for 4 min. Then, if needed, may repeat load and increase to 0.1mg/kg/min.	**W/P:** Hypotension may occur; monitor BP and reduce dose or discontinue if needed. May cause cardiac failure; withdraw at 1st sign of impending cardiac failure. Caution with supraventricular arrhythmias when patient is compromised hemodynamically or is taking other drugs that decrease peripheral resistance, myocardial filling/contractility, and/or electrical impulse propagation in the myocardium. Not for HTN associated with hypothermia. Caution in bronchospastic diseases; titrate to lowest possible effective dose and terminate immediately in the event of bronchospasm. Caution in diabetics; may mask tachycardia occurring with hypoglycemia. Caution in impaired renal function. Avoid concentrations >10mg/mL and infusions into small veins or through butterfly catheters. Sloughing of skin and necrosis reported with infiltration and extravasation. Use caution when discontinuing infusion in CAD patients. **Contra:** Sinus bradycardia, heart block greater than first degree, cardiogenic shock or overt heart failure. **P/N:** Category C, caution in nursing.	Hypotension, dizziness, diaphoresis, somnolence, confusion, headache, agitation, nausea, infusion site reactions.

*Scored.   †Bold entries denote special dental considerations.

NAME	FORM/ STRENGTH	DOSAGE	WARNINGS/PRECAUTIONS & CONTRAINDICATIONS	ADVERSE EFFECTS†
Metoprolol (Toprol-XL, Lopressor)	**Tab, ER** 25mg*, 50mg*, 100mg*, 200mg*; **Inj:** 1mg/mL	***Adults:* HTN: Initial:** 25-100mg qd. **Titrate:** May increase weekly. **Max:** 400mg/day. **Angina: Initial:** 100mg qd. **Titrate:** May increase weekly. **Max:** 400mg/day. **Heart Failure: Initial:** (NYHA Class II) 25mg qd for 2 weeks. (Severe Heart Failure) 12.5mg qd for 2 weeks. **Titrate:** Double dose every 2 weeks as tolerated. **Max:** 200mg/day. **(Lopressor) MI (Early Phase):** 5mg IV every 2 minutes for 3 doses (monitor BP, HR, and ECG). If tolerated, give 50mg PO q6h (25-50mg q6h depending on IV dose intolerance) for 48 hrs. **MI (Late Phase):** 100mg bid for at least 3 months. Take with meals.	**W/P:** Exacerbation of angina pectoris and MI reported following abrupt withdrawal; taper over 1-2 weeks. Caution with heart failure, bronchospastic disease, DM, hepatic dysfunction, hyperthyroidism, or peripheral vascular disease. May mask symptoms of hyperthyroidism and hypoglycemia. Withdrawal prior to surgery is controversial. **Contra:** Severe bradycardia, >1st-degree heart block, cardiogenic shock, sick sinus syndrome (unless a pacemaker is present), decompensated cardiac failure. **P/N:** Category C, caution with nursing.	Bradycardia, shortness of breath, fatigue, dizziness, depression, diarrhea, pruritus, rash, hepatitis, arthralgia.

β-BLOCKERS, NONSELECTIVE

NAME	FORM/ STRENGTH	DOSAGE	WARNINGS/PRECAUTIONS & CONTRAINDICATIONS	ADVERSE EFFECTS†
Nadolol (Corgard)	**Tab:** 20mg*, 40mg*, 80mg*, 120mg*, 160mg*	***Adults:* Angina Pectoris: Initial:** 40mg qd. **Titrate:** Increase by 40-80mg every 3-7 days. **Usual:** 40-80mg qd. **Max:** 240mg/day. **HTN: Initial:** 40mg qd. **Titrate:** Increase by 40-80mg. **Max:** 320mg/day. **CrCl 31-50mL/min:** Dose q24-36h. **CrCl 10-30mL/min:** Dose q24-48h. **CrCl <10mL/min:** Dose q40-60h.	**W/P:** Caution in well-compensated cardiac failure, nonallergic bronchospasm, renal dysfunction. Exacerbation of ischemic heart disease with abrupt withdrawal. Withdrawal before surgery is controversial. May mask hyperthyroidism or hypoglycemia symptoms. Can cause cardiac failure. **Contra:** Bronchial asthma, sinus bradycardia and >1st-degree conduction block, cardiogenic shock, overt cardiac failure. **P/N:** Category C, not for use in nursing.	Bradycardia, peripheral vascular insufficiency, dizziness, fatigue.
Penbutolol Sulfate (Levatol)	**Tab:** 20mg*	***Adults:*** 20mg qd.	**W/P:** Caution with well-compensated heart failure, elderly, nonallergic bronchospasm, renal impairment. Can cause cardiac failure. Avoid abrupt withdrawal. Withdrawal before surgery is controversial. May mask hypoglycemia or hyperthyroidism symptoms. **Contra:** Cardiogenic shock, sinus bradycardia, 2nd- and 3rd-degree AV block, bronchial asthma. **P/N:** Category C, caution in nursing.	Diarrhea, nausea, dyspepsia, dizziness, fatigue, headache, insomnia, cough.
Pindolol	**Tab:** 5mg, 10mg	***Adults:* Initial:** 5mg bid. **Titrate:** May increase by 10mg/day after 3-4 weeks. **Max:** 60mg/day.	**W/P:** Caution with well-compensated heart failure, nonallergic bronchospasm, renal or hepatic impairment. Can cause cardiac failure. Avoid abrupt withdrawal. Withdrawal before surgery is controversial. May mask hypoglycemia or hyperthyroidism symptoms. **Contra:** Bronchial asthma, overt cardiac failure, cardiogenic shock, 2nd- and 3rd-degree heart block, severe bradycardia. **P/N:** Category B, not for use in nursing.	Dizziness, fatigue, insomnia, nervousness, dyspnea, edema, joint pain, muscle cramps/pain.
Propranolol Hydrochloride (Inderal, Inderal LA, InnoPran XL)	**(Inderal) Inj:** 1mg/mL; **Tab:** 10mg*, 20mg*, 40mg*, 60mg*, 80mg*; **(Inderal LA) Cap, ER:** 60mg, 80mg, 120mg, 160mg; **(InnoPran XL) Cap, ER:** 80mg, 120mg	***Adults:* (Inderal) HTN: (Tab) Initial:** 40mg bid. **Titrate:** Increase gradually. **Maint:** 120-240mg/day. **Angina: (Tab)** 80-320mg/day, given bid-qid. **Arrhythmia: (Inj)** 1-3mg IV at 1 mg/min. **(Tab)** 10-30mg tid-qid ac and qhs. **MI: (Tab)** 180-240mg/day, given bid-tid. **Migraine: (Tab) Initial:** 80mg/day in divided doses. **Usual:** 160-240mg/day in divided doses. **Tremor: (Tab) Initial:** 40mg bid. **Maint:** 120mg/day. **Max:** 320mg/day. **Hypertrophic Subaortic**	**W/P:** Caution with well-compensated cardiac failure, nonallergic bronchospasm, Wolff-Parkinson-White syndrome, hepatic or renal dysfunction. Withdrawal before surgery is controversial. May mask hypoglycemia or hyperthyroidism symptoms. Avoid abrupt discontinuation. May reduce IOP. Can cause cardiac failure. **Contra:** Cardiogenic shock, sinus bradycardia and >1st-degree block, bronchial asthma, CHF (unless failure is secondary to tachyarrhythmia treatable with propranolol). **P/N:** Category C, caution in nursing.	Bradycardia, CHF, hypotension, light-headedness, mental depression, nausea, vomiting, allergic reactions, agranulocytosis.

Table 14.1 PRESCRIBING INFORMATION FOR CARDIOVASCULAR DRUGS (cont.)

NAME	FORM/ STRENGTH	DOSAGE	WARNINGS/PRECAUTIONS & CONTRAINDICATIONS	ADVERSE EFFECTS†
β-BLOCKERS, NONSELECTIVE (cont.)				
Propranolol Hydrochloride (cont.)		**Stenosis: (Tab)** 20-40mg tid-qid, ac and qhs. **Pheochromocytoma: (Tab)** 60mg/day in divided doses for 3 days before surgery with α-blocker. **Inoperable Tumor: (Tab)** 30mg/day in divided doses. **Pediatrics: HTN (Tab): Initial:** 1mg/kg/day PO. **Usual:** 1-2mg/kg bid. **Max:** 16mg/kg/day. **(Inderal LA) HTN: Initial:** 80mg qd. **Maint:** 120-160mg qd. **Angina: Initial:** 80mg qd. **Titrate:** Increase gradually every 3-7 days. **Maint:** 160mg qd. **Max:** 320mg/day. **Migraine: Initial:** 80mg qd. **Maint:** 160-240mg qd. Discontinue gradually if no response within 4-6 weeks. **Hypertrophic Subaortic Stenosis:** 80-160mg qd. **(InnoPran XL) Initial:** 80mg qhs (approximately 10 PM) consistently either on an empty stomach or with food. **Titrate:** Based on response may titrate to a dose of 120mg.		
Sotalol Hydrochloride (Betapace)	**Tab:** 80mg*, 120mg*, 160mg*, 240mg*	**Adults: Initial:** 80mg bid. **Titrate:** Increase to 120-160mg bid if needed. Allow 3 days between dose increments. **Usual:** 160-320mg/day given bid-tid. **Refractory Patients:** 480-640mg/day. **CrCl 30-59mL/min:** Dose q24h. **CrCl 10-29mL/min:** Dose q36-48h. **CrCl <10mL/min:** Individualize dose. May increase dose with renal impairment after at least 5-6 doses. **Pediatrics: ≤2 yrs: Initial:** 30mg/m² tid. **Titrate:** Wait at least 36 hrs between dose increases. Guide dose by response, heart rate and QTc. **Max:** 60mg/m². **<2 yrs:** See dosing chart in labeling. Reduce dose or discontinue if QTc >550msec. **Renal Impairment:** Reduce dose or increase interval. **Preparation of 5mg/mL Oral Solution:** Add five 120mg tabs to 120mL simple syrup in a 6oz plastic, amber bottle. Shake bottle to wet all tabs. Allow tabs to hydrate for 2 hrs then shake bottle intermittently over 2 hrs until tabs are completely disintegrated. Shake before administration. Store at room temp for 3 months.	**BB:** To minimize risk of arrhythmia, place patients initiated or reinitiated on therapy for minimum of 3 days in a facility that can provide ECG monitoring and cardiac resuscitation. Perform CrCl before therapy. Do not substitute Betapace for Betapace AF. **W/P:** Caution with heart failure controlled by digitalis and/or diuretics, DM, left ventricular dysfunction, nonallergic bronchospasm, sick sinus syndrome, renal impairment, 2-weeks post-MI. Avoid with hypokalemia, hypomagnesemia, excessive QT interval prolongation (>550msec). Correct electrolyte imbalances before therapy. May provoke new or worsen ventricular arrhythmias. Avoid abrupt withdrawal. Use in surgery is controversial. May mask hypoglycemia, hyperthyroidism symptoms. Proarrhythmic events reported. **Contra:** Bronchial asthma, sinus bradycardia, 2nd- and 3rd-degree AV block (unless a functioning pacemaker is present), long QT syndromes, cardiogenic shock, uncontrolled CHF. **P/N:** Category B, not for use in nursing.	Dyspnea, fatigue, dizziness, bradycardia, chest pain, palpitation, ECG, hypotension, headache, lightheadedness, edema
Timolol Maleate	**Tab:** 5mg, 10mg*, 20mg*	**Adults: HTN: Initial:** 10mg qd. **Maint:** 20-40mg/day. Wait at least 7 days between dose increases. **Max:** 60mg/day given bid. **MI:** 10mg bid. **Migraine: Initial:** 10mg bid. **Maint:** 20mg qd. **Max:** 30mg/day in divided doses. May decrease to 10 mg qd. Discontinue if inadequate response after 6-8 weeks with max dose.	**W/P:** Caution with well-compensated cardiac failure, DM, mild to moderate COPD, bronchospastic disease, dialysis, hepatic/renal impairment, or cerebrovascular insufficiency. Exacerbation of ischemic heart disease with abrupt cessation. May mask hyperthyroidism or hypoglycemia symptoms. Withdrawal before surgery is controversial. May potentiate weakness with myasthenia gravis. Can cause cardiac failure. Caution and consider monitoring renal function in elderly. **Contra:** Active or history of bronchial asthma, severe COPD, sinus bradycardia, 2nd- and 3rd-degree AV block, overt cardiac failure, cardiogenic shock. **P/N:** Category C, not for use in nursing.	Fatigue, headache, nausea, arrhythmia, pruritus, dizziness, dyspnea, asthenia, bradycardia, dizziness.

*Scored.   †Bold entries denote special dental considerations.

NAME	FORM/ STRENGTH	DOSAGE	WARNINGS/PRECAUTIONS & CONTRAINDICATIONS	ADVERSE EFFECTS†
β-BLOCKERS & α-BLOCKERS (combined)				
Carvedilol (Coreg)	**Tab:** 3.125mg, 6.25mg, 12.5mg, 25mg	***Adults:* CHF: Initial:** 3.125mg bid for 2 weeks. **Titrate:** Double dose every 2 weeks as tolerated. **Max:** 50mg bid if >85kg. Reduce dose if HR <55 beats/min. **HTN: Initial:** 6.25mg bid for 7-14 days. **Titrate:** May double dose at 7-14 day intervals. **Max:** 50mg/day. **LVD Post-MI: Initial:** 6.25mg bid. Double dose every 3-10 days to target of 25mg bid. May begin with 3.125mg bid and slow rate of up-titration if clinically indicated. Take with food. Monitor dose increases.	**W/P:** Hepatic injury reported; discontinue and do not restart if develop hepatic injury. Hypotension reported with uptitration; avoid driving. May mask hypoglycemia and hyperthyroidism. May potentiate insulin-induced hypoglycemia and delay recovery of glucose levels. Avoid abrupt withdrawal; taper over 1-2 weeks. Decrease dose if pulse <55 beats/min. Monitor renal function during uptitration with low BP (SBP <100mmHg), ischemic heart disease, and/or renal insufficiency. Worsening cardiac failure or fluid retention with uptitration. Caution in pheochromocytoma, peripheral vascular disease, major surgery with anesthesia, prinzmetal's variant angina, and broncho-spastic disease. **Contra:** Decompensated cardiac failure requiring IV inotropic therapy, bronchial asthma or related bronchospastic conditions, 2nd- or 3rd-degree AV block, cardiogenic shock, hepatic impairment, sick sinus syndrome or severe bradycardia (without permanent pacemaker). **P/N:** Category C, not for use in nursing.	Bradycardia, edema, hypotension, syncope, AV block, dizziness, diarrhea, nausea, hyperglycemia, weight increase, abnormal vision, dyspnea, anemia.
Labetalol Hydrochloride (Normodyne, Trandate)	**Inj:** 5mg/mL; **Tab:** 100mg*, 200mg*, 300mg	***Adults:* (Tab) HTN: Initial:** 100mg bid. **Titrate:** 100mg bid every 2-3 days. **Maint:** 200-400mg bid. **Severe HTN:** 1200-2400mg/day given bid-tid. Increments should not exceed 200mg bid for titration. **(Inj) Severe HTN:** Administer in supine position. **Repeated IV Infusion: Initial:** 20mg over 2 minutes. **Titrate:** Give additional 40-80mg at 10 minute intervals if needed. **Max:** 300mg. **Slow Continuous Infusion:** 200mg at a rate of 2mg/min. May adjust dose according to BP. Switch to tabs when BP is stable while in hospital. **Initial:** 200mg, then 200-400mg 6-12 hrs later on Day 1. **Titrate:** May increase at 1 day interval. **(Trandate) Elderly: Initial:** 100mg bid. **Titrate:** May increase by 100mg bid. **Maint:** 100-200mg bid. **IV: Repeated IV Injection:** 20mg over 2 minutes. **Slow IV Infusion:** Titrate to response.	**W/P:** Severe hepatocellular injury reported; caution with hepatic dysfunction. Monitor LFTs periodically; discontinue at 1st sign of hepatic injury. Caution with well-compensated heart failure. Can cause heart failure. Exacerbation of ischemic heart disease with abrupt withdrawal. Caution in nonallergic bronchospasm patients refractory to or intolerant to other antihypertensives. May mask hypoglycemia symptoms. Withdrawal before surgery is controversial. Paradoxical HTN may occur with pheochromocytoma. Death reported during surgery. Avoid injection with low cardiac indices and elevated systemic vascular resistance. **Contra:** Bronchial asthma, obstructive airway disease, overt cardiac failure, >1st-degree heart block, cardiogenic shock, severe bradycardia, other conditions associated with severe and prolonged hypotension. **P/N:** Category C, caution in nursing.	Fatigue, dizziness, dyspepsia, nausea, nasal stuffiness.
β-BLOCKERS, CARDIOSELECTIVE/DIURETICS				
Atenolol/ Chlorthalidone (Tenoretic)	**Tab:** (Atenolol-Chlorthalidone) 50mg-25mg*, 100mg-25mg	***Adults:* Initial:** 50mg-25mg tab qd. May increase to 100mg-25mg tab qd. **CrCl 15-35mL/min: Max:** 50mg atenolol/day. **CrCl <15mL/min: Max:** 50mg atenolol every other day.	**W/P:** Withdrawal before surgery is not recommended. Caution with bronchospastic disease, conduction abnormalities, left ventricular dysfunction, heart failure controlled by digitalis and/or diuretics, renal dysfunction. Can cause heart failure with prolonged use. May mask hypoglycemia or hyperthyroidism symptoms. Avoid abrupt discontinuation. Avoid with untreated pheochromocytoma. Possible fetal harm in pregnancy. May aggravate peripheral arterial circulatory disorders. Enhanced effects in postsympathectomy patient. Neonates born to mothers receiving atenolol may be at risk of hypoglycemia and bradycardia.	Bradycardia, hypotension, dizziness, fatigue, nausea, depression, dyspnea, blood dyscrasias.

Table 14.1 PRESCRIBING INFORMATION FOR CARDIOVASCULAR DRUGS (cont.)

NAME	FORM/STRENGTH	DOSAGE	WARNINGS/PRECAUTIONS & CONTRAINDICATIONS	ADVERSE EFFECTS†
β-BLOCKERS, CARDIOSELECTIVE/DIURETICS (cont.)				
Atenolol/ Chlorthalidone (cont.)			**Contra:** Sinus bradycardia, >1st-degree heart block, cardiogenic shock, overt cardiac failure, anuria, sulfonamide hypersensitivity. **P/N:** Category C (1st trimester) and D (2nd and 3rd trimesters), not for use in nursing.	
Bisoprolol Fumarate/ Hydrochloro-thiazide (Ziac)	**Tab: (Biso-prolol-HCTZ)** 2.5mg-6.25mg, 5mg-6.25mg, 10mg-6.25mg	**Adults: Initial:** 2.5mg-6.25mg tab qd. **Maint:** May increase every 14 days. **Max:** 20mg bisoprolol-12.5mg HCTZ/day. **Renal/Hepatic Dysfunction:** Caution in dosing/titrating.	**W/P:** Caution with compensated cardiac failure, DM, bronchospastic disease, hepatic/renal impairment, or peripheral vascular disease. Avoid abrupt withdrawal. Photosensitivity reactions, hypokalemia, hypercalcemia, hypophosphatemia reported. May activate/exacerbate SLE. Enhanced effects in post-sympathectomy patients. May mask hyperthyroidism or hypoglycemia symptoms. Monitor for fluid/electrolyte imbalance. May precipitate hyperuricemia, acute gout, cardiac failure. **Contra:** Cardiogenic shock, overt cardiac failure, 2nd- or 3rd-degree AV block, marked sinus bradycardia, anuria, sulfonamide hypersensitivity. **P/N:** Category C, not for use in nursing.	Cough, diarrhea, myalgia, headache, dizziness, fatigue, upper respiratory infection.
Metoprolol Tartrate/ Hydrochloro-thiazide (Lopressor HCT)	**Tab: (Metoprolol-HCTZ)** 50mg-25mg*, 100-25mg*, 100mg-50mg*	**Adults: Usual:** 100-450mg metoprolol/day and 12.5-50mg HCTZ/day. **Max:** 50mg HCTZ/day.	**W/P:** Avoid abrupt withdrawal; taper over 1-2 weeks. Withdrawal before surgery is controversial. May mask hyperthyroidism and of hypoglycemia symptoms. May cause cardiac failure. Caution with hepatic dysfunction, CHF controlled by digitalis, bronchospastic disease, severe renal disease, allergy or asthma history. Monitor for fluid/electrolyte imbalance. May manifest latent DM. Hypokalemia, hyperuricemia, hypercalcemia, hypophosphatemia, and hypomagnesemia may occur. May exacerbate SLE. Enhanced effects in post-sympathectomy patient. **Contra:** Sinus bradycardia, >1st-degree heart block, cardiogenic shock, overt cardiac failure, anuria, sulfonamide hypersensitivity. **P/N:** Category C, not for use in nursing.	Fatigue, dizziness, flu syndrome, drowsiness, hypokalemia, headache, bradycardia.
β-BLOCKERS, NONSELECTIVE/DIURETICS				
Nadolol/ Bendroflume-thiazide (Corzide)	**Tab: (Nadolol-Bendroflu-methiazide)** 40mg-5mg*, 80mg-5mg*	**Adults: Initial:** 40mg-5mg tab qd. **Max:** 80mg-5mg tab qd. **CrCl >50mL/min:** Dose q24h. **CrCl 31-50mL/min:** Dose q24-36h. **CrCl 10-30mL/min:** Dose q24-48h. **CrCl <10mL/min:** Dose q40-60h.	**W/P:** Caution in well-compensated cardiac failure, nonallergic bronchospasm, progressive hepatic disease, and renal or hepatic dysfunction. Exacerbation of ischemic heart disease with abrupt withdrawal. Withdrawal before surgery is controversial. May mask hyperthyroidism or hypoglycemia symptoms. Can cause cardiac failure, sensitivity reactions, hypokalemia, hyperuricemia, hypomagnesemia, hypophosphatemia. May activate or exacerbate SLE. Monitor for fluid/electrolyte imbalance. Enhanced effects in postsympathectomy patient. May manifest latent DM. May decrease PBI levels. **Contra:** Bronchial asthma, sinus bradycardia and >1st-degree conduction block, cardiogenic shock, overt cardiac failure, anuria, sulfonamide hypersensitivity. **P/N:** Category C, not for use in nursing.	Bradycardia, peripheral vascular insufficiency, dizziness, fatigue, nausea, vomiting, blood dyscrasias, hypersensitivity reactions.

*Scored.   †Bold entries denote special dental considerations.

NAME	FORM/ STRENGTH	DOSAGE	WARNINGS/PRECAUTIONS & CONTRAINDICATIONS	ADVERSE EFFECTS†
Propranolol Hydrochloride/ Hydrochloro-thiazide (Inderide)	**(Propranolol-HCTZ) Tab: (Inderide)** 40mg-25mg*, 80mg-25mg*; **Cap, Extended Release: (Inderide LA)** 80mg-50mg	***Adults:* Initial:** 80-160mg propranolol/day; 25mg-50mg HCTZ/day. **Max: (Propranolol-HCTZ)** 160mg-50mg/day. **Elderly:** Start at low end of dosing range. Do not substitute mg-for-mg of extended release cap for immediate release tab plus HCTZ. Dose tab bid and extended release cap qd.	**W/P:** Caution with well-compensated cardiac failure, nonallergic bronchospasm, Wolff-Parkinson-White syndrome, hepatic or renal dysfunction. Withdrawal before surgery is controversial. May mask hypoglycemia or hyperthyroidism symptoms. Avoid abrupt discontinuation. May reduce IOP. Can cause cardiac failure, hypokalemia, hyperuricemia, hypercalcemia, hypophosphatemia. May exacerbate or activate SLE. Monitor for fluid/electrolyte imbalance. May manifest latent DM. Enhanced effect in postsympathectomy patient. **Contra:** Cardiogenic shock, sinus bradycardia and >1st-degree block, bronchial asthma, CHF (unless failure is secondary to tachyarrhythmia treatable with propranolol), anuria, sulfonamide hypersensitivity. **P/N:** Category C, not for use in nursing.	Bradycardia, CHF, hypotension, light-headedness, mental depression, nausea, vomiting, allergic reactions, blood dyscrasias, pancreatitis.
Timolol Maleate/ Hydrochlorothia-zide (Timolide)	**Tab: (Timolol-HCTZ)** 10mg-25mg	***Adults:*** 1 tab bid or 2 tabs qd.	**W/P:** Caution with well-compensated cardiac failure, DM, mild to moderate COPD, bronchospastic disease, dialysis, hepatic/renal impairment, or cerebrovascular insufficiency. Exacerbation of ischemic heart disease with abrupt cessation. May mask hyperthyroidism or hypoglycemia symptoms. Withdrawal before surgery is controversial. May potentiate weakness with myasthenia gravis. Can cause cardiac failure. Hypomagnesemia, hypokalemia, hypercalcemia, hypophosphatemia, hyperuricemia may occur. Monitor for fluid/electrolyte imbalance. May increase cholesterol and TG levels. May exacerbate or activate SLE. Enhanced effects in post-sympathectomy patient. **Contra:** Active or history of bronchial asthma, severe COPD, sinus bradycardia, 2nd- and 3rd-degree AV block, overt cardiac failure, cardiogenic shock, anuria, sulfonamide hypersensitivity. **P/N:** Category C, not for use in nursing.	Fatigue/tiredness, asthenia, hypotension, bradycardia, dizziness, bronchial spasm, dyspnea.

CALCIUM CHANNEL BLOCKERS

NAME	FORM/ STRENGTH	DOSAGE	WARNINGS/PRECAUTIONS & CONTRAINDICATIONS	ADVERSE EFFECTS†
Amlodipine Besylate (Norvasc)	**Tab:** 2.5mg, 5mg, 10mg	***Adults:* HTN: Initial:** 5mg qd. **Titrate** over 7-14 days. **Max:** 10mg qd. **Small, Fragile, or Elderly/Hepatic Dysfunction/Concomitant Antihypertensive: Initial:** 2.5mg qd. **Angina:** 10mg qd. **Elderly/Hepatic Dysfunction:** 5mg qd. ***Pediatrics:* 6-17 yrs: HTN:** 2.5-5mg qd.	**W/P:** May increase angina or MI with severe obstructive CAD. Caution with severe aortic stenosis, CHF, severe hepatic impairment, and in elderly. **P/N:** Category C, not for use in nursing.	Edema, flushing, palpitation, dizziness, headache, fatigue.
Diltiazem Hydrochloride (Cardizem LA, Cardizem CD, Dilacor XR, Diltiazem CD, Tiazac)	**(Dilacor XR) Cap, ER:** 120mg, 180mg, 240mg;. **(Tiazac) Cap, ER:** 120mg, 180mg, 240mg, 300mg, 360mg, 420mg; **Cap, ER: (Cardizem CD, Cartia XT)** 120mg, 180mg, 240mg, 300mg; **(Cardizem CD)**	***Adults:* HTN: Initial:** 180-240mg qd. **Usual:** 180-480mg qd. **Max:** 540mg qd. >60 yrs: **Initial:** 120mg qd. **Angina: Initial:** 120mg qd. **Titrate:** Adjust at 1-2 week intervals. **Max:** 480mg/day. Swallow whole on an empty stomach in the am. **(Tiazac) HTN: Initial:** 120-240mg qd. **Titrate:** Adjust at 2 week intervals. **Usual:** 120-540mg qd. **Max:** 540mg qd. **Angina: Initial:** 120-180mg qd **Titrate:** Increase over 7-14 days. **Max:** 540mg qd. **HTN: (CD,**	**W/P:** Caution in renal, hepatic, or ventricular dysfunction. Monitor LFTs and renal function with prolonged use. Discontinue if persistent rash occurs. Symptomatic hypotension may occur. Acute hepatic injury reported. **Contra:** Sick sinus syndrome, 2nd- or 3rd-degree AV block (except with functioning pacemaker), hypotension (<90mmHg systolic), acute MI, pulmonary congestion. **P/N:** Category C, not for use in nursing.	(Dilacor XR) Rhinitis, pharyngitis, cough, flu syndrome, peripheral edema, myalgia, vomiting, sinusitis, asthenia, nausea, vasodilation, headache, constipation, diarrhea. (Tiazac) Headache, peripheral edema, vasodilation, dizziness, rash, dyspepsia. (Cardizem) Headache, dizziness,

Table 14.1 PRESCRIBING INFORMATION FOR CARDIOVASCULAR DRUGS *(cont.)*

NAME	FORM/ STRENGTH	DOSAGE	WARNINGS/PRECAUTIONS & CONTRAINDICATIONS	ADVERSE EFFECTS†
CALCIUM CHANNEL BLOCKERS *(cont.)*				
Diltiazem Hydrochloride *(cont.)*	360mg; **Tab, ER: (Cardizem LA)** 120mg, 180mg, 240mg, 300mg, 360mg, 420mg; **(Cardizem): Tab:** 30mg, 60mg*, 90mg*, 120mg*	**Cartia XT) Initial (monotherapy):** 180-240mg qd. **Titrate:** Adjust at 2 week intervals. **Usual:** 240-360mg qd. **Max:** 480mg qd. **(LA) Initial:** 180-240mg qd. Adjust at 2 week intervals. **Max:** 540mg qd. **Angina: (CD, Cartia XT) Initial:** 120-180mg qd. Adjust at 1-2 week intervals. **Max:** 480mg/day. **(LA) Initial:** 180mg qd. Adjust at 1-2 week intervals. **(Cardizem) Initial:** 30mg qid (before meals and qhs). Adjust at 1-2 day intervals. **Usual:** 180-360mg/day.		asthenia, flushing, 1st-degree AV block, edema, nausea, bradycardia, rash.
Felodipine (Plendil)	**Tab, Extended Release:** 2.5mg, 5mg, 10mg	**Adults: Initial:** 5mg qd. **Titrate:** Adjust at no less than 2 week intervals. **Maint:** 2.5-10mg qd. **Elderly/Hepatic Dysfunction: Initial:** 2.5mg qd. Take without food or with a light meal. Swallow tab whole.	**W/P:** May cause hypotension and lead to reflex tachycardia with precipitation of angina. Caution with heart failure or ventricular dysfunction, especially with concomitant β-blockers. Monitor dose adjustment with hepatic dysfunction or elderly. Peripheral edema reported. Maintain good dental hygiene; gingival hyperplasia reported. **P/N:** Category C, not for use in nursing.	Peripheral edema, headache, flushing, dizziness.
Isradipine (DynaCirc)	**Cap:** 2.5mg, 5mg; **Tab, CR:** 5mg, 10mg	**Adults: Initial: (Cap)** 2.5mg bid or **(Tab, CR)** 5mg qd alone or with a thiazide diuretic. **Titrate:** May adjust by 5mg/day at 2-4 week intervals. **Max:** 20mg/day. Swallow CR tabs whole.	**W/P:** May produce symptomatic hypotension. Caution in CHF, especially with concomitant β-blockers. Caution with CR tab in pre-existing severe GI narrowing. Peripheral edema reported. Increased bioavailability in elderly. **P/N:** Category C, not for use in nursing.	Headache, edema, dizziness, constipation, fatigue, flushing, abdominal discomfort.
Nicardipine Hydrochloride (Cardene IV)	**Inj:** 2.5mg/mL	**Adults: IV:** Dosage must be individualized depending on severity of HTN and response of patient. Administer by slow continuous infusion at a concentration of 0.1mg/mL. **Initial:** 50mL/hr (5mg/hr). **Titrate:** May increase by 25mL/hr (2.5mg/hr) q5-15min. **Max:** 150mL/hr (15mg/hr). With rapid BP reduction, decrease rate to 30mL/hr (3mg/hr) after BP reduction is achieved. **Equiv PO/IV Dose:** 20mg q8h ≤0.5mg/hr, 30mg q8h ≤1.2mg/hr, 40mg q8h ≤2.2mg/hr.	**W/P:** May induce or exacerbate angina. Caution with CHF, significant left ventricular dysfunction, or pheochromocytoma. Change IV site every 12 hrs to minimize risk of peripheral venous irritation. Monitor BP during administration. Caution with impaired liver function or reduced hepatic blood flow; consider lower doses. Caution with portal hypertension. Careful dose titration is advised with renal impairment. **Contra:** Advanced aortic stenosis. **P/N:** Category C, not for use in nursing.	Headache, hypotension, tachycardia, nausea/vomiting.
Nifedipine (Adalat CC, Procardia XL)	**Tab, ER:** 30mg, 60mg, 90mg. **Cap:** 10mg, 20mg	**Adults: (Adalat CC) Initial:** 30mg qd. Titrate over 7-14 days. **Max:** 90mg/day. Take on empty stomach. Swallow tab whole. **(Nifedipine) Initial:** 10mg tid. Titrate over 7-14 days. **Usual:** 10-20mg tid. **Max:** 180mg/day. **Elderly:** Start at low end of dosing range. **(Procardia XL) Angina/HTN: Initial:** 30-60mg qd. Titrate over 7-14 days. **Max:** 120mg/day. Caution if dose >90mg with angina.	**W/P:** May cause hypotension; monitor BP initially or with titration. May exacerbate angina from β-blocker withdrawal. CHF risk, especially with aortic stenosis or β-blockers. Peripheral edema reported. May increase angina or MI with severe obstructive CAD. Caution in elderly. **P/N:** Category C, not for use in nursing.	Headache, flushing, heat sensation, dizziness, peripheral edema, fatigue, asthenia.
Nimodipine (Nimotop)	**Cap:** 30mg	**Adults:** 60mg q4h for 21 days, 1 hr before or 2 hrs after meals. **Hepatic Cirrhosis:** 30mg q4h for 21 days. Start therapy within 96 hrs of SAH. If cannot swallow cap, extract contents into syringe and empty into NG tube, then flush with 30mL of 0.9% NaCl.	**W/P:** Carefully monitor BP; monitor BP and heart rate with hepatic dysfunction. Do not administer contents of caps parenterally. **P/N:** Category C, not for use in nursing.	Decreased BP, headache, rash, diarrhea, bradycardia, nausea, abnormal LFTs.

*Scored.   †Bold entries denote special dental considerations.

NAME	FORM/ STRENGTH	DOSAGE	WARNINGS/PRECAUTIONS & CONTRAINDICATIONS	ADVERSE EFFECTS†
Nisoldipine (Sular)	**Tab, ER:** 10mg, 20mg, 30mg, 40mg	***Adults:*** **Initial:** 20mg qd. **Titrate:** Increase by 10mg weekly or longer. **Maint:** 20-40mg qd. **Max:** 60mg/ day. **Elderly (>65 yrs)/Hepatic Dysfunction: Initial:** Do not exceed 10mg/day. Do not chew, divide, or crush tabs.	**W/P:** May increase angina or MI with severe obstructive CAD. May cause hypotension; monitor BP initially or with titration. Caution with heart failure or compromised ventricular function, especially with concomitant β-blockers. Caution with severe hepatic dysfunction or in elderly. **P/N:** Category C, not for use in nursing.	Peripheral edema, headache, dizziness, pharyngitis, vasodilation, sinusitis, palpitations.
Verapamil Hydrochloride (Calan, Calan SR, Covera-HS, Isoptin SR, Verelan, Verelan PM)	**(Calan) Tab:** 40mg, 80mg*, 120mg*; **(Calan SR) Tab, ER:** 120mg, 180mg*, 240mg*; **(Covera-HS) Tab, ER:** 180mg, 240mg; **(Isoptin SR) Tab, ER:** 120mg, 180mg*, 240mg*; **(Verelan) Cap, ER:** 120mg, 180mg, 240mg, 360mg; **(Verelan PM) Cap, ER:** 100mg, 200mg, 300mg	***Adults:*** **HTN: Initial:** 80mg tid. **Usual:** 360-480mg/day. **Elderly/Small Stature: Initial:** 40mg tid. **Angina: Usual:** 80-120mg tid. **Elderly/Small Stature: Initial:** 40mg tid. **Titrate:** Increase daily or weekly. **A-Fib (Digitalized): Usual:** 240-320mg/day given tid-qid. **PSVT Prophylaxis (Non-Digitalized): Usual:** 240-480mg/day given tid-qid. **Max:** 480mg/day. **Severe Hepatic Dysfunction:** Give 30% of normal dose. **(Calan SR) ≥18 yrs: Initial:** 180mg qam. **Titrate:** If inadequate response, increase to 240mg qam, then 180mg bid; or 240mg qam plus 120mg qpm, then 240mg q12h. **(Covera-HS) Initial:** 180mg qhs. **Titrate:** May increase to 240mg qhs, then 360mg qhs, then 480mg qhs, if needed. Swallow tab whole. **(Isoptin SR) Initial:** 180mg qam. **Titrate:** If inadequate response, increase to 240mg qam, then 180mg bid; or 240mg qam plus 120mg qpm, then 240mg q12h. **Elderly/Small Stature: Initial:** 120mg qam. Take with food. **(Verelan) Usual:** 240mg qam. **Titrate:** May increase by 120mg qam. Max: 480mg qam. **Elderly/Small Stature: Initial:** 120mg qam. **Titrate:** May increase to 180mg qam, then 240mg qam, then 360mg qam, then 480mg qam. May sprinkle on applesauce; do not crush or chew. **(Verelan PM) Usual:** 200mg qhs. **Titrate:** May increase to 300mg qhs, then 400mg qhs. **Renal or Hepatic Dysfunction/Elderly/Small Stature: Initial:** 100mg qhs. **Max:** 400mg qhs. May sprinkle on applesauce; do not crush or chew.	**W/P:** Avoid with moderate to severe cardiac failure, and ventricular dysfunction if taking a β-blocker. May cause hypotension, AV block, transient bradycardia, PR interval prolongation. Monitor LFTs periodically; hepatocellular injury reported. Give 30% of normal dose with severe hepatic dysfunction. Caution with hypertrophic cardiomyopathy, renal or hepatic dysfunction. Decrease dose with decreased neuromuscular transmission. **Contra:** Severe ventricular dysfunction, hypotension, cardiogenic shock, sick sinus syndrome or 2nd- or 3rd-degree AV block (except with functioning ventricular pacemaker), A-Fib/Flutter with an accessory bypass tract. **P/N:** Category C, not for use in nursing.	Constipation, dizziness, nausea, hypotension, headache, edema, CHF, fatigue, elevated liver enzymes, dyspnea, bradycardia, AV block, rash, flushing.

CALCIUM CHANNEL BLOCKERS/ACE INHIBITORS

Amlodipine Besylate/ Benazepril Hydrochloride (Lotrel)	**Cap: (Amlodipine-Benazepril)** 2.5mg-10mg, 5mg-10mg, 5mg-20mg, 10mg-20mg	***Adults:*** **Usual:** 2.5-10mg amlodipine and 10-80mg benazepril per day. **Small/Elderly/Frail/Hepatic Impairment: Initial:** 2.5mg amlodipine.	**ACE inhibitors can cause death/injury to developing fetus during 2nd and 3rd trimesters. Stop therapy if pregnancy detected.** **W/P:** Discontinue if angioedema, jaundice, or if marked LFT elevation occurs. Risk of hyperkalemia with DM, renal dysfunction. Persistent nonproductive cough reported. Monitor WBCs in collagen vascular disease. Anaphylactoid reactions reported. Fetal/neonatal morbidity and death reported. Monitor for hypotension in high risk patients (heart failure, surgery/anesthesia, volume and/or salt depletion,etc.). Caution with CHF, severe hepatic or renal dysfunction, and renal artery stenosis. Avoid if CrCl ≥30mL/min. **P/N:** Category C (1st trimester) and D (2nd and 3rd trimesters), not for use in nursing.	Cough, headache, dizziness, edema.

Table 14.1 PRESCRIBING INFORMATION FOR CARDIOVASCULAR DRUGS *(cont.)*

NAME	FORM/ STRENGTH	DOSAGE	WARNINGS/PRECAUTIONS & CONTRAINDICATIONS	ADVERSE EFFECTS†
CALCIUM CHANNEL BLOCKERS/ACE INHIBITORS *(cont.)*				
Trandolapril/ Verapamil Hydrochloride (Tarka)	Tab: (Trandol- april-Verapamil) 2mg-180mg, 1mg-240mg, 2mg-240mg, 4mg-240mg	*Adults:* **Replacement Therapy:** 1 tab qd with food. **Severe Hepatic Dysfunction:** Give 30% of normal dose.	**ACE inhibitors can cause death/injury to developing fetus during 2nd and 3rd trimesters. Stop therapy if pregnancy detected.** **W/P:** Monitor for hypotension with surgery or anesthesia. Risk of hyperkalemia with renal insufficiency, DM. Discontinue if develop jaundice. Avoid with moderate to severe cardiac failure, and ventricular dysfunction if taking a β-blocker. May cause angioedema, cough, fetal/neonatal morbidity, hypotension, AV block, anaphylactoid reactions, transient bradycardia, PR interval prolongation. Monitor LFTs periodically. Give 30% of normal dose with severe hepatic dysfunction. Caution with CHF, hypertrophic cardiomyopathy, renal or hepatic dysfunction. Decrease dose in those with decreased neuromuscular transmission. Monitor WBC with collagen-vascular disease and/or renal disease. **Contra:** Severe ventricular dysfunction, hypotension, cardiogenic shock, sick sinus syndrome or 2nd- or 3rd-degree AV block (except with functioning ventricular pacemaker), A-Fib/ Flutter with an accessory bypass tract, history of ACE inhibitor associated angioedema. **P/N:** Category C (1st trimester) and D (2nd and 3rd trimesters), not for use in nursing.	AV block, constipation, cough, dizziness, fatigue, headache, increased hepatic enzymes, chest pain, upper respiratory tract infection/congestion.
CALCIUM CHANNEL BLOCKERS/HMG-CoA REDUCTASE INHIBITORS				
Amlodipine Besylate/ Atorvastatin Calcium (Caduet)	Tab: (amlodipine-atorvastatin) 2.5mg-10mg, 2.5mg-20mg, 2.5mg-40mg, 5mg-10mg, 5mg-20mg, 5mg-40mg, 5mg-80mg, 10mg-10mg, 10mg-20mg, 10mg-40mg, 10mg-80mg	*Adults:* Dosing should be individualized and based on the appropriate combination of recommendations for the monotherapies. **(Amlodipine): HTN: Initial:** 5mg qd. Titrate over 7-14 days. **Max:** 10mg qd. **Small, Fragile, or Elderly/Hepatic Dysfunction/Concomitant Antihypertensive: Initial:** 2.5mg qd. **Angina:** 5-10mg qd. **Elderly/Hepatic Dysfunction:** 5mg qd. **(Atorvastatin): Hypercholesterolemia/Mixed Dyslipidemia: Initial:** 10-20mg qd (or 40mg qd for LDL-C reduction >45%). **Titrate:** Adjust dose if needed at 2-4 week intervals. **Usual:** 10-80mg qd. **Homozygous Familial Hypercholesterolemia:** 10-80mg qd. *Pediatrics:* **≥10 yrs (postmenarchal): (Amlodipine): HTN:** 2.5-5mg qd. **10-17 yrs (postmenarchal): (Atorvastatin): Heterozygous Familial Hypercholesterolemia: Initial:** 10mg/day. **Titrate:** Adjust dose if needed at intervals of ≥4 weeks. **Max:** 20mg/day.	**W/P:** May, rarely, increase angina or MI with severe obstructive CAD. Monitor LFTs prior to therapy, at 12 weeks after initiation, with dose elevation, and periodically thereafter. Reduce dose or withdraw if AST or ALT >3X ULN persist. Caution with heavy alcohol use and/or history of hepatic disease, severe aortic stenosis, CHF. Discontinue if markedly elevated CPK levels occur, if myopathy is diagnosed or suspected, or if predisposition to renal failure secondary to rhabdomyolysis. **Contra:** Active liver disease, unexplained persistent elevations of serum transaminases, pregnancy, nursing mothers. **P/N:** Category X, not for use in nursing.	Headache, edema, palpitation, dizziness, fatigue, constipation, flatulence, dyspepsia, abdominal pain.
VASODILATORS				
Hydralazine Hydrochloride	Inj: 20mg/mL; Tab: 10mg, 25mg, 50mg, 100mg	*Adults:* **Initial:** 10mg qid for 2-4 days. **Titrate:** Increase to 25mg qid for the rest of the week, then increase to 50mg qid. **Maint:** Use lowest effective dose. **Resistant Patients:** 300mg/day or titrate to lower dose	**W/P:** Discontinue if SLE symptoms occur. May cause angina and ECG changes of MI. Caution with suspected CAD, CVA, advanced renal impairment. May increase pulmonary artery pressure in mitral valvular disease. Postural hypotension reported. Add pyridoxine	Headache, anorexia, nausea, vomiting, diarrhea, tachycardia, angina.

*Scored. †Bold entries denote special dental considerations.

NAME	FORM/ STRENGTH	DOSAGE	WARNINGS/PRECAUTIONS & CONTRAINDICATIONS	ADVERSE EFFECTS†
Hydralazine Hydrochloride *(cont.)*		combined with thiazide diuretic and/or reserpine, or β-blocker. ***Pediatrics:* Initial:** 0.75mg/kg/day given qid. **Titrate:** Increase gradually over 3-4 weeks to a max of 7.5mg/kg/day or 200mg/day.	if develop peripheral neuritis. Monitor CBC and ANA titer before and periodically during therapy. **Contra:** CAD and mitral valvular rheumatic heart disease. **P/N:** Category C, safety in nursing not known.	
Hydralazine Hydrochloride/ Isosorbide Dinitrate (BiDil)	**Tab:** (Hydralazine/Isosorbide) 37.5mg-20mg	***Adults:* Initial:** 1 tab tid. **Max:** 2 tabs tid.	**W/P:** May produce a clinical picture simulating systemic lupus erythematosus including glomerulonephritis. May cause symptomatic hypotension, tachycardia, peripheral neuritis. Caution in patients with acute MI, hemodynamic and clinical monitoring recommended. May aggravate angina associated with hypertrophic cardiomyopathy. **Contra:** Allergies to organic nitrates. **P/N:** Category C, caution in nursing.	Headache, dizziness, chest pain, asthenia, nausea, bronchitis, hypotension, sinusitis, ventricular tachycardia, palpitations, hyperglycemia, rhinitis, paresthesia, vomiting, amblyopia, hyperlipidemia.
Isosorbide Mononitrate (Imdur, Ismo, Monoket)	**Tab, Extended Release:** 30mg*, 60mg*, 120mg; **Ismo, Tab:** 20mg*	***Adults:* Initial:** 30-60mg qd in the am. **Titrate:** May increase after several days to 120mg/day. Swallow whole with fluids. **Elderly:** Start at lower end of dosing range. **(Ismo)** 20mg bid; 1st dose on awakening then 7 hrs later.	**W/P:** Not for use with acute MI or CHF. Severe hypotension may occur; caution with volume depletion and hypotension. Hypotension may increase angina pectoris. May aggravate angina caused by hypertrophic cardiomyopathy. Monitor for tolerance. May interfere with cholesterol test. **P/N:** Category B, caution with nursing. (Ismo) Category C, caution in nursing.	Headache, dizziness, hypotension.
Isosorbide Dinitrate (Dilatrate-SR, Isochron, Isordil Titradose)	**Tab:** 2.5mg, 5mg*, 10mg*, 20mg*, 30mg*, 40mg*	***Adults:* Prevention: Initial:** 5-20mg bid-tid. **Maint:** 10-40mg bid-tid. Allow a dose-free interval of at least 14 hrs for both formulations. **Elderly:** Start at low end of dosing range.	**W/P:** Not for use with acute MI or CHF. Severe hypotension may occur. May aggravate angina caused by hypertrophic cardiomyopathy. Caution with volume depletion, hypotension, elderly. Monitor for tolerance. **P/N:** Category C, caution in nursing.	Headache, lightheadedness, hypotension.
Minoxidil	**Tab:** 2.5mg, 10mg	***Adults:* Initial:** 5mg qd. **Titrate:** Increase by no less than 3 days; may increase every 6 hrs if closely monitored. Usual: 10-40mg/day. **Max:** 100mg/day. **Frequency:** Give qd if diastolic BP is reduced to <30 mmHg and bid if reduced to >30 mmHg. Give with a diuretic (eg, hydrochlorothiazide 50mg bid, furosemide 40mg bid) and a β-blocker (equivalent to propranolol 80-160mg/day) or methyldopa (250-750mg bid starting 24 hrs before therapy). **Renal Failure/Dialysis:** Reduce dose. ***Pediatrics:* >12 yrs:** Initial: 5mg qd. **Titrate:** Increase by no less than 3 days; may increase every 6 hrs if closely monitored. **Usual:** 10-40mg/day. **Max:** 100mg/day. **Frequency:** Give qd if diastolic BP is reduced to <30 mmHg and bid if reduced to >30 mmHg. Give with a diuretic (eg, hydrochlorothiazide 50mg bid, furosemide 40mg bid) and a β-blocker (equivalent to propranolol 80-160mg/day) or methyldopa (250-750mg bid starting 24 hrs before therapy). **<12 yrs:** 0.2mg/kg qd. **Titrate:** May increase by 50-100% increments. **Usual:** 0.25-1mg/kg/day. **Max:** 50mg/day. **Renal Failure/Dialysis:** Reduce dose.	**W/P:** Administer with a diuretic and β-blocker. Pericarditis, pericardial effusion and tamponade reported. With renal failure or dialysis, reduce dose to prevent renal failure exacerbation and precipitation of cardiac failure. Avoid rapid control with severe HTN. Monitor body weight, fluid and electrolyte balance. Use extreme caution with post-MI. Hypersensitivity reactions reported. **Contra:** Pheochromocytoma. **P/N:** Category C, not for use in nursing.	Salt and water retention, pericarditis, pericardial effusion, tamponade, hypertrichosis, nausea, vomiting, rash, ECG changes, hemodilution effects.

Table 14.1 PRESCRIBING INFORMATION FOR CARDIOVASCULAR DRUGS *(cont.)*

NAME	FORM/STRENGTH	DOSAGE	WARNINGS/PRECAUTIONS & CONTRAINDICATIONS	ADVERSE EFFECTS[†]

VASODILATORS *(cont.)*

NAME	FORM/STRENGTH	DOSAGE	WARNINGS/PRECAUTIONS & CONTRAINDICATIONS	ADVERSE EFFECTS[†]
Nitroglycerin (Nitro-Bid, Nitro-Dur, Nitrolingual Spray, Nitrostat)	**Oint:** 2% (15mg/inch); **Patch: (Mini-tran)** 0.1mg/hr, 0.2mg/hr, 0.4mg/hr, 0.6mg/hr [30^S]; **(Nitrek)** 0.2mg/hr, 0.4mg/hr, 0.6mg/hr [30^S]; **(Nitro-Dur)** 0.1mg/hr, 0.2mg/hr, 0.3mg/hr, 0.4mg/hr, 0.6mg/hr, 0.8mg/hr [30^S]; **Spray:** 0.4mg/spray. **Tab, Sublingual:** 0.3mg, 0.4mg, 0.6mg	**Adults: (Oint) Initial:** Apply 0.5 inch bid (once in the am and 6 hrs later). **Titrate:** May increase to 1 inch bid, then to 2 inches bid. Should have 10-12 hr nitrate-free period. **(Patch) Initial:** 0.2-0.4mg/hr for 12-14 hrs. Remove for 10-12 hrs. **(Spray) Acute:** 1-2 sprays at onset of attack onto or under tongue. **Max:** 3 sprays/15 minutes. **Prophylaxis:** 1-2 sprays onto or under tongue 5-10 minutes before activity that may cause acute attack. Do not expectorate medication or rinse mouth for 5-10 minutes after administration. **(Tab, SL) Treatment:** 1 tab SL or in buccal pouch at onset of attack. May repeat in 5 minutes. **Max:** 3 tabs in 15 minutes. **Prophylaxis:** Take 5-10 minutes before activity that may cause acute attack.	**W/P:** Monitor with acute MI or CHF. Severe hypotension may occur; caution with volume depletion and hypotension. May aggravate angina caused by hypertrophic cardiomyopathy. Tolerance to other nitrates may decrese effects. Vasodilatory effects with phosphodiesterase inhibitors (eg, sildenafil) can result in severe hypotension. (Nitrostat) Do not swallow tabs. **Contra:** Allergy to adhesives in NTG patches. (Nitrostat) Early MI, severe anemia, increased intracranial pressure, concomitant sildenafil. **P/N:** Category C, caution in nursing.	Headache, lightheadedness, hypotension, flushing, syncope.

VASODILATORS USED FOR ERECTILE DYSFUNCTION

NAME	FORM/STRENGTH	DOSAGE	WARNINGS/PRECAUTIONS & CONTRAINDICATIONS	ADVERSE EFFECTS[†]
Sildenafil (Revatio, Viagra)	**(Revatio) Tab:** 20mg; **(Viagra) Tab:** 25mg, 50mg, 100mg	**Adults: (Revatio)** 20mg tid 4-6 hrs apart. **(Viagra) Usual:** 50mg 1 hr (range 0.5-4 hrs) prior to sexual activity at frequency of up to once daily. **Titrate:** May decrease to 25mg qd or increase to 100mg qd. **Max:** 100mg qd. **Elderly/Hepatic Impairment/CrCl <30mL/min/Concomitant CYP450 3A4 Inhibitors** (eg, ketoconazole, itraconazole, erythromycin, saquinavir): **Initial:** 25mg qd. **Concomitant Ritonavir: Max:** 25mg q48h. **Concomitant α-blocker:** Avoid doses >25mg sildenafil within 4 hrs of an α-blocker.	**W/P:** Caution with MI, stroke, or life-threatening arrhythmia within last 6 months; with resting hypotension (BP<90/50), fluid depletion, severe left ventricular outflow obstruction, autonomic dysfunction, or HTN (BP>170/110); unstable angina due to cardiac failure or CAD; anatomical penile deformation; predisposition to priapism; and retinitis pigmentosa. Avoid in patients with veno-occlvusive disease. Decrease in supine BP reported. **Contra:** Organic nitrates taken regularly and/or intermittently. **P/N:** Category B, caution in nursing.	Epistaxis, headache, flushing, dyspepsia, insomnia, erythema, dyspnea, rhinitis, diarrhea, myalgia, pyrexia, gastritis, sinusitis, paresthesia, abnormal vision (eg, color tinge, increased light sensitivity, blurred vision), cardiovascular events.
Tadalafil (Cialis)	**Tab:** 5mg, 10mg, 20mg	**Adults:** Take once daily prior to sexual activity. **Initial:** 10mg. **Range:** 5-20mg. **Renal Impairment: CrCl 31-50mL/min: Initial:** 5mg. **Max:** 10mg/48hrs. **CrCl <30mL/min/ Hemodialysis: Max:** 5mg. **Hepatic Impairment: Mild/Moderate: Max:** 10mg. **With Potent CYP3A4 Inhibitors (eg, ketoconazole, itraconazole, ritonavir): Max:** 10mg/72hrs.	**W/P:** Avoid in men for whom sexual activity is inadvisable due to underlying cardiovascular status. Increased sensitivity to vasodilatory effect with left ventricular outflow obstruction. Avoid with MI (within last 90 days), unstable angina or angina occurring during sexual intercourse, NYHA Class 2 or greater heart failure (in the last 6 months), uncontrolled arrhythmias, hypotension (<90/50 mmHg), or uncontrolled HTN (>170/100 mmHg), stroke within the last 6 months, severe hepatic impairment (Childs-Pugh Class C), degenerative retinal disorders, including retinitis pigmentosa. Caution with predisposition to priapism (eg, sickle cell anemia, multiple myeloma, leukemia), anatomical deformation of the penis, bleeding disorders or active peptic ulceration. May cause transient decrease in blood pressure. Caution with coadministration of phosphodiesterase type 5 inhibitors (PDE5) and α-blockers. May cause additive hypotensive effect. Initiate at lowest dose once patient is stable on either therapy. Rare	Headache, dyspepsia, back pain, myalgia, nasal congestion, flushing, limb pain.

*Scored.   †Bold entries denote special dental considerations.

NAME	FORM/ STRENGTH	DOSAGE	WARNINGS/PRECAUTIONS & CONTRAINDICATIONS	ADVERSE EFFECTS†
Tadalafil (cont.)			reports of nonarteritic anterior ischemic optic neuropathy with PDE5 inhibitors. **Contra:** Concomitant nitrates. **P/N:** Category B, not for use in nursing.	
Vardenafil Hydrochloride (Levitra)	**Tab:** 2.5mg, 5mg, 10mg, 20mg	**Adults: Initial:** 10mg one hour prior to sexual activity at frequency of up to once daily. **Titrate:** May decrease to 5mg or increase to max of 20mg based on response. **Elderly: ≥65 yrs:** Initial: 5mg. **Moderate Hepatic Impairment: Initial:** 5mg; **Max:** 10mg. **Concomitant Ritonavir: Max:** 2.5mg/72 hrs. **Concomitant Indinavir, Ketoconazole 400mg daily/Itraconazole 400mg daily: Max:** 2.5mg/24 hrs. **Concomitant Ketoconazole 200mg daily/Itraconazole 200mg daily/Erythromycin: Max:** 5mg/24hrs.	**W/P:** Avoid when sexual activity is inadvisable due to underlying cardiovascular status. Increased sensitivity to vasodilation effects with left ventricular outflow obstruction. Decrease in supine BP reported. Avoid with unstable angina, hypotension (SBP<90mmHg), uncontrolled HTN (>170/100 mmHg), recent history of stroke, life-threatening arrhythmia, myocardial infarction (within last 6 months), severe cardiac failure, severe hepatic impairment (Childs-Pugh Class C), end-stage renal disease requiring dialysis, hereditary degenerative retinal disorders including retinitis pigmentosa, congenital QT prolongation. Caution with bleeding disorders, peptic ulcers, anatomical deformation of the penis, or predisposition to priapism. Rare reports of nonarteritic anterior ischemic optic neuropathy with phosphodiesterase type 5 inhibitors. **Contra:** Concomitant nitrates or nitric oxide donors. **P/N:** Category B, not for use in nursing.	Headache, flushing, rhinitis, dyspepsia, sinusitis, flu syndrome.

MISCELLANEOUS

NAME	FORM/ STRENGTH	DOSAGE	WARNINGS/PRECAUTIONS & CONTRAINDICATIONS	ADVERSE EFFECTS†
Amyl Nitrite	**Sol:** 300mg/ 10mL	**Adults: Angina Pectoris, Acute:** 0.18-0.3mL by INH (1-6 inhalations of the vapors); may be repeated in 3-5 min. **Cyanide Poisoning:** INH for 30-60 seconds every 5 min until the patient is conscious, then repeated at longer intervals for 24 hr.	**W/P:** Anemia, avoid abrupt withdrawal, avoid alcohol (increased hypotension), geriatrics (othostatic hypotension), hyperthyroidism, hypertrophic cardiomyopathy, hypotension, myocardial infarction. **P/N:** Safety in pregnancy and nursing not known. **Contra:** cerebral hemorrhage, glaucoma, recent head trauma.	Hypotension, tachyarrhythmia, nausea, vomiting, dyspnea, syncope, hemolytic anemia, methemoglobinemia.
Aspirin/ Pravastatin Sodium (Pravigard PAC)	**Tab: (Buffered Aspirin-Pravastatin):** 81mg-20mg; 325mg-20mg; 81mg-40mg; 325mg-40mg; 81mg-80mg; 325mg-80mg. [30 tabs of each]	**Adults: (Buffered Aspirin-Pravastatin): Usual:** 81mg-40mg or 325mg-40mg qd. If desired cholesterol levels not achieved, may increase to 81mg-80mg or 325mg-80mg qd.	**W/P:** Perform LFTs before therapy, before dose increase, and if clinically indicated. Risk of myopathy, myalgia, and rhabdomyolysis. May elevate CPK and transaminase levels. Discontinue if AST or ALT ≥3X ULN persists, if elevated CPK levels occur, or if myopathy diagnosed or suspected. Less effective with homozygous familial hypercholesterolemia. Caution with heavy alcohol use, coagulation abnormalities. Avoid with peptic ulcer disease, severe renal failure, severe hepatic insufficiency, recent history or signs of hepatic disease, or renal dysfunction. Associated with elevated BUN and serum creatinine, hyperkalemia, proteinuria, and prolonged bleeding time. **Contra:** Active liver disease, unexplained persistent elevations of LFTs, pregnancy, nursing mothers, NSAID allergy, viral infections in children or teenagers with or without fever, syndrome of asthma, rhinitis, and nasal polyps. **P/N:** Category X, not for use in nursing.	Headache, rash, fatigue, chest pain, heartburn, myalgia, cough, increased ALT/AST/CPK, dyspepsia, GI bleeding, nausea, vomiting.
Bosentan (Tracleer)	**Tab:** 62.5mg, 125mg	**Adults: Initial:** 62.5mg bid. **Titrate/Maint:** Increase to 125mg bid after 4 weeks. **Low Weight (<40kg): Initial/Maint:** 62.5mg bid. **Adjust if Develop LFT Abnormality: >3 to >5X ULN:** Reconfirm LFTs. Reduce	**Potential liver injury; monitor LFTs before therapy, then monthly. Contraindicated in pregnancy; obtain monthly pregnancy tests. Prescribe through Tracleer Access Program. W/P:** May decrease Hgb and Hct; monitor 1 and 3 months after initiation, then	Headache, nasopharyngitis, flushing, hepatic dysfunction, lower limb edema, hypotension, palpitations, dyspepsia, edema, fatigue, pruritus.

Table 14.1 PRESCRIBING INFORMATION FOR CARDIOVASCULAR DRUGS *(cont.)*

NAME	FORM/ STRENGTH	DOSAGE	WARNINGS/PRECAUTIONS & CONTRAINDICATIONS	ADVERSE EFFECTS†
MISCELLANEOUS *(cont.)*				
Bosentan *(cont.)*		dose or interrupt therapy. Monitor LFTs every 2 weeks. If LFTs return to pre-treatment levels, reintroduce or continue therapy. **>5 to ≤8X ULN:** Reconfirm LFTs. Stop treatment and monitor LFTs every 2 weeks. If LFTs return to pre-treatment values, may reintroduce therapy. **>8X ULN:** Stop treatment, do not reintroduce. *Pediatrics:* **>12 yrs: <40kg: Initial/ Maint:** 62.5mg bid.	every 3 months. Caution in elderly or mild hepatic impairment. Avoid with moderate to severe hepatic impairment, or LFTs >3X ULN. Discontinue gradually. **Contra:** Pregnancy, cyclosporine A, glyburide. **P/N:** Category X, not for use in nursing.	
Digoxin (Digitek, Lanoxin, Lanoxin Pediatric)	**Cap: (Lanoxicaps)** 0.1mg, 0.2mg; **Inj: (Pediatric Inj)** 0.1mg/mL, 0.25mg/mL; **Sol: (Pediatric Sol)** 0.05mg/mL [60mL]; **Tab:** 0.125mg*, 0.25mg*	*Adults:* **Rapid Digitalization: LD: (Cap/Inj)** 0.4-0.6mg PO/IV or **(Tab)** 0.5-0.75mg PO, may give additional **(Cap/Inj)** 0.1-0.3mg or **(Tab)** 0.125-0.375mg at 6-8 hr intervals until clinical effect. **Maint: (Tab)** 0.125-0.5mg qd. **Elderly (>70 yrs)/Renal Dysfunction: Initial:** 0.125mg qd. **Marked Renal Dysfunction: Initial:** 0.0625mg qd. **Titrate:** Increase every 2 weeks based on response. **A-Fib:** Titrate to minimum effective dose for desired response. *Pediatrics:* **(Ped Sol) Oral Digitalizing Dose: Premature Infants:** 20-30µg/kg. **Full-Term Infants:** 25-35µg/kg. **1-24 months:** 35-60µg/kg. **2-5 yrs:** 30-40µg/kg. **5-10 yrs:** 20-35µg/kg. **>10 yrs:** 10-15µg/kg. **Maint: Premature Infants:** 20-30% of PO digitalizing dose/day. **Full-Term Infants to >10 yrs:** 25-35% of PO digitalizing dose. **(Ped Inj) IV Digitalizing Dose: Premature Infants:** 15-25µg/kg. **Full-Term Infants:** 20-30µg/kg. **1-24 months:** 30-50µg/kg. **2-5 yrs:** 25-35µg/kg. **5-10 yrs:** 15-30µg/kg. **>10 yrs:** 8-12µg/kg. **Maint: Premature Infants:** 20-30% of IV digitalizing dose. **Full-Term Infants to >10 yrs:** 25-35% of IV digitalizing dose/day. **(Cap) Oral Digitalizing Dose: 2-5 yrs:** 25-35µg/kg. **5-10 yrs:** 15-30µg/kg. **>10 yrs:** 8-12µg/kg. **Maint: ≥2 yrs:** 25-25% of PO or IV digitalizing dose. **(Tab) Maint: 2-5 yrs:** 10-15µg/kg. **5-10 yrs:** 7-10µg/kg. **>10 yrs:** 3-5µg/kg. **A-Fib:** Titrate to minimum effective dose for desired response.	**W/P:** May cause severe sinus bradycardia or sinoatrial block with pre-existing sinus node disease. May cause advanced or complete heart block with pre-existing incomplete AV block. May cause very rapid ventricular response or ventricular fibrillation. Caution with thyroid disorders, AMI, hypermetabolic states, restrictive cardiomyopathy, constrictive pericarditis, amyloid heart disease, elderly, acute cor pulmonale, and idiopathic hypertrophic subaortic stenosis. Caution with renal dysfunction; high risk for toxicity. Caution with hypokalemia, hypomagnesemia, or hypercalcemia; toxicity may occur. Hypocalcemia can nullify effects of digoxin. Monitor electrolytes and renal function periodically. Risk of ventricular arrhythmia with electrical cardioversion. Bioavailability is different between dosage forms. **Contra:** Ventricular fibrillation, digitalis. **P/N:** Category C, caution in nursing. hypersensitivity.	Heart block, rhythm disturbances, anorexia, nausea, vomiting, diarrhea, visual disturbances, headache, weakness, dizziness, mental disturbances.
Enalapril Maleate/ Felodipine (Lexxel)	**Tab, Extended Release: (Enalapril-Felodipine)** 5mg-5mg	*Adults:* **For Combination Therapy from Monotherapy (felodipine or enalapril): Initial:** One 5mg-5mg tab qd. **Titrate:** If inadequate control, may increase after 1-2 weeks to two 5mg-5mg tabs qd, and then to four 5mg-2.5mg tabs qd. If receiving both felodipine and enalapril separately, may give same component doses. **Elderly/Hepatic Impairment: Initial:** 2.5mg felodipine qd. **CrCl ≤30mL/min: Initial:** 2.5mg enalapril qd. Take without	**ACE inhibitors can cause death/injury to developing fetus during 2nd and 3rd trimesters. Stop therapy if pregnancy detected. W/P:** Discontinue if angioedema, jaundice, or if marked LFT elevation occurs. Risk of hyperkalemia with DM, renal dysfunction. ACE inhibitor-induced cough reported. Monitor WBCs in renal or collagen vascular disease. Anaphylactoid reactions reported. Fetal/neonatal morbidity and death reported. Monitor for hypotension in high risk patients (heart failure, surgery/anesthesia, hyponatremia,	Edema, headache, dizziness, cough.

*Scored.   †Bold entries denote special dental considerations.

NAME	FORM/ STRENGTH	DOSAGE	WARNINGS/PRECAUTIONS & CONTRAINDICATIONS	ADVERSE EFFECTS†
Enalapril Maleate/ Felodipine *(cont.)*		food or with a light meal. Swallow tab whole.	high dose diuretic therapy, severe volume and/or salt depletion, etc.). Caution with CHF, obstruction to left ventricle outflow tract, renal dysfunction, and renal artery stenosis. More reports of angioedema in blacks than nonblacks. Peripheral edema reported with felodipine. Caution with hepatic dysfunction or elderly; increased felodipine levels. Mild gingival hyperplasia reported. **Contra:** History of ACE inhibitor associated angioedema and hereditary or idiopathic angioedema. **P/N:** Category C (1st trimester) and D (2nd and 3rd trimesters), not for use in nursing.	
Epoprostenol Sodium (Flolan)	**Inj:** 0.5mg, 1.5mg	***Adults:* Initial:** 2ng/kg/min IV chronic infusion. **Titrate:** Increase by 2ng/kg/min every 15 minutes until no further increases are clinically warranted. May use a lower initial infusion rate if not tolerated.	**W/P:** Abrupt withdrawal or large dose reductions may result in symptoms associated with rebound pulmonary HTN (eg, dyspnea, dizziness, and asthenia); avoid abrupt withdrawal. Unless contraindicated, administer anticoagulant therapy to reduce risk of pulmonary thromboembolism or systemic embolism through a patent foramen ovale. Monitor standing and supine BP and heart rate for several hours after dose adjustments. **Contra:** Chronic use in CHF due to left ventricular systolic dysfunction, chronic therapy in patients who develop pulmonary edema during dose initiation. **P/N:** Category B, caution in nursing.	Flushing, headache, nausea, vomiting, hypotension, anxiety, nervousness, agitation, chest pain, dizziness, bradycardia, abdominal pain.
Fenoldopam Mesylate (Corlopam)	**Inj:** 10mg/mL	***Adults:* Range: Initial:** 0.01-0.8 µg/kg/min IV. **Titrate:** Increase/decrease by 0.05-0.1µg/kg/min no more frequently than every 15 minutes. May use for up to 48 hrs. Refer to prescribing information for detailed dosing information.	**W/P:** Contains sodium metabisulfite; may cause allergic-type reactions especially in asthmatics. Caution in glaucoma or intraocular HTN. Dose-related tachycardia reported. Symptomatic hypotension may occur; monitor BP. Avoid hypotension with acute cerebral infarction or hemorrhage. Hypokalemia reported; monitor serum electrolytes. **P/N:** Category B, caution in nursing.	Headache, nausea, flushing, extrasystoles, palpitations, bradycardia, heart failure, elevated BUN/glucose/transaminase, chest pain, leukocytosis, bleeding, dyspnea.
Methyldopa/ Hydrochloro-thiazide (Aldoril 25)	**Tab: (HCTZ-Methyldopa)** 15mg-250mg, 25-250mg, 30mg-500mg	***Adults:* Initial:** 250mg-15mg tab bid-tid, 250mg-25mg tab bid, or 500mg-30mg qd. **Max:** 50mg HCTZ/day or 3g methyldopa/day.	Not for initial therapy of HTN. **W/P:** Positive Coombs test, hemolytic anemia, liver disorders, sensitivity reactions, hypokalemia, hyperuricemia, hyperglycemia, hypomagnesemia, hypercalcemia may occur. Fever reported within the 1st 3 weeks of therapy. HTN has recurred after dialysis. Caution with liver disease or dysfunction, severe renal disease. Discontinue if develop signs of heart failure, progressive renal dysfunction, or involuntary choreoathetotic movements. Edema and weight gain reported. Blood count, Coombs test and LFTs before therapy and periodically thereafter. Monitor electrolytes. May exacerbate or activate SLE. May increase cholesterol and TG levels. Enhanced effects in postsympathectomy patient. **Contra:** Active hepatic disease, anuria, sulfonamide allergy, concomitant MAOIs, history of methyldopa associated liver disorder. **P/N:** Category C, not for use in nursing.	Weakness, asthenia, headache, pancreatitis, diarrhea, vomiting, constipation, nausea, blood dyscrasias, rash, electrolyte imbalance, renal failure, impotence, vertigo.
Mecamylamine Hydrochloride (Inversine)	**Tab:** 2.5mg	***Adults:* Initial:** 2.5mg bid after meals. **Titrate:** Increase by 2.5mg/day at intervals of not less than 2 days. **Usual:** 25mg/day given tid. Give larger doses at noontime and	**W/P:** Caution with renal, cerebral, or cardiovascular dysfunction, marked cerebral or coronary insufficiency, prostatic hypertrophy, bladder neck obstruction, urethral stricture. Large doses in cerebral or renal insufficiency	Ileus, constipation, vomiting, nausea, anorexia, dryness of mouth, syncope, postural hypotension,

Table 14.1 PRESCRIBING INFORMATION FOR CARDIOVASCULAR DRUGS *(cont.)*

NAME	FORM/ STRENGTH	DOSAGE	WARNINGS/PRECAUTIONS & CONTRAINDICATIONS	ADVERSE EFFECTS†
MISCELLANEOUS *(cont.)*				
Mecamylamine Hydrochloride *(cont.)*		evening. Reduce dose by 50% with thiazides.	may produce CNS effects. Withdraw gradually and add other antihypertensives. May be potentiated by excessive heat, fever, infection, hemorrhage, pregnancy, anesthesia, surgery, vigorous exercise, other antihypertensive drugs, alcohol, salt depletion. Discontinue if paralytic ileus occurs. **Contra:** Coronary insufficiency, recent MI, uremia, glaucoma, organic pyloric stenosis, uncooperative patients, mild to moderate or labile HTN, with antibiotics or sulfonamides. Administer with great discretion in renal insufficiency. **P/N:** Category C, not for use in nursing.	convulsions, tremor, interstitial pulmonary edema, urinary retention, impotence, blurred vision.
Metyrosine (Demser)	**Cap:** 250mg	**Adults: Initial:** 250mg qid. **Titrate:** May increase by 250-500mg/day. **Max:** 4g/day. Titrate based on clinical symptoms and catecholamine excretion. **Usual:** 2-3g/day. **Preoperative Preparation:** Take 5-7 days before surgery. **Pediatrics: >12 yrs: Initial:** 250mg qid. **Titrate:** May increase by 250-500mg/day. **Max:** 4g/day. Titrate based on clinical symptoms and catecholamine excretion. **Usual:** 2-3g/day. **Preoperative Preparation:** Take 5-7 days before surgery.	**W/P:** When used preoperatively or with α-adrenergic blockers, maintain intravascular volume intra- and postoperatively to avoid hypotension and decreased perfusion. Maintain adequate water intake to achieve urine volume of ≤2000mL to prevent crystalluria. Risk of hypertensive crisis or arrhythmias during tumor manipulation. Monitor BP and ECG continuously during surgery. **P/N:** Category C, caution in nursing.	Sedation, EPS, anxiety, depression, hallucinations, disorientation, confusion, diarrhea.
Polythiazide/ Prazosin Hydrochloride (Minizide)	**Cap: (Polythia- zide-Prazosin)** 0.5mg-1mg, 0.5mg-2mg, 0.5mg-5mg	**Adults:** 1 cap bid-tid. Determine strength by individual component titration.	**Not for initial therapy of HTN. W/P:** Syncope may occur, usually after initial dose or dose increase. Excessive postural hypotensive effects. Avoid driving for 24 hrs after 1st dose or dose increase. Always start on 1mg prazosin. Caution with severe renal disease, hepatic dysfunction, or progressive liver disease. Sensitivity reactions may occur with history of allergy or bronchial asthma. May exacerbate or activate SLE. Hyperuricemia, hypokalemia or frank gout may occur. Monitor electrolytes. May manifest latent DM. Enhanced effects in the post-sympathectomy patient. May decrease serum protein-bound iodine levels. False (+) for pheochromocytoma. **Contra:** Anuria, thiazide or sulfonamide sensitivity. **P/N:** Category C, not for use in nursing.	Dizziness, headache, drowsiness, lack of energy, weakness, palpitations, nausea, blood dyscrasias, rash.
Reserpine	**Tab:** 0.1mg, 0.25mg	**Adults: HTN: Initial:** 0.5mg/day for 1-2 weeks. **Maint:** Reduce to 0.1-0.25mg/day. **Psychotic Disorders: Initial:** 0.5mg/day. **Range:** 0.1-1mg/day.	**W/P:** Caution with renal insufficiency. May cause depression; discontinue at 1st sign. Caution with history of peptic ulcer, ulcerative colitis, or gallstones. **Contra:** Active or history of mental depression, active peptic ulcer, ulcerative colitis, current electroconvulsive therapy. **P/N:** Category C, not for use in nursing.	GI effects, **dry mouth**, hypersecretion, arrhythmia, syncope, edema, dyspnea, muscle aches, dizziness, depression, nervousness, impotence, gynecomastia, rash.

CHOLESTEROL-LOWERING DRUGS

BILE ACID SEQUESTRANTS

NAME	FORM/ STRENGTH	DOSAGE	WARNINGS/PRECAUTIONS & CONTRAINDICATIONS	ADVERSE EFFECTS†
Cholestyramine (Questran, Questran Light)	**Pow:** 4g/packet [60§, 378g]; **(Light)** 4g/ scoopful [60§, 268g]	**Adults: Initial:** 1 packet or scoopful qd or bid. **Maint:** 2-4 packets or scoopfuls/day, given bid. **Titrate:** Adjust at no less than 4 week intervals. **Max:** 6 packets/day or 6 scoopfuls/day. May also give	**W/P:** May produce hyperchloremic acidosis with prolonged use. Caution in renal insufficiency, volume depletion. Chronic use may produce or worsen constipation. Avoid constipation with symptomatic CAD. May increase bleeding tendency due to	Constipation, heartburn, nausea, vomiting, abdominal pain, flatulence, diarrhea, anorexia, osteoporosis, rash, hyperchloremic

*Scored.   †Bold entries denote special dental considerations.

NAME	FORM/ STRENGTH	DOSAGE	WARNINGS/PRECAUTIONS & CONTRAINDICATIONS	ADVERSE EFFECTS†
Cholestyramine *(cont.)*		as 1-6 doses/day. Mix with fluid or highly fluid food. ***Pediatrics***: **Usual:** 240mg/kg/day of anhydrous cholestyramine resin in 2-3 divided doses. **Max:** 8g/day.	vitamin K deficiency. Serum or red cell folate reduced with chronic use. Constipation may aggravate hemorrhoids. Light formulation contains phenylalanine. Measure cholesterol during 1st few months; periodically thereafter. Measure TG periodically. **Contra:** Complete biliary obstruction. **P/N:** Category C, caution in nursing.	acidosis (children), vitamin A and D deficiency, steatorrhea, hypoprothrombinemia (vitamin K deficiency).
Colesevelam Hydrochloride (WelChol)	**Tab:** 625mg	***Adults***: 3 tabs bid or 6 tabs qd. **Max:** 7 tabs/day. Take with liquids and a meal.	**W/P:** Exclude secondary causes of hypercholesterolemia and perform a lipid profile. Monitor cholesterol and TG based on NCEP guidelines. Caution if TG levels >300mg/dL, dysphagia, swallowing disorders, GI motility disorders, major GI tract surgery, and those susceptible to vitamin K or fat soluble vitamin deficiencies. **Contra:** Bowel obstruction. **P/N:** Category B, safety not known for nursing.	Asthenia, constipation, dyspepsia, pharyngitis, myalgia.
Colestipol Hydrochloride (Colestid)	**Granules:** 5g/packet [30ˢ, 90ˢ], 5g/scoopful [300g, 500g]; **Tab:** 1g	***Adults***: **Initial:** 2g, 1 packet or 1 scoopful qd-bid. **Titrate:** Increase by 2g qd or bid at 1-2 month intervals. **Usual:** 2-16g/day **(Tab)** or 1-6 packets or scoopfuls qd or in divided doses. Always mix granules with liquid. Swallow tabs whole with plenty of liquid.	**W/P:** Exclude secondary causes of hypercholesterolemia and perform a lipid profile. May produce hyperchloremic acidosis with prolonged use. Monitor cholesterol and TG based on NCEP guidelines. May cause hypothyroidism. May interfere with normal fat absorption. Chronic use may produce or worsen constipation. Avoid constipation with symptomatic CAD. May increase bleeding tendency due to vitamin K deficiency. **P/N:** Safety in pregnancy not known, caution in nursing.	Constipation, musculoskeletal pain, headache, migraine headache, sinus headache.

Fibric Acid Derivatives

NAME	FORM/ STRENGTH	DOSAGE	WARNINGS/PRECAUTIONS & CONTRAINDICATIONS	ADVERSE EFFECTS†
Fenofibrate (Tricor, Triglide, Antara)	**Tab:** 48mg, 145mg. **Cap:** 43mg, 130mg	***Adults***: **Hypercholesterolemia/ Mixed Dyslipidemia: Initial:** 145mg qd. **Hypertriglyceridemia: Initial:** 48-145mg/day. **Titrate:** Adjust if needed after repeat lipid levels at 4-8 week intervals. **Max:** 145mg/day. **Renal Dysfunction/Elderly: Initial:** 48mg/day. Take without regards to meals. **Hypercholesterolemia/ Mixed Dyslipidemia: Initial:** 130mg qd. **Hypertriglyceridemia: Initial:** 43-130mg/day. **Titrate:** Adjust if needed after repeat lipid levels at 4-8 week intervals. **Max:** 130mg/day. **Renal Dysfunction/Elderly: Initial:** 43mg/day. Take with meals.	**W/P:** Monitor LFTs regularly; discontinue if >3X ULN. May cause cholelithiasis; discontinue if gallstones found. Discontinue if myopathy or marked CPK elevation occurs. Decreased Hgb, Hct, WBCs, thrombocytopenia, and agranulocytosis reported; monitor CBCs during first 12 months of therapy. Acute hypersensitivity reactions (rare) and pancreatitis reported. Monitor lipids periodically initially, discontinue if inadequate response after 2 months on 145mg/day. Minimize dose in severe renal impairment. Caution in elderly. **Contra:** Pre-existing gallbladder disease, unexplained persistent hepatic function abnormality, hepatic or severe renal dysfunction (including primary biliary cirrhosis). **P/N:** Category C, not for use in nursing.	Abdominal pain, back pain, headache, abnormal LFTs, respiratory disorder, increased creatinine phosphokinase. Increased SGPT/SGOT.
Gemfibrozil (Lopid)	**Tab:** 600mg*	***Adults***: 600mg bid. Give 30 minutes before morning and evening meals.	**W/P:** Abnormal LFTs reported; monitor periodically. Only use if indicated and discontinue if significant lipid response not obtained. Associated with myositis. Discontinue if suspect or diagnose myositis, if abnormal LFTs persists, or develop gallstones. Cholelithiasis reported. Monitor blood counts periodically during first 12 months. May worsen renal insufficiency. **Contra:** Hepatic or severe renal dysfunction, including primary biliary cirrhosis; pre-existing gallbladder disease, concomitant cerivastatin. **P/N:** Category C, not for use in nursing.	Dyspepsia, abdominal pain, diarrhea, fatigue, bacterial and viral infections, musculoskeletal symptoms, abnormal LFTs, hematologic changes, hypesthesia, paresthesia, **taste perversion**.

Table 14.1 PRESCRIBING INFORMATION FOR CARDIOVASCULAR DRUGS (cont.)

NAME	FORM/ STRENGTH	DOSAGE	WARNINGS/PRECAUTIONS & CONTRAINDICATIONS	ADVERSE EFFECTS†
HMG-CoA Reductase Inhibitors				
Atorvastatin Calcium (Lipitor)	**Tab:** 10mg, 20mg, 40mg, 80mg	*Adults:* **Hypercholesterolemia/ Mixed Dyslipidemia: Initial:** 10-20mg qd (or 40mg qd for LDL-C reduction >45%). **Titrate:** Adjust dose if needed at 2-4 week intervals. **Usual:** 10-80mg qd. **Homozygous Familial Hypercholesterolemia:** 10-80mg qd. *Pediatrics:* **Heterozygous Familial Hypercholesterolemia: 10-17 yrs (postmenarchal): Initial:** 10mg/day. **Titrate:** Adjust dose if needed at intervals of ≤4 weeks. **Max:** 20mg/day.	**W/P:** Monitor LFTs prior to therapy, at 12 weeks or with dose elevation, and periodically thereafter. Reduce dose or withdraw if AST or ALT >3X ULN persist. Caution with heavy alcohol use and/or history of hepatic disease. Discontinue if markedly elevated CPK levels occur, if myopathy is diagnosed or suspected, or if predisposition to renal failure secondary to rhabdomyolysis. **Contra:** Active liver disease, unexplained persistent elevations of serum transaminases, pregnancy, nursing mothers. **P/N:** Category X, not for use in nursing.	Constipation, flatulence, dyspepsia, abdominal pain.
Fluvastatin Sodium (Lescol, Lescol XL)	**Cap:** 20mg, 40mg; **Tab, Extended Release:** 80mg	*Adults:* ≥18 yrs: (For LDL-C reduction of <25%) **Initial:** 20mg cap qpm. (For LDL-C reduction of ≥25%) **Initial:** 40mg cap qpm or 80mg XL tab qpm (or 40mg cap bid). **Usual:** 20-80mg/day. **Severe Renal Impairment:** Caution with dose >40mg/day. Take 2 hrs after bile-acid resins qhs.	**W/P:** Monitor LFTs prior to therapy, at 12 weeks or with dose elevation. Discontinue if AST or ALT >3X ULN on 2 consecutive occasions. Risk of myopathy and/or rhabdomyolysis reported. Discontinue if markedly elevated CPK levels occur, if myopathy is diagnosed or suspected, or if predisposition to renal failure secondary to rhabdomyolysis. Less effective with homozygous familial hypercholesterolemia. Caution with heavy alcohol use and/or history of hepatic disease. Evaluate if develop endocrine dysfunction. **Contra:** Active liver disease, unexplained persistent elevations of serum transaminases, pregnancy, nursing mothers. **P/N:** Category X, not for use in nursing.	Dyspepsia, abdominal pain, headache, nausea, diarrhea, abnormal LFTs, myalgia, flu-like symptoms.
Lovastatin (Altoprev, Mevacor)	**Tab, ER:** 10mg, 20mg, 40mg, 60mg; **(Mevacor) Tab:** 20mg, 40mg	*Adults:* **Initial:** 20, 40, or 60mg qhs. Consider 10mg/day in patients requiring smaller reductions. May adjust at intervals of >4 weeks. Concomitant **Cyclosporine: Initial:** 10mg/day. **Max:** 20mg/day. **Concomitant Fibrates/Niacin (≥1g/day):** Try to avoid. **Max:** 20mg/day. Concomitant **Amiodarone/ Verapamil: Max:** 40mg/day. **CrCl ≥30mL/min:** Consider dose increase of >20mg/day carefully and implement cautiously. Swallow whole; do not chew or crush.	**W/P:** May increase serum transaminases and CPK levels; consider in differential diagnosis of chest pain. Discontinue if AST or ALT >3X ULN persist, if myopathy diagnosed or suspected, and a few days before major surgery. Monitor LFTs prior to therapy, at 6 weeks, 12 weeks, then periodically or with dose elevation. Caution with heavy alcohol use and/or history of hepatic disease. Caution with dose escalation in renal insufficiency. Lovastatin immediate-release found to be less effective with homozygous familial hypercholesterolemia. Rhabdomyolysis (rare), myopathy reported. **Contra:** Active liver disease, unexplained persistent elevations of serum transaminases, pregnancy, nursing mothers. **P/N:** Category X, not for use in nursing.	Nausea, abdominal pain, insomnia, dyspepsia, headache, asthenia, myalgia.
Pravastatin Sodium (Pravachol)	**Tab:** 10mg, 20mg, 40mg, 80mg	*Adults:* ≥18 yrs: **Initial:** 40mg qd. Perform lipid tests within 4 weeks and adjust according to response and guidelines. **Titrate:** May increase to 80mg qd if needed. **Significant Renal/Hepatic Dysfunction: Initial:** 10mg qd. **Concomitant Immunosuppressives: Initial:** 10mg qd. **Max:** 20mg/day. *Pediatrics:* **Heterozygous Familial Hypercholesterolemia: 14-18 yrs: Initial:** 40mg qd. **8-13 yrs:** 20mg qd. **Concomitant Immunosuppressives: Initial:** 10mg qhs. **Max:** 20mg/day.	**W/P:** Perform LFTs before therapy, before dose increases, and if clinically indicated. Risk of myopathy, myalgia, and rhabdomyolysis. Discontinue if AST or ALT >3X ULN persists, if elevated CPK levels occur, or if myopathy diagnosed or suspected. Less effective with homozygous familial hypercholesterolemia. Monitor for endocrine dysfunction. Closely monitor with heavy alcohol use, recent history or signs of hepatic disease, or renal dysfunction. **Contra:** Active liver disease, unexplained persistent elevations of LFTs, pregnancy, nursing mothers. **P/N:** Category X, not for use in nursing.	Rash, nausea, vomiting, diarrhea, headache, chest pain, influenza, abdominal pain, dizziness, increases ALT, AST, CPK.

*Scored.   †Bold entries denote special dental considerations.

NAME	FORM/ STRENGTH	DOSAGE	WARNINGS/PRECAUTIONS & CONTRAINDICATIONS	ADVERSE EFFECTS†
Rosuvastatin Calcium (Crestor)	Tab: 5mg, 10mg, 20mg, 40mg	*Adults:* **Hypercholesterolemia/ Mixed Dyslipidemia: Initial:** 10mg qd (or 5mg qd for less aggressive LDL-C reductions; 20mg qd with LDL-C >190mg/dL). **Titrate:** Adjust dose if needed at 2-4 week intervals. **Range:** 5-40mg qd. **Homozygous Familial Hypercholesterolemia:** 20mg qd. **Max:** 40mg qd. **Concomitant Cyclosporine: Max:** 5mg qd. **Concomitant Gemfibrozil: Max:** 10mg qd. **Severe Renal Impairment: CrCl <30mL/min (not on hemodialysis): Initial:** 5mg qd. **Max:** 10mg qd.	**W/P:** Rare cases of rhabdomyolysis with acute renal failure secondary to myoglobinuria have been reported. Monitor LFTs prior to therapy, at 12 weeks or with dose elevation, and periodically thereafter. Reduce dose or withdraw if AST or ALT >3X ULN persist. Caution with heavy alcohol use, history of hepatic disease, renal impairment, hypothyroidism, elderly. Discontinue if markedly elevated CPK levels occur, if myopathy is diagnosed or suspected, or if predisposition to renal failure secondary to rhabdomyolysis. Approximately 2-fold elevation in median exposure in Asian subjects. **Contra:** Active liver disease, unexplained persistent elevations of serum transaminases, pregnancy, nursing mothers. **P/N:** Category X, not for use in nursing.	**Pharyngitis**, headache, diarrhea, dyspepsia, nausea.
Simvastatin (Zocor)	Tab: 5mg, 10mg, 20mg, 40mg, 80mg	*Adults:* **Initial:** 20-40mg qpm. **Usual:** 5-80mg/day. **Titrate:** Adjust at ≥4-week intervals. **High Risk for CHD Events: Initial:** 40mg/day. **Homozygous Familial Hypercholesterolemia:** 40mg qpm or 80mg/day given as 20mg bid plus 40mg qpm. **Concomitant Cyclosporine: Initial:** 5mg/day. **Max:** 10mg/day. **Concomitant Gemfibrozil (try to avoid): Max:** 10mg/day. **Concomitant Amiodarone/Verapamil: Max:** 20mg/day. **Severe Renal Insufficiency:** 5mg/day; monitor closely. *Pediatrics:* **Heterozygous Familial Hypercholesterolemia: 10-17 yrs (at least 1yr postmenarchal): Initial:** 10mg qpm. **Usual:** 10-40mg/day. **Titrate:** Adjust at ≥4-week intervals. **Max:** 40mg/day.	**W/P:** Caution with heavy alcohol use, severe renal insufficiency or history of hepatic disease. Monitor LFTs prior to therapy, periodically thereafter for 1st year, or until 1 year after last dose elevation (additional test at 3 months for 80mg dose). Discontinue if AST or ALT >3X ULN persist, if myopathy is suspected or diagnosed, a few days prior to major surgery. Rhabdomyolysis (rare), myopathy reported. **Contra:** Active liver disease, unexplained persistent elevations of serum transaminases, pregnancy, nursing mothers. **P/N:** Category X, not for use in nursing.	Abdominal pain, headache, CK and transaminase elevations.

MISCELLANEOUS CHOLESTEROL-LOWERING DRUGS

NAME	FORM/ STRENGTH	DOSAGE	WARNINGS/PRECAUTIONS & CONTRAINDICATIONS	ADVERSE EFFECTS†
Ezetimibe (Zetia)	Tab: 10mg	*Adults:* 10mg qd. May give with statin for incremental effect. **Concomitant Bile Sequestrant:** Give either ≥2 hrs before or ≥4 hrs after bile acid sequestrant.	**W/P:** Monitor LFTs with concurrent statin therapy. Not recommended with moderate or severe hepatic insufficiency. **Contra:** When used with a statin, refer to the HMG-CoA reductase inhibitor monographs. **P/N:** Category C, contraindicated in nursing.	Back pain, arthralgia, diarrhea, sinusitis, abdominal pain, myalgia.
Ezetimibe/ Simvastatin (Vytorin)	Tab: (ezetimibe-simvastatin) 10mg/10mg, 10mg/20mg, 10mg/40mg, 10mg/80mg	*Adults:* Take once daily in the evening. **Initial:** 10mg/20mg qd. **Less aggressive LDL-C reductions:** 10mg/10mg qd. **LDL-C reduction >55%: initial:** 10mg/40mg qd. **Titrate:** Adjust at ≥2 weeks. **Homozygous Familial Hypercholesterolemia:** 10mg/40mg or 10mg/80mg qd. **Severe Renal Insufficiency:** Avoid unless tolerant of ≥5mg of simvastatin; monitor closely. **Concomitant Bile Acid Sequestrant:** Take either ≥2 hours before or ≥4 hours after bile acid sequestrant. **Concomitant Cyclosporine:** Avoid unless tolerant of ≥5mg of simvastatin. **Max:** 10mg/10mg/ day. **Concomitant Amiodarone/Verapamil: Max:** 10mg/20mg/day.	**W/P:** Rhabdomyolysis (rare), myopathy reported. Discontinue therapy if myopathy is suspected or diagnosed, if AST or ALT >3X ULN persist, a few days prior to major surgery or when any major medical or surgical condition supervenes. Monitor LFTs prior to therapy and thereafter when clinically indicated. With 10mg/80mg dose, monitor LFTs prior to titration, 3 months after titration and periodically thereafter for the first year. Caution with heavy alcohol use, severe renal insufficiency, or history of hepatic disease. Avoid use in moderate or severe hepatic insufficiency. **Contra:** Active liver disease, unexplained persistent elevations in serum transaminases, pregnancy, lactation. **P/N:** Category X, not for use in nursing.	Headache, upper respiratory tract infection, myalgia, CK and transaminase elevations.

Table 14.1 PRESCRIBING INFORMATION FOR CARDIOVASCULAR DRUGS *(cont.)*

NAME	FORM/ STRENGTH	DOSAGE	WARNINGS/PRECAUTIONS & CONTRAINDICATIONS	ADVERSE EFFECTS†
MISCELLANEOUS CHOLESTEROL-LOWERING DRUGS *(cont.)*				
Lovastatin/ Niacin (Advicor)	**Tab: (Niacin Extended Release-Lovastatin)** 500mg-20mg, 750mg-20mg, 1000mg-20mg	***Adults:*** ≥18 yrs: **Initial:** 500mg-20mg qhs. **Titrate:** Increase by no more than 500mg of niacin every 4 weeks. **Max:** 2000mg-40mg. Concomitant **Cyclosporine/Fibrates: Max:** 1000mg-20mg. Swallow tab whole. Take with low-fat snack.	**W/P:** Do not substitute for equivalent dose of immediate-release niacin. Myopathy, rhabdomyolysis, severe hepatotoxicity reported. Caution with history of liver disease or jaundice, heavy alcohol use, hepatobilliary disease, peptic ulcer, diabetes, unstable angina, acute phase of MI, gout, renal dysfunction. Monitor LFTs prior to therapy, every 6-12 weeks for 1st 6 months, and periodically thereafter. May elevate PT, uric acid levels. Discontinue if AST or ALT ≥3X ULN persist, if myopathy diagnosed or suspected, and a few days before surgery. May reduce phosphorous levels. **Contra:** Active liver disease, unexplained persistent elevations in serum transaminases, active PUD, arterial bleeding, pregnancy, nursing mothers. **P/N:** Category X, not for use in nursing.	Flushing, asthenia, flu syndrome, headache, infection, pain, GI effects, hyperglycemia, pruritus, rash.
Niacin (Niaspan, Niacor)	**Tab, Extended Release:** 500mg, 750mg, 1000mg	***Adults:*** Take qhs after low-fat snack. **Initial:** 500mg qhs. **Titrate:** Increase by 500mg every 4 weeks. **Maint:** 1-2g qhs. **Max:** 2g/day. Take ASA or NSAIDs 30 minutes before to reduce flushing. Do not chew, crush, or break; swallow whole. Women may respond to lower doses than men.	**W/P:** Do not substitute with equivalent doses of immediate-release niacin (severe hepatic toxicity may occur). Associated with abnormal LFTs; monitor LFTs before therapy, every 6-12 weeks during 1st year, then periodically thereafter. Discontinue if LFTs ≥3X ULN persists or develop signs of hepatotoxicity. Monitor for rhabdomyolysis. Observe closely with history of jaundice, hepatobiliary disease, and peptic ulcer; monitor LFTs and blood glucose frequently. Dose-related rise in glucose tolerance in diabetics. Caution with history of hepatic disease, heavy alcohol use, renal dysfunction, unstable angina, and acute phase of MI. Elevated uric acid levels reported. May reduce platelet and phosphorous levels. **Contra:** Unexplained or significant hepatic dysfunction, active peptic ulcer disease, arterial bleeding. **P/N:** Category C, not for use in nursing.	Flushing episodes (eg, warmth, redness, itching, tingling), dizziness, tachycardia, shortness of breath, sweating, chills, edema.
DIURETICS				
CARBONIC ANHYDRASE INHIBITORS				
Acetazolamide (Diamoz Sequels)	**Cap, Extended Release:** 500mg	***Adults:*** **Glaucoma:** 500mg bid. **Acute Mountain Sickness:** 500mg-1g/day in divided doses; 1g for rapid ascent. Initiate 24-48 hrs before ascent and continue for 48 hrs while at high altitude or longer as needed.	**W/P:** Rare reports of fatal sulfonamide hypersensitivity reactions (eg, Stevens-Johnson syndrome, toxic epidermal necrolysis, fulminant hepatic necrosis, anaphylaxis, agranulocytosis, aplastic anemia, other blood dyscrasias) have occurred. Discontinue drug if this occurs. Sensitizations may recur despite route of administration. A dose increase does not increase diuresis and may result in a decrease in diuresis and increased drowsiness. Use with caution if patient is predisposed to acid/base imbalances (elderly with renal impairment), diabetes mellitus, or impaired alveolar ventilation. Monitor serum electrolytes. Obtain CBC and platelet count before therapy and at regular intervals during therapy. **Contra:** In sodium or potassium depleted patients, marked hepatic or kidney impairment, cirrhosis, suprarenal gland failure, hyperchloremic acidosis, (with long-term therapy) chronic noncongestive angle-closure glaucoma. **P/N:** Category C, not for use in nursing.	Paresthesia, hearing dysfunction, tinnitus, loss of appetite, **taste alteration,** GI disturbances, polyuria, drowsiness, confusion, metabolic acidosis, electrolyte imbalance, transient myopia.

*Scored.   †Bold entries denote special dental considerations.

NAME	FORM/ STRENGTH	DOSAGE	WARNINGS/PRECAUTIONS & CONTRAINDICATIONS	ADVERSE EFFECTS†
Methazolamide (Neptazane)	**Tab:** 25mg, 50mg	**Adults:** 50-100mg bid-tid.	**W/P:** Caution with concomitant high dose aspirin, concomitant steroid therapy, hepatic insufficiency, pulmonary obstruction or emphysema (impaired alveolar ventilation). Increased dose does not increase and may decrease diuresis, yet may increase drowsiness and/or paresthesia. **Contra:** Adrenal gland failure, cirrhosis (use may precipitate development of hepatic encephalopathy), hyperchloremic acidosis, hyponatremia/hypokalemia, marked renal or hepatic impairment, angle-closure glaucoma (long-term use). **P/N:** Category C, not for use in nursing.	Fatigue, malaise, paresthesia, diarrhea, loss of appetite, **metallic taste,** nausea, vomiting.

LOOP DIURETICS

NAME	FORM/ STRENGTH	DOSAGE	WARNINGS/PRECAUTIONS & CONTRAINDICATIONS	ADVERSE EFFECTS†
Bumetanide (Bumex)	**Inj:** 0.25mg/mL; **Tab:** 0.5mg*, 1mg*, 2mg*	**Adults:** ≥18 yrs: **PO:** Usual: 0.5-2mg qd. **Maint:** May give every other day or every 3-4 days. **Max:** 10mg/day. **IV/IM:** Initial: 0.5-1mg over 1-2 minutes, may repeat every 2-3 hrs for 2-3 doses. **Max:** 10mg/day. **Elderly:** Start at low end of dosing range.	**Can lead to profound water and electrolyte depletion with excessive use. W/P:** Monitor for volume/electrolyte depletion, hypokalemia, blood dyscrasias, hepatic damage. Elderly are prone to volume/electrolyte depletion. Caution in elderly, hepatic cirrhosis and ascites. Associated with ototoxicity, hypocalcemia, thrombocytopenia, hypomagnesemia, hypokalemia, and hyperuricemia. Hypersensitivity with sulfonamide allergy. Discontinue if marked increase in BUN or creatinine or if develop oliguria with progressive renal disease. **Contra:** Anuria, hepatic coma, severe electrolyte depletion. **P/N:** Category C, not for use in nursing.	Muscle cramps, dizziness, hypotension, headache, nausea, hyperuricemia, hypokalemia, hyponatremia, hyperglycemia, azotemia, increase serum creatinine.
Ethacrynate Sodium (Edecrin, Edecrin Sodium)	**(Edecrin) Inj:** 50mg; **(Edecrin Sodium) Tab:** 25mg*, 50mg*	**(Edecrin) Adults:** 50mg or 0.5-1mg/kg IV single dose. May give 2nd dose if necessary. **(Edecrin Sodium) Adults:** Initial: 50-100mg qd. **Titrate:** 25-50mg increments. **Usual:** 50-200mg/day. After diuresis achieved, give smallest effective dose continuously or intermittently. **Pediatrics:** Initial: 25mg. **Titrate:** Increase by 25mg increments. **Maint:** Reduce dose and frequency once dry weight achieved; may give intermittently.	**W/P:** Caution in advanced liver cirrhosis. Monitor serum electrolytes, CO_2, BUN early in therapy and periodically during active diuresis. Vigorous diuresis may induce acute hypotensive episode and in elderly cardiac patients, hemoconcentration resulting in thromboembolic disorders. Ototoxicity reported with severe renal dysfunction. Hypomagnesemia and transient increase in serum urea nitrogen may occur. Reduce dose or withdraw if excessive electrolyte loss occurs. Initiate therapy in the hospital for cirrhotic patients with ascites. Liberalize salt intake and supplement with K+ if needed. Reduced responsiveness in renal edema with hypoproteinemia; use salt poor albumin. **Contra:** Anuria, infants. Discontinue if increasing electrolyte imbalance, azotemia, or oliguria develops during treatment of severe, progressive renal disease. Discontinue if severe, watery diarrhea occurs. **P/N:** Category B, not for use in nursing.	Anorexia, malaise, abdominal discomfort, gout, deafness, tinnitus, vertigo, headache, fatigue, rash, chills.
Furosemide (Lasix)	**Inj:** 10mg/mL; **Sol:** 10mg/mL, 40mg/5mL; **Tab:** 20mg, 40mg*, 80mg	**Adults: (PO) HTN: Initial:** 40mg bid. **Edema: Initial:** 20-80mg PO. May repeat or increase by 20-40mg after 6-8 hrs. **Max:** 600mg/day. **Alternative Regimen:** Dose on 2-4 consecutive days each week. Closely monitor if on >80mg/day. **(Inj) Edema: Initial:** 20-40mg IV/IM. May repeat or increase by 20mg after 2 hrs. **Acute Pulmonary Edema: Initial:** 40mg IV. May increase to 80mg IV after 1 hr.	**Can lead to profound water and electrolyte depletion with excessive use. W/P:** Monitor for fluid/electrolyte imbalance (eg, hypokalemia), renal or hepatic dysfunction. Initiate in hospital with hepatic cirrhosis and ascites. Tinnitus, hearing impairment, hyperglycemia, hyperuricemia reported. May activate SLE. Cross-sensitivity with sulfonamide allergy. Avoid excessive diuresis, especially in elderly. **Contra:** Anuria. **P/N:** Category C, caution in nursing.	Pancreatitis, jaundice, anorexia, paresthesias, ototoxicity, blood dyscrasias, dizziness, rash, urticaria, photosensitivity, fever, thrombophlebitis, restlessness.

Table 14.1 PRESCRIBING INFORMATION FOR CARDIOVASCULAR DRUGS *(cont.)*

NAME	FORM/ STRENGTH	DOSAGE	WARNINGS/PRECAUTIONS & CONTRAINDICATIONS	ADVERSE EFFECTS†
LOOP DIURETICS *(cont.)*				
Furosemide *(cont.)*		***Pediatrics:* Edema: (PO) Initial:** 2mg/kg single dose. May increase by 1-2mg/kg after 6-8 hrs. **Max:** 6mg/kg. **(Inj) Initial:** 1mg/kg IV/IM single dose. May increase by 1mg/kg IV/IM after 2 hrs. **Max:** 6mg/kg.		
Torsemide (Demadex)	**Inj:** 10mg/mL; **Tab:** 5mg*, 10mg*, 20mg*, 100mg*	***Adults:* PO/IV (bolus over 2 minutes or continuous): CHF: Initial:** 10-20mg qd. **Max:** 200mg single dose. **Chronic Renal Failure: Initial:** 20mg qd. **Max:** 200mg single dose. **Hepatic Cirrhosis: Initial:** 5-10mg qd with aldosterone antagonist or K+ sparing diuretic. **Titrate:** Double dose. **Max:** 40mg single dose. **HTN: Initial:** 5mg qd. **Titrate:** May increase to 10mg qd in 4-6 weeks, then may add additional antihypertensive agent.	**W/P:** Caution with cirrhosis and ascites in hepatic disease. Tinnitus and hearing loss (usually reversible) reported. Avoid excessive diuresis, especially in elderly. Caution with brisk diuresis, inadequate oral intake of electrolytes, and cardiovascular disease, especially with digitalis glycosides. Monitor for electrolyte/volume depletion. Hyperglycemia, hypokalemia, hypermagnesemia, hypercalcemia, gout reported. May increase cholesterol and TG. **Contra:** Anuria, sulfonamide hypersensitivity. **P/N:** Category B, caution in nursing.	Headache, excessive urination, dizziness, cough, ECG abnormality, asthenia, rhinitis, diarrhea.
POTASSIUM-SPARING DIURETICS				
Amiloride Hydrochloride (Midamor)	**Tab:** 5mg	***Adults:* Initial:** 5mg qd. **Titrate:** Increase to 10mg/day. If hyperkalemia persists, may increase to 15mg/day then to 20mg/day with careful monitoring. Take with food.	**W/P:** Risk of hyperkalemia (>5.5 mEq/L) especially with renal impairment, elderly, DM; monitor levels frequently. Discontinue if hyperkalemia occurs. Caution in severely ill in whom respiratory or metabolic acidosis may occur; monitor acid-base balance frequently. Hepatic encephalopathy reported with severe hepatic disease. Increased BUN reported. Discontinue at least 3 days before glucose tolerance test. Monitor electrolytes and renal function in DM. **Contra:** Hyperkalemia, anuria, acute or chronic renal insufficiency, diabetic neuropathy, K+-sparing agents (eg, diuretics), and K+ supplements, K+ salt substitutes, K+-rich diet (except with severe hypokalemia). **P/N:** Category B, not for use in nursing.	Headache, nausea, anorexia, vomiting, elevated serum potassium, diarrhea.
Spironolactone (Aldactone)	**Tab:** 25mg, 50mg*, 100mg*	***Adults:* Hyperaldosteronism: (Diagnostic)** 400mg/day for 3-4 weeks or 400mg/day for 4 days. **(Preoperative)** 100-400mg/day. **Maint:** Lowest effective dose. **Edema: Initial:** 100mg/day given qd or in divided doses for at least 5 days. **Maint:** 25-200mg/day given qd-bid. **HTN: Initial:** 50-100mg/day given qd or in divided doses. **Titrate:** Adjust at 2 week intervals. **Hypokalemia:** 25-100mg/day.	**Tumorigenic in chronic toxicity animal studies; avoid unnecessary use. W/P:** Monitor for fluid/electrolyte imbalance. Caution with renal and hepatic dysfunction. Hyperchloremic metabolic acidosis reported with decompensated hepatic cirrhosis. Mild acidosis, gynecomastia, transient BUN elevation may occur. Discontinue and monitor ECG if hyperkalemia occurs. Risk of dilutional hyponatremia. **Contra:** Anuria, acute renal insufficiency, significantly impaired renal excretory function, hyperkalemia. **P/N:** Category C, not for use in nursing.	Gastric bleeding, ulceration, gynecomastia, impotence, agranulocytosis, fever, urticaria, confusion, ataxia, renal dysfunction.
Triamterene (Dyrenium)	**Cap:** 50mg, 100mg	***Adults:* Initial:** 100mg bid pc. **Max:** 300mg/day.	**W/P:** Risk of hyperkalemia (≥5.5mEq/L) especially with renal impairment, elderly, DM or severely ill; monitor levels frequently. Check ECG if hyperkalemia occurs. May cause decreased alkali reserve with possibility of metabolic acidosis, mild nitrogen retention. Monitor BUN periodically. May contribute to megaloblastosis in folic acid deficiency. Caution with gouty arthritis; may elevate uric acid levels. May aggravate or cause electrolyte imbalances in CHF, renal	Hypersensitivity reactions, hyper- or hypokalemia, azotemia, renal stones, jaundice, nausea, vomiting, diarrhea, weakness, dizziness.

*Scored. †Bold entries denote special dental considerations.

NAME	FORM/ STRENGTH	DOSAGE	WARNINGS/PRECAUTIONS & CONTRAINDICATIONS	ADVERSE EFFECTS†
Triamterene *(cont.)*			disease, or cirrhosis. Caution with history of renal stones. **Contra:** Anuria, severe or progressive kidney disease or dysfunction (except with nephrosis), severe hepatic disease, hyperkalemia, K+ supplements, K+ salt substitutes, K+-sparing agents (eg, diuretics). **P/N:** Category C, not for use in nursing.	

THIAZIDE DIURETICS

NAME	FORM/ STRENGTH	DOSAGE	WARNINGS/PRECAUTIONS & CONTRAINDICATIONS	ADVERSE EFFECTS†
Chlorothiazide (Diuril)	**Inj:** 0.5g; **Sus:** 250mg/5mL [237mL]; **Tab:** 250mg*, 500mg*	*Adults:* **(PO/IV) Edema:** 0.5-1g qd-bid. May give every other day or 3-5 days/week. Substitute IV for oral using same dosage. **(PO) HTN:** 0.5-1g qd or in divided doses. **Max:** 2g/day. *Pediatrics:* **(PO) Diuresis/HTN: Usual:** 10-20mg/kg/ day given qd-bid. **Max: Infants ≤2 yrs:** 375mg/day. **2-12 yrs:** 1g/day. **<6 months:** Up to 15mg/kg bid may be required.	**W/P:** Caution in severe renal disease, liver dysfunction, electrolyte/fluid imbalance. Monitor electrolytes. Hyperuricemia, hyperglycemia, hypokalemia, hyponatremia, hypomagnesemia, hypercalcemia may occur. Increases in cholesterol and triglyceride levels reported. May exacerbate SLE. Sensitivity reactions reported. Discontinue prior to parathyroid test. Enhanced effects in post-sympathectomy patient. IV use not recommended in infants or children. **Contra:** Anuria, sulfonamide hypersensitivity. **P/N:** Category C, not for use in nursing.	Weakness, hypotension, pancreatitis, jaundice, diarrhea, vomiting, blood dyscrasias, rash, photosensitivity, electrolyte imbalance, impotence.
Chlorthalidone (Thalitone)	**Tab:** 15mg	*Adults:* **HTN: Initial:** 15mg qd. **Titrate:** May increase to 30mg qd, then to 45-50mg qd. **Edema: Initial:** 30-60mg/day or 60mg every other day, up to 90-120mg/day. **Maint:** May be lower than initial; adjust to patient. Take in the morning with food.	**W/P:** Caution in severe renal disease, liver dysfunction, allergy history, asthma. May exacerbate or activate SLE. Monitor for fluid and electrolyte imbalance. Hyperuricemia, hypomagnesemia, hypokalemia, hypercalcemia, hypophosphatemia, and hyperglycemia may occur. May manifest latent DM. **Contra:** Anuria, sulfonamide hypersensitivity. **P/N:** Category B, not for use in nursing.	Pancreatitis, jaundice, diarrhea, vomiting, constipation, nausea, blood dyscrasias, rash, photosensitivity, electrolyte disturbance, impotence.
Hydrochloro- thiazide (Microzide)	**Cap:** 12.5mg	*Adults:* **Initial:** 12.5mg qd. **Max:** 50mg/day.	**W/P:** Caution in severe renal disease, liver dysfunction, electrolyte/fluid imbalance. Monitor electrolytes. Hyperuricemia, hyperglycemia, hypokalemia, hyponatremia, hypomagnesemia, hypercalcemia may occur. Increases in cholesterol and triglyceride levels reported. May exacerbate SLE. Sensitivity reactions reported. Discontinue prior to parathyroid test. Enhanced effects in post-sympathectomy patient. **Contra:** Anuria, sulfonamide hypersensitivity. **P/N:** Category B, not for use in nursing.	Weakness, hypotension, pancreatitis, jaundice, diarrhea, vomiting, blood dyscrasias, rash, photosensitivity, electrolyte imbalance, impotence.
Indapamide (Lozol)	**Tab:** 1.25mg	*Adults:* **HTN:** 1.25mg qam. **Titrate:** May increase to 2.5mg qd after 4 weeks, then to 5mg qd after another 4 weeks. **Max:** 5mg/day. **CHF:** 2.5mg qam. **Titrate:** May increase to 5mg qd after 1 week. **Max:** 5mg/day.	**W/P:** Caution in severe renal disease, liver dysfunction. May exacerbate or activate SLE. Monitor for fluid/electrolyte imbalance. Hyperuricemia, hypercalcemia, hypokalemia, hypophosphatemia, and hyperglycemia may occur. Monitor renal function, serum uric acid levels periodically. May precipitate gout. May manifest latent DM. Enhanced effects in post-sympathectomy patient. **Contra:** Anuria, sulfonamide hypersensitivity. **P/N:** Category B, not for use in nursing.	Headache, infection, pain, back pain, dizziness, rhinitis, fatigue, muscle cramps, nervousness, numbness of extremities, electrolyte imbalance, anxiety, agitation.
Metolazone (Zaroxolyn)	**Tab:** 2.5mg, 5mg, 10mg	*Adults:* **Edema:** 5-20mg qd. **HTN:** 2.5-5mg qd. **Elderly:** Start at low end of dosing range.	**Do not interchange rapid and complete bioavailability metolazone formulations for other slow and incomplete bioavailability metolazone formulations; they are not therapeutically equivalent. W/P:** Risk of hypokalemia, orthostatic hypotension, hypercalcemia, hyperuricemia, azotemia and rapid onset hyponatremia. Cross-allergy with sulfonamide-derived drugs, thiazides,	Chest pain/discomfort, orthostatic hypotension, syncope, neuropathy, necrotizing angiitis, hepatitis,

Table 14.1 PRESCRIBING INFORMATION FOR CARDIOVASCULAR DRUGS *(cont.)*

NAME	FORM/ STRENGTH	DOSAGE	WARNINGS/PRECAUTIONS & CONTRAINDICATIONS	ADVERSE EFFECTS†
THIAZIDE DIURETICS *(cont.)*				
Metolazone *(cont.)*			or quinethazone. Sensitivity reactions may occur with 1st dose. Monitor electrolytes. May cause hyperglycemia and glycosuria in diabetics. Caution in elderly or severe renal impairment. May exacerbate or activate SLE. **Contra:** Anuria, hepatic coma or precoma. **P/N:** Category B, not for use in nursing.	jaundice, pancreatitis, blood dyscrasias, joint pain.
COMBINATIONS				
Amiloride Hydrochloride/ Hydrochloro- thiazide (Moduretic 5-50)	**Tab: (Amiloride-HCTZ)** 5mg-50mg*	**Adults: Initial:** 1 tab qd. **Titrate:** May increase to 2 tabs qd or in divided doses. **Max:** 2 tabs/day. May give intermittently once diuresis is achieved. Take with food.	**W/P:** Risk of hyperkalemia (≥5.5mEq/L) especially with renal impairment or DM; discontinue if hyperkalemia occurs. Monitor for fluid/electrolyte imbalance. Caution in severely ill (risk of respiratory or metabolic acidosis). Increases BUN, cholesterol, and TG levels. Discontinue at least 3 days before glucose tolerance test. May precipitate gout or exacerbate SLE. **Contra:** Hyperkalemia, anuria, sulfonamide hypersensitivity, acute or chronic renal insufficiency, diabetic neuropathy. Concomitant K⁺-sparing agents (eg, spironolactone, triamterene), K⁺ supplements, salt substitutes, K⁺- rich diet (except with severe hypokalemia). **P/N:** Category B, not for use in nursing.	Nausea, anorexia, rash, headache, weakness, hyperkalemia, dizziness.
Hydrochloro- thiazide/ Spironolactone (Aldactazide)	**Tab: (Spirono-lactone-HCTZ)** 25mg-25mg, 50mg-50mg*	**Adults: Edema:** 100mg/day per component qd or in divided doses. **Maint:** 25-200mg/day per component. **HTN:** 50-100mg/day per component qd or in divided doses.	**Tumorigenic in chronic toxicity animal studies; avoid unnecessary use. Not for initial therapy. W/P:** Monitor for fluid/ electrolyte imbalance. Caution with renal and hepatic dysfunction. Hyperchloremic metabolic acidosis reported with decompensated hepatic cirrhosis. Mild acidosis, gynecomastia, transient BUN elevation, hypercalcemia, hyperglycemia, hyperuricemia, hypomagnesemia, and sensitivity reactions may occur. Discontinue if hyperkalemia occurs. Risk of dilutional hyponatremia. Enhanced effects in post-sympathectomy patient. May increase cholesterol and TG levels. May manifest latent DM. **Contra:** Acute renal impairment, significantly impaired renal excretory function, hyperkalemia, acute or severe hepatic dysfunction, anuria, sulfonamide hypersensitivity. **P/N:** Category C, not for use in nursing.	Gastric bleeding, ulceration, gynecomastia, impotence, agranulocytosis, fever, urticaria, confusion, ataxia, renal dysfunction, blood dyscrasias, electrolyte disturbances, weakness.
Hydrochloro- thiazide/ Triamterene (Dyazide, Maxzide)	**(Dyazide) (Triamterene-HCTZ)Cap:** 37.5mg-25mg; **(Maxzide) (Triamterene-HCTZ) Tab: (Maxzide)** 75mg-50mg*, **(Maxzide-25)** 37.5mg-25mg*	**(Dyazide) Adults:** 1-2 caps qd. **(Maxzide) Adults:** (37.5mg-25mg tab) 1-2 tabs qd. (75mg-50mg tab) 1 tab qd.	**W/P:** Risk of hyperkalemia (≥5.5mEq/L) especially with renal impairment, elderly, DM or severely ill; monitor levels frequently. Caution in severely ill in whom respiratory or metabolic acidosis may occur; monitor acid-base balance frequently. May manifest DM. Caution with hepatic dysfunction, history of renal stones. Increases uric acid levels, BUN, creatinine. May decrease PBI levels. D/C before parathyroid function tests. May potentiate electrolyte imbalance with heart failure, renal disease, cirrhosis. **Contra:** Hyperkalemia, anuria, acute or chronic renal insufficiency, sulfonamide hypersensitivity, diabetic neuropathy, K⁺-sparing agents (eg, diuretics), K⁺ supplements (except with severe hypokalemia), K⁺ salt substitutes, K⁺-rich diet. **P/N:** Category C, not for use in nursing.	Muscle cramps, GI effects, weakness, blood dyscrasias, arrhythmia, impotence, **dry mouth**, jaundice, paresthesia, renal stones, hypersensitivity reactions.

*Scored.   †Bold entries denote special dental considerations.

Table 14.2: DRUG INTERACTIONS FOR CARDIOVASCULAR DRUGS

ACE INHIBITORS

Benazepril Hydrochloride (Lotensin)

Diuretics	Hypotension risk with diuretics.
K⁺-sparing diuretics	Increase risk of hyperkalemia with K⁺-sparing diuretics, K⁺-containing salt substitutes, or K⁺ supplements.
Lithium	May increase lithium levels.

Captopril (Capoten)

Antihypertensives	Augmented effect by antihypertensives that cause renin release (eg, thiazides).
Diuretics	Hypotension risk with diuretics.
K⁺-sparing diuretics	Increased risk of hyperkalemia with K⁺-sparing diuretics, K⁺-containing salt substitutes, or K⁺ supplements.
Lithium	May increase lithium levels.
NSAIDs	NSAIDs may decrease antihypertensive effects.
Vasodilators	Caution with vasodilators or agents affecting sympathetic activity.

Enalapril Maleate (Vasotec)

Antihypertensives	Augmented effect by antihypertensives that cause renin release (eg, thiazides).
Diuretics	Hypotension risk with diuretics.
K⁺-sparing diuretics	Increase risk of hyperkalemia with K⁺-sparing diuretics, K⁺-containing salt substitutes or K⁺ supplements.
Lithium	May increase lithium levels.
NSAIDs	May further decrease renal dysfunction with NSAIDs and diminish antihypertensive effect.

Fosinopril Sodium (Monopril)

Antacids	Decreased absorption with antacids; space dosing by 2hrs.
Diuretics	Hypotension risk with diuretics.
K⁺-sparing diuretics	Increase risk of hyperkalemia with K⁺-sparing diuretics, K⁺-containing salt substitutes or K⁺ supplements.
Lithium	May increase lithium levels.

Lisinopril (Zestril, Prinivil)

Indomethacin	Indomethacin may reduce effects.
Diuretics	Hypotension risk with diuretics.
K⁺-sparing diuretics	Increase risk of hyperkalemia with K⁺-sparing diuretics, K⁺-containing salt substitutes or K⁺ supplements.
Lithium	May increase lithium levels.

Table 14.2: DRUG INTERACTIONS FOR CARDIOVASCULAR DRUGS *(cont.)*

ACE INHIBITORS *(cont.)*

Moexipril Hydrochloride (Univasc)

Diuretics	Hypotension risk with diuretics.
K+-sparing diuretics	Increase risk of hyperkalemia with K+-sparing diuretics, K+-containing salt substitutes or K+ supplements.
Lithium	May increase lithium levels.

Perindopril Erbumine (Aceon)

Diuretics	Hypotension risk with diuretics.
Gentamicin	Caution with gentamicin.
K+-sparing diuretics	Increase risk of hyperkalemia with K+-sparing diuretics, K+-containing salt substitutes or K+ supplements.
Lithium	May increase lithium levels.

Quinapril Hydrochloride (Accupril)

Diuretics	Hypotension risk with diuretics.
K+-sparing diuretics	Increase risk of hyperkalemia with K+-sparing diuretics, K+-containing salt substitutes or K+ supplements.
Lithium	May increase lithium levels.
Tetracycline	Decreases tetracycline absorption (possibly due to magnesium content in quinapril); consider interaction with drugs that interact with magnesium.

Ramipril (Altace)

Diuretics	Hypotension risk with diuretics.
K+-sparing diuretics	Increase risk of hyperkalemia with K+-sparing diuretics, K+-containing salt substitutes or K+ supplements.
Lithium	May increase lithium levels.
NSAIDs	NSAIDs may worsen renal failure and increase serum potassium.

Trandolapril (Mavik)

Diuretics	Hypotension risk with diuretics.
K+-sparing diuretics:	Increase risk of hyperkalemia with K+-sparing diuretics, K+-containing salt substitutes or K+ supplements.
Lithium	May increase lithium levels.

ACE INHIBITORS/DIURETICS

Benazepril Hydrochloride/Hydrochlorothiazide (Lotensin HCT)

Cholestyramine/ Colestipol	Cholestyramine, colestipol decrease absorption.
Insulin	Insulin may need adjustment.

ACE INHIBITORS/DIURETICS *(cont.)*

Benazepril Hydrochloride/Hydrochlorothiazide (Lotensin HCT) *(cont.)*

K+-sparing diuretics	Increase risk of hyperkalemia with K+-sparing diuretics, K+-containing salt substitutes or K+ supplements.
Lithium	Risk of lithium toxicity.
Norepinephrine	May decrease arterial responsiveness to norepinephrine.
NSAIDs	NSAIDs reduce effects.
Tubocurarine	May increase responsiveness to tubocurarine.

Captopril/Hydrochlorothiazide (Capozide)

ACTH	ACTH deplete electrolytes.
Alcohol	Potentiates orthostatic hypotension with alcohol.
Amines	May decrease response to pressor amines.
Amphotericin B	Amphotericin B deplete electrolytes.
Anesthetics/muscle relaxants	May potentiate non-depolarizing skeletal muscle relaxants, anesthetics.
Anticoagulants	Adjust anticoagulants agents.
Antidiabetic	Adjust antidiabetic agents.
Antigout	Adjust antigout drugs.
Antihypertensives	Adjust other antihypertensives agents.
Barbiturates	Potentiates orthostatic hypotension with barbiturates.
Calcium salts	Monitor serum calcium levels with calcium salts.
Cholestyramine/ Colestipol	Reduced absorption with cholestyramine, colestipol.
Corticosteroids	Corticosteroids deplete electrolytes.
Diazoxide	Diazoxide enhances hyperglycemic, hyperuricemic and antihypertensive effects.
Glycosides	Monitor potassium levels with cardiac glycosides.
Lithium	Risk of lithium toxicity.
MAOIs	Enhanced hypotensive effects with MAOIs.
Methenamine	May decrease methenamine effects.
Narcotics	Potentiates orthostatic hypotension with narcotics.
NSAIDs	NSAIDs (eg, indomethacin) reduce effects.
Probenecid	Probenecid may need dose increase.
Sulfinpyrazone	Sulfinpyrazone may need dose increase.
Vasodilators	Discontinue vasodilators before therapy. Caution and decrease vasodilator dose if resumed during therapy.

Table 14.2: DRUG INTERACTIONS FOR CARDIOVASCULAR DRUGS (cont.)

ACE INHIBITORS/DIURETICS (cont.)

Enalapril Maleate/Hydrochlorothiazide (Vaseretic)

ACTH	ACTH deplete electrolytes.
Alcohol	Potentiates orthostatic hypotension with alcohol.
Amines	May decrease response to pressor amines.
Anesthetics/muscle relaxants	May potentiate non-depolarizing skeletal muscle relaxants, anesthetics.
Antihypertensives	Adjust other antihypertensives agents.
Barbiturates	Potentiates orthostatic hypotension with barbiturates.
Calcium salts	Monitor serum calcium levels with calcium salts.
Cholestyramine/ Colestipol	Reduced absorption with cholestyramine, colestipol.
Corticosteroids	Corticosteroids deplete electrolytes.
Lithium	Risk of lithium toxicity.
Narcotics	Potentiates orthostatic hypotension with narcotics.
NSAIDs	NSAIDs (eg, indomethacin) reduce effects.

Fosinopril Sodium/Hydrochlorothiazide (Monopril HCT)

Antacids	Decreased absorption with antacids; space dosing by 2 hrs.
K^+-sparing diuretics	Increase risk of hyperkalemia with K^+-sparing diuretics, K^+-containing salt substitutes or K^+ supplements.
Diuretics	Hypotension risk with diuretics.
Lithium	Risk of lithium toxicity.

Hydrochlorothiazide/Lisinopril (Prinzide)

ACTH	ACTH deplete electrolytes.
Alcohol	Potentiates orthostatic hypotension with alcohol.
Amines	May decrease response to pressor amines.
Anesthetics/muscle relaxants	May potentiate non-depolarizing skeletal muscle relaxants, anesthetics.
Antidiabetic	Adjust antidiabetic agents.
Antihypertensives	Adjust other antihypertensives agents.
Barbiturates	Potentiates orthostatic hypotension with barbiturates.
Cholestyramine/ Colestipol	Reduced absorption with cholestyramine, colestipol.
Corticosteroids	Corticosteroids deplete electrolytes.
K^+-sparing diuretics	Increase risk of hyperkalemia with K^+-sparing diuretics, K^+-containing salt substitutes or K^+ supplements.

ACE INHIBITORS/DIURETICS *(cont.)*

Hydrochlorothiazide/Lisinopril (Zestoretic)

Lithium	Risk of lithium toxicity.
Narcotics	Potentiates orthostatic hypotension with narcotics.
NSAIDs	NSAIDs reduce effects and worsen renal dysfunction.

Hydrochlorothiazide/Lisinopril (Zestoretic)

ACTH	ACTH deplete electrolytes.
Alcohol	Potentiates orthostatic hypotension with alcohol.
Amines	May decrease response to pressor amines.
Anesthetics/muscle relaxants	May potentiate non-depolarizing skeletal muscle relaxants, anesthetics.
Antidiabetic	Adjust antidiabetic agents.
Antihypertensives	Adjust other antihypertensives agents.
Barbiturates	Potentiates orthostatic hypotension with barbiturates.
Cholestyramine/ Colestipol	Reduced absorption with cholestyramine, colestipol.
Corticosteroids	Corticosteroids deplete electrolytes.
K+-sparing diuretics	Increase risk of hyperkalemia with K+-sparing diuretics, K+-containing salt substitutes or K+ supplements.
Lithium	Risk of lithium toxicity.
Narcotics	Potentiates orthostatic hypotension with narcotics.
NSAIDs	NSAIDs reduce effects and worsen renal dysfunction.

Hydrochlorothiazide/Moexipril Hydrochloride (Uniretic)

ACTH	ACTH deplete electrolytes.
Alcohol	Potentiates orthostatic hypotension with alcohol.
Amines	May decrease response to pressor amines.
Anesthetics/muscle relaxants	May potentiate non-depolarizing skeletal muscle relaxants, anesthetics.
Antidiabetic	Adjust antidiabetic agents.
Antihypertensives	Adjust other antihypertensives agents.
Barbiturates	Potentiates orthostatic hypotension with barbiturates.
Cholestyramine/ Colestipol	Reduced absorption with cholestyramine, colestipol.
Corticosteroids	Corticosteroids deplete electrolytes.
K+-sparing diuretics	Increase risk of hyperkalemia with K+-sparing diuretics, K+-containing salt substitutes or K+ supplements.

Table 14.2: DRUG INTERACTIONS FOR CARDIOVASCULAR DRUGS (cont.)

ACE INHIBITORS/DIURETICS (cont.)

Hydrochlorothiazide/Quinapril Hydrochloride (Accuretic)

Lithium	Risk of lithium toxicity.
Narcotics	Potentiates orthostatic hypotension with narcotics.
NSAIDs	NSAIDs reduce effects.
HCTZ	Increased absorption of HCTZ with guanabenz and propantheline.
ACTH	ACTH deplete electrolytes.
Alcohol	Potentiates orthostatic hypotension with alcohol.
Amines	May decrease response to pressor amines.
Anesthetics/muscle relaxants	May potentiate non-depolarizing skeletal muscle relaxants, anesthetics.
Antidiabetic	Adjust antidiabetic agents.
Antihypertensives	Adjust other antihypertensives agents.
Barbiturates	Potentiates orthostatic hypotension with barbiturates.
Cholestyramine/ Colestipol	Reduced absorption with cholestyramine, colestipol.
Corticosteroids	Corticosteroids deplete electrolytes.
K+-sparing diuretics	Increase risk of hyperkalemia with K+-sparing diuretics, K+-containing salt substitutes or K+ supplements.
Lithium	Risk of lithium toxicity.
Narcotics	Potentiates orthostatic hypotension with narcotics.
NSAIDs	NSAIDs decrease diuretic effects.
Tetracycline	Decreases tetracycline absorption (possibly due to magnesium content in quinapril); consider interaction with drugs that interact with magnesium.

α₂-ADRENERGIC AGONISTS, CENTRALLY ACTING

Clonidine Hydrochloride (Catapres)

β-blockers	Additive bradycardia and AV block with β-blocker agents that affect sinus node function or AV nodal conduction.
Calcium channel blockers	Additive bradycardia and AV block with calcium channel blockers that affect sinus node function or AV nodal conduction.
Digitalis	Additive bradycardia and AV block with digitalis that affect sinus node function or AV nodal conduction.
Sedatives	May potentiate CNS depression with alcohol, barbiturates, or other sedatives.
TCAs	Hypotensive effect reduced by TCAs.

α_2-ADRENERGIC AGONISTS, CENTRALLY ACTING *(cont.)*

Guanfacine Hydrochloride (Tenex)

CNS depressants	Additive sedation with other CNS depressants.
CYP450 inducers	Caution with CYP450 inducers (eg, phenobarbital, phenytoin) in renal dysfunction.

Methyldopa, Methyldopate Hydrochloride

Anesthetics	Anesthetics may need dose reduction.
Antihypertensives	May potentiate other antihypertensives.
Iron	Ferrous sulfate and ferrous gluconate decrease bioavailability; avoid coadministration.
Lithium	Risk of lithium toxicity.
MAOIs	Avoid MAOIs.

α-ADRENERIC BLOCKERS

Doxazosin Mesylate (Cardura)

CYP3A4 inhibitors	Caution with potent CYP3A4 inhibitors (eg, atanazavir, clarithromycin, indinavir, itraconazole, ketoconazole, nefazodone, nelfinavir, ritonavir, saquinavir, telithromycin, voriconazole).

Phenoxybenzamine Hydrochloride (Dibenzyline)

α- and β-adrenergic stimulants	Exaggerated hypotensive response and tachycardia with agents that stimulate both α- and β-adrenergic receptors (eg, epinephrine).
Levarterenol	Blocks hyperthermia production by levarterenol.
Reserpine	Blocks hypothermia production by reserpine.

Prazosin Hydrochloride (Minipress)

Alcohol	Dizziness or syncope may occur with alcohol.
Antihypertensives	Additive hypotensive effects with diuretics, β-blockers, or other antihypertensives.

Terazosin Hydrochloride (Hytrin)

Antihypertensives	Possibility of significant hypotension with other antihypertensives; may need dose reduction or retitration of either agent.
Verapamil	Increased levels with verapamil.

ANGIOTENSIN II RECEPTOR ANTAGONISTS

Candesartan Cilexetil (Atacand)

Lithium	Increases lithium levels.

Eprosartan Mesylate (Teveten)

Diuretics	Risk of hypotension with diuretics.

Table 14.2: DRUG INTERACTIONS FOR CARDIOVASCULAR DRUGS (cont.)

α-ADRENERIC BLOCKERS (cont.)

Losartan Potassium (Cozaar)

K+-sparing diuretics	K+-sparing diuretics (eg, spironolactone, triamterene, amiloride), K+ supplements, or K+-containing salt substitutes may increase serum K+.

Olmesartan Medoxomil (Benicar)

Diuretics	Risk of hypotension with high-dose diuretics.

Telmisartan (Micardis)

Warfarin	May alter warfarin levels.
Digoxin	Increases digoxin levels.

Valsartan (Diovan)

ACE inhibitors	Avoid with concomitant ACE inhibitors with heart failure.
β-blockers	Avoid with concomitant β-blockers with heart failure.
K+-sparing diuretics	Potassium-sparing diuretics, potassium supplements, or salt substitutes containing potassium may increase serum potassium levels, and in heart failure patients increase serum creatinine.

ANGIOTENSIN II RECEPTOR ANTAGONISTS/DIURETICS

Candesartan Cilexetil/Hydrochlorothiazide (Atacand HCT)

Lithium	Increases lithium levels.

Eprosartan Mesylate/Hydrochlorothiazide (Teveten HCT)

ACTH	ACTH deplete electrolytes.
Alcohol	Potentiates orthostatic hypotension with alcohol.
Amines	May decrease response to pressor amines (eg, norepinephrine).
Antidiabetic/insulin	Adjust antidiabetic agents.
Antihypertensives	Adjust other antihypertensives agents.
Barbiturates	Potentiates orthostatic hypotension with barbiturates.
Cholestyramine/ Colestipol	Reduced absorption with cholestyramine, colestipol.
Corticosteroids	Corticosteroids deplete electrolytes.
K+-sparing diuretics	Increased risk of hyperkalemia with potassium-sparing diuretics, potassium supplements, or potassium-containing salt substitutes.
Lithium	Increases lithium levels.
Muscle relaxants	May potentiate non-depolarizing skeletal muscle relaxants (eg, tubocurarine).
Narcotics	Potentiates orthostatic hypotension with narcotics.
NSAIDs	NSAIDs may decrease diuretic/antihypertensive effects.

ANGIOTENSIN II RECEPTOR ANTAGONISTS/DIURETICS *(cont.)*

Hydrochlorothiazide/Irbesartan (Avalide)

ACTH	ACTH deplete electrolytes.
Alcohol	Potentiates orthostatic hypotension with alcohol.
Amines	May decrease response to pressor amines (eg, norepinephrine).
Amines	May decrease response to pressor amines.
Antidiabetic/Insulin	Adjust antidiabetic agents.
Antihypertensives	Adjust other antihypertensives agents.
Barbiturates	Potentiates orthostatic hypotension with barbiturates.
Cholestyramine/Colestipol	Reduced absorption with cholestyramine, colestipol.
Corticosteroids	Corticosteroids deplete electrolytes.
Lithium	Increases lithium levels.
Muscle relaxants	May potentiate non-depolarizing skeletal muscle relaxants.
Narcotics	Potentiates orthostatic hypotension with narcotics.
NSAIDs	NSAIDs may decrease diuretic effects.

Hydrochlorothiazide/Losartan Potassium (Hyzaar)

Rifampin	Decreased levels with rifampin.
ACTH	ACTH deplete electrolytes.
Alcohol	Potentiates orthostatic hypotension with alcohol.
Amines	May decrease response to pressor amines (eg, norepinephrine).
Antidiabetic/Insulin	Adjust antidiabetic agents.
Antihypertensives	Adjust other antihypertensives agents.
Barbiturates	Potentiates orthostatic hypotension with barbiturates.
Cholestyramine/Colestipol	Reduced absorption with cholestyramine, colestipol.
Corticosteroids	Corticosteroids deplete electrolytes.
Fluconazole	Increased levels with fluconazole.
K+-sparing diuretics	Increased risk of hyperkalemia with potassium-sparing diuretics, potassium supplements, or potassium-containing salt substitutes.
Lithium	Increases lithium levels.
Muscle relaxants	May potentiate non-depolarizing skeletal muscle relaxants (eg, tubocurarine).
Narcotics	Potentiates orthostatic hypotension with narcotics.
NSAIDs	NSAIDs may decrease diuretic/antihypertensive effects.

Table 14.2: DRUG INTERACTIONS FOR CARDIOVASCULAR DRUGS *(cont.)*

ANGIOTENSIN II RECEPTOR ANTAGONISTS/DIURETICS *(cont.)*

Hydrochlorothiazide/Olmesartan Medoxomil (Benicar HCT)

ACTH	ACTH deplete electrolytes.
Alcohol	Potentiates orthostatic hypotension with alcohol.
Amines	May decrease response to pressor amines (eg, norepinephrine).
Antidiabetic	Adjust antidiabetic agents.
Antihypertensives	Adjust other antihypertensives agents.
Barbiturates	Potentiates orthostatic hypotension with barbiturates.
Cholestyramine/ Colestipol	Reduced absorption with cholestyramine, colestipol.
Corticosteroids	Corticosteroids deplete electrolytes.
Lithium	Increases lithium levels.
Muscle relaxants	May potentiate non-depolarizing skeletal muscle relaxants.
Narcotics	Potentiates orthostatic hypotension with narcotics.
NSAIDs	NSAIDs may decrease diuretic effects.

Hydrochlorothiazide/Telmisartan (Micardis HCT)

ACTH	ACTH deplete electrolytes.
Alcohol	Potentiates orthostatic hypotension with alcohol.
Amines	May decrease response to pressor amines (eg, norepinephrine).
Antidiabetic	Adjust antidiabetic agents.
Antihypertensives	Adjust other antihypertensives agents.
Barbiturates	Potentiates orthostatic hypotension with barbiturates.
Cholestyramine/ Colestipol	Reduced absorption with cholestyramine, colestipol.
Corticosteroids	Corticosteroids deplete electrolytes.
Digoxin	Increases digoxin levels.
Lithium	Increases lithium levels.
Muscle relaxants	May potentiate non-depolarizing skeletal muscle relaxants.
Narcotics	Potentiates orthostatic hypotension with narcotics.
NSAIDs	NSAIDs may decrease diuretic effects.
Warfarin	May alter warfarin levels.

Hydrochlorothiazide/Valsartan (Diovan HCT)

ACTH	ACTH deplete electrolytes.
Alcohol	Potentiates orthostatic hypotension with alcohol.

ANGIOTENSIN II RECEPTOR ANTAGONISTS/DIURETICS *(cont.)*

Hydrochlorothiazide/Valsartan (Diovan HCT) *(cont.)*

Amines	May decrease response to pressor amines (eg, norepinephrine).
Antidiabetic	Adjust antidiabetic agents.
Antihypertensives	Adjust other antihypertensives agents.
Barbiturates	Potentiates orthostatic hypotension with barbiturates.
Cholestyramine/ Colestipol	Reduced absorption with cholestyramine, colestipol.
Corticosteroids	Corticosteroids deplete electrolytes.
Lithium	Increases lithium levels.
Muscle relaxants	May potentiate non-depolarizing skeletal muscle relaxants.
Narcotics	Potentiates orthostatic hypotension with narcotics.
NSAIDs	NSAIDs may decrease diuretic effects.

ANTIARRHYTHMICS

Disopyramide Phosphate (Norpace)

Alcohol	Monitor blood glucose with alcohol.
Antiarrhythmics	Avoid type IA and IC antiarrhythmics except in unresponsive, life-threatening arrhythmias.
β-blockers	Monitor blood glucose with β-blockers.
CYP3A4 inhibitors	Possible fatal interactions with CYP3A4 inhibitors.
Enzyme inducers	Hepatic enzyme inducers may lower levels.
Propranolol	Avoid propranolol except in unresponsive, life-threatening arrhythmias.
Verapamil	Avoid within 48 hrs before or 24 hrs after verapamil.

Flecainide Acetate (Tambocor)

Amiodarone	Potentiated by amiodarone.
β-blockers	Additive negative inotropic effects with β-blockers (eg, propranolol).
Carbamazepine	Increased elimination with carbamazepine.
Cimetidine	Potentiated by cimetidine.
CYP2D6 inhibitors	Potentiated by CYP2D6 inhibitors (eg, quinidine).
Digoxin	Increases digoxin levels.
Diltiazem	Diltiazem not recommended.
Disopyramide	Disopyramide not recommended.
Nifedipine	Nifedipine not recommended.
Phenobarbital	Increased elimination with phenobarbital.

Table 14.2: DRUG INTERACTIONS FOR CARDIOVASCULAR DRUGS *(cont.)*

ANTIARRHYTHMICS *(cont.)*

Flecainide Acetate (Tambocor) *(cont.)*

Phenytoin	Increased elimination with phenytoin.
Verapamil	Verapamil not recommended.

Ibutilide Fumarate (Corvert)

Antiarrhythmics	Avoid Class IA (eg, disopyramide, quinidine, procainamide) and other Class III (eg, amio-darone, sotalol) antiarrhythmics with or within 4 hrs postinfusion of ibutilide.
Digoxin	Supraventricular arrhythmias may mask cardiotoxicity associated with excessive digoxin levels.
Phenothiazines	Increase proarrhythmia potential with phenothiazines that prolong the QT interval.
TCAs	Increase proarrhythmia potential with TCAs that prolong the QT interval.

Mexiletine Hydrochloride

Enzyme inducers	Enzyme inducers (eg, rifampin, phenobarbital, phenytoin) lower plasma levels.
Caffeine	Decreases caffeine clearance.
Cimetidine	Cimetidine may alter levels.
Theophylline	May increase theophylline levels.

Procainamide Hydrochloride (Procanbid, Pronestyl)

Alcohol	Alcohol decreases half-life.
Amiodarone	Potentiated by amiodarone.
Antiarrhythmics	Additive cardiac effects with other class 1A drugs (quinidine, disopyramide).
Anticholinergics	Additive antivagal effects with anticholinergics.
Cimetidine	Potentiated by cimetidine.
Neuromuscular blockers	May require less than usual dose of neuromuscular blockers.
Ranitidine	Potentiated by ranitidine.
Trimethoprim	Potentiated by trimethoprim.

Propafenone Hydrochloride (Rythmol, Rythmol SR)

Anesthetics	Local anesthetics may increase CNS side effects.
Cimetidine	Cimetidine increases plasma levels.
Desipramine	Increases levels of desipramine.
Digoxin	Increases levels of digoxin.
Quinidine	Avoid quinidine.
Rifampin	Decreased effects with rifampin.
Theophylline	Increases levels of theophylline.

ANTIARRHYTHMICS *(cont.)*

Propafenone Hydrochloride (Rythmol, Rythmol SR) *(cont.)*

β-blockers	Increases levels of β-blockers.
Warfarin	Increases levels of warfarin.

Quinidine Gluconate, Quinidine Sulfate

Amiodarone	Increased levels with amiodarone.
Anticholinergics	Additive effects with anticholinergics.
β-blockers	β-blockers decrease clearance.
Cimetidine	Increased levels with cimvetidine.
CYP3A4 inducers	CYP3A4 inducers may accelerate elimination.
CYP3A4 and 2D6 metabolizers	Caution with drugs metabolized by CYP3A4 and 2D6.
Dietary salt	Dietary salt may affect absorption.
Digoxin	Digoxin may need dose reduction.
Diltiazem	Diltiazem decrease clearance.
Grapefruit juice	Avoid grapefruit juice.
Haloperidol	Increases levels of haloperidol.
Ketoconazole	Increased levels with ketoconazole.
Negative inotropics	Additive effects with negative inotropics.
Neuromuscular blockers	Potentiates depolarizing and nondepolarizing neuromuscular blockers.
Procainamide	Increases levels of procainamide.
Urine alkalinizers	Urine alkalinizers (eg, carbonic anhydrase inhibitors, sodium bicarbonate, thiazide diuretics) reduce renal elimination.
Vasodilators	Additive effects with vasodilators.
Verapamil	Verapamil decrease clearance.
Warfarin	Potentiates warfarin.

β-BLOCKERS, CARDIOSELECTIVE

Atenolol (Tenormin)

Anesthetics	Caution with drugs that depress the myocardium (eg, anesthesia).
Atenolol	Serious adverse reactions with IV atenolol use.
Calcium channel blockers	Additive effects with calcium channel blockers.

Table 14.2: DRUG INTERACTIONS FOR CARDIOVASCULAR DRUGS (cont.)

β-BLOCKERS, CARDIOSELECTIVE (cont.)

Atenolol (Tenormin) (cont.)

Catecholamine-depleting drugs	Additive effects with catecholamine-depleting drugs (eg, reserpine).
Clonidine	Exacerbates rebound HTN with clonidine withdrawal.
Digitalis	Additive effects with digitalis.
Diltiazem	Bradycardia, heart block, and left ventricular end diastolic pressure can rise with diltiazem.
Epinephrine	May block epinephrine effects.
Prostaglandin synthase inhibitors	Prostaglandin synthase inhibitors (eg, indomethacin) may decrease hypotensive effects.
Verapamil	Serious adverse reactions with IV verapamil. Bradycardia, heart block, and left ventricular end diastolic pressure can rise with verapamil.

Bisoprolol Fumarate (Zebeta)

Anesthetics	Caution with anesthetics that depress myocardial function.
Antiarrhythmics	Caution with antiarrhythmics (eg, disopyramide).
Antidiabetic	Antidiabetic agents may need adjustment.
β-blockers	Avoid other β-blockers.
Catecholamine-depleting drugs	Excessive reduction of sympathetic activity with catecholamine-depleting drugs.
Calcium channel blockers	Caution with calcium channel blockers (eg, verapamil, diltiazem) that depress myocardial function.
Clonidine	Caution with clonidine withdrawal.
Epinephrine	May block epinephrine effects.
Rifampin	Rifampin increases clearance.

Esmolol Hydrochloride (Brevibloc)

Catecholamine-depleting agents	Additive effects with catecholamine-depleting agents (eg, reserpine); monitor for hypotension or bradycardia.
Digoxin	May increase digoxin levels; titrate with caution.
Morphine	Levels increased by morphine titrate with caution.
Succinylcholine	May prolong effects of succinylcholine titrate with caution.
Vasoconstrictive/inotropic agents	Do not use to control supraventricular tachycardia with vasoconstrictive and inotropic agents (eg, dopamine, epinephrine, norepinephrine) because of the danger of blocking cardiac contractility when systemic vascular resistance is high.
Verapamil	Caution when using with verapamil in depressed myocardial function; fatal cardiac arrest may occur.
Warfarin	Levels increased by warfarin titrate with caution.

β-BLOCKERS, CARDIOSELECTIVE (cont.)

Metoprolol (Toprol-XL, Lopressor)

Catecholamine-depleting drugs	Additive effects with catecholamine-depleting drugs (eg, reserpine).
Epinephrine	May block epinephrine effects.
Digitalis	Caution with digitalis; both agents slow AV conduction.

β-BLOCKERS, NONSELECTIVE

Nadolol (Corgard)

Catecholamine-depleting drugs	Additive hypotension and/or bradycardia with catecholamine-depleting drugs.
Antidiabetics	Antidiabetic agents may need adjustment.
Anesthetics	General anesthetics may exaggerate hypotension.
Epinephrine	May block epinephrine effects.

Penbutolol Sulfate (Levatol)

Alcohol	Caution with alcohol.
Anesthetics	Caution with anesthetics that depress the myocardium.
Catecholamine-depleting drugs	Avoid catecholamine-depleting drugs.
Calcium channel blockers	Synergistic hypotensive effects, bradycardia, and arrhythmias with oral calcium channel blockers.
Epinephrine	May antagonize epinephrine.
Lidocaine	Increases volume of distribution of lidocaine; may need larger LD.

Pindolol

Catecholamine-depleting drugs	Additive hypotension and/or bradycardia with catecholamine-depleting drugs.
Thioridazine	Both thioridazine and pindolol levels may increase when used concomitantly.

Propranolol Hydrochloride (Inderal, Inderal LA, InnoPran XL)

Alcohol	Alcohol decreases absorption rate.
Aluminum hydroxide gel	Aluminum hydroxide gel reduces intestinal absorption.
Antipyrine	Reduces clearance of antipyrine.
Catecholamine-depleting drugs	Additive hypotension and/or bradycardia with catecholamine-depleting drugs.
Calcium channel blockers	May increase cardiac effects of calcium channel blockers.
Chlorpromazine	Potentiated by chlorpromazine.

Table 14.2: DRUG INTERACTIONS FOR CARDIOVASCULAR DRUGS *(cont.)*

β-BLOCKERS, NONSELECTIVE *(cont.)*

Propranolol Hydrochloride (Inderal, Inderal LA, InnoPran XL) *(cont.)*

Cimetidine	Potentiated by cimetidine.
Epinephrine	May block epinephrine effects.
Haloperidol	Hypotension and cardiac arrest reported with haloperidol.
Lidocaine	Reduces clearance of lidocaine.
NSAIDs	Antagonized by NSAIDs.
Phenobarbital	Antagonized by phenobarbital.
Phenytoin	Antagonized by phenytoin.
Rifampin	Antagonized by rifampin.
Theophylline	Reduces clearance of theophylline.
Thyroxine	May block thyroxine effects.

Sotalol Hydrochloride (Betapace)

Antacids	Avoid within 2 hrs of aluminum- or magnesium-containing antacids.
Antiarrhythmics	Caution with drugs that prolong the QT interval (eg, Class I and III antiarrhythmics), potential to prolong refractoriness.
Antidiabetic	Antidiabetic agents may need adjustment.
Astemizole	Caution with drugs that prolong the QT interval (eg, astemizole).
β$_2$-agonists	β$_2$-agonists (eg, terbutaline) may need dose increase.
β-blockers	Additive Class II effects with β-blockers.
Bepridil	Caution with drugs that prolong the QT interval (eg, bepridil).
Catecholamine-depleting drugs	Additive effects with catecholamine-depleting drugs (eg, reserpine).
Calcium channel blockers	Additive conduction abnormalities with calcium channel blockers.
Clonidine	Potentiates rebound HTN with clonidine withdrawal.
Digoxin	Additive conduction abnormalities with digoxin.
Diuretics	Caution with diuretics.
Epinephrine	May block epinephrine effects.
Macrolides	Caution with oral macrolides that prolong the QT interval.
Phenothiazines	Caution with phenothiazines that prolong the QT interval.
Quinolones	Caution with certain quinolones that prolong the QT interval.
TCAs	Caution with TCAs that prolong the QT interval.

β-BLOCKERS, NONSELECTIVE *(cont.)*

Timolol Maleate

β-blockade	Quinidine may potentiate β-blockade.
Calcium antagonists	Hypotension, AV conduction disturbances, left ventricular failure reported with oral calcium antagonists.
Catecholamine-depleting drugs	Possible additive effects and hypotension and/or marked bradycardia with catecholamine-depleting drugs.
Clonidine	Exacerbates rebound HTN with clonidine withdrawal.
Digitalis	AV conduction time prolonged with digitalis and either diltiazem or verapamil.
Diltiazem	AV conduction time prolonged with digitalis and either diltiazem or verapamil.
Epinephrine	May block epinephrine effects.
Hypoglycemics	Caution with oral hypoglycemics.
Insulin	Caution with insulin.
NSAIDs	NSAIDs may reduce antihypertensive effects.
Verapamil	AV conduction time prolonged with digitalis and either diltiazem or verapamil.

β-BLOCKERS & α-BLOCKERS (COMBINED)

Carvedilol *(Coreg)*

Catecholamine-depleting agents	Monitor for hypotension and bradycardia with catecholamine-depleting agents (eg, reserpine, MAOIs).
Calcium channel blockers	Monitor ECG and BP with calcium channel blockers (eg, verapamil, diltiazem).
Cimetidine	Cimetidine increases AUC.
Clonidine	Clonidine may potentiate BP and heart-rate-lowering effects.
Cyclosporin	Monitor with cyclosporin.
CYP2D6 inhibitors	CYP2D6 inhibitors (eg, quinidine, fluoxetine, paroxetine, and propafenone) may increase levels.
Digoxin	Monitor with digoxin.
Hypoglycemics/insulin	Monitor with insulin and oral hypoglycemics.
Rifampin	Rifampin increases clearance.

Labetalol Hydrochloride *(Normodyne, Trandate)*

Antidiabetic	Antidiabetic agents may need dose adjustment.
Calcium antagonists	Caution with calcium antagonists.
Cimetidine	Potentiated by cimetidine.

Table 14.2: DRUG INTERACTIONS FOR CARDIOVASCULAR DRUGS *(cont.)*

β-BLOCKERS & α-BLOCKERS (COMBINED) *(cont.)*

Labetalol Hydrochloride (Normodyne, Trandate) *(cont.)*

β-agonists	Antagonizes bronchodilator effect of β-agonists.
Epinephrine	May block epinephrine effects.
Halothane	(Inj) Synergistic with halothane; do not use ≥3% halothane.
NTG	Blunts reflex tachycardia of NTG without preventing hypotensive effect.
TCAs	Increased tremors with TCAs.

β-BLOCKERS, CARDIOSELECTIVE/DIURETICS

Atenolol/Chlorthalidone (Tenoretic)

ACTH	Possible hypokalemia with ACTH.
Anesthetic	Caution with anesthetic agents.
Catecholamine-depleting drugs	Additive effects with catecholamine-depleting drugs (eg, reserpine).
Calcium channel blockers	Additive effects with calcium channel blockers.
Clonidine	Exacerbates rebound HTN with clonidine withdrawal.
Corticosteroids	Possible hypokalemia with corticosteroids.
Digitalis	Additive effects digitalis.
Diltiazem	Bradycardia, heart block, and left ventricular end diastolic pressure can rise with diltiazem.
Epinephrine	May block epinephrine effects.
Insulin	May alter insulin requirements.
Lithium	Increases risk of lithium toxicity.
Norepinephrine	May decrease arterial response to norepinephrine.
Prostaglandin synthase inhibitors	Prostaglandin synthase inhibitors (eg, indomethacin) may decrease hypotensive effects.
Verapamil	Bradycardia, heart block, and left ventricular end diastolic pressure can rise with verapamil.

Bisoprolol Fumarate/Hydrochlorothiazide (Ziac)

ACTH	ACTH intensify electrolyte imbalance.
Alcohol	Alcohol potentiate orthostatic hypotension.
Amines	Decreased arterial responsiveness with pressor amines.
Anesthesia	Caution with anesthesia.
Anesthetics	General anesthetics may exaggerate hypotension.

β-BLOCKERS, CARDIOSELECTIVE/DIURETICS *(cont.)*

Bisoprolol Fumarate/Hydrochlorothiazide (Ziac) *(cont.)*

Antiarrhythmics	Caution with antiarrhythmics.
Antidiabetics	Antidiabetic agents may need adjustment.
Antihypertensives	Other antihypertensives may need adjustment.
β-blockers	Avoid other β-blockers.
Barbiturates	Barbiturates potentiate orthostatic hypotension.
Catecholamine-depleting drugs	Excessive reduction of sympathetic activity with catecholamine-depleting drugs.
Calcium channel blockers	Caution with calcium channel blockers.Caution with calcium channel blockers.
Cholestyramine/colestipol	Cholestyramine and colestipol may delay or decrease absorption and colestipol may delay or decrease absorption.
Clonidine	Exacerbates rebound HTN with clonidine withdrawal.
Corticosteroids	Corticosteroids intensify electrolyte imbalance.
Epinephrine	May block epinephrine effects.
Lithium	Lithium toxicity.
Myocardial depressants	Caution with myocardial depressants. Caution with myocardial depressants.
Narcotics	Narcotics potentiate orthostatic hypotension.
NSAIDs	NSAIDs may decrease effects.
Rifampin	Increased clearance with rifampin.

Metoprolol Tartrate/Hydrochlorothiazide (Lopressor HCT)

ACTH	ACTH may increase risk of hypokalemia.
Alcohol	Alcohol potentiate orthostatic hypotension.
Antihypertensives	Other antihypertensives may need adjustment.
Barbiturates	Barbiturates potentiate orthostatic hypotension.
Catecholamine-depleting drugs	Excessive reduction of sympathetic activity with catecholamine-depleting drugs.
Cholestyramine/colestipol	Cholestyramine and colestipol may delay or decrease absorption.Cholestyramine and colestipol may delay or decrease absorption.
Corticosteroids	Corticosteroids may increase risk of hypokalemia.
Digitalis	Additive effects digitalis.
Epinephrine	May block epinephrine effects.
Insulin	Insulin agents may need adjustment.

Table 14.2: DRUG INTERACTIONS FOR CARDIOVASCULAR DRUGS (cont.)

β-BLOCKERS, CARDIOSELECTIVE/DIURETICS (cont.)

Metoprolol Tartrate/Hydrochlorothiazide (Lopressor HCT) (cont.)

Lithium	Lithium toxicity.
Narcotics	Narcotics potentiate orthostatic hypotension.
Norepinephrine	May decrease arterial responsiveness to norepinephrine.
NSAIDs	NSAIDs may decrease effects.
Tubocurarine	May increase responsiveness to tubocurarine.

β-BLOCKERS, NONSELECTIVE/DIURETICS

Nadolol/Bendroflumethiazide (Corzide)

Catecholamine-depleting drugs	Additive effects with catecholamine-depleting drugs (eg, reserpine).
ACTH	ACTH intensify electrolyte imbalance.
Alcohol	Alcohol potentiate orthostatic hypotension.
Amines	Decreased arterial responsiveness with pressor amines.
Amphotericin B	Amphotericin B intensify electrolyte imbalance.
Anesthetics	General anesthetics may exaggerate hypotension. May potentiate nondepolarizing muscle relaxants, preanesthetics, and anesthetics.
Anticoagulants	Anticoagulants may need adjustment.
Antidiabetics	Antidiabetic agents may need adjustment.
Antigout	Antigout agents may need adjustment.
Antihypertensives	Other antihypertensives may need adjustment.
Barbiturates	Barbiturates potentiate orthostatic hypotension.
Calcium salts	Monitor calcium levels with calcium salts.
Cholestyramine/colestipol	Cholestyramine and colestipol may delay or decrease absorption.
Corticosteroids	Corticosteroids intensify electrolyte imbalance.
Diazoxide	Enhanced hyperglycemic, hyperuricemic, and antihypertensive effects with diazoxide.
Digoxin	Monitor digoxin.
Epinephrine	May block epinephrine effects.
Lithium	Lithium toxicity.
MAOIs	Enhanced hypotensive effects with MAOIs.
Methenamine	Possible decreased effectiveness with methenamine.
Narcotics	Narcotics potentiate orthostatic hypotension.
NSAIDs	NSAIDs may decrease effects.

β-BLOCKERS, NONSELECTIVE/DIURETICS *(cont.)*

Nadolol/Bendroflumethiazide (Corzide)

Probenecid	Probenecid may need dose increase.
Sulfinpyrazone	Sulfinpyrazone may need dose increase.

Propranolol Hydrochloride/Hydrochlorothiazide (Inderide)

Narcotics	Narcotics potentiate orthostatic hypotension.
ACTH	ACTH may increase risk of hypokalemia.
Adrenergic-blockers	Potentiation with ganglionic or peripheral adrenergic-blockers.
Alcohol	Alcohol potentiate orthostatic hypotension.
Aluminum hydroxide gel	Aluminum hydroxide gel reduces intestinal absorption.
Antipyrine	Reduces clearance of antipyrine.
Barbiturates	Barbiturates potentiate orthostatic hypotension.
Catecholamine-depleting drugs	Excessive reduction of sympathetic activity with catecholamine-depleting drugs.
Calcium channel blockers	May increase cardiac effects of calcium channel blockers.
Chlorpromazine	Potentiated by chlorpromazine.
Cimetidine	Potentiated by cimetidine.
Corticosteroids	Corticosteroids may increase risk of hypokalemia.
Digoxin	Monitor digoxin.
Epinephrine	May block epinephrine effects.
Haloperidol	Hypotension and cardiac arrest reported with haloperidol.
Insulin	Insulin agents may need adjustment.
Lidocaine	Reduces clearance of lidocaine.
Norepinephrine	May decrease arterial responsiveness to norepinephrine.
NSAIDs	Antagonized by NSAIDs.
Phenobarbital	Antagonized by phenobarbital.
Phenytoin	Antagonized by phenytoin.
Rifampin	Antagonized by rifampin.
Theophylline	Reduces clearance of theophylline.
Thyroxine	May block thyroxine effects.
Tubocurarine	May increase responsiveness to tubocurarine.

Timolol Maleate/Hydrochlorothiazide (Timolide)

Antihypertensives	Other antihypertensives may need adjustment.
ACTH	ACTH may increase risk of hypokalemia.

Table 14.2: DRUG INTERACTIONS FOR CARDIOVASCULAR DRUGS *(cont.)*

β-BLOCKERS, NONSELECTIVE/DIURETICS *(cont.)*

Timolol Maleate/Hydrochlorothiazide (Timolide) *(cont.)*

Antidiabetics	Antidiabetic agents may need adjustment.
Calcium antagonists	Hypotension, AV conduction disturbances, and left ventricular failure reported with oral calcium antagonists.
Catecholamine-depleting drugs	Excessive reduction of sympathetic activity with catecholamine-depleting drugs.
Clonidine	May exacerbate rebound hypertension following clonidine withdrawal.
Corticosteroids	Corticosteroids may increase risk of hypokalemia.
Digitalis	AV conduction time prolonged with digitalis and diltiazem or verapamil.
Diltiazem	AV conduction time prolonged with digitalis and diltiazem or verapamil.
Epinephrine	May block epinephrine effects.
Lithium	Lithium toxicity.
Norepinephrine	May decrease arterial response to norepinephrine.
NSAIDs	NSAIDs may decrease effects.
Quinidine	Quinidine may potentiate β-blockade.
Tubocurarine	May increase responsiveness to tubocurarine.
Verapamil	AV conduction time prolonged with digitalis and diltiazem or verapamil.

CALCIUM CHANNEL BLOCKERS

Diltiazem Hydrochloride (Cardizem LA, Cardizem CD, Dilacor XR, Diltiazem CD, Tiazac)

Anesthetics	Potentiates the depression of cardiac contractility, conductivity, automaticity and vascular dilation with anesthetics.
Carbamazepine	Increased levels of carbamazepine; monitor closely.
Cimetidine	Increased levels of diltiazem with cimetidine.
Cyclosporine	Increased levels of cyclosporine; monitor closely.
CYP3A4 inducers	Avoid with CYP3A4 inducers.
Digitalis	Additive cardiac conduction effects with digitalis.
Digoxin	Increased levels of digoxin; monitor closely.
Diltiazem	Increased levels of diltiazem with cimetidine.
Midazolam/triazolam	May increase levels of midazolam/triazolam.
Propranolol	Increased levels of propranolol; monitor closely.

Felodipine (Plendil)

Anticonvulsants	Levels decreased with long-term anticonvulsant therapy.
CYP3A4 inhibitors	CYP3A4 inhibitors (eg, itraconazole, ketoconazole, erythromycin, grapefruit juice, cimetidine) may increase plasma levels.

CALCIUM CHANNEL BLOCKERS *(cont.)*

Felodipine (Plendil)

Metoprolol	May increase metoprolol levels.

Isradipine (DynaCirc)

β-blockers	Severe hypotension possible with β-blockers.
Fentanyl	Severe hypotension possible with fentanyl.
HCTZ	Additive effects with HCTZ.
Propranolol	Increases AUC and C_{max} of propranolol.
Rifampicin	Decreased levels with rifampicin.

Nicardipine Hydrochloride (Cardene IV)

β-blocker	With β-blocker withdrawal, gradually reduce over 8-10 days.
Cimetidine	Increased levels with cimetidine.
Cyclosporine	Elevates cyclosporine levels.
Digoxin	Monitor digoxin levels.
Fentanyl	Caution with fentanyl anesthesia.

Nifedipine (Adalat CC, Procardia XL)

β-blockers	β-blockers may increase risk of CHF, severe hypotension, or angina exacerbation.
Cimetidine	Potentiated by cimetidine.
Coumarin	Monitor coumarin.
Digoxin	Potentiates digoxin.
Fentanyl	Possible hypotension with fentanyl.
Grapefruit juice	Avoid grapefruit juice due to risk of potentiation.
Quinidine	Monitor quinidine.

Nimodipine (Nimotop)

Antihypertensives	May intensify effects of antihypertensives.
Calcium channel blockers	May intensify effects of antihypertensives. May enhance cardiovascular effects of other calcium channel blockers.
Cimetidine	Increased serum levels with cimetidine.

Nisoldipine (Sular)

Cimetidine	Increased AUC and C_{max} with cimetidine.
CYP3A4 inducers	Avoid CYP3A4 inducers.
Grapefruit juice	Avoid grapefruit juice.
High fat meals	High fat meals increase peak drug levels.
Phenytoin	Avoid phenytoin.

Table 14.2: DRUG INTERACTIONS FOR CARDIOVASCULAR DRUGS *(cont.)*

CALCIUM CHANNEL BLOCKERS *(cont.)*

Nisoldipine (Sular) *(cont.)*

Quinidine	Decreased bioavailability with quinidine.

Verapamil Hydrochloride (Calan, Calan SR, Covera-HS, Isoptin SR, Verelan, Verelan PM)

Alcohol	May increase alcohol levels.
Anesthetics	Caution with inhalation anesthetics.
Antihypertensives	Potentiates other antihypertensives.
ASA	Increased bleeding time with ASA.
β-blockers	Additive negative effects on HR, AV conduction, and contractility with β-blockers.
Carbamazepine	May increase carbamazepine levels.
Cyclosporine	May increase cyclosporine levels.
CYP3A4 inducers	CYP3A4 inducers (eg, rifampin) may lower levels.
CYP3A4 inhibitors	CYP3A4 inhibitors (eg, erythromycin, ritonavir) may increase levels.
Grapefruit juice	May increase levels.
Cytotoxic drugs	Reduced absorption with COPP and VAC cytotoxic drug regimens.
Digoxin	May increase digoxin levels.
Disopyramide	Avoid disopyramide within 48 hrs before or 24 hrs after verapamil.
Doxorubicin	Increased efficacy of doxorubicin.
Flecainide	Additive negative inotropic effects and AV conduction prolongation with flecainide.
Lithium	Monitor lithium levels.
Neuromuscular blockers	May potentiate neuromuscular blockers; both agents may need dose reduction.
Paclitaxel	May decrease clearance of paclitaxel.
Phenobarbital	Increased clearance with phenobarbital.
Quinidine	Avoid quinidine with hypertrophic cardiomyopathy.
Rifampin	Rifampin may reduce oral bioavailability.
Theophylline	May increase theophylline levels.

CALCIUM CHANNEL BLOCKERS/ACE INHIBITORS

Amlodipine Besylate/Benazepril Hydrochloride (Lotrel)

Diuretics	Hypotension risk with diuretics.
K+-sparing diuretics	Increase risk of hyperkalemia with K+-sparing diuretics, K+ supplements, or K+-containing salt substitutes.
Lithium	May increase lithium levels.
Vasodilators	Caution with other peripheral vasodilators.

CALCIUM CHANNEL BLOCKERS/ACE INHIBITORS *(cont.)*

Trandolapril/Verapamil Hydrochloride (Tarka)

Alcohol	May increase alcohol blood levels and prolong effects.
Antihypertensives	Potentiates other antihypertensives.
β-blockers	Additive effects on HR, AV conduction, and contractility with β-blockers.
Carbamazepine	May increase carbamazepine levels.
Cyclosporine	May increase cyclosporine levels.
Digoxin	May increase digoxin.
Disopyramide	Avoid disopyramide within 48 hrs before or 24 hrs after verapamil.
Flecainide	Additive negative inotropic effects and AV conduction prolongation with flecainide.
K+-sparing diuretics	Increase risk of hyperkalemia with K+-sparing diuretics, K+ supplements, or K+-containing salt substitutes.
Lithium	Monitor lithium.
Neuromuscular blockers	May potentiate neuromuscular blockers; both agents may need dose reduction.
Phenobarbital	Increased clearance with phenobarbital.
Quinidine	Avoid quinidine with hypertrophic cardiomyopathy.
Rifampin	Rifampin may reduce oral bioavailability.
Theophylline	May increase theophylline levels.

CALCIUM CHANNEL BLOCKERS/HMG-CoA REDUCTASE INHIBITORS

Amlodipine Besylate/Atorvastatin Calcium (Caduet)

Azole antifungals	Azole antifungals may increase risk of myopathy.
Colestipol	Colestipol decreases levels when coadministered, but greater LDL-C reduction with coadministration than when each given alone.
Cyclosporine	Increases levels of cyclosporine.
Digoxin	Increases levels of digoxin.
Erythromycin	Increases levels with erythromycin; increase risk of myopathy.
Fibrates	Avoid fibrates.
Fibric acid derivatives	Fibric acid derivatives may increase risk of myopathy.
Maalox	Decreased levels with Maalox TC, but LDL-C reduction not altered.
Niacin	Niacin may increase risk of myopathy.
Oral contraceptives	Increases levels of oral contraceptives (norethindrone, ethinyl estradiol).
Steroids	Caution with drugs that decrease levels or activity of endogenous steroid hormones (eg, ketoconazole, spironolactone, cimetidine).

Table 14.2: DRUG INTERACTIONS FOR CARDIOVASCULAR DRUGS *(cont.)*

VASODILATORS

Hydralazine Hydrochloride

Antihypertensives	Profound hypotension with potent parenteral antihypertensives (eg, diazoxide).
Epinephrine	May reduce pressor response to epinephrine.
MAOIs	Caution with MAOIs.

Hydralazine Hydrochloride/Isosorbide Dinitrate (BiDil)

Antihypertensive	Increased risk of hypotension with potent parenteral antihypertensive agents.
MAOIs	Caution with MAOIs.
Phosphodiesterase inhibitors	Increased vasodilatory effects with phosphodiesterase inhibitors (sildenafil, vardenafil, tadalafil).

Isosorbide Mononitrate (Imdur, Ismo, Monoket)

Calcium channel blockers	Orthostatic hypotension with calcium channel blockers.
Sildenafil	Severe hypotension with sildenafil.
Vasodilators	Additive vasodilation with other vasodilators (eg, alcohol).

Minoxidil

Guanethidine	Severe orthostatic hypotension with guanethidine.

Nitroglycerin (Nitro-Bid, Nitro-Dur, Nitrolingual Spray, Nitrostat)

Calcium channel blockers	Orthostatic hypotension with calcium channel blockers.
Sildenafil	Severe hypotension with sildenafil.
Vasodilators	Additive vasodilation with other vasodilators (eg, alcohol).

VASODILATORS USED FOR ERECTILE DYSFUNCTION

Sildenafil (Revatio, Viagra)

α-blockers	Simultaneous administration with α-blockers may lead to symptomatic hypotension. Sildenafil dose should not exceed 25mg and should not be taken within 4 hrs of taking an α-blocker.
Amlodipine	Additional supine BP reduction with amlodipine reported.
CYP2C9 inhibitors	CYP2C9 inhibitors may decrease sildenafil clearance.
CYP3A4 inducers	Decreased levels with CYP3A4 inducers (eg, bosentan; more potent inducers such as barbiturates, carbamazepine, phenytoin, efavirenz, nevirapine, rifampin, rifabutin).
CYP3A4 inhibitors	Increased levels with CYP3A4 inhibitors (eg, cimetidine, ketoconazole, itraconazole, erythromycin, saquinavir).
ED drugs	Do not combine with other drugs used for erectile dysfunction.

VASODILATORS USED FOR ERECTILE DYSFUNCTION *(cont.)*

Sildenafil (Revatio, Viagra) *(cont.)*

Nitrates	Use with organic nitrates taken regularly and/or intermittently is contraindicated
Protease inhibitors	Increased levels with protease inhibitors (eg, ritonavir).
Vitamin K antagonists	Reports of bleeding (epistaxis) with vitamin K antagonists.

Tadalafil (Cialis)

α-blockers	Caution with α-blockers; may cause additive hypotensive effects.
Alcohol	Additive hypotensive effects with alcohol.
Antihypertensives	Additive hypotensive effects with antihypertensives (eg, amlodipine, metoprolol, bendrofluazide, enalapril, angiotensin II receptor blockers).
CYP3A4 inducers	Decreased levels with CYP3A4 inducers (eg, rifampin, carbamazepine, phenytoin, phenobarbital).
CYP3A4 inhibitors	Increased levels with CYP3A4 inhibitors (eg, ketoconazole, HIV protease inhibitors, erythromycin, itraconazole, grapefruit juice).
ED drugs	Do not combine with other drugs used for erectile dysfunction.

Vardenafil Hydrochloride (Levitra)

α-blockers	Avoid use with α-blockers.
Antiarrhythmics	Avoid use with Class IA (eg, quinidine, procainamide) or Class III (eg, amiodarone, sotalol) antiarrhythmics.
CYP3A4 inhibitors	Increased levels with CYP3A4 inhibitors (eg, ketoconazole, HIV protease inhibitors, erythromycin, itraconazole, grapefruit juice).
ED drugs	Do not combine with other drugs used for erectile dysfunction.
Nifedipine	May have additive hypotensive effect with nifedipine.
Nitrates	Avoid use with nitrates.

MISCELLANEOUS

Amyl Nitrite

Sildenafil	Potentiation of hypotensive effects with sildenafil.

Aspirin/Pravastatin Sodium (Pravigard PAC)

ACE inhibitors	Diminished hypotensive and hyponatremic effects of ACE inhibitors.
Acetazolamide	May increase levels of acetazolamide.
β-blockers	Decreased hypotensive effects of β-blockers.
Cholestyramine/ colestipol	Decreased levels with concomitant cholestyramine/colestipol; take 1 hr before or 4 hrs after resins.
Cyclosporine	Increases levels of cyclosporine.

Table 14.2: DRUG INTERACTIONS FOR CARDIOVASCULAR DRUGS *(cont.)*

MISCELLANEOUS *(cont.)*

Aspirin/Pravastatin Sodium (Pravigard PAC) *(cont.)*

Diuretics	Decreased diuretic effects with renal or cardiovascular disease.
Erythromycin	Erythromycin may increase risk of myopathy.
Fibrates	Avoid fibrates unless benefit outweighs risk.
Fibric acid derivatives	Fibric acid derivatives may increase risk of myopathy.
Gemfibrozil	Increased levels with gemfibrozil.
Heparin	Increased bleeding risk with heparin.
hypoglycemic agents	Increased effects of hypoglycemic agents.
Itraconazole	Increased levels with itraconazole.
Methotrexate	Decreased methotrexate clearance; increased risk of bone marrow toxicity.
Niacin	Niacin may increase risk of myopathy.
NSAIDs	Avoid NSAIDs.
Phenytoin	Decreased levels of phenytoin.
Steroids	Caution with drugs that decrease levels or activity of endogenous steroid hormones (eg, ketoconazole, spironolactone, cimetidine).
Uricosuric agents	Antagonizes uricosuric agents.
Valproic acid	May increase levels of valproic acid.
Warfarin	Increased bleeding risk with warfarin.

Bosentan (Tracleer)

Contraception	Do not rely on hormonal contraception alone.
Cyclosporine	Cyclosporine A increases levels.
CYP450 inhibitors	May decrease levels of drugs metabolized by CYP450 3A4 (eg, statins) and 2C9. CYP450 3A4 inhibitors (eg, ketoconazole) increase levels.
Glyburide	Glyburide increases risk of elevated LFTs.
Statin	May reduce statin efficacy; monitor cholesterol levels.

Digoxin (Digitek, Lanoxin, Lanoxin Pediatric)

Alprazolam	Increased serum levels with alprazolam; monitor for toxicity.
Amiodarone	Increased serum levels with amiodarone; monitor for toxicity.
Antacids	Decreased intestinal absorption with antacids.
Anticancer drugs	Decreased intestinal absorption with certain anticancer drugs.
β-blockers	Additive effects on AV node conduction with β-blockers.
Calcium	Increased risk of arrhythmias with calcium.

MISCELLANEOUS *(cont.)*

Digoxin (Digitek, Lanoxin, Lanoxin Pediatric) *(cont.)*

Calcium channel blockers	Additive effects on AV node conduction with calcium channel blockers.Additive effects on AV node conduction with calcium channel blockers.
Cholestyramine	Decreased intestinal absorption with cholestyramine.
Diphenoxylate	Increased absorption with diphenoxylate; monitor for toxicity.
Indomethacin	Increased serum levels with indomethacin; monitor for toxicity.
Itraconazole	Increased serum levels with itraconazole; monitor for toxicity.
K⁺-depleting diuretics	Risk of toxicity with K⁺-depleting diuretics.
Kaolin-pectin	Decreased intestinal absorption with kaolin-pectin.
Macrolides	Increased absorption with macrolides; monitor for toxicity.
Metoclopramide	Decreased intestinal absorption with metoclopramide.
Neomycin	Decreased intestinal absorption with neomycin.
Propafenone	Increased serum levels with propafenone; monitor for toxicity.
Propantheline	Increased absorption with propantheline; monitor for toxicity.
Quinidine	Increased serum levels with quinidine; monitor for toxicity.
Rifampin	Decreased serum levels with rifampin.
Spironolactone	Increased serum levels with spironolactone; monitor for toxicity.
Succinylcholine	Increased risk of arrhythmias with succinylcholine.
Sulfasalazine	Decreased intestinal absorption with sulfasalazine.
Sympathomimetics	Increased risk of arrhythmias with sympathomimetics.
Tetracycline	Increased absorption with tetracycline; monitor for toxicity.
Thyroid supplements	Increased digoxin dose requirement with thyroid supplements.
Verapamil	Increased serum levels with verapamil; monitor for toxicity.

Enalapril Maleate/Felodipine (Lexxel)

Anticonvulsants	Levels decreased with long-term anticonvulsant therapy.
Antihypertensives	Augmented effect by antihypertensives that cause renin release (eg, diuretics).
CYP3A4 inhibitors	CYP3A4 inhibitors (eg, itraconazole, ketoconazole, erythromycin, grapefruit juice, cimetidine) may increase plasma levels.
Diuretics	Hypotension risk with diuretics.
Food	Peak levels doubled and trough levels halved when taken with food.
K⁺-sparing diuretics	Risk of hyperkalemia with K⁺-sparing diuretics, K⁺-containing salt substitutes, or K⁺ supplements.

Table 14.2: DRUG INTERACTIONS FOR CARDIOVASCULAR DRUGS *(cont.)*

MISCELLANEOUS *(cont.)*

Enalapril Maleate/Felodipine (Lexxel) *(cont.)*

Lithium	May increase lithium levels.
Metoprolol	May increase metoprolol levels.
NSAIDs	May further decrease renal function with NSAIDs.

Epoprostenol Sodium (Flolan)

Antihypertensives	Potentiates BP reduction with antihypertensives.
Anticoagulants	Increased risk of bleeding with anticoagulants.
Antiplatelets	Increased risk of bleeding with antiplatelets.
Diuretics	Potentiates BP reduction with diuretics.
Vasodilators	Potentiates BP reduction with vasodilators.

Fenoldopam Mesylate (Corlopam)

β-blockers	Avoid β-blockers; unexpected hypotension may occur.

Methyldopa/Hydrochlorothiazide (Aldoril 25)

ACTH	ACTH deplete electrolytes.
Alcohol	Potentiates orthostatic hypotension with alcohol.
Anesthetics	Anesthetics may need dose reduction.
Antidiabetics	Adjust antidiabetic drugs.
Antihypertensives	May potentiate nondepolarizing antihypertensives.
Antihypertensives	May potentiate other antihypertensives.
Barbiturates	Potentiates orthostatic hypotension with barbiturates.
Cholestyramine/ Colestipol	Reduced absorption with cholestyramine, colestipol.
Corticosteroids	Corticosteroids deplete electrolytes.
Iron	Ferrous sulfate and ferrous gluconate decrease bioavailability; avoid coadministration.
Lithium	Risk of lithium toxicity.
MAOIs	Avoid MAOIs.
Muscle relaxants	May potentiate nondepolarizing skeletal muscle relaxants.
Narcotics	Potentiates orthostatic hypotension with narcotics.
NSAIDs	NSAIDs decrease diuretic effects.
Pressor amines	May decrease response to pressor amines.

Mecamylamine Hydrochloride (Inversine)

Alcohol	Alcohol may potentiate effect.
Anesthesia	Anesthesia may potentiate effect.

MISCELLANEOUS *(cont.)*
Mecamylamine Hydrochloride (Inversine) *(cont.)*

Antibiotics	Avoid with antibiotics.
Antihypertensives	Other antihypertensives may potentiate effect.
Sulfonamides	Avoid with sulfonamides.

Metyrosine (Demser)

CNS depressants	Additive sedative effects with alcohol and other CNS depressants (eg, hypnotics, sedatives, tranquilizers).
Haloperidol	May potentiate EPS with haloperidol.
Phenothiazines	May potentiate EPS with phenothiazines.

Nesiritide (Natrecor)

ACE inhibitors	Increased risk of hypotension with drugs that cause hypotension such as oral ACE inhibitors.
Heparin	Do not co-administer through the same IV catheter with heparin. Flush catheter between uses with incompatible drugs.
Insulin	Do not co-administer through the same IV catheter with insulin. Flush catheter between uses with incompatible drugs.
Ethacrynate sodium	Do not co-administer through the same IV catheter with ethacrynate sodium. Flush catheter between uses with incompatible drugs.
Bumetamide	Do not co-administer through the same IV catheter with bumetamide. Flush catheter between uses with incompatible drugs.
Enalaprilat	Do not co-administer through the same IV catheter with enalaprilat. Flush catheter between uses with incompatible drugs.
Hydralazine	Do not co-administer through the same IV catheter with hydralazine. Flush catheter between uses with incompatible drugs.

Polythiazide/Prazosin Hydrochloride (Minizide)

Antihypertensives	Additive effects with other antihypertensives.
Adrenergic blockers	Potentiation with ganglionic or peripheral adrenergic blockers.
Narcotics	Potentiates orthostatic hypotension with narcotics.
ACTH	Increased risk of hypokalemia with ACTH.
Tubocurarine	May increase responsiveness to tubocurarine.
Alcohol	Potentiates orthostatic hypotension with alcohol.
Barbiturates	Potentiates orthostatic hypotension with barbiturates.
Insulin	May alter insulin requirements.
Corticosteroids	Increased risk of hypokalemia with corticosteroids.
Norepinephrine	May decrease arterial responsiveness to norepinephrine.

Table 14.2: DRUG INTERACTIONS FOR CARDIOVASCULAR DRUGS *(cont.)*

MISCELLANEOUS *(cont.)*

Reserpine

Antihypertensives	Titrate carefully with other antihypertensives.
Digoxin	Risk of arrhythmia with digoxin.
MAOIs	Avoid MAOIs or use extreme caution.
Quinidine	Risk of arrhythmia with quinidine.
Sympathomimetics	Prolonged effect of direct-acting sympathomimetics (eg, epinephrine, isoproterenol). May inhibit effects of indirect-acting sympathomimetics (eg, ephedrine, tyramine).
TCAs	Decreased effect with TCAs.

CHOLESTEROL-LOWERING DRUGS

BILE ACID SEQUESTRANTS

Cholestyramine (Questran, Questran Light)

Digitalis	May reduce or delay absorption of digitalis.
Diuretics	May reduce or delay absorption of thiazide diuretics.
Estrogens	May reduce or delay absorption of estrogens.
HMG-CoA reductase inhibitors	Additive effects with HMG-CoA reductase inhibitors.
Nicotinic acid	Additive effects with nicotinic acid.
Penicillin G	May reduce or delay absorption of penicillin G.
Phenobarbital	May reduce or delay absorption of phenobarbital.
Phenylbutazone	May reduce or delay absorption of phenylbutazone.
Progestins	May reduce or delay absorption of progestins.
Propranolol	May reduce or delay absorption of propranolol.
Spironolactone	Caution with spironolactone.
Tetracycline	May reduce or delay absorption of tetracycline.
Thyroid agents	May reduce or delay absorption of thyroid and thyroxine agents.
Vitamins (fat-soluble)	May interfere with absorption of fat-soluble vitamins (A, D, E, K), drugs that undergo enterohepatic circulation, and oral phosphate supplements.
Warfarin	May reduce or delay absorption of warfarin.

Colesevelam Hydrochloride (WelChol)

Verapamil	Decreases levels of sustained-release verapamil.

Colestipol Hydrochloride (Colestid)

Chlorothiazide	Reduces absorption of chlorothiazide.
Digitalis	Caution with digitalis agents.

BILE ACID SEQUESTRANTS *(cont.)*

Colestipol Hydrochloride (Colestid) *(cont.)*

Folic acid	May interfere with absorption of folic acid.
Furosemide	Reduces absorption of furosemide.
Gemfibrozil	Reduces absorption of gemfibrozil.
Hydrochlorothiazide	Reduces absorption of hydrochlorothiazide.
Hydrocortisone	May interfere with absorption of hydrocortisone.
Oral drugs	May delay or reduce absorption of concomitant oral medication; take other drugs 1 hr before or 4 hrs after colestipol.
Penicillin G	May reduce or delay absorption of penicillin G.
Phosphate	May interfere with absorption of oral phosphate supplements.
Propranolol	Caution with propranolol.
Tetracycline	Reduces absorption of tetracycline.
Vitamins (fat soluble)	May interfere with absorption of fat soluble vitamins (eg, A, D, K).

FIBRIC ACID DERIVATIVES

Fenofibrate (Tricor, Triglide, Antara)

Anticoagulant	Potentiates coumarin anticoagulants; reduce anticoagulant dose and monitor PT/INR.
Bile acid sequestrants	Bile acid sequestrants may impede absorption; take at least 1 hr before or 4-6 hrs after the resin.
HMG-CoA reductase inhibitors	Avoid HMG-CoA reductase inhibitors unless benefits outweigh risks.
Nephrotoxic agents	Evaluate benefits/risks with immunosuppressants (eg, cyclosporine) and other nephrotoxic agents.

Gemfibrozil (Lopid)

Anticoagulant	Potentiates coumarin anticoagulants; reduce anticoagulant dose and monitor PT/INR.
HMG-CoA reductase inhibitors	Increased risk of myopathy and rhabdomyolysis with HMG-CoA reductase inhibitors. Avoid unless benefits outweigh risks.
Repaglinide	Avoid initiating therapy with repaglinide. If already on repaglinide therapy, monitor levels and adjust repaglinide dose.
Itraconazole	Avoid itraconazole in patients taking gemfibrozil and repaglinide.

HMG-CoA REDUCTASE INHIBITORS

Atorvastatin Calcium (Lipitor)

Antifungals, azole	Azole antifungals may increase risk of myopathy.
Colestipol	Colestipol decreases levels when coadministered, but greater LDL-C reduction with coadministration than when each given alone.

Table 14.2: DRUG INTERACTIONS FOR CARDIOVASCULAR DRUGS *(cont.)*

HMG-CoA Reductase Inhibitors *(cont.)*

Atorvastatin Calcium (Lipitor) *(cont.)*

Contraceptives, oral	Increases levels of oral contraceptives (norethindrone, ethinyl estradiol).
Cyclosporine	Cyclosporine may increase risk of myopathy.
Digoxin	Increases levels of digoxin. Monitor digoxin.
Erythromycin	Erythromycin may increase risk of myopathy.
Fibrates	Avoid fibrates.
Fibric acid derivatives	Fibric acid derivatives may increase risk of myopathy.
Maalox	Decreases levels with Maalox TC, but LDL-C reduction not altered.
Niacin	Niacin may increase risk of myopathy.
Steroid hormones	Caution with drugs that decrease levels or activity of endogenous steroid hormones (eg, ketoconazole, spironolactone, cimetidine).

Fluvastatin Sodium (Lescol, Lescol XL)

Anticoagulants	Monitor anticoagulants.
Cholestyramine	Cholestyramine given within 4 hrs decreases serum levels but has additive effects when given 4 hrs after fluvastatin (immediate-release).
Cimetidine	Increase serum levels with cimetidine.
Diclofenac	Increases levels of diclofenac.
Digoxin	Monitor digoxin.
Erythromycin	Erythromycin may increase risk of myopathy.
Fibrates	Avoid fibrates.
Fibric acid derivatives	Fibric acid derivatives may increase risk of myopathy.
Glyburide	Increases levels of glyburide.
Niacin	Niacin may increase risk of myopathy.
Omeprazole	Increase serum levels with omeprazole.
Phenytoin	Increases levels of phenytoin.
Ranitidine	Increase serum levels with ranitidine.
Rifampicin	Rifampicin significantly decreases serum levels.
Steroid hormones	Caution with drugs that decrease levels or activity of endogenous steroid hormones (eg, ketoconazole, spironolactone, cimetidine).

Lovastatin (Altoprev, Mevacor)

Anticoagulants	Monitor anticoagulants.
CYP3A4 inhibitors	Increased risk of myopathy with CYP3A4 inhibitors (eg, cyclosporine, itraconazole, ketoconazole, erythromycin, clarithromycin, telithromycin, protease inhibitors, nefazodone, >1 quart/day of grapefruit juice).

HMG-CoA Reductase Inhibitors *(cont.)*

Lovastatin (Altoprev, Mevacor) *(cont.)*

Steroid hormones	Caution with drugs that decrease levels or activity of endogenous steroid hormones (eg, ketoconazole, spironolactone, cimetidine).

Pravastatin Sodium (Pravachol)

Cholestyramine/ colestipol	Decreased levels with concomitant cholestyramine/colestipol; take 1 hr before or 4 hrs after resins.
Cyclosporine	Risk of myopathy with cyclosporine.
Erythromycin	Erythromycin may increase risk of myopathy.
Fibric acid derivatives	Fibric acid derivatives may increase risk of myopathy. Avoid unless benefit outweighs drug combination risk.
Gemfibrozil	Increased levels with gemfibrozil.
Itraconazole	Increased levels with itraconazole.
Niacin	Niacin may increase risk of myopathy.
Steroid hormones	Caution with drugs that decrease levels or activity of endogenous steroid hormones (eg, ketoconazole, spironolactone, cimetidine).

Rosuvastatin Calcium (Crestor)

Antacid	Space antacid dosing by 2 hours.
Contraceptives, oral	Increases levels of oral contraceptives (norgestrel, ethinyl estradiol).
Cyclosporine	Risk of myopathy with cyclosporine.
Fibric acid derivatives	Fibric acid derivatives may increase risk of myopathy. Avoid unless benefit outweighs drug combination risk.
Gemfibrozil	Increased levels with gemfibrozil.
Niacin	Niacin may increase risk of myopathy.
Steroid hormones	Caution with drugs that decrease levels or activity of endogenous steroid hormones (eg, ketoconazole, spironolactone, cimetidine).
Warfarin	Increases INR with warfarin.

Simvastatin (Zocor)

Amiodarone	Max 20mg/day with amiodarone.
Clarithromycin	Avoid use with concomitant clarithromycin increased risk of myopathy/rhabdomyolysis.
Cyclosporin	Max 10mg/day with cyclosporin.
Danazol	Max 10mg/day with danazol.
Digoxin	Monitor digoxin.
Erythromycin	Avoid use with concomitant erythromycin, increased risk of myopathy/rhabdomyolysis.
Gemfibrozil	Max 10mg/day with gemfibrozil.

Table 14.2: DRUG INTERACTIONS FOR CARDIOVASCULAR DRUGS *(cont.)*

HMG-CoA Reductase Inhibitors *(cont.)*

Simvastatin (Zocor) *(cont.)*

Grapefruit juice	Avoid use with concomitant grapefruit juice (>1quart/day); increased risk of myopathy/rhabdomyolysis.
Itraconazole	Avoid use with concomitant itraconazole increased risk of myopathy/rhabdomyolysis.
Ketoconazole	Avoid use with concomitant ketoconazole increased risk of myopathy/rhabdomyolysis.
Nefazodone	Avoid use with concomitant nefazodone, increased risk of myopathy/rhabdomyolysis.
Niacin	Caution with other fibrates, ≥1g/day of niacin.
Protease inhibitors	Avoid use with concomitant HIV protease inhibitors, increased risk of myopathy/rhabdomyolysis.
Telithromycin	Avoid use with concomitant telithromycin, increased risk of myopathy/rhabdomyolysis.
Verapamil	Max 20mg/day with verapamil.
Warfarin	Monitor warfarin.

MISCELLANEOUS CHOLESTEROL-LOWERING DRUGS

Ezetimibe (Zetia)

Cholestyramine	Incremental LDL-C reduction may be reduced with concomitant cholestyramine.
Fibrates	Fibrates may increase cholesterol excretion into the bile; concurrent use is not recommended.
Fenofibrate	Increased levels with fenofibrate.
Gemfibrozil	Increased levels with gemfibrozil.
Cyclosporine	Monitor cyclosporine levels with concomitant use.
Warfarin	Monitor INR when administered with warfarin.

Ezetimibe/Simvastatin (Vytorin)

Itraconazole	Avoid use with concomitant itraconazole increased risk of myopathy/rhabdomyolysis.
Amiodarone	Max 10/20mg daily with amiodarone.
Cholestyramine	Incremental LDL-C reductions with concomitant cholestyramine.
Clarithromycin	Avoid use with concomitant clarithromycin increased risk of myopathy/rhabdomyolysis.
Cyclosporin	Max 10/10mg daily with cyclosporin.
Danazol	Max 10/10mg daily with danazol.
Digoxin	Monitor digoxin.
Erythromycin	Avoid use with concomitant erythromycin, increased risk of myopathy/rhabdomyolysis.
Gemfibrozil	Max 10/10mg daily with gemfibrozil.
Grapefruit juice	Avoid use with concomitant grapefruit juice (>1 quart/day); increased risk of myopathy/rhabdomyolysis.

MISCELLANEOUS CHOLESTEROL-LOWERING DRUGS *(cont.)*

Ezetimibe/Simvastatin (Vytorin) *(cont.)*

Ketoconazole	Avoid use with concomitant ketoconazole increased risk of myopathy/rhabdomyolysis.
Nefazodone	Avoid use with concomitant nefazodone, increased risk of myopathy/rhabdomyolysis.
Niacin	Caution with other fibrates, ≥1g/day of niacin.
Protease inhibitors	Avoid use with concomitant HIV protease inhibitors, increased risk of myopathy/rhabdomyolysis.
Telithromycin	Avoid use with concomitant telithromycin, increased risk of myopathy/rhabdomyolysis.
Verapamil	Max 10/20mg daily with verapamil.
Warfarin	Monitor warfarin.

Lovastatin/Niacin (Advicor)

Adrenergic blockers	Caution with acute MI adrenergic blockers.
Alcohol	Avoid concomitant alcohol and hot drinks; may increase flushing and pruritus.
Antidiabetic	Antidiabetic agents may need adjustment.
ASA	Decreased niacin clearance with ASA.
Bile acid sequestrants	Separate bile acid sequestrants by 4-6 hrs
Calcium channel blockers	Caution with acute MI calcium channel blockers.
CYP3A4 inhibitors	Increased risk of skeletal muscle disorders with CYP3A4 inhibitors (eg, cyclosporine, itraconazole, ketoconazole, erythromycin, clarithromycin, protease inhibitors, nefazodone, >1 quart/day of grapefruit juice), verapamil, fibrates (eg, gemfibrozil).
Ganglionic blockers	May potentiate ganglionic blockers.
Niacin	Caution with niacin-containing nutritional supplements.
Nitrates	Caution with acute MI and nitrates.
Steroid hormones	Caution with drugs that decrease levels or activity of endogenous steroid hormones (eg, ketoconazole, spironolactone, cimetidine).
Vasoactive drugs	May potentiate vasoactive drugs.
Warfarin	Monitor warfarin.

Niacin (Niaspan, Niacor)

Alcohol	Avoid concomitant alcohol and hot drinks; may increase flushing and pruritus.
Antidiabetic	Antidiabetic agents may need adjustment.
HMG-CoA reductase inhibitors	Rhabdomyolysis may occur with HMG-CoA reductase inhibitors.
Antihypertensives	May potentiate antihypertensives (eg, ganglionic blockers, vasoactive drugs).
Bile acid	Separate dosing from bile acid resins by at least 4-6 hrs.

Table 14.2: DRUG INTERACTIONS FOR CARDIOVASCULAR DRUGS *(cont.)*

MISCELLANEOUS CHOLESTEROL-LOWERING DRUGS *(cont.)*

Niacin (Niaspan, Niacor) *(cont.)*

Anticoagulants	Caution with anticoagulants.
Niacin	High dose niacin or nicotinamide may potentiate adverse effects.

DIURETICS

CARBONIC ANHYDRASE INHIBITORS

Acetazolamide (Diamoz Sequels)

Amphetamine	Increased effects of amphetamine.
Aspirin	Caution with high-dose aspirin.
Carbonic anhydrase inhibitors	Increased effects of other carbonic anhydrase inhibitors.
Cyclosporine	Increased levels of cyclosporine.
Folic acid antagonists	Increased effects of folic acid antagonists.
Lithium	Decreased levels of lithium.
Methenamine	May prevent urinary antiseptic effect of methenamine.
Phenytoin	Increased phenytoin levels; may increase occurrence of osteomalacia.
Primidone	Decreased levels of primidone.
Quinidine	Increased effects of quinidine.
Sodium bicarbonate	Increased risk of renal calculus formation with sodium bicarbonate.

LOOP DIURETICS

Bumetanide (Bumex)

Aminoglycosides	Avoid aminoglycosides.
Antihypertensives	Potentiates antihypertensives.
Indomethacin	Avoid concomitant indomethacin.
Lithium	May cause lithium toxicity.
Nephrotoxic drugs	Avoid nephrotoxic drugs.
Ototoxic drugs	Avoid ototoxic drugs.
Probenecid	Probenecid reduces effects.

Ethacrynate Sodium (Edecrin Sodium)

Aminoglycosides	May increase ototoxic potential of aminoglycosides.
Antihypertensives	Orthostatic hypotension may occur with antihypertensives.
Cephalosporins	May increase ototoxic potential of some cephalosporins.
Corticosteroids	Increased risk of gastric hemorrhage with corticosteroids.

LOOP DIURETICS *(cont.)*

Ethacrynate Sodium (Edecrin Sodium) *(cont.)*

Digitalis	Excessive K+ loss may precipitate digitalis toxicity.
K+-depleting steroids	Excessive K+ loss may precipitate digitalis toxicity. Caution with K+-depleting steroids.
Lithium	Risk of lithium toxicity.
NSAIDs	NSAIDs may decrease effects.
Warfarin	Displaces warfarin from plasma protein; may need dose reduction.

Ethacrynic Acid (Edecrin)

Aminoglycosides	May increase ototoxic potential of aminoglycosides.
Antihypertensives	Orthostatic hypotension may occur with antihypertensives.
Cephalosporins	May increase ototoxic potential of some cephalosporins.
Corticosteroids	Increased risk of gastric hemorrhage with corticosteroids.
Digitalis	Excessive K+-loss may precipitate digitalis toxicity.
K+-depleting steroids	Excessive K+-loss may precipitate digitalis toxicity. Caution with K+-depleting steroids.
Lithium	Risk of lithium toxicity.
NSAIDs	NSAIDs may decrease effects.
Warfarin	Displaces warfarin from plasma protein; may need dose reduction.

Furosemide (Lasix)

ACTH	Hypokalemia with ACTH.
Alcohol	Orthostatic hypotension may be aggravated by alcohol.
Aminoglycosides	Ototoxicity with aminoglycosides.
Antihypertensives	Potentiates antihypertensives.
Barbiturates	Orthostatic hypotension may be aggravated by barbiturates.
Corticosteroids	Hypokalemia with corticosteroids.
Ethacrynic acid	Ototoxicity with ethacrynic acid.
Ganglionic adrenergic blockers	Potentiates ganglionic adrenergic blockers.
Indomethacin	Indomethacin may decrease effects.
Lithium	Risk of lithium toxicity.
Narcotics	Orthostatic hypotension may be aggravated by narcotics.
Norepinephrine	Decreases arterial response to norepinephrine.
NSAIDs	Renal changes with NSAIDs.
Peripheral adrenergic blockers	Potentiates peripheral adrenergic blockers.

Table 14.2: DRUG INTERACTIONS FOR CARDIOVASCULAR DRUGS (cont.)

LOOP DIURETICS (cont.)

Furosemide (Lasix) (cont.)

Salicylates	Caution with high dose salicylates.
Succinylcholine	Potentiates succinylcholine.
Sucralfate	Separate sucralfate dose by 2 hrs.
Tubocurarine	Antagonizes tubocurarine.

Torsemide (Demadex)

ACTH	Risk of hypokalemia with ACTH.
Aminoglycosides	Caution with high dose aminoglycosides.
Cholestyramine	Avoid simultaneous cholestyramine administration.
Corticosteroids	Risk of hypokalemia with corticosteroids.
Indomethacin	Indomethacin partially inhibits natriuretic effect.
Lithium	Risk of lithium toxicity.
NSAIDs	Possible renal dysfunction with NSAIDs.
Probenecid	Probenecid decreases effects.
Salicylates	Caution with high dose salicylates.
Spironolactone	Reduces spironolactone clearance.

POTASSIUM-SPARING DIURETICS

Amiloride Hydrochloride (Midamor)

ACE inhibitors	Increased risk of hyperkalemia with ACE inhibitors.
Angiotensin II receptor antagonists	Increased risk of hyperkalemia with angiotensin II receptor antagonists.
Cyclosporine	Increased risk of hyperkalemia with cyclosporine.
Diuretics	Hyponatremia and hypochloremia with other diuretics.
Indomethacin	Increased risk of hyperkalemia with indomethacin.
Lithium	Risk of lithium toxicity.
NSAIDs	Decreased effects with NSAIDs.
Tacrolimus	Increased risk of hyperkalemia with tacrolimus.

Spironolactone (Aldactone)

ACE inhibitors	Risk of hyperkalemia with ACE inhibitors.
ACTH	ACTH may intensify electrolyte depletion.
Alcohol	Alcohol potentiate orthostatic hypotension.

POTASSIUM-SPARING DIURETICS *(cont.)*

Spironolactone (Aldactone)

Barbiturates	Barbiturates potentiate orthostatic hypotension.
Corticosteroids	Corticosteroids may intensify electrolyte depletion.
Digoxin	Risk of digoxin toxicity.
K^+-sparing diuretics	Risk of hyperkalemia with K^+-sparing diuretics.
K^+ supplements	Risk of hyperkalemia with K^+ supplements.
Lithium	Risk of lithium toxicity.
Narcotics	Narcotics potentiate orthostatic hypotension.
Nondepolarizing skeletal muscle relaxants	Increased response to nondepolarizing skeletal muscle relaxants.
Norepinephrine	Reduced vascular response to norepinephrine.
NSAIDs	Risk of hyperkalemia with NSAIDs. NSAIDs may reduce effects.

Triamterene (Dyrenium)

ACE inhibitors	Increased risk of hyperkalemia with ACE inhibitors.
Anesthetics	May potentiate anesthetics.
Antidiabetic agents	May cause hyperglycemia; adjust antidiabetic agents.
Antihypertensives	May potentiate antihypertensives.
Blood from blood bank	Avoid blood from a blood bank; may potentiate serum K^+ levels.
Chlorpropamide	Chlorpropamide may increase risk of severe hyponatremia.
Diuretics	May potentiate diuretics.
Indomethacin	Indomethacin may cause renal failure.
K^+-containing agents	Avoid K^+-containing agents; may potentiate serum K^+ levels.
K^+-sparing diuretics	Avoid K^+-sparing diuretics; may potentiate serum K^+ levels.
K^+ supplements	Avoid K^+ supplements; may potentiate serum K^+ levels.
Lithium	Risk of lithium toxicity.
Low-salt milk	Avoid low-salt milk; may potentiate serum K^+ levels.
Nondepolarizing muscle relaxants	May potentiate nondepolarizing muscle relaxants.
NSAIDs	Caution with NSAIDs.
Preanesthetics	May potentiate preanesthetics.
Salt substitutes	Avoid salt substitutes; may potentiate serum K^+ levels.

Table 14.2: DRUG INTERACTIONS FOR CARDIOVASCULAR DRUGS *(cont.)*

THIAZIDE DIURETICS

Chlorothiazide (Diuril)

ACTH	ACTH increases electrolyte depletion.
Alcohol	May potentiate orthostatic hypotension with alcohol.
Antidiabetic drugs	Adjust antidiabetic drugs.
Antihypertensives	May potentiate antihypertensives.
Barbiturates	May potentiate orthostatic hypotension barbiturates.
Cholestyramine	Decreased PO absorption with cholestyramine.
Colestipol	Decreased PO absorption with colestipol.
Corticosteroids	Corticosteroids increase electrolyte depletion.
Lithium	Risk of lithium toxicity.
Narcotics	May potentiate orthostatic hypotension with narcotics.
Nondepolarizing skeletal muscle relaxants	May potentiate nondepolarizing skeletal muscle relaxants.
NSAIDs	NSAIDs decrease effects.
Pressor amines	Possible decreased response to pressor amines.

Chlorthalidone (Thalitone)

Alcohol	Orthostatic hypotension aggravated by alcohol.
Antidiabetic agents	Antidiabetic agents may need adjustment.
Antihypertensive drugs	Potentiates action of other antihypertensive drugs.
Barbiturates	Orthostatic hypotension aggravated by barbiturates.
Lithium	Risk of lithium toxicity.
Narcotics	Orthostatic hypotension aggravated by narcotics.
Norepinephrine	May decrease arterial effectiveness of norepinephrine.
Tubocurarine	May increase responsiveness to tubocurarine.

Indapamide (Lozol)

ACTH	Increases risk of hypokalemia with ACTH.
Antidiabetic agents	Antidiabetic agents may need adjustment.
Antihypertensives	May potentiate other antihypertensives.
Corticosteroids	Increases risk of hypokalemia with corticosteroids.
Lithium	Risk of lithium toxicity.
Norepinephrine	May decrease arterial responsiveness to norepinephrine.

THIAZIDE DIURETICS *(cont.)*

Metolazone (Zaroxolyn)

ACTH	ACTH increases hypokalemia and salt and water retention.
Alcohol	Potentiates hypotensive effects of alcohol.
Anticoagulants	Adjust anticoagulants.
Antidiabetics	Adjust antidiabetics.
Antihypertensives	Adjust dose of other antihypertensives.
Barbiturates	Potentiates hypotensive effects of barbiturates.
Corticosteroids	Corticosteroids increase hypokalemia and salt and water retention.
Curariform drugs	Enhanced neuromuscular blocking effects of curariform drugs.
Digitalis	Digitalis toxicity.
Furosemide	Furosemide prolongs fluid and electrolyte loss.
Lithium	Risk of lithium toxicity.
Loop diuretics	Loop diuretics prolong fluid and electrolyte loss.
Methenamine	Decrease in methenamine efficacy.
Narcotics	Potentiates hypotensive effects of narcotics.
Norepinephrine	Decreased arterial response to norepinephrine.
NSAIDs	NSAIDs decrease effects.
Salicylates	Salicylates decrease effects.

COMBINATIONS

Amiloride Hydrochloride/Hydrochlorothiazide (Moduretic 5-50)

ACE inhibitors	Increased risk of hyperkalemia with ACE inhibitors.
ACTH	ACTH intensifies electrolyte depletion.
Alcohol	Alcohol may potentiate orthostatic hypotension.
Angiotensin II receptor antagonists	Increased risk of hyperkalemia with angiotensin II receptor antagonists.
Antidiabetic	Antidiabetic agents may need adjustment.
Antihypertensives	May potentiate other antihypertensives.
Barbiturates	Barbiturates may potentiate orthostatic hypotension.
Cholestyramine	Cholestyramine impairs absorption.
Colestipol	Colestipol impairs absorption.
Corticosteroids	Corticosteroids intensify electrolyte depletion.

Table 14.2: DRUG INTERACTIONS FOR CARDIOVASCULAR DRUGS *(cont.)*

COMBINATIONS *(cont.)*

Amiloride Hydrochloride/Hydrochlorothiazide (Moduretic 5-50) *(cont.)*

Cyclosporine	Increased risk of hyperkalemia with cyclosporine.
Indomethacin	Increased risk of hyperkalemia with indomethacin.
Lithium	Risk of lithium toxicity.
Narcotics	Narcotics may potentiate orthostatic hypotension.
Nondepolarizing muscle relaxants	Increased response to nondepolarizing muscle relaxants.
Norepinephrine	May decrease response to norepinephrine.
NSAIDs	NSAIDs may decrease effects.
Tacrolimus	Increased risk of hyperkalemia with tacrolimus.

Hydrochlorothiazide/Spironolactone (Aldactazide)

ACTH	ACTH may intensify electrolyte depletion.
ACE inhibitors	ACE inhibitors potentiate orthostatic hypotension. Risk of hyperkalemia with ACE inhibitors.
Alcohol	Alcohol potentiates orthostatic hypotension.
Antidiabetic	Antidiabetic agents may need adjustment.
Barbiturates	Barbiturates potentiate orthostatic hypotension.
Corticosteroids	Corticosteroids may intensify electrolyte depletion.
Digoxin	Risk of digoxin toxicity.
K^+-sparing diuretics	Risk of hyperkalemia with K^+-sparing diuretics.
K^+-supplements	Risk of hyperkalemia with K^+-supplements.
Lithium	Risk of lithium toxicity.
Narcotics	Narcotics potentiate orthostatic hypotension.
Nondepolarizing skeletal muscle relaxants	Increased response to nondepolarizing skeletal muscle relaxants.
Norepinephrine	Reduced vascular response to norepinephrine.
NSAIDs	NSAIDs may reduce effects. Risk of hyperkalemia with NSAIDs.

Hydrochlorothiazide/Triamterene (Dyazide, Maxzide)

ACTH	ACTH intensifies electrolyte depletion.
ACE inhibitors	Hyperkalemia risk with ACE inhibitors.
Alcohol	Alcohol may potentiate orthostatic hypotension.
Amphotericin B	Amphotericin B intensifies electrolyte depletion.
Anticoagulants drugs	Adjust oral anticoagulants.

COMBINATIONS *(cont.)*

Hydrochlorothiazide/Triamterene (Dyazide, Maxzide) *(cont.)*

Antidiabetic drugs	Adjust antidiabetic drugs.
Antigout drugs	Adjust antigout drugs.
Antihypertensives	Increases effects of antihypertensives.
Barbiturates	Barbiturates may potentiate orthostatic hypotension.
Blood from blood bank	Hyperkalemia risk with blood from blood bank.
Chlorpropamide	Increased risk of hyponatremia with chlorpropamide.
Corticosteroids	Corticosteroids intensify electrolyte depletion.
Indomethacin	Indomethacin may cause renal failure.
Insulin	May alter insulin requirements.
K^+-containing agents	Hyperkalemia risk with K^+-containing agents (eg, parenteral penicillin G potassium).
Laxatives	Overuse of laxatives reduces K^+ levels.
Lithium	Risk of lithium toxicity.
Low-salt milk	Hyperkalemia risk with low-salt milk.
Methenamine	Reduces methenamine effects.
Narcotics	Narcotics may potentiate orthostatic hypotension.
Nondepolarizing muscle relaxants	Increases effects of nondepolarizing muscle relaxants.
Norepinephrine	May decrease arterial responsiveness to norepinephrine.
NSAIDs	Possible renal dysfunction with NSAIDs.
Salt substitutes	Hyperkalemia risk with salt substitutes.
Sodium polystyrene sulfonate	Overuse of sodium polystyrene sulfonate reduces K^+ levels. of sodium polystyrene sulfonate reduces K^+ levels.
Tubocurarine	May increase responsiveness to tubocurarine.

Chapter 15

Respiratory Drugs

Martha Somerman, D.D.S., Ph.D.

A significant number of people in the general population have respiratory disorders that require the use of medications. Bronchial asthma is the most common respiratory disease the dentist encounters; therefore, he or she should be particularly familiar with drugs taken by patients with such conditions.

Asthma is characterized physiologically by reversible airway obstruction that results from constriction of the bronchial and bronchiolar muscles and hypersecretion of viscous mucus. Factors that can precipitate an asthmatic attack include respiratory infection, physical exertion, exposure to cold air or irritating gases, allergy and stress.

There are three major approaches to the treatment of asthma:

- use of anti-inflammatory drugs (and more recently, diet-related products) to reduce symptoms and bronchial hyperactivity;
- use of agents that reverse or inhibit bronchoconstriction;
- avoidance of causative factors.

Causative factors include indoor allergens and stress; thus, the dentist must be sensitive to the possibility of these factors provoking an asthmatic attack in a susceptible person while he or she is in the dental office. If a patient is using metered-dose inhalants, these inhalants should be readily accessible at his or her dental appointment.

The information in this chapter will provide summary data on special dental considerations for, use of, interactions of, adverse effects of and contraindications for drugs taken by and potentially given to people who have respiratory conditions.

When treating a patient with a respiratory condition, the dentist must determine the nature of the condition and which, if any, drugs the patient is taking for these conditions. The American Society of Anesthesiologists classification of asthma is provided in Table 15.1.

Corticosteroids are covered in more detail in Chapter 5, while β-blockers are covered in Chapter 14.

Tables 15.2 and 15.3 provide general information on drugs used for respiratory diseases, including typical dosage ranges and interactions with other drugs.

Special Dental Considerations

When it comes to treating patients with respiratory conditions, practitioners should keep the following important points in mind.

First, chronic obstructive pulmonary disease (COPD) is a respiratory disease of major medical concern; bronchial obstruction in this disease is irreversible, resulting in severe infections, heart disease and respiratory failure. Respiratory conditions and the use of inhalants can result in decreased salivary flow and associated problems, including caries and candidiasis. Therefore, patients should use fluoride rinses and should be observed for the need to use antifungal agents.

Reduction of stress may require the use of sedatives, especially when complex procedures are being performed. Stress reduction methods, including medications, may be required to prevent an asthmatic attack.

NSAIDs and aspirin are contraindicated in patients with respiratory conditions, as they may prompt an asthmatic attack.

A semisupine chair position should be used for patients with respiratory diseases, especially for patients with COPD. To prevent orthostatic hypotension, patients should sit upright for a few minutes before being dismissed.

Inhalants that patients are using should be easily accessible during the dental appointment.

With patients receiving chronic steroid therapy, there is an enhanced concern about stress situations—such as the possibility of adrenal crisis—as well as increased susceptibility to infections.

With patients using β-adrenergic agonists, there is a concern about cardiovascular side effects. Most of the drugs in this category used to treat asthma are selective β_2 adrenergic agonists and thus act as bronchodilators. However, they do have some β_1 side effects, so there is a need to be aware of possible cardiovascular side effects (for example, tachycardia and hypertension).

In addition to the concerns above, patients with cystic fibrosis may be using inhalants containing pancreatic enzymes and tobramycin (or tablets/capsules with similar formulas). Beyond high risk of respiratory infections in individuals with cystic fibrosis, caution must be taken in administration of other antibiotics in patients receiving the aminoglycoside antibiotic tobramycin (see Table 15.3).

Drug Interactions of Dental Interest
Avoid drugs that may precipitate an asthmatic attack: aspirin, NSAIDs and narcotics.

Special Patients
As a rule, inhalants are not recommended for use in children aged < 5 years. Also, these drugs may have hepatic and renal side effects that often are of more concern with children and older adults.

Adverse Effects, Precautions and Contraindications
Table 15.2 describes adverse effects, precautions and contraindications associated with

steroids and β_2-adrenergic blockers (whether taken orally or inhaled).

Pharmacology

Inhibitors of Chemical Mediators/ Anti-Inflammatory Drugs
Cromolyn sulfate
Cromolyn sulfate is thought to act by stabilizing mast cells. In addition, cromolyn also may inhibit mast cell release of histamine, leukotrienes and other inflammatory mediators and inhibit calcium influx into mast cells. The result is decreased stimuli for bronchospasm. However, as it has no bronchodilating activity, cromolyn is useful only for prophylactic treatment and not for acute situations.

Leukotriene antagonists and inhibitors
These drugs act by blocking the synthesis of leukotriene from arachidonic acid (eg, zileuton [Zyflo]) or by acting as leukotriene receptor antagonists (eg, montelukast [Singulair], zafirlukast [Accolate]), thereby decreasing leukotriene levels and associated increased inflammatory activity. Antileukotriene approaches are recommended as maintenance therapies for persistent asthma requiring daily bronchodilator treatment.

Corticosteroids
See Chapter 5 for details.

Bronchodilators
β-adrenergic agonists
β-adrenergic agonists are used for treatment of acute bronchospasm. Ideal drugs act predominantly on β_2-adrenergic receptors and stimulate dilation of bronchial smooth muscles. This relaxes the airway's smooth muscle. β-adrenergic agents also inhibit release of substances from mast cells and thus prevent bronchoconstriction. Most adrenergic drugs have some β_1 activity; therefore, there is a need to monitor patients for cardiovascular

effects, including increased force and rate of cardiac contraction. This is especially true of epinephrine. **Note:** Epinephrine usually is used for emergency situations such as rapid/acute asthmatic attack, in which case 0.2-0.5 mL of 1:1,000 solution is administered subcutaneously or intramuscularly.

Intramuscular injection of epinephrine into the buttocks should be avoided, because it could cause gas gangrene. The subcutaneous route is recommended for bronchodilatory purposes; for anaphylactic reactions, either the subcutaneous or the intramuscular route could be used.

Xanthines

Xanthines relax bronchial smooth muscle (in both acute and chronic situations, and often in combination with other drugs). Several mechanisms for this activity have been proposed, but none have been definitively proven. These mechanisms include inhibition of phosphodiesterase, mobilization of calcium pools, inhibition of prostaglandin activity and decreased uptake of catecholamines.

Anticholinergic agents

Anticholinergic agents act on receptors to prevent smooth muscle contraction. They are marketed for inhalant treatment of chronic obstructive pulmonary disease, but this use is still under investigation.

Evolving Respiratory Therapies

New therapies continue to be targeted at decreasing inflammation. DNase inhibitors are thought to act by breaking up long extracellular DNA into smaller fragments. DNA is considered to contribute to thick sputum,

especially in patients with cystic fibrosis. Omalizumab (Xolair injection) is a recombinant DNA-derived monoclonal antibody that selectively binds to human IgE, resulting in decreased IgE binding to receptors on mast cells and basophils. In recent years nutrition/diet control for many diseases, including cardiovascular, gastrointestinal and pulmonary diseases, has received much attention. There is some indication that the inflammatory state in the airways, often associated with increased oxygen species and free radical-mediated reactions, can be controlled by foods/supplements that are able to control oxidant insult, ie antioxidants. In the area of allergen avoidance, there have been efforts to develop products that can control dust-mite allergens and that can denature allergens.

Suggested Readings

Kips JC, Pauwels RA. Long-acting inhaled β_2-agonist therapy in asthma. Am J Respir Crit Care Med 2001;164: 923-32.

Laube BL. The expanding role of aerosols in systemic drug delivery, gene therapy and vaccination. Respir Care 2005;50(9):1161-76.

Lukacs NW. Role of chemokines in the pathogenesis of asthma. Nat Rev Immunol 2001;1(2):108-16.

Malamed SE. Medical emergencies in the dental office. 5th ed. St Louis: Mosby; 2000:169-243.

Peebles RS, Hartert TV. Highlights from the annual scientific assembly: patient-centered approaches to asthma management—strategies for the treatment and management of asthma. South Med J 2002;95:775-9.

Riccioni G, Di Ilio C, D'Orazio N. Review: An update of the leukotriene modulators for treatment of asthma. Expert Opin Investig Drugs 2004;13(7):763-76.

Riccioni G, D'Orazio N. The role of selenium, zinc and antioxidant vitamin supplementation in the treatment of bronchial asthma: adjuvant therapy or not? Expert Opin Investig Drugs. 2005;14(9):1145-55.

Table 15.1: AMERICAN SOCIETY OF ANESTHESIOLOGISTS CLASSIFICATION: ASTHMA

ASA CLASS*	DESCRIPTION	DENTAL TREATMENT MODIFICATIONS
II	**Typical extrinsic or intrinsic asthma**	Reduce stress as needed
	• Easily managed	Determine triggering factors
	• Characterized by infrequent episodes	Avoid triggering factors
	• Does not require emergency care or hospitalization	Have bronchodilators available during dental treatment
III	**Exercise-induced asthma**	Follow ASA II modifications
	• Often accompanied by fear	Administer sedation-inhalation with nitrous oxide, oxygen or oral benzodiazepines, if indicated
	• Patient with Class III asthma usually has history of emergency care or hospitalization	
IV	**Chronic asthma**	Obtain medical consultation before beginning treatment
	• Signs and symptoms of asthma present at rest	Provide only emergency care in office
		Defer elective care until respiratory status improves or until patient can be treated in controlled environment

*Class I represents a healthy person with no asthma.

Adapted with permission of the publisher from Malamed SF. Medical emergencies in the dental office. 5th ed. St. Louis: Mosby; 2000:213. Copyright © 2000 C.V. Mosby Co.

Table 15.2: PRESCRIBING INFORMATION FOR RESPIRATORY DRUGS

NAME	FORM/ STRENGTH	DOSAGE	WARNINGS/PRECAUTIONS & CONTRAINDICATIONS	ADVERSE EFFECTS†
α/β-ADRENERGIC AGONISTS				
Epinephrine (Epipen)	**Inj: (Epipen Jr)** 0.5mg/mL, **(Epipen)** 1mg/mL	**Adults:** 0.3mg IM in thigh. May repeat with severe anaphylaxis. **Pediatrics:** 0.15mg or 0.3mg (0.01mg/kg) IM in thigh. May repeat with severe anaphylaxis.	**W/P:** Not for IV use. Contains sulfites. Extreme caution with heart disease. Anginal pain may be induced with coronary insufficiency. Increased risk of adverse reactions with hyperthyroidism, CVD, HTN, DM, elderly, pregnancy, pediatrics <30kg with Epipen and <15kg with Epipen, Jr. **P/N:** Category C, safety in nursing not known.	Palpitations, tachycardia, sweating, nausea, vomiting, respiratory difficulty, pallor, dizziness, weakness, tremor, headache, apprehension, anxiety.
ANTICHOLINERGICS				
Ipratropium Bromide (Atrovent, Atrovent HFA)	**MDI:** 0.018mg/ inh [14g], **(HFA)** 0.017mg/inh [12.9g]; **Sol (neb):** 0.02% [2.5mL, 25ˢ]	**Adults: (MDI, HFA MDI) Initial:** 2 inh qid. **Max:** 12 inh/24hrs. **(Sol)** 1 vial (500µg/2.5mL) nebulized tid-qid; separate doses by 6-8 hrs. **Pediatrics: ≥12 yrs: (MDI) Initial:** 2 inh qid. **Max:** 12 inh/24hrs. **(Sol)** 1 vial (500µg/2.5mL) nebulized tid-qid; separate doses by 6-8 hrs.	**W/P:** Not for acute episodes. Immediate hypersensitivity reaction reported. Caution with narrow-angle glaucoma, prostatic hypertrophy or bladder-neck obstruction. **Contra:** Hypersensitivity to atropine or its derivatives. (MDI) History of hypersensitivity to soya lecithin or related food products (eg, soybeans, peanuts). **P/N:** Category B, caution in nursing.	Nervousness, bronchitis, dyspnea, dizziness, headache, nausea, blurred vision, **dry mouth**, exacerbation of symptoms.
Tiotropium Bromide (Spiriva)	**Cap, Inhalation:** 18µg [6ˢ, 30ˢ]	**Adults:** Inhale the contents of one capsule (18µg) qd, with the HandiHaler device.	**W/P:** Not for the initial treatment of acute episodes. Discontinue if hypersensitivity (eg, angioedema) or paradoxical bronchospasm occurs. Caution with narrow-angle glaucoma, prostatic hyperplasia, bladder-neck obstruction. Monitor with moderate to severe renal impairment (CrCl ≤50mL/min). **Contra:** Hypersensitivity to atropine or its derivatives (eg, ipratropium). **P/N:** Category C, caution in nursing.	**Dry mouth**, arthritis, cough, flu-like symptoms, sinusitis, constipation, abdominal pain, urinary tract infection, moniliasis, rash.
β-ADRENERGIC AGONISTS				
Albuterol Sulfate (AccuNeb, Proventil, Proventil HFA, Ventolin HFA)	**(Accuneb) Sol:** 1.25mg/3mL, 0.63mg/3mL [3mL, 25ˢ] **(Proventil/Proventil HFA) Aerosol:** 0.09mg/inh [17g], **(HFA)** 0.09mg/inh [6.7g]; **Sol (Neb):** 0.083% [3mL, 25ˢ], 0.5% [20mL]; **Syrup:** 2mg/5mL; **Tab:** 2mg*, 4mg*; **Tab, Extended Release (Repetabs):** 4mg* **(Ventolin HFA) MDI:** 0.09mg/inh [18g]	**(AccuNeb) Pediatrics: 2-12 yrs: Initial:** 0.63mg or 1.25mg tid-qid via nebulizer. **6-12 yrs with severe asthma or >40kg or 11-12 yrs: Initial:** 1.25mg tid-qid. **(Proventil/Proventil HFA) Adults: Bronchospasm: (Aerosol, HFA Aerosol)** 2 inh q4-6h or 1 inh q4h. **(Repetabs) Initial:** 4-8mg q12h. **Max:** 32mg/day. **(Sol)** 2.5mg tid-qid by nebulizer. **(Syrup, Tabs)** 2-4mg tid-qid. **Max:** 32mg/day. **Elderly/Beta-Adrenergic Sensitivity: (Syrup, Tabs) Initial:** 2mg tid-qid. **Max: (Tabs)** 8mg tid-qid. **Exercise-Induced Bronchospasm: (Aerosol, HFA Aerosol)** 2 inh 15 minutes (up to 30 minutes for HFA) before activity. **Pediatrics: Bronchospasm:** >14 yrs: **(Syrup) Initial:** 2-4mg tid-qid. **Max:** 8mg qid. **≥12 yrs: (Aerosol, HFA Aerosol)** 2 inh q4-6h or 1 inh q4h. **(Sol)** 2.5mg tid-qid by nebulizer. **(Tabs) Initial:** 2-4mg tid-qid. **Max:** 8mg qid. >12 yrs: **(Repetabs) Initial:** 4-8mg q12h. **Max:** 32mg/day. **6-14 yrs: (Syrup) Initial:** 2mg tid-qid. **Max:** 24mg/day. **6-12 yrs: (Repetabs) Initial:** 4mg q12h. **Max:** 24mg/day. **(Tabs) Initial:** 2mg tid-qid. **Max:** 24mg/day.	**W/P: (Accuneb)** Hypersensitivity reactions reported. Fatalities reported with excessive use. Caution with cardiovascular disorders, especially coronary insufficiency, arrhythmias and HTN. May need concomitant anti-inflammatory agents. Can produce paradoxical bronchospasm. Caution with DM. May cause hypokalemia. (Proventil/Proventil HFA/Ventolin HFA) Discontinue if paradoxical bronchospasm or cardiovascular events occur. Avoid excessive use. Caution with coronary insufficiency, arrhythmias, HTN, DM, hyperthyroidism, seizures, sensitivity to sympathomimetics. Hypersensitivity reactions may occur. May cause transient hypokalemia. **P/N:** Category C, not for use in nursing.	Asthma exacerbation, otitis media, allergic reaction, gastroenteritis, cold symptoms, **throat irritation**, viral respiratory infections, upper respiratory inflammation, cough, musculoskeletal pain.

*Scored.   †Bold entries denote special dental considerations

Table 15.2: PRESCRIBING INFORMATION FOR RESPIRATORY DRUGS *(cont.)*

NAME	FORM/ STRENGTH	DOSAGE	WARNINGS/PRECAUTIONS & CONTRAINDICATIONS	ADVERSE EFFECTS†
β-ADRENERGIC AGONISTS *(cont.)*				
Albuterol Sulfate *(cont.)*		**2-5 yrs: (Syrup) Initial:** 0.1mg/kg tid (not to exceed 2mg tid). **Titrate:** May increase to 0.2mg/kg/day. **Max:** 4mg tid. **≥4 yrs: (HFA Aerosol)** 2 inh q4-6h or 1 inh q4h. **Exercise-induced Bronchospasm: ≥12 yrs: (Aerosol)** 2 inh 15 minutes before activity. **≥4 yrs: (HFA Aerosol)** 2 inh 15-30 minutes before activity. **(Ventolin HFA)** *Adults:* **Broncho-spasm:** 2 inh q4-6h or 1 inh q4h. **EIB:** 2 inh 15-30 minutes before activity. *Pediatrics:* **≥4 yrs: Bronchospasm:** 2 inh q4-6h or 1 inh q4h. **EIB:** 2 inh 15-30 minutes before activity.		
Formoterol Fumarate (Foradil)	**Cap, Inh:** 12µg [12ˢ, 60ˢ]	*Adults:* Do not swallow cap; give only by inhalation with Aerolizer™; Inhaler. **Asthma/COPD:** 12µg q12h. **Max:** 24µg/day. **EIB:** 12µg 15 minutes before exercise (do not give added dose if already on q12h dose). *Pediatrics:* **≥5 yrs:** Do not swallow cap; give only by inhalation with Aerolizer™; Inhaler. Asthma/COPD: 12µg q12h. **Max:** 24µg/day. **EIB:** 12µg 15 minutes q12h dose). before exercise (do not give added dose if already on q12h dose).	**W/P:** Do not discontinue inhaled corticosteroids. Continue to use short-acting beta²-agonist inhaler for acute symptoms. Discontinue if paradoxical bronchospasm occurs. Discontinue if ECG changes, QT interval increases, or ST depression occurs. Caution with cardiovascular disorders (eg, HTN, arrhythmias), thyrotoxicosis and convulsive disorders. Anaphylactic and other allergic reactions reported. Not for use in acute asthmatic conditions. May cause hypokalemia. **P/N:** Category C, caution in nursing.	Viral infection, dyspnea, chest pain, tremor, dizziness, insomnia, rash, dysphonia, HTN, hypotension, tachycardia, arrhythmias, **dry mouth**, headache, nausea, vomiting, fatigue, hypokalemia, hyperglycemia.
Levalbuterol Hydrochloride (Xopenex)	**Sol:** 0.31mg/ 3mL, 0.63mg/ 3mL, 1.25mg/ 3mL [3mL, 24ˢ]	*Adults:* **Initial:** 0.63mg tid, q6-8h. **Severe Asthma:** 1.25mg tid, q6-8h. Administer by nebulizer. *Pediatrics:* **≥12 yrs: Initial:** 0.63mg tid, q6-8h. **Severe Asthma:** 1.25mg tid, q6-8h. 6-11 yrs: 0.31mg tid. **Max:** 0.63mg tid. Administer by nebulizer.	**W/P:** Hypersensitivity reactions reported. Discontinue immediately if paradoxical bronchospasm occurs. May produce ECG changes; caution with cardiovascular disorders, oronary insufficiency, arrhythmias, and HTN. Caution with convulsive disorders, hyperthyroidism, and DM. May produce transient hypokalemia. **P/N:** Category C, not for use in nursing.	Tachycardia, migraine, dyspepsia, leg cramps, nervousness, dizziness, tremor, rhinitis, increased cough, chest pain, HTN, hypotention, diarrhea, **dry mouth**, anxiety, insomnia, paresthesia, wheezing.
Levalbuterol Tartrate (Xopenex HFA)	**MDI:** 45µg/inh [15g]	*Adults:* 2 inh (90µg) q 4-6 hrs or 1 inh (45µg) q 4 hrs may be sufficient. *Pediatrics:* **≥4 yrs:** 2 inh (90µg) q 4-6 hrs or 1 inh (45µg) q 4 hrs may be sufficient.	**W/P:** Discontinue immediately if paradoxical bronchospasm occurs. May produce ECG changes; caution with cardiovascular disorders, coronary insufficiency, arrhythmias, and HTN. Caution with convulsive disorders, hyperthyroidism, and DM. May produce transient hypokalemia. **P/N:** Category C, not for use in nursing.	Asthma, **pharyngitis**, rhinitis, pain, vomiting.
Metaproterenol Sulfate (Alupent)	**MDI:** 0.65mg/ inh [14g]; **Sol, Inhalation:** 0.4% [2.5mL], 0.6% [2.5mL]; **Syr:** 10mg/5mL [480mL]; **Tab:** 10mg, 20mg	*Adults:* **(MDI)** 2-3 inh q3-4h. **Max:** 12 inh/day. **(Sol 5%) Nebulizer or IPPB:** 0.2-0.3mL (dilute in 2.5mL saline) tid-qid. **Hand-bulb Nebulizer:** 5-15 inh (undiluted) tid-qid. **(Sol 0.4%, 0.6%)** 2.5mL by IPPB tid-qid, up to q4h. **(Syr, Tab)** 20mg tid-qid. *Pediatrics:* **(MDI) ≥12 yrs:** 2-3 inh q3-4h. **Max:** 12 inh/day. **(Sol 5%) ≥12 yrs: Nebulizer or IPPB:** 0.2-0.3mL (dilute in 2.5mL saline) tid-qid. **Hand-bulb Nebulizer:** 5-15 inh (undiluted) tid-qid. **6-12 yrs: Nebulizer:** 0.1-0.2mL (dilute in 3mL saline) tid-qid. **(Sol 0.4%, 0.6%) ≥12 yrs:** 2.5mL by IPPB tid-qid, up to q4h. **(Syr, Tab) >9 yrs or >60 lbs:** 20mg tid-qid. **6-9 yrs or <60 lbs:** 10mg tid-qid.	**W/P:** Caution with CVD, (eg, ischemic heart disease, HTN, arrhythmias) hyperthyroidism, diabetes, convulsive disorders. Fatalities reported with excessive use. Can produce paradoxical bronchospasm. Monitor BP. Nebulized solution single dose may not abort an asthma attack. **Contra:** Cardiac arrhythmias associated with tachycardia. **P/N:** Category C, caution in nursing.	Headache, dizziness, HTN, GI distress, **throat irritation**, cough, asthma exacerbation, nervousness, tremor, nausea, vomiting.

*Scored.   †Bold entries denote special dental considerations

NAME	FORM/ STRENGTH	DOSAGE	WARNINGS/PRECAUTIONS & CONTRAINDICATIONS	ADVERSE EFFECTS†
Pirbuterol Acetate (Maxair)	**Autohaler:** 0.2mg/inh [14g, 25.6g]; **MDI:** 0.2mg/inh [14g]	**Adults:** 1-2 inh q4-6h. **Max:** 12 inh/day. **Pediatrics: 12 yrs:** 1-2 inh q4-6h. **Max:** 12 inh/day.	**W/P:** Caution with cardiovascular disorders, (eg, ischemic heart disease, HTN, arrhythmias), hyperthyroidism, diabetes, convulsive disorders. Fatalities reported with excessive use. Can produce paradoxical bronchospasm. Monitor BP. **P/N:** Category C, caution in nursing.	Nervousness, tremor, headache, dizziness, palpitations, tachycardia, cough, nausea.
Salmeterol Xinafoate (Serevent)	**Disk:** 50µg [28, 60 blisters]	**Adults: Asthma/COPD:** 1 inh bid, am and pm (12 hrs apart). **EIB Prevention:** 1 inh 30 minutes before exercise (do not give preventive doses if already on bid dose). **Pediatrics: ≥4 yrs: Asthma:** 1 inh bid, am and pm (12 hrs apart). **EIB Prevention:** 1 inh 30 minutes before exercise (do not give preventive doses if already on bid dose).	**BB:** Small increase in asthma-related deaths reported with use, especially in African-Americans. **W/P:** Avoid with significantly worsening or acutely deteriorating asthma. Not for acute treatment or substitute for oral/inhaled corticosteroids. Monitor for increasing use of inhaled beta$_2$ agonists. QTc interval prolongation reported when exceeded recommended dose. D/C if paradoxical bronchospasm occurs. Immediate hypersensitivity and upper airway symptom reactions reported. Caution with cardiovascular disorder (eg, coronary insufficiency, arrhythmia, HTN), convulsive disorders, thyrotoxicosis, if usually unresponsive to sympathomimetic amines. May cause hypokalemia. **P/N:** Category C, not for use in nursing.	Nasal/sinus congestion, pallor, rhinitis, headache, tracheitis/bronchitis, influenza, **throat irritation**.
Terbutaline Sulfate (Brethine)	**Inj:** 1mg/mL [1mL]; **Tab:** 2.5mg*, 5mg*	**Adults: (PO) Usual:** 5mg tid. May reduce to 2.5mg tid. **Max:** 15mg/24hrs. **(Inj) Usual:** 0.25mg SC into lateral deltoid area. May repeat within 15-30 minutes if no improvement. **Max:** 0.5mg/4hrs. **Pediatrics: (PO) 12-15 yrs: Usual:** 2.5mg tid. **Max:** 7.5mg/24hrs. **(Inj) ≥12 yrs: Usual:** 0.25mg SC into lateral deltoid area. May repeat within 15-30 minutes if no improvement. **Max:** 0.5mg/4hrs.	**W/P:** Caution with ischemic heart disease, HTN, arrhythmias, hyperthyroidism, DM, seizures. Not approved for tocolysis. Hypersensitivity and exacerbation of bronchospasm reported. Monitor for transient hypokalemia. **Contra:** Hypersensitivity to sympathomimetic amines. **P/N:** Category B, caution in nursing.	Nervousness, tremor, headache, somnolence, palpitations, dizziness, tachycardia, nausea.

BRONCHODILATOR COMBINATIONS

NAME	FORM/ STRENGTH	DOSAGE	WARNINGS/PRECAUTIONS & CONTRAINDICATIONS	ADVERSE EFFECTS†
Albuterol Sulfate/Ipratropium Bromide (Combivent, Duoneb)	**(Combivent) MDI:** (Albuterol-Ipratropium) 0.09mg-0.018mg/inh [14.7g]; **(Duoneb) Sol, Inh:** (Albuterol-Ipratropium) 3mg-0.5mg/ 3mL [3mL, 30ˢ 60ˢ]	**(Combivent) Adults:** 2 inh qid. **Max:** 12 inh/24 hrs. **(Duoneb) Adults:** 3mL qid via nebulizer. May give 2 additional doses/day.	**W/P:** Paradoxical bronchospasm reported. Hypersensitivity reactions reported. Caution with coronary insufficiency, arrhythmias, narrow-angle glaucoma, prostatic hypertrophy, bladder-neck obstruction, HTN, DM, hyperthyroidism, seizures, renal or hepatic dysfunction, and in those unusually responsive to sympathomimetic amines. May produce transient hypokalemia. Fatalities reported with excessive use. **Contra:** (Combivent) History of hypersensitivity to soya lecithin or related food products (eg, soybeans, peanuts). (Duoneb) Hypersensitivity to atropine and its derivatives. **P/N:** Category C, not for use in nursing.	Headache, cough, respiratory disorders, pain, dyspnea, bronchitis, nausea, diarrhea, **pharyngitis,** pneumonia.
Fluticasone Propionate/ Salmeterol Xinafoate (Advair Diskus)	**Disk Inh:** (Fluticasone-Salmeterol) (100/50) 0.1mg-0.05mg/inh, (250/50)	**Adults: Asthma:** 1 inh q12h. **Without Prior Inhaled Corticosteroid: Initial:** 100/50 bid. **Max:** 500/50 bid. **Current Inhaled Corticosteroid: Beclomethasone:** ≤420µg/day use 100/50 bid, 462-840 µg/day use 250/50 bid. **Budesonide:** ≤400µg/day use 100/50	**W/P:** Deaths due to adrenal insufficiency have occurred with transfer from systemic corticosteroids to inhaled corticosteroids. Resume oral corticosteroids during stress or severe asthma attack. Observe for adrenal insufficiency, systemic	Upper respiratory tract inflammation, **pharyngitis**, sinusitis, cough, **hoarseness**, headaches, GI effects, musculoskeletal pain, palpitations.

Table 15.2: PRESCRIBING INFORMATION FOR RESPIRATORY DRUGS *(cont.)*

NAME	FORM/ STRENGTH	DOSAGE	WARNINGS/PRECAUTIONS & CONTRAINDICATIONS	ADVERSE EFFECTS†
BRONCHODILATOR COMBINATIONS *(cont.)*				
Fluticasone Propionate/ Salmeterol Xinafoate *(cont.)*	0.25mg-0.05mg/inh, (500/50) 0.5mg-0.05mg/inh [60 blisters]	bid, 800-1200 µg/day use 250/50 bid, 1600µg/day use 500/50 bid. **Flunisolide:** ≤1000µg/day use 100/50 bid, 1250-2000µg/day use 250/50 bid. **Fluticasone Aerosol:** ≤176µg/day use 100/50 bid, 440µg/day use 250/50 bid, 660-880µg/day use 500/50 bid. **Fluticasone Powder:** ≤200µg/day use 100/50 bid, 500µg/day use 250/50 bid, 1000µg/day use 500/50 bid. **Triamcinolone:** ≤1000µg/day use 100/50 bid, 1100-1600µg/day use 250/50 bid. If no response within 2 weeks, increase to higher strength. **COPD:** (250/50µg only): 1 inh q12h. Rinse mouth after use. **Pediatrics:** **Asthma: ≥12 yrs:** 1 inh q12h. **Without Prior Inhaled Corticosteroid: Initial:** 100/50 bid. **Max:** 500/50 bid. **Current Inhaled Corticosteroid: Beclo-methasone:** ≤420µg/day use 100/50 bid, 462-840µg/day use 250/50 bid. **Budesonide:** ≤400µg/day use 100/50 bid, 800-1200µg/day use 250/50 bid, 1600µg/day use 500/50 bid. **Flunisolide:** ≤1000µg/day use 100/50 bid, 1250-2000µg/day use 250/50 bid. **Fluticasone Aerosol:** ≤176µg/day use 100/50 bid, 440µg/day use 250/50 bid, 660-880µg/day use 500/50 bid. **Fluticasone Powder:** ≤200µg/day use 100/50 bid, 500µg/day use 250/50 bid, 1000µg/day use 500/50 bid. **Triam-cinolone:** ≤1000µg/ day use 100/50 bid, 1100-1600µg/day use 250/50 bid. If no response within 2 weeks, increase to higher strength. **4-11 yrs: (100/50µg only): Symptomatic on Inhaled Corticosteroid:** 1 inh q12h. Rinse mouth after use.	corticosteroid withdrawal effects, hypercorticism, reduction in growth velocity (pediatrics). More susceptible to infection. Not for acute bronchospasm. Discontinue if bronchospasm occurs after dosing. Caution with TB; untreated systemic fungal, bacterial, viral or parasitic infections; or ocular herpes simplex. *Candida* infection of mouth and pharynx, glaucoma, hypersensitivity reactions, increased IOP, cataracts reported. Monitor for increasing use of beta^2 agonists. QTc interval prolongation reported with large doses. Discontinue if paradoxical bronchospasm occurs. Caution with cardiovascular disorders. **Contra:** Status asthmaticus or other acute asthma or COPD episodes. **P/N:** Category C, caution in nursing.	
CORTICOSTEROIDS (INHALED)				
BRONCHIAL				
Beclomethasone Dipropionate (Qvar)	**MDI:** 40µg/inh, 80µg/inh [7.3g]	***Adults: Previous Bronchodilator Only:*** 40-80µg bid. **Max:** 320µg bid. **Previous Inhaled Corticosteroid Therapy:** 40-160µg bid. **Max:** 320µg bid. **Maint With Oral Corticosteroids:** May attempt gradual reduction of oral dose after 1 week on inhaled therapy. ***Pediatrics:*** **Adolescents: Previous Bronchodila-tor Only:** 40-80µg bid. **Max:** 320µg bid. **Previous Inhaled Corticosteroid Therapy:** 40-160µg bid. **Max:** 320µg bid. **5-11 yrs: Previous Bronchodila-tor Only or Inhaled Corticosteroid Therapy:** 40µg bid. Max: 80µg bid. **≥5 yrs: Maint With Oral Corticosteroids:** May attempt gradual reduction of oral dose after 1 week on inhaled therapy.	**W/P:** Deaths due to adrenal insuf-ficiency have occurred with transfer from systemic corticosteroids to inhaled corticosteroids. Resume oral corticosteroids during stress or severe asthma attack. Risk of adrenal insufficiency and withdrawal symptoms when replacing systemic corticosteroids. May unmask allergic conditions previously suppressed by systemic steroid therapy. Caution with TB, ocular herpes simplex, or untreated systemic bacterial, fungal, parasitic or viral infections. May sup-press growth in children. Exposure to chickenpox or measles requires prophylaxis treatment. Not for rapid relief of bronchospasm. **Contra:** Status asthmaticus, acute asthmatic attacks. **P/N:** Category C, not for use in nursing.	Headache, **pharyngitis**, upper respiratory tract in-fection, rhinitis, increased asthma symptoms, sinusitis.

*Scored.   †Bold entries denote special dental considerations

NAME	FORM/ STRENGTH	DOSAGE	WARNINGS/PRECAUTIONS & CONTRAINDICATIONS	ADVERSE EFFECTS†
Budesonide (Pulmicort Respules, Pulmicort Turbuhaler)	**Pow, Inh:** **(Turbuhaler)** 200µg/inh. **Sus,** **Inh: (Respules)** 0.25mg/2mL; 0.5mg/2mL [2mL, 30ˢ]	***Adults:*** **(Turbuhaler) Previous Bron-** **chodilator Only: Initial:** 200-400µg bid. **Max:** 400µg bid. **Previous Inhaled** **Corticosteroid: Initial:** 200-400µg bid [mild-to-moderate asthma patients may use 200-400µg qd]. **Max:** 800µg bid. **Previous Oral Corticosteroid: Initial:** 400-800µg bid. **Max:** 800µg bid. Gradu- ally reduce PO corticosteroid after 1 week of budesonide. ***Pediatrics:*** **(Turbu-** **haler) ≥6 yrs: Previous Bronchodilator** **Only/Inhaled Corticosteroid: Initial:** 200µg bid. [mild-to-moderate asthma patients previously controlled on inhaled steroids may use 200-400µg qd]. **Max:** 400µg bid. Oral Corticosteroid: **Max:** 400µg bid. **(Respules) 1-8 yrs: Previous** **Bronchodilator Only: Initial:** 0.5mg qd or 0.25mg bid. Administer via jet nebulizer. **Max:** 0.5mg/day. **Previous** **Inhaled Corticosteroid:** 0.5mg qd or 0.25mg bid. **Max:** 1mg/day. **Previous** **Oral Corticosteroid:** 1mg qd or 0.5mg bid. **Max:** 1mg/day. Gradually reduce PO corticosteroid after 1 week of budesonide.	**W/P:** Deaths due to adrenal insuf- ficiency have occurred with transfer from systemic corticosteroids to inhaled corticosteroids. Resume oral corticosteroids during stress or severe asthma attack. Transferring from oral to inhalation therapy may unmask allergic conditions (eg, rhinitis, conjunctivitis, eczema). Observe for adrenal insufficiency, systemic corticosteroid withdrawal effects, and growth suppression (children). More susceptible to infec- tions. Not for acute bronchospasm. Discontinue if bronchospasm occurs after dosing. Caution with tuberculosis of the respiratory tract; untreated systemic fungal, bacterial, viral or parasitic infections; or ocular herpes simplex. *Candida* infection of the mouth and pharynx reported**.** **Contra:** Primary treatment of status asthmaticus or other acute asthma attacks. **P/N:** (Respules) .Category B, caution in nursing; (Turbuhaler) Category B, not for use in nursing.	**Pharyngitis**, headache, fever, sinusitis, pain, bronchospasm, bronchi- tis, respiratory infection, **moniliasis**.
Flunisolide (Aerobid, Aerobid-M)	**MDI:** 0.25mg/ inh [7g]	***Adults:* Initial:** 2 inh bid. **Max:** 4 inh bid. Rinse mouth after use. ***Pediatrics:*** **6-15 yrs:** 2 inh bid. Rinse mouth after use.	**W/P:** Deaths due to adrenal insuf- ficiency have occurred with transfer from systemic corticosteroids to inhaled corticosteroids. Resume oral corticosteroids during stress or severe asthma attack. Observe for adrenal insufficiency, systemic cor- ticosteroid withdrawal effects, and growth suppression (children). More susceptible to infections. Not for acute bronchospasm. Discontinue if bronchospasm occurs after dosing. Caution with tuberculosis of the respiratory tract; untreated systemic fungal, bacterial, viral or parasitic infections; or ocular herpes simplex. *Candida* infection of the mouth and pharynx reported. **Contra:** Primary treatment of status asthmaticus or other acute asthma attacks. **P/N:** Category C, caution with nursing.	Upper respiratory infec- tion, diarrhea, stomach upset, cold symptoms, nasal congestion, head- ache, nausea, vomiting, **sore throat, unpleasant** **taste**.
Fluticasone **Propionate** (Flovent, Flovent HFA, Flovent Rotadisk)	**MDI:** 44µg/inh [7.9g, 13g], 110µg/inh [7.9g, 13g], 220µg/inh [7.9g, 13g], **(HFA)** 44µg/inh [10.6g], 110µg/ inh [12g], 220µg/inh [12g]; **Rotadisk:** 50µg/dose, 100µg/dose, 250µg/dose [15 x 4 blisters]	***Adults:* (MDI, HFA MDI) Previous** **Bronchodilator Only: Initial:** 88µg bid. **Max:** 440µg bid. **Previous Inhaled** **Corticosteroids: Initial:** 88-220µg bid. **Max:** 440µg bid. **Previous Oral Cor-** **ticosteroids: Initial/Max:** 880µg bid. **(Rotadisk) Previous Bronchodilator** **Only: Initial:** 100µg bid. **Max:** 500µg bid. **Previous Inhaled Corticosteroids:** **Initial:** 100-250µg bid. **Max:** 500µg bid. **Previous Oral Corticosteroids:** **(Rotadisk) Initial/Max:** 1000µg bid. Reduce PO prednisone no faster than 2.5mg/day weekly, beginning at least 1 week after starting fluticasone. Rinse mouth after use. ***Pediatrics:* ≥12 yrs:** **(MDI, HFA MDI) Previous Bronchodila-** **tor Only: Initial:** 88µg bid. **Max:** 440µg bid. **Previous Inhaled Corticosteroids:**	**W/P:** Deaths due to adrenal insuf- ficiency have occurred with transfer from systemic corticosteroids to inhaled corticosteroids. Resume oral corticosteroids during stress or severe asthma attack. Wean slowly from systemic corticosteroid therapy. Observe for adrenal insufficiency, systemic corticosteroid withdrawal effects, hypercorticism, adrenal sup- pression (including adrenal crisis), reduction in growth velocity (children and adolescents). May increase susceptibility to infections. Not for acute bronchospasm. Discontinue if bronchospasm occurs after dosing. Caution with TB of the respiratory tract; untreated systemic fungal, bacterial, viral or parasitic infections; or ocular herpes simplex. *Candida*	**Pharyngitis**, nasal congestion, sinusitis, rhinitis, dysphonia, **oral candidiasis**, upper respiratory infection, influenza, headache, nasal discharge, allergic rhinitis, fever, osteoporosis, para- doxical bronchospasm, pneumonia.

Table 15.2: PRESCRIBING INFORMATION FOR RESPIRATORY DRUGS *(cont.)*

NAME	FORM/ STRENGTH	DOSAGE	WARNINGS/PRECAUTIONS & CONTRAINDICATIONS	ADVERSE EFFECTS†
CORTICOSTEROIDS (INHALED) *(cont.)*				
Fluticasone Propionate *(cont.)*		**Initial:** 88-220µg bid. **Max:** 440 µg bid. **Previous Oral Corticosteroids: Initial/Max:** 880µg bid. **(Rotadisk) Previous Bronchodilator Only: Initial:** 100µg bid. **Max:** 500µg bid. **Previous Inhaled Corticosteroids: Initial:** 100-250µg bid. Max: 500µg bid. **Previous Oral Corticosteroids: (Rotadisk) Initial/Max:** 1000µg bid. **4-11 yrs: (Rotadisk) Previous Bronchodilator Only/Inhaled Corticosteroids: Initial:** 50µg bid. **Max:** 100µg bid. Reduce PO prednisone no faster than 2.5mg/day weekly, beginning at least 1 week after starting fluticasone. Rinse mouth after use.	infection of the mouth and pharynx reported. Glaucoma, increased IOP and cataracts reported. **Contra:** Primary treatment of status asthmaticus or other acute asthma attacks. **P/N:** Category C, caution in nursing.	
Mometasone Furoate (Asmanex Twisthaler)	**Twisthaler:** 220µg/inh	***Adults:* Previous Therapy with Bronchodilators Alone or Inhaled Corticosteroids: Initial:** 220µg qpm. **Max:** 440µg qpm or 220µg bid. **Previous Therapy with Oral Corticosteroids: Initial:** 440µg bid. **Max:** 880µg/day. Titrate to lowest effective dose once asthma stability is achieved. ***Pediatrics:*** **≥12 yrs: Previous Therapy with Bronchodilators Alone or Inhaled Corticosteroids: Initial:** 220µg qpm. **Max:** 440µg qpm or 220µg bid. **Previous Therapy with Oral Corticosteroids: Initial:** 440µg bid. **Max:** 880µg/day. Titrate to lowest effective dose once asthma stability is achieved.	**W/P:** Deaths due to adrenal insufficiency have occurred with transfer from systemic corticosteroids to inhaled corticosteroids. Wean slowly from systemic corticosteroid therapy. Resume oral corticosteroids during stress or severe asthma attack. May unmask allergic conditions previously suppressed by systemic corticosteroid therapy. May increase susceptibility to infections. Not for rapid relief of bronchospasm or other acute episodes of asthma. Discontinue if bronchospasm occurs after dosing. Observe for systemic corticosteroid withdrawal effects, hypercorticism, reduced bone mineral density, and adrenal suppression; reduce dose slowly if needed. Decreased growth velocity may occur in pediatric patients. Candida infections in the mouth and pharynx reported. Caution with active or quiescent TB infection of the respiratory tract; untreated systemic fungal, bacterial, viral, or parasitic infections; or ocular herpes simplex. Glaucoma, increased IOP, and cataracts reported. **Contra:** Primary treatment of status asthmaticus or other acute episodes of asthma where intensive measures are required. **P/N:** Category C, caution in nursing.	Headache, allergic rhinitis, **pharyngitis,** upper respiratory tract infection, sinusitis, **oral candidiasis,** dysmenorrhea, musculoskeletal pain, back pain, dyspepsia, myalgia, abdominal pain, nausea.
Triamcinolone Acetonide (Azmacort)	**MDI:** 100µg/inh [20g]	***Adults:*** 2 inh tid-qid or 4 inh bid. **Severe Asthma: Initial:** 12-16 inh/day. **Max:** 16 inh/day. **Rinse mouth after use.** *Pediatrics:* **>12 yrs:** 2 inh tid-qid or 4 inh bid. **Severe Asthma: Initial:** 12-16 inh/day. **Max:** 16 inh/day. 6-12 yrs: 1-2 inh tid-qid or 2-4 inh bid. **Max:** 12 inh/day. Rinse mouth after use.	**W/P:** Deaths due to adrenal insufficiency have occurred with transfer from systemic corticosteroids to inhaled corticosteroids. Resume oral corticosteroids during stress or severe asthma attack. Observe for adrenal insufficiency, systemic corticosteroid withdrawal effects, hypercorticism and growth suppression (children). More susceptible to infections. Not for acute bronchospasm. Discontinue if bronchospasm occurs after dosing. Caution with TB of the	**Pharyngitis,** sinusitis, headache, flu syndrome.

*Scored.   †Bold entries denote special dental considerations

NAME	FORM/ STRENGTH	DOSAGE	WARNINGS/PRECAUTIONS & CONTRAINDICATIONS	ADVERSE EFFECTS†
Triamcinolone Acetonide *(cont.)*			respiratory tract; untreated systemic fungal, bacterial, viral or parasitic infections; or ocular herpes simplex. *Candida* infection of the mouth and pharynx reported. **Contra:** Primary treatment of status asthmaticus or other acute asthma attacks. **P/N:** Category C, caution in nursing.	

NASAL

NAME	FORM/ STRENGTH	DOSAGE	WARNINGS/PRECAUTIONS & CONTRAINDICATIONS	ADVERSE EFFECTS†
Beclomethasone Dipropionate Monohydrate (Beconase AQ)	**Aerosol: (Beconase)** 0.042mg/inh [6.7g, 16.8g]; **Spray: (Beconase AQ)** 0.042mg/inh [25g]	***Adults:*** **(Inhaler):** 1 spray per nostril bid-qid. **(Spray)** 1-2 sprays per nostril bid. ***Pediatrics:*** **(Inhaler)** ≥12 yrs: 1 spray per nostril bid-qid. **6-12 yrs:** 1 spray per nostril tid. **(Spray)** ≥6 yrs: 1-2 sprays per nostril bid.	**W/P:** Risk of adrenal insufficiency and withdrawal symptoms when replacing systemic corticosteroids with a topical corticosteroid. Caution with active or quiescent TB, ocular herpes simplex, or untreated bacterial, fungal and systemic viral infections. Avoid with recent nasal trauma, surgery or septum ulcers. Risk for more severe/fatal course of infections (eg, chickenpox, measles) and for Candida infection of the nose and pharynx. Potential for growth velocity reduction in pediatrics. **P/N:** Category C, caution in nursing.	**Nasopharyngeal irritation**, sneezing, headache, nausea, lightheadedness, **irritated/dry nose and throat, unpleasant taste/smell**.
Budesonide (Rhinocort Aqua)	**Spray:** 32µg/inh [8.6g]	***Adults:*** 1 spray per nostril qd. **Max:** 4 sprays/nostril/day. ***Pediatrics:*** ≥6 **yrs:** 1 spray per nostril qd. **Max: 6-12 yrs:** 2 sprays/nostril/day. **>12 yrs:** 4 sprays/nostril/day	**W/P:** Risk of adrenal insufficiency and withdrawal symptoms when replacing systemic corticosteroids with a topical corticosteroid. Caution with active or quiescent TB, ocular herpes simplex, or untreated bacterial, fungal and systemic viral infections. Avoid with recent nasal trauma, surgery or septum ulcers. Risk for more severe/fatal course of infections (eg, chickenpox, measles) and for *Candida* infection of the nose and pharynx. Potential for growth velocity reduction in pediatrics. **P/N:** Category B, caution in nursing.	Nasal irritation, **pharyngitis**, cough, epistaxis.
Flunisolide (Nasarel)	**Spray:** 0.029mg/ inh [25mL]	***Adults:*** **Initial:** 2 sprays per nostril bid. **Titrate:** May increase to 2 sprays per nostril tid. **Max:** 8 sprays per nostril/day. ***Pediatrics:*** **6-14 yrs: Initial:** 1 spray per nostril tid or 2 sprays per nostril bid. **Max:** 4 sprays per nostril/day.	**W/P:** Risk of adrenal insufficiency and withdrawal symptoms when replacing systemic corticosteroids with a topical corticosteroid. Caution with active or quiescent TB, ocular herpes simplex, or untreated bacterial, fungal and systemic viral infections. Avoid with recent nasal trauma, surgery or septum ulcers. Risk for more severe/fatal course of infections (eg, chickenpox, measles) and for *Candida* infection of the nose and pharynx. Potential for growth velocity reduction in pediatrics. **Contra:** Untreated localized infection of the nasal mucosa. **P/N:** Category C, caution in nursing.	**Aftertaste**, nasal burning/ stinging, cough, epistaxis, nasal dryness.
Fluticasone Propionate (Flonase)	**Spray:** 0.05mg/ inh [16g]	***Adults:*** **Initial:** 2 sprays per nostril qd or 1 spray per nostril bid. **Maint:** 1 spray per nostril qd. May dose as 2 sprays per nostril qd as needed for seasonal allergic rhinitis. ***Pediatrics:*** ≥4 yrs: **Initial:** 1 spray per nostril qd. If inadequate response, may increase to 2 sprays per nostril. **Maint:** 1 spray per nostril qd. **Max:** 2 sprays per	**W/P:** Risk of adrenal insufficiency and withdrawal symptoms when replacing systemic corticosteroids with a topical corticosteroid. Caution with active or quiescent TB, ocular herpes simplex, or untreated bacterial, fungal and systemic viral infections. Avoid with recent nasal trauma, surgery or septum ulcers.	Headache, **pharyngitis**, epistaxis, nasal burning/irritation, asthma symptoms, nausea/vomiting, cough.

Table 15.2: PRESCRIBING INFORMATION FOR RESPIRATORY DRUGS (cont.)

NAME	FORM/ STRENGTH	DOSAGE	WARNINGS/PRECAUTIONS & CONTRAINDICATIONS	ADVERSE EFFECTS†
CORTICOSTEROIDS (INHALED) *(cont.)*				
Fluticasone Propionate *(cont.)*		nostril/day. **≥12 yrs:** May dose as 2 sprays per nostril qd as needed for seasonal allergic rhinitis.	Risk for more severe/fatal course of infections (eg, chickenpox, measles); avoid exposure in patients who have not had disease or been properly immunized. *Candida* infection of nose and pharynx reported (rare). Potential for growth velocity reduction in pediatrics. Excessive use may cause signs of hypercorticism or HPA suppression. **P/N:** Category C, caution with nursing.	
Mometasone Furoate Monohydrate (Nasonex)	**Spray:** 0.05mg/ inh [17g]	***Adults:* Allergic Rhinitis:** Treatment/Prophylaxis: 2 sprays per nostril qd. For prophylaxis, start 2-4 weeks before allergy season. **Nasal Polyps:** 2 sprays per nostril bid. ***Pediatrics:* ≥12 yrs: Treatment/Prophylaxis:** 2 sprays per nostril qd. For prophylaxis, start 2-4 weeks before allergy season. **2-11 yrs: Treatment:** 1 spray per nostril qd	**W/P:** Risk of adrenal insufficiency and withdrawal symptoms when replacing systemic corticosteroids with a topical corticosteroid. Caution with active or quiescent TB, ocular herpes simplex, or untreated bacterial, fungal and systemic viral infections. Avoid with recent nasal trauma, surgery or septum ulcers. Risk for more severe/fatal course of infections (eg, chickenpox, measles) and for *Candida* infection of the nose and pharynx. Potential for growth velocity reduction in pediatrics. **P/N:** Category C, caution with nursing	Headache, viral infection, **pharyngitis**, epistaxis, cough, upper respiratory tract infection, dysmenorrhea, myalgia, sinusitis.
Triamcinolone Acetonide (Nasacort AQ)	**AQ Spray:** 55µg/ inh [16.5g]; **HFA Aerosol:** 55µg/inh [9.3g]	***Adults:* (AQ Spray) Initial/Max:** 2 sprays per nostril qd. May reduce dose with improvement to 1 spray per nostril qd. **(HFA Aerosol) Initial:** 2 sprays per nostril qd. **Max:** 4 sprays per nostril qd. ***Pediatrics:* 6-12 yrs: (AQ Spray) Initial:** 1 spray per nostril qd. **Max:** 2 sprays per nostril qd. **≥12 yrs: Initial/Max:** 2 sprays per nostril qd. May reduce dose with improvement to 1 spray per nostril qd. **(HFA Aerosol) ≥6 yrs:** 2 sprays per nostril qd.	**W/P:** Risk of adrenal insufficiency and withdrawal symptoms when replacing systemic corticosteroids with a topical corticosteroid. Caution with active or quiescent TB, ocular herpes simplex, or untreated bacterial, fungal and systemic viral infections. Avoid with recent nasal trauma, surgery or septum ulcers. Risk for more severe/fatal course of infections (eg, chickenpox, measles) and for *Candida* infection of the nose and pharynx. Potential for growth velocity reduction in pediatrics. **P/N:** Category C, caution in nursing.	**Pharyngitis**, epistaxis, infection, otitis media, headache, sneezing, rhinitis, nasal irritation, cough, sinusitis, vomiting.
LEUKOTRIENE MODIFIERS				
Montelukast Sodium (Singulair)	**Granules:** 4mg/packet; **Tab, Chewable:** 4mg, 5mg; **Tab:** 10mg	***Adults:* Asthma:** 10mg qpm. **Allergic Rhinitis:** 10mg qd. ***Pediatrics:* Asthma:** **≥15 yrs:** 10mg qpm. **6-14 yrs:** 5mg qpm. **2-5 yrs:** 4mg qpm. **12 to 23 months:** 4mg qpm. **Allergic Rhinitis:** **≥15 yrs:** 10mg qd. **6-14 yrs:** 5mg qd. **2-5 yrs:** 4mg qd. **Perennial Allergic Rhinitis: 6 to 23 months:** 4mg qd. Granules may be mixed with applesauce, carrots, rice or ice cream; give within 15 minutes of opening packet.	**W/P:** Not for treatment of acute asthma attacks or monotherapy in excercise-induced bronchospasm. Do not abruptly substitute for inhaled or oral corticosteroids. Eosinophilic conditions reported (rare). **P/N:** Category B, caution in nursing.	(Adults, Pediatrics) Headache, cough. (Pediatrics) **Pharyngitis**, fever, flu, nausea, diarrhea, dyspepsia, rhinorrhea, upper respiratory infection.
Zafirlukast (Accolate)	**Tab:** 10mg, 20mg	***Adults:*** 20mg bid. Administer 1 hr ac or 2 hrs pc. ***Pediatrics:* ≥12 yrs:** 20mg bid. **5-11 yrs:** 10mg bid. Administer 1 hr ac or 2 hrs pc.	**W/P:** Not for treatment of acute asthma attacks. Bioavailability decreases with food. Hepatic dysfunction and systemic eosinophilia reported. **P/N:** Category B, not for use in nursing.	Headache, infection, nausea, diarrhea, hypersensitivity reactions including angioedema.
Zileuton (Zyflo)	**Tab:** 600mg	***Adults/Pediatrics:* ≥12 yrs:** 600mg qid.	**W/P:** Not for treatment of acute asthma attacks. Hepatic dysfunction reported. **Contra:** Acute liver disease. **P/N:** Category C, not for use in nursing.	Abdominal pain, asthenia, accidental injury, dyspepsia, nausea.

*Scored.   †Bold entries denote special dental considerations

NAME	FORM/ STRENGTH	DOSAGE	WARNINGS/PRECAUTIONS & CONTRAINDICATIONS	ADVERSE EFFECTS†
MAST CELL STABILIZERS				
Cromolyn Sodium (Intal)	**MDI:** 0.8mg/inh [8.1g, 14.2g]; **Sol (Neb):** 10mg/mL [2mL, 10⁵ 60⁵]	***Adults:* Asthma: (Inhaler) Usual/Max:** 2 inh qid. **(Sol)** 20mg nebulized qid. **Acute Bronchospasm Prevention: (Inhaler) Usual:** 2 inh 10-60 minutes before exposure to precipitant. **(Sol)** 20mg nebulized shortly before exposure to precipitant. **Renal/Hepatic Dysfunction:** Decrease inhaler dose. ***Pediatrics:* Asthma: (Inhaler)** ≥5 yrs: **Usual/Max:** 2 inh qid. **(Sol)** ≥2 yrs: 20mg nebulized qid. **Acute Bronchospasm Prevention: (Inhaler)** ≥5 yrs: **Usual:** 2 inh 10-60 minutes before exposure to precipitant. **(Sol)** ≥2 yrs: 20mg nebulized shortly before exposure to precipitant. **Renal/Hepatic Dysfunction:** Decrease inhaler dose.	**W/P:** Not for treatment of acute attack. Severe anaphylaxis may occur. Discontinue if develop eosinophilic pneumonia or pulmonary infiltrates with eosinophilia. May experience cough and/or bronchospasm. Caution with inhaler in coronary artery disease or history of cardiac arrhythmias. Decrease dose or discontinue with renal/hepatic dysfunction. **P/N:** Category B, caution in nursing.	**Throat irritation/dryness**, **bad taste**, cough, nausea, bronchospasm, sneezing, wheezing.
Nedocromil Sodium (Tilade)	**MDI:** 1.75mg/ inh [16.2g]	***Adults:*** 2 inh qid. May reduce to bid-tid once desired response is observed. ***Pediatrics:*** ≥6 yrs: 2 inh qid. May reduce to bid-tid once desired response is observed.	**W/P:** Not for treatment of acute bronchospasm or status asthmaticus. Monitor when reducing systemic or inhaled steroid therapy. Stop therapy if bronchospasm occurs. **P/N:** Category B, caution with nursing.	**Unpleasant taste**, nausea, vomiting, dyspepsia, abdominal pain, **pharyngitis**, headache, cough, rhinitis.
XANTHINE DERIVATIVES				
Aminophylline	**Inj:** 25mg/mL; **Sol:** 105mg/5mL; **Tab:** 100mg, 200mg	***Adults:* Initial:** 16mg/kg/24hr PO or 400mh/24hr PO of theophylline given q6-8h. **Titrate:** Increase by 25% q3d as tolerated & adjust to 10-20mg/mL. ***Pediatrics:* 9 to <16 yrs: Initial:** 6.3mg/kg. **Maint:** 0.8mg/kg/hr. **1 to <9 yr: Initial:** 6.3mg/kg. **Maint:** 1mg/kg/hr.	**W/P:** Extreme caution in peptic ulcer disease, seizure disorders and/or cardiac arrhythmias (except bradycardia). Caution in neonates, children <1 yr, and the elderly. Caution in pulmonary edema, CHF, fever =102°F for 24 hrs, cor-pulmonale, hypothyroidism, liver disease, reduced renal function, sepsis, shock, and HTN. If toxicity develops (eg, repetitive vomiting) monitor serum levels and adjust dosage. **P/N:** Category C, not for use in nursing.	Diarrhea, nausea, vomiting, abdominal pain, nervousness, headache, insomnia, seizures, dizziness, tremor, tachycardia, arrhythmias, restlessness, tremor, transient diuresis.
Theophylline (Theo-24, Theolair, Uniphyl)	**(Theo-24) Cap, Extended Release:** 100mg, 200mg, 300mg, 400mg; **(Theolair) Tab:** 125mg*, 250mg*; **(Uniphyl) Tab, Extended Release:** 400mg*, 600mg*	**(Theo-24)** ***Adults:* Initial:** 300-400mg/ day. **Titrate:** After 3 days increase to 400-600mg/day if tolerated. May increase to >600mg/day if needed and tolerated after 3 more days. **Renal/Liver Dysfunction/Elderly/CHF: Max:** 400mg/ day. May give in divided doses q12h in fast metabolizers. Swallow tab whole with full glass of water, do not crush. Dose should be titrated based on serum levels. **(Theolair)** ***Adults:* Initial:** 300mg/ day divided q6-8h. **Titrate:** if tolerated, after 3 days, increase to 400mg/day divided q6-8h. May increase to 600mg/day divided q6-8h if needed and tolerated after 3 more days. ***Pediatrics:*** ≥1 yr and <45kg: **Initial:** 12-14mg/kg/day divided q4-6h. **Max:** 300mg/day. **Titrate:** If tolerated after 3 days, increase to 16mg/ kg/day divided q6-8h. **Max:** 400mg/day. May increase to 20mg/kg/day divided q6-8h if tolerated and needed after 3 more days. **Max:** 600mg/day. ≥1 yr and >45kg: Follow adult dosage schedule. **(Uniphyl)** ***Adults:* Initial:** 300-400mg qd for 3 days with meals. **Titrate:** Increase to 400-600mg qd. After 3 days	**W/P:** Extreme caution in peptic ulcer disease, seizure disorders and/or cardiac arrhythmias (except bradycardia). Caution in neonates, children <1 yr, and the elderly. Caution in pulmonary edema, CHF, fever =102°F for 24 hrs, cor-pulmonale, hypothyroidism, liver disease, reduced renal function, sepsis, shock, and HTN. If toxicity develops (eg, repetitive vomiting) monitor serum levels and adjust dosage. **P/N:** Category C, caution in nursing.	Diarrhea, nausea, vomiting, abdominal pain, nervousness, headache, insomnia, seizures, dizziness, tremor, tachycardia, arrhythmias, restlessness, tremor, transient diuresis.

Table 15.2: PRESCRIBING INFORMATION FOR RESPIRATORY DRUGS *(cont.)*

NAME	FORM/ STRENGTH	DOSAGE	WARNINGS/PRECAUTIONS & CONTRAINDICATIONS	ADVERSE EFFECTS†
XANTHINE DERIVATIVES *(cont.)*				
Theophylline *(cont.)*		and if needed/tolerated, increase dose according to blood levels. Tab may be split in half; do not chew or crush. **Renal Dysfunction/Elderly (>60 yrs): Max:** 400mg/day. **Conversion from Immediate-Release Theophylline:** Give same daily dose as once daily. ***Pediatrics:* 12-15 yrs: (<45kg): Initial:** 12-14mg/kg/day up to 300mg qd for 3 days with meals. **Titrate:** Increase to 16mg/kg/day up to 400mg qd. After 3 days if needed/tolerated increase to 20mg/kg/day up to 600mg qd. **(>45kg):** Follow adult dose schedule. Tab may be split in half; do not chew or crush. **Conversion from Immediate-Release Theophylline: ≥12 yrs:** Give same daily dose as once daily. **Renal Dysfunction: Max:** 400mg qd. ***Pediatrics:* 12-15 yrs: <45kg: Initial:** 12-14mg/kg/day. **Max:** 300mg/day. **Titrate:** After 3 days increase to 16mg/kg/day. **Max:** 400mg/ day. May increase to 20mg/kg/day if tolerated and needed after 3 more days. **Max:** 600mg/day. **12-15 yrs (>45kg):** Follow adult dose schedule. **Renal/Liver Dysfunction/CHF: Max:** 16mg/kg/day or 400mg/day. May give in divided doses q12h in fast metabolizers. Swallow tab whole with full glass of water, do not crush. Dose should be titrated based on serum levels.		
MISCELLANEOUS				
Dornase alfa (Pulmozyme)	**Sol:** 2.5mg/ 2.5mL [2.5mL, 1ˢ, 30ˢ]	***Adults:*** 2.5mg qd-bid via nebulizer. ***Pediatrics:* ≥5 yrs:** 2.5mg qd-bid via nebulizer.	**W/P:** Use with standard therapies of cystic fibrosis. **Contra:** Hypersensitivity to Chinese hamster ovary cell products. **P/N:** Category B, caution in nursing.	**Voice alteration, pharyngitis,** rash, **laryngitis,** chest pain, conjunctivitis, rhinitis.
Omalizumab (Xolair)	**Inj.:** 150mg [5mL]	***Adults:*** 150-375mg SC every 2 or 4 weeks based on body weight and pre-treatment serum total IgE level. **Max:** 150mg/site. **30-90kg & IgE ≥30-100 IU/mL:** 150mg q4 weeks. **>90-150kg & IgE ≥30-100 IU/mL OR 30-90kg & IgE >100-200 IU/mL OR 30-60kg & IgE >200-300 IU/mL:** 300mg q4 weeks. **>90-150kg & IgE ≥100-200 IU/mL OR >60-90kg & IgE >200-300 IU/mL OR 30-70kg & IgE >300-400 IU/mL:** 225mg q2 weeks. **>90-150kg & IgE >200-300 IU/mL OR >70-90kg & IgE >300-400 IU/mL OR 30-70kg & IgE >400-500 IU/mL OR 30-60kg & IgE >500-600 IU/mL:** 300mg q2 weeks. **>70-90kg & IgE >400-500 IU/mL OR >60-70kg & IgE >500-600 IU/mL OR 30-60kg & IgE >600-700 IU/mL:** 375mg q2 weeks. ***Pediatrics:* ≥12 yrs:** 150-375mg SC 150mg/site. **30-90kg & IgE ≥30-100 IU/mL:** 150mg q4 weeks. **>90-150kg & IgE ≥30-100 IU/mL OR 30-90kg & IgE >100-200 IU/mL OR 30-60kg & IgE >200-300 IU/mL:** 300mg q4 weeks.	**W/P:** Malignant neoplasms and anaphylaxis reported. Not for use in treatment of acute bronchospasm or status asthmaticus. Systemic or inhaled corticosteroids should not be abruptly discontinued when initiating therapy. **P/N:** Category B, caution in nursing.	Injection site reactions, viral infections, upper respiratory infection, sinusitis, headache, **pharyngitis,** pain, arthralgia, leg pain.

*Scored.   †Bold entries denote special dental considerations

NAME	FORM/ STRENGTH	DOSAGE	WARNINGS/PRECAUTIONS & CONTRAINDICATIONS	ADVERSE EFFECTS†
Omalizumab *(cont.)*		>90-150kg & IgE >100-200 IU/mL OR >60-90kg & IgE >200-300 IU/mL OR 30-70kg & IgE >300-400 IU/mL: 225mg q2 weeks. >90-150kg and IgE >200-300 IU/mL OR >70-90kg & IgE >300-400 IU/mL OR 30-70kg & IgE >400-500 IU/mL OR 30-60kg & IgE >500-600 IU/mL: 300mg q2 weeks. >70-90kg & IgE >400-500 IU/mL OR >60-70kg & IgE >500-600 IU/mL OR 30-60kg & IgE >600-700 IU/mL: 375mg q2 weeks.		
Tobramycin (Tobi)	**Sol:** 60mg/mL (300mg/ampule)	*Adults:* Inhale via nebulizer 300mg q12h for 28 days, then stop for 28 days. Resume therapy for next 28 day on/28 day off cycle. *Pediatrics:* ≥6 yrs: Inhale via nebulizer 300mg q12h for 28 days, then stop for 28 days. Resume therapy for next 28 day on/28 day off cycle.	**W/P:** Caution with muscular disorders (eg, myasthenia gravis, Parkinson's disease), and renal, auditory, vestibular, or neuromuscular dysfunction. May cause hearing loss, bronchospasm. Can cause fetal harm in pregnancy. Discontinue if nephrotoxicity occurs until serum level <2µg/mL. **P/N:** Category D, not for use in nursing.	**Voice alteration, taste perversion,** tinnitus.

Table 15.3: DRUG INTERACTIONS FOR RESPIRATORY DRUGS

α/β-ADRENERGIC AGONISTS

Epinephrine (Epipen)

Digitalis	Increased risk of arrhythmias with digitalis.
MAOIs	Potentiated by MAOIs.
Mercurial diuretics	Increased risk of arrhythmias with mercurial diuretics.
Quinidine	Increased risk of arrhythmias with quinidine.
Tricyclic antidepressants	Potentiated by TCAs.
Vasodilators, rapidly acting	Pressor effects may be counteracted by rapidly acting vasodilators.

ANTICHOLINERGICS

Ipratropium Bromide (Atrovent, Atrovent HFA)

Anticholinergics	Caution with anticholinergic-containing drugs.

Tiotropium Bromide (Spiriva)

Anticholinergics	Avoid use with other anticholinergics (eg, ipratropium).

β-ADRENERGIC AGONISTS

Albuterol Sulfate (AccuNeb, Proventil, Proventil HFA, Ventolin HFA)

β-blockers	May cause severe bronchospasm with β-blockers.
Digoxin	Decreases digoxin levels; monitor digoxin.
Epinephrine	Avoid epinephrine.
MAOIs	Extreme caution with MAOIs during or within 2 weeks of discontinuation.
Nonpotassium-sparing diuretics	ECG changes and/or hypokalemia with nonpotassium-sparing diuretics.
Sympathomimetic bronchodilators, short-acting	Avoid other short-acting sympathomimetic bronchodilators.
Sympathomimetics, oral	Caution with oral sympathomimetics
Tricyclic antidepressants	Extreme caution with TCAs during or within 2 weeks of discontinuation.

Formoterol Fumarate (Foradil)

β-blockers	Antagonized effect with β-blockers.
MAOIs	Extreme caution with MAOIs.
Nonpotassium-sparing diuretics	Hypokalemia potentiated by non-potassium sparing diuretics.

β-ADRENERGIC AGONISTS *(cont.)*

Formoterol Fumarate (Foradil) *(cont.)*

QT interval enhancers	Extreme caution with drugs known to prolong QT interval.
Steroids	Hypokalemia potentiated by steroids.
Sympathomimetics	Potentiates other sympathomimetics.
Tricyclic antidepressants	Extreme caution with MAOIs.
Xanthine derivatives	Hypokalemia potentiated by xanthine derivatives (eg, theophylline).

Levalbuterol Hydrochloride (Xopenex)

β-blockers	Antagonized by β-blockers.
Digoxin	Monitor digoxin.
MAOIs	Extreme caution with MAOIs.
Nonpotassium-sparing diuretics	ECG changes and/or hypokalemia with nonpotassium-sparing diuretics.
Sympathomimetics	Avoid other sympathomimetic agents.
Tricyclic antidepressants	Extreme caution with MAOIs.

Levalbuterol Tartrate (Xopenex HFA)

β-blockers	Antagonized by β-blockers.
Digoxin	Monitor digoxin.
MAOIs	Extreme caution with MAOIs.
Nonpotassium-sparing diuretics	ECG changes and/or hypokalemia with nonpotassium-sparing diuretics.
Sympathomimetics	Avoid other sympathomimetic agents.
Tricyclic antidepressants	Extreme caution with MAOIs.

Metaproterenol Sulfate (Alupent)

β$_2$-agonists, aerosol	Avoid other aerosol β$_2$-agonists.
MAOIs	Vascular effects may be potentiated by MAOIs.
Sympathomimetics	Vascular effects may be potentiated by sympathomimetics.
Tricyclic antidepressants	Vascular effects may be potentiated by TCAs.

Pirbuterol Acetate (Maxair)

β$_2$-agonists, aerosol	Avoid other aerosol β$_2$-agonists.
β-blockers	Decreased effect with β-blockers.

Table 15.3: DRUG INTERACTIONS FOR RESPIRATORY DRUGS *(cont.)*

β-ADRENERGIC AGONISTS *(cont.)*

Pirbuterol Acetate (Maxair) *(cont.)*

MAOIs	Vascular effects may be potentiated by MAOIs.
Nonpotassium-sparing diuretics	ECG changes and/or hypokalemia may occur with nonpotassium-sparing diuretics.
Sympathomimetics	Vascular effects may be potentiated by sympathomimetics.
Tricyclic antidepressants	Vascular effects may be potentiated by TCAs.

Salmeterol Xinafoate (Serevent)

β_2-agonists, short-acting	Caution with >8 inhalations of short-acting β_2-agonists.
MAOIs	Extreme caution within 14 days of using MAOIs.
Nonpotassium-sparing diuretics	Caution with non-potassium-sparing diuretics.
Tricyclic antidepressants	Extreme caution within 14 days of using TCAs.

Terbutaline Sulfate (Brethine)

β-blockers	Decreased effect with β-blockers.
Diuretics, loop	Possible ECG changes and hypokalemia with loop diuretics.
Diuretics, thiazide	Possible ECG changes and hypokalemia with thiazide diuretics.
MAOIs	Extreme caution with MAOIs during or within 14 days of treatment.
Sympathomimetics	Avoid other sympathomimetic agents (except aerosol bronchodilators).
Tricyclic antidepressants	Extreme caution with TCAs during or within 14 days of treatment.

BRONCHODILATOR COMBINATIONS

Albuterol Sulfate/Ipratropium Bromide (Combivent, Duoneb)

Anticholinergics	Potential additive interactions with other anticholinergic drugs.
β-blockers	β-blockers and albuterol inhibit effects of each other.
β_1-selective blockers	Use β_1-selective blockers with hyperactive airways.
MAOIs	Avoid MAOI's. Caution with or within 2 weeks of discontinuation of MAOIs.
Non-K+-sparing diuretics	ECG changes and/or hypokalemia may occur with non-K+-sparing diuretics.
Sympathomimetics	Increased risk of cardiovascular effects with other sympathomimetics.
Tricyclic antidepressants	Avoid TCA's. Caution with or within 2 weeks of discontinuation of TCA's.

BRONCHODILATOR COMBINATIONS *(cont.)*

Fluticasone Propionate/Salmeterol Xinafoate (Advair Diskus)

β-blockers	Antagonized by β-blockers.
CYP3A4 inhibitors	Potentiated by other CYP3A4 inhibitors.
Ketoconazole	Potentiated by ketoconazole.
MAOIs	Extreme caution with MAOIs during or within 14 days of use.
Nonpotassium-sparing diuretics	Caution with non-potassium sparing diuretics; ECG changes, hypokalemia may develop.
Tricyclic antidepressants	Extreme caution with TCAs during or within 14 days of use.

INHALED GLUCOCORTICOIDS

Beclomethasone Dipropionate Monohydrate (Beconase AQ)

Corticosteroids	Concomitant systemic corticosteroids increases risk of hypercorticism and/or HPA axis suppression.

Budesonide (Pulmicort Respules, Pulmicort Turbuhaler, Rhinocort Aqua)

Cimetidine	Cimetidine increases plasma levels. (Respules) Slight decrease in clearance and increase in oral bioavailabilty with cimetidine.
Corticosteroids	Concomitant systemic corticosteroids increases risk of hypercorticism and/or HPA axis suppression.
CYP3A4 inhibitors	CYP3A4 inhibitors (eg, itraconazole, clarithromycin, erythromycin) may inhibit metabolism and increase systemic exposure.
Ketoconazole, oral	Oral ketoconazole increases plasma levels.

Flunisolide (Aerobid, Aerobid-M, Nasarel)

Corticosteroids	Concomitant systemic corticosteroids increases risk of hypercorticism and/or HPA axis suppression.

Fluticasone Propionate (Flonase, Flovent HFA)

Ketoconazole	Caution with ketoconazole, may increase serum fluticasone levels.
CYP3A4 inhibitors	Caution with other potent CYP3A4 inhibitors, may increase serum fluticasone levels.
Corticosteroids, inhaled	Concomitant inhaled corticosteroids increases risk of hypercorticism and/or HPA axis suppression.
Ritonavir	Increased levels with ritonavir; avoid use.

Mometasone Furoate (Asmanex Twisthaler)

Ketoconazole	Ketoconazole may increase plasma levels.

Triamcinolone Acetonide (Azmacort, Nasacort AQ)

Prednisone	Caution with prednisone.

Table 15.3: DRUG INTERACTIONS FOR RESPIRATORY DRUGS (cont.)

LEUKOTRIENE MODIFIERS

Montelukast Sodium (Singulair)

CYP450 inducers	Monitor with potent CYP450 inducers (eg, phenobarbital, rifampin).

Zafirlukast (Accolate)

ASA	Increased levels with ASA.
CYP2C9 metabolized drugs	Caution with drugs metabolized by CYP2C9 (eg, tolbutamide, phenytoin, carbamazepine).
CYP3A4 metabolized drugs	Caution with drugs metabolized by CYP3A4 (eg, dihydropyridine calcium-channel blockers, cyclosporine, cisapride, astemizole).
Erythromycin	Decreased levels by erythromycin.
Theophylline	Decreased levels by theophylline. May increase theophylline levels.
Warfarin	Potentiates warfarin.

Zileuton (Zyflo)

Astemizole	Cardiotoxicity (QT interval prolongation, torsades de pointes, cardiac arrest).
β-blockers	Significant increase in β-adrenergic blockade.
Ergoloid Mesylates	Increased risk of ergotism (nausea, vomiting, vasospastic ischemia).
Pimozide	Increased risk of cardiotoxicity (QT prolongation, torsades de pointes, cardiac arrest).
Terfenadine	Increased risk of terfenadine cardiotoxicity (QT prolongation, torsades de pointes, cardiac arrest).
Theophylline	Increased possibility of theophylline toxicity (nausea, vomiting, palpitations, seizures).
Warfarin	Significant increase in prothrombin time.

MAST CELL STABILIZERS

Cromolyn Sodium (Intal)

Isoproterenol	Avoid with isoproterenol during pregnancy.

XANTHINE DERIVATIVES

Theophylline (Theo-24, Theolair, Uniphyl)

Adenosine	Diminishes the effects of adenosine.
Alcohol	Alcohol may increase levels.
Allopurinol	Potentiated by allopurinol.
Aminoglutethimide	Diminished effects with aminoglutethimide.
β-adrenergic blockers	Potentiated by β-adrenergic blockers.
Barbiturates	Diminished effects with barbiturates.

XANTHINE DERIVATIVES *(cont.)*

Theophylline (Theo-24, Theolair, Uniphyl) *(cont.)*

Calcium channel blockers	Potentiated by calcium channel blockers.
Carbamazepine	Diminished effects with carbamazepine. Potentiated by carbamazepine.
Charcoal broiled food	Diminished effects with charcoal broiled food.
Cimetidine	Potentiated by cimetidine.
Ciprofloxacin	Potentiated by ciprofloxacin.
Clarithromycin	Potentiated by clarithromycin.
Contraceptives, oral	Potentiated by oral contraceptives.
Corticosteroids	Potentiated by corticosteroids.
Diazepam	Diminishes the effects of diazepam.
Disulfiram	Potentiated by disulfiram.
Diuretics	Potentiated by diuretics. Diminished effects with diuretics.
Enoxacin	Potentiated by enoxacin.
Ephedrine	Potentiated by ephedrine. Synergistic CNS effects with ephedrine.
Erythromycin	Potentiated by erythromycin.
Estrogen-containing oral contraceptives	May increase levels.
Flurazepam	Diminishes the effects of flurazepam.
Fluvoxamine	Potentiated by fluvoxamine.
Halothane	Increased risk of ventricular arrhythmias with halothane.
High protein/low carbohydrate diet	Diminished effects with high protein/low carbohydrate diet.
Hydantoins	Diminished effects with hydantoins.
Influenza virus vaccine	Potentiated by influenza virus vaccine.
INH	Diminished effects with INH.
Interferon	Potentiated by interferon.
Isoniazid	Potentiated by isoniazid.
Isoproterenol	Diminished effects with isoproterenol.
Ketamine	May lower theophylline seizure threshold.
Ketoconazole	Diminished effects with ketoconazole.

Table 15.3: DRUG INTERACTIONS FOR RESPIRATORY DRUGS (cont.)

XANTHINE DERIVATIVES (cont.)

Theophylline (Theo-24, Theolair, Uniphyl) (cont.)

Lithium	Diminishes the effects of lithium.
Lorazepam	Diminishes the effects of lorazepam.
Macrolides	Potentiated by macrolides.
Methotrexate	Potentiated by methotrexate.
Mexiletine	Potentiated by mexiletine.
Midazolam	Diminishes the effects of midazolam.
Moricizine	Moricizine may decrease levels.
Pancuronium	Diminishes the effects of pancuronium.
Pentoxifylline	Potentiated by pentoxifylline.
Phenobarbital	Diminished effects with phenobarbital.
Phenytoin	Diminished effects with phenytoin.
Propafenone	Propafenone may increase levels.
Propranolol	Potentiated by propranolol.
Quinolone antibiotics	Potentiated by quinolone antibiotics.
Rifampin	Diminished effects with rifampin.
Ritonavir	Diminished effects with ritonavir.
St. John's wort	Diminished effects with St. John's wort.
Sulfinpyrazone	Diminished effects with sulfinpyrazone.
Sympathomimetics	Diminished effects with sympathomimetics.
Tacrine	Potentiated by tacrine.
Thiabendazole	Potentiated by thiabendazole.
Thyroid hormones	Potentiated by thyroid hormones.
Ticlopidine	Potentiated by ticlopidine.
Troleandomycin	Potentiated by troleandomycin.
Verapamil	Verapamil may increase levels.

MISCELLANEOUS

Tobramycin (Tobi)

Aminoglycosides	Hearing loss reported with previous or concomitant systemic aminoglycosides.
Ethacrynic acid	Avoid ethacrynic acid.
Furosemide	Avoid furosemide.

MISCELLANEOUS *(cont.)*

Tobramycin (Tobi) *(cont.)*

Mannitol	Avoid mannitol.
Neurotoxics	Avoid neurotoxic drugs.
Ototoxics	Avoid ototoxic drugs.
Urea	Avoid urea.

Chapter 16

Gastrointestinal Drugs

B. Ellen Byrne, R.Ph., D.D.S., Ph.D.

"Heartburn" occurs daily in approximately 7% of the population. It is a symptom of reflux esophagitis, an irritation and inflammation of the esophageal mucosa caused by the reflux of acidic stomach or duodenal contents retrograde into the esophagus. Reflux esophagitis is commonly seen in gastroesophageal reflux disease (GERD) and peptic ulcer disease (PUD), which are considered together in this chapter because the same drugs are used to treat them. Other symptoms associated with GERD include regurgitation, dysphagia, bleeding and chest pain. Regurgitation is the most specific symptom of GERD and may result in morning hoarseness, laryngitis and pulmonary aspiration.

PUD is a heterogeneous group of disorders characterized by ulceration of the upper gastrointestinal tract. Peptic ulcer disease can occur at any place in the gastrointestinal (GI) tract that is exposed to the erosive action of pepsin and acid. It can be exacerbated by stress, alcohol, cigarette smoking, some foods, aspirin and aspirin-like drugs. Medical therapy for GERD and PUD consists mainly of neutralizing the stomach contents or reducing gastric acid secretions and using promotility agents to enhance peristalsis. Infections with a bacterium, *Helicobacter pylori*, also have been implicated in the pathogenesis of PUD, and eradication of this organism with antibiotics, bismuth compounds and an antisecretory agent has been shown to alter the natural course of peptic ulcer disease. Although the optimal regimen to eradicate *H. pylori* and cure PUD has not been established, a number of combinations are effective. An antisecretory drug often is added to achieve more rapid relief from ulcer symptoms as well as ulcer healing. Antibiotics used in PUD therapy include amoxicillin, clarithromycin, metronidazole and tetracycline. The antisecretory drugs include H_2 receptor antagonists such as cimetidine and proton pump inhibitors such as omeprazole. Bismuth subsalicylate, the third drug in this triad, is found in Pepto-Bismol.

Diarrhea is usually caused by infection, toxins or drugs. Antidiarrheal agents can be sold over the counter or by prescription only. Virally or bacterially induced diarrhea is usually transient and requires only a clear liquid diet and increased fluid intake. Antimicrobial therapy may be indicated. Intravenous fluids may be required if dehydration occurs.

Drug- or toxin-induced diarrhea is best treated by discontinuing the causative agent when possible. Chronic diarrhea may be caused by laxative abuse, lactose intolerance, inflammatory bowel disease, malabsorption syndromes, endocrine disorders or irritable bowel syndrome. Treatment of chronic diarrhea should be aimed at correcting the cause of diarrhea rather than alleviating the symptoms.

"Gastroparesis" is the term for disorders causing gastric stasis. Nausea, vomiting, bloating, fullness and early satiety are signs of gastroparesis. Treatment is aimed at accelerating gastric emptying. This condition is often associated with diabetes.

Crohn's disease and ulcerative colitis are considered together because the same drugs are used to treat these disorders. Crohn's disease is a chronic inflammatory disease that can affect any part of the gastrointestinal system, from mouth to anus. The etiology is unknown. The most common symptoms are abdominal pain and diarrhea. Perirectal fissure with sinus formation and strictures is common.

Ulcerative colitis is an inflammatory disease of the gastrointestinal tract that is limited to the colon and rectum. Typically, patients with ulcerative colitis present with bloody diarrhea. The disease primarily affects young adults. The etiology is unknown. Management of both Crohn's disease and ulcerative colitis is aimed at decreasing the inflammation and providing symptomatic relief.

Nausea and vomiting usually are self-limiting events without serious sequelae. Protracted vomiting may result in dehydration, malnutrition, metabolic alkalosis, hyponatremia, hypokalemia and hypochloremia. Infants and children are at greatest risk.

Nausea and vomiting may occur in patients with inferior myocardial infarction or diabetic ketoacidosis, Addisonian crisis, acute pancreatitis or acute appendicitis.

Drug-induced nausea and vomiting are common in cancer chemotherapy. However, numerous other drugs—such as narcotics, antibiotics (erythromycin, quinolones, flucytosine, nitrofurantoin and tetracyclines), digoxin and theophylline—also may cause nausea and vomiting.

Viral gastroenteritis is the most common cause of nausea and vomiting. Bacterial infections, motion sickness and pregnancy are other frequently encountered etiologies of nausea and vomiting.

Treatment of nausea and vomiting can include removal or treatment of the underlying cause. Antiemetic therapy is indicated in patients with electrolyte disturbances secondary to vomiting, severe anorexia or weight loss. Antiemetic drugs are available over the counter and by prescription. If a patient is unable to retain oral medication, rectal and injectable routes of administration may be preferable. Many classes of drugs have been used to treat nausea and vomiting, including antihistamines, anticholinergics, seratonin antagonists, dopamine antagonists, phenothiazines, cannabinoids and butyrophenones.

Antidiarrheal Agents

Special Dental Considerations

There are no contraindications to the dental treatment of patients with diarrhea.

Most acute diarrhea is self-limiting. The opioids and anticholinergics used to treat diarrhea produce xerostomia; therefore, meticulous oral hygiene should be stressed. These drugs also produce drowsiness and this effect is additive with other CNS depressants, thereby producing greater drowsiness. For general prescribing information on antidiarrheal agents, see Tables 16.1 (Rx) and 16.2 (OTC).

Drug Interactions of Dental Interest

Drugs used to treat diarrhea include opioids and absorbents. Drug interactions of concern with opioids (narcotics) would occur if the patient took another CNS depressant drug, such as alcohol, antidepressants, antianxiety agents, anticholinergics, antihistamines or barbiturates. This combination of drugs may seriously increase the side effect of either drug.

Adsorbent drugs such as bismuth salts and cholestyramine can bind with various drugs resulting in decreased adsorption of the drug and a decreased therapeutic response. If these drugs must be taken together it is best to space dosing by 6 hours.

For information on drug interactions with antidiarrheal agents, see Tables 16.3 (Rx) and 16.4 (OTC).

Pharmacology

Antidiarrheal agents can be divided into antibiotic and nonantibiotic drugs. Antibiotics are the mainstay of treatment of acute bacterial diarrhea. Whenever possible, antibiotics should be directed toward specific microorganisms either identified by culture or clinically suspected.

There are many commercial preparations sold for symptomatic relief of diarrhea. Controlled clinical trials have not proven the safety and effectiveness of most of them.

Adsorbents have been shown to increase stool consistency but do not decrease stool water content.

Anticholinergics relieve cramps by reducing contractile activity but have no effect on diarrhea.

Bismuth subsalicylate binds toxins and prevents bacteria from attaching to intestinal epithelium.

Cholestyramine has been shown to effectively bind *Clostridium difficile* toxins and perhaps other bacterial toxins.

The opioids have a profound effect on motility. These agents are generally contraindicated in dysentery.

In general, these nonspecific antidiarrheal agents should not be used as a substitute for oral rehydration and directed antibiotics.

Crohn's Disease and Ulcerative Colitis Drugs

Special Dental Considerations

There are no contraindications to the dental treatment of patients with Crohn's disease. The leukopenic and thrombocytopenic effects of sulfasalazine may increase the incidence of certain microbial infections, delay healing and increase gingival bleeding. If a patient has leukopenia or thrombocytopenia, dental treatment should be deferred until laboratory counts have returned to normal. Patients treated with glucocorticoids are likely to have a decreased resistance to infection and a poor wound healing response. Actual and potential sources of infection in the mouth should be treated promptly. If surgical procedures are necessary, they should be as atraumatic, conservative and aseptic as possible. Prophylactic antibiotic coverage should be considered in most cases. Adrenal suppression owing to the administration of glucocorticoids is also a consideration. Depending on the dose and length of treatment, the patient may require an increased dose of glucocorticoids before undergoing stressful dental treatment.

For patients with ulcerative colitis, use of antibiotics may aggravate the problem. Antibiotics most often associated with ulcerative colitis are broad-spectrum penicillins.

See Table 16.1 for general prescribing information on Crohn's disease and ulcerative colitis drugs.

Drug Interactions of Dental Interest

See Table 16.3 for drug interaction information on Crohn's disease and ulcerative colitis drugs.

Pharmacology

Crohn's disease is a chronic inflammatory condition of the gastrointestinal tract. Current therapy is directed at reducing inflammation and providing systematic relief. Initial treatment includes sulfasalazine antibiotics and nutritional support. Sulfasalazine (through its active component 5-aminosalicylic acid [5ASA]) exerts an anti-inflammatory effect on the colon. Metronidazole is most commonly used and likely functions by reducing bacterial endotoxin and granuloma formation.

Second-line therapy includes the use of glucocorticoids for reduction of inflammation followed by the use of immunomodulating drugs, such as azothioprine, which also reduce inflammation.

Gastric Motility Disorder (Gastroparesis) Drug

Special Dental Considerations

There are no contraindications to the dental treatment of patients with gastroparesis. See Table 16.1 for general prescribing information on the gastric motility drug metoclopramide.

Drug Interactions of Dental Interest

Drugs that treat gastroparesis increase gastrointestinal mobility and decrease gastric emptying time. Oral absorption from the stomach may be decreased while absorption from the small intestine may be enhanced. See Table 16.3 for drug interaction information on the gastric motility drug metoclopramide.

Pharmacology

Diabetic gastroparesis is a common GI complication of diabetes mellitus. Caused by delayed gastric emptying, the symptoms range from early satiety and bloating to severe gastric retention with nausea, vomiting and abdominal pain. Impaired gastric emptying is caused by abnormal motility of the stomach or a reduction in motor activity in the intestine. Metoclopramide affects gut motility through indirect cholinergic stimulation of the gut muscle.

Gastroesophageal Reflux Disease and Peptic Ulcer Disease Drugs

Special Dental Considerations

There are no contraindications to the dental treatment of patients with GERD or PUD; however, drugs that cause gastrointestinal injury should be avoided in patients with GERD or PUD. These drugs include erythromycin, aspirin, corticosteroids and nonsteroidal anti-inflammatory agents. Dental patients with GERD should be kept in a semi-supine chair position for patient comfort because of the reflux effects of this disease. Xerostomia is a common side effect of the anticholinergic agents and meticulous oral hygiene must be emphasized. Many anticholinergic agents also induce orthostatic or postural hypotension. Therefore, dental patients treated with one of these agents should remain in the dental chair in an upright position for several minutes before being dismissed.

For general prescribing information on GERD and PUD drugs, see Tables 16.1 (Rx) and 16.2 (OTC).

Drug Interactions of Dental Interest

Drugs used to treat GERD and PUD include antacids, H_2 histamine receptor antagonists, anticholinergics and promotility agents.

Antacids potentially interfere with the absorption of many drugs by forming a complex with these drugs or by altering gastric pH. Antacids containing metal cations (Mg^{2+}, Ca^{2+}, Al^{3+}) have a strong affinity for tetracycline, and response to the antibiotic can vary according to the extent of the complex.

Antacids increase the intragastric pH, and this can decrease the absorption of drugs that require an acidic environment for dissolution and absorption. Conversely, enteric-coated drugs such as erythromycin may be released prematurely.

Most of these drug-antacid interactions can be minimized by administering each drug 2 hours from the other.

The H_2 histamine receptor antagonist cimetadine can bind to the cytochrome P450 mixed-function oxidase system and can inhibit the biotransformation of drugs by the liver. This results in inhibition of metabolism and increased serum drug concentrations of the drug not metabolized. Serum levels of some benzodiazepines (diazepam, alprazolam, chlorodiazepoxide, midazolam, triazolam) have been shown to increase, resulting in enhanced sedation.

Anticholinergics can decrease gastric emptying time, which can increase the amount of drug absorbed or increase the degradation of a drug in the stomach, thus decreasing the amount of drug absorbed. Overall, this interaction appears to have minor significance.

For drug interaction information on GERD and PUD drugs, see Tables 16.3 (Rx) and 16.4 (OTC).

Pharmacology

H_2 histamine receptor antagonists are effective for short-term treatment of GERD and PUD. These agents prevent histamine-induced acid release by competing with histamine for H_2 receptors.

Proton-pump inhibitors (such as omeprazole) act by irreversibly blocking the H^+/ K^+-ATPase pump. It markedly inhibits both basal and stimulated gastric acid secretion.

Antacids act by neutralizing gastric acid and thus raising the gastric pH. This has the effect of inhibiting peptic activity, which practically ceases at pH 5. The antacids in common use are salts of magnesium and aluminum. Magnesium salts cause diarrhea and aluminum salts cause constipation, so mixtures of the two are used to maintain bowel function.

Drugs that protect the mucosa can do so by either forming a protective physical barrier over the surface of the ulcer (sucralfate) or enhancing or augmenting endogenous prostaglandins (misoprostol) to promote bicarbonate and mucin release, and inhibit acid secretion.

Anticholinergic agents (such as propantheline bromide) have played a limited role in the treatment of PUD by inhibiting vagally stimulated gastric acid secretion. These agents are not considered first-line agents for treatment of PUD.

Antiemetic Drugs

Special Dental Considerations

The dentist should be aware of why the patient is taking a drug for nausea and vomiting. If the patient is receiving the drug for cancer chemotherapy, he or she may require palliative therapy for stomatitis. Patients with cancer may be taking chronic opioids for pain. The dentist should not prescribe additional drugs for pain without reviewing the patient's medication profile. Also, the dentist should avoid procedures or drugs that could promote nausea and vomiting. An increased gag reflex makes it difficult for the patient to undergo dental procedures such as obtaining radiographs or impressions. Many antiemetic drugs cause xerostomia, so these patients should avoid mouthrinses containing alcohol because of its drying effects. They also should use sugarless gum or saliva substitutes or take sips of water.

For general prescribing information on antiemetic drugs, see Tables 16.1 (Rx) and 16.2 (OTC).

Drug Interactions of Dental Interest

Antacids can decrease the absorption of many drugs, including tetracycline, digoxin, benzodiazepines, iron salts and indomethacin. Antihistamines, phenothiazines and butyrophenones cause drowsiness. This drowsiness may be additive with that caused by other CNS depressants.

For drug interaction information on antiemetic drugs, see Tables 16.3 (Rx) and 16.4 (OTC).

Pharmacology

Numerous pathways are capable of stimulating the vomiting center and chemoreceptor trigger zone in the brain, so it is not surprising that a wide variety of drugs can be used in treating nausea and vomiting. Phenothiazines and butyrophenones block dopamine receptors and are believed to act at the chemoreceptor trigger zone. Antihistamines and anticholinergics are effective in managing vomiting associated with vestibular disturbances by blocking acetylcholine receptors in the vestibular center. Metoclopramide is a dopamine antagonist that has both peripheral and central antiemetic actions. This drug accelerates gastric emptying, inhibits gastric relaxation and appears to block the chemoreceptor trigger zone. Ondansetron is a highly selective and potent antagonist of 5-HT$_3$ (serotonin) receptors. Cannabinoids such as dronabinol are believed to inhibit emesis by blocking descending impulses from the cerebral cortex. Glucocorticoids have demonstrated antiemetic activity in patients receiving cancer chemotherapy. Their mechanism of action is unknown.

Laxatives

Constipation generally is defined as a decrease in the frequency of fecal elimination and is characterized by the difficult passage of hard, dry stools. By definition, laxatives facilitate the passage and elimination of feces from the large intestine (colon) and rectum.

Laxatives can be divided into bulk products, lubricants, osmotics, saline laxatives, stimulants and stool softeners.

Bulk laxatives work by absorbing water and expanding to increase moisture content and bulk in the stool. Lubricants increase water retention in the stool, causing reabsorption of water in the bowel. Stimulants act by increasing peristalsis by direct effect on the intestines. Saline draws water into the intestinal lumen. Osmotics increase distension and promote peristalsis. Stool softeners, also known as emollients, reduce surface tension of liquids in the bowel.

For general prescribing information on laxatives, see Tables 16.1 (Rx) and 16.2 (OTC). For information on drug interactions, see Tables 16.3 (Rx) and 16.4 (OTC).

Suggested Readings

Anderson PO, Knoben JE, eds. Handbook of clinical drug data. 8th ed. Stamford, Conn.: Appleton & Lange; 1997.

Berardi RR. GI disorders. In: Allen LV, ed. Handbook of nonprescription drugs. 12th ed. Washington: American Pharmaceutical Association; 2000:241–737.

Tatro DS, ed. Drug interactions facts: facts and comparisons. St. Louis: Facts and Comparisons; 1995.

Wells BG, DiPiro JT, Schwinghammer TL, Hamilton CW. Pharmacotherapy handbook. Stamford, Conn.: Appleton & Lange; 1998.

Young LY, Koda-Kimble MA, eds. Applied therapeutics: the clinical use of drugs. 6th ed. Vancouver, Wash.: Applied Therapeutics; 1995.

Table 16.1: PRESCRIBING INFORMATION FOR RX GASTROINTESTINAL DRUGS

NAME	FORM/ STRENGTH	DOSAGE	WARNINGS/PRECAUTIONS & CONTRAINDICATIONS	ADVERSE EFFECTS†
ANTIDIARRHEAL				
Atropine Sulfate/ Diphenoxylate Hydrochloride (Lomotil)	**Sol:** 2.5mg-0.025/5mL [60mL]; **Tab:** 2.5mg-0.025mg	***Adults*: Initial:** 2 tabs or 10mL qid. **Titrate:** Reduce dose after symptoms are controlled. **Maint:** 2 tabs or 10mL qd. **Max:** 20mg/day diphenoxylate. Discontinue if symptoms are not controlled after 10 days of max dose 20mg/day (diphenoxylate). ***Pediatrics*: 2-12 yrs: Initial:** 0.3-0.4mg/kg/day of solution given qid. **13-16 yrs: Initial:** 2 tabs or 10mL tid. **Titrate:** Reduce dose after symptoms are controlled. **Maint:** 25% of initial dose. Discontinue if no improvement within 48 hrs.	**W/P:** May induce toxic megacolon in ulcerative colitis; discontinue if abdominal distention occurs. May cause intestinal fluid retention. Avoid use with diarrhea associated with organisms that penetrate the intestinal mucosa, and with pseudomembranous enterocolitis. Caution in pediatrics, especially with Down's syndrome. Extreme caution advanced hepatorenal disease and liver dysfunction. Do not use with severe dehydration or electrolyte imbalance until corrective therapy is initiated. **Contra:** Obstructive jaundice, diarrhea associated with pseudomembranous enterocolitis or enterotoxin-producing bacteria. **P/N:** Category C, caution in nursing.	Numbness of extremities, dizziness, anaphylaxis, hyperthermia, tachycardia, urinary retention, flushing, drowsiness, toxic megacolon, nausea, vomiting.
ANTIEMETICS				
Arepitant (Emend)	**Cap:** 80mg, 125mg [Tri-Pak]	***Adults*: Day 1:** 125mg 1 hr prior to chemotherapy. **Days 2 and 3:** 80mg qam. Regimen should include a corticosteroid and a 5-HT₃ antagonist. **Concomitant Corticosteroid:** Reduce dexamethasone PO or methylprednisolone PO by 50% and methylprednisolone IV by 25%.	**W/P:** Chronic continuous use is not recommended. Caution with severe hepatic insufficiency. **Contra:** Concurrent treatment with pimozide, terfenadine, astemizole, or cisapride. **P/N:** Category B, not for use in nursing.	Asthenia/fatigue, nausea, constipation, diarrhea, hiccups, anorexia, headache, vomiting, dizziness, dehydration, heartburn, abdominal pain, epigastric discomfort, gastritis, tinnitis, neutropenia.
Benzocaine/ Trimethobenzamide Hydrochloride (Tigan)	**Sup:** (Benzocaine-Trimethobenzamide) 2%-200mg (Sup, Pediatric), 2%-100mg	***Adults*: (Sup)** 200mg tid-qid. ***Pediatrics*: (Sup, Pediatric) 30-90 lbs:** 100-200mg tid-qid. **<30 lbs:** 100mg tid-qid.	**W/P:** Caution in children; may cause EPS, which may be confused with CNS signs of undiagnosed primary disease (eg, Reye's syndrome) and may unfavorably alter the course of Reye's syndrome due to hepatotoxic potential. Caution with acute febrile illness, encephalitides, gastroenteritis, dehydration, electrolyte imbalance, and in elderly; CNS reactions reported. May produce drowsiness. **Contra:** Injection in children, suppositories in premature or newborn infants, suppositories if hypersensitive to similar local anesthetics. **P/N:** Safety in pregnancy and nursing not known.	Hypersensitivity reactions, Parkinson-like symptoms, hypotension (inj), blood dyscrasias, blurred vision, coma, convulsions, mood depression, diarrhea, disorientation, dizziness, drowsiness, headache, jaundice, muscle cramps, opisthotonos.
Chlorpromazine (Thorazine)	**Cap, Extended Release:** 30mg, 75mg, 150mg; **Tab:** 10mg, 25mg, 50mg, 100mg, 200mg; **Inj:** 25mg/mL; **Syr:** 10mg/5mL [120mL]; **Sup:** 25mg, 100mg	***Adults*: Severe Behavioral Problems: Inpatient: Acute Schizophrenic/ Manic State:** 25mg IM, then 25-50mg IM in 1 hr if needed. **Titrate:** Increase over several days up to 400mg q4-6h until controlled then switch to PO. **Usual:** 500mg/day PO. **Max:** 1000mg/day PO. **Less Acutely Disturbed:** 25mg PO tid. **Titrate:** Increase gradually to 400mg/day. **Outpatient:** 10mg PO tid-qid or 25mg PO bid-tid. **More Severe:** 25mg PO tid. **Titrate:** After 1-2 days, increase by 20-50mg twice weekly until calm. **Prompt Control of Severe Symptoms:** 25mg IM, may repeat in 1 hr then 25-50mg PO tid. **Nausea/Vomiting: Usual:** 10-25mg PO q4-6h prn; 25mg IM then, if no hypotension,	**W/P:** Tardive dyskinesia, NMS may occur. Caution with chronic respiratory disorders, acute respiratory infections (especially in children), glaucoma, cardiovascular, hepatic, or renal disease, history of hepatic encephalopathy due to cirrhosis. Suppresses cough reflex; aspiration of vomitus possible. Caution if exposed to extreme heat or organophosphates. Avoid in children/adolescents with signs of Reye's syndrome. Lowers seizure threshold. Reduce dose gradually to prevent side effects. May mask signs of overdoses to other drugs and obscure diagnosis of other conditions (eg, intestinal obstruction, brain tumor, Reye's syndrome). May produce false-positive PKU test. May elevate prolactin levels. Injection	Drowsiness, jaundice, agranulocytosis, hypotensive effects, EKG changes, dystonias, motor restlessness, pseudo-parkinsonism, tardive dyskinesia, anticholinergic effects, NMS, ocular changes.

*Scored.   †Bold entries denote special dental considerations.

Table 16.1: PRESCRIBING INFORMATION FOR RX GASTROINTESTINAL DRUGS (cont.)

NAME	FORM/ STRENGTH	DOSAGE	WARNINGS/PRECAUTIONS & CONTRAINDICATIONS	ADVERSE EFFECTS†
ANTIEMETICS (cont.)				
Chlorpromazine (cont.)		25-50mg q3-4h prn until vomiting stops then switch to PO; 100mg rectally q6-8h prn. **Nausea/Vomiting in Surgery:** 12.5mg IM, may repeat in 1/2 hr; 2mg IV per fractional injection at 2 minute intervals. **Max:** 25mg. **Presurgical Apprehension:** 25-50mg PO 2-3 hrs pre-op; 12.5-25mg IM 1-2 hrs pre-op. **Intractable Hiccups:** 25-50mg PO tid-qid; if symptoms persist after 2-3 days, give 25-50mg IM; if symptoms still persist, give 25-50mg slow IV. **Porphyria:** 25-50mg PO tid-qid; 25mg IM tid-qid until PO therapy. **Tetanus:** 25-50mg IM tid-qid; 25-50mg IV. **Elderly:** Use lower doses, increase dose more gradually, monitor closely. *Pediatrics:* **6 months-12 yrs: Severe Behavioral Problems: Outpatient:** 0.25mg/lb PO q4-6h prn; 0.5mg/lb sup rectally q6-8h prn; 0.25mg/lb IM q6-8h prn. **Inpatient:** Start low and increase gradually to 50-100mg/day; ≥200mg/day in older children. **Max:** 500mg/day. **<5 yrs (<50lbs): Max:** ≤40mg/day **IM: 5-12 yrs (50-100lbs): Max:** ≤75mg/day IM. **Nausea/Vomiting:** 0.25mg/lb PO q4-6h; 0.5mg/lb sup rectally q6-8 prn. 0.25mg/lb IM q6-8h prn. **Max: 6 months-5 yrs (or 50 lbs):**<40mg/day. **5-12 yrs (or 50-100lbs):** <75mg/day except in severe cases. **During Surgery:** 0.125mg/lb IM repeat in 1/2 hr if needed; 1mg IV per fractional injection at 2-minute intervals and not exceeding recommended IM dosage. **Presurgical Apprehension:** 0.25mg/lb PO 2-3 hrs (or IM 1-2 hrs) before operation. **Tetanus:** 0.25mg/lb IM/IV q6-8h. **<50lbs: Max:** <40mg/day. **50-100lbs: Max:** <75mg/day.	contains sulfites. **Contra:** Comatose states, or with large amounts of CNS depressants. Hypersensitivity to phenothiazines. **P/N:** Safety in pregnancy not known. Not for use in nursing.	
Dolasetron Mesylate (Anzemet)	Tab: 50mg, 100mg; Inj: 20mg/mL	*Adults:* (Inj) **Prevention of Chemotherapy Nausea/Vomiting:** 1.8mg/kg IV single dose or 100mg IV 30 minutes before chemotherapy. **Prevention/Treatment of Post-op Nausea/Vomiting:** 12.5mg IV single dose 15 minutes before cessation of anesthesia or as soon as nausea/vomiting presents. **(Tab) Prevention of Chemotherapy Induced Nausea/Vomiting:** 100mg PO within 1 hr before chemotherapy. **Prevention of Postoperative Nausea/Vomiting:** 100mg PO within 2 hrs before surgery. *Pediatrics:* **2-16 yrs: (Inj) Prevention of Chemotherapy Nausea/Vomiting:** 1.8mg/kg IV single dose 30 minutes before	**W/P:** Caution in patients with or may develop cardiac conduction interval prolongation, especially those with congenital QT syndrome, hypokalemia and hypomagnesemia. Cross sensitivity may occur with other 5-HT$_3$ antagonists. Can cause ECG interval changes. **P/N:** Category B, caution in nursing.	Headache, diarrhea, fever, fatigue, dizziness, abnormal hepatic function, chills/shivering, urinary retention, abdominal pain, HTN.

*Scored.   †Bold entries denote special dental considerations.

NAME	FORM/ STRENGTH	DOSAGE	WARNINGS/PRECAUTIONS & CONTRAINDICATIONS	ADVERSE EFFECTS†
Dolasetron Mesylate (cont.)		chemotherapy. **Max:** 100mg. May mix Injection in apple or grape juice and take orally within 1 hr before chemotherapy. **Prevention/Treatment of Post-op Nausea/Vomiting:** 0.35mg/kg IV single dose 15 minutes before cessation of anesthesia or as soon as nausea/vomiting presents. **Max:** 12.5mg single dose. May mix 1.2mg/kg inj in apple or grape juice and take orally within 2 hrs before surgery. **Max:** 100mg/dose. **(Tab) Prevention of Chemotherapy Induced Nausea/Vomiting:** 1.8mg/kg PO within 1 hr before chemotherapy. **Max:** 100mg. **Prevention of Postoperative Nausea/Vomiting:** 1.2mg/kg PO within 2 hrs before surgery. **Max:** 100mg.		
Dronabinol (Marinol)	**Cap:** 2.5mg, 5mg, 10mg	***Adults*: Appetite Stimulation: Initial:** 2.5mg bid before lunch and supper or 2.5mg qpm or qhs if 5mg/day is intolerable. **Max:** 20mg/day in divided doses. **Antiemetic: Initial:** 5mg/m² given 1-3 hrs before chemotherapy, then q2-4h after chemotherapy, up to 4-6 doses/day. **Titrate:** May increase by 2.5mg/m² increments. **Max:** 15mg/m²/dose.	**W/P:** Do not engage in any hazardous activity until ability to tolerate drug is established. Caution with cardiac disorders due to possible HTN/hypotension, syncope, tachycardia. Caution with history of substance abuse. Monitor with mania, depression, schizophrenia; may exacerbate illness. Caution in elderly due to increased sensitivity to the psychoactive effects. Initial dose and adjustments should be supervised by responsible adult. **Contra:** Hypersensitivity to sesame oil. **P/N:** Category C, not for use in nursing.	Euphoria, dizziness, paranoid reaction, somnolence, abnormal thinking, abdominal pain, nausea, vomiting, diarrhea, conjunctivitis, hypotension, flushing.
Droperidol (Inapsine)	**Inj:** 2.5mg/mL	***Adults*: Initial (Max):** 2.5mg IM/IV. May give additional 1.25mg cautiously to achieve desired effect. Lower initial doses in elderly, debilitated, poor-risk patients. ***Pediatrics*: 2-12 yrs: Initial (Max):** 0.1 mg/kg IM/IV. May give additional dose cautiously. Lower initial doses in debilitated, poor-risk patients.	**BB:** QT prolongation, torsade de pointes, arrhythmias reported. Use in patients resistant or intolerant to other therapies. Monitor ECG before and 2-3 hrs after treatment. Extreme caution if at risk for developing prolonged QT syndrome. **W/P:** Caution with renal/hepatic impairment. HTN, tachycardia reported with pheochromocytoma. Risk of prolonged QT syndrome with CHF, cardiac disease, bradycardia, cardiac hypertrophy, electrolyte imbalances (eg, hypokalemia, hypomagnesemia), >65 yrs, alcohol abuse. NMS reported; give dantrolene with increased temperature, heart rate, or carbon dioxide production. May decrease pulmonary arterial pressure. **Contra:** Known or suspected QT prolongation, including congenital long QT syndrome. **P/N:** Category C, caution in nursing.	QT interval prolongation, torsade de pointes, cardiac arrest, hypotension, tachycardia, dysphoria, post-op drowsiness, restlessness, hyperactivity, anxiety, depression, syncope, irregular cardiac rhythm.
Meclizine Hydrochloride (Antivert)	**Tab:** 12.5mg, 25mg, 50mg*	***Adults*: Motion Sickness:** 25-50mg 1 hr prior to trip/departure, repeat q24h prn. Vertigo: 25-100mg/day in divided doses. ***Pediatrics*: ≥12 yrs: Motion Sickness:** 25-50mg 1 hr prior to trip/departure, repeat q24h prn. **Vertigo:** 25-100mg/day in divided doses.	**W/P:** Caution with asthma, glaucoma, prostatic hypertrophy. **P/N:** Category B, safety in nursing is not known.	Drowsiness, **dry mouth**, blurred vision (rare).

Table 16.1: PRESCRIBING INFORMATION FOR RX GASTROINTESTINAL DRUGS (cont.)

NAME	FORM/ STRENGTH	DOSAGE	WARNINGS/PRECAUTIONS & CONTRAINDICATIONS	ADVERSE EFFECTS†
ANTIEMETICS (cont.)				
Granisetron Hydrochloride (Kytril)	**Inj:** 0.1mg/ml, 1mg/mL; **Sol:** 2mg/10mL; **Tab:** 1mg	**Adults: Prevention with Chemotherapy:** (PO) 2mg qd up to 1 hr before chemotherapy or 1mg bid (up to 1 hr before chemotherapy and 12 hrs later). (IV) 10µg/kg within 30 minutes before chemotherapy. **Prevention with Radiation:** (PO) 2mg within 1 hr of radiation. **Post-Op Prevention:** (IV) Administer 1 mg over 30 seconds before induction of anesthesia or immediately before anesthesia reversal. **Post-Op Treatment:** (IV) Administer 1mg over 30 seconds. **Pediatrics: 2-16 yrs: Prevention with Chemotherapy:** 10µg/kg IV within 30 minutes before chemotherapy.	**W/P:** (Inj) Does not stimulate gastric or intestinal peristalsis. Do not use instead of nasogastric suction. May mask progressive ileus or gastric distension. **P/N:** Category B, caution in nursing.	Headache, asthenia, somnolence, diarrhea, constipation, abdominal pain, dizziness, insomnia, decreased appetite, fever.
Metoclopramide Hydrochloride (Reglan)	**Inj:** 5mg/mL; **Syr:** 5mg/5mL; **Tab:** 5mg, 10mg*	**Adults: GERD: PO:** 10-15mg qid 30 minutes ac and hs. **Elderly:** 5 mg qid. **Max:** 12 weeks of therapy. **Intermittent Symptoms:** Up to 20mg single dose prior to provoking situation. **Gastroparesis:** 10mg PO 30 minutes ac and hs for 2-8 weeks. **Severe Gastroparesis:** May give same doses IV/IM for up to 10 days if needed. **Antiemetic:** (Postoperative) 10-20mg IM near end of surgery. (Chemotherapy-Induced) 1-2mg/kg 30 minutes before chemotherapy then q2h for two doses, then q3h for three doses. Give 2mg/kg for highly emetogenic drugs for initial 2 doses. **Small Bowel Intubation/Radiological Exam:** 10mg IV single dose. **CrCl <40mL/min:** 50% of normal dose. **Pediatrics: Small Bowel Intubation: 6-14 yrs:** 2.5-5mg IV single dose. **<6 yrs:** 0.1mg/kg IV single dose. **CrCl <40mL/min:** 50% of normal dose.	**W/P:** Caution with HTN, Parkinson's disease, depression. EPS, tardive dyskinesia, Parkinsonian-like symptoms, neuroleptic malignant syndrome reported. Administer IV injection slowly. Risk of developing fluid retention and volume overload especially with cirrhosis or CHF; discontinue if these occur. May increase pressure of suture lines. **Contra:** Where GI mobility stimulation is dangerous (eg, perforation, obstruction, hemorrhage), pheochromocytoma, seizure disorder, concomitant drugs that cause EPS effects. **P/N:** Category B, caution with nursing.	Restlessness, drowsiness, fatigue, EPS effects (acute dystonic reactions), galactorrhea, hyperprolactinemia, hypotension, arrhythmia, diarrhea, dizziness, urinary frequency.
Ondansetron (Zofran, Zofran ODT)	**Inj:** 2mg/mL, 32mg/50mL; **Sol:** 4mg/5mL [50mL]; **Tab:** 4mg, 8mg, 24mg; **Tab, Disintegrating:** 4mg, 8mg	**Adults: Prevention of Chemotherapy-Induced Nausea/Vomiting: (Inj)** 32mg single dose or three 0.15mg/kg doses, 1st dose 30 minutes before chemotherapy, then 4 and 8 hours after the 1st dose. **Prevention of Nausea/Vomiting Associated With Highly Emetogenic Cancer Chemotherapy: (Tab)** 24mg single dose tab 30 minutes before chemotherapy. **Prevention of Nausea/Vomiting Associated With Moderately Emetogenic Cancer Chemotherapy: (Sol/Tab)** 8mg bid, 1st dose 30 minutes before chemotherapy, then 8 hrs later, then bid for 1-2 days after chemotherapy. **Prevention of Post-Op Nausea/Vomiting: (Inj)** 4mg IM/IV immediately before anesthesia or post-op after surgery if nausea or vomiting occurs. **(Sol/Tab)** 16mg 1 hr before anesthesia. **Prevention of Nausea/Vomiting Associated with Radiation Therapy: (Sol/Tab)**	**W/P:** Hypersensitivity reactions have been reported in those hypersensitive to other 5-HT$_3$ receptor antagonists. May mask a progressive ileus or gastric distension. Orally disintegrating tablets contain phenylalanine; caution in phenylketonurics. **P/N:** Category B, caution in nursing.	Headache, diarrhea, dizziness, drowsiness, malaise/fatigue, constipation, LFT abnormalities.

*Scored.   †Bold entries denote special dental considerations.

NAME	FORM/ STRENGTH	DOSAGE	WARNINGS/PRECAUTIONS & CONTRAINDICATIONS	ADVERSE EFFECTS†
Ondansetron (cont.)		**Usual:** 8mg tid. **Total Body Irradiation:** 8mg 1-2 hrs before therapy daily. **Single High-Dose Therapy To Abdomen:** 8mg 1-2 hrs before therapy then q8h after 1st dose for 1-2 days after completion of therapy. **Daily Fractionated Therapy To Abdomen:** 8mg 1-2 hrs before therapy then q8h after 1st dose. **Severe Hepatic Dysfunction (Child-Pugh2 ≥10): Max:** 8mg/day IV single dose infused over 15 minutes, start 30 minutes before chemotherapy or 8mg/day PO. *Pediatrics:* **Prevention of Chemotherapy-Induced Nausea/ Vomiting: (Inj) 6 months-18 yrs:** Three 0.15mg/kg doses, 1st dose 30 minutes before chemotherapy, then 4 and 8 hrs after the 1st dose. **(Sol/Tab) Prevention of Nausea/Vomiting Associated With Moderately Emetogenic Cancer Chemotherapy: ≥12 yrs:** 8mg bid, 1st dose 30 minutes before chemotherapy, then 8mg 8 hrs later, then bid for 1-2 days. **4-11 yrs:** 4mg tid, 1st dose 30 minutes before chemotherapy, then 4 and 8 hrs after 1st dose, then tid for 1-2 days. **Prevention of Post-Op Nausea/Vomiting: (Inj) >12 yrs:** 4mg IM/IV immediately before anesthesia or post-op after surgery if nausea or vomiting occurs. **1 month-12 yrs: ≤40kg:** 0.1mg/kg single dose. **>40kg:** 4mg single dose. **Severe Hepatic Dysfunction: Max:** 8mg/day IV single dose infused over 15 minutes, start 30 minutes before chemotherapy or 8mg/day PO.		
Palonosetron Hydrochloride (Aloxi)	**Inj:** 0.25mg/5mL	*Adults:* 0.25mg IV single dose 30 minutes before start of chemotherapy. Repeated dosing within a 7-day interval is not recommended.	**W/P:** Caution with, or at risk of developing, prolongation of cardiac conduction intervals, particulary QTc (eg, hypokalemia, hypomagnesemia, congenital QT syndrome). Caution with diuretics which induce electrolyte abnormalities, drugs which cause QT prolongation (eg, antiarrhythmics), and cumulative high-dose anthracycline therapy. **P/N:** Category B, not for use in nursing.	Headache, constipation, diarrhea, dizziness.
Prochlorperazine (Compazine)	**Inj:** (as edisylate) 5mg/mL; **Sup:** (as edisylate) 2.5mg; **Tab:** (as maleate) 5mg, 10mg	*Adults:* **Nausea/Vomiting: (Tab) Usual:** 5-10mg tid-qid. **Max:** 40mg/day. **(IM)** 5-10mg IM q3-4h prn. **Max:** 40mg/day. **(IV)** 2.5-10mg IV **(not bolus). Max:** 10mg single dose and 40mg/day. **Nausea/Vomiting with Surgery:** 5-10mg IM 1-2 hrs or 5-10mg IV 15-30 minutes before anesthesia, or during or after surgery; repeat once if needed. **Non-Psychotic Anxiety: (Tab)** 5mg tid-qid. **Psychosis: Mild/Outpatient:** 5-10mg PO tid-qid. **Moderate-Severe/Hospitalized: Initial:** 10mg PO tid-qid. May increase in small increments every 2-3 days. **Severe: (PO)** 100-150mg/day. **(IM)** 10-20mg,	**W/P:** Secondary extrapyramidal symptoms can occur. Tardive dyskinesia, NMS may develop. Caution with activities requiring alertness. May mask symptoms of overdose of other drugs. May obscure diagnosis of intestinal obstruction, brain tumor, and Reye's syndrome. May interfere with thermoregulation. Caution with glaucoma, cardiac disorders. Caution in children with dehydration or acute illness and the elderly. Discontinue 48 hrs before myelography and may resume after 24 hrs post-procedure. **Contra:** Comatose states, concomitant large dose CNS depressants(alcohol, barbiturates, narcotics), pediatric surgery,	Drowsiness, dizziness, amenorrhea, blurred vision, skin reactions, hypotension, neuroleptic malignant syndrome, cholestatic jaundice.

Table 16.1: PRESCRIBING INFORMATION FOR RX GASTROINTESTINAL DRUGS (cont.)

NAME	FORM/ STRENGTH	DOSAGE	WARNINGS/PRECAUTIONS & CONTRAINDICATIONS	ADVERSE EFFECTS†
ANTIEMETICS (cont.)				
Prochlorpera-zine (cont.)		may repeat q2-4 hrs if needed. Switch to oral after obtain control or if needed, 10-20mg IM q4-6h. **Elderly:** Use lower dosing range and titrate more gradually. *Pediatrics:* **Nausea/Vomiting: >2 yrs and >20lbs: (PO/PR) 20-29 lbs:** Usual: 2.5mg qd-bid. **Max:** 7.5mg/day. **30-39 lbs:** 2.5mg bid-tid. **Max:** 10mg/day. **40-85 lbs:** 2.5mg tid or 5mg bid. **Max:** 15mg/day. **(IM)** 0.06mg/lb, usually single dose for control. **Psychosis: (PO/PR) 2-12 yrs: Initial:** 2.5mg bid-tid, up to 10mg/day on 1st day. **Max:** 2-5 yrs: 20mg/day. **6-12 yrs:** 25mg/day. **(IM) <12 yrs:** 0.06mg/lb single dose. Switch to oral after obtain control.	pediatrics <2 yrs or <20 lbs. **P/N:** Safety in pregnancy is not known; caution in nursing.	
Promethazine Hydrochloride (Phenergan)	**Inj:** 25mg/mL, 50mg/mL; **Sup:** 12.5mg, 25mg, 50mg; **Tab:** 12.5mg*, 25mg*, 50mg	*Adults:* **Allergy:** 25mg qhs or 12.5mg ac and hs. **Motion Sickness: Initial:** 25mg 30-60 minutes before travel, then 25mg 8-12 hrs later if needed. **Maint:** 25mg bid. **Prevention/Control of Nausea/Vomiting:** 25mg initially, then 12.5-25mg q4-6h prn. **Sedation:** 25-50mg qhs. **Preoperative:** 50mg night before surgery, then 50mg preoperatively. **Postoperative:** 25-50mg. *Pediatrics:* **≥2 yrs: Allergy:** 25mg or 0.5mg/lb qhs or 6.25-12.5 tid. **Motion Sickness:** 12.5-25mg bid. **Prevention/Control of Nausea/Vomiting:** 25mg or 0.5mg/lb initially then 12.5-25mg or 0.5mg/lb q4-6h prn. **Sedation:** 12.5-25mg hs. **Preoperative:** 12.5-25mg night before surgery, then 0.5mg/lb preoperatively. **Postoperative:** 12.5-25mg.	**W/P:** Potential for fatal respiratory depression in pediatric patients <2 yrs. Caution in patients ≥2 yrs. Avoid with compromised respiratory function (eg, COPD, sleep apnea). Caution with bone marrow depression, narrow-angle glaucoma, stenosing peptic ulcer, bladder or pyloroduodenal obstruction, prostatic hypertrophy, CVD, hepatic dysfunction. Cholestatic jaundice reported. Alters HCG pregnancy tests. May lower seizure threshold, increase blood glucose, cause sun sensitivity. May impair mental/physical abilities. **Contra:** Treatment of lower respiratory tract symptoms (eg, asthma). Pediatric patients <2 yrs. **P/N:** Category C, not for use in nursing.	Drowsiness, sedation, blurred vision, dizziness, increased or decreased blood pressure, urticaria, **dry mouth**, nausea, vomiting.
Trimethoben-zamide Hydrochloride (Tigan)	**Cap:** 300mg; **Inj:** 100mg/mL; **Sup: (Benzocaine-Trimetho-benzamide)** 2%-200mg; **(Sup, Pediatric)**, 2%-100mg	*Adults:* **(Cap)** 300mg tid-qid. **(Inj)** 200mg IM tid-qid. **(Sup)** 200mg tid-qid. *Pediatrics:* **(Sup; Sup, Pediatric) 30-90 lbs:** 100-200mg tid-qid. **<30 lbs:** 100mg tid-qid	**W/P:** Caution in children; may cause EPS, which may be confused with CNS signs of undiagnosed primary disease (eg, Reye's syndrome) and may unfavorably alter the course of Reye's syndrome due to hepatotoxic potential. Caution with acute febrile illness, encephalitides, gastroenteritis, dehydration, electrolyte imbalance, and in elderly; CNS reactions reported. May produce drowsiness. **Contra:** Injection in children, suppositories in premature or newborn infants, suppositories if hypersensitive to similar local anesthetics. **P/N:** Safety in pregnancy and nursing not known.	Hypersensitivity reactions, parkinson-like symptoms, hypotension (inj), blood dyscrasias, blurred vision, coma, convulsions, mood depression, diarrhea, disorientation, dizziness, drowsiness, headache, jaundice, muscle cramps, opisthotonos.
ANTISPASMODICS				
Alosetron Hydrochloride (Lotronex)	**Tab:** 0.5mg, 1mg	*Adults:* **Initial:** 1mg qd for 4 weeks. **Titrate:** If tolerated and IBS symptoms not controlled, may increase to 1mg bid. Discontinue after 4 weeks if symptoms not controlled on 1mg bid.	**BB:** Serious GI adverse events, some fatal, reported (eg, ischemic colitis, serious constipation complications). Physicians must enroll in GlaxoSmithKline's Prescribing Program for Lotronex and patients must sign the	Constipation, abdominal discomfort/pain, nausea, GI discomfort/pain.

*Scored.   †Bold entries denote special dental considerations.

NAME	FORM/ STRENGTH	DOSAGE	WARNINGS/PRECAUTIONS & CONTRAINDICATIONS	ADVERSE EFFECTS†
Alosetron Hydrochloride *(cont.)*			Patient-Physician Agreement. Discontinue immediately if constipation or symptoms of ischemic colitis develop (rectal bleeding, bloody diarrhea, abdominal pain); do not resume therapy. W/P: Increased risk of constipation and ischemic colitis. Caution with hepatic insufficiency. **Contra:** Current constipation or diverticulitis. History of chronic/severe constipation or sequelae of constipation, intestinal obstruction/stricture, toxic megacolon, GI perforation/adhesions, ischemic colitis, impaired intestinal circulation, thrombophlebitis, hypercoagulable state, Crohn's disease, ulcerative colitis, diverticulitis. Inability to understand/comply with Patient-Physician Agreement. **P/N:** Category B, caution in nursing.	
Atropine Sulfate/Hyoscyamine Sulfate/Phenobarbital (Donnatal)	**Tab:** 0.0194mg-0.1037mg-16.2mg-0.0065mg; **Tab, Extended Release: (Extentabs)** 0.0582mg-0.3111mg-48.6mg-0.0195mg; **Elixir:** 0.0194mg-0.1037mg-16.2mg-0.0065mg/5mL	***Adults:*** **Elixir:** 5-10mL tid-qid. **Hepatic Disease:** Use lower doses. ***Pediatrics:*** **4.5kg:** 0.5mL q4h or 0.75mL q6h. **9.1kg:** 1mL q4h or 1.5mL q6h. **13.6kg:** 1.5mL q4h or 2mL q6h. **22.7kg:** 2.5mL q4h or 3.75mL q6h. **34kg:** 3.75mL q4h or 5mL q6h. **45.4kg:** 5mL q4h or 7.5mL q6h. **Hepatic Disease:** Use lower doses. **Tab:** 1-2 tabs. **Extentabs:** 1 tab q8-12h. **Hepatic Disease:** Use lower doses.	**W/P:** Inconclusive whether anticholinergic/antispasmodic drugs aid in duodenal ulcer healing, decrease recurrence rate, or prevent complications. Heat prostration can occur with high environmental temperatures. Avoid with intestinal obstruction. May be habit forming; caution with history of physical and/or psychological drug dependence. Caution with hepatic disease, renal disease, autonomic neuropathy, hyperthyroidism, coronary heart disease, CHF, arrhythmias, tachycardia, HTN. May delay gastric emptying. Diarrhea may be an early symptom of incomplete intestinal obstruction, especially with ileostomy or colostomy; treatment would be inappropriate. **Contra:** Glaucoma, obstructive uropathy, obstructive GI disease, paralytic ileus, intestinal atony in elderly or debilitated, unstable cardiovascular status in acute hemorrhage, severe ulcerative colitis, myasthenia gravis, hiatal hernia with reflux esophagitis, intermittent porphyria, and for patients in whom phenobarbital produces restlessness and/or excitement. **P/N:** Category C, caution in nursing.	**Dry mouth**, urinary hesitancy/retention, blurred vision, tachycardia/palpitation, mydriasis, cycloplegia, increased ocular tension, **loss of taste**, headache, nervousness, drowsiness, weakness, dizziness, insomnia, nausea, vomiting, impotence, suppression of lactation, constipation, bloated feeling, musculoskeletal pain, allergic reaction/drug idiosyncrasies, decreased sweating.
Chlordiazepoxide Hydrochloride/ Methscopolamine (Librax)	**Cap:** (Chlordiazepoxide-Methscopolamine) 5mg-2.5mg	***Adults:*** **Usual/Maint:** 1-2 caps tid-qid ac and hs. **Elderly/Debilitated: Initial:** 2 caps/day and increase gradually, if needed.	**W/P:** Risk of congenital malformations during first trimester of pregnancy; avoid use. Avoid abrupt withdrawal. Paradoxical reactions reported in psychiatric patients. Caution with depression, renal or hepatic dysfunction, the elderly. Inhibition of lactation may occur. **Contra:** Glaucoma, prostatic hypertrophy, benign bladder neck obstruction. **P/N:** Not for use in pregnancy; safety in nursing is not known.	Drowsiness, ataxia, confusion, skin eruptions, extrapyramidal symptoms, **dry mouth**, nausea, constipation, altered libido, blood dyscrasias, jaundice, hepatic dysfunction.
Dicyclomine Hydrochloride (Bentyl)	**Cap:** 10mg; **Tab:** 20mg; **Inj:** 10mg/mL; **Syr:** 10mg/5mL	***Adults:*** **(Tab/Syr) Initial:** 20mg qid. **Usual:** 40mg qid if tolerated. Discontinue if no improvement after 2 weeks or if doses ≥80mg/day are not tolerated. **(Inj)** 20mg IM qid for 1-2 days,	**W/P:** Caution in autonomic neuropathy, hepatic/renal impairment, ulcerative colitis, hyperthyroidism, HTN, CHF, cardiac tachyarrhythmia, coronary heart disease, hiatal hernia,	**Dry mouth**, nausea, vomiting, blurred vision, dizziness, drowsiness, nervousness, mental confusion/excitement

Table 16.1: PRESCRIBING INFORMATION FOR RX GASTROINTESTINAL DRUGS *(cont.)*

NAME	FORM/ STRENGTH	DOSAGE	WARNINGS/PRECAUTIONS & CONTRAINDICATIONS	ADVERSE EFFECTS†

ANTISPASMODICS *(cont.)*

NAME	FORM/ STRENGTH	DOSAGE	WARNINGS/PRECAUTIONS & CONTRAINDICATIONS	ADVERSE EFFECTS†
Dicylomine Hydrochloride *(cont.)*		followed by oral dicyclomine. Not for IV use.	and prostatic hypertrophy. Heat prostration may occur in high environmental temperature. Monitor for diarrhea, may be the early symptom of intestinal obstruction. Psychosis reported. Serious respiratory symptoms, seizures, syncope and death reported in infants. **Contra:** GI tract obstruction, obstructive uropathy, severe ulcerative colitis, reflux esophagitis, glaucoma, myasthenia gravis, unstable cardiovascular status and in acute hemorrhage, nursing mothers, infants <6 months of age. P/N: Category B, contraindicated in nursing	(especially in the elderly), mydriasis, increased ocular tension, urinary retention, dyspnea, apnea, tachycardia, decreased sweating, lactation suppression, impotence.
Hyoscyamine Sulfate (Levbid, Levsin, Levsinex)	**(Levbid) Tab, Extended Release:** 0.375mg*. **(Levsin) Drops:** 0.125mg/mL [15mL]; **Elixir:** 0.125mg/5mL [473mL]; **Inj:** 0.5mg/mL; **Tab:** 0.125mg*; **Tab, SL:** 0.125mg*. **(Levsinex) Cap, Extended Release:** 0.375mg	*Adults:* May also chew or swallow SL tab. **(Drops, Eli, Tab, and Tab, SL)** 0.125-0.25mg q4h or prn. **Max:** 1.5mg/24hrs. **(Cap and Tab, Extended Release)** 0.375-0.75mg q12h; or 1 cap q8h. **Max:** 1.5mg/24hrs. Do not crush or chew. **(Inj) GI Disorders:** 0.25-0.5mg IM/IV/SC as single dose or up to qid at 4 hr intervals. **Diagnostic Procedures:** 0.25-0.5mg IV 5-10 minutes before procedure. **Anesthesia:** 5μg/kg IM/IV/SC 30-60 minutes before anesthesia or with narcotic/sedative administration. **Drug-Induced Bradycardia (Surgery):** Increments of 0.25mL IV; repeat prn. **Neuromuscular Blockade Reversal:** 0.2mg for every 1mg neostigmine or equal dose of physostigmine or pyridostigmine.	**W/P:** Risk of heat prostration with high environmental temperature. Avoid activities requiring mental alertness. Psychosis has been reported. Caution with diarrhea, autonomic neuropathy, hyperthyroidism, coronary heart disease, CHF, arrhythmias/tachycardia, HTN, renal disease, and hiatal hernia associated with reflux esophagitis. **Contra:** Glaucoma, obstructive uropathy, GI tract obstructive disease, paralytic ileus, intestinal atony of elderly/debilitated, unstable cardiovascular status in acute hemorrhage, severe ulcerative colitis, toxic megacolon, myasthenia gravis. **P/N:** Category C, caution in nursing.	Anticholinergic effects, drowsiness, headache, nervousness.
Hyoscyamine Sulfate (Nulev)	**Tab, Disintegrating:** 0.125mg	*Adults:* 0.125-0.25mg q4h or prn. **Max:** 1.5mg/24hrs. Take with or without water. *Pediatrics:* ≥**12 yrs:** 0.125-0.25mg q4h or prn. **Max:** 1.5mg/24hrs. **2 to <12 yrs:** 0.0625-0.125mg q4h or prn. **Max:** 0.75mg/24hrs. Take with or without water.	**W/P:** Risk of heat prostration with high environmental temperature. Avoid activities requiring mental alertness. Psychosis has been reported in sensitive patients. Caution with diarrhea, autonomic neuropathy, hyperthyroidism, coronary heart disease, CHF, arrhythmias/tachycardia, HTN, renal disease, and hiatal hernia associated with reflux esophagitis. Contains phenylalanine. **Contra:** Glaucoma, obstructive uropathy, GI tract obstruction, paralytic ileus; intestinal atony of elderly/debilitated, unstable cardiovascular status in acute hemorrhage, toxic megacolon complicating ulcerative colitis, myasthenia gravis. **P/N:** Category C, caution in nursing.	Anticholinergic effects, drowsiness, headache, nervousness.
Tegaserod Maleate (Zelnorm)	**Tab:** 2mg, 6mg	*Adults:* **IBS:** 6mg bid before meals for 4-6 weeks. If response to therapy, may consider an additional 4-6 week course. **Chronic Idiopathic Constipation:** 6mg bid before meals.	**W/P:** Do not initiate in patients currently experiencing or frequently experiencing diarrhea. Discontinue if new or sudden worsening of abdominal pain, hypotension, syncope, or symptoms of ischemic colitis develop. **Contra:** Severe renal impairment, moderate or severe hepatic impairment, history of bowel obstruction,	Abdominal pain, diarrhea, nausea, flatulence, headache, dizziness, back pain, diarrhea.

*Scored.   †Bold entries denote special dental considerations.

NAME	FORM/ STRENGTH	DOSAGE	WARNINGS/PRECAUTIONS & CONTRAINDICATIONS	ADVERSE EFFECTS†
Tegaserod Maleate (cont.)			symptomatic gallbladder disease, suspected sphincter of Oddi dysfunction, abdominal adhesions. **P/N:** Category B, not for use in nursing.	

ANTIULCER AGENTS

NAME	FORM/ STRENGTH	DOSAGE	WARNINGS/PRECAUTIONS & CONTRAINDICATIONS	ADVERSE EFFECTS†
Cimetidine (Tagamet)	**Tab:** 200mg, 300mg, 400mg	*Adults:* **(PO) Active DU:** 800mg qhs or 300mg qid or 400mg bid for 4-8 weeks. **Maint:** 400mg qhs. **Active Benign GU:** 800mg qhs or 300mg qid for 6 weeks. **GERD:** 800mg bid or 400mg qid for 12 weeks. **Hypersecretory Conditions:** 300mg qid. **Max:** 2400mg/day. *Pediatrics:* ≥16 yrs: **(PO) Active DU:** 800mg qhs or 300mg qid or 400mg bid for 4-8 weeks. **Maint:** 400mg qhs. **Active Benign GU:** 800mg qhs or 300mg qid for 6 weeks. **GERD:** 800mg bid or 400mg qid for 12 weeks. **Hypersecretory Conditions:** 300mg qid. **Max:** 2400mg/day.	**W/P:** Cardiac arrhythmias and hypotension reported following rapid IV administration (rare). Symptomatic response does not preclude presence of gastric malignancy. Reversible confusional states reported, especially in severely ill patients. Elderly, renal and/or hepatic impairment are risk factors for confusional states. Risk of hyperinfection of strongyloidiasis in immunocompromised patients. **P/N:** Category B, not for use in nursing.	Diarrhea, headache, dizziness, somnolence, reversible confusional states, impotence, increased serum transaminases, rash, gynecomastia, blood dyscrasias.
Esomeprazole Magnesium (Nexium)	**Cap, Delayed Release:** 20mg, 40mg; **Inj:** 20mg, 40mg	*Adults:* **Capsules: Erosive Esophagitis: Healing:** 20-40mg qd for 4-8 weeks; may extend treatment for 4-8 weeks if not healed. **Maint:** 20mg qd for up to 6 months. **Risk Reduction of NSAID-Associated Gastric Ulcer:** 20-40mg qd for up to 6 months. **Symptomatic GERD:** 20mg qd for 4 weeks; may extend treatment for 4 weeks if symptoms do not resolve. **H. pylori: Triple Therapy:** 40mg qd + amoxicillin 1000mg bid + clarithromycin 500mg bid, all for 10 days. **Severe Hepatic Dysfunction: Max:** 20mg/day. Take 1hr before meals. Swallow capsule whole. Contents may be mixed with soft food (eg, applesauce, yogurt) that does not require chewing. **(Injection)** 20mg or 40mg qd IV injection (no less than 3 minutes) or infusion (10-30 minutes). Discontinue as soon as patient is able to resume oral therapy.	**W/P:** Atrophic gastritis may occur. Symptomatic response does not preclude gastric malignancy. **Contra:** Hypersensitivity to substituted benzimidazoles. Clarithromycin is contraindicated with pimozide. **P/N:** Category B, not for use in nursing.	Headache, diarrhea, abdominal pain, constipation, nausea, flatulence, **dry mouth**.
Famotidine (Pepcid, Pepcid AC)	**Inj:** 0.4mg/mL, 10mg/mL; **Sus:** 40mg/5mL [50mL]; **Tab:** 20mg, 40mg; **Tab, Disintegrating: (RPD)** 20mg, 40mg	*Adults:* **(PO) Acute DU, Pepcid:** 40mg qhs or 20mg bid for 4-8 weeks. **Maint DU:** 20mg qhs. **GU:** 40mg qhs. **GERD:** 20mg bid up to 6 weeks. **GERD with Esophagitis:** 20-40mg bid up to 12 weeks. **Hypersecretory Conditions: Initial:** 20mg q6h. **Max:** 160mg q6h. **(Inj)** 20mg IV q12h, hypersecretory conditions may require higher doses. **CrCl <50mL/min:** Reduce to 1/2 dose, or increase interval to q36-48h. **Pepcid AC: Relief:** 1 tab/cap prn. **Max:** 2 doses/24 hrs. **Prevention:** 1 tab/cap 15-60 minutes before food or beverages that cause heartburn. **Max:** 2 doses/24 hrs. *Pediatrics:* **1-16 yrs: (PO) DU/GU: Usual:** 0.5mg/kg/day qhs or divided bid. **Max:** 40mg/day.	**W/P:** CNS adverse effects reported with moderate to severe renal insufficiency; adjust dose. Disintegrating tabs contain phenylalanine; caution in phenylketonurics. Symptomatic response does not preclude the presence of gastric malignancy. **Contra:** Hypersensitivity to other H_2 antagonists. **P/N:** Category B, not for use in nursing.	Headache, dizziness, constipation, diarrhea.

Table 16.1: PRESCRIBING INFORMATION FOR RX GASTROINTESTINAL DRUGS (cont.)

NAME	FORM/ STRENGTH	DOSAGE	WARNINGS/PRECAUTIONS & CONTRAINDICATIONS	ADVERSE EFFECTS†
ANTIULCER AGENTS (cont.)				
Famotidine (cont.)		**GERD With or Without Esophagitis:** 0.5mg/kg PO bid. **Max:** 40mg bid. **(Inj)** 0.25mg/kg IV q12h up to 40mg/day. Base duration of therapy on clinical response, and/or pH, and endoscopy. **(PO) GERD: 3 months-1 yr:** 0.5mg/kg bid for up to 8 weeks. **<3 months:** 0.5mg/kg qd for up to 8 weeks. **CrCl <50mL/min:** Reduce to 1/2 dose, or increase interval to q36-48h.		
Glycopyrrolate (Robinul, Robinul Forte)	**Tab:** 1mg*, **(Forte)** 2mg*	**Adults:** Usual: **(Tab)** 1mg tid (am, pm and hs); may increase to 2mg qhs if needed. **Maint:** 1mg bid. **(Forte)** 2mg bid-tid. **Max:** 8mg/day. **Pediatrics:** ≥12 yrs: Usual: **(Tab)** 1mg tid (am, pm & hs); may increase to 2mg qhs if needed. **Maint:** 1mg bid. **(Forte)** 2mg bid-tid. **Max:** 8mg/day.	**W/P:** May produce drowsiness and blurred vision; avoid operating machinery. Risk of heat prostration with high environmental temperature. Diarrhea may be early symptom of incomplete intestinal obstruction especially with ileostomy or colostomy. Caution in elderly, autonomic neuropathy, hepatic/renal disease, ulcerative colitis, hyperthyroidism, coronary heart disease, CHF, tachyarrhythmias, tachycardia, HTN, prostatic hypertrophy, hiatal hernia associated with reflux esophagitis. **Contra:** Glaucoma, obstructive uropathy, GI tract obstruction, paralytic ileus, intestinal atony of elderly or debilitated, unstable cardiovascular status in acute hemorrhage, severe ulcerative colitis, toxic megacolon complicating ulcerative colitis, myasthenia gravis. **P/N:** Safety in pregnancy is not known; not for use in nursing.	Blurred vision, **dry mouth**, urinary retention and hesitancy, increased ocular tension, tachycardia, decreased sweating, **loss of taste**, headache.
Lansoprazole (Prevacid)	**Cap, Delayed Release:** 15mg, 30mg; **Inj:** 30mg; **Sus:** 15mg, 30mg (granules/ packet); **Tab, Disintegrating (SoluTab):** 15mg, 30mg	**Adults:** >17 yrs: **(PO) DU:** 15mg qd for 4 weeks. **Maint:** 15mg qd. **GU:** 30mg qd up to 8 weeks. **GERD:** 15mg qd up to 8 weeks. **Erosive Esophagitis:** 30mg qd up to 8 weeks. May repeat for 8 weeks if needed. **Maint:** 15mg qd. **NSAID Induced GU:** 30mg qd for 8 weeks. **Reduce Risk of NSAID Induced GU:** 15mg qd for 12 weeks. **Hypersecretory Conditions: Initial:** 60mg qd, then adjust. **Max:** 90mg qd. Divide dose if >120mg/day. **H. pylori: Triple Therapy:** 30mg + clarithromycin 500mg + amoxicillin 1000mg, all bid (q12h) for 10-14 days. **Dual Therapy:** 30mg + amoxicillin 1000mg both tid (q8h) for 14 days. Take before eating. **(Caps)** Swallow whole or sprinkle cap contents on 1 tbsp of applesauce, Ensure pudding, cottage cheese, yogurt, strained pears, or in 60mL orange juice or tomato juice; swallow immediately. **(Sus)** Do not chew or crush. Mix packet with 30mL of water; stir well and drink immediately; not for use with NG tube. **(Solutab)** Place on tongue with or without water. **(Oral Syringe) (SoluTab)** Place 15mg tab in oral syringe and draw up 4mL of water, or 30mg tab	**W/P:** Symptomatic response does not preclude the presence of gastric malignancy. Adjust dose with hepatic impairment. **P/N:** Category B, not for use in nursing.	Abdominal pain, constipation, diarrhea, nausea.

*Scored.   †Bold entries denote special dental considerations.

NAME	FORM/ STRENGTH	DOSAGE	WARNINGS/PRECAUTIONS & CONTRAINDICATIONS	ADVERSE EFFECTS†
Lansoprazole (cont.)		in oral syringe and draw up 10mL of water. Shake contents and administer after tablet has dispersed within 15 min. Refill syringe with 2mL (5mL for 30mg tab) of water, shake, and give any remaining contents. **NG Tube: (Cap)** Mix cap contents with 40mL apple juice and inject into NG tube; flush with additional juice to clear tube. **(SoluTab)** Place 15mg tab and draw up 4mL of water, or 30mg tab and draw up 10mL of water. Shake contents and after tablet has dispersed, inject through NG tube into stomach within 15 min. Refill syringe with 5mL of water, shake, and flush NG tube. **(Inj) Erosive Esophagitis:** 30mg IV qd over 30 min for 7 days. May switch to PO formulation for total of 6 to 8 weeks of therapy once patient is able to take oral medications. **Severe Hepatic Impairment:** Adjust dose. ***Pediatrics:* 12-17 yrs: Short-Term Symptomatic GERD:** 15mg qd for up to 8 weeks. **Erosive Esophagitis:** 30mg qd for up to 8 weeks. **1-11 yrs: Short-Term Symptomatic GERD/Erosive Esophagitis: ≥30kg:** 15mg qd for up to 12 weeks. **>30kg:** 30mg qd for up to 12 weeks. **Titrate:** May increase up to 30mg bid after 2 weeks if symptomatic. **Severe Hepatic Impairment:** Adjust dose. Take before eating. **(Caps)** Swallow whole or sprinkle contents on 1 tbsp of applesauce, pudding, cottage cheese, yogurt, strained pears, or in 60mL orange juice or tomato juice; swallow immediately. **(Sus)** Do not chew or crush. Mix packet with 30mL water; stir well and drink immediately; not for use with NG tube. **(SoluTab)** Place on tongue with or without water. **(Oral Syringe) (SoluTab)** Place 15mg tab in oral syringe and draw up 4mL of water, or 30mg tab in oral syringe and draw up 10mL of water. Shake contents and administer after tablet has dispersed within 15 mins. Refill syringe with 2mL (5mL for 30mg tab) of water, shake, and give any remaining contents. **NG Tube: (Cap)** Mix cap contents with 40mL apple juice and inject into NG tube; flush with additional juice to clear tube. **(SoluTab)** Place 15mg tab and draw up 4mL of water, or 30mg tab and draw up 10mL of water. Shake contents and after tablet has dispersed, inject through NG tube into stomach within 15 min. Refill syringe with 5mL of water, shake, and flush NG tube.		
Methscopolamine Bromide (Pamine, Pamine Forte)	**Tab:** 2.5mg; **(Forte)** 5mg	***Adults:*** 2.5mg tid 30 minutes ac and 2.5-5mg qhs. **Severe Symptoms:** 5mg 30 minutes ac and qhs. **Max:** 30mg/day.	**W/P:** Heat prostration may occur with high environmental temperatures. Avoid or discontinue use if diarrhea develops, especially with ileostomy or colostomy. Caution in elderly,	Constipation, decreased sweating, headache, drowsiness, dizziness.

Table 16.1: PRESCRIBING INFORMATION FOR RX GASTROINTESTINAL DRUGS (cont.)

NAME	FORM/ STRENGTH	DOSAGE	WARNINGS/PRECAUTIONS & CONTRAINDICATIONS	ADVERSE EFFECTS†
ANTIULCER AGENTS (cont.)				
Methscopol-amine Bromide (cont.)			autonomic neuropathy, hepatic/renal disease, ulcerative colitis, hyperthy-roidism, coronary heart disease, CHF, tachyrhythmia, tachycardia, HTN, or prostatic hypertrophy. May impair mental/physical abilities. **Contra:** Glaucoma, obstructive uropathy, obstructive GI disease, paralytic ileus, intestinal atony of the elderly or debilitated, unstable cardiovascular status in acute hemorrhage, severe ulcerative colitis, toxic megacolon, myasthenia gravis. **P/N:** Category C, caution in nursing.	
Misoprostol (Cytotec)	**Tab:** 100µg, 200µg*	**Adults:** 200µg qid, or if not tolerated, 100µg qid. Take for the duration of NSAID therapy. Take with meals; last dose at bedtime.	**BB:** Can cause abortion, premature birth, or birth defects. Uterine rupture reported when used to induce labor or induce abortion beyond 8th week of pregnancy. Not for use by pregnant women to reduce risk of NSAID-induced ulcers. Only use in women of childbearing age if at high risk of GI ulcers or complications with NSAID therapy; patient must then have nega-tive serum pregnancy test within 2 weeks before therapy, maintain contra-ceptive measures, and begin therapy on 2nd or 3rd day of menstrual period. **Contra:** Pregnant women to reduce risk of NSAID-induced ulcers, prosta-glandin allergy. **P/N:** Category X, not for use in nursing.	Diarrhea, abdominal pain, nausea, flatulence, headache, dyspepsia.
Nizatidine (Axid)	**Cap:** 150mg, 300mg; **Sol:** 15mg/mL	**Adults: Active DU/Active Benign GU: Usual:** 300mg qhs or 150mg bid up to 8 weeks. **Healed DU: Maint:** 150mg qhs, up to 1 year. **GERD:** 150mg bid up to 12 weeks. **Renal Impairment: Treat-ment: CrCl 20-50mL/min:** 150mg/day. **CrCl <20mL/min:** 150mg every other day. **Maint: CrCl 20-50mL/min:** 150mg every other day. **CrCl <20mL/min:** 150mg every 3 days. **Pediatrics: ≥12 yrs: (Sol) Erosive Esophagitis/GERD:** 150mg bid up to 8 weeks. **Max:** 300mg/day. **Renal Impairment: Treat-ment: CrCl 20-50mL/min:** 150mg/day. **CrCl <20mL/min:** 150mg every other day. **Maint: CrCl 20-50mL/min:** 150mg every other day. **CrCl <20mL/min:** 150mg every 3 days.	**W/P:** Caution with renal dysfunction; reduce dose. Symptomatic response does not preclude the presence of gastric malignancy. False positive tests for urobilinogen with Multistix[174]. **P/N:** Category B, not for use in nursing.	Headache, abdominal pain, pain, asthenia, diarrhea, nausea, flatulence, vomit-ing, dyspepsia, rhinitis, pharyngitis, dizziness.
Omeprazole (Prilosec)	**Cap, Delayed Release: (Prilosec)** 10mg, 20mg, 40mg; **(Prilosec OTC)** 20mg	**Adults: Duodenal Ulcer:** 20mg qd for 4-8 weeks. **Gastric Ulcer:** 40mg qd for 4-8 weeks. **GERD:** 20mg qd up to 4 weeks without esophageal lesions and 4-8 weeks with erosive esopha-gitis. **Treatment Erosive Esophagitis with GERD:** 20mg qd for 4-8 weeks. **Maint:** 20mg qd. **Hypersecretory Conditions: Initial:** 60mg qd, then adjust if needed. Divide dose	**W/P:** Atrophic gastritis reported with long-term use. Symptomatic response does not preclude the presence of gastric malignancy. **P/N:** Category C, not for use in nursing.	Headache, diarrhea, abdominal pain, asthenia, nausea, vomiting.

*Scored.   †Bold entries denote special dental considerations.

NAME	FORM/ STRENGTH	DOSAGE	WARNINGS/PRECAUTIONS & CONTRAINDICATIONS	ADVERSE EFFECTS†
Omeprazole (cont.)		if >80mg/day. Doses up to 120mg tid have been given. **H. pylori Triple Therapy:** 20mg + clarithromycin 500mg + amoxicillin 1g, all bid for 10 days. Give additional 18 days of omeprazole 20mg every morning if ulcer present initially. **Dual Therapy:** 40mg qd + clarithromycin 500mg tid for 14 days. Give additional 14 days of omeprazole 20mg every morning if ulcer present initially. Do not crush or chew. Take before eating. Can add contents of caps to applesauce if difficulty swallowing; swallow immediately without chewing. *Pediatrics:* **≥2 yrs: GERD/Erosive Esophagitis: >20kg:** 20mg qd. **<20kg:** 10mg qd. Do not crush or chew. Take before eating. Can add contents of caps to applesauce if difficulty swallowing; swallow immediately without chewing.		
Pantoprazole Sodium (Protonix)	**Inj:** 40mg; **Tab, Delayed Release:** 20mg, 40mg	*Adults:* **(Tab) Erosive Esophagitis Treatment:** 40mg qd for up to 8 weeks. May repeat for 8 weeks if needed. **Maintenance:** 40mg qd. **Hypersecretory Conditions: Initial:** 40mg bid. Adjust to patient's needs. **Max:** 240mg/day. **(Inj) GERD:** 40mg IV qd for 7-10 days. **Pathological Hypersecretion:** 80mg IV q12h. May adjust up to 80mg IV q8h based on acid output. **Max:** 240mg/day. Duration >6 days not studied. Do not split, crush or chew tabs.	**W/P:** Symptomatic response does not preclude the presence of gastric malignancy. False (+) urine screening test for THC reported. (Inj) Immediate hypersensitivity reactions reported (eg, thrombophlebitis, LFT elevation). **P/N:** Category B, not for use in nursing.	(Inj) Abdominal pain, headache, constipation, dyspepsia, nausea. (Tab) Headache, flatulence, diarrhea, abdominal pain.
Ranitidine (Zantac)	**Inj:** 1mg/mL, 25mg/mL; **Syr:** 15mg/mL; **Tab:** 150mg, 300mg; **Tab, Effervescent:** 25mg, 150mg	*Adults:* **(PO) DU/GU:** 150mg bid or (DU) 300mg after evening meal or qhs. **Maint:** 150mg qhs. **GERD:** 150mg bid. **Erosive Esophagitis:** 150mg qid. **Maint:** 150mg bid. **Hypersecretory Conditions:** 150mg bid. May give up to 6g/day with severe disease. **(Inj) Usual:** 50mg IV/IM q6-8 hrs or 6.25mg/hr continuous IV. **Max:** 400mg/day. **Zollinger-Ellison: Initial:** 1mg/kg/hr. **Titrate:** May increase after 4 hrs by 0.5mg/kg/hr increments. **Max:** 2.5mg/kg/hr or 220mg/hr. **CrCl <50mL/min:** 50mg IV q18-24 hrs or 150mg PO q24h. Give more frequent (q12h) if necessary. **Hemodialysis:** Give dose at end of treatment. Dissolve each 150mg effervescent tab in 6-8oz of water before administration. *Pediatrics:* **1 month-16 yrs:** (PO) **DU/GU:** 2-4mg/kg bid. **Max:** 300mg/day. **Maint:** 2-4mg/kg qd. **Max:** 150mg/day. **GERD/Erosive Esophagitis:** 2.5-5mg/kg bid. **(Inj) DU:** 2-4mg/kg/day IV given q6-8 hrs. **Max:** 50mg q6-8 hrs. **CrCl <50mL/min:** 50mg IV q18-24 hrs or 150mg PO q24h. Give more frequent (q12h) if necessary. **Hemodialysis:** Give dose at end of treatment. Dissolve each 25mg effervescent tab in 5mL of water before administration.	**W/P:** Do not exceed recommended infusion rates; bradycardia reported with rapid infusion. Caution with liver and renal dysfunction. Monitor SGPT if on IV therapy for ≥5 days at dose >100mg qid. Avoid use with history of acute porphyria. Symptomatic response does not preclude the presence of gastric malignancy. May cause false (+) urine protein test. Granules and effervescent tablets contain phenylalanine. **P/N:** Category B, caution with nursing.	Headache, constipation, diarrhea, nausea, abdominal discomfort, vomiting, hepatitis, blood dyscrasias, rash, injection site reactions (IV/IM).

Table 16.1: PRESCRIBING INFORMATION FOR RX GASTROINTESTINAL DRUGS *(cont.)*

NAME	FORM/ STRENGTH	DOSAGE	WARNINGS/PRECAUTIONS & CONTRAINDICATIONS	ADVERSE EFFECTS†
ANTIULCER AGENTS *(cont.)*				
Sucralfate (Carafate)	**Sus:** 1g/10mL [414mL]; **Tab:** 1g*	***Adults:*** **Active Ulcer: (Sus/Tab)** 1g qid for 4-8 weeks. **Maint: (Tab)** 1g bid. Take on empty stomach.	**W/P:** Caution with chronic renal failure and dialysis. **P/N:** Category B, caution with nursing.	Constipation, diarrhea, nausea, vomiting, pruritus, rash, dizziness, insomnia, back pain, headache.
COLORECTAL AGENTS				
Balasalazide Disodium (Colazal)	**Cap:** 750mg	***Adults:*** 3 caps tid for 8 weeks (up to 12 weeks if needed).	**W/P:** May exacerbate symptoms of colitis. Prolonged gastric retention with pyloris stenosis. Caution with renal dysfunction or history of renal disease. **Contra:** Hypersensitivity to salicylates. **P/N:** Category B, caution in nursing.	Headache, abdominal pain, diarrhea, nausea, vomiting, respiratory problems, arthralgia, rhinitis, insomnia, fatigue, rectal bleeding, flatulence, fever, dyspepsia.
Hydrocortisone Acetate (Cortifoam)	**Foam:** 10% [15g]	***Adults:*** 1 applicatorful rectally qd-bid for 2-3 weeks, and every 2nd day thereafter. **Maint:** Decrease in small amounts to lowest effective dose. Discontinue if no improvement within 2-3 weeks.	**W/P:** Absorption may be greater than from other corticosteroid enemas. May elevate BP, cause salt and water retention, IOP, or increase potassium and calcium excretion. Caution with recent MI, hypo- or hyperthyroidism, Strongyloides infestation, TB, CHF, HTN, renal insufficiency, peptic ulcers, diverticulitis, nonspecific ulcerative colitis, cirrhosis, risk of osteoporosis. May produce reversible HPA axis suppression, posterior subcapsular cataracts, glaucoma with possible optic nerve damage. May mask signs of infection or cause new infections. Kaposi's sarcoma reported with chronic use. Avoid with cerebral malaria, systemic fungal infections, active ocular herpes simplex, postoperative ileorectostomy. Rule out latent or active amebiasis. Avoid exposure to chickenpox and/or measles. Observe growth in pediatrics. Withdraw gradually. Acute myopathy observed with high steroid doses. May aggravate existing emotional instability or psychosis. Discontinue if severe reaction occurs. **Contra:** Obstruction, abscess, perforation, peritonitis, fresh intestinal anastomoses, extensive fistulas and sinus tracts. **P/N:** Category C, caution in nursing.	Bradycardia, acne, abdominal distention, convulsions, depression, abnormal fat deposits, fluid/electrolyte disturbances, muscle weakness, osteoporosis, peptic ulcer, pancreatitis, **impaired wound healing**, headache, psychic disturbances, suppression of growth in children, glaucoma, hyperglycemia, weight gain, thromboembolism, malaise, hypersensitivity reactions.
Mesalamine (Asacol)	**Tab, Delayed Release:** 400mg	***Adults:*** **Mild-Moderate Active Ulcerative Colitis: Usual:** 800mg tid for 6 weeks. **Maintenance of Remission:** 1.6g/day in divided doses.	**W/P:** Exacerbation of colitis reported upon initiation of therapy; symptoms abate with discontinuation. Caution with sulfasalazine hypersensitivity. Caution with renal dysfunction or history of renal disease. Monitor renal function prior to therapy and periodically after. Pyloric stenosis could delay mesalamine release in the colon. **Contra:** Hypersensitivity to salicylates. **P/N:** Category B, caution in nursing.	Diarrhea, headache, nausea, pharyngitis, abdominal pain, pain, eructation, dizziness, asthenia, fever, dysmenorrhea, arthralgia, dyspepsia, vomiting.
Mesalamine (Canasa)	**Sup:** 500mg, 1000mg	***Adults:*** 500mg rectally bid for 3-6 weeks, depending on symptoms and sigmoidoscopy results. May increase to tid after 2 weeks if needed. 1000mg rectally qhs. Retain suppository for at least 1-3 hrs.	**W/P:** Discontinue if acute intolerance syndrome develops (eg, cramping, bloody diarrhea, abdominal pain, headache); consider sulfasalazine hypersensitivity. If rechallenge is considered, perform under careful	Dizziness, rectal pain, fever, acne, colitis, rash, hair loss.

*Scored. †Bold entries denote special dental considerations.

NAME	FORM/ STRENGTH	DOSAGE	WARNINGS/PRECAUTIONS & CONTRAINDICATIONS	ADVERSE EFFECTS†
Mesalamine *(cont.)*			observation. Caution with sulfasalazine hypersensitivity. Carefully monitor with renal dysfunction. Pancolitis, pericarditis (rare) reported. **Contra:** Hypersensitivity to suppository vehicle (eg, saturated vegetable fatty acid esters). **P/N:** Category B, caution in nursing.	
Mesalamine (Pentasa)	**Cap, Extended Release:** 250mg, 500mg	**Adults:** 1g qid. Can be given up to 8 weeks.	**W/P:** Caution with hepatic and renal dysfunction; monitor closely. Discontinue if acute intolerance syndrome develops (eg, cramping, bloody diarrhea, abdominal pain, headache). If rechallenge is considered, perform under careful observation. **Contra:** Hypersensitivity to salicylates. **P/N:** Category B, caution in nursing.	Diarrhea, headache, nausea, abdominal pain.
Mesalamine (Rowasa)	**Enema:** 4g/60mL	**Adults:** Use 1 enema rectally qhs for 3-6 weeks. Retain for 8 hrs. Empty bowel prior to administration.	**W/P:** Discontinue if acute intolerance syndrome develops (eg, cramping, bloody diarrhea, abdominal pain, headache); consider sulfasalazine hypersensitivity. If rechallenge is considered, perform under careful observation. Caution with sulfasalazine hypersensitivity. Carefully monitor with renal dysfunction. Contains potassium metabisulfite; caution with sulfite sensitivity especially in asthmatics. Pancolitis, pericarditis (rare) reported. **P/N:** Category B, not for use in nursing.	Abdominal problems, headache, flatulence, flu, fever, nausea, malaise/fatigue.
Olsalazine Sodium (Dipentum)	**Cap:** 250mg	**Adults:** 500mg bid with food.	**W/P:** May exacerbate colitis symptoms. Diarrhea may be dose related, or an underlying symptom of the disease. Caution with renal dysfunction; monitor urinalysis, BUN, creatinine levels. **Contra:** Salicylate hypersensitivity. **P/N:** Category C, caution with nursing.	Diarrhea, abdominal pain, nausea, dyspepsia, headache, rash/itching, arthralgia.
Sulfasalazine (Azulfidine)	**Tab:** 500mg*	**Adults: Initial:** 3-4g/day in divided doses. May initiate at 1-2g/day to reduce GI intolerance. **Maint:** 2g/day. **Pediatrics: ≥2 yrs:** 40-60mg/kg/day divided into 3-6 doses. **Maint:** 7.5mg/kg qid.	**W/P:** Caution with hepatic/renal impairment, blood dyscrasias, severe allergy, bronchial asthma, G6PD deficiency. Monitor CBC, WBC, LFTs, at baseline, every 2nd week for 1st 3 months, monthly for next 3 months, and every 3 months thereafter. Monitor renal function periodically. Maintain adequate fluid intake to prevent crystalluria and stone formation. Discontinue if hypersensitivity or toxic reaction occurs. **Contra:** Intestinal or urinary obstruction, porphyria, hypersensitivity to sulfonamides, salicylates. **P/N:** Category B, caution in nursing.	Anorexia, headache, nausea, vomiting, gastric distress, reversible oligospermia.

DIGESTIVE ENZYMES

NAME	FORM/ STRENGTH	DOSAGE	WARNINGS/PRECAUTIONS & CONTRAINDICATIONS	ADVERSE EFFECTS†
Ursodiol (Actigall)	**Cap:** 300mg	**Adults: Treatment:** 8-10mg/kg/day given bid-tid. Obtain ultrasound at 6 month intervals for 1 year. Continue therapy after stones have dissolved and confirm with repeat ultrasound within 1-3 months. **Prevention:** 300mg bid.	**W/P:** Therapy is not associated with liver damage. Monitor LFTs at the initiation of therapy and periodically thereafter. Caution in elderly. **Contra:** Calcified cholesterol stones, radiopaque stones, radiolucent bile pigment stones, unremitting acute cholecystitis, cholangitis, biliary obstruction, gallstone pancreatitis,	Abdominal pain, constipation, diarrhea, dyspepsia, flatulence, nausea, arthralgia, coughing, viral infection, vomiting, bronchitis, pharyngitis, back pain, myalgia, headache, sinusitis, upper respiratory tract infection.

Table 16.1: PRESCRIBING INFORMATION FOR RX GASTROINTESTINAL DRUGS (cont.)

NAME	FORM/ STRENGTH	DOSAGE	WARNINGS/PRECAUTIONS & CONTRAINDICATIONS	ADVERSE EFFECTS†
DIGESTIVE ENZYMES (cont.)				
Ursodiol (cont.)			biliary-gastrointestinal fistula, bile acid hypersensitivity. **P/N:** Category B, caution in nursing.	
Ursodiol (Urso 250, Urso Forte)	**Tab: (Urso 250)** 250mg, **(Urso Forte)** 500mg	**Adults: Usual:** 13-15mg/kg/day given bid-qid with food.	**W/P:** Administer appropriate specific treatment with variceal bleeding, hepatic encephalopathy, ascites, or when in need of urgent liver transplant. **P/N:** Category B, caution in nursing.	Diarrhea, leukopenia, peptic ulcer, hyperglycemia, skin rash, increased creatinine.
LAXATIVES				
Polyethylene Glycol/ Potassium Chloride/ Sodium Bicarbonate/ Sodium Chloride (NuLYTELY)	**Sol: (Polyethylene Glycol-Potassium Chloride-Sodium Bicarbonate-Sodium Chloride)** 420g-1.48g-5.72g-11.2g [4000mL]	**Adults: Oral:** 240mL every 10 minutes until fecal discharge is clear or 4L is consumed. **Nasogastric Tube:** 20-30mL/minute (1.2-1.8L/hr). Patient should fast at least 3-4 hours before administration. **Pediatrics: ≥6 months: Oral/Nasogastric Tube:** 25mL/kg/hr until fecal discharge is clear. Patient should fast at least 3-4 hours before administration.	**W/P:** Do not add additional ingredients (eg, flavorings). Caution with severe ulcerative colitis. Monitor therapy with impaired gag reflex, unconsciousness/semiconsciousness and patients prone to regurgitation and aspiration. Temporarily discontinue if develop severe bloating, distention, or abdominal pain. Monitor for hypoglycemia in pediatrics <2 yrs of age. **Contra:** GI obstruction, gastric retention, bowel perforation, toxic colitis, toxic megacolon, ileus. **P/N:** Category C, caution in nursing.	Nausea, abdominal fullness/cramps, bloating, vomiting, anal irritation.
Polyethylene Glycol/ Potassium Chloride/ Sodium Bicarbonate/ Sodium Chloride/ Sodium Sulfate (Colyte)	**Sol: (Polyethylene Glycol-Potassium Chloride-Sodium Bicarbonate-Sodium Chloride-Sodium Sulfate)** 60g-0.745g-1.68g-1.46g-5.68g/L [3754mL, 4000mL]	**Adults: Oral:** 240mL every 10 minutes until fecal discharge is clear. **Nasogastric Tube:** 20-30mL/minute (1.2-1.8L/hr). Patient should fast at least 3 hrs before administration, except for clear liquids.	**W/P:** Caution with severe ulcerative colitis. Monitor therapy with impaired gag reflex, semi- or unconsciousness, and risk of regurgitation or aspiration especially with NG tube. **Contra:** Ileus, gastric retention, GI obstruction, bowel perforation, toxic colitis, toxic megacolon. **P/N:** Category C, safety in nursing is unknown.	Nausea, abdominal fullness/cramps, bloating, anal irritation, vomiting.
Polyethylene Glycol/ Potassium Chloride/ Sodium Bicarbonate/ Sodium Chloride/ Sodium Sulfate (GoLYTELY)	**Sol: (Polyethylene Glycol-Potassium Chloride-Sodium Bicarbonate-Sodium Chloride-Sodium Sulfate)** 236g-2.97g-6.74g-5.86g-22.74g [4000mL]	**Adults: Oral:** 240mL every 10 minutes until fecal discharge is clear or 4L is consumed. **Nasogastric Tube:** 20-30mL/minute (1.2-1.8L/hr). Patient should fast at least 3-4 hours before administration.	**W/P:** Do not add additional ingredients (eg, flavorings). Caution with severe ulcerative colitis. Monitor therapy with impaired gag reflex, unconsciousness/semiconsciousness and patients prone to regurgitation or aspiration. Slow administration or temporarily discontinue if severe bloating, distention, or abdominal pain develops. **Contra:** GI obstruction, gastric retention, bowel perforation, toxic colitis, toxic megacolon, ileus. **P/N:** Category C, caution in nursing.	Nausea, abdominal fullness, cramping, bloating, vomiting, anal irritation.
PANCREATIC ENZYME SUPPLEMENTS				
Amylase/ Lipase/ Protease (Creon 5, Creon 10, Creon 20)	**Cap, Delayed Release: (Amylase-Lipase-Protease) (Creon 5)** 16,600U-5000U-18,750U,	**Adults: Initial: (Creon 5)** 2-4 caps per meal/snack. **(Creon 10)** 1-2 caps per meal/snack. **(Creon 20)** 1 cap per meal/snack. **CF: Usual:** 1500-3000U lipase/kg/meal. Adjust dose to disease severity, control of steatorrhea, and maintenance of good nutritional status.	**W/P:** Strictures in the ileocecal region and/or ascending colon reported with ≥20,000U lipase/cap in CF patients. Caution if >6000U lipase/kg/meal fails to resolve symptoms especially with history of intestinal complications. Maintain adequate fluid	Nausea, vomiting, bloating, cramping, constipation, diarrhea.

*Scored. †Bold entries denote special dental considerations.

NAME	FORM/ STRENGTH	DOSAGE	WARNINGS/PRECAUTIONS & CONTRAINDICATIONS	ADVERSE EFFECTS†
Amylase/ Lipase/ Protease (cont.)	(Creon 10) 33,200U-10,000U-37,500U, (Creon 20) 66,400U-20,000U-75,000U	Do not chew/crush caps. May add capsule contents to soft food (pH <5.5) and swallow immediately without chewing; take with water. **Pediatrics:** **<6 yrs: Initial: (Creon 5)** 1-2 caps per meal/snack. (Creon 10) 1 cap per meal/snack. **(Creon 20)** Dose based on clinical experience for age group. **>6 yrs: Initial: (Creon 5)** 2-4 caps per meal/snack. **(Creon 10)** 1-2 caps per meal/snack. **(Creon 20)** 1 cap per meal/snack. **CF: Usual:** 1500-3000U lipase/kg/meal. Adjust dose to disease severity, control of steatorrhea, and maintenance of good nutritional status. **Max:** 6000U lipase/kg/meal. Do not chew/crush caps. May add capsule contents to soft food (pH <5.5) and swallow immediately without chewing; take with water.	intake. Discontinue if hypersensitivity occurs. **Contra:** Pork protein hypersensitivity and early stages of acute pancreatitis. **P/N:** Category C, caution in nursing.	
Amylase/Lipase/Protease (Kutrase)	Cap: 30,000U-10,0000U-37500U	**Adults:** Use as directed.	**W/P:** Strictures in the ileo-cecal region and/or ascending colon reported with ≥20,000U lipase/cap in CF patients. Caution if >6000U lipase/kg/meal fails to resolve symptoms especially with history of intestinal complications. Maintain adequate fluid intake. Discontinue if hypersensitivity occurs. **Contra:** Pork protein hypersensitivity and early stages of acute pancreatitis. **P/N:** Category C, caution in nursing.	Nausea, vomiting, bloating, cramping, constipation, diarrhea.
Amylase/ Lipase/ Protease (Ku-zyme)	Cap: 15,000U-1200U-15,000U	**Adults:** Use as directed.	**W/P:** Strictures in the ileo-cecal region and/or ascending colon reported with ≥20,000U lipase/cap in CF patients. Caution if >6000U lipase/kg/meal fails to resolve symptoms especially with history of intestinal complications. Maintain adequate fluid intake. Discontinue if hypersensitivity occurs. **Contra:** Pork protein hypersensitivity and early stages of acute pancreatitis. **P/N:** Category C, caution in nursing.	Nausea, vomiting, bloating, cramping, constipation, diarrhea.
Amylase/ Lipase/ Protease (Pancrease MT 4, MT 10, MT 16, MT 20; Pancrecarb MS-4, MS 8, MS 16; Ultrase MT 12, MT 18, MT 20)	Cap, Extended Release: (Amylase-Lipase-Protease) 20,000U-4500U-25,000U, (MT 4) 12,000U-4000U-12,000U, (MT 10) 30,000U-10,000U-30,000U, (MT 16) 48,000U-16,000U-48,000U, (MT 20) 56,000U-20,000U-44,000U; Cap: 25,000U-4000U-25,000U (MS-4),	**Adults: Initial:** 400U lipase/kg/meal. **Max:** 2500U lipase/kg/meal. Adjust dose based on 3-day fecal fat studies. Take with plenty of water. Do not chew/crush caps. May add capsule contents to soft food (pH <7.3) and swallow immediately without chewing. **Pediatrics: ≤12 months:** 2000-4000U lipase/120mL formula or per breast feeding. **13 months-3 yrs: Initial:** 1000U lipase/kg/meal. **Max:** 2500U lipase/kg/meal. **≥4 yrs: Initial:** 400U lipase/kg/meal. **Max:** 2500U lipase/kg/meal. Adjust dose based on 3-day fecal fat studies. Take with plenty of water. Do not chew/crush caps. May add capsule contents to soft food (pH <7.3) and swallow immediately without chewing.		Diarrhea, abdominal pain, intestinal obstruction, vomiting, flatulence, nausea, constipation, melena, perianal irritation, weight loss, pain.

Table 16.1: PRESCRIBING INFORMATION FOR RX GASTROINTESTINAL DRUGS *(cont.)*

NAME	FORM/ STRENGTH	DOSAGE	WARNINGS/PRECAUTIONS & CONTRAINDICATIONS	ADVERSE EFFECTS†
PANCREATIC ENZYME SUPPLEMENTS *(cont.)*				
Amylase/ Lipase/ Protease *(cont.)*	40,000U-8000U-45000U(MS-8), 52000-16,000U-52,000 (MS-16); **Cap:** 20,000U-4500U-25,000, 39,000U-12,000U-39,000U (MT 12), 58,500U-18,000U-58,500 (MT 18), 65,000U-20,000U-65,000 (MT 20)	*Pediatrics:* ≤**12 months:** 2000-4000U lipase/120mL formula or per breast feeding. **13 months-3 yrs: Initial:** 1000U lipase/kg/meal. **Max:** 2500U lipase/kg/meal. ≥**4 yrs: Initial:** 400U lipase/kg/meal. **Max:** 2500U lipase/kg/meal. Adjust dose based on 3-day fecal fat studies. Take with plenty of water. Do not chew/crush caps. May add capsule contents to soft food (pH <7.3) and swallow immediately without chewing.		
Amylase/ Lipase/ Protease (Zymase)	**Cap, Delayed Release: (Amylase-Lipase-Protease)** 24,000U-12,000U-24,000U	*Adults:* 1-2 caps with each meal or snack. Contents of cap may be mixed with liquids or soft foods that do not require chewing. *Pediatrics:* 1-2 caps with each meal or snack. Contents of cap may be mixed with liquids or soft foods that do not require chewing.	**W/P:** Do not chew or crush contents of capsules. High doses can cause hyperuricemia and hyperuricosuria. **Contra:** Pork protein hypersensitivity. **P/N:** Safety in pregnancy and nursing not known.	Diarrhea, abdominal pain, intestinal obstruction, vomiting, flatulence, nausea, constipation, melena, perianal irritation, weight loss, pain.
Amylase/ Lipase/ Protease (Viokase)	**(Amylase-Lipase-Protease) Powder:**70,000U-16,800U-70,000U/0.7g [240g]; **Tab: (Viokase 8)** 30,000U-8,000U-30,000U; **(Viokase 16)** 60,000U-16,000U-60,000U	*Adults:* **(Powder) Cystic Fibrosis:** 0.7g (1/2 tsp) with meals. **(Tab) Cystic Fibrosis/Pancreatitis:** 8,000-32,000U Lipase with meals. **Pancreatectomy/Pancreatic Duct Obstruction:** 8,000-16,000U Lipase q2h. *Pediatrics:* **(Powder) Cystic Fibrosis:** 0.7g (1/2 tsp) with meals. **(Tab) Cystic Fibrosis/Pancreatitis:** 8,000-32,000U Lipase with meals. **Pancreatectomy/Pancreatic Duct Obstruction:** 8,000-16,000U Lipase q2h.	**W/P:** May have allergic reactions if previously sensitized to trypsin, pancreatin or pancrelipase. Irritating to oral mucosa if held in mouth. Inhalation of powder can cause an asthma attack. High doses can cause hyperuricemia and hyperuricosuria. **Contra:** Pork protein hypersensitivity. **P/N:** Category C, caution in nursing.	Irritation to nasal mucosa and respiratory tract with inhaled powder.

*Scored. †Bold entries denote special dental considerations.

Table 16.2: PRESCRIBING INFORMATION FOR OTC GASTROINTESTINAL DRUGS

NAME	FORM/BRAND/ STRENGTH	DOSAGE	WARNINGS/PRECAUTIONS & CONTRAINDICATIONS	ADVERSE EFFECTS
ACTIVATED CHARCOAL				
	Capsules: Charcoal Plus DS 260mg **Powder:** E-Z-Char 25g/20.4g **Suspension:** Actidose-Aqua 15g/72mL, 25g/120mL; Kerr Insta-Char 25g/120mL **Tablet:** Charcoal Plus DS 250mg	**Adults: Diarrhea:** 520mg after meals or at the first sign of discomfort. **Max:** 4160mg/day. **Dyspepsia:** 520mg after meals or at the first sign of discomfortt. **Max:** 4160mg/day. **Poisoning-Selective Decontamination of the Digestive Tract: Initial:** 30-100g or 1-2g/kg; repeat initial dose as soon as possible or 20-50g q2-6hr. **Pediatrics: Poisoning-Selective Decontamination of the Digestive Tract:** ≤1 yr: As slurry in water 1g/kg; may repeat half the initial dose q2-6hr prn. **1-12yr:** As slurry in water, 25-50g or 1-2g/kg; may repeat half the initial dose q 2-6 hr prn.	**W/P:** If symptoms persist more than 72 hours consult your physician. Consult a physician if taking other drugs as this medication may interfere with their effectiveness. It is suggested to allow 2 hours before or after taking any medication. May cause temporary darkening of the stool. Keep this and all drugs out of reach of children. **Contra:** Absence of bowel sounds, gastrointestinal perforation, intestinal obstruction, recent surgery, risk of GI hemorrhage.	Black feces, diarrhea, vomiting, pulmonary aspiration.
ACTIVATED CHARCOAL/SIMETHICONE				
	Tablet: Bicarsim 250mg-80mg, Bicarsim Forte 250mg-125mg; Flatulex 250mg-80mg, Flatulex Max 250mg-125mg	Use as directed.	**W/P:** If symptoms persist more than 72 hours consult your physician. Consult a physician if taking other drugs as this medication may interfere with their effectiveness. It is suggested to allow 2 hours before or after taking any medication. May cause temporary darkening of the stool. Keep this and all drugs out of reach of children. **Contra:** Absence of bowel sounds, gastrointestinal perforation, intestinal obstruction, recent surgery, risk of GI hemorrhage.	Black feces, diarrhea, vomiting, pulmonary aspiration.
ACTIVATED CHARCOAL/SORBITOL				
	Suspension: Actidose w/Sorbitol; 25g/120mL	Use as directed.	**W/P:** If symptoms persist more than 72 hours consult your physician. Consult a physician if taking other drugs as this medication may interfere with their effectiveness. It is suggested to allow 2 hours before or after taking any medication. May cause temporary darkening of the stool. Keep this and all drugs out of reach of children. **Contra:** Absence of bowel sounds, gastrointestinal perforation, intestinal obstruction, recent surgery, risk of GI hemorrhage.	Black feces, diarrhea, vomiting, pulmonary aspiration.
ALPHA-D-GALACTOSIDASE				
	Tablet: Beano; 150 IU; **Drops:** Beano; 30U/drop	**Adults:** About 5 drops per food serving or 3 tablets per meal (1 tablet per ½ cup serving) of 3 servings of problem foods; higher levels depending on symptoms.	**W/P:** If you are pregnant or nursing, ask your doctor before product use. Beano is made from a safe, food-grade mold. However, if a rare sensitivity occurs, discontinue use. Galactosemics should not use without physician's advice, since one of the breakdown sugars is galactose.	NA
ALUMINUM HYDROXIDE				
	Suspension: Alternagel 320mg/5mL, 600mg/5mL	**Adults:** Take 1-2 tsp between meals, at bedtime or as directed.	**W/P:** Antacid use may mask the symptoms of internal bleeding secondary to nonsteroidal antiinflammatory drugs.	Fluid retention, dementia, aluminum toxicity, metabolic alkalosis,

NA = not available.

Table 16.2: PRESCRIBING INFORMATION FOR OTC GASTROINTESTINAL DRUGS (cont.)

NAME	FORM/BRAND/ STRENGTH	DOSAGE	WARNINGS/PRECAUTIONS & CONTRAINDICATIONS	ADVERSE EFFECTS
ALUMINUM HYDROXIDE (cont.)				
			Antacids decrease the absorption of some drugs (eg, tetracyclines, quinolones, propranolol, atenolol, captopril, ranitidine, famotidine, and aspirin); avoid concomitant use of these drugs. Caution in renal disease.	hypercalcemia, uremia, calcinosis, hypophosphatemia, hypermagnesemia, trace element deficiency, constipation, diarrhea, gastrointestinal obstruction, nephrotoxicity, aspiration pneumonia, and osteomalacia.
ALUMINUM HYDROXIDE/MAGNESIUM CARBONATE				
	Sus: Gaviscon 5mg/15mL-358mg/ 15mL, Gaviscon ES 254mg/5mL- 237.5mg/5mL; **Tab:** Gaviscon 80mg-20mg, Gaviscon ES 160mg-105mg	**Adults:** Take 2 to 4 tsp or tabs qid or as directed.	**W/P:** Antacid use may mask the symptoms of internal bleeding secondary to nonsteroidal antiinflammatory drugs. Antacids decrease the absorption of some drugs (eg, tetracyclines, quinolones, propranolol, atenolol, captopril, ranitidine, famotidine, and aspirin); avoid concomitant use of these drugs. Caution in renal disease.	Fluid retention, dementia, aluminum toxicity, metabolic alkalosis, hypercalcemia, uremia, calcinosis, hypophosphatemia, hypermagnesemia, trace element deficiency, constipation, diarrhea, gastrointestinal obstruction, nephrotoxicity, aspiration pneumonia, and osteomalacia.
ALUMINUM HYDROXIDE/MAGNESIUM HYDROXIDE				
	Suspension: Maalox, Maalox TC, Alamag: 225mg/ 5mL-200mg/5mL; **Tablet:** Alamag 300mg-15-mg	**Adults/Pediatrics (Sus):** >12yrs: 2 tbsp (30 mL) every 1/2 hour to 1 hour, as required, not to exceed 8 tablespoons (120 mL) in 24 hours. **(Tab):** As directed.	**W/P:** Antacid use may mask the symptoms of internal bleeding secondary to nonsteroidal antiinflammatory drugs. Antacids decrease the absorption of some drugs (eg, tetracyclines, quinolones, propranolol, atenolol, captopril, ranitidine, famotidine, and aspirin); avoid concomitant use of these drugs. Caution in renal disease.	Fluid retention, dementia, aluminum toxicity, metabolic alkalosis, hypercalcemia, uremia, calcinosis, hypophosphatemia, hypermagnesemia, trace element deficiency, constipation, diarrhea, gastrointestinal obstruction, nephrotoxicity, aspiration pneumonia, and osteomalacia.
ALUMINUM HYDROXIDE/MAGNESIUM HYDROXIDE/SIMETHICONE				
	Suspension: 200mg-200mg- 20mg; **Maximum Strength:** 400mg- 400mg-40mg **Tablet:** Gelusil 200mg-200mg- 25mg	**Adults:** 2-4 tsp or tabs after meals or at bedtime as directed.	**W/P:** Antacid use may mask the symptoms of internal bleeding secondary to nonsteroidal antiinflammatory drugs. Antacids decrease the absorption of some drugs (eg, tetracyclines, quinolones, propranolol, atenolol, captopril, ranitidine, famotidine, and aspirin); avoid concomitant use of these drugs. Caution in renal disease.	Fluid retention, dementia, aluminum toxicity, metabolic alkalosis, hypercalcemia, uremia, calcinosis, hypophosphatemia, hypermagnesemia, trace element deficiency, constipation, diarrhea, gastrointestinal obstruction, nephrotoxicity, aspiration pneumonia, and osteomalacia.
ATTAPULGITE				
	Tablet: Kaopectate 750mg **Suspension:** Kaopectate Advanced Formula 750mg/15mL, Kaopectate Children's Liquid 600mg/15mL	**Adults/Pediatrics:** >12yrs: 30mL or 2 tbsp. **Pediatrics:** 9 to 11 yrs: 15 mL or 1 tbsp. 6 to 8 yrs: 10mL or 2 tsp. 3 to 5 years: 5mL or 1 tsp.	**W/P:** Suspected bowel obstruction, caution in infants and children under 3 years of age, dehydration, elderly patients, fever, prolonged use or excessive doses of attapulgite can lead to severe constipation or fecal impactionm 2- to 3-hr interval should separate the oral administration of attapulgite and other drugs. **Contra:** Hypersensitivity to	Constipation, dyspepsia, flatulence, nausea.

NA = not available.

NAME	FORM/BRAND/ STRENGTH	DOSAGE	WARNINGS/PRECAUTIONS & CONTRAINDICATIONS	ADVERSE EFFECTS
			attapulgite products, suspected bowel obstruction. **P/N:** Safety in pregnancy and nursing not known.	

BETAINE HYDROCHLORIDE

	Tablet: Betaine 300mg, 325mg	**Adults:** 3gm bid. **Pediatrics:** >3yrs: 3gm bid. <3yrs: **Initial:**100mg/kg/day; may increase weekly by 100mg/kg increments.	**Contra:** Hypersensitivity to betaine. **P/N:** Category C, safety in nursing not known.	Diarrhea, drug-induced gastrointestinal disturbance, nausea.

BISACODYL

	Tablets: Dulcolax, Correctol, Fleet Biscadoyl, Modane: 5mg (delayed release) **Suppository:** Dulcolax, Fleet Biscodyl: 10mg **Enema:** Fleet Biscadoyl 10mg	**Adults:** **(Tab)** Take 2-3 tabs qd. Do not crush/chew. **(Sup)** Insert 1 sup rectally; retain for 15-20 minutes. May coat tip with petroleum jelly with anal fissures or hemorrhoids. **X-Ray Endoscopy For Barium Enema:** Avoid food after tab administration. Insert 1 sup rectally 1-2 hrs before exam. **(Enema)** Use 1 rectally single dose qd. **Pediatrics:** ≥12 yrs: **(Tab)** 2-3 tabs qd. **6-12 yrs:** 1 tab qd. Do not crush/chew. **(Sup)** ≥12 yrs: Insert 1 sup rectally; retain for 15-20 minutes. **6-12 yrs:** Insert 1/2 sup rectally qd. May coat tip with petroleum jelly with anal fissures or hemorrhoids. **X-Ray Endoscopy For Barium Enema:** ≥6 yrs: Avoid food after tab administration. Insert 1 sup 1-2 hrs before exam. **<6 yrs:** Avoid tab. Insert 1/2 sup rectally 1-2 hrs before exam. ≥12 yrs: **(Enema)** Use 1 rectally single dose qd.	**W/P:** Avoid with abdominal pain, nausea, or vomiting. Not for long-term use (>7 days). Discontinue with rectal bleeding or fail to have bowel movement. **Contra:** Acute abdominal surgery, appendicitis, rectal bleeding, gastroenteritis, intestinal obstruction. **P/N:** Safety in pregnancy and nursing not known.	Abdominal discomfort.

BISACODYL/SODIUM PHOSPHATE

	Kit: Fleet Prep Kit 1, Fleet Prep Kit 2, Fleet Prep Kit 3	Use as directed.	**W/P:** Avoid with abdominal pain, nausea, or vomiting. Not for long-term use (>7 days). Discontinue with rectal bleeding or fail to have bowel movement. **Contra:** Acute abdominal surgery, appendicitis, rectal bleeding, gastroenteritis, intestinal obstruction. **P/N:** Safety in pregnancy and nursing not known.	Abdominal discomfort.

BISMUTH SUBSALICYLATE

	Tablet: Pepto Bismol **Tab:** 262mg; **Tab, Chewable:** 262mg **Suspension:** PeptoBismol, Kaopectate: 262mg/15mL; **(Maximum Strength)** 525mg/15mL	**Adults:** **(Sus)** 30mL every 0.5-1 hr prn. **Max:** 8 doses/24hrs. **(Sus, Max Strength)** 30mL hourly prn. **Max:** 4 doses/24 hrs. **(Tab; Tab, Chewable)** 2 tabs every 0.5-1 hr prn. **Max:** 8 doses/24hrs. Drink plenty of clear fluids. **Pediatrics:** **(Sus)** 9-12 yrs: 15mL every 0.5-1 hr prn. **6-9 yrs:** 10mL every 0.5-1 hr prn. **3-6 yrs:** 5mL every 0.5-1 hr. **Max:** 8 doses/24hrs. **(Sus, Max Strength)** 9-12 yrs: 15mL hourly prn. **6-9 yrs:** 10mL hourly prn. **3-6 yrs:** 5mL hourly prn. **Max:** 4 doses/24hrs. **(Tab; Tab, Chewable)**	**W/P:** Avoid in children and teenagers with or recovering from chickenpox or flu. Do not give to patients with aspirin or nonaspirin salicylate allergy. May cause temporary darkening of tongue or stool. Product may contain small amounts of naturally occurring lead. **P/N:** Safety in pregnancy and nursing not known.	NA

Table 16.2: PRESCRIBING INFORMATION FOR OTC GASTROINTESTINAL DRUGS (cont.)

NAME	FORM/BRAND/ STRENGTH	DOSAGE	WARNINGS/PRECAUTIONS & CONTRAINDICATIONS	ADVERSE EFFECTS
BISMUTH SUBSALICYLATE (cont.)				
		9-12 yrs: 1 tab every 0.5-1 hr prn. **6-9 yrs:** 2/3 tab every 0.5-1 hr prn. **3-6 yrs:** 1/3 tab every 0.5-1 hr prn. **Max:** 8 doses/24 hrs. Drink plenty of clear fluids.		
CALCIUM CARBONATE				
	Tablet: Chewable: 220mg **(Rolaids),** 400mg **(Mylanta Children's),** 420 **(Titralac),** 500mg **(Chooz, Tums),** 750mg **(Titralac ES, Tums E-X),** 850mg **(Alka-Mints),** 1000mg **(Tums Ultra)**	**Adults:** Chew 2-4 tablets as symptoms occur.	**W/P:** Antacids may interact with certain prescription drugs. Do not take more than 12 tablets in a 24-hour period, or use the maximum dosage for more than 2 weeks, except under the advice and supervision of a physician. **P/N:** Safety in pregnancy and nursing not known.	Hypercalcemia, constipation.
CALCIUM POLYCARBOPHIL				
	Tablet: 625mg **(Equalactin, Fibercon, Konsyl Fiber, Perdiem);** 1250mg **(Fiberall)**	**Adults:** 625mg daily; chew and swallow 1-4 times daily as needed up to a maximum of 5000mg/day.	**W/P:** Abdominal pain, nausea, vomiting or sudden, persistent change in bowel habits may occur, adequate water (8oz) must accompany calcium polycarbophil administration, consult a physician for children under 6 years. Concomitant tetracyclines should be administered 1 hours after or 2 hours before calcium polycarbophil. **Contra:** Difficulty swallowing, intestinal obstruction, fecal impaction. **P/N:** Safety in pregnancy and nursing not known.	Epigastric fullness, flatulence.
CASCARA SAGRADA				
	Liquid: Cascara Sagrada 50mg/15mL; **Tablet:** Cascara Sagrada 325mg; **Capsules:** Cascara Sagrada 425mg	Use as directed.	**Contra:** Fecal impaction, bowel obstruction, appendicitis, hypersensitivity to Cascara or anthraquinone laxatives, inflammatory conditions of the intestines (appendicitis, colitis, Crohn's disease, irritable bowel), lactation, nausea, vomiting, abdominal pain, or other symptoms of appendicitis. **P/N:** Category C, nursing not known.	Abdominal pain, nausea, vomiting, diarrhea, electrolyte abnormalities, melanotic pigmentation, urine discoloration.
CASTOR OIL				
	Oil: Castor Oil USP 100%	**Adults:** 15-60 mL, dose varies depending on product. **Pediatrics:** >12yrs: 15-60 mL. **2-12 yrs:** 5-15 mL. **<2yrs:** 1-2mL.	**W/P:** Caution in pregnancy. **Contra:** Abdominal pain. intestinal obstruction, nausea, vomiting, symptoms of appendicitis. **P/N:** Pregnancy and nursing not known.	Abdominal pain, nausea, vomiting, cramps.
CITRIC ACID/POTASSIUM BICARBONATE				
	Tablet: Alka-Seltzer 1000mg/1940mg	**Adults:** Fully dissolve tablets in 4 ounces of water before taking. **Pediatrics:** >12 yrs: 2 tablets every 4 hours, or as directed.	**W/P:** Large doses may cause alkalosis, especially in presence of renal disease, caution in concurrent administration of potassium-containing medications, potassium-sparing diuretics, angiotensin-converting enzyme (ACE) inhibitors,	Abnormal ECG, alkalosis, hyperkalemia.

NA = not available.

NAME	FORM/BRAND/ STRENGTH	DOSAGE	WARNINGS/PRECAUTIONS & CONTRAINDICATIONS	ADVERSE EFFECTS
			or cardiac glycosides. **Contra:** Addison's disease, untreated adynamia episodica hereditaria, anuria, dehydration, acute heat cramps, hyperkalemia myocardial damage, severe renal impairment with oliguria or azotemia **P/N:** Pregnancy and nursing unknown.	

DIMENHYDRINATE

	FORM/BRAND/ STRENGTH	DOSAGE	WARNINGS/PRECAUTIONS & CONTRAINDICATIONS	ADVERSE EFFECTS
	Tablets: Drama-mine, Triptone: 50mg	**Adults:** 50-100 mg 30 min prior to travel; repeat every 4-6hrs. **Max:** 400 mg/day. **Pediatrics: 6-12 yrs:** 25-50 mg q6-8 hrs. **Max:** 150 mg/day.	**W/P:** Caution in asthma, avoid alcoholic beverages, caution in chronic bronchitis, emphysema, enlarged prostate. nar-row-angle glaucoma, may cause marked drowsiness. **Contra:** Hypersensitivity to dimenhydrinate or diphenhydramine. **P/N:** Pregnancy and nursing unknown.	Nausea, vomiting, xero-stomia, drowsiness.

DOCUSATE SODIUM

	FORM/BRAND/ STRENGTH	DOSAGE	WARNINGS/PRECAUTIONS & CONTRAINDICATIONS	ADVERSE EFFECTS
	Capsule: Colace 50mg, 100mg; **Liquid:** Colace 100mg/mL; **Syrup:** Colace 20mg/5mL; **Tablet:** Fleet Sof-Lax, Ex-Lax Stool Softener, Phillip's Stool Softener Laxa-tive: 100mg	**Adults:** 50-200mg/day. **Retention or Flushing Enema:** Add 5-10mL of liquid to enema fluid. Mix liq/syr into 6-8 oz of milk or juice. **Pediatrics: ≥12 yrs:** 50-200mg/day. **6-12 yrs:** 40-120mg/day liq. **3-6 yrs:** 2mL liq tid. Mix liq/syr into 6-8 oz of milk, juice or formula. **Retention/Flushing Enema:** Add 5-10mL of liquid to enema fluid.	**W/P:** Avoid with abdominal pain, nausea, or vomiting. Discontinue enema if rectal bleeding occurs or fail to have a bowel movement. **P/N:** Safety in pregnancy and nursing not known.	Bitter taste, throat irrita-tion, nausea, rash.

DOCUSATE SODIUM/SENNOSIDES A AND B

	FORM/BRAND/ STRENGTH	DOSAGE	WARNINGS/PRECAUTIONS & CONTRAINDICATIONS	ADVERSE EFFECTS
	Tablet: Peri-colace, Senokot S: 50mg-8.6mg	**Adults:** Take 2-4 tablets daily.	**W/P:** Avoid with abdominal pain, nausea, or vomiting. Discontinue enema if rectal bleeding occurs or fail to have a bowel movement. **P/N:** Safety in pregnancy and nursing not known.	Bitter taste, throat irrita-tion, nausea, rash.

GLYCERIN

	FORM/BRAND/ STRENGTH	DOSAGE	WARNINGS/PRECAUTIONS & CONTRAINDICATIONS	ADVERSE EFFECTS
	Suppository: Fleet Glycerin 1g, 2g, 3g	**Adults:** 1 suppository (2g or 3g) rectally. **Pediatrics: 2-5 yrs:** 1 suppository (1g) rectally. **≥6 yrs:** 1 suppository (2g or 3g) rectally.	**W/P:** Rectal irritation may occur. Do not use with nausea, vomiting, or abdominal pain. Rectal bleeding or failure to have a bowel movement after use may indicate a serious condition. Do not use longer than 1 week. **P/N:** Safety in pregnancy and nursing in not known.	Rectal discomfort, burning sensation.

IPECAC SYRUP

	FORM/BRAND/ STRENGTH	DOSAGE	WARNINGS/PRECAUTIONS & CONTRAINDICATIONS	ADVERSE EFFECTS
	Syrup: Ipecac Syrup: 7mg/5mL	**Adults:** Repeat dose if patient does not vomit within 30 min.	**W/P:** Caution in cardiac conditions. **Contra:** Ingestion of petroleum distillate, strong acids or bases, strychnine, un-consciousness or absence of gag reflex. **P/N:** Pregnancy and nursing unknown.	Diarrhea, stomach cramps, myalgia, lethargy.

LACTASE

	FORM/BRAND/ STRENGTH	DOSAGE	WARNINGS/PRECAUTIONS & CONTRAINDICATIONS	ADVERSE EFFECTS
	Tablet: Lactaid 3300U, Lactain ES 4500U, Lactain Ultra 9000U	**Adults:** Swallow 1 caplet with your first bite of dairy foods. If neces-sary, you may swallow 2 caplets at one time. If you continue to eat foods containing dairy after 30-45 minutes, take another caplet.	**W/P:** Caution if your symptoms continue after using the product or if your symp-toms are unusual and seem unrelated to eating dairy. **P/N:** Pregnancy and nursing unknown.	NA

Table 16.2: PRESCRIBING INFORMATION FOR OTC GASTROINTESTINAL DRUGS (cont.)

NAME	FORM/BRAND/ STRENGTH	DOSAGE	WARNINGS/PRECAUTIONS & CONTRAINDICATIONS	ADVERSE EFFECTS
LACTOBACILLUS ACIDOPHILUS				
	Capsules: Various brands/strengths; **Powder:** Various brands/strengths	**Adults:** 1 to 2 capsules or 1/4 tsp powder twice daily before meals.	**W/P:** Caution if your symptoms continue after using the product or if your symptoms are unusual and seem unrelated to eating dairy. **Contra:** Hypersensitivity to lactose or milk. Patients sensitive to milk should not use lactobacillus products **P/N:** Pregnancy and nursing unknown.	Burping, diarrhea, gas, hiccups, vomiting.
LOPERAMIDE HYDROCHLORIDE				
	Solution: Imodium A-D 1mg/5mL; **Tablet:** Imodium A-D 2mg	**Adults: ≥12 yrs:** Initial: 4mg after the first loose bowel movement then 2mg after each additional loose bowel with plenty of liquid. **Max:** 8mg/day for no more than 2 days. **Pediatrics: <9-11 yrs (60-95 lbs):** 2mg after the first loose bowel movement then 1mg after each additional loose bowel with plenty of liquid. **Max:** 6mg/day for no more than 2 days. **6-8 yrs (48-59 lbs):** 2mg after the first loose bowel movement then 1mg after each additional loose bowel. **Max:** 4mg/day for no more than 2 days. **2-5 yrs (24-47 lbs):** 1mg after the first loose bowel movement then 1mg after each additional loose bowel. **Max:** 3mg/day.	**W/P:** Do not use if diarrhea is accompanied with high fever, blood, or mucus in stool. Caution with history of liver disease. **P/N:** Safety in pregnancy and nursing is not known.	NA
MAGNESIUM HYDROXIDE				
	Suspension: Phillips Milk of Magnesia 400mg/5mL	**Adults/Pediatrics: >12 yrs:** 2-4 tbs at bedtime or upon arising, followed by a full glass (8 oz) of liquid.	**W/P:** Prolonged use of aluminum-containing antacids in patients with renal failure may result in or worsen dialysis osteomalacia. Elevated tissue aluminum levels contribute to the development of the dialysis encephalopathy and osteomalacia syndromes. Small amounts of aluminum are absorbed from the gastrointestinal tract and renal excretion of aluminum is impaired in renal failure. Aluminum is not well removed by dialysis because it is bound to albumin and transferrin, which do not cross dialysis membranes. As a result, aluminum is deposited in bone, and dialysis osteomalacia may develop when large amounts of aluminum are ingested orally by patients with impaired renal function. **P/N:** Pregnancy and nursing unknown.	NA
MINERAL OIL				
	Oil: Fleet Mineral Oil Enema, Kondremul	**Adults: Constipation:** 15-45mL qhs. **Max:** 45mL. **Fecal Impaction:** 15-45mL qhs. **Max:** 45 mL. **Irrigation of Bowel After Barium Sulfate Administration:** 118mL rectally once daily as an enema.	**W/P:** Caution if you experience nausea, vomiting, or abdominal pain, sudden change in bowel habits persisting for 2 wks, and use in any young children **Contra:** Appendicitis, children less than 2 yr of age (rectal administration),	Anal irritation, pruritus ani, incontinence of feces, intestinal malabsorption, rectal discharge.

NA = not available.

NAME	FORM/BRAND/ STRENGTH	DOSAGE	WARNINGS/PRECAUTIONS & CONTRAINDICATIONS	ADVERSE EFFECTS
		Pediatrics: **Constipation: 6-12 yrs:** 5-15mL qhs. **>12 yrs:** Use adult dose. **2-11 yrs:** 59mL rectally once daily as an enema.	children less than 6 yrs of age (oral administration), colostomy/ileostomy, diverticulitis, hypersensitivity to mineral oil products, ulcerative colitis, rectal bleeding. **P/N:** Pregnancy and nursing unknown.	

PSYLLIUM

NAME	FORM/BRAND/ STRENGTH	DOSAGE	WARNINGS/PRECAUTIONS & CONTRAINDICATIONS	ADVERSE EFFECTS
	Powder: Metamucil, Konsyl-Orange, Fiberall: 3.4g/dose; **Wafers:** Metamucil, Fiberall: 3.4g/dose	*Adults:* **(Powder)** 1 rounded tsp in 8 oz of liquid 3 times daily. **(Wafer)** 2 wafers with 8 oz of your favorite hot or cold beverage at the first sign of irregularity. Can take up to 3 doses daily if needed.	**Contra:** Difficulty swallowing, esophageal narrowing, fecal impaction, hypersensitivity to Psyllium, intestinal obstruction. **P/N:** Pregnancy and nursing unknown.	Abdominal distention and flatulence, potentially severe (but rare) allergic reactions, anaphylaxis, and asthma.

SCOPOLAMINE

NAME	FORM/BRAND/ STRENGTH	DOSAGE	WARNINGS/PRECAUTIONS & CONTRAINDICATIONS	ADVERSE EFFECTS
	Patch: Transderm Scop 0.33mg/24hr; **Capsule:** Scopodex 0.5mg; **Solution:** Scopolamine 0.4mg/mL; **Tablet:** Scopace 0.4mg	*Adults:* **(Patch) Motion Sickness:** Apply 1 patch 4 hrs before travel. Replace after 3 days. **Post-OP N/V:** Apply 1 patch the evening before surgery or 1 hr prior to cesarean section. Keep in place for 24 hrs. Apply patch to a hairless area behind the ear. Do not cut patch in half. **(Cap, Sol, Tab)** Use as directed.	**W/P:** Monitor IOP with open-angle glaucoma. Not for use in children. Caution with pyloric obstruction, urinary bladder neck or intestinal obstruction, elderly. Increased CNS effects with liver or kidney dysfunction. May aggravate seizures or psychosis. Idiosyncratic reactions reported (rare). **Contra:** Angle-closure (narrow angle) glaucoma, hypersensitivity to belladonna alkaloids. **P/N:** Category C, caution in nursing.	Dry mouth, drowsiness, blurred vision, dilation of pupils, dizziness, disorientation, confusion.

SENNA

NAME	FORM/BRAND/ STRENGTH	DOSAGE	WARNINGS/PRECAUTIONS & CONTRAINDICATIONS	ADVERSE EFFECTS
	Granules: Senokot 15mg/dose; **Tablet:** Sennoside A and B: Senokot 8.6mg, SenokotXTRA 17mg; Docusate Sodium-Sennoside A and B: Senokot-S: 50mg-8.6mg	*Adults:* Take at bedtime. (Senokot/Senokot-S) 2 tabs qd. **Max:** 4 tabs bid. **(SenokotXTRA)** 1 tab qd. **Max:** 2 tabs bid. **(Granules)** 5mL qd. **Max:** 15mL bid. Granules may be eaten plain, mixed with liquids, or sprinkled on food. *Pediatrics:* Take at bedtime. **(Senokot/Senokot-S)** ≥**12 yrs:** 2 tabs qd. **Max:** 4 tabs bid. **6-12 yrs:** 1 tab qd. **Max:** 2 tabs bid. **2-6 yrs:** 1/2 tab qd. **Max:** 1 tab bid. **(SenokotXTRA)** ≥**12 yrs:** 1 tab qd. **Max:** 2 tabs bid. **6-12 yrs:** 1/2 tab qd. **Max:** 1 tab bid. **(Granules)** ≥**12 yrs:** 1 tsp qd. **Max:** 2 tsp bid. **6-12 yrs:** 1/2 tsp qd. **Max:** 1 tsp bid. **2-6 yrs:** 1/4 tsp qd. **Max:** 1/2 tsp bid. Granules may be eaten plain, mixed with liquids, or sprinkled on food.	**W/P:** Do not use with abdominal pain, nausea, or vomiting. Should not be used for longer than 1 week. Rectal bleeding or failure to have a bowel movement after use may indicate serious condition. **P/N:** Safety in pregnancy and nursing not known.	NA

SENNOSIDES A AND B

NAME	FORM/BRAND/ STRENGTH	DOSAGE	WARNINGS/PRECAUTIONS & CONTRAINDICATIONS	ADVERSE EFFECTS
	Tablet: Senokot 8.6mg; Ex-Lax, Perdiem: 15mg; Ex-Lax Maximum Strength 25mg	*Adults:* 2 tablets once or twice daily.	**W/P:** Do not use with abdominal pain, nausea, or vomiting. Should not be used for longer than 1 week. Rectal bleeding or failure to have a bowel movement after use may indicate serious condition. **P/N:** Safety in pregnancy and nursing not known.	NA

Table 16.2: PRESCRIBING INFORMATION FOR OTC GASTROINTESTINAL DRUGS (cont.)

NAME	FORM/BRAND/ STRENGTH	DOSAGE	WARNINGS/PRECAUTIONS & CONTRAINDICATIONS	ADVERSE EFFECTS
SIMETHICONE				
	Tablet: Chewable **Tablet:** 80mg (Gas-X, Maalox Anti-Gas, Mylanta Gas); 125mg (Gas-X ES, Mylanta Gas MS, Phazyme); 150mg (Maalox ES)	**Adults**: 40-360 mg qid after meals and at bedtime as needed. **Max:** 500 mg/day. **Pediatrics**: **<2yrs:** 20 mg qid. **Max:** 240 mg/day. **2-12yrs:** 40mg qid after meals and at bedtime. **Max:** 12 doses/day (240 mg/day).	**W/P:** Do not exceed recommended dosage. **Contra:** Hypersensitivity to simethicone products, Known or suspected intestinal perforation and obstruction **P/N:** Safety in pregnancy and nursing not known.	Diarrhea (mild), nausea, regurgitation, vomiting.

NA = not available.

Table 16.3: DRUG INTERACTIONS FOR RX GASTROINTESTINAL DRUGS

ANTIDIARRHEAL

Atropine Sulfate/Diphenoxylate Hydrochloride (Lomotil)

Alcohol	May potentiate alcohol.
Barbituates	May potentiate barbituates.
MAOIs	May precipitate hypertensive crisis.
Tranquilizers	May potentiate tranquilizers.

ANTIEMETICS

Arepitant (Emend)

Astemizole	Avoid use with astemizole.
Cisapride	Avoid use with cisapride.
CYP2C9	May decrease levels of drugs metabolized by CYP2C9.
CYP3A4	May increase levels of drugs metabolized by CYP3A4; caution with strong CYP3A4 inhibitors; decreased efficacy with CYP3A4 inducers.
Oral contraceptives	May reduce efficacy of oral contraceptives; use alternative contraception during treatment and for 1 month after last dose.
Paroxetine	Concomitant use with paroxetine may decrease levels of both drugs.
Pimozide	Avoid use with pimozide.
Terfenadine	Avoid use with terfenadine.

Benzocaine/Trimethobenzamide Hydrochloride (Tigan)

Alcohol	Adverse drug interactions reported with alcohol.
CNS agents	Caution with CNS agents in acute febrile illness, encephalitides, gastroenteritis, dehydration, and electrolyte imbalance.

Chlorpromazine (Thorazine)

Amipaque	Discontinue at least 48 hrs before myelography and resume at least 24 hrs after.
Anitcoagulants	May decrease effects of oral anticoagulants.
Anticonvulsants	May need dose adjustment.
Atropine	Caution with atropine or related drugs.
CNS depressants	Potentiates effects of CNS depressants; reduce doses of these drugs by 1/4 to 1/2.
Guanethidine	May decrease effects of guanethidine.
Lithium	Encephalopathic syndrome reported with lithium.
Phenytoin	Toxicity reported; may need dose adjustment.
Propanolol	May increase levels of chlorpromazine and propanolol.
Thiazide diuretics	May potentiate orthostatic hypotension.

Table 16.3: DRUG INTERACTIONS FOR RX GASTROINTESTINAL DRUGS *(cont.)*

ANTIEMETICS *(cont.)*

Dolasetron Mesylate (Anzemet)

Antiarrhythmics	Increased risk of prolongation of cardiac conduction intervals with antiarrhytmics.
Anthracycline	Increased risk of prolongation of cardiac conduction intervals with anthracycline.
Atenolol	Decreased clearance with IV atenolol.
Cimetidine	Increased levels with cimetidine.
Diuretics	Increased risk of prolongation of cardiac conduction intervals with diuretics.
QT interval prolonging drugs	Increased risk of prolongation of cardiac conduction intervals with drugs that prolong QT interval.
Rifampin	Decreased levels with rifampin.

Dronabinol (Marinol)

Alcohol	Additive effects with alcohol.
Amphetamines	Additive HTN, tachycardia, and possible cardiotoxicity with amphetamines.
Antipyrine	Decreases clearance of antipyrine.
Anticholinergics	Increased tachycardia and drowsiness.
Barbituates	Decreases clearance of barbituates.
Cocaine	Additive HTN, tachycardia, and possible cardiotoxicity with cocaine.
CNS depressants	Potentiates effects of CNS depressants.
Hyponotics	Additive effects with hypnotics.
Protein bound drugs	Highly protein bound drugs may require dosage changes.
Psychoactive drugs	Additive effects with psychoactive drugs.
Sedatives	Additive effects with sedatives.
Sympathomimetics	Additive HTN, tachycardia, and possible cardiotoxicity with sympathomimetics.
TCAs	Potentiates effects of TCAs.

Droperidol (Inapsine)

Alcohol	Caution with alcohol.
Antiarrhythmics	Avoid class I and class III antiarrhythmics.
Antidepressants	Avoid antidepressants.
Antihistamines	Avoid antihistamines.
CNS depressants	Potentiates effects of CNS depressants; may be potenentiated by CNS depressants; use lower doses.
Conduction anesthesia	Caution with conduction anesthesia (spinal, peridural).
Diuretics	Caution with diuretics.

ANTIEMETICS *(cont.)*

Droperidol (Inapsine) *(cont.)*

Epinephrine	May paradoxically decrease BP.
Fentanyl	Increased BP with fentanyl citrate or other parenteral analgesics.
MAOIs	Caution with MAOIs.
Neuroleptics	Avoid neuroleptics.
QT interval prolonging drugs	Avoid drugs that prolong QT intervals.

Meclizine Hydrochloride (Antivert)

Alcohol	Avoid alcohol.

Granisetron Hydrochloride (Kytril)

CYP450 enzyme inducers	May alter clearance of granistetron.
CYP450 enzyme inhibitors	May alter clearance of granisetron.

Metoclopramide (Reglan)

Alcohol	Additive sedation with alcohol.
Anticholinergics	Antagonized by anticholinergics.
APAP	May increase intestinal absorption of APAP.
Cyclosporine	May increase intestinal absorption of cyclosporine.
Digoxin	May decrease gastric absorption of digoxin.
Ethanol	May increase intestinal absorption of ethanol.
Hypnotics	Additive sedation with hypnotics.
Insulin	Insulin dose or timing of dose may need adjustment to prevent hypoglycemia.
Levodopa	May increase intestinal absorption of levodopa.
MAOIs	Caution with MAOIs.
Narcotics	Additive sedation with narcotics; antagonized by narcotics.
Tranquilizers	Additive sedation with tranquilizers.

Ondansetron (Zofran, Zofran ODT)

CYP450	Inducers and inhibitors of these enzymes may changes the clearance and half-life of ondansetron.

Prochlorperazine (Compazine)

Anticoagulants	Decreases oral anticoagulant effects.
Anticonvulsants	May need dose adjustment.
Guanethidine	Antagonizes antihypertensive effects of guanethidine and related compounds.

Table 16.3: DRUG INTERACTIONS FOR RX GASTROINTESTINAL DRUGS (cont.)

ANTIEMETICS (cont.)

Prochlorperazine (Compazine) (cont.)

LIthium	Encephalopathic syndrome reported with lithium.
Propanolol	May increase levels of prochlorperazine and propanolol.

Promethazine Hydrochloride (Phenergan)

Anesethetics (local)	Caution with drugs that alter seizure threshold.
Analgesics	Reduce dose by one-quarter to one-half with analgesic depressants.
Anticholinergics	Caution with anticholinergics.
Barbiturates	Reduce barbiturate dose by one-half.
CNS depressants	Added sedative effects with CNS depressants; reduce dose or eliminate these agents.
Epinephrine	Do not use epinephrine for promethazine injection overdose.
MAOIs	Caution with MAOIs.
Narcotics	Caution with drugs that alter seizure threshold.

Trimethobenzamide Hydrochloride (Tigan)

Alcohol	Adverse drug reactions reported with alcohol.
CNS agents	Caution with CNS agents in acute febrile illness, encephalitidies, gasterneteritis, dehydration, and electrolyte imbalance.

ANTISPASMODICS

Alosetron Hydrochloride (Lotronex)

Cimetidine	Avoid use of cimetidine.
Clarithromycin	Avoid use with clarithromycin.
CYP450	Inducers and inhibitors of hepatic CYP450 drug metabolizing enzymes may change the clearance of alosetron.
Fluvoxamine	Increase AUC of alosetron; avoid use of fluvoxamine.
Itriconazole	Avoid use with itriconazole.
Ketoconazole	Avoid use with ketoconazole.
Protease Inhibitors	Avoid use with protease inhibitors.
Quinolone antibiotics	Avoid use of quinolone antibiotics.
Telithromycin	Avoid use with telithromycin.
Voriconazole	Avoid use with voriconazole.

Atropine Sulfate/Hyoscyamine Sulfate/Phenobarbital (Donnatal)

Anticoagulants	Phenobarbital may decrease anticoagulant effects; adjust dose.

ANTISPASMODICS *(cont.)*

Chlordiazepoxide Hydrochloride/Methscopolamine (Librax)

Alcohol	Use caution with alcohol.
Anticoagulants	Altered coagulation effects with oral anticoagulants.
CNS depressants	Use caution with CNS depressants.
Psychotropics	Avoid use with other psychotropics; if combination is indicated, use caution especially with MAOIs and phenothiazines.

Dicylomine Hydrochloride (Bentyl)

Amantadine	Potentiated by amantadine.
Antacids	Decreased absorption with antacids.
Antiglaucoma agents	Antagonized the effects of antiglaucoma agents.
Antihistamines	Potentiated by antihistamines.
Antipsychotics	Potentiated by antipsychotics.
Benzodiazepines	Potentiated by benzodiazepines.
Corticosteroid	Do not give with corticosteroid eye drops.
Digoxin	May effect the GI absorption of delayed release digoxin.
MAOIs	Potentiated by MAOIs.
Metoclopramide	Antagonized the effect of metoclopramide.
Narcotics analgesics	Potentiated by narcotic analgesics.
Nitrates	Potentiated by nitrates.
Quinidine	Potentiated by quinidine (Class I antiarrhytmics).
Sympathomimetics	Potentiated by sympathomimetics.
TCAs	Potentiated by TCAs.

Hyoscyamine Sulfate (Levbid, Nulev)

Amantadine	Additive effects with amantadine.
Antimuscarinics	Additive effects with other antimuscarinics.
Antacids	Antacids intefere with absorption; take ac and antacids pc.
Haloperidol	Additive effects with haloperidol.
MAOIs	Additive effects with MAOIs.
Phenothiazines	Additive effects with phenothiazines.
TCAs	Additive effects with TCAs.

Table 16.3: DRUG INTERACTIONS FOR RX GASTROINTESTINAL DRUGS *(cont.)*

ANTIULCER AGENTS

Cimetidine (Tagamet)

Antacids	May interfere with absorption of cimetidine; space dosing.
Chlordiazepoxide	Reduces metabolism of chlordiazepoxide.
Diazepam	Reduces metabolism of diazepam.
Lidocaine	Reduces metabolsim of lidocaine; adverse effects with lidocaine; monitor levels.
Metronidazole	Reduces metabolism of metronidazole.
Nifedipine	Reduces metabolism of nifedipine.
Phenytoin	Reduces metabolism of phenytoin; adverse effects with phenytoin.
Propanolol	Reduces metabolism of propanolol.
Theophylline	Reduces metabolism of theophylline; adverse effects with theophylline; monitor levels.
TCAs	Reduces metabolism of certain TCAs.
Warfarin	Reduces metabolism of warfarin-type anticoagulants.

Esomeprazole Magnesium (Nexium)

Amoxicillin	Increased levels with amoxicillin.
Clarithromycin	Avoid use with clarithromycin; Clarithromycin is contraindicated with pimozide.
Diazepam	Potentiates diazepam.
pH-dependent drugs	May alter absorption of pH-dependent drugs.

Famotidine (Pepcid, Pepcid AC)

Antacids	May give with antacids.

Lansoprazole (Prevacid)

pH-dependent drugs	May alter absorption of pH-dependent drugs.
Sucralfate	Give at least 30 minutes prior to sucralfate.
Theophylline	Theophylline may need adjustment.

Methscopolamine Bromide (Pamine, Pamine Forte)

Antacids	Antacids may intefere with absorption.
Antipsychotics	Additive anticholinergic effects with antipsychotics.
TCAs	Additive anticholinergic effects with TCAs.

Misoprostol (Cytotec)

Antacids	Avoid magnesium-containing antacids to decrease incidence of diarrhea.

Nizatidine (Axid)

Aspirin	May elevate serum salicylate levels with high dose ASA.

ANTISPASMODICS *(cont.)*

Omeprazole (Prilosec)

Clarithromycin	Increased levels with clarithromycin; Increases levels of clarithromycin.
CYP450	Monitor drugs metabolized by CYP450.
Diazepam	May potentiate diazepam.
pH-dependent drugs	May alter absorption of pH-dependent drugs.
Phenytoin	May potentiate phenytoin.
Warfarin	May potentiate warfarin.

Pantoprazole Sodium (Protonix)

pH-dependent drugs	May alter absorption of pH-dependent drugs.

Ranitidine (Zantac)

Anticoagulants	Monitor anticoagulants.
Triazolam	Increases plasma levels of triazolam.

Sucralfate (Carafate)

Aluminium	Additive aluminum absorption with aluminum-containing products.
Antacids	Antacids should not be taken within 1/2 hr before or after sucralfate.
Cimetidine	Reduced absorption of cimetidine.
Digoxin	Reduced absorption of digoxin.
Fluoroquinolones	Reduced absorption of fluoroquinolones.
Ketoconazole	Reduced absorption with ketoconazole.
Levothyroxine	Reduced absorption with levothyroxine.
Phenytoin	Reduced absorption with phenytoin.
Quinidine	Reduced absorption with quinidine.
Ranitidine	Reduced absorption with ranitidine.
Sucralfate	Dose concomitant drugs 2 hrs before sucralfate.
Tetracycline	Reduced absorption with tetracycline.
Theophylline	Reduced absorption with theophylline.
Warfarin	Monitor warfarin.

COLORECTAL AGENTS

Balasalazide Disodium (Colazal)

Oral antibiotics	May interfere with the release of mesalamine in the colon.

Table 16.3: DRUG INTERACTIONS FOR RX GASTROINTESTINAL DRUGS *(cont.)*

COLORECTAL AGENTS *(cont.)*

Hydrocortisone Acetate (Cortifoam)

Aminoglutethimide	Caution with aminoglutethimide.
Amphotericin B	Risk of hypokalemia with amphotericin B injection.
Anticholinesterase agents	Withdraw anticholinesterase agents 24 hrs prior to initiation.
Antidiabetic agents	May increase blood glucose levels; may need to adjust antidiabetic agent.
Aspirin	Caution with aspirin in hypoprothrombinemia; increased risk of GI side effects.
Cholestyramine	Increased clearance with cholestyramine.
Cyclosporine	Cyclosporine may increase activity of both drugs; convulsions reported with concomitant use.
Digitalis glycosides	Risk of hypokalemia with digitalis glycosides.
Estrogens	Decreased clearance or metabolism with estrogens.
Hepatic enzyme inducers	Increased metabolism with hepatic enzyme inducers.
Isoniazid	May decrease isoniazid levels.
Ketoconazole	Decreased clearance or metabolism with ketoconazole.
Immunsuppresive doses	Avoid with immunosupressive doses.
Live vaccines	Avoid live vaccines.
Macrolide antibiotics	Decreased clearance or metabolism with macrolide antibiotics.
Neuromuscular blockers	Caution with neuromuscular blockers.
NSAIDs	Increased risk of GI side effects.
Potassium-depleting agents	Risk of hypokalemia with potassium-depleting agents.
Salicylate	May decrease salicylate levels.
Warfarin	Inhibits response to warfarin; monitor PT/INR.

Olsalazine Sodium (Dipentum)

Warfarin	Increased PT time with warfarin.

Sulfasalazine (Azulfidine)

Digoxin	Reduces absorption digoxin.
Folic acid	Reduces absorption of folic acid.

DIGESTIVE ENZYME

Ursodiol (Actigall, Urso 250, Urso Forte)	
Antacids (aluminum-based)	Decreased absorption with aluminum-based antacids.
Bile acid sequestrants	Decreased absorption with bile acid sequestrants.
Clofibrate	Encourage gallstone formation.
Estrogens	Encourage gallstone formation.
Oral contraceptives	Encourage gallstone formation.

LAXATIVES

Polyethylene Glycol/Potassium Chloride/Sodium Bicarbonate/Sodium Chloride (NuLYTELY)	
Oral medications	Taken within 1 hr of start of administration; may not be absorbed from GI tract.

Polyethylene Glycol/Potassium Chloride/Sodium Bicarbonate/Sodium Chloride/Sodium Sulfate (Colyte)	
Oral medications	Taken within 1 hr of start of administration; may not be absorbed from GI tract.

Polyethylene Glycol/Potassium Chloride/Sodium Bicarbonate/Sodium Chloride/Sodium Sulfate (GoLYTELY)	
Oral medications	Taken within 1 hr of start of administration; may not be absorbed from GI tract.

PANCREATIC ENZYME SUPPLEMENT

Amylase/Lipase/Protease (Creon 5, Creon 10, Creon 10)	
Food with pH >5.5	Do not add capsule contents to food with pH >5.5.

Table 16.4: DRUG INTERACTIONS FOR OTC GASTROINTESTINAL DRUGS

Activated Charcoal (Charcoal Plus DS, EZ-Char, Actidose-Aqua, Kerr Insta-Char, Charcoal Plus DS)

Acarbose	Reduced effects of acarbose.
Carbamazepine	Decreased carbamazepine effectiveness.
Digoxin	Decreased digoxin effectiveness.
Furosemide	Decreased furosemide effectiveness.
Leflunomide	Reduced leflunomide efficacy.
Miglitol	Reduced effectiveness of miglitol.
Mycophenolate	Reduced exposure of mycophenolic acid (MPA), the active metabolite of mycophenolate mofetil.
Olanzapine	Decreased bioavailability of olanzapine.

Activated Charcoal/Simethicone (Bicarsim, Bicarsim Forte, Flatulex, Flatulex Max)

Acarbose	Reduced effects of acarbose.
Carbamazepine	Decreased carbamazepine effectiveness.
Digoxin	Decreased digoxin effectiveness.
Furosemide	Decreased furosemide effectiveness.
Leflunomide	Reduced leflunomide efficacy.
Miglitol	Reduced effectiveness of miglitol.
Mycophenolate	Reduced exposure of mycophenolic acid (MPA), the active metabolite of mycophenolate mofetil.
Olanzapine	Decreased bioavailability of olanzapine.

Activated Charcoal/Sorbitol (Actidose w/Sorbitol)

Acarbose	Reduced effects of acarbose.
Carbamazepine	Decreased carbamazepine effectiveness.
Digoxin	Decreased digoxin effectiveness.
Furosemide	Decreased furosemide effectiveness.
Leflunomide	Reduced leflunomide efficacy.
Miglitol	Reduced effectiveness of miglitol.
Mycophenolate	Reduced exposure of mycophenolic acid (MPA), the active metabolite of mycophenolate mofetil.
Olanzapine	Decreased bioavailability of olanzapine.

Aluminum Hydroxide (Alternagel)

Alendronate	Decreased alendronate absorption.
Allopurnol	Decreased allopurinol effectiveness.
Aluminum	Increased risk of aluminum toxicity.

Aluminum Hydroxide (Alternagel) *(cont.)*

Ascorbic acid	Aluminum toxicity (personality changes, seizures, coma) may occur.
Aspirin	Decreased salicylate effectiveness.
Atazanavir	Reduced plasma concentrations of atazanavir.
Atenolol	Reduced effectiveness of atenolol.
Ateviridine	Decreased atevirdine absorption.
Azithromycin	Decreased azithromycin effectiveness.
Bismuth subcitrate	Decreased bismuth subcitrate efficacy.
Cefdinir	Decreased cefdinir efficacy.
Cefditoren	Decreased cefditoren effectiveness.
Cefpodoxime	Decreased cefpodoxime effectiveness.
Chlorpromazine	Decreased phenothiazine effectiveness.
Cholecalciferol	Aluminum toxicity (personality changes, seizures, coma) may occur.
Cinoxacin	Decreased cinoxacin effectiveness.
Ciprofloxacin	Decreased ciprofloxacin effectiveness.
Citric acid	Aluminum toxicity (encephalopathy) may occur.
Clofazimine	Decreased clofazimine plasma concentrations.
Deferasirox	Decreased deferasirox effectiveness.
Delaviridine	Decreased delavirdine bioavailability.
Didanosine	An increased risk of adverse effects from the antacid.
Digoxin	Decreased digoxin levels.
Doxycycline	Decreased effectiveness of tetracyclines.
Enoxacin	Decreased enoxacin efficacy.
Ethambutol	Decreased ethambutol serum concentrations.
Etidronate	Decreased etidronate absorption.
Fexofenadine	Decreased fexofenadine efficacy.
Gemifloxacin	Decreased gemifloxacin effectiveness.
Hyoscyamine	Decreased hyoscyamine efficacy.
Ibandronate	Decreased ibandronate effectiveness.
Iron	Decreased iron effectiveness.
Isoniazid	Decreased isoniazid effectiveness.
Itraconazole	Loss of itraconazole efficacy.
Ketoconazole	Decreased ketoconazole effectiveness.
Levofloxacin	Decreased levofloxacin effectiveness.

Table 16.4: DRUG INTERACTIONS FOR OTC GASTROINTESTINAL DRUGS *(cont.)*

Aluminum Hydroxide (Alternagel) *(cont.)*

Levothyroxine	Decreased levothyroxine absorption.
Lomefloxacin	Decreased lomefloxacin effectiveness.
Methenamine	Decreased methenamine effectiveness.
Minocycline	Decreased effectiveness of tetracyclines.
Moxifloxacin	Decreased moxifloxacin effectiveness.
Mycophenolate	Decreased mycophenolate mofetil efficacy.
Nalidixic acid	Decreased nalidixic acid effectiveness.
Norfloxacin	Decreased norfloxacin efficacy.
Ofloxacin	Decreased ofloxacin efficacy.
Pefloxacin	Decreased pefloxacin effectiveness.
Polystyrene sulfonate	Increased risk of metabolic alkalosis.
Potassium phosphate	Reduced phosphate absorption.
Propanolol	Decreased propranolol bioavailability.
Qunidine	Quinidine toxicity (ventricular arrhythmias, hypotension, exacerbation of heart failure) may occur.
Risedronate	Decreased risedronate absorption.
Rosuvastatin	Decreased rosuvastatin effectiveness.
Sodium phosphate	Reduced phosphate absorption.
Sotalol	Decreased sotalol serum concentrations and efficacy.
Sparfloxacin	Decreased sparfloxacin efficacy.
Sucralfate	Decreased sucralfate effectiveness.
Tacrolimus	Increased tacrolimus exposure.
Temafloxacin	Decreased temafloxacin effectiveness.
Tetracyclines	Decreased effectiveness of tetracyclines.
Ticlodipine	Decreased ticlopidine effectiveness.
Tiludronate	Decreased tiludronate absorption.
Trovafloxacin	Reduced efficacy of trovafloxacin.
Zalcatibine	Reduced zalcitabine efficacy.

Aluminum Hydroxide/Magnesium Carbonate (Gaviscon, Gaviscon ES)

Alendronate	Decreased alendronate absorption.
Allopurnol	Decreased allopurinol effectiveness.

Aluminum Hydroxide/Magnesium Carbonate (Gaviscon, Gaviscon ES) *(cont.)*

Aluminum	Increased risk of aluminum toxicity.
Ascorbic Acid	Aluminum toxicity (personality changes, seizures, coma) may occur.
Aspirin	Decreased salicylate effectiveness.
Atazanavir	Reduced plasma concentrations of atazanavir.
Atenolol	Reduced effectiveness of atenolol.
Ateviridine	Decreased atevirdine absorption.
Azithromycin	Decreased azithromycin effectiveness.
Bismuth subcitrate	Decreased bismuth subcitrate efficacy.
Cefdinir	Decreased cefdinir efficacy.
Cefditoren	Decreased cefditoren effectiveness.
Cefpodoxime	Decreased cefpodoxime effectiveness.
Chlorpromazine	Decreased phenothiazine effectiveness.
Cholecalciferol	Aluminum toxicity (personality changes, seizures, coma) may occur.
Cinoxacin	Decreased cinoxacin effectiveness.
Ciprofloxacin	Decreased ciprofloxacin effectiveness.
Citric acid	Aluminum toxicity (encephalopathy) may occur.
Clofazimine	Decreased clofazimine plasma concentrations.
Deferasirox	Decreased deferasirox effectiveness.
Delaviridine	Decreased delavirdine bioavailability.
Didanosine	Increased risk of adverse effects from the antacid.
Digoxin	Decreased digoxin levels.
Doxycycline	Decreased effectiveness of tetracyclines.
Enoxacin	Decreased enoxacin efficacy.
Ethambutol	Decreased ethambutol serum concentrations.
Etidronate	Decreased etidronate absorption.
Fexofenadine	Decreased fexofenadine efficacy.
Gemifloxacin	Decreased gemifloxacin effectiveness.
Hyoscyamine	Decreased hyoscyamine efficacy.
Ibandronate	Decreased ibandronate effectiveness.
Iron	Decreased iron effectiveness.
Isoniazid	Decreased isoniazid effectiveness.
Itraconazole	Loss of itraconazole efficacy.

Table 16.4: DRUG INTERACTIONS FOR OTC GASTROINTESTINAL DRUGS *(cont.)*

Aluminum Hydroxide/Magnesium Carbonate (Gaviscon, Gaviscon ES) *(cont.)*

Ketoconazole	Decreased ketoconazole effectiveness.
Levofloxacin	Decreased levofloxacin effectiveness.
Levothyroxine	Decreased levothyroxine absorption.
Lomefloxacin	Decreased lomefloxacin effectiveness.
Methenamine	Decreased methenamine effectiveness.
Minocycline	Decreased effectiveness of tetracyclines.
Moxifloxacin	Decreased moxifloxacin effectiveness.
Mycophenolate	Decreased mycophenolate mofetil efficacy.
Nalidixic acid	Decreased nalidixic acid effectiveness.
Norfloxacin	Decreased norfloxacin efficacy.
Ofloxacin	Decreased ofloxacin efficacy.
Pefloxacin	Decreased pefloxacin effectiveness.
Polystyrene sulfonate	Increased risk of metabolic alkalosis.
Potassium phosphate	Reduced phosphate absorption.
Propanolol	Decreased propranolol bioavailability.
Qunidine	Quinidine toxicity (ventricular arrhythmias, hypotension, exacerbation of heart failure) may occur.
Risedronate	Decreased risedronate absorption.
Rosuvastatin	Decreased rosuvastatin effectiveness.
Sodium phosphate	Reduced phosphate absorption.
Sotalol	Decreased sotalol serum concentrations and efficacy.
Sparfloxacin	Decreased sparfloxacin efficacy.
Sucralfate	Decreased sucralfate effectiveness.
Tacrolimus	Increased tacrolimus exposure.
Temafloxacin	Decreased temafloxacin effectiveness.
Tetracyclines	Decreased effectiveness of tetracyclines.
Ticlodipine	Decreased ticlopidine effectiveness.
Tiludronate	Decreased tiludronate absorption.
Trovafloxacin	Reduced efficacy of trovafloxacin.
Zalcatibine	Reduced zalcitabine efficacy.

Aluminum Hydroxide/Magnesium Hydroxide (Maalox, Maalox TC, Alamag)

Alendronate	Decreased alendronate absorption.

Aluminum Hydroxide/Magnesium Hydroxide (Maalox, Maalox TC, Alamag) *(cont.)*

Allopurnol	Decreased allopurinol effectiveness.
Aluminum	Increased risk of aluminum toxicity.
Ascorbic Acid	Aluminum toxicity (personality changes, seizures, coma) may occur.
Aspirin	Decreased salicylate effectiveness.
Atazanavir	Reduced plasma concentrations of atazanavir.
Atenolol	Reduced effectiveness of atenolol.
Ateviridine	Decreased atevirdine absorption.
Azithromycin	Decreased azithromycin effectiveness.
Bismuth subcitrate	Decreased bismuth subcitrate efficacy.
Cefdinir	Decreased cefdinir efficacy.
Cefditoren	Decreased cefditoren effectiveness.
Cefpodoxime	Decreased cefpodoxime effectiveness.
Chlorpromazine	Decreased phenothiazine effectiveness.
Cholecalciferol	Aluminum toxicity (personality changes, seizures, coma) may occur.
Cinoxacin	Decreased cinoxacin effectiveness.
Ciprofloxacin	Decreased ciprofloxacin effectiveness.
Citric acid	Aluminum toxicity (encephalopathy) may occur.
Clofazimine	Decreased clofazimine plasma concentrations.
Deferasirox	Decreased deferasirox effectiveness.
Delaviridine	Decreased delavirdine bioavailability.
Didanosine	An increased risk of adverse effects from the antacid.
Digoxin	Decreased digoxin levels.
Doxycycline	Decreased effectiveness of tetracyclines.
Enoxacin	Decreased enoxacin efficacy.
Ethambutol	Decreased ethambutol serum concentrations.
Etidronate	Decreased etidronate absorption.
Fexofenadine	Decreased fexofenadine efficacy.
Gemifloxacin	Decreased gemifloxacin effectiveness.
Hyoscyamine	Decreased hyoscyamine efficacy.
Ibandronate	Decreased ibandronate effectiveness.
Iron	Decreased iron effectiveness.
Isoniazid	Decreased isoniazid effectiveness.
Itraconazole	Loss of itraconazole efficacy.

Table 16.4: DRUG INTERACTIONS FOR OTC GASTROINTESTINAL DRUGS *(cont.)*

Aluminum Hydroxide/Magnesium Hydroxide (Maalox, Maalox TC, Alamag) *(cont.)*

Ketoconazole	Decreased ketoconazole effectiveness.
Levofloxacin	Decreased levofloxacin effectiveness.
Levothyroxine	Decreased levothyroxine absorption.
Lomefloxacin	Decreased lomefloxacin effectiveness.
Methenamine	Decreased methenamine effectiveness.
Minocycline	Decreased effectiveness of tetracyclines.
Moxifloxacin	Decreased moxifloxacin effectiveness.
Mycophenolate	Decreased mycophenolate mofetil efficacy.
Nalidixic acid	Decreased nalidixic acid effectiveness.
Norfloxacin	Decreased norfloxacin efficacy.
Ofloxacin	Decreased ofloxacin efficacy.
Pefloxacin	Decreased pefloxacin effectiveness.
Polystyrene sulfonate	Increased risk of metabolic alkalosis.
Potassium phosphate	Reduced phosphate absorption.
Propanolol	Decreased propranolol bioavailability.
Qunidine	Quinidine toxicity (ventricular arrhythmias, hypotension, exacerbation of heart failure) may occur.
Risedronate	Decreased risedronate absorption.
Rosuvastatin	Decreased rosuvastatin effectiveness.
Sodium phosphate	Reduced phosphate absorption.
Sotalol	Decreased sotalol serum concentrations and efficacy.
Sparfloxacin	Decreased sparfloxacin efficacy.
Sucralfate	Decreased sucralfate effectiveness.
Tacrolimus	Increased tacrolimus exposure.
Temafloxacin	Decreased temafloxacin effectiveness.
Tetracyclines	Decreased effectiveness of tetracyclines.
Ticlodipine	Decreased ticlopidine effectiveness.
Tiludronate	Decreased tiludronate absorption.
Trovafloxacin	Reduced efficacy of trovafloxacin.
Zalcatibine	Reduced zalcitabine efficacy.

Aluminum Hydroxide/Magnesium Hydroxide/Simethicone (Mylanta, Maalox, DI-Gel, Gelusil)

Alendronate	Decreased alendronate absorption.
Allopurnol	Decreased allopurinol effectiveness.
Aluminum	Increased risk of aluminum toxicity.
Ascorbic acid	Aluminum toxicity (personality changes, seizures, coma) may occur.
Aspirin	Decreased salicylate effectiveness.
Atazanavir	Reduced plasma concentrations of atazanavir.
Atenolol	Reduced effectiveness of atenolol.
Ateviridine	Decreased atevirdine absorption.
Azithromycin	Decreased azithromycin effectiveness.
Bismuth subcitrate	Decreased bismuth subcitrate efficacy.
Cefdinir	Decreased cefdinir efficacy.
Cefditoren	Decreased cefditoren effectiveness.
Cefpodoxime	Decreased cefpodoxime effectiveness.
Chlorpromazine	Decreased phenothiazine effectiveness.
Cholecalciferol	Aluminum toxicity (personality changes, seizures, coma) may occur.
Cinoxacin	Decreased cinoxacin effectiveness.
Ciprofloxacin	Decreased ciprofloxacin effectiveness.
Citric acid	Aluminum toxicity (encephalopathy) may occur.
Clofazimine	Decreased clofazimine plasma concentrations.
Deferasirox	Decreased deferasirox effectiveness.
Delaviridine	Decreased delavirdine bioavailability.
Didanosine	An increased risk of adverse effects from the antacid.
Digoxin	Decreased digoxin levels.
Doxycycline	Decreased effectiveness of tetracyclines.
Enoxacin	Decreased enoxacin efficacy.
Ethambutol	Decreased ethambutol serum concentrations.
Etidronate	Decreased etidronate absorption.
Fexofenadine	Decreased fexofenadine efficacy.
Gemifloxacin	Decreased gemifloxacin effectiveness.
Hyoscyamine	Decreased hyoscyamine efficacy.
Ibandronate	Decreased ibandronate effectiveness.

Table 16.4: DRUG INTERACTIONS FOR OTC GASTROINTESTINAL DRUGS *(cont.)*

Aluminum Hydroxide/Magnesium Hydroxide/Simethicone (Mylanta, Maalox, DI-Gel, Gelusil)*(cont.)*

Iron	Decreased iron effectiveness.
Isoniazid	Decreased isoniazid effectiveness.
Itraconazole	Loss of itraconazole efficacy.
Ketoconazole	Decreased ketoconazole effectiveness.
Levofloxacin	Decreased levofloxacin effectiveness.
Levothyroxine	Decreased levothyroxine absorption.
Lomefloxacin	Decreased lomefloxacin effectiveness.
Methenamine	Decreased methenamine effectiveness.
Minocycline	Decreased effectiveness of tetracyclines.
Moxifloxacin	Decreased moxifloxacin effectiveness.
Mycophenolate	Decreased mycophenolate mofetil efficacy.
Nalidixic acid	Decreased nalidixic acid effectiveness.
Norfloxacin	Decreased norfloxacin efficacy.
Ofloxacin	Decreased ofloxacin efficacy.
Pefloxacin	Decreased pefloxacin effectiveness.
Polystyrene sulfonate	Increased risk of metabolic alkalosis.
Potassium phosphate	Reduced phosphate absorption.
Propanolol	Decreased propranolol bioavailability.
Qunidine	Quinidine toxicity (ventricular arrhythmias, hypotension, exacerbation of heart failure) may occur.
Risedronate	Decreased risedronate absorption.
Rosuvastatin	Decreased rosuvastatin effectiveness.
Sodium phosphate	Reduced phosphate absorption.
Sotalol	Decreased sotalol serum concentrations and efficacy.
Sparfloxacin	Decreased sparfloxacin efficacy.
Sucralfate	Decreased sucralfate effectiveness.
Tacrolimus	Increased tacrolimus exposure.
Temafloxacin	Decreased temafloxacin effectiveness.
Tetracyclines	Decreased effectiveness of tetracyclines.
Ticlodipine	Decreased ticlopidine effectiveness.
Tiludronate	Decreased tiludronate absorption.

Aluminum Hydroxide/Magnesium Hydroxide/Simethicone (Mylanta, Maalox, DI-Gel, Gelusil) *(cont.)*

Trovafloxacin	Reduced efficacy of trovafloxacin.
Zalcatibine	Reduced zalcitabine efficacy.

Bisacodyl (Dulcolax, Correctol, Fleet Biscadoyl, Modane, Dulcolax, Fleet Biscodyl, Fleet Biscodyl)

Aluminum	Decreased effectiveness of bisacodyl.
Calcium	Decreased effectiveness of bisacodyl.
Cimetidine	Decreased effectiveness of bisacodyl.
Dihydroxyaluminum aminoacetate	Decreased effectiveness of bisacodyl.
Dihydroxyaluminum sodium carbonate	Decreased effectiveness of bisacodyl.
Famotidine	Decreased effectiveness of bisacodyl.
Magaldrate	Decreased effectiveness of bisacodyl.
Magnesium	Decreased effectiveness of bisacodyl.
Nizatidine	Decreased effectiveness of bisacodyl.

Bisacodyl/Sodium Phosphate (Fleet Prep Kit 1, Fleet Prep Kit 2, Fleet Prep Kit 3)

Aluminum	Decreased effectiveness of bisacodyl; decreased phosphate absorption.
Calcium	Decreased effectiveness of bisacodyl; decreased phosphate absorption.
Cimetidine	Decreased effectiveness of bisacodyl.
Colestipol	Decreased phosphate absorption.
Dihydroxyaluminum aminoacetate	Decreased effectiveness of bisacodyl.
Dihydroxyaluminum sodium carbonate	Decreased effectiveness of bisacodyl.
Famotidine	Decreased effectiveness of bisacodyl.
Magaldrate	Decreased effectiveness of bisacodyl; decreased phosphate absorption.
Magnesium	Decreased effectiveness of bisacodyl; decreased phosphate absorption.
Nizatidine	Decreased effectiveness of bisacodyl.

Bismuth Subsalicylate (Pepto Bismol, Kaopectate)

Aluminum	Decreased bismuth subcitrate efficacy.
Calcium	Decreased bismuth subcitrate efficacy.
Doxycycline	Decreased doxycycline effectiveness.

Table 16.4: DRUG INTERACTIONS FOR OTC GASTROINTESTINAL DRUGS (cont.)

Bismuth Subsalicylate (Pepto Bismol, Kaopectate) (cont.)

Magaldrate	Decreased bismuth subcitrate efficacy.
Magnesium	Decreased bismuth subcitrate efficacy.
Methacycline	Decreased methacycline effectiveness.
Methotrexate	Methotrexate toxicity (hemorrhage, anemia, septicemia) may occur.
Minocycline	Decreased effectiveness of tetracyclines.
Probenecid	Decreased uricosuric effects with probenecid.
Sulfinpyrazone	Decreased uricosuric effects with sulfinpyrazone.
Tamarind	Increased salicylate toxicity.
Tetracyclines	Decreased effectiveness of tetracyclines.
Warfarin	An increased risk of bleeding with warfarin.

Calcium Carbonate (Alka-Minta, Chooz, Mylanta Children's, Rolaids, Titralac, Tums, Tums E-X, Tums Ultra)

Alendronate	Decreased alendronate absorption.
Aspirin	Decreased salicylate effectiveness.
Atazanavir	Reduced plasma concentrations of atazanavir.
Atenolol	Reduced effectiveness of atenolol.
Azithromycin	Decreased azithromycin effectiveness.
Bemetizide	Milk-alkali syndrome (hypercalcemia, metabolic alkalosis, renal failure) may occur.
Benzthiazide	Milk-alkali syndrome (hypercalcemia, metabolic alkalosis, renal failure) may occur.
Bismuth subcitrate	Decreased bismuth subcitrate efficacy.
Buthiazide	Milk-alkali syndrome (hypercalcemia, metabolic alkalosis, renal failure) may occur.
Cefpodoxime	Decreased cefpodoxime effectiveness.
Chlorothiazide	Milk-alkali syndrome (hypercalcemia, metabolic alkalosis, renal failure) may occur.
Chlorthalidone	Milk-alkali syndrome (hypercalcemia, metabolic alkalosis, renal failure) may occur.
Ciprofloxacin	Decreased ciprofloxacin effectiveness.
Clopamide	Milk-alkali syndrome (hypercalcemia, metabolic alkalosis, renal failure) may occur.
Doxycycline	Decreased effectiveness of tetracyclines.
Enoxacin	Decreased enoxacin efficacy.
Gemifloxacin	Decreased gemifloxacin effectiveness.
Hydrochlorothiazide	Milk-alkali syndrome (hypercalcemia, metabolic alkalosis, renal failure) may occur.
Hyoscyamine	Decreased hyoscyamine efficacy.
Ibandronate	Decreased ibandronate effectiveness.

Calcium Carbonate (Alka-Minta, Chooz, Mylanta Children's, Rolaids, Titralac, Tums, Tums E-X, Tums Ultra) *(cont.)*

Indapamide	Milk-alkali syndrome (hypercalcemia, metabolic alkalosis, renal failure) may occur.
Iron	Decreased iron effectiveness.
Itraconazole	Loss of itraconazole efficacy.
Ketoconazole	Decreased ketoconazole effectiveness.
Levofloxacin	Decreased levofloxacin effectiveness.
Levothyroxine	Decreased levothyroxine absorption.
Lomefloxacin	Decreased lomefloxacin effectiveness.
Metolazone	Milk-alkali syndrome (hypercalcemia, metabolic alkalosis, renal failure) may occur.
Minocycline	Decreased effectiveness of tetracyclines.
Moxifloxacin	Decreased moxifloxacin effectiveness.
Nalidixic acid	Decreased nalidixic acid effectiveness.
Norfloxacin	Decreased norfloxacin efficacy.
Ofloxacin	Decreased ofloxacin efficacy.
Polystyrene sulfonate	Increased risk of metabolic alkalosis.
Potassium phosphate	Reduced phosphate absorption.
Sodium phosphate	Reduced phosphate absorption.
Sparfloxacin	Decreased sparfloxacin efficacy.
Sucralfate	Decreased sucralfate effectiveness.
Tetracyclines	Decreased effectiveness of tetracyclines.
Thiazide	Thiazide/thiazide-like diuretics may cause milk-alkali syndrome (hypercalcemia, metabolic alkalosis, renal failure) may occur.
Ticlodipine	Decreased ticlopidine effectiveness.
Zalcitabine	Reduced zalcitabine efficacy.

Calcium Polycarbophil (Equalactin, Fiberall, Fibercon, Konsyl Fiber, Perdiem)

Alendronate	Decreased alendronate absorption.
Aspirin	Decreased salicylate effectiveness.
Atazanavir	Reduced plasma concentrations of atazanavir.
Atenolol	Reduced effectiveness of atenolol.
Azithromycin	Decreased azithromycin effectiveness.
Bemetizide	Milk-alkali syndrome (hypercalcemia, metabolic alkalosis, renal failure) may occur.
Benzthiazide	Milk-alkali syndrome (hypercalcemia, metabolic alkalosis, renal failure) may occur.

Table 16.4: DRUG INTERACTIONS FOR OTC GASTROINTESTINAL DRUGS *(cont.)*

Calcium Polycarbophil (Equalactin, Fiberall, Fibercon, Konsyl Fiber, Perdiem) *(cont.)*

Bismuth subcitrate	Decreased bismuth subcitrate efficacy.
Buthiazide	Milk-alkali syndrome (hypercalcemia, metabolic alkalosis, renal failure) may occur.
Cefpodoxime	Decreased cefpodoxime effectiveness.
Chlorothiazide	Milk-alkali syndrome (hypercalcemia, metabolic alkalosis, renal failure) may occur.
Chlorthalidone	Milk-alkali syndrome (hypercalcemia, metabolic alkalosis, renal failure) may occur.
Ciprofloxacin	Decreased ciprofloxacin effectiveness.
Clopamide	Milk-alkali syndrome (hypercalcemia, metabolic alkalosis, renal failure) may occur.
Doxycycline	Decreased effectiveness of tetracyclines.
Enoxacin	Decreased enoxacin efficacy.
Gemifloxacin	Decreased gemifloxacin effectiveness.
Hydrochlorothiazide	Milk-alkali syndrome (hypercalcemia, metabolic alkalosis, renal failure) may occur.
Hyoscyamine	Decreased hyoscyamine efficacy.
Ibandronate	Decreased ibandronate effectiveness
Indapamide	Milk-alkali syndrome (hypercalcemia, metabolic alkalosis, renal failure) may occur.
Iron	Decreased iron effectiveness.
Itraconazole	Loss of itraconazole efficacy.
Ketoconazole	Decreased ketoconazole effectiveness.
Levofloxacin	Decreased levofloxacin effectiveness.
Levothyroxine	Decreased levothyroxine absorption.
Lomefloxacin	Decreased lomefloxacin effectiveness.
Metolazone	Milk-alkali syndrome (hypercalcemia, metabolic alkalosis, renal failure) may occur.
Minocycline	Decreased effectiveness of tetracyclines.
Moxifloxacin	Decreased moxifloxacin effectiveness.
Nalidixic acid	Decreased nalidixic acid effectiveness.
Norfloxacin	Decreased norfloxacin efficacy.
Ofloxacin	Decreased ofloxacin efficacy.
Polystyrene sulfonate	Increased risk of metabolic alkalosis.
Potassium phosphate	Reduced phosphate absorption.
Sodium phosphate	Reduced phosphate absorption.
Sparfloxacin	Decreased sparfloxacin efficacy.

Calcium Polycarbophil (Equalactin, Fiberall, Fibercon, Konsyl Fiber, Perdiem) *(cont.)*	
Sucralfate	Decreased sucralfate effectiveness.
Tetracyclines	Decreased effectiveness of tetracyclines.
Thiazide	Thiazide/thiazide-like diuretics may cause milk-alkali syndrome (hypercalcemia, metabolic alkalosis, renal failure) may occur.
Ticlodipine	Decreased ticlopidine effectiveness.
Zalcitabine	Reduced zalcitabine efficacy.

Cascara Sagrada	
Digoxin	Associated with potassium loss.

Castor Oil	
Droperidol	Increased risk of cardiotoxicity (QT prolongation, torsades de pointes, cardiac arrest).
Levomethadyl	Increased risk of QT prolongation.
Licorice	Increased risk of hypokalemia.

Citric Acid/Potassium Bicarbonate (Alka-Seltzer)	
Aluminium	Aluminum toxicity (encephalopathy) may occur.
Magaldrate	Aluminum toxicity (encephalopathy) may occur.
Trovafloxacin	Reduced efficacy of trovafloxacin.

Dimenhydrinate (Dramamine, Triptone)	
Procarbazine	CNS depression may occur.

Docusate Sodium (Colace, Fleet Sof-Lax, Ex-Lax Stool Softener, Phillip's Stool Softener Laxative)	
Droperidol	Increased risk of cardiotoxicity (QT prolongation, torsades de pointes, cardiac arrest).
Levomethadyl	Increased risk of QT prolongation.
Licorice	Increased risk of hypokalemia.
Mineral oil	Inflammation of intestinal mucosa, liver, spleen, and lymph nodes.

Docusate Sodium/Sennosides A and B (Peri-Colace, Senokot S)	
Droperidol	Increased risk of cardiotoxicity (QT prolongation, torsades de pointes, cardiac arrest).
Levomethadyl	Increased risk of QT prolongation.
Licorice	Increased risk of hypokalemia.
Mineral oil	Inflammation of intestinal mucosa, liver, spleen, and lymph nodes.

Glycerin (Fleet Glycerin, Colace, Colace Infant/Child)	
Arsenic trioxide	Increased risk of QT prolongation.
Licorice	Increased risk of hypokalemia and/or reduced effectiveness of the diuretic.

Table 16.4: DRUG INTERACTIONS FOR OTC GASTROINTESTINAL DRUGS *(cont.)*

Loperamide (Imodium A-D)

St. John's wort	Delirium with symptoms of confusion, agitation, and disorientation.
Valerian	Delirium with symptoms of confusion, agitation, and disorientation.

Magnesium Hydroxide (Phillips Milk of Magnesia)

Alendronate	Decreased alendronate absorption.
Allopurnol	Decreased allopurinol effectiveness.
Aluminum	Increased risk of aluminum toxicity.
Ascorbic Acid	Aluminum toxicity (personality changes, seizures, coma) may occur.
Aspirin	Decreased salicylate effectiveness.
Atazanavir	Reduced plasma concentrations of atazanavir.
Atenolol	Reduced effectiveness of atenolol.
Ateviridine	Decreased atevirdine absorption.
Azithromycin	Decreased azithromycin effectiveness.
Bismuth subcitrate	Decreased bismuth subcitrate efficacy.
Cefdinir	Decreased cefdinir efficacy.
Cefditoren	Decreased cefditoren effectiveness.
Cefpodoxime	Decreased cefpodoxime effectiveness.
Chlorpromazine	Decreased phenothiazine effectiveness.
Cholecalciferol	Aluminum toxicity (personality changes, seizures, coma) may occur.
Cinoxacin	Decreased cinoxacin effectiveness.
Ciprofloxacin	Decreased ciprofloxacin effectiveness.
Citric acid	Aluminum toxicity (encephalopathy) may occur.
Clofazimine	Decreased clofazimine plasma concentrations.
Deferasirox	Decreased deferasirox effectiveness.
Delaviridine	Decreased delavirdine bioavailability.
Didanosine	An increased risk of adverse effects from the antacid.
Digoxin	Decreased digoxin levels.
Doxycycline	Decreased effectiveness of tetracyclines.
Enoxacin	Decreased enoxacin efficacy.
Ethambutol	Decreased ethambutol serum concentrations.
Etidronate	Decreased etidronate absorption.
Fexofenadine	Decreased fexofenadine efficacy.
Gemifloxacin	Decreased gemifloxacin effectiveness.

Magnesium Hydroxide (Phillips Milk of Magnesia) *(cont.)*

Hyoscyamine	Decreased hyoscyamine efficacy.
Ibandronate	Decreased ibandronate effectiveness.
Iron	Decreased iron effectiveness.
Isoniazid	Decreased isoniazid effectiveness.
Itraconazole	Loss of itraconazole efficacy.
Ketoconazole	Decreased ketoconazole effectiveness.
Levofloxacin	Decreased levofloxacin effectiveness.
Levothyroxine	Decreased levothyroxine absorption.
Lomefloxacin	Decreased lomefloxacin effectiveness.
Methenamine	Decreased methenamine effectiveness.
Minocycline	Decreased effectiveness of tetracyclines.
Moxifloxacin	Decreased moxifloxacin effectiveness.
Mycophenolate	Decreased mycophenolate mofetil efficacy.
Nalidixic acid	Decreased nalidixic acid effectiveness.
Norfloxacin	Decreased norfloxacin efficacy.
Ofloxacin	Decreased ofloxacin efficacy.
Pefloxacin	Decreased pefloxacin effectiveness.
Polystyrene sulfonate	Increased risk of metabolic alkalosis.
Potassium phosphate	Reduced phosphate absorption.
Propanolol	Decreased propranolol bioavailability.
Qunidine	Quinidine toxicity (ventricular arrhythmias, hypotension, exacerbation of heart failure) may occur.
Risedronate	Decreased risedronate absorption.
Rosuvastatin	Decreased rosuvastatin effectiveness.
Sodium phosphate	Reduced phosphate absorption.
Sotalol	Decreased sotalol serum concentrations and efficacy.
Sparfloxacin	Decreased sparfloxacin efficacy.
Sucralfate	Decreased sucralfate effectiveness.
Tacrolimus	Increased tacrolimus exposure.
Temafloxacin	Decreased temafloxacin effectiveness.
Tetracyclines	Decreased effectiveness of tetracyclines.

Table 16.4: DRUG INTERACTIONS FOR OTC GASTROINTESTINAL DRUGS *(cont.)*

Magnesium Hydroxide (Phillips Milk of Magnesia) *(cont.)*

Ticlodipine	Decreased ticlopidine effectiveness.
Tiludronate	Decreased tiludronate absorption.
Trovafloxacin	Reduced efficacy of trovafloxacin.
Zalcatibine	Reduced zalcitabine efficacy.

Mineral Oil (Fleet Mineral Oil Enema, Kondremul)

Cholecalciferol	Decreased systemic cholecalciferol (vitamin D) concentrations.
Docusate	Inflammation of intestinal mucosa, liver, spleen, and lymph nodes.

Psyllium (Metamucil, Konsyl-Orange, Fiberall)

Antidiabetic agents	Increased risk of hypoglycemia.
Carbamazepine	Decreased absorption and concentration of carbamazepine.
Lithium	Decreased plasma levels and effectiveness of lithium.

Scopolamine (Transderm Scop, Scopodex, Scopolamine, Scopace)

Alcohol	Increased CNS effects with alcohol.
Anticholinergics	Use with caution with anticholinergics.
Antihistamine	Use with caution with antihistamines.
Muscle relaxants	Use with caution with muscle relaxants.
Sedatives	Increased CNS effects with sedatives.
TCAs	Use with caution with TCAs.
Tranquilizers	Increased CNS effects with tranquilizers.

Chapter 17

Neurological Drugs

Steven Ganzberg, D.M.D., M.S.

Patients who are receiving ongoing treatment of neurological conditions may consult the dentist for oral health care. One of the more common neurological conditions dentists see among these patients is seizure disorders; they also may encounter other conditions such as Parkinson's disease, multiple sclerosis, Alzheimer's disease, myasthenia gravis and other myopathies, spasticity resulting from spinal cord injury, and poststroke syndrome. Long-term medication management is common. The dentist also may prescribe neurological drugs for treatment of orofacial pains of neuropathic origin as well as for primary headache syndromes, such as migraine, cluster and tension-type headaches. The dentist who undertakes treatment of these disorders is presumed to have advanced training or experience in diagnosis and management of these disorders. For general information on neurological drugs, see Tables 17.1 and 17.2.

Clinicians should review the condition and level of disease control (for example, quality of seizure control) of patients who have neurological conditions. If warranted, delay in elective dental treatment may be prudent pending medical consultation. Vital signs, including respiratory status, should be evaluated preoperatively. Adverse effects and precautions/contraindications are provided in Table 17.1.

Anticonvulsant Drugs

Anticonvulsant drugs typically are used to control epilepsy, a convulsive disorder characterized by intermittent excessive discharges of neurons. This dysregulation of neural function is frequently associated with altered or lost consciousness. Seizure disorders have been characterized as generalized, including tonic-clonic (grand mal) seizures, absence, partial, atonic and other forms. Specific anticonvulsant agents have been shown to be superior for some types of seizures.

In orofacial pain management, anticonvulsants are useful in treating trigeminal neuralgia and other posttraumatic trigeminal neuropathies. Carbamazepine, phenytoin, valproic acid and its derivatives, clonazepam, gabapentin and lamotrigine (as well as baclofen, an antispastic) have been reported to be useful. Other newer agents are being investigated in this regard. Certain anticonvulsants have been reported to provide some benefit for migraine headache as well. These medications have numerous side effects, some life-threatening. The dentist prescribing an anticonvulsant drug is presumed to be fully aware of the drug's interactions, adverse effects, monitoring requirements and contraindications.

See Tables 17.1 and 17.2 for basic information on anticonvulsant drugs, both commonly and rarely used (owing to pronounced side effects or inferior efficacy compared to that of newer agents).

Special Dental Considerations

Many commonly prescribed anticonvulsants can cause blood dyscrasias, especially carbamazepine, phenytoin and valproic acid. Stevens-Johnson syndrome can occur with many anticonvulsants, especially lamotrigine. Xerostomia and taste changes are common with many anticonvulsants. Topiramate can cause gingivitis. Consider these agents in the differential diagnosis of oral complaints if signs or symptoms warrant. Valproic acid/divalproex sodium may inhibit platelet aggregation.

Drug Interactions of Dental Interest

Anticonvulsants are frequently sedating. Sedative agents, including opioids, may potentiate this effect. Meperidine, especially when used in multiple doses, can promote seizures in patients with otherwise well-controlled seizure disorders due to accumulation of its metabolite.

Many anticonvulsants induce hepatic microsomal enzymes, causing decreased effectiveness or shorter duration of action of certain concomitantly prescribed drugs. Patients taking anticonvulsants may experience increased metabolism of concomitantly administered corticosteroids, benzodiazepines and barbiturates, a situation that leads to decreased effectiveness of these agents.

Prolonged use of acetaminophen may increase the risk of anticonvulsant-induced hepatic toxicity.

Propoxyphene, erythromycin and clarithromycin may result in decreased metabolism of carbamazepine and increased risk of toxicity.

Fluconazole, ketaconazole and metronidazole may result in decreased metabolism of phenytoin and related hydantoins and increased risk of toxicity. Aspirin may increase plasma concentrations of hydantoins, thereby leading to toxicity. For phenytoin, high doses of lidocaine may have additive cardiac depressant effects.

Laboratory Value Alterations

- With most anticonvulsants (except benzodiazepines, acetazolamide and gabapentin): leukopenia, thrombocytopenia, anemia or pancytopenia is possible.
- With hydantoin derivatives: increase in serum glucose is possible.

- With acetazolamide: increase in serum glucose is possible.
- With valproic acid/divalproex sodium: bleeding time may be increased.

Special Patients
Pediatric patients
Pediatric patients taking hydantoin derivatives are more prone than adults to gingival enlargement, coarsening of facial features (widening of nasal tip, thickening of lips) and facial hair growth.

Pharmacology

Anticonvulsants' primary action is to prevent the spread of abnormal neuronal depolarization from an epileptic focus without completely suppressing that focus. The pharmacological mechanisms of action are varied but generally involve, alone or in combination, stabilization of neuronal sodium channels, increasing γ–aminobutyric acid (GABA) tone, alteration of excitatory amino acid neurotransmission and alteration of calcium ion influx.

Antimyasthenic and Alzheimer's-Type Dementia Drugs

Myasthenia gravis is a progressive disease characterized by a decreased number of functional acetylcholine receptors at the neuromuscular junction, resulting in muscular weakness. Drugs to combat this disease impair acetylcholinesterase, the enzyme that degrades acetylcholine, thus increasing the relative concentration of available acetylcholine.

The Alzheimer's-type dementia drugs are included in this discussion, as they are reversible centrally acting anticholinesterase drugs. Current theories of Alzheimer's disease attribute some of the symptoms to a deficiency in central nervous system (CNS) cholinergic transmission. The use of these drugs for mild to moderate Alzheimer's disease shows variable, but clinically measurable, improvement in some patients.

See Tables 17.1 and 17.2 for basic information on antimyasthenic and Alzheimer's-type dementia drugs.

Special Dental Considerations

The dentist should monitor vital signs, including respiratory status, before beginning dental treatment.

The dentist should evaluate the patient for possible postural hypotension by having him or her sit in the dental chair for a minute or two after being in a supine position and then evaluating him or her when standing.

These drugs may cause decreased salivation.

Drug Interactions of Dental Interest

There may be a reduced rate of metabolism of ester local anesthetics.

High doses of local anesthetic may depress muscle function.

CNS depressants should be used with caution.

Pharmacology

Antimyasthenic drugs increase the amount of acetylcholine present at the neuromuscular junction by inhibition of acetylcholinesterase, the enzyme that degrades acetylcholine. The increase in acetylcholine concentration improves muscular function.

The anti–Alzheimer's-type-dementia drugs increase CNS cholinergic function by inhibiting the cholinesterase enzyme. In some patients, cognitive indices are improved.

Antiparkinsonism Drugs

Parkinson's disease is a CNS disorder characterized by compromised cognition, resting tremor, frequently accompanied by involuntary mouth and tongue movements, rigidity of the limbs and trunk, postural instability and bradykinesia, including loss of facial expressions (masklike facies). Drooling is common owing to swallowing incoordination. A relative imbalance between dopamine, acetylcholine and GABA neurotransmission in the basal ganglia and related areas plays a significant role in the pathophysiology of this disorder. Antiparkinsonism drugs attempt to alter this neurotransmitter imbalance.

See Tables 17.1 and 17.2 for basic information on antiparkinsonism drugs.

Special Dental Considerations

Many of these drugs can cause xerostomia. The dentist should consider them in the differential diagnosis of caries, periodontal disease or oral candidiasis.

If newly diagnosed mouthing movements (involuntary mouth and tongue movements and/or drooling) are seen, which may indicate a serious medication side effect, consultation with the patient's physician may be appropriate.

Selegiline may cause circumoral burning.

The dentist should monitor the patient's vital signs during all dental visits. The dentist should have the patient sit upright in the dental chair for a minute or two after being in a supine position and then monitor the patient when standing.

Sedation or general anesthesia may be required for dental care.

Drug Interactions of Dental Interest

Patients taking levodopa, entacapone, tolcapone and high doses of selegiline may produce an exaggerated hemodynamic response to vasoconstrictors in local anesthetic solutions. The dentist should employ careful aspiration technique with limited vasoconstrictor (0.04 mg epinephrine). Additional vasoconstrictor may be used after monitoring of vital signs.

Dopamine antagonist medications, such as chlorpromazine, metoclopramide, and promethazine, which may be prescribed for nausea, are contraindicated in patients with Parkinson's disease.

Anticholinergics may have an additive oral drying effect and should be used with caution.

In patients taking high doses of selegiline, meperidine (and possibly other opioids) may cause a hyperthermic and possibly hypertensive crisis.

Pharmacology

Parkinson's disease is classically characterized by an imbalance in dopaminergic and cholinergic neurotransmission with contributions involving GABA neurotransmission in the nigrastriatum. Medications that act on dopamine increase its availability either by increasing the concentration of dopamine precursors (levodopa), decreasing the breakdown of precursors (carbidopa), acting as agonists at the dopamine receptor (bromocriptine, pergolide and amantadine) or decreasing the degradation of dopamine by MAO-B (selegiline). The catechol-O-methyl-transferase (COMT) inhibitor drugs entacapone and tolcapone are used with carbidopa-levodopa (Sinemet) to decrease levodopa degradation, thus increasing levodopa plasma levels. Centrally acting anticholinergic drugs, or antihistamines with some degree of anticholinergic activity, decrease cholinergic tone by blocking cholinergic receptors and improving the balance between dopaminergic and cholinergic transmission. GABA agonists, such as clonazepam, and other drugs, such as β-blockers, are also useful in some cases.

Muscle Relaxants and Antispastic Drugs

Muscle relaxants are generally used for acute muscle spasm, including that associated with temporomandibular disorders. The efficacy in chronic muscular disorders is not well established. Patients taking antispastic drugs typically have spinal cord or other CNS lesions. Spasticity can occur in some neurological disorders, such as multiple sclerosis.

Baclofen also may be effective for the treatment of trigeminal neuralgia and other trigeminal neuropathies.

See Tables 17.1 and 17.2 for basic information on antispastic drugs.

Special Dental Considerations

Baclofen and orphenadrine may cause dry mouth. Carisoprodol has some potential for abuse and abstinence syndrome on discontinuation. Carisoprodol should be used for no more than 2 weeks except for those dentists with training and/or experience in chronic pain management. Dantrolene can infrequently cause blood dyscrasias. The dentist should consider these drugs in the differential diagnosis if oral signs and symptoms warrant it. Tizanidine may cause hypotension.

Drug Interactions of Dental Interest

These drugs may be sedating. Sedative agents, including opioids, may potentiate this effect.

Laboratory Value Alterations

- Dantrolene may infrequently cause blood dyscrasias.

Pharmacology

Muscle relaxants do not produce any direct effect on muscle. Muscle-relaxing effects are due to either generalized sedative effects or effects on CNS motor or reflex activity. Orphenadrine citrate may have mild analgesic effects. Antispastic drugs work directly on the muscle by decreasing calcium release from the sarcoplasmic reticulum (dantrolene), in the CNS by increasing GABA tone (baclofen) or by a CNS α_2 agonist effect (tizanidine).

Vascular Headache Suppressants

There are numerous conditions that cause headache or facial pain. The majority of patients who list headache as a primary condition on the medical history will be diagnosed with migraine, tension-type or cluster headache. Numerous drugs are used to treat these conditions. They can be divided into symptomatic medications, abortive medications and preventive medications. Symptomatic medications include analgesics and antiemetics, both of which have been covered in other chapters and will not be listed here. These drugs generally are taken intermittently for severe head pain, as continued use can aggravate headache conditions.

Abortive medications include those drugs which, when taken at onset of or during a severe headache (such as migraine or cluster headache), will arrest the headache process and in some cases the associated symptoms (such as nausea and photophobia). These medications include ergotamines, triptans, isometheptene mucate combinations and, in some cases, phenothiazines. These medications can have adverse cardiovascular consequences, but because they generally are taken on an intermittent basis not associated with a dental visit, they should not be of concern in dental care.

Preventive medications are varied and frequently draw from other drug categories. Various cardiovascular medications—including calcium channel blockers and β-blockers—are used for management of chronic headache. Likewise, most antidepressants and some anticonvulsants have been used for headache prevention.

Neuropathic facial pains, if they respond to medical treatment, are usually treated with anticonvulsant or antidepressant medications. Specific conditions may respond to baclofen, α-blockers or clonidine.

See Tables 17.1 and 17.2 for basic information on vascular headache supressants. A thorough discussion of the pharmacological management of headache and facial pain is beyond the scope of this book. Headache suppressant medications, which have not been covered elsewhere in this text, will be presented.

Special Dental Considerations

Abortive headache medications are used only when needed for moderate-to-severe headache and generally not on the day of a dental appointment. If ergot preparations or a triptan are used within 12-24 hours of a dental procedure, vasoconstrictor precautions similar to those for hypertensive patients should be followed. For preventive medications—for example, antidepressants, anticonvulsants or antihypertensives—the dentist should follow precautions listed for that specific category of drug.

The dentist who undertakes primary treatment of head and face pain is presumed to have established a proper diagnosis and to be fully aware of the interactions, adverse effects and contraindications of headache medications.

Drug Interactions of Dental Interest

Ergot derivatives may have hypertensive effects, in which case vasoconstrictors in local anesthetic solutions should be used cautiously.

For preventive medications, see the appropriate drug category.

Laboratory Value Alterations

- For preventive medications, see the appropriate drug category.

• Methysergide may cause blood dyscrasias and fibrotic disorders.

Pharmacology

Numerous drugs are used for the management of headache and facial pain. The pharmacology reflects the condition that is to be treated. For example, migraine headache is thought to involve abnormal serotonergic transmission. Varied medications, such as antidepressants, ergots and specific antihistamines, alter serotonin neurotransmission and can be effective in the acute or preventive treatment of migraine. Trigeminal neuralgia responds to anticonvulsant medications by decreasing hyperactive neuronal function.

Treatment of headache and facial pain is beyond the scope of this text. For a more complete review of the pharmacological basis of headache and facial pain management, consult appropriate references.

Adverse Effects, Precautions and Contraindications

Table 17.1 presents adverse effects and precautions/contraindications of neurological drugs.

Suggested Readings

Calne DB. Treatment of Parkinson's disease. New Engl J Med 1993;329:1021-7.

Fraser AD. New drugs for the treatment of epilepsy. Clinical Biochem 1996:29(2):97-110.

McQuay H, Carrol D, et al. Anticonvulsant drugs for the management of pain: a systematic review. Br Med J 1995;311(7012):1047-52.

Millard CB, Broomfield CA. Anticholinesterases: medical applications of neuro-chemical principles. J Neurochem 1995;64(5):1909-18.

Saper JR, Siberstein S, et al. Handbook of headache management. Baltimore: Williams & Wilkins; 1993.

The United States Pharmacopeial Convention, Inc. Drug information for the health care professional. 23rd ed. Rockville, Md.: The United States Pharmacopeial Convention, Inc.; 2003.

Table 17.1 PRESCRIBING INFORMATION FOR NEUROLOGICAL AGENTS

NAME	FORM/ STRENGTH	DOSAGE	WARNINGS/PRECAUTIONS & CONTRAINDICATIONS	ADVERSE EFFECTS†
ALZHEIMER'S DRUGS				
Donepezil Hydrochloride (Aricept)	**Sol:** 1mg/mL; **Tab:** 5mg, 10mg; **Tab, Disintegrating:** 5mg, 10mg	**Adults: Initial:** 5mg qhs. **Titrate:** May increase to 10mg after 4-6 weeks.	**W/P:** May exaggerate succinylcho-line-type muscle relaxation during anesthesia. May have vagotonic effects on sinoatrial and atrioventricular node; may cause bradycardia or heart block. May increase gastric acid secretion; monitor for GI bleeding. May cause bladder outflow obstruction or sei-zures. Caution with asthma or COPD. **Contra:** Hypersensitivity to piperidine derivatives. **P/N:** Category C, not for use in nursing.	Nausea, diarrhea, insomnia, vomiting, muscle cramps, fatigue, anorexia, dizziness, depression, somnolence, weight decrease.
Ergoloid Mesylates (Gerimal, Hydergine)	**Tab:** 1mg; **Tab, Sublingual:** 1mg	**Adults: Usual:** 1mg tid.	**W/P:** Since symptoms are of unknown etiology, careful diagnosis should be attempted before prescribing. **Contra:** Acute or chronic psychosis. **P/N:** Safety in pregnancy and nursing is not known.	Transient nausea, gastric disturbances.
Galantamine (Razadyne, Rayadyne ER)	**(Razadyne) Sol:** 4mg/mL [100mL]; **Tab:** 4mg, 8mg, 12mg; **(Razadyne ER) Tab, Extended-Release:** 8mg, 16mg, 24mg	**Adults: (Sol, Tab) Initial:** 4mg bid with am and pm meals. **Titrate:** Increase to 8mg bid after 4 weeks if tolerated, then increase to 12mg bid after 4 weeks if tolerated. **Usual:** 16-24mg/day. **Max:** 24mg/day. **(Tab, ER) Initial:** 8mg qd with am meal. **Titrate:** Increase to 16mg qd after 4 weeks, then increase to 24mg qd after 4 weeks if tolerated. **Usual:** 16-24mg/day. **Max:** 24mg/day. If therapy is in-terrupted, restart at lowest dose and increase to current dose. **Moderate Renal/Hepatic Impairment (Child-Pugh: 7-9):** Caution during dose titration. **Max:** 16mg/day. Avoid use with severe renal (CrCl <9mL/min) and severe hepatic impairment (Child-Pugh: 10-15).	**W/P:** Vagotonic effects; caution with supraventricular conduction disorder. Caution with asthma or obstructive pulmonary disease. Monitor for active or occult GI bleeding and ulcers due to increased gastric acid secretion. Risk of generalized convulsions or bladder outflow obstruction. Ensure adequate fluid intake during treatment. Deaths reported with mild cognitive impairment. **P/N:** Category B, not for use in nursing.	Nausea, vomiting, diarrhea, anorexia, weight loss, fatigue, dizziness, headache, depression, insomnia, abdominal pain, dyspepsia, urinary tract infection.
Memantine Hydrochloride (Namenda)	**Sol:** 2mg/mL; **Tab:** 5mg, 10mg; **Titra-tion-Pak:** 5mg [28ˢ], 10mg [21ˢ]	**Adults: Initial:** 5mg qd. **Titrate:** Increase at intervals of at least one week to 5mg bid, then 5mg and 10mg as separate doses, then to 10mg bid. **Severe Renal Impairment:** Reduce dose.	**W/P:** Use not evaluated with seizure disorders. Alkalinized urine (eg, renal tubular acidosis, severe urinary tract infections) may increase levels. Reduce dose with severe renal impair-ment. **P/N:** Category B, caution in nursing.	Dizziness, confusion, headache, constipation, coughing, HTN, pain, vomiting, somnolence, hal-lucinations.
Rivastigmine (Exelon)	**Cap:** 1.5mg, 3mg, 4.5mg, 6mg; **Sol:** 2mg/mL [120mL]	**Adults: Initial:** 1.5mg bid. **Titrate:** May increase by 1.5mg bid every 2 weeks. **Max:** 12mg/ day. Take with food in am and pm. If not tolerating, suspend therapy for several doses and restart at same or next lower dose. If interrupted longer than several days, reinitiate with lowest daily dose and titrate as above. May mix solution with water, cold fruit juice or soda.	**W/P:** Significant GI intolerance (eg, nausea, vomiting, anorexia, and weight loss); always follow dosing guidelines. Vagotonic effect on heart rate (bradycardia), especially in "sick sinus syndrome" or supraventricular conduction abnormalities. May cause urinary obstruction and seizures. Moni-tor for peptic ulcers/GI bleeds. Caution in asthma and COPD. **Contra:** Hypersensitivity to carbamate derivatives. **P/N:** Category B, not for use in nursing.	Nausea, vomiting, abdominal pain, dyspepsia, constipa-tion, somnolence, anorexia, asthenia, headache, dizzi-ness, fatigue, diarrhea.

*Scored.   †Bold entries denote special dental considerations.

Table 17.1 PRESCRIBING INFORMATION FOR NEUROLOGICAL AGENTS *(cont.)*

NAME	FORM/STRENGTH	DOSAGE	WARNINGS/PRECAUTIONS & CONTRAINDICATIONS	ADVERSE EFFECTS†
ALZHEIMER'S DRUGS *(cont.)*				
Tacrine (Cognex)	**Cap:** 10mg, 20mg, 30mg, 40mg	**Adults: Initial:** 10mg qid. **Titrate:** Increase to 20mg qid after 4 weeks, then increase at 4-week intervals to 30mg qid then to 40mg qid. **ALT/SGPT: >3 to ≤5X ULN:** Reduce dose by 40mg/day and resume dose titration when levels are normal. **>5X ULN:** Stop therapy and monitor; may rechallenge when ALT/SGPT levels are normal. Discontinue and do not rechallenge if jaundice and/or signs of hypersensitivity. **Rechallenge:** 10mg qid, may titrate if normal ALT/SGPT after 6 weeks. Monitor weekly for 16 weeks, then monthly for 2 months, and every 3 months thereafter. Take between meals.	**W/P:** Vagotonic effects; caution with conduction abnormalities, bradyarrhythmia, sick sinus syndrome. May increase risk of developing ulcers. Monitor LFTs every other week from weeks 4-16 from start of therapy, then every 3 months. Modify LFT monitoring based on LFTs (see dosage). Higher incidence of LFTs elevation in females. May cause seizures, bladder outflow obstruction, neutrophil abnormalities. May worsen cognitive function with abrupt withdrawal. Caution with liver disease, ulcers, asthma. Discontinue with clinical jaundice or hypersensitivity with ALT/SGPT elevations. **Contra:** Hypersensitivity to acridine derivatives, history of tacrine-associated jaundice (bilirubin >3mg/dL) or signs of hypersensitivity associated with ALT/SGPT elevations. **P/N:** Category C, caution in nursing.	Elevated LFTs, nausea, vomiting, diarrhea, dyspepsia, myalgia, anorexia, ataxia.
ANTICONVULSANTS				
Carbamazepine (Carbatrol, Tegretol, Tegretol-XR)	**(Carbatrol) Cap, ER:** 200mg, 300mg; **(Tegretol, Tegretol-XR) Sus:** 100mg/5mL; **Tab:** 200mg*; **Tab, Chewable:** 100mg*; **Tab, Extended Release:** 100mg, 200mg, 400mg	**(Carbatrol) Adults: Epilepsy: Initial:** 200mg bid. **Titrate:** May increase weekly by 200mg/day. **Maint:** 800-1200mg/day. **Max:** 1200mg/day. **Trigeminal Neuralgia: Initial (Day 1):** 200mg qd. **Titrate:** May increase by 200mg/day q12h. **Maint:** 400-800mg/day. **Max:** 1200mg/day. Re-evaluate every 3 months. **Pediatrics: Epilepsy: >12 yrs: Initial:** 200mg bid. **Titrate:** May increase weekly by 200mg/day. **Max: 12-15 yrs:** 1000mg/day. **>15 yrs:** 1200mg/day. **6 months-12 yrs:** May convert immediate-release dose ≥400mg/day to equal daily dose using bid regimen. **Usual/Max:** ≤35mg/kg/day. **(Tegretol, Tegretol-XR) Adults: Epilepsy: Initial: (Immediate or Extended Release Tabs)** 200mg bid or **(Sus)** 100mg qid. **Titrate: (Immediate Release Tabs/Sus)** Increase weekly by 200mg/day given tid-qid. **(Extended Release Tabs)** Increase weekly by 200mg/day given bid. **Maint:** 800-1200mg/day. **Max:** 1200mg/day. **Trigeminal Neuralgia: Initial (Day 1): (Immediate or Extended Release Tabs)** 100mg bid or **(Sus)** 50mg qid. **Titrate:** May increase by 100mg q12h **(Tabs)** or 50mg qid **(Sus)**. **Maint:** 400-800mg/day.	**Aplastic anemia and agranulocytosis reported. Obtain complete pretreatment hematological testing as a baseline. Discontinue if develop evidence of bone marrow depression. W/P:** Lyell's syndrome and Stevens-Johnson syndrome, multi-organ hypersensitivity reactions reported. Caution with history of adverse hematologic reaction to any drug, increased IOP, the elderly, mixed seizure with atypical absence seizure. Fetal harm with pregnancy. May activate latent psychosis. Caution with cardiac, hepatic, or renal damage. Perform eye exam and monitor LFTs and renal function at baseline and periodically. **Contra:** History of bone marrow depression, MAOI use within 14 days, sensitivity to TCAs. **P/N:** Category D, not for use in nursing.	Dizziness, drowsiness, unsteadiness, nausea, vomiting, bone marrow depression, hypersensitivity reactions, photosensitivity reactions, CHF, edema, HTN, hypotension.

*Scored.   †Bold entries denote special dental considerations.

NAME	FORM/ STRENGTH	DOSAGE	WARNINGS/PRECAUTIONS & CONTRAINDICATIONS	ADVERSE EFFECTS†
Carbamazepine *(cont.)*		**Max:** 1200mg/day. Re-evaluate every 3 months. Swallow extended release tabs whole; do not crush or chew. ***Pediatrics:* Epilepsy: >12 yrs: Initial: (Immediate or Extended Release Tabs)** 200mg bid or **(Sus)** 100mg qid. **Titrate: (Immediate Release Tabs/Sus)** Increase weekly by 200mg/day given tid-qid. **(Extended Release Tabs)** Increase weekly by 200mg/day given bid. **Max: 12-15 yrs:** 1000mg/day. **>15 yrs:** 1200mg/day. **6-12 yrs: Initial: (Immediate or Extended Release Tabs)** 100mg bid or **(Sus)** 50mg qid. **Titrate: (Immediate Release Tabs/Sus)** Increase weekly by 100mg/day given tid-qid. **(Extended Release Tabs)** Increase weekly by 100mg/day given bid. **Maint:** 400-800mg/day. **Max:** 1000mg/day. **6 months-6 yrs: Initial: (Immediate Release Tabs)** 10-20mg/kg/day given bid-tid or **(Sus)** 10-20mg/kg/day given qid. **Titrate: (Immediate Release Tabs/Sus)** Increase weekly tid-qid. **Max:** 35mg/kg/day. Swallow extended release tabs whole; do not crush or chew.		
Clonazepam[CIV] (Klonopin, Klonopin Wafers)	**Tab:** 0.5mg*, 1mg, 2mg; **Tab, Disintegrating (Wafer):** 0.125mg, 0.25mg, 0.5mg, 1mg, 2mg	***Adults:* Seizure Disorders: Initial:** Not to exceed 1.5mg/day given tid. **Titrate:** May increase by 0.5-1mg every 3 days. **Max:** 20mg qd. **Panic Disorder: Initial:** 0.25mg bid. **Titrate:** Increase to 1mg/day after 3 days, then may increase by 0.125-0.25mg bid every 3 days. **Max:** 4mg/day. **Wafer:** Dissolve in mouth with or without water. ***Pediatrics:* <10 yrs or 30kg: Seizure Disorders: Initial:** 0.01-0.03mg/kg/day up to 0.05mg/kg/day given bid-tid. **Titrate:** Increase by no more than 0.25-0.5mg every 3 days. **Maint:** 0.1-0.2mg/kg/day given tid. **Wafer:** Dissolve in mouth with or without water.	**W/P:** May increase incidence of generalized tonic-clonic seizures. Monitor blood counts and LFT's periodically with long-term therapy. Caution with renal dysfunction, chronic respiratory depression. Increased fetal risks during pregnancy. Avoid abrupt withdrawal. Hypersalivation reported. **Contra:** Significant liver disease, acute narrow angle glaucoma, untreated open angle glaucoma. **P/N:** Category D, not for use in nursing.	Somnolence, depression, ataxia, CNS depression, upper respiratory tract infection, fatigue, dizziness, sinusitis, colpitis.
Diazepam [CIV] (Valium)	**Tab:** 2mg*, 5mg*, 10mg*	***Adults:* Anxiety:** 2-10mg bid-qid. **Alcohol Withdrawal:** 10mg tid-qid for 24 hours. **Maint:** 5mg tid-qid prn. **Skeletal Muscle Spasm:** 2-10mg tid-qid. **Seizure Disorders:** 2-10mg bid-qid. **Elderly/Debilitated:** 2-2.5mg qd-bid initially; may increase gradually as needed and tolerated. ***Pediatrics:* ≥6 months:** 1-2.5mg tid-qid initially; may increase gradually as needed and tolerated	**W/P:** Monitor blood counts and LFTs in long-term use. Neutropenia and jaundice reported. Increase in grand mal seizures reported. Avoid abrupt withdrawal. Caution with kidney or hepatic dysfunction. **Contra:** Acute narrow angle glaucoma, untreated open angle glaucoma, patients ≥6 months. **P/N:** Not for use during pregnancy, safety in nursing not known.	Drowsiness, fatigue, ataxia, paradoxical reactions, minor EEG changes.

Table 17.1 PRESCRIBING INFORMATION FOR NEUROLOGICAL AGENTS (cont.)

NAME	FORM/ STRENGTH	DOSAGE	WARNINGS/PRECAUTIONS & CONTRAINDICATIONS	ADVERSE EFFECTS†
ANTICONVULSANTS (cont.)				
Divalproex Sodium (Depakote, Depakote ER, Depakote Sprinkles)	**(Depakote/Depakote Sprinkles) Cap, Delayed Release: (Sprinkle)** 125mg; **Tab, Delayed Release:** 125mg, 250mg, 500mg; **(Depakote ER) Tab, Extended Release:** 250mg, 500mg	**(Depakote/Depakote Sprinkles)** *Adults:* (Cap/Tab) **Complex Partial Seizures: Initial:** 10-15mg/kg/day. **Titrate:** Increase by 5-10mg/kg/week. **Max:** 60mg/kg/day. **Absence Seizures: Initial:** 15mg/kg/day. **Titrate:** Increase weekly by 5-10mg/kg/day. **Max:** 60mg/kg/day. Give in divided doses if >250mg/day. **(Tab) Migraine: Initial:** ≥16 yrs: 250mg bid. **Max:** 1000mg/day. **Mania:** 750mg in divided doses. **Titrate:** Increase dose rapidly to clinical effect. **Max:** 60mg/ kg/day. **Elderly:** Reduce initial dose and titrate slowly. Decrease dose or discontinue if decreased food or fluid intake or if excessive somnolence occurs. *Pediatrics:* ≥10 yrs: (Cap/Tab) **Complex Partial Seizures: Initial:** 10-15mg/kg/day. **Titrate:** Increase by 5-10mg/kg/week. **Max:** 60mg/kg/day. **Absence Seizures: Initial:** 15mg/kg/day. **Titrate:** Increase weekly by 5-10mg/kg/day. **Max:** 60mg/kg/day. Give in divided doses if >250mg/day. **(Depakote ER)** *Adults:* For qd dosing. **Migraine: Initial:** 500mg qd for 1 week. **Titrate:** Increase to 1000mg qd. **Max:** 1000mg/day. **Complex Partial Seizures: Monotherapy/Adjunct Therapy: Initial:** 10-15mg/kg/day. **Titrate:** Increase by 5-10mg/ kg/week to optimal response. **Usual:** Less than 60mg/kg/day (accepted therapeutic range 50-100mcg/mL). When converting to monotherapy, reduce concomitant antiepilepsy drug by 25% every 2 weeks starting at initiation or delay 1-2 weeks after start of therapy. **Simple and Complex Absence Seizures: Initial:** 15mg/kg/day. **Titrate:** Increase weekly by 5-10mg/kg/day to optimal response. **Max:** 60mg/kg/day. **Mania: Initial:** 25mg/kg/day given once daily. **Titrate:** Increase dose rapidly to clinical effect. **Max:** 60mg/kg/day. **Conversion from Depakote:** Administer Depakote ER qd using a dose 8-20% higher than the total daily dose of Depakote.	**Fatal hepatic failure (<2 yrs at considerable risk), teratogenic effects (eg, neural tube defects), and life-threatening pancreatitis reported. W/P:** Hyperammonemic encephalopathy in UCD patients; discontinue if this occurs. Prior to therapy, evaluate for UCD in high risk patients (eg, history of unexplained encephalopathy, coma, etc). Measure ammonia levels if develop unexplained lethargy, vomiting, or mental status changes. Caution with hepatic disease. Check LFTs prior to therapy, then frequently during first 6 months. Dose-related thrombocytopenia and elevated liver enzymes reported. Monitor platelet and coagulation tests prior to therapy, then periodically. Altered thyroid function tests and urine ketone test. May stimulate replication of HIV and CMV viruses. Avoid abrupt discontinuation. **Contra:** Hepatic disease, significant hepatic dysfunction, known urea cycle disorders (UCD). **P/N:** Category D, not for use in nursing.	Nausea, vomiting, diarrhea, somnolence, dyspepsia, thrombocytopenia, asthenia, abdominal pain, tremor, headache, anorexia, diplopia, blurred vision, weight gain, ataxia, nystagmus.

*Scored.   †Bold entries denote special dental considerations.

NAME	FORM/ STRENGTH	DOSAGE	WARNINGS/PRECAUTIONS & CONTRAINDICATIONS	ADVERSE EFFECTS†
Divalproex Sodium (cont.)		If cannot directly convert to Depakote ER, consider increasing to next higher Depakote total daily dose before converting to appropriate total dsaily Depakote ER dose. **Elderly:** Give lower initial dose and titrate slowly. Decrease dose or discontinue if decreased food or fluid intake or if excessive somnolensce occurs. Swallow whole; do not crush or chew. **Pediatrics: ≥10yrs:** For qd dosing. **Complex Partial Seizures: Monotherapy/Adjunct Therapy: Initial:** 10-15mg/kg/day. **Titrate:** Increase by 5-10mg/kg/week to optimal response. **Usual:** Less than 60mg/kg/day (accepted therapeutic range 50-100mcg/mL). When converting to monotherapy, reduce concomitant antiepilepsy drug by 25% every 2 weeks starting at initiation or delay 1-2 weeks after start of therapy. **Simple and Complex Absence Seizures: Initial:** 15mg/kg/day. **Titrate:** Increase weekly by 5-10mg/kg/day to optimal response. **Max:** 60mg/kg/day. **Conversion from Depakote:** Administer Depakote ER qd using a dose 8-20% higher than the total daily dose of Depakote. If cannot directly convert to Depakote ER, consider increasing to next higher Depakote total daily dose before converting to appropriate total daily Depakote ER dose. Swallow whole; do not crush or chew.		
Ethosuximide (Zarontin)	**Cap:** 250mg; **Syrup:** 250mg/5mL	**Adults:** 500mg qd. **Titrate:** May increase daily dose by 250mg every 4-7 days. **Max:** 1.5g/day. **Pediatrics: Initial: 3-6 yrs:** 250mg qd. **≥6 yrs:** 500mg qd. **Titrate:** May increase daily dose by 250mg every 4-7 days. **Usual:** 20mg/kg/day. **Max:** 1.5g/day.	**W/P:** Extreme caution in liver and renal dysfunction. Monitor blood counts, liver and renal function periodically. SLE, blood dyscrasias reported. Adjust dose slowly and avoid abrupt withdrawal. May increase grand mal seizures in mixed types of epilepsy when used alone. Caution with mental/physical activities. **P/N:** Safety in pregnancy and nursing not known.	Anorexia, nausea, vomiting, abdominal pain, blood dyscrasias, drowsiness, headache, urticaria, SLE, myopia.
Felbamate (Felbatol)	**Sus:** 600mg/5mL [240mL, 960mL]; **Tab:** 400mg*, 600mg*	**Adults: Initial Monotherapy:** 300mg qid or 400mg tid. **Titrate:** Increase by 600mg every 2 weeks to 2.4g/day. **Max:** 3.6g/day. **Initial Monotherapy Conversion/Adjunct Therapy:** 300mg qid or 400mg tid while reducing present AED (see literature). **Titrate:** For conversion, increase at week 2 to 2.4g/day, at week 3 up to 3.6g/day. **Adjunct Therapy:** Increase by 1.2g/day every week up to 3.6mg/day.	**Associated with aplastic anemia and fatal hepatic failure. Monitor blood, LFTs. Avoid in history of hepatic dysfunction. W/P:** Avoid abrupt discontinuation. Caution with renal dysfunction. Obtain written, informed consent. Obtain full hematologic evaluations and LFTs before, during and after discontinuation. Discontinue if bone marrow depression or liver abnormalities occur. **Contra:** History of blood dyscrasias, hepatic dysfunction. **P/N:** Category C, safety in nursing not known.	Anorexia, vomiting, insomnia, nausea, headache, anemias, hepatic failure.

Table 17.1 PRESCRIBING INFORMATION FOR NEUROLOGICAL AGENTS *(cont.)*

NAME	FORM/ STRENGTH	DOSAGE	WARNINGS/PRECAUTIONS & CONTRAINDICATIONS	ADVERSE EFFECTS†
ANTICONVULSANTS *(cont.)*				
Felbamate *(cont.)*		**Renal Dysfunction:** May need to reduce dose with concomitant AEDs. **Pediatrics: ≥14 yrs: Initial Monotherapy:** 300mg qid or 400mg tid. **Titrate:** Increase by 600mg every 2 weeks to 2.4g/day. **Max:** 3.6g/day. **Initial Monotherapy Conversion/Adjunct Therapy:** 300mg qid or 400mg tid while reducing present AED (see literature **Titrate:** For conversion, increase at week 2 to 2.4g/day, at week 3 up to 3.6g/day. **Adjunct Therapy:** Increase by 1.2g/day every week up to 3.6mg/day. **2-14 yrs: Lennox-Gastaut Adjunct Therapy: Initial:** 15mg/kg/day in 3-4 divided doses. **Titrate:** Increase by 15mg/kg/day every week to 45mg/kg/day. **Renal Dysfunction:** May need to reduce dose with concomitant AEDs.		
Fosphenytoin Sodium (Cerebyx)	**Inj:** 50mg PE/mL (2mL, 10mL)	**Adults:** Doses, concentration in dosing solutions, and infusion rates are expressed as phenytoin sodium equivalents (PE). **Status Epilepticus: LD:** 15-20 PE/kg IV at 100-150mg PE/min then switch to maintenance dose. **Non-Emergent Cases: LD:** 10-20mg PE/kg IV (max 150mg PE/min) or IM. **Maint: Initial:** 4-6mg PE/kg/day. May substitute for oral phenytoin sodium at the same total daily dose.	**W/P:** Avoid abrupt discontinuation. Not for use in absence seizures. Hypotension and severe cardiovascular reactions and fatalities reported; continuously monitor ECG, BP, and respiration during and for at least 20 minutes after IV infusion and monitor phenytoin levels at least 2 hours after IV infusion or 4 hours after IM injection. Caution with severe myocardial insufficiency, porphyria, hepatic/renal dysfunction, hypoalbuminemia, elderly, and diabetes. Acute hepatotoxicity, lymphadenopathy, hemopoietic complications, hyperglycemia reported. Discontinue if rash or acute hepatotoxicity occurs. Neonatal postpartum bleeding disorder, congenital malformations and increased seizure frequency reported with use during pregnancy. Avoid use with seizures due to hypoglycemia or other metabolic causes. Caution with phosphate restriction because of phosphate load (0.0037 mmol phosphate/mg PE). May lower folate levels. **Contra:** Sinus bradycardia, sino-atrial block, 2nd- and 3rd-degree AV block, Adams-Stokes syndrome. **P/N:** Category D, not for use in nursing.	Cardiovascular collapse and/or CNS depression, nystagmus, dizziness, pruritus, paresthesia, headache, somnolence, ataxia, tinnitus, stupor, nausea, hypotension, vasodilation, tremor, incoordination.
Gabapentin (Neurontin)	**Cap:** 100mg, 300mg, 400mg; **Sol:** 250mg/5mL; **Tab:** 600mg*, 800mg*	**Adults: Epilepsy: Initial:** 300mg tid. **Titrate:** Increase up to 1800mg/day. **Max:** 3600mg/day. **PHN:** 300mg single dose on Day 1, then 300mg bid on Day 2, and 300mg tid on Day 3. Increase further prn pain. **Max:** 600mg tid.	**W/P:** Avoid abrupt withdrawal. Possible tumorigenic potential. Sudden and unexplained deaths reported. Neuropsychiatric adverse events in pediatrics (3-12 yrs). **P/N:** Category C, caution in nursing.	Somnolence, dizziness, ataxia, nystagmus, fatigue, tremor, rhinitis, weight gain, nausea, vomiting, viral infection, fever, dysarthria, diplopia.

*Scored.   †Bold entries denote special dental considerations.

NAME	FORM/ STRENGTH	DOSAGE	WARNINGS/PRECAUTIONS & CONTRAINDICATIONS	ADVERSE EFFECTS†
Gabapentin (cont.)		**Renal Impairment: CrCl 30-59mL/min:** 400-1400 mg/day. **CrCl 15-29mL/min:** 200-700 mg/day. **CrCl 15mL/min:** 100-300mg/ day. **CrCl <15 mL/min:** Reduce dose in proportion to CrCl. **Hemodialysis: Maint:** Base on CrCl. Give supplemental dose (125-350mg) after 4 hrs of hemodialysis. Refer to prescribing information for dose-adjustment. *Pediatrics:* **Epilepsy: >12 yrs: Initial:** 300mg tid. **Titrate:** Increase up to 1800mg/day. **Max:** 3600mg/day. **3-12 yrs: Initial:** 10-15mg/kg/day given tid. **Titrate:** Increase over 3 days. **Usual: 3-4 yrs:** 40mg/kg/day given tid. **≥5 yrs:** 25-35mg/ kg/day given tid. **Max:** 50mg/ kg/day. **Renal Impairment: ≥12 yrs: CrCl 30-59mL/min:** 400-1400 mg/day. **CrCl 15-29mL/min:** 200-700 mg/day. **CrCl 15mL/min:** 100-300mg/ day. **CrCl <15 mL/min:** Reduce dose in proportion to CrCl. **Hemodialysis: Maint:** Base on CrCl. Give supplemental dose (125-350 mg) after 4 hrs of hemodialysis. Refer to prescribing information for dose-adjustment.		
Lamotrigine (Lamictal, Lamictal CD)	**Tab:** 25mg*, 100mg*, 150mg*, 200mg*; **Tab, Chewable:** (Lamictal CD) 2mg, 5mg, 25mg	*Adults:* **Epilepsy: Concomitant AEDs with valproate (VPA): Weeks 1 and 2:** 25mg every other day. **Weeks 3 and 4:** 25mg qd. **Titrate:** Increase every 1-2 weeks by 25-50mg/day. **Maint:** 100-400mg/day, given qd or bid; 100-200mg/day when added to VPA alone. **Concomitant EIAEDs without VPA: Weeks 1 and 2:** 50mg qd. **Weeks 3 and 4:** 50mg bid. **Titrate:** Increase every 1-2 weeks by 100mg/day. **Maint:** 150-250mg bid. **Conversion to Monotherapy From Single EIAED: ≥16 yrs: Weeks 1 and 2:** 50mg qd. **Weeks 3 and 4:** 50mg bid. **Titrate:** Increase every 1-2 weeks by 100mg/day. **Maint:** 250mg bid. Withdraw EIAED over 4 weeks. **Conversion to Monotherapy From VPA: ≥16 yrs: Step 1:** Follow Concomitant AEDs with VPA dosing regimen to achieve Lamictal dose of 200mg/day. Maintain previous VPA dose.	**Serious life threatening rash including Stevens-Johnson syndrome and toxic epidermal necrolysis reported. Occurs more often in pediatrics than adults. Discontinue at 1st sign of rash.** **W/P:** Risk of serious life-threatening rash; discontinue if rash occurs. Multiorgan failure, sudden unexplained death, hypersensitivity reactions, and pure red cell aplasia reported. Avoid abrupt withdrawal. Caution with renal, hepatic, or cardiac functional impairment. May cause ophthalmic toxicity. Do not exceed recommended initial dose and dose escalations. Caution in elderly. Chewable tabs may be swallowed whole, chewed (with water/diluted fruit juice) or dispersed in water/diluted fruit juice; do administer partial quantities. **P/N:** Category C, not for use in nursing.	Serious rash, dizziness, ataxia, somnolence, headache, diplopia, blurred vision, nausea, vomiting, insomnia, back/abdominal pain, fatigue, **xerostomia**, rhinitis.

Table 17.1 PRESCRIBING INFORMATION FOR NEUROLOGICAL AGENTS *(cont.)*

NAME	FORM/ STRENGTH	DOSAGE	WARNINGS/PRECAUTIONS & CONTRAINDICATIONS	ADVERSE EFFECTS†
ANTICONVULSANTS *(cont.)*				
Lamotrigine *(cont.)*		**Step 2:** Maintain Lamictal 200mg/day. Decrease VPA to 500mg/day by decrements of ≤500mg/day per week. Maintain VPA 500mg/day for 1 week. **Step 3:** Increase to Lamictal 300mg/day for 1 week. Decrease VPA simultaneously to 250mg/day for 1 week. **Step 4:** Discontinue VPA. Increase Lamictal 100mg/day every week to maint dose of 500mg/day. **Bipolar Disorder: Patients not taking carbamazepine, other enzyme-inducing drugs (EIDs) or VPA: Weeks 1 and 2:** 25mg qd. **Weeks 3 and 4:** 50mg qd. **Week 5:** 100mg qd. **Weeks 6 and 7:** 200mg qd. **Patients taking VPA: Weeks 1 and 2:** 25mg every other day. **Weeks 3 and 4:** 25mg qd. **Week 5:** 50mg qd. **Weeks 6 and 7:** 100mg qd. **Patients taking carbamazepine (or other EIDs) and not taking VPA: Weeks 1 and 2:** 50mg qd. **Weeks 3 and 4:** 100mg qd (divided doses). **Week 5:** 200mg qd (divided doses). **Week 6:** 300mg qd (divided doses). **Week 7:** up to 400mg qd (divided doses). **After discontinuation of psychotropic drugs excluding VPA, carbamazepine, or other EIDs:** Maintain current dose. **After discontinuation of VPA and current lamotrigine dose of 100mg qd: Week 1:** 150mg qd. **Week 2 and onward:** 200mg qd. **After discontinuation of carbamazepine or other EIDs and current lamotrigine dose of 400mg qd: Week 1:** 400mg qd. **Week 2:** 300mg qd. **Week 3 and onward:** 200mg qd. **Hepatic Impairment: Initial/Titrate/ Maint:** Reduce by 50% for moderate (Child-Pugh Grade B) and 75% for severe (Child-Pugh Grade C) impairment. **Significant Renal Impairment: Maint:** Reduce dose. **Elderly:** Start at low end of dosing range. *Pediatrics:* Round dose down to nearest whole tab. **2-12 yrs: ≥6.7kg: Lennox-Gastaut/Partial Seizures: Concomitant AEDs with VPA: Weeks 1 and 2:** 0.15mg/kg/day given qd-bid. **Weeks 3 and 4:** 0.3mg/kg/day given qd or bid. **Titrate:** Increase every 1-2 weeks by 0.3mg/kg/day.		

*Scored.   †Bold entries denote special dental considerations.

NAME	FORM/ STRENGTH	DOSAGE	WARNINGS/PRECAUTIONS & CONTRAINDICATIONS	ADVERSE EFFECTS†
Lamotrigine (cont.)		**Maint:** 1-5mg/kg/day given qd or bid; 1-3mg/kg/day when added to VPA alone. **Max:** 200mg/day. **Concomitant EIAEDs without VPA: Weeks 1 and 2:** 0.3mg/kg bid. **Weeks 3 and 4:** 0.6mg/kg bid. **Titrate:** Increase every 1-2 weeks by 1.2mg/kg/day. **Maint:** 2.5-7.5mg/kg bid. **Max:** 400mg/day. **>12 yrs: Concomitant AEDs with VPA: Weeks 1 and 2:** 25mg every other day. **Weeks 3 and 4:** 25mg qd. **Titrate:** Increase every 1-2 weeks by 25-50mg/day. **Maint:** 100-400mg/day, given qd or bid; 100-200mg/day when added to VPA alone. **Concomitant EIAEDs without VPA: Weeks 1 and 2:** 50mg qd. **Weeks 3 and 4:** 50mg bid. **Titrate:** Increase every 1-2 weeks by 100mg/day. **Maint:** 150-250mg bid. **Hepatic Impairment: Initial/Titrate/ Maint:** Reduce by 50% for moderate (Child-Pugh Grade B) and 75% for severe (Child-Pugh Grade C) impairment. **Significant Renal Impairment: Maint:** Reduce dose.		
Levetiracetam (Keppra)	**Sol:** 100mg/mL; **Tab:** 250mg*, 500mg*, 750mg*	**Adults: Initial:** 500mg bid. **Titrate:** Increase by 1000mg/day every 2 weeks. **Max:** 3000mg/day. **CrCl 50-80mL/min:** 500-1000mg q12h. **CrCl 30-50mL/min:** 250-750mg q12h. **CrCl <30mL/min:** 250-500mg q12h. **ESRD with Dialysis:** 500-1000mg q24h; supplemental 250-500mg after dialysis. **Pediatrics: ≥16 yrs: Initial:** 500mg bid. **Titrate:** Increase by 1000mg/day every 2 weeks. **Max:** 3000mg/day. **CrCl 50-80mL/min:** 500-1000mg q12h. **CrCl 30-50mL/min:** 250-750mg q12h. **CrCl <30mL/min:** 250-500mg q12h. **ESRD with Dialysis:** 500-1000mg q24h; supplemental 250-500mg after dialysis. **4-16 yrs: Initial:** 10mg/kg bid. **Titrate:** Increase by 20mg/kg/ day every 2 weeks. **Max:** 60mg/kg/day.	**W/P:** Associated with somnolence, fatigue, coordination difficulties, and behavioral abnormalities. Avoid abrupt withdrawal. Hematologic abnormalities reported. Caution in renal dysfunction. **P/N:** Category C, caution in nursing.	Somnolence, asthenia, headache, infection, pain, anorexia, dizziness, nervous- ness, vertigo, ataxia, vertigo, pharyngitis, rhinitis.
LorazepamCIV (Ativan)	**Tab:** 0.5mg, 1mg*, 2mg*	**Adults: Initial:** 2-3mg/day given bid-tid. **Usual:** 2-6mg/day in divided doses. **Insomnia:** 2-4mg qhs. **Elderly/Debilitated:** 1-2mg/day in divided doses. **Pediatrics: >12 yrs: Initial:** 2-3mg/day given bid-tid.	**W/P:** Avoid with primary depression or psychosis. Withdrawal symptoms with abrupt discontinuation. Careful supervision if addiction-prone. Caution with elderly, and renal or hepatic dysfunction. Monitor for GI disease with prolonged therapy. Periodic blood counts and LFTs recommended with	Sedation, dizziness, weakness, unsteadiness, transient amnesia, memory impairment.

Table 17.1 PRESCRIBING INFORMATION FOR NEUROLOGICAL AGENTS *(cont.)*

NAME	FORM/ STRENGTH	DOSAGE	WARNINGS/PRECAUTIONS & CONTRAINDICATIONS	ADVERSE EFFECTS†
ANTICONVULSANTS *(cont.)*				
LorazepamCIV *(cont.)*		**Usual:** 2-6mg/day in divided doses. **Insomnia:** 2-s4mg qhs.	long-term therapy. **Contra:** Acute narrow-angle glaucoma. **P/N:** Not for use in pregnancy or nursing.	
Magnesium Sulfate	**Inj:** 40mg/mL, 80mg/mL	***Pediatrics:*** 20-40mg/kg IM to control seizures.	**W/P:** Caution with renal impairment. **Contra:** Parenteral administration is contraindicated in heart block and myocardial damage. **P/N:** Category A, caution in nursing.	Decreased heart rate, vasodilation, hypotension, excessive sweating, flushing, nausea, vomiting, muscle weakness.
Mephobarbital CIV (Mebaral)	**Tab:** 32mg, 50mg, 100mg	***Adults: Epilepsy:*** 400-600mg/day. Start with small dose, gradually increase over 4-5 days until optimum dose. **Elderly/ Debilitated/Renal or Hepatic Dysfunction:** Reduce dose. **Concomitant Phenobarbital:** Give 50% of each drug. **Concomitant Phenytoin:** Reduce phenytoin dose. **Sedation:** 32-100mg tid-qid. **Optimum Dose:** 50mg tid-qid. ***Pediatrics: Epilepsy:*** **>5 yrs:** 32-64mg tid-qid. **<5 yrs:** 16-32mg tid-qid. Start with small dose, gradually increase over 4-5 days until optimum dose. **Sedation:** 16-32mg tid-qid.	**W/P:** May be habit forming; tolerance and dependence may occur with continued use. Avoid abrupt withdrawal. Caution in acute/chronic pain; paradoxical excitement may occur or symptoms masked. Can cause fetal damage. May cause marked excitement, depression and confusion in elderly or debilitated. Reduce initial dose with hepatic damage. Careful adjustment in impaired renal, cardiac, or respiratory function, myasthenia gravis, and myxedema. May increase vitamin D requirements. Caution with depression, suicidal tendencies and history of drug abuse. **Contra:** Manifest or latent porphyria. **P/N:** Category D, caution with nursing.	Somnolence, agitation, confusion, hyperkinesia, ataxia, CNS depression, hypoventilation, apnea, bradycardia, hypotension, syncope, nausea, vomiting, headache.
Methsuximide (Celontin Kapseals)	**Cap:** 150mg, 300mg	***Adults:*** **Initial:** 300mg qd for 7 days. **Titrate:** Increase weekly by 300mg/day for 3 weeks if needed. **Max:** 1.2g/day. ***Pediatrics:*** **Initial:** 300mg qd for 7 days. **Titrate:** Increase weekly by 300mg/day for 3 weeks if needed. **Max:** 1.2g/day. Use 150mg caps in small children.	**W/P:** Fatal blood dyscrasias reported; monitor blood counts periodically or if signs of infection. SLE reported. Withdraw slowly if altered behavior appears. May increase frequency of grand mal seizures if given alone in mixed type of seizures. Avoid abrupt withdrawal. Caution with renal/hepatic disease. **P/N:** Safety in pregnancy and nursing not known.	GI effects, blood dyscrasias, dermatologic manifestations, drowsiness, ataxia, dizziness, hyperemia, proteinuria, periorbital edema.
Oxcarbazepine (Trileptal)	**Sus:** 300mg/5mL [250mL]; **Tab:** 150mg*, 300mg*, 600mg*	***Adults: Monotherapy:*** **Initial:** 300mg bid. **Titrate:** Increase by 300mg/day every 3rd day. **Maint:** 1200mg/day. **Adjunct Therapy: Initial:** 300mg bid. **Titrate:** Increase weekly by a maximum of 600mg/day. **Maint:** 600mg bid. **Conversion to Monotherapy: Initial:** 300mg bid while reducing other AEDs.	**W/P:** Risk of hyponatremia. Cross sensitivity with carbamazepine. Avoid abrupt withdrawal. Adjust dose in renal impairment. Reports of serious dermatologic reactions (eg, Stevens-Johnson syndrome, toxic epidermal necrolysis). CNS effects reported (eg, psychomotor slowing, concentration difficulty, speech or language problems, somnolence or fatigue, coordination abnormalities). Reports of multi-organ hypersensitivity reactions in close temporal association to initiation of therapy. **P/N:** Category C, not for use in nursing.	Dizziness, somnolence, diplopia, nausea, vomiting, asthenia, nystagmus, ataxia, abnormal vision, tremor, abnormal gait, headache.

*Scored.   †Bold entries denote special dental considerations.

NAME	FORM/ STRENGTH	DOSAGE	WARNINGS/PRECAUTIONS & CONTRAINDICATIONS	ADVERSE EFFECTS[†]
Oxcarbazepine *(cont.)*	·	**Titrate:** Increase weekly by 600mg/day. Withdraw other AEDs over 3-6 weeks. **Maint:** 2400mg/day. Renal Impairment: **CrCl <30mL/min: Initial:** 300mg qd. **Titrate:** Increase gradually. *Pediatrics:* **4-16yrs: Monotherapy: Initial:** 4-5mg/kg bid. **Titrate:** Increase by 5mg/kg/day every 3rd day. **Maint (mg/day): 20kg: Initial:** 600mg. **Max:** 900mg. **25-30kg: Initial:** 900mg. **Max:** 1200mg. 35-40kg: **Initial:** 900mg. **Max:** 1500mg. 45kg: **Initial:** 1200mg. **Max:** 1500mg. **50-55kg: Initial:** 1200mg. **Max:** 1800mg. **60-65kg: Initial:** 1200mg. **Max:** 2100mg. **70kg: Initial:** 1500mg. **Max:** 2100mg. **Adjunct Therapy: Initial:** 4-5mg/kg bid. **Max:** 600mg/day. **Titrate:** Increase over 2 weeks. **Maint (mg/day): 20-29kg:** 900mg. **29.1-39kg:** 1200mg. **>39kg:** 1800mg. **Conversion to Monotherapy: Initial:** 4-5mg/kg bid while reducing other AEDs. **Titrate:** Increase weekly by max of 10mg/kg/day to target dose. Withdraw other AEDs over 3-6 weeks. **Renal Impairment: CrCl <30mL/min: Initial:** 300mg qd. **Titrate:** Increase gradually.		
Pentobarbital Sodium[CII] (Nembutal Sodium)	**Inj:** 50mg/mL	*Adults:* **Usual:** 150-200mg as a single IM injection. **IV:** 100mg (commonly used initial dose for 70kg adult); if needed additional small increments may be given up to 200-500mg total dose. Rate of IV injection should not exceed 50mg/min. **Elderly/Debilitated/Renal or Hepatic Impairment:** Reduce dose. *Pediatrics:* 2-6mg/kg as a single IM injection. **Max:** 100mg. **IV:** Proportional reduction in dosage. Slow IV injection is essential.	**W/P:** May be habit forming; avoid abrupt cessation after prolonged use. Avoid rapid administration. Tolerance to hypnotic effect can occur. Prehepatic coma use not recommended. Use with caution in patients with chronic or acute pain, mental depression, suicidal tendencies, history of drug abuse or hepatic impairment. Monitor blood, liver and renal function. May impair mental/physical abilities. Avoid alcohol. **Contra:** History of manifest or latent porphyria. **P/N:** Category D, caution with nursing.	Agitation, confusion, hyperkinesia, ataxia, CNS depression, somnolence, bradycardia, hypotension, nausea, vomiting, constipation, headache, hypersensitivity reactions, liver damage.

Table 17.1 PRESCRIBING INFORMATION FOR NEUROLOGICAL AGENTS *(cont.)*

NAME	FORM/ STRENGTH	DOSAGE	WARNINGS/PRECAUTIONS & CONTRAINDICATIONS	ADVERSE EFFECTS†
ANTICONVULSANTS *(cont.)*				
Phenobarbital^{CIV}	**Elixir:** 20mg/5mL; **Tab:** 15mg, 30mg, 32.4mg, 60mg, 64.8mg, 100mg	*Adults:* **Sedation:** 30-120mg/day given bid-tid. **Max:** 400mg/24h. **Hypnotic:** 100-200mg. **Seizures:** 60-200mg/day. **Elderly/Debilitated/Renal or Hepatic Dysfunction:** Reduce dosage. *Pediatrics:* **Seizures:** 3-6mg/kg/day.	**W/P:** May be habit forming. Avoid abrupt withdrawal. Caution with acute or chronic pain; may mask symptoms or paradoxical excitement may occur. Cognitive deficits reported in children with febrile seizures. May cause excitement in children and excitement, depression or confusion in elderly, debilitated. Caution with hepatic dysfunction, borderline hypoadrenal function, depression. **Contra:** Respiratory disease with dyspnea or obstruction, porphyria, severe liver dysfunction. Large doses with nephritic patients. **P/N:** Category D, caution in nursing.	Drowsiness, residual sedation, lethargy, vertigo, somnolence, respiratory depression, hypersensitivity reactions, nausea, vomiting, headache.
Phenytoin (Dilantin Infatabs, Dilantin-125)	**Cap, Extended Release (CER):** 30mg, 100mg; **Sus:** 125mg/5mL [237mL]; **Tab, Chewable (CTB):** 50mg*	*Adults:* **(CER) Initial:** 100mg tid. **Titrate:** May increase at 7-10 day intervals. **Max:** 200mg tid. May give once daily with extended release if controlled on 300mg daily. **LD (clinic/hospital):** 1g in 3 divided doses (400mg, 300mg, 300mg) given 2 hrs apart. Start maintenance 24 hrs later. **(CTB) Initial:** 100mg tid. **Titrate:** May increase at 7-10 day intervals. **Usual:** 300-400mg/day. **Max:** 600mg/day. May chew or swallow tab whole. Not for once daily dosing. **(Sus) Initial:** 125mg tid. **Titrate:** May increase at 7-10 day intervals. **Max:** 625mg/day. *Pediatrics:* **(CER, CTB, Sus) Initial:** 5mg/kg/day given bid-tid. **Titrate:** May increase at 7-10 day intervals. **Maint:** 4-8mg/kg/day. **Max:** 300mg/day. **>6 yrs:** May require the minimum adult dose (300mg/day).	**W/P:** Avoid abrupt discontinuation. Caution with porphyria, hepatic dysfunction, elderly, diabetes, debilitated. Discontinue if rash occurs. Lymphadenopathy reported. Serum sickness may occur with lymph node involvement. Gingival hyperplasia reported; maintain proper dental hygiene. Hyperglycemia, birth defects and osteomalacia reported. Monitor levels. Confusional states reported with increased levels. Increased seizure frequency during pregnancy. Neonatal coagulation defects reported within first 24 hrs of birth. Give Vitamin K to mother before delivery and to neonate after birth. Avoid use with seizures due to hypoglycemia or other metabolic causes. **P/N:** Possibly teratogenic, weigh benefits versus risk; not for use in nursing.	Nystagmus, ataxia, slurred speech, decreased coordination, confusion, dizziness, insomnia, transient nervousness, motor twitchings, headaches, nausea, vomiting, constipation, rash, hypersensitivity reactions.
Phenytoin Sodium, Extended (Phenytek)	**Cap, Extended Release:** 200mg, 300mg	*Adults:* **No Previous Treatment: Initial:** 100mg extended phenytoin sodium capsule tid. **Titrate:** May increase at 7-10 day intervals. **Usual:** 100mg tid-qid. May increase up to 200mg Phenytek tid.	**W/P:** Avoid abrupt discontinuation. Caution with porphyria, hepatic dysfunction, elderly, diabetes, debilitated. Discontinue if rash occurs. Lymphadenopathy reported. Serum sickness may occur with lymph node involvement. Gingival hyperplasia reported; maintain proper dental hygiene. Hyperglycemia, birth defects and osteomalacia reported. Monitor levels within first 24 hrs of birth;	Nystagmus, ataxia, slurred speech, decreased coordination, confusion, dizziness, insomnia, transient nervousness, motor twitchings, headaches, nausea, vomiting, constipation, rash, hypersensitivity reactions.

*Scored.   †Bold entries denote special dental considerations.

NAME	FORM/ STRENGTH	DOSAGE	WARNINGS/PRECAUTIONS & CONTRAINDICATIONS	ADVERSE EFFECTS†
Phenytoin Sodium, Extended *(cont.)*	**Once Daily Dosing:** 300mg Phenytek qd may replace 100mg extended phenytoin sodium capsule tid if seizures are controlled.	Confusional states reported with toxic levels. Increased seizure frequency during pregnancy. Neonatal coagulation defects reported. **LD (clinic/ hospital):** 1g in 3 divided doses (400mg, 300mg, 300mg) given 2 hrs apart. Start maintenance 24 hrs later. Avoid LD with renal and hepatic disease. ***Pediatrics:* Initial:** 5mg/kg/day given bid-tid. **Titrate:** May increase at 7-10 day intervals. **Maint:** 4-8mg/kg/day. **Max:** 300mg/day. **>6 yrs:** May require the minimum adult dose (300mg/day).	give Vitamin K to mother before delivery and to neonate after birth. Avoid use with seizures due to hypoglycemia or other metabolic causes. **P/N:** Possibly teratogenic, weigh benefits versus risk; not for use in nursing.	
PregabalinCV (Lyrica)	**Cap:** 25mg, 50mg, 75mg, 100mg, 150mg, 200mg, 225mg, 300mg	***Adults:* Neuropathic Pain: Initial:** 50mg tid (150mg/day). **Titrate:** May increase to 300mg/day within 1 week. **Max:** 100mg tid (300mg/day). **Postherpetic Neuralgia: Initial:** 150mg/day divided bid or tid. **Max:** 600mg/ day divided bid or tid. **Epilepsy: Initial:** 150mg/ day divided bid-tid. **Max:** 600mg/day. **Renal Impairment: CrCl 30-60mL/min:** 75-300mg/day divided bid or tid. **CrCl 15-30mL/min:** 25-150mg/day divided qd or bid. **CrCl <15mL/min:** 25-75mg/day given qd. Give supplemental dose (25-150mg) immediately after every 4-hour hemodialysis treatment. Refer to prescribing information. Discontinue over 1 week.	**W/P:** Avoid abrupt withdrawal. Gradually taper over 1 week. Possible tumorigenic potential. May impair physical/mental abilities. May cause weight gain; blurred vision, monitor for ophthalmic changes; peripheral edema, caution in heart failure; elevated creatine kinase, discontinue if myopathy or markedly elevated creatine kinase levels occur; decreased platelet count; and mild PR interval prolongation. **P/N:** Category C, not for use in nursing.	Somnolence, dizziness, **dry mouth**, edema, blurred vision, weight gain, abnormal thinking (difficulty with concentration/attention).
Primidone (Mysoline)	**Tab:** 50mg*, 250mg*	***Adults:* Initial: Day 1-3:** 100-125mg qhs. **Day 4-6:** 100-125mg bid. **Day 7-9:** 100-125mg tid. **Day 10-Maint:** 250mg tid. **Max:** 500mg qid. Effective serum level is 5-12mcg/mL. **Prior Anticonvulsant Therapy: Initial:** 100-125mg qhs. **Titrate:** Increase gradually to maintenance dose as other drug is discontinued over 2 weeks. ***Pediatrics:* ≥8 yrs: Initial: Day 1-3:** 100-125mg qhs. **Day 4-6:** 100-125mg bid. **Day 7-9:** 100-125mg tid. **Day 10-Maint:** 250mg tid.	**W/P:** Avoid abrupt withdrawal. May take several weeks to assess therapeutic efficacy. Pregnant women should receive prophylactic vitamin K₁ therapy for one month prior to, and during delivery. Perform CBC and a SMA-12 test every 6 months. Phenobarbital is a metabolite of primidone. **Contra:** Porphyria, phenobarbital hypersensitivity. **P/N:** Safety in pregnancy not known, caution in nursing.	Ataxia, vertigo, nausea, anorexia, vomiting, fatigue, hyperirritability, emotional disturbances, sexual impotency, diplopia, nystagmus, drowsiness, morbilliform skin eruptions.

Table 17.1 PRESCRIBING INFORMATION FOR NEUROLOGICAL AGENTS *(cont.)*

NAME	FORM/STRENGTH	DOSAGE	WARNINGS/PRECAUTIONS & CONTRAINDICATIONS	ADVERSE EFFECTS†
ANTICONVULSANTS *(cont.)*				
Primidone *(cont.)*		**Max:** 500mg qid. **<8 yrs: Day 1-3:** 50mg qhs. **Day 4-6:** 50mg bid. **Day 7-9:** 100mg bid. **Day 10-Maint:** 125-250mg tid or 10-25mg/kg/day in divided doses. Effective serum level is 5-12mcg/mL. **Prior Anticonvulsant Therapy: Initial:** 100-125mg qhs. **Titrate:** Increase gradually to maintenance dose as other drug is discontinued over 2 weeks.		
Tiagabine Hydrochloride (Gabitril)	**Tab:** 2mg, 4mg, 12mg, 16mg	***Adults:* Initial:** 4mg qd. **Titrate:** May increase weekly by 4-8mg/day until clinical response. **Max:** 56mg/day given bid-qid. Take with food. ***Pediatrics:* ≥12 yo: Initial:** 4mg qd. **Titrate:** May increase to 8mg qd at beginning of week 2, then increase weekly by 4-8mg/day until clinical response. **Max:** 32mg/day. Take with food.	**W/P:** Reports of new onset seizure or status epilepticus in patients without epilepsy. Discontinue and evaluate for underlying seizure disorder. Avoid abrupt withdrawal. Monitor during initial titration for impaired concentration, speech problem, somnolence, fatigue; may require hospitalization if reaction is severe. May exacerbate EEG abnormalities; adjust dose. Status epilepticus and sudden death reported. Reduce dose or discontinue if generalized weakness occurs. Reduce dose with hepatic impairment. Serious skin rash reported. **P/N:** Category C, caution in nursing.	Dizziness, asthenia, somnolence, nausea, vomiting, nervousness, tremor, abdominal pain, abnormal thinking, depression, confusion, **pharyngitis**, rash.
Topiramate (Topamax)	**Cap:** 15mg, 25mg; **Tab:** 25mg, 50mg, 100mg, 200mg	***Adults:* Seizures: Monotherapy: Initial:** 25mg qam and qpm for one week. **Titrate:** Increase am and pm dose by 25mg every week until 200mg/day, then increase by 50mg every week until 400mg/day. **Adjunct Therapy: ≥17 yrs: Initial:** 25-50mg/day. **Titrate:** Increase by 25-50mg/week. **Usual: Partial:** 100-200mg bid. **Tonic-Clonic:** 200mg bid. **Max:** 1600mg/day. **Migraine Prophylaxis: Titrate: Week 1:** 25mg qpm. **Week 2:** 25mg bid. **Week 3:** 25mg qam and 50mg qpm. **Week 4:** 50mg bid. **Usual:** 50mg bid. **Renal Dysfunction:** 50% of usual dose. Swallow caps whole or sprinkle over food. ***Pediatrics:* Seizures: Monotherapy: ≥10 yrs: Initial:** 25mg qam and qpm for one week. **Titrate:** Increase am and pm dose by 25mg every week until 200mg/day,	**W/P:** Hyperchloremic, non-anion gap, metabolic acidosis reported; obtain baseline and periodic serum bicarbonate levels. Withdraw gradually. Psychomotor slowing, difficulty with concentration, speech/language problems, paresthesia, acute myopia with secondary angle closure glaucoma, oligohydrosis, hyperthermia reported. Risk of kidney stones; maintain adequate fluid intake. Caution with renal or hepatic dysfunction. **P/N:** Category C, caution in nursing.	Somnolence, fatigue, dizziness, ataxia, speech disorders, psychomotor slowing, abnormal vision, memory difficulty, paresthesia, diplopia, depression, anorexia, anxiety, mood problems, pancreatitis, hepatic failure.

*Scored.   †Bold entries denote special dental considerations.

NAME	FORM/ STRENGTH	DOSAGE	WARNINGS/PRECAUTIONS & CONTRAINDICATIONS	ADVERSE EFFECTS†
Topiramate *(cont.)*		then increase by 50mg every week until 400mg/day. **Adjunct Therapy: 2-16 yrs: Initial:** 1-3mg/kg nightly for 1 week. **Titrate:** Increase by 1-3mg/kg/day every 1-2 weeks. **Usual:** 2.5-4.5mg/kg bid. Swallow caps whole or sprinkle over food.		
Valproate Sodium (Depacon)	**Inj:** 100mg/mL	***Adults:*** **Simplex/Complex Absence Seizure: Initial:** 15mg/kg/day. **Titrate:** Increase weekly by 5-10mg/kg/day until optimal response. **Max:** 60mg/kg/day. **Complex Partial Seizure: Initial:** 10-15mg/kg/day. **Titrate:** Increase weekly by 5-10mg/kg/day until optimal response. **Max:** 60mg/kg/day. **Elderly:** Reduce initial dose and titrate slowly. If dose >250mg/day, give in divided doses. Administer as 60 minute IV infusion, not >20mg/min. Not for use >14 days; switch to oral route as soon as clinically feasible. Decrease dose or discontinue if decreased food or fluid intake or if excessive somnolence occurs. ***Pediatrics:*** **≥2 yrs: Simplex/Complex Absence Seizure: Initial:** 15mg/kg/day. **Titrate:** Increase weekly by 5-10mg/kg/day until optimal response. **Max:** 60mg/kg/day. **≥10 yrs: Complex Partial Seizure: Initial:** 10-15mg/kg/day. **Titrate:** Increase weekly by 5-10mg/kg/day until optimal response. **Max:** 60mg/kg/day. If dose >250mg/day, give in divided doses. Administer as 60 minute IV infusion, not >20mg/min. Not for use >14 days; switch to oral route as soon as clinically feasible. Decrease dose or discontinue with decreased food or fluid intake and if excessive somnolence.	**Fatal hepatic failure (<2 yrs at considerable risk), teratogenic effects (eg, neural tube defects), and life-threatening pancreatitis reported.** **W/P:** Hyperammonemic encephalopathy in UCD patients; discontinue if this occurs. Prior to therapy, evaluate for UCD in high risk patients (eg, history of unexplained encephalopathy, coma, etc). Measure ammonia levels if develop unexplained lethargy, vomiting, or mental status changes. Caution in elderly; monitor for fluid/nutritional intake, dehydration, somnolence. Monitor LFTs before therapy and during 1st 6 months. Discontinue if develop hepatic dysfunction, pancreatitis. Increased risk of hepatotoxicity with multiple anticonvulsants, congenital metabolic disorders, severe seizure disorder with mental retardation, organic brain disease, children <2 yrs. Avoid abrupt withdrawal. Monitor platelets and coagulation tests before therapy and periodically thereafter. Elevated liver enzymes and thrombocytopenia may be dose-related. Not for prophylaxis of post-traumatic seizures in acute head trauma. May interfere with urine ketone and thyroid function tests. **Contra:** Hepatic disease, significant hepatic dysfunction, known urea cycle disorders (UCD). **P/N:** Category D, not for use in nursing.	Dizziness, headache, nausea, local reactions.
Valproic Acid (Depakene)	**Cap:** 250mg; **Syrup:** 250mg/5mL	***Adults:*** **Simplex/Complex Absence Seizure: Initial:** 15mg/kg/day. **Titrate:** Increase weekly by 5-10mg/kg/day until optimal response.	**Fatal hepatic failure (<2 yrs at considerable risk), teratogenic effects (eg, neural tube defects), and life-threatening pancreatitis reported. W/P:** Hyperammonemic encephalopathy in UCD patients; discontinue if this occurs.	Headache, asthenia, nausea, vomiting, diarrhea, abdominal pain, somnolence, tremor, dizziness, thrombocytopenia, ecchymosis, nystagmus, alopecia.

Table 17.1 PRESCRIBING INFORMATION FOR NEUROLOGICAL AGENTS *(cont.)*

NAME	FORM/ STRENGTH	DOSAGE	WARNINGS/PRECAUTIONS & CONTRAINDICATIONS	ADVERSE EFFECTS†
ANTICONVULSANTS *(cont.)*				
Valproic Acid *(cont.)*		**Max:** 60mg/kg/day. **Complex Partial Seizure: Initial:** 10-15mg/kg/day. **Titrate:** Increase weekly by 5-10mg/kg/day until optimal response. **Max:** 60mg/kg/day. If dose >250mg/day, give in divided doses. **Elderly:** Reduce initial dose. Swallow caps whole, do not chew. ***Pediatrics:* ≥10 yrs: Complex Partial Seizure: Initial:** 10-15mg/kg/day. **Titrate:** Increase weekly by 5-10mg/kg/day until optimal response. **Max:** 60mg/kg/day. If dose >250mg/day, give in divided doses. Swallow caps whole, do not chew.	Prior to therapy, evaluate for UCD in high risk patients (eg, history of unexplained encephalopathy, coma, etc). Measure ammonia levels if develop unexplained lethargy, vomiting, or mental status changes. Caution in elderly; monitor for fluid/nutritional intake, dehydration, somnolence. Monitor LFTs before therapy and during 1st 6 months. Discontinue if develop hepatic dysfunction, pancreatitis. Increased risk of hepatotoxicity with multiple anticonvulsants, congenital metabolic disorders, severe seizure disorder with mental retardation, organic brain disease, children <2 yrs. Avoid abrupt withdrawal. Monitor platelets and coagulation tests before therapy and periodically thereafter. Elevated liver enzymes and thrombocytopenia may be dose-related. Not for prophylaxis of post-traumatic seizures in acute head trauma. May interfere with urine ketone and thyroid function tests. **Contra:** Hepatic disease, significant hepatic dysfunction, known urea cycle disorders (UCD). **P/N:** Category D, not for use in nursing.	
Zonisamide (Zonegran)	**Cap:** 25mg, 50mg, 100mg	***Adults:* Initial:** 100mg qd for 2 weeks. **Titrate:** Increase to 200mg/day for 2 weeks, then increase to 300mg/day, then to 400mg/day at 2 week intervals. **Max:** 400mg/day. ***Pediatrics:* ≥16 yrs: Initial:** 100mg qd for 2 weeks. **Titrate:** Increase to 200mg/day for 2 weeks, then increase to 300mg/day, then to 400mg/day at 2 week intervals. **Max:** 400mg/day.	**W/P:** Sulfonamide hypersensitivity reactions (eg, Stevens-Johnson syndrome, toxic epidermal necrolysis, fulminant hepatic necrosis, blood dyscrasias), cognitive/neuropsychiatric effects, kidney stones, sudden death reported. Discontinue with unexplained rash. Increased risk of oligohydrosis and hyperthermia in pediatrics; monitor for decreased sweating and increased body temperature. Advise females to use contraceptives to prevent pregnancy. Caution with renal/hepatic impairment. Avoid abrupt withdrawal. **Contra:** Sulfonamide hypersensitivity. **P/N:** Category C, not for use in nursing.	Somnolence, anorexia, dizziness, tremor, convulsion, dry mouth, incoordination, amblyopia, tinnitus, GI effects, flu syndrome, ataxia, nystagmus, pruritus.
ANTIPARKINSONISM DRUGS				
Amantadine Hydrochloride (Symmetrel)	**Syrup:** 50mg/5mL; **Tab:** 100mg	***Adults:* Influenza A Virus Prophylaxis/Treatment:** 200mg qd or 100mg bid. **Elderly: ≥65 yrs:** 100mg qd. **Parkinsonism: Initial:** 100mg bid. **Serious Associated Illness/Concomitant High Dose Antiparkinson Agent: Initial:** 100mg qd. **Titrate:** May increase to 100mg bid after 1 to several weeks.	**W/P:** Deaths reported from overdose. Suicide attempts, NMS reported. Caution with CHF, peripheral edema, orthostatic hypotension, renal or hepatic dysfunction, recurrent eczematoid rash, uncontrolled psychosis or severe psychoneurosis. Avoid in untreated angle closure glaucoma. Do not discontinue abruptly in Parkinson's disease. May increase seizure activity. **P/N:** Category C, not for use in nursing.	Nausea, dizziness, insomnia, depression, anxiety, hallucinations, confusion, anorexia, **dry mouth**, constipation, ataxia, livedo reticularis, peripheral edema, orthostatic hypotension, headache.

*Scored. †Bold entries denote special dental considerations.

NAME	FORM/ STRENGTH	DOSAGE	WARNINGS/PRECAUTIONS & CONTRAINDICATIONS	ADVERSE EFFECTS[†]
Amantadine Hydrochloride *(cont.)*		**Max:** 400mg/day. **Drug-Induced Extrapyramidal Reactions:** 100mg bid. **Titrate:** May increase to 300mg/day in divided doses. **CrCl 30-50mL/min:** 200mg on day 1, then 100mg qd. **CrCl 15-29mL/min:** 200mg on day 1, then 100mg every other day. **CrCl <15mL/min/Hemodialysis:** 200mg every 7 days. *Pediatrics:* **Influenza A Virus Prophylaxis/Treatment: 9-12 yrs:** 100mg bid. **1-9 yrs:** 4.4-8.8mg/kg/day. **Max:** 150mg/day.		
Benztropine Mesylate (Cogentin)	**Inj:** 1mg/mL; **Tab:** 0.5mg, 1mg, 2mg	*Adults:* **Parkinsonism: Initial:** 0.5-1mg PO/IV/IM qhs. **Titrate:** May increase every 5-6 days by 0.5mg. **Usual:** 1-2mg PO/IV/IM qhs. **Max:** 6mg/day. **Extrapyramidal Disorders:** 1-4mg PO/IV/IM qd-bid. **Acute Dystonic Reactions:** 1-2mg IM/IV, then 1-2mg PO bid.	**W/P:** May produce anhydrosis, caution in hot weather. Muscle weakness and dysuria may occur. Caution in pediatrics >3 years of age. Not recommended for tardive dyskinesia. Avoid with angle-closure glaucoma. Caution with CNS disease, mental disorders, tachycardia, prostatic hypertrophy, alcoholics, chronically ill, those exposed to hot environments. **Contra:** Patients <3 yrs. **P/N:** Safety in pregnancy and nursing not known.	Tachycardia, paralytic ileus, constipation, vomiting, nausea, **dry mouth**, confusion, blurred vision, urinary retention, heat stroke, hyperthermia, fever.
Bromocriptine Mesylate (Parlodel)	**Cap:** 5mg; **Tab:** 2.5mg*	*Adults:* Take with food. **Parkinson's Disease: Initial:** 1.25mg bid. **Titrate:** if needed, increase by 2.5mg/day every 2-4 weeks. **Max:** 100mg/day. **Hyperprolactinemia: Initial:** 1.25mg-2.5mg qd. **Titrate:** If needed, increase by 2.5mg every 2-7 days. **Usual:** 2.5-15mg/day. **Acromegaly: Initial:** 1.25-2.5mg qhs for 3 days. **Titrate:** Increase by 1.25-2.5mg every 3-7 days until optimal response. **Usual:** 20-30mg/day. **Max:** 100mg/day. Withdraw for 4-8 weeks every year in patients treated with pituitary irradiation. *Pediatrics:* Take with food. **11-15 yrs: Prolactin-Secreting Pituitary Adenomas: Initial:** 1.25-2.5mg/day. **Titrate:** Increase as tolerated. **Usual:** 2.5-10mg/day.	**W/P:** Caution with renal or hepatic dysfunction, psychosis, CVD, peptic ulcer, dementia. Discontinue with macroadenomas associated with rapid regrowth of tumor and increased prolactin levels and if severe headache or HTN develops. Risk of pulmonary infiltrates, pleural effusion, thickening of pleura, and retroperitoneal fibrosis with long-term use. Not for prevention of physiological lactation. Monitor BP for symptomatic hypotension and HTN. **Contra:** Uncontrolled HTN, ergot alkaloid sensitivity, postpartum with CVD unless withdrawal is medically contraindicated, pregnancy if treating hyperprolactinemia, HTN in pregnancy. **P/N:** Category B, not for use in nursing.	Headache, dizziness, GI effects, orthostatic hypotension, fatigue, arrhythmia, insomnia, hallucinations, abnormal involuntary movements, depression, syncope.

Table 17.1 PRESCRIBING INFORMATION FOR NEUROLOGICAL AGENTS *(cont.)*

NAME	FORM/ STRENGTH	DOSAGE	WARNINGS/PRECAUTIONS & CONTRAINDICATIONS	ADVERSE EFFECTS†
ANTIPARKINSONISM DRUGS *(cont.)*				
Carbidopa/ Entacapone/ Levodopa (Stalevo 50, Stalevo 100, Stalevo 150)	**Tab:** (Carbidopa/Levodopa/Entacapone): **Stalevo 50:** 12.5mg/50mg/200mg; **Stalevo 100:** 25mg/100mg/200mg; **Stalevo 150:** 37.5mg/150mg/200mg	**Adults: Currently Taking Carbidopa/Levodopa and Entacapone:** May switch directly to corresponding strength of levodopa/carbidopa. **Currently Taking Carbidopa/Levodopa but not Entacapone:** First titrate individually with carbidopa/levodopa product and entacapone product then transfer to corresponding dose. **Max:** 8 tabs/day.	**W/P:** Dyskinesia, mental disturbances, hypotension/syncope, hallucinations, rhabdomyolysis, hyperpyrexia, confusion, and fibrotic complications reported. Caution with biliary obstruction, severe cardiovascular or pulmonary disease, bronchial asthma, renal, hepatic or endocrine disease, chronic wide-angle glaucoma, history of MI with residual arrhythmias, peptic ulcer. Neuroleptic malignant syndrome reported with dose reductions or withdrawal. Avoid rapid withdrawal or abrupt dose reduction. May cause dark color to appear in saliva, urine, or sweat. May cause false (+) ketonuria, false (-) glucosuria (glucose-oxidase method), elevated LFTs, abnormal BUN, positive Coombs test. May depress prolactin secretion and increase growth hormone levels. **Contra:** MAOIs during or within 14 days of use, narrow-angle glaucoma, undiagnosed skin lesions, history of melanoma. **P/N:** Category C, caution in nursing.	Dyskinesia, hyperkinesia, hypokinesia, dizziness, nausea, diarrhea, abdominal pain, constipation, vomiting, urine discoloration, back pain, fatigue.
Carbidopa/Levodopa (Parcopa, Sinemet 10-100, Sinemet 25-100, Sinemet 25-250, Sinemet CR)	**(Parcopa) Tab, Disintegrating:** (Carbidopa-Levodopa) 10mg-100mg*, 25mg-100mg*, 25mg, 250mg*; **(Sinemet) Tab:** (Carbidopa-Levodopa) 10mg-100mg*, 25mg-100mg*, 25mg-250mg*; **Tab, Extended Release:** (Carbidopa-Levodopa) 25mg-100mg, 50mg-200mg*	**(Parcopa) Adults: ≥18yrs: 25mg-100mg tab: Initial:** 1 tab tid. **Titrate:** Increase by 1 tab qd or qod until 8 tabs/day. **10mg-100mg tab: Initial:** 1 tab tid-qid. **Titrate:** Increase 1 tab qd or qod until 2 tabs qid. 70-100mg/day carbidopa required. **Max:** 200mg/day carbidopa. Levodopa must be discontinued 12 hrs before starting carbidopa-levodopa. **(Sinemet) Adults: ≥18 yrs: Initial:** (25mg-100mg tab) 1 tab tid. **Titrate:** Increase by 1 tab qd or every other day until 8 tabs/day. 10mg-100mg **Tab: Initial:** 1 tab tid-qid. **Titrate:** Increase 1 tab qd or every other day until 2 tabs qid. 70-100mg/day carbidopa required. **Max:** 200mg/day carbidopa. **(Tab, Extended-Release) No Prior Levodopa Use: Initial:** 1 tab 50mg-200mg bid at intervals >6 hrs. **Titrate:** Increase or decrease dose or interval accordingly. Adjust dose every 3 days. **Usual:** 400-1600mg/day levodopa, given in 4-8 hr intervals while awake. **Conversion to Extended-Release Tabs:** see labeling.	**W/P:** Dyskinesias and mental disturbances may occur. Caution with severe cardiovascular or pulmonary disease, bronchial asthma, renal or hepatic disease, endocrine disease, chronic wide-angle glaucoma, peptic ulcer, and MI with residual arrhythmias. NMS reported during dose reduction or withdrawal. Dark color may appear in saliva, urine, or sweat. May cause false (+) ketonuria or false (-) glucosuria (glucose-oxidase method). **Contra:** MAOIs during or within 14 days of use, narrow-angle glaucoma, suspicious, undiagnosed skin lesions, history of melanoma. **P/N:** Category C, caution in nursing.	Dyskinesias, choreiform, dystonic, other involuntary movements, nausea, **dark saliva**, GI bleeding, confusion, agitation, dizziness, somnolence, dream abnormalities.

*Scored.   †Bold entries denote special dental considerations.

NAME	FORM/ STRENGTH	DOSAGE	WARNINGS/PRECAUTIONS & CONTRAINDICATIONS	ADVERSE EFFECTS†
Entacapone (Comtan)	**Tab:** 200mg	***Adults:*** 200mg with each levodopa/carbidopa dose. **Max:** 1600mg/day. Withdraw slowly for discontinuation.	**W/P:** Hypotension/syncope, diarrhea, hallucinations, dyskinesia, rhabdomyolysis, hyperpyrexia, confusion, and fibrotic complications may occur due to increased dopaminergic activity. Caution with hepatic impairment, biliary obstruction. Avoid rapid withdrawal or abrupt dose reduction. May impair mental and/or motor performance. **P/N:** Category C, caution with nursing.	Sweating, back pain, dyskinesia, hyperkinesia, hypokinesia, nausea, diarrhea, abdominal pain, urine discoloration.
Pergolide Mesylate (Permax)	**Tab:** 0.05mg*, 0.25mg*, 1mg*	***Adults:*** **Initial:** 0.05mg/ day for first 2 days. **Titrate:** Increase by 0.1- 0.15mg/day every 3rd day over next 12 days, then increase dose by 0.25mg/ day every 3rd day. **Max:** 5mg/day. Give in 3 divided doses. May reduce levodopa/carbidopa dose during titration.	**W/P:** Somnolence reported; discontinue if significant daytime sleepiness or sleeping episodes develop during daily activities. Symptomatic hypotension, hallucinosis reported. Caution and monitor with history of pleuritis, pleural effusion/fibrosis, pericarditis, pericardial effusion, cardiac valvulopathy or retroperitoneal fibrosis or if prone to arrhythmias. Avoid abrupt discontinuation. **P/N:** Category B, not for use in nursing.	Dyskinesia, hallucinations, somnolence, insomnia, nausea, constipation, diarrhea, dyspepsia, rhinitis.
Pramipexole Dihydrochloride (Mirapex)	**Tab:** 0.125mg, 0.25mg*, 0.5mg*, 1mg*, 1.5mg*	***Adults:*** **Initial:** 0.125mg tid. **Titrate:** Increase every 5-7 days according to dose titration table. **Maint:** 0.5-1.5mg tid. **CrCl >60mL/min: Initial:** 0.125mg tid. **Max:** 1.5mg tid. **CrCl 35-59mL/min: Initial:** 0.125mg bid. **Max:** 1.5mg bid. **CrCl 15-34mL/min: Initial:** 0.125mg qd. **Max:** 1.5mg qd.	**W/P:** Somnolence, symptomatic hypotension, hallucinations and rhabdomyolysis reported. Caution with renal insufficiency. May potentiate dyskinesia. May cause retinal pathology, fibrotic complications, withdrawal-emergent hyperpyrexia and confusion. Consider discontinuation if significant daytime sleepiness or sudden onset of sleep occurs during daily activities. **P/N:** Category C, not for use in nursing.	Nausea, dizziness, somnolence, insomnia, constipation, asthenia, hallucinations.
Ropinirole Hydrochloride (Requip)	**Tab:** 0.25mg, 0.5mg, 1mg, 2mg, 3mg, 4mg, 5mg	***Adults:*** **Parkinson's: Initial:** 0.25mg tid. **Titrate:** May increase weekly by 0.25mg/day (0.75mg/day) for 4 weeks. After week 4, may increase weekly by 1.5mg/day up to 9mg/day, then by 3mg/day weekly to 24mg/day. **Max:** 24mg/day. **Withdrawal:** Decrease dose to bid for 4 days, then qd for 3 days. **RLS: Initial:** 0.25mg qd, 1-3 hours before bedtime. **Titrate:** 0.5mg qd days 3-7, 1mg qd week 2, then increase by 0.5mg weekly. **Max:** 4mg.	**W/P:** Falling asleep during activities of daily living reported; if significant, discontinue or warn patient to refrain from dangerous activities. Syncope, symptomatic hypotension, and hallucinations reported. Caution with severe renal or hepatic dysfunction. May cause or exacerbate pre-existing dyskinesia. Augmentation and rebound in RLS reported. Avoid abrupt withdrawal. **P/N:** Category C, not for use in nursing.	Neuralgia, increased BUN, hallucinations, somnolence, vomiting, headache, sweating, asthenia, edema, fatigue, syncope, orthostatic symptoms.
Selegiline Hydrochloride (Eldepryl)	**Cap:** 5mg	***Adults:*** 5mg bid, at breakfast and lunch. **Max:** 10mg/day. May reduce levodopa/carbidopa by 10-30% after 2-3 days of therapy. May reduce further with continued therapy.	**W/P:** Do not exceed 10mg/day due to non-selective MAO inhibition. Decrease levodopa/carbidopa by 10-30% to prevent exacerbation of levodopa side effects. **Contra:** Concomitant meperidine, other opioids. **P/N:** Category C, not for use in nursing.	Nausea, dizziness, lightheadedness, fainting, abdominal pain, confusion, hallucinations, **dry mouth**.

Table 17.1 PRESCRIBING INFORMATION FOR NEUROLOGICAL AGENTS *(cont.)*

NAME	FORM/ STRENGTH	DOSAGE	WARNINGS/PRECAUTIONS & CONTRAINDICATIONS	ADVERSE EFFECTS†
ANTIPARKINSONISM DRUGS *(cont.)*				
Tolcapone (Tasmar)	**Tab:** 100mg, 200mg	**Adults: Initial:** 100mg tid. Use 200mg tid only if clinical benefit is justified. May need to decrease levodopa dose.	**W/P:** Risk of fatal, acute fulminant liver failure. Withdraw if patients fail to show benefit within 3 weeks of initiation. Discontinue if develop hepatotoxicity, and do not consider retreatment. Perform LFTs before therapy, then every 2 weeks for 1st year, every 4 weeks for next 6 months, then every 8 weeks thereafter. Perform LFTs before increase dose to 200mg tid. Avoid with liver disease or if LFTs ≥2X ULN. Caution with severe dyskinesia or dystonia. Hypotension/ syncope, rhabdomyolysis, hallucinations, confusion, diarrhea, hematuria reported. Fibrotic complications can occur. Avoid with liver dysfunction. Caution with severe renal dysfunction. Closely monitor when discontinuing therapy. **Contra:** Liver disease, patients withdrawn from therapy due to drug-induced hepatocellular injury. History of non-traumatic rhabdomyolysis, hyperpyrexia or confusion related to medication. **P/N:** Category C, caution in nursing.	Dyskinesia, nausea, dystonia, excessive dreaming, anorexia, muscle cramps, orthostatic complaints, diarrhea, confusion, hallucination, vomiting, constipation, fatigue, increased sweating, xerostomia, urine discoloration, hepatotoxicity.
Trihexyphenidyl Hydrochloride	**Sol:** 2mg/5mL; **Tab:** 2mg, 5mg	**Adults: Idiopathic Parkinsonism:** 1mg on Day 1. **Titrate:** Increase by 2mg every 3-5 days. **Usual:** 6-10mg/day. **Max:** 15mg/day. **Drug-Induced Parkinsonism: Initial:** 1mg. If extrapyramidal manifestations not controlled in a few hrs, increase dose until achieve control. **Usual:** 5-15mg/day. **Concomitant Levodopa:** Trihexyphenidyl dose may need reduction. **Usual:** 3-6mg/day. Divide total daily dose into 3 doses. May divide doses >10mg/day into 4 doses. Take with meals and at bedtime.	**W/P:** Monitor IOP. Caution with exposure in hot weather (esp. alcoholics), glaucoma, obstructive disease of GI or GU tract, prostatic hypertrophy, HTN, and cardiac, liver, or kidney disorders. Angle-closure glaucoma reported with long-term treatment. Neuroleptic Malignant Syndrome (NMS) reported with dose reduction or discontinuation. Avoid in tardive dyskinesia except in Parkinson's Disease. Use low initial dose with history of idiosyncrasy to other drugs or arteriosclerosis. Avoid abrupt withdrawal. **Contra:** Narrow angle glaucoma. **P/N:** Safety in pregnancy not known, caution in nursing.	**Dry mouth,** blurred vision, dizziness, nausea, nervousness, constipation, drowsiness, urinary hesitancy/retention, tachycardia, pupil dilation, increased intraocular tension, vomiting.
MUSCLE RELAXANTS AND ANTISPASTICS				
Aspirin/Carisoprodol (Soma Compound)	**Tab:** (Carisoprodol-ASA) 200mg-325mg	**Adults:** 1-2 tabs qid. **Pediatrics: ≥12 yrs:** 1-2 tabs qid.	**W/P:** First-dose idiosyncratic reactions reported (rare). Caution with liver or renal dysfunction, elderly, peptic ulcer, gastritis, addiction-prone patients and anticoagulant therapy. **Contra:** Acute intermittent porphyria, bleeding disorders. **P/N:** Category C, not for use in nursing.	Drowsiness, dizziness, vertigo, ataxia, nausea, vomiting, gastritis, occult bleeding, constipation, diarrhea.
Baclofen (Kemstro)	**Tab: (Generic)** 10mg, 20mg; **Tab: Disintegrating (ODT): (Kemstro)** 10mg, 20mg	**Adults: Initial:** 5mg tid for 3 days. **Titrate:** May increase dose by 5mg tid every 3 days. **Usual:** 40-80mg/day. **Max:** 80 mg/day (20mg qid). **Renal Impairment:** Reduce dose.	**W/P:** Caution with psychosis, schizophrenia, confusional states; may exacerbate conditions. Caution with bladder sphincter hypertonia, peptic ulceration, seizures, elderly, cerebrovascular disorder, respiratory failure, hepatic or renal failure.	Drowsiness, dizziness, weakness, fatigue, confusion, daytime sedation, headache, insomnia, hypotension, nausea, constipation, urinary frequency.

*Scored.   †Bold entries denote special dental considerations.

NAME	FORM/ STRENGTH	DOSAGE	WARNINGS/PRECAUTIONS & CONTRAINDICATIONS	ADVERSE EFFECTS†
Baclofen *(cont.)*		***Pediatrics:*** **≥12 yrs: Initial:** 5mg tid for 3 days. **Titrate:** May increase dose by 5mg tid every 3 days. **Usual:** 40-80mg/ day. **Max:** 80 mg/day (20mg qid). **Renal Impairment:** Reduce dose.	Abnormal AST, alkaline phosphatase and blood glucose reported. Caution when used to maintain locomotion or to obtain increased function. Decreased alertness with operating machinery. Has not significantly benefited stroke patients. Avoid abrupt discontinuation; reduce dose slowly over 1-2 weeks. **P/N:** Category C, caution in nursing.	
Carisoprodol (Soma)	**Tab:** 350mg	***Adults:*** 350mg tid and hs. ***Pediatrics:*** **≥12 yrs:** 350mg tid and hs.	**W/P:** First-dose idiosyncratic reactions reported (rare). Caution in addiction-prone patients. Caution with liver or renal dysfunction. **Contra:** Acute intermittent porphyria. **P/N:** Safety in pregnancy and nursing not known.	Drowsiness, dizziness, nausea, vomiting, tachycardia, postural hypotension, idiosyncratic reactions.
Chlorzoxazone (Parafon Forte DSC)	**Tab:** 500mg*	***Adults:*** **Usual:** 500mg tid-qid. **Titrate:** May increase to 750mg tid-qid.	**W/P:** Serious (including fatal) hepatocellular toxicity reported. Discontinue if develop signs of hepatotoxicity. Caution with history of drug allergies. **P/N:** Safety in pregnancy and nursing not known.	Drowsiness, dizziness, malaise, lightheadedness, overstimulation.
Cyclobenzaprine Hydrochloride (Flexeril)	**Tab:** 5mg, 10mg	***Adults:*** **Usual:** 5mg tid. Titrate: May increase to 10mg tid.**Mild Hepatic Dysfunction/Elderly: Initial:** 5mg qd, then slowly increase. **Moderate/Severe Hepatic Dysfunction:** Avoid use. Treatment should not exceed 2-3 weeks. ***Pediatrics:*** **≥15 yrs:** Usual: 5mg tid. **Titrate:** May increase to 10mg tid. **Mild Hepatic Dysfunction/Elderly: Initial:** 5mg qd, then slowly increase. **Moderate/Severe Hepatic Dysfunction:** Avoid use. Treatment should not exceed 2-3 weeks.	**W/P:** Caution with history of urinary retention, angle-closure glaucoma, increased IOP, hepatic dysfunction. Caution in elderly due to increased risk of CNS effects. May produce arrhythmias, sinus tachycardia and conduction time prolongation. May impair ability to drive. **Contra:** Acute recovery phase of MI, arrhythmias, heart block or conduction disturbances, CHF, hyperthyroidism, MAOI use during or within 14 days. **P/N:** Category B, caution in nursing.	Drowsiness, **dry mouth**, headache, fatigue.
Dantrolene Sodium (Dantrium)	**Cap:** 25mg, 50mg, 100mg	***Adults:*** **Chronic Spasticity: Initial:** 25mg qd for 7 days. **Titrate:** Increase to 25mg tid for 7 days, then 50mg tid for 7 days, then 100mg tid. **Max:** 100mg qid. If no further benefit at next higher dose, decrease to previous lower dose. **Malignant Hyperthermia: Pre-Op:** 4-8mg/kg/day given tid-qid for 1-2 days before surgery, with last dose given 3-4 hrs before surgery. **Post-Op Following Malignant Hyperthermia Crisis:** 4-8mg/kg/day given qid for 1-3 days. ***Pediatrics:*** **≥5 yrs: Chronic Spasticity: Initial:** 0.5mg/kg qd for 7 days.	**W/P:** Monitor LFTs at baseline, then periodically. Increased risk of hepatocellular disease in females and patients >35 yrs. Caution with pulmonary, cardiac, and liver dysfunction. Photosensitivity reaction may occur; limit sunlight exposure. **Contra:** Active hepatic disease, where spasticity is utilized to sustain upright posture and balance in locomotion, when spasticity is utilized to obtain or maintain increased function. **P/N:** Safety in nursing not known. Not for use in nursing.	Drowsiness, dizziness, weakness, malaise, fatigue, diarrhea, hepatitis, tachycardia, aplastic anemia, thrombocytopenia, depression, seizure.

Table 17.1 PRESCRIBING INFORMATION FOR NEUROLOGICAL AGENTS *(cont.)*

NAME	FORM/ STRENGTH	DOSAGE	WARNINGS/PRECAUTIONS & CONTRAINDICATIONS	ADVERSE EFFECTS†
MUSCLE RELAXANTS AND ANTISPASTICS *(cont.)*				
Dantrolene Sodium *(cont.)*		**Titrate:** Increase to 0.5mg/kg tid for 7 days, then 1mg/kg tid for 7 days, then 2mg/kg tid. **Max:** 100mg qid. If no further benefit at next higher dose, decrease to previous lower dose.		
Metaxalone (Skelaxin)	**Tab:** 800mg*	***Adults:*** 800mg tid-qid. ***Pediatrics:* >12 yrs:** 800mg tid-qid	**W/P:** Caution with pre-existing liver damage. Monitor hepatic function. False-positive Benedict's test reported. **Contra:** Tendency for drug-induced, hemolytic, and other anemias. Significant renal or hepatic impairment. **P/N:** Not for use in pregnancy or nursing.	Nausea, vomiting, GI upset, drowsiness, dizziness, headache, nervousness, leukopenia, hemolytic anemia, jaundice.
Methocarbamol (Robaxin)	**Inj:** 100mg/mL; **Tab:** 500mg, 750mg	***Adults:* (PO) Initial:** (500mg tab) 1500mg qid for 2-3 days. **Maint:** 1000mg qid. **Initial:** (750mg tab) 1500mg qid for 2-3 days. **Maint:** 750mg q4h or 1500mg tid. **Max:** 6gm/d for 2-3 days; 8gm/d if severe. **(Inj) Moderate Symptoms:** 10mL IV/IM. **IV Max Rate:** 3mL undiluted drug/min. **IM Max:** 5mL into each gluteal region. **Severe/ Post-Op Condition: Max:** 20-30mL/day up to 3 consecutive days. If feasible, continue with PO. **Tetanus:** 10-20mL up to 30mL. May repeat q6h until NG tube can be inserted. Continue with crushed tabs. **Max:** 24g/day PO. ***Pediatrics:* Tetanus: Initial:** 15mg/kg. Repeat q6h prn. Administer through tubing or IV. Safety and effctiveness in pediatric patients have not been established except tetanus.	**W/P:** May cause color interference in certain screening tests for 5-hydroxy-indoleacetic acid (5-HIAA) and vanillylmandelic acid (VMA). Caution in epilepsy with the injection. Injection rate should not exceed 3mL/min. Avoid extravasation with injection. **Contra:** (Inj) Renal pathology with injection due to propylene glycol content. **P/N:** Category C, caution in nursing.	Lightheadedness, dizziness, drowsiness, nausea, urticaria, pruritus, rash, conjunctivitis, nasal congestion, blurred vision, headache, fever, seizures, syncope, flushing.
Orphenadrine Citrate (Norflex)	**Inj:** 30mg/mL; **Tab, Extended Release:** 100mg	***Adults:* (Tab)** 100mg bid, in the am and pm. **(Inj)** 60mg IM/IV q12h.	**W/P:** Caution with tachycardia, cardiac decompensation, coronary insufficiency, cardiac arrhythmias. Monitor blood, urine, and LFTs periodically with prolonged use. Injection contains sodium bisulfite. **Contra:** Glaucoma, pyloric or duodenal obstruction, stenosing peptic ulcers, prostatic hypertrophy, bladder neck obstruction, cardiospasm, myasthenia gravis. **P/N:** Category C, safety in nursing not known.	**Dry mouth**, tachycardia, palpitation, urinary hesitancy/retention, blurred vision, pupil dilation, increased ocular tension, weakness, dizziness, constipation.

*Scored. †Bold entries denote special dental considerations.

NAME	FORM/ STRENGTH	DOSAGE	WARNINGS/PRECAUTIONS & CONTRAINDICATIONS	ADVERSE EFFECTS†
Tizanidine Hydrochloride (Zanaflex)	**Cap:** 2mg, 4mg, 6mg; **Tab:** 2mg*, 4mg*	**Adults: Initial:** 4mg single dose q6-8h. **Titrate:** Increase by 2-4mg. **Usual:** 8mg single dose q6-8h. **Max:** 3 doses/24h or 36mg/day.	**W/P:** May prolong QT interval. May cause liver damage; monitor baseline LFTs and at 1, 3, and 6 months. Retinal degeneration and corneal opacities reported. Caution with renal impairment or elderly. May cause hypotension; caution with antihypertensives. **P/N:** Category C, caution in nursing.	**Dry mouth**, somnolence, asthenia, dizziness, UTI, urinary frequency, flu-like syndrome, rhinitis.

VASCULAR HEADACHE SUPPRESSANTS

NAME	FORM/ STRENGTH	DOSAGE	WARNINGS/PRECAUTIONS & CONTRAINDICATIONS	ADVERSE EFFECTS†
Acetaminophen/ Dichloralphena-zone/Isometheptene Mucate (Midrin)	**Cap:** (APAP-Dichloral-phenazone-Isomethep-tene) 325mg-100mg-65mg	**Adults: Migraine:** 2 caps, then 1 cap every hr until relieved. **Max:** 5 caps/12hrs. **Tension Headache:** 1-2 caps q4h. **Max:** 8 caps/day.	**W/P:** Caution with HTN, periph-eral vascular disease, or recent cardiovascular attacks. **Contra:** Glaucoma, severe renal disease, HTN, organic heart disease, hepatic disease, concomitant MAOI therapy. **P/N:** Safety in pregnancy and nursing are not known.	Transient dizziness, skin rash.
Almotriptan Malate (Axert)	**Tab:** 6.25mg, 12.5mg	**Adults: ≥18 yrs: Initial:** 6.25-12.5mg at onset of headache. May repeat after 2 hrs. **Max:** 2 doses/24 hrs. **Hepatic/Renal Impair-ment:** 6.25mg at onset of headache. **Max:** 12.5mg/24 hrs. Safety of treating >4 headaches/30 days not known.	**W/P:** Confirm diagnosis. Supervise first dose and monitor cardiac function in those at risk of CAD (eg, HTN, hypercholesterolemia, smoker, obesity, diabetes, CAD family history, postmenopausal women, males >40 yrs). Monitor cardiovascular function with long term intermittent use. May cause vasospastic reactions or cerebrovascular events. Caution with renal or hepatic dysfunction. Avoid in elderly. **Contra:** Ischemic heart disease, coronary artery vasospasm, other significant CVD, uncontrolled HTN, within 24 hrs of another 5-HT₁ agonist or ergot type agent, hemiple-gic or basilar migraine. **P/N:** Category C, caution in nursing.	Nausea, somnolence, headache, paresthesia, **dry mouth**, coronary artery vasospasm, MI, ventricular tachycardia, fibrillation.
Aspirin/Caffeine/Or-phenadrine Citrate (Norgesic, Norgesic Forte)	**Tab:** (Orphenadrine-ASA-Caffeine) 25mg-385mg-30mg; **Tab:** (Forte) 50mg-770mg-60mg*	**Adults:** 1-2 tabs tid-qid. **(Forte)** 1/2-1 tab tid-qid.	**W/P:** Reye's syndrome may develop with chickenpox, influenza, or flu symptoms. Extreme caution with peptic ulcers and coagulation abnormalities. Monitor blood, urine, and LFT's periodically with prolonged use. **Contra:** Glaucoma, pyloric or duodenal obstruction, achalasia, prostatic hypertrophy, bladder neck obstruction, myasthenia gravis. **P/N:** Safety in pregnancy and nursing not known.	Tachycardia, urinary hesi-tancy/retention, **dry mouth**, blurred vision, increased intraocular tension, nausea, vomiting, headache, dizziness, constipation, drowsiness, urticaria, GI hemorrhage.
Caffeine/Ergotamine Tartrate (Cafergot)	**Sup:** (Ergotamine-Caf-feine) 2mg-100mg; **Tab:** (Ergotamine-Caf-feine) 1mg-100mg	**Adults: (Sup)** Insert 1 sup rectally at start of attack. Repeat after 1 hr if needed for full relief. **Max:** 2 sups/attack and 5 sups/week. May give at bedtime as short-term preventive measure. **(Tab)** 2 tabs at start of attack. Repeat 1 tab every 1/2 hr prn. **Max:** 6 tabs/attack, 10 tabs/week. May give at bedtime as short-term preventive measure.	**(Sup) Serious and life-threatening peripheral ischemia associated with concomitant potent CYP450 3A4 inhibitors (eg, protease inhibi-tors, macrolide antibiotics). W/P: (Sup)** Do not exceed recommended dosage. Ergotism manifested by intense arterial vaso-constriction producing peripheral vascular ischemia; progression can lead to gangrene. Rectal or anal ulcers reported with abuse or long-term use. **(Tab)** Do not exceed recommended dosage.	Precordial distress, transient tachycardia or bradycardia, nausea, vomiting, localized edema, itching, numbness/tingling of fingers/toes, muscle pains, leg weakness.

Table 17.1 PRESCRIBING INFORMATION FOR NEUROLOGICAL AGENTS *(cont.)*

NAME	FORM/ STRENGTH	DOSAGE	WARNINGS/PRECAUTIONS & CONTRAINDICATIONS	ADVERSE EFFECTS†
VASCULAR HEADACHE SUPPRESSANTS *(cont.)*				
Caffeine/Ergotamine Tartrate *(cont.)*			**Contra:** Concomitant use with potent CYP3A4 inhibitors (eg, ritonavir, nelfinavir, indinavir, erythromycin, clarithromycin, troleandomycin, ketoconazole, itraconazole). Pregnancy, peripheral vascular disease, CHD, HTN, hepatic or renal dysfunction, sepsis. **P/N:** Safety in pregnancy and nursing not known.	
Dihydroergotamine Mesylate (D.H.E. 45)	**Inj:** 1mg/mL	***Adults:*** 1mL IV/IM/SC. May repeat at 1 hr intervals. **Max:** 3mL/24hrs IM/SC or 2mL/24hrs IV and 6mL/week.	**Serious and life-threatening peripheral ischemia reported with potent CYP450 3A4 inhibitors (eg, protease inhibitors, macrolides). Elevated levels of dihydroergotamine increases risk of vasospasm leading to cerebral ischemia or ischemia of the extremities. Concomitant use with CYP450 3A4 inhibitors is contraindicated.** **W/P:** Confirm migraine diagnosis. Risk of adverse cardiac, cerebrovascular, and vasospastic events and fatalities. Avoid with cardiac risk factors (eg, HTN, hypercholesterolemia, smoker, obesity, DM, strong family history of CAD, females who are surgically/physiologically postmenopausal, or males >40 yrs) unless cardiovascular evaluation is done. Perform cardiovascular monitoring with long-term use. Significant BP elevations reported. **Contra:** Ergot alkaloids hypersensitivity, ischemic heart disease, coronary artery vasospasm (eg, Prinzmetal's variant angina), uncontrolled HTN, hemiplegic or basilar migraine, peripheral artery disease, sepsis, following vascular surgery, severe renal/hepatic dysfunction, pregnancy, nursing, with potent CYP3A4 inhibitors (eg, ritonavir, nelfinavir, indinavir, erythromycin, clarithromycin, troleandomycin, ketoconazole, itraconazole), concomitant peripheral and central vasoconstrictors, and within 24 hrs after taking 5-HT₁ agonists, methysergide, ergotamine-containing, or ergot-type agents. **P/N:** Category X, contraindicated in nursing.	Vasospasm, angina, paraesthesia, HTN, dizziness, anxiety, dyspnea, headache, flushing, diarrhea, rash, increased sweating.
Eletriptan Hydrobromide (Relpax)	**Tab:** 20mg, 40mg	***Adults:*** ≥18 yrs: **Initial:** 20 or 40mg at onset of headache. If recurs after initial relief, may repeat after 2 hrs. **Max:** 40mg/dose or 80mg/day. Safety of treating >3 headaches/30 days not known. **Severe Hepatic Impairment:** Avoid use. Avoid within 72 hrs of potent CYP3A4 inhibitors.	**W/P:** Confirm diagnosis. Supervise 1st dose and monitor cardiac function in those at risk of CAD (eg, HTN, hypercholesterolemia, smoker, obesity, diabetes, CAD family history, postmenopausal women, males >40 yrs). Consider ECG during interval immediately following initial administration in patients with CAD risk factors. Monitor cardiac function in intermittent long-term users with CAD risk factors. Serious adverse cardiac events, increased BP, cerebrovascular events, vasospastic reactions reported.	Asthenia, chest tightness, dizziness, **dry mouth**, headache, nausea, paresthesia, somnolence, **pain/pressure/heaviness in precordium/throat/jaw.**

*Scored. †Bold entries denote special dental considerations.

NAME	FORM/ STRENGTH	DOSAGE	WARNINGS/PRECAUTIONS & CONTRAINDICATIONS	ADVERSE EFFECTS†
Eletriptan Hydrobromide *(cont.)*			Caution in elderly. Possible long-term ophthalmic effects. **Contra:** Ischemic heart disease, coronary artery vasospasm (eg, Prinzmetal's angina) or other significant underlying cardio-vascular disease, peripheral vascular disease, cerebrovascular syndromes, uncontrolled HTN, hemiplegic or basilar migraine, use within 24 hrs of other 5-HT$_1$ agonist or ergot-type agent (eg, dihydroergotamine, methy-sergide), severe hepatic impairment. **P/N:** Category C, caution in nursing.	
Frovatriptan Succinate (Frova)	**Tab:** 2.5mg	***Adults:*** **≥18 yrs:** 2.5mg with fluids. If headache recurs after initial relief, may repeat after 2 hrs. **Max:** 7.5mg/day. Safety of treating >4 headaches/30 days not known.	**W/P:** Confirm diagnosis. Supervise 1st dose and monitor cardiac function in those at risk of CAD (eg, HTN, hypercholesterolemia, smoker, obesity, diabetes, CAD family history, postmenopausal women, males >40 yrs). Serious adverse cardiac events, cerebrovascular events, vasospastic reactions reported with 5-HT$_1$ ago-nists. May bind to melanin in the eye; possibility of long-term effects. **Con-tra:** Ischemic heart disease, coronary artery vasospasm (eg, Prinzmetal's angina), significant cardiovascular disease, cerebrovascular syndromes, peripheral vascular disease, uncontrolled HTN, hemiplegic or basilar migraine, use within 24 hrs of treatment with another 5-HT$_1$ agonist or ergot-type agent. **P/N:** Category C, caution in nursing.	Dizziness, headache, paresthesia, **dry mouth**, dyspepsia, fatigue, hot or cold sensation, chest pain, skeletal pain, flushing.
Naratriptan Hydrochloride (Amerge)	**Tab:** 1mg, 2.5mg	***Adults:*** **≥18 yrs:** 1mg or 2.5mg taken with fluids; may repeat dose once after 4 hrs. **Max:** 5mg/24 hrs. **Mild-Moderate Re-nal/Hepatic Impairment: Initial:** Lower dose. **Max:** 2.5mg/24 hrs. Safety of treating >4 headaches/30 days not known.	**W/P:** Confirm diagnosis. Supervise 1st dose and monitor cardiac function in those at risk of CAD (eg, HTN, hypercholesterolemia, smoker, obesity, diabetes, CAD family history, postmenopausal women, males >40 yrs). Monitor cardiovascular function with long term intermittent use. May cause vasospastic reactions or cerebrovascular events. Caution with renal or hepatic dysfunction. Avoid in elderly. **Contra:** Uncontrolled HTN, ischemic cardiac, cerebrovascular or peripheral vascular syndromes, other significant CVD, severe renal or hepatic impairment and basilar or hemiplegic migraine. Within 24 hrs of another 5-HT$_1$ agonist, ergotamine-containing or ergot containing drug (dihydroergotamine or methysergide). **P/N:** Category C, caution in nursing.	Paresthesias, dizziness, drowsiness, malaise/fa-tigue, **throat and neck symptoms (eg, pain/pres-sure sensation)**.
Rizatriptan Benzoate (Maxalt, Maxalt-MLT)	**Tab:** 5mg, 10mg; **Tab, Disintegrating: (MLT)** 5mg, 10mg	***Adults:*** **≥18 yrs:** 5-10mg, may repeat q2h. **Max:** 30mg/24 hrs. Safety of treating >4 headaches/30 days not known. **MLT:** Dissolve on tongue without water. **Concomitant Proprano-lol:** 5mg, up to 3 doses/24 hrs.	**W/P:** Confirm diagnosis. Supervise 1st dose and monitor cardiac function in those at risk of CAD (eg, HTN, hypercholesterolemia, smoker, obesity, diabetes, CAD family history, postmenopausal women, males >40 yrs). Serious adverse cardiac events, cerebrovascular events, vasospastic reactions, hypertensive crisis, and fatalities reported with 5-HT$_1$ ago-nists. Disintegrating tabs contain	Paresthesia, **dry mouth**, nausea, dizziness, somno-lence, asthenia/fatigue.

Table 17.1 PRESCRIBING INFORMATION FOR NEUROLOGICAL AGENTS *(cont.)*

NAME	FORM/ STRENGTH	DOSAGE	WARNINGS/PRECAUTIONS & CONTRAINDICATIONS	ADVERSE EFFECTS[†]
VASCULAR HEADACHE SUPPRESSANTS *(cont.)*				
Rizatriptan Benzoate *(cont.)*			phenylalanine. Caution with renal dialysis and hepatic dysfunction. **Contra:** Ischemic heart disease, coronary artery vasospasm (eg, Prinzmetal's angina), uncontrolled HTN, significant cardiovascular disease, hemiplegic or basilar migraine, MAOI use within 14 days, other 5-HT$_1$ agonist or ergot-type agent use within 24 hrs. **P/N:** Category C, caution in nursing.	
Sumatriptan (Imitrex)	**Inj:** 6mg/0.5mL; **Nasal Spray:** 5mg, 20mg [0.1mL 6^s]; **Tab:** 25mg, 50mg, 100mg [9^s]	**Adults: ≥18 yrs: (Inj) Initial:** 6mg SC; may repeat after 1 hr. **Max:** 12mg/24 hrs. **(Spray)** 5mg, 10mg, or 20mg single dose; may repeat after 2 hrs. **Max:** 40mg/24 hrs. **(Tab) Initial:** 25-100mg; may repeat after 2 hrs. **Max:** 200mg/24 hrs. May give up to 100mg/day of tabs after initial inj dose. **Hepatic Disease: Max:** 50mg/single dose. Safety of treating >4 headaches/30 days not known.	**W/P:** Confirm diagnosis. Supervise first dose and monitor cardiac function in those at risk of CAD (eg, HTN, hypercholesterolemia, smoker, obesity, diabetes, CAD family history, postmenopausal women, males >40 yrs). Monitor cardiac function in intermittent long-term users with CAD risk factors. Serious adverse cardiac events, cerebrovascular events, vasospastic reactions reported. Avoid in elderly. Caution with hepatic or renal impairment, history of seizures or brain lesions. Possible long-term ophthalmic effects. Reconsider diagnosis before 2nd dose. **Contra:** History, symptoms, or signs of ischemic cardiac, cerebrovascular, or peripheral vascular syndromes. Other significant CVD, uncontrolled HTN, hemiplegic or basilar migraine, severe hepatic impairment, MAOIs during or within 2 weeks of use, within 24 hrs of ergotamine-containing agents, ergot-type agents, or other 5-HT$_1$ agonists. **P/N:** Category C, caution in nursing.	Tingling, burning sensation, flushing, **chest/mouth/ tongue discomfort**, injection site reaction, numbness, weakness, neck pain/stiffness.
Zolmitriptan (Zomig, Zomig-ZMT)	**Nasal Spray:** 5mg [0.1mL 6^s]; **Tab:** 2.5mg*; 5mg; **Tab, Disintegrating:** (ZMT) 2.5mg, 5mg	**Adults: ≥18 yrs: (Spray)** 5mg single dose; may repeat once after 2 hours. **Max:** 10mg/24 hrs. Safety of treating >4 headaches/30 days unknown. **(Tab) Initial:** 2.5mg or lower (2.5mg tab may be broken in 1/2), may repeat after 2 hrs. **Max:** 10mg/24 hrs. Safety of treating >3 headaches in 30 days is unknown. **(ZMT)** Dissolve on tongue without water. **Hepatic Impairment:** Use low dose and monitor blood pressure.	**W/P:** Confirm diagnosis. Supervise 1st dose and monitor cardiac function in those at risk of CAD (eg, HTN, hypercholesterolemia, smoker, obesity, diabetes, CAD family history, postmenopausal women, males >40 yrs). Serious adverse cardiac events, cerebrovascular events, vasospastic reactions reported with 5-HT$_1$ agonists. Disintegrating tabs contain phenylalanine. Caution with hepatic dysfunction. Reconsider diagnosis before 2nd dose. **Contra:** Ischemic heart disease, coronary artery vasospasm (eg, Prinzmetal's angina), uncontrolled HTN, other significant cardiovascular disease, hemiplegic or basilar migraine, MAOI use during or within 14 days, other 5-HT$_1$ agonist or ergot-type agent use within 24 hrs. **P/N:** Category C, caution in nursing.	Paresthesia, asthenia, warm/cold sensation, **neck/throat/jaw pain**, **dry mouth**, nausea, dizziness, somnolence, **unusual taste** (nasal spray).

*Scored.   †Bold entries denote special dental considerations.

Table 17.2: DRUG INTERACTIONS FOR NEUROLOGICAL AGENTS

ALZHEIMER'S DRUGS

Donepezil Hydrochloride (Aricept)

Anticholinergic medications	May interfere with anticholinergic medications.
Cholinergic agonists	Synergistic effect with cholinergic agonists (eg, bethanechol).
CYP2D6 inducers	CYP2D6 inducers (eg, phenytoin, carbamazepine, dexamethasone, rifampin, phenobarbital) may increase elimination rate.
CYP3A4 inducers	CYP3A4 inducers (eg, phenytoin, carbamazepine, dexamethasone, rifampin, phenobarbital) may increase elimination rate.
Neuromuscular blockers	Synergistic effect with neuromuscular blocking agents (eg, succinylcholine).

Galantamine (Razadyne, Razadyne ER)

Anticholinergics	Potential to interfere with anticholinergics.
Cholinergic agonists	Synergistic effect with cholinergic agonists (eg, bethanechol).
Cholinesterase inhibitors	Synergistic effect with other cholinesterase inhibitors.
Cimetidine	Increased levels with cimetidine, ketoconazole, and paroxetine.
Drugs that slow heart rate	Caution with drugs that slow heart rate due to vagotonic effects.
Ketoconazole	Increased levels ketoconazole.
Neuromuscular blockers	Synergistic effect with similar neuromuscular blockers.
NSAIDs	Monitor for GI bleed with NSAIDs.
Paroxetine	Increased levels with paroxetine.
Succinylcholine	Synergistic effect with succinylcholine.

Memantine Hydrochloride (Namenda)

NMDA antagonists	Caution with other NMDA antagonists (eg, amantadine, ketamine, dextromethorphan).
Renally-excreted drugs	Other renally-excreted drugs (eg, HCTZ, triamterene, metformin, cimetidine, ranitidine, quinidine, nicotine) may alter levels of both agents.
Urinary alkalinizers	Caution with urinary alkalinizers (eg, carbonic anhydrase inhibitors, sodium bicarbonate).

Rivastigmine (Exelon)

Anticholinergics	May block effects of anticholinergics.
Cholinergic agonists	May be synergistic with cholinergic agonists (eg, bethanechol).
Neuromuscular blockers	May be synergistic with similar neuromuscular blockers.
Succinylcholine	May be synergistic with succinylcholine. May exaggerate succinylcholine-type muscle relaxation during anesthesia.

Tacrine (Cognex)

Anticholinergics	May antagonize anticholinergics.

Table 17.2: DRUG INTERACTIONS FOR NEUROLOGICAL AGENTS *(cont.)*

ALZHEIMER'S DRUGS *(cont.)*

Tacrine (Cognex) *(cont.)*

Cholinergic agonists	May potentiate cholinergic agonists.
Cholinesterase inhibitors	May potentiate cholinesterase inhibitors.
Cimetidine	Increased levels with cimetidine.
CYP450	May interact with drugs metabolized by CYP450.
Fluvoxamine	Fluvoxamine increases levels.
NSAIDs	Monitor for GI disease with NSAIDs.
Succinylcholine	May potentiate succinylcholine.
Theophylline	May potentiate theophylline.

ANTICONVULSANTS

Carbamazepine (Carbatrol, Tegretol, Tegretol-XR)

Alprazolam	Decreases levels of alprazolam.
APAP	Decreases levels of APAP.
Clomipramine	Increases plasma levels of clomipramine.
Clonazepam	Decreases levels of clonazepam.
Clozapine	Decreases levels of clozapine.
Contraceptives, oral	Decreases oral contraceptive levels and effectiveness.
CYP3A4 inhibitors	Metabolism is inhibited by CYP3A4 inhibitors (eg, cimetidine, macrolides, etc.).
CYP3A4 inducers	Metabolism is induced by CYP3A4 inducers (eg, rifampin, phenytoin, etc.).
Dicumarol	Decreases levels of dicumarol.
Diluents	Do not give suspension with diluents.
Doxycycline	Decreases levels of doxycycline.
Ethosuximide	Decreases levels of ethosuximide.
Haloperidol	Decreases levels of haloperidol.
Lamotrigine	Decreases levels of lamotrigine.
Lithium	Increased risk of neurotoxic side effects with lithium.
MAOIs	Avoid MAOIs.
Medicinal liquids	Do not give suspension with other medicinal liquids.
Methsuximide	Decreases levels of methsuximide.
Phensuximide	Decreases levels of phensuximide.
Phenytoin	Increases/decreases plasma levels of phenytoin.
Primidone	Increases plasma levels of primidone.
Theophylline	Decreases levels of theophylline.

ANTICONVULSANTS *(cont.)*

Carbamazepine (Carbatrol, Tegretol, Tegretol-XR) *(cont.)*

Tiagabine	Decreases levels of tiagabine.
Topiramate	Decreases levels of topiramate.
Valproate	Decreases levels of valproate.
Warfarin	Decreases levels of warfarin.

Clonazepam[CIV] (Klonopin, Klonopin Wafers)

Alcohol	Alcohol potentiates CNS-depressant effects.
Antianxiety agents	Antianxiety agents potentiate CNS-depressant effects.
Anticonvulsant drugs	Anticonvulsant drugs potentiate CNS-depressant effects.
Barbiturates	Barbiturates potentiate CNS-depressant effects.
Butyrophenone antipsychotics	Butyrophenone antipsychotics potentiate CNS-depressant effects.
CYP3A inhibitors	Caution with CYP3A inhibitors (eg, oral antifungals).
CYP450 inducers	Decreased serum levels with CYP450 inducers (eg, phenytoin, carbamazepine, phenobarbital).
MAOIs	MAOIs potentiate CNS-depressant effects.
Narcotics	Narcotics potentiate CNS-depressant effects.
Nonbarbiturate hypnotics	Nonbarbiturate hypnotics potentiate CNS-depressant effects.
Phenothiazines	Phenothiazines potentiate CNS-depressant effects.
TCAs	TCAs potentiate CNS-depressant effects.
Thioxanthene	Thioxanthene potentiates CNS-depressant effects.

Diazepam[CIV] (Diastat, Valium)

Alcohol	Avoid alcohol.
Antidepressants	Other antidepressants may potentiate effects.
Barbiturates	Barbiturates may potentiate effects.
Cimetidine	Delayed clearance with cimetidine.
CNS depressants	Avoid other CNS-depressants.
Flumazenil	Risk of seizure with flumazenil.
MAOIs	MAOIs may potentiate effects.
Narcotics	Narcotics may potentiate effects.
Phenothiazines	Phenothiazines may potentiate effects.

Divalproex Sodium (Depakote, Depakote ER, Depakote Sprinkles)

Alcohol	CNS depression with alcohol.
Amitriptyline	Potentiates amitriptyline.

Table 17.2: DRUG INTERACTIONS FOR NEUROLOGICAL AGENTS *(cont.)*

ANTICONVULSANTS *(cont.)*

Divalproex Sodium (Depakote, Depakote ER, Depakote Sprinkles) *(cont.)*

ASA	Efficacy potentiated by ASA.
Carbamazepine	Potentiates carbamazepine. Efficacy reduced by carbamazepine.
Clonazepam	Clonazepam may induce absence status in patients with absence type seizures.
CNS depressants	CNS depression with other CNS depressants.
Diazepam	Potentiates diazepam.
Ethosuximide	Potentiates ethosuximide.
Felbamate	Efficacy potentiated by felbamate.
Lamotrigine	Potentiates lamotrigine.
Lorazepam	Potentiates lorazepam.
Nortriptyline	Potentiates nortriptyline.
Phenobarbital	Potentiates phenobarbital. Efficacy reduced by phenobarbital.
Phenytoin	Potentiates phenytoin. Efficacy reduced by phenytoin.
Primidone	Potentiates primidone. Efficacy reduced by primidone.
Rifampin	Efficacy reduced by rifampin.
Tolbutamide	Potentiates tolbutamide.
Warfarin	Monitor PT/INR with warfarin.
Zidovudine	Potentiates zidovudine.

Ethosuximide (Zarontin)

Phenytoin	May increase phenytoin levels.
Valproic acid	Valproic acid may alter levels.

Felbamate (Felbatol)

Carbamazepine metabolite	Increases plasma levels of active carbamazepine metabolite. Decreases carbamazepine levels. Decreased felbamate levels with carbamazepine.
Contraceptives, oral	Caution with oral contraceptives.
Phenobarbital	Increases plasma levels of phenobarbital. Decreased felbamate levels with phenobarbital.
Phenytoin	Increases plasma levels of phenytoin. Decreased felbamate levels with phenytoin.
Valproate	Increases plasma levels of valproate.

Fosphenytoin Sodium (Cerebyx)

Alcohol	Increased levels with acute alcohol intake. Decreased levels with chronic alcohol abuse.
Amiodarone	Increased levels with amiodarone.
Anticoagulants	Decreases efficacy of anticoagulants.

ANTICONVULSANTS *(cont.)*

Fosphenytoin Sodium (Cerebyx) *(cont.)*

Carbamazepine	Decreased levels with carbamazepine.
Chloramphenicol	Increased levels with chloramphenicol.
Chlordiazepoxide	Increased levels with chlordiazepoxide.
Cimetidine	Increased levels with cimetidine.
Contraceptives, oral	Decreases efficacy of oral contraceptives.
Corticosteroids	Decreases efficacy of corticosteroids.
Coumarin	Decreases efficacy of coumarin.
Diazepam	Increased levels with diazepam.
Dicumarol	Increased levels with dicumarol.
Digitoxin	Decreases efficacy of digitoxin.
Disulfiram	Increased levels with disulfiram.
Doxycycline	Decreases efficacy of doxycycline.
Estrogens	Increased levels with estrogens. Decreases efficacy of estrogens.
Ethosuximide	Increased levels with ethosuximide.
Fluoxetine	Increased levels with fluoxetine.
Furosemide	Decreases efficacy of furosemide.
H_2-antagonists	Increased levels with H_2-antagonists.
Halothane	Increased levels with halothane.
Isoniazid	Increased levels with isoniazid.
Methylphenidate	Increased levels with methylphenidate.
Phenobarbital	Variable effects (increase or decrease levels) with phenobarbital.
Phenothiazines	Increased levels with phenothiazines.
Phenylbutazone	Increased levels with phenylbutazone.
Quinidine	Decreases efficacy of quinidine.
Reserpine	Decreased levels with reserpine.
Rifampin	Decreases efficacy of rifampin.
Salicylates	Increased levels with salicylates.
Serum albumin	Caution with drugs highly bound to serum albumin.
Sodium valproate	Variable effects (increase or decrease levels) with sodium valproate.
Succinimides	Increased levels with succinimides.
Sulfonamides	Increased levels with sulfonamides.
Theophylline	Decreases efficacy of theophylline.
Tolbutamide	Increased levels with tolbutamide.
Trazodone	Increased levels with trazodone.

Table 17.2: DRUG INTERACTIONS FOR NEUROLOGICAL AGENTS *(cont.)*

ANTICONVULSANTS *(cont.)*

Fosphenytoin Sodium (Cerebyx) *(cont.)*

Tricyclic antidepressants	TCAs may precipitate seizures.
Valproic acid	Variable effects (increase or decrease levels) with valproic acid.
Vitamin D	Decreases efficacy of vitamin D.

Gabapentin (Neurontin)

Antacids	Take 2 hrs after antacids.
Morphine	Increased levels with controlled-release morphine.

Lamotrigine (Lamictal, Lamictal CD)

Carbamazepine	Decreased levels with carbamazepine.
Dihydrofolate reductase	Inhibits dihydrofolate reductase.
Folate inhibitors	May potentiate folate inhibitors.
Phenobarbital	Decreased levels with phenobarbital.
Phenytoin	Decreased levels with phenytoin.
Primidone	Decreased levels with primidone.
Valproic acid	Risk of life-threatening rash with valproic acid. Lamotrigine decreases valproic acid levels; valproic acid increases lamotrigine levels.

Lorazepam[CIV] (Ativan)

Alcohol	CNS-depressant effects with alcohol. Diminished tolerance to alcohol.
Barbiturates	CNS-depressant effects with barbiturates.
CNS depressants	Diminished tolerance to other CNS depressants.

Mephobarbital (Mebaral)

Alcohol	Additive CNS depression with alcohol.
Anticoagulants, oral	Decreases effects of oral anticoagulants.
CNS depressants	Additive CNS depression with other CNS depressants.
Contraceptives, oral	Decreases effects of oral contraceptives.
Corticosteroids	Increases corticosteroid metabolism.
Doxycycline	Decreases half-life of doxycycline.
Griseofulvin	Interferes with griseofulvin absorption.
MAOIs	MAOIs may prolong effects.
Phenytoin	May alter phenytoin metabolism.
Sodium valproate	Sodium valproate decreases metabolism.
Valproic acid	Valproic acid decreases metabolism.

ANTICONVULSANTS *(cont.)*

Methsuximide (Celontin Kapseals)

Anticonvulsants	May interact with other anticonvulsants; monitor serum levels periodically.

Oxcarbazepine (Trileptal)

Alcohol	Additive sedative effect with alcohol.
Carbamazepine	Carbamazepine may decrease levels.
Felodipine	Decreased plasma levels of felodipine.
Contraceptives, oral	Decreased plasma levels of oral contraceptives.
Phenobarbital	Phenobarbital may decrease levels. Increased plasma levels of phenobarbital.
Phenytoin	Phenytoin may decrease levels. Increased plasma levels of phenytoin.
Verapamil	Verapamil may decrease levels.
Valproic acid	Valproic acid may decrease levels.

Pentobarbital Sodium[CII] (Nembutal Sodium)

Anticoagulants, oral	May decrease levels of oral anticoagulants. Dosage adjustments may be required for anticoagulants.
CNS depressants	May produce additive CNS depression with other CNS depressants (eg, other sedatives/hypnotics, antihistamines, tranquilizers, alcohol).
Corticosteroids	May decrease levels of corticosteroids. Dosage adjustments may be required for corticosteroids.
Doxycycline	May decrease levels of doxycycline.
Estradiol	May decrease effects of estradiol; alternative contraceptive method should be suggested.
Griseofulvin	May decrease levels of griseofulvin.
MAOIs	Prolonged effect with MAOIs.
Phenytoin	Variable effects on phenytoin; monitor blood levels and adjust dose appropriately.
Sodium valproate	Increased levels with sodium valproate; monitor blood levels and adjust dose appropriately.
Valproic acid	Increased levels with valproic acid; monitor blood levels and adjust dose appropriately.

Phenobarbital[CIV]

Alcohol	May be potentiated by alcohol.
Anticoagulants, oral	Decreases effects of oral anticoagulants.
Antihistamines	May be potentiated by antihistamines.
CNS depressants	May be potentiated by other CNS depressants.

Table 17.2: DRUG INTERACTIONS FOR NEUROLOGICAL AGENTS (cont.)

ANTICONVULSANTS (cont.)

Phenobarbital[CIV] (cont.)

Contraceptives, oral	Decreases effects of oral contraceptives.
Corticosteroids	Increases corticosteroid metabolism.
Doxycycline	Decreases half-life of doxycycline.
Griseofulvin	Decreases absorption of griseofulvin.
MAOIs	May be potentiated by MAOIs.
Phenytoin	May alter phenytoin metabolism.
Sedative/hypnotics	May be potentiated by sedative/hypnotics.
Sodium valproate	Increased levels with sodium valproate.
Tranquilizers	May be potentiated by tranquilizers.
Valproic acid	Increased levels with valproic acid.

Phenytoin (Dilantin Infatabs, Dilantin-125, Dilantin Kapseals, Phenytek) and Phenytoin Sodium, Extended (Dilantin

Alcohol	Increased levels with acute alcohol intake. Decreased levels with chronic alcohol abuse.
Amiodarone	Increased levels with amiodarone.
Barbiturates	Increased risk of phenytoin hypersensitivity with barbiturates.
Calcium antacids	Calcium antacids decrease absorption; space dosing.
Carbamazepine	Decreased levels with carbamazepine.
Chloramphenicol	Increased levels with chloramphenicol.
Chlordiazepoxide	Increased levels with chlordiazepoxide.
Contraceptives, oral	Decreases effects of oral contraceptives.
Corticosteroids	Decreases effects of corticosteroids.
Coumarin anticoagulants	Decreases effects of coumarin anticoagulants.
Diazepam	Increased levels with diazepam.
Dicumarol	Increased levels with dicumarol.
Digitoxin	Decreases effects of digitoxin.
Disulfiram	Increased levels with disulfiram.
Doxycycline	Decreases effects of doxycycline.
Estrogens	Increased levels with estrogens. Decreases effects of estrogens.
Furosemide	Decreases effects of furosemide.
H_2-antagonists	Increased levels with H_2-antagonists
Halothane	Increased levels with halothane.

ANTICONVULSANTS *(cont.)*

Phenytoin (Dilantin Infatabs, Dilantin-125) and **Phenytoin Sodium, Extended** (Dilantin Kapseals, Phenytek) *(cont.)*

Isoniazid	Increased levels with isoniazid.
Methylphenidate	Increased levels with methylphenidate.
Moban	Contains calcium ions that interfere with absorption.
Oxazolidinediones	Increased risk of phenytoin hypersensitivity with oxazolidinediones.
Phenobarbital	May increase or decrease levels of phenobarbital or phenytoin.
Phenothiazines	Increased levels with phenothiazines.
Phenylbutazone	Increased levels with phenylbutazone.
Quinidine	Decreases effects of quinidine.
Reserpine	Decreased levels with reserpine.
Rifampin	Decreases effects of rifampin.
Salicylates	Increased levels with salicylates.
Sodium valproate	May increase or decrease levels of sodium valproate or phenytoin.
Succinamides	Increased levels with succinamides. Increased risk of phenytoin hypersensitivity with succinamides.
Sucralfate	Decreased levels with sucralfate.
Sulfonamides	Increased levels with sulfonamides.
Theophylline	Decreases effects of theophylline.
Tolbutamide	Increased levels with tolbutamide.
Trazodone	Increased levels with trazodone.
Tricyclic antidepressants	TCAs may precipitate seizures.
Valproic acid	Valproic acid may increase or decrease levels. May increase or decrease levels of valproic acid.
Vitamin D	Decreases effects of vitamin D.

Pregabalin[CV] (Lyrica)

Alcohol	May potentiate the impairment of motor skills and sedation of alcohol; avoid consumption of alcohol during therapy.
CNS depressants	Additive CNS side effects with CNS depressants (eg, opiates, benzodiazepines).

Tiagabine Hydrochloride (Gabitril)

Alcohol	Additive CNS depression with alcohol.
Carbamazepine	Diminished effects with carbamazepine.
CNS depressants	Additive CNS depression with CNS depressants.
Phenytoin	Diminished effects with phenytoin.

Table 17.2: DRUG INTERACTIONS FOR NEUROLOGICAL AGENTS *(cont.)*

ANTICONVULSANTS *(cont.)*

Tiagabine Hydrochloride (Gabitril) *(cont.)*

Triazolam	Additive CNS depression with triazolam.
Valproate	May reduce valproate levels.

Topiramate (Topamax)

Alcohol	May potentiate CNS depression with alcohol.
Carbamazepine	Carbamazepine decrease levels.
Carbonic anhydrase inhibitors	Increased risk of kidney stones with carbonic anhydrase inhibitors.
CNS depressants	May potentiate CNS depression with other CNS depressants.
Digoxin	May decrease AUC of digoxin.
Metformin	May increase metformin levels; monitor diabetics regularly.
Phenytoin	Phenytoin decrease levels. Increases phenytoin levels.
Valproic acid	Valproic acid decrease levels. Decreases valproic acid levels.

Valproate Sodium (Depacon)

Amitriptyline	Potentiates amitriptyline.
ASA	Potentiated by ASA.
Carbamazepine	Potentiates carbamazepine. Antagonized by carbamazepine.
Clonazepam	Clonazepam may induce absence status in patients with absence seizures.
CNS depressants	Additive CNS depression with other CNS depressants (eg, alcohol).
Diazepam	Potentiates diazepam.
Ethosuximide	Potentiates ethosuximide.
Felbamate	Potentiated by felbamate.
Lamotrigine	Potentiates lamotrigine.
Nortriptyline	Potentiates nortriptyline.
Phenobarbital	Potentiates phenobarbital. Antagonized by phenobarbital.
Phenytoin	Potentiates phenytoin. Antagonized by phenytoin.
Primidone	Potentiates primidone.
Rifampin	Antagonized by rifampin.
Tolbutamide	Potentiates tolbutamide.
Warfarin	Potentiates warfarin.
Zidovudine	Potentiates zidovudine.

Valproic Acid (Depakene)

Amitriptyline	Potentiates amitriptyline.

ANTICONVULSANTS *(cont.)*

Valproic Acid (Depakene) *(cont.)*

ASA	Potentiated by ASA.
Carbamazepine	Potentiates carbamazepine. Antagonized by carbamazepine.
Clonazepam	Clonazepam may induce absence status in patients with absence seizures.
CNS depressants	Additive CNS depression with other CNS depressants (eg, alcohol).
Diazepam	Potentiates diazepam.
Ethosuximide	Potentiates ethosuximide.
Felbamate	Potentiated by felbamate.
Lamotrigine	Potentiates lamotrigine.
Nortriptyline	Potentiates nortriptyline.
Phenobarbital	Potentiates phenobarbital. Antagonized by phenobarbital.
Phenytoin	Potentiates phenytoin. Antagonized by phenytoin.
Primidone	Potentiates primidone.
Rifampin	Antagonized by rifampin.
Tolbutamide	Potentiates tolbutamide.
Warfarin	Potentiates warfarin.
Zidovudine	Potentiates zidovudine.

Zonisamide (Zonegran)

Enzyme inducers	Enzyme inducers increase metabolism and clearance.

ANTIPARKINSONISM DRUGS

Amantadine Hydrochloride (Symmetrel)

Anticholinergic agents	Anticholinergic agents may potentiate the anticholinergic side effects.
CNS stimulants	Caution with CNS stimulants.
Thioridazine	Increased tremor in elderly Parkinson's disease patients with thioridazine.
Trimethoprim-sulfamethoxazole	Increased plasma levels with trimethoprim-sulfamethoxazole.
Quinine	Increased plasma levels with quinine.
Quinidine	Increased plasma levels with quinidine.

Benztropine Mesylate (Cogentin)

Atropine-like agents	Caution with other atropine-like agents.
Phenothiazines	Paralytic ileus, hyperthermia and heat stroke reported with phenothiazines.
Tricyclic antidepressants	Paralytic ileus, hyperthermia and heat stroke reported with TCAs.

Table 17.2: DRUG INTERACTIONS FOR NEUROLOGICAL AGENTS *(cont.)*

ANTIPARKINSONISM DRUGS *(cont.)*

Bromocriptine Mesylate (Parlodel)

Alcohol	Alcohol may potentiate side effects.
Antihypertensives	Caution with antihypertensives.
Dopamine antagonists	Decreased effects with dopamine antagonists (eg, butyrophenones, haloperidol, phenothiazines, pimozide, metoclopramide).
Ergot alkaloids	Not for use with other ergot alkaloids.
Levodopa	Levodopa may cause hallucinations.

Carbidopa/Entacapone/Levodopa (Stalevo 50, Stalevo 100, Stalevo 150)

Antibiotics	Some antibiotics (eg, erythromycin, rifampicin, ampicillin, chloramphenicol) may interfere with biliary excretion.
Antihypertensives	Risk of postural hypotension with antihypertensives.
Cholestyramine	Cholestyramine may interfere with biliary excretion.
Dopamine D_2 antagonists	Reduced effect with dopamine D_2 antagonists (eg, phenothiazines, butyrophenones, risperidone).
Drugs metabolized by COMT	Increased HR, arrhythmias, and BP changes with drugs metabolized by COMT (eg, isoproterenol, epinephrine, norepinephrine, dopamine, dobutamine, alpha-methyldopa, apomorphine, isoetherine, bitolterol).
Epinephrine	Increased HR, arrhythmias, and BP changes.
Iron salts	Reduced bioavailability with iron salts.
Isoniazid	Reduced effect with isoniazid.
Metoclopramide	Reduced effect with metoclopramide.
Papaverine	Reduced effect with papaverine.
Phenytoin	Reduced effect with phenytoin.
Probenecid	May interfere with biliary excretion.
Protein-bound drugs, highly	Caution with highly protein-bound drugs (eg, warfarin, salicylic acid, phenylbutazone, diazepam).
Selegiline	Risk of postural hypotension with selegiline.
Tricyclic antidepressants	HTN and dyskinesia may occur with TCAs.

Carbidopa/Levodopa (Parcopa, Sinemet 10-100, Sinemet 25-100, Sinemet 25-250, Sinemet CR)

Antihypertensives	Risk of postural hypotension with antihypertensives.
Dopamine D_2 antagonists	Reduced effect with dopamine D_2 antagonists (eg, phenothiazines, butyrophenones, risperidone).
Iron salts	Reduced bioavailability with iron salts.
Metoclopramide	Antagonized by metoclopramide.

ANTIPARKINSONISM DRUGS *(cont.)*

Carbidopa/Levodopa (Parcopa, Sinemet 10-100, Sinemet 25-100, Sinemet 25-250, Sinemet CR) *(cont.)*

Papaverine	Antagonized by papaverine.
Phenytoin	Antagonized by phenytoin.
High-protein diets	Reduced bioavailability with high-protein diets.
Selegiline	Risk of postural hypotension with selegiline.
Tricyclic antidepressants	HTN and dyskinesia may occur with TCAs.

Entacapone (Comtan)

Antibiotics, some	Some antibiotics (eg, erythromycin, rifampicin, ampicillin, chloramphenicol) may interfere with biliary excretion.
Cholestyramine	Cholestyramine may interfere with biliary excretion.
CNS depressants	Additive sedative effects with CNS depressants.
Drugs metabolized by COMT	Caution with drugs metabolized by COMT (eg, isoproterenol, epinephrine, norepinephrine, dopamine, dobutamine, alpha-methyldopa, apomorphine, isoetherine, bitolterol); increased heart rate, arrhythmias, and BP changes may occur.
Nonselective MAOIs	Avoid nonselective MAOIs (eg, phenelzine, tranylcypromine).
Probenecid	May interfere with biliary excretion.

Pergolide Mesylate (Permax)

CNS depressants	Additive sedative effects may occur with other CNS depressants.
Dopamine antagonists	Decreased effects with dopamine antagonists (eg, phenothiazines, butyrophenones, thioxanthines, metoclopramide); avoid concurrent use.
Protein-bound drugs, highly	Caution with highly protein-bound drugs.

Pramipexole Dihydrochloride (Mirapex)

Cimetidine	Cimetidine may decrease clearance.
Diltiazem	May decrease clearance.
Dopamine antagonists	Dopamine antagonists (eg, phenothiazines, butyrophenones, thioxanthenes, metoclopramide) may decrease effects.
Ranitidine	Ranitidine may decrease clearance.
Triamterene	May decrease clearance.
Verapamil	May decrease clearance.
Quinidine	May decrease clearance.
Quinine	May decrease clearance.

Ropinirole Hydrochloride (Requip)

Alcohol	Caution with alcohol.
Ciprofloxacin	Potentiated by ciprofloxacin.

Table 17.2: DRUG INTERACTIONS FOR NEUROLOGICAL AGENTS *(cont.)*

ANTIPARKINSONISM DRUGS *(cont.)*

Ropinirole Hydrochloride (Requip) *(cont.)*

CYP1A2 inhibitor	Adjust dose if CYP1A2 inhibitor is stopped or started during treatment.
Dopamine antagonists	Decreased effects with dopamine antagonists (eg, phenothiazines, butyrophenones, thioxanthines, metoclopramide). Caution with dopamine antagonists.
Estrogen	Adjust dose if estrogen is stopped or started during treatment.
Sedatives	Drowsiness increased with sedatives.

Selegiline Hydrochloride (Eldepryl)

Fluoxetine	Allow 5 weeks for fluoxetine due to a longer half-life.
Meperidine	Stupor, muscular rigidity, severe agitation, and elevated temperature reported with meperidine; avoid concomitant use.
Selective serotonin reuptake inhibitors	Avoid SSRIs; severe toxicity reported. Allow 2 weeks between discontinuation of selegiline and initiation of SSRIs.
Sympathomimetics	Caution with sympathomimetics.
Tricyclic antidepressants	Avoid TCAs; severe toxicity reported. Allow 2 weeks between discontinuation of selegiline and initiation of TCAs.
Tyramine-containing food	Caution with tyramine-containing food.

Tolcapone (Tasmar)

Apomorphine	Apomorphine may need a dose reduction.
Desipramine	Caution with desipramine.
Dobutamine	Dobutamine may need a dose reduction.
Isoproterenol	Isoproterenol may need a dose reduction.
Levodopa	May increase risk of orthostatic hypotension and dyskinesia with levodopa.
MAOIs, nonselective	Avoid nonselective MAOIs (eg, phenelzine, tranylcypromine).
Tolbutamide	Caution with tolbutamide.
Warfarin	Caution with warfarin.

Trihexyphenidyl Hydrochloride

Alcohol	Additive effects with alcohol.
Barbiturates	Additive effects with barbiturates.
Cannabinoids	Additive effects with cannabinoids.
CNS depressants	Additive effects with other CNS depressants.
Levodopa	May need to reduce concomitant levodopa dose.
MAOIs	MAOIs may intensify anticholinergic effects.
Neuroleptics	Increased risk of tardive dyskinesia with neuroleptics.

ANTIPARKINSONISM DRUGS *(cont.)*

Trihexyphenidyl Hydrochloride *(cont.)*

Opiates	Additive effects with opiates.
Tricyclic antidepressants	TCAs may intensify anticholinergic effects.

MUSCLE RELAXANTS

Aspirin/Carisoprodol (Soma Compound)

Alcohol	Increases GI bleeding risk with alcohol. Additive effects with alcohol.
Antacids	Antacids decrease plasma levels.
Anticoagulants	Increases bleeding risk with anticoagulants.
Antidiabetics, oral	Enhances methotrexate toxicity and hypoglycemia with oral antidiabetics.
CNS depressants	Additive effects with other CNS depressants.
Corticosteroids	Corticosteroids decrease plasma levels.
Probenecid	Antagonizes uricosuric effects of probenecid.
Psychotropic drugs	Additive effects with psychotropic drugs.
Sulfinpyrazone	Antagonizes uricosuric effects of sulfinpyrazone.
Urine acidifiers	Potentiated by urine acidifiers (eg, ammonium chloride).

Baclofen

Alcohol	Additive CNS effects with alcohol.
Antidiabetic agents	May increase blood glucose and require dosage adjustment of antidiabetic agents.
Antihypertensives	May potentiate antihypertensives.
CNS depressants	Additive CNS effects with other CNS depressants.
Levodopa plus carbidopa	Mental confusion, hallucinations and agitation with levodopa plus carbidopa therapy.
Magnesium sulfate	Synergistic effects with magnesium sulfate.
MAOIs	May increase CNS depressant effects with MAOIs.
Neuromuscular blockers	Synergistic effects with other neuromuscular blockers.
Tricyclic antidepressants	Potentiated by TCAs.

Carisoprodol (Soma)

Alcohol	Additive effects with alcohol.
CNS depressants	Additive effects with other CNS depressants.
Psychotropic drugs	Additive effects with psychotropic drugs.

Cyclobenzaprine Hydrochloride (Flexeril)

Alcohol	Enhances effects of alcohol.

Table 17.2: DRUG INTERACTIONS FOR NEUROLOGICAL AGENTS *(cont.)*

MUSCLE RELAXANTS *(cont.)*

Cyclobenzaprine Hydrochloride (Flexeril) *(cont.)*

Anticholinergic medication	Caution with anticholinergic medication.
Barbiturates	Enhances effects of barbiturates.
CNS depressants	Enhances effects of other CNS depressants.
Guanethidine	May block antihypertensive action of guanethidine and similar compounds.
MAOIs	Contraindicated with MAOIs.
Tramadol	May enhance seizure risk with tramadol.

Dantrolene Sodium (Dantrium)

Calcium channel blockers	Avoid with calcium channel blockers; risk of cardiovascular collapse.
CNS depressants	Increased drowsiness with CNS depressants.
Estrogen	Caution with estrogens; risk of hepatotoxicity.
Vecuronium	May potentiate vecuronium-induced neuromuscular block.

Metaxalone (Skelaxin)

Alcohol	May enhance the effects of alcohol.
Barbiturates	May enhance the effects of barbiturates.
CNS depressants	May enhance the effects of other CNS depressants.

Methocarbamol (Robaxin, Robaxin-750)

Alcohol	Additive adverse effects with alcohol.
Anticholinergics	Caution in patients with myasthemia gravis receiving anticholinergics.
CNS depressants	Additive adverse effects with other CNS depressants.
Pyridostigmine	May inhibit effect of pyridostigmine.

Orphenadrine Citrate (Norflex)

Propoxyphene	Confusion, anxiety, and tremors reported with propoxyphene.

Tizanidine Hydrochloride (Zanaflex)

Alcohol	Potentiated depressant effect with alcohol.
Alpha-adrenergic agonists	Avoid alpha-adrenergic agonists.
Oral contraceptives	Potentiated by oral contraceptives.

VASCULAR HEADACHE SUPPRESSANTS

Almotriptan Malate (Axert)

5-HT$_1$ agonist drugs	Avoid other 5-HT$_1$ agonist drugs within 24 hr period.
CYP3A4 inhibitors	Increased levels possible with CYP3A4 inhibitors (eg, ketoconazole).
Ergotamines	Additive vasospastic reactions with ergotamines.

VASCULAR HEADACHE SUPPRESSANTS *(cont.)*

Almotriptan Malate (Axert) *(cont.)*

MAOIs	Clearance may be decreased by MAOIs.
Selective Serotonin Reuptake Inhibitors	SSRIs may cause weakness, hyperreflexia, and incoordination.

Aspirin/Caffeine/Orphenadrine Citrate (Norgesic, Norgesic Forte)

Propoxyphene	Confusion, tremor, anxiety reported with propoxyphene.

Caffeine/Ergotamine Tartrate (Cafergot)

CYP3A4 inhibitors	Increased risk of toxicity including vasospasm with less potent CYP3A4 inhibitors (eg, saquinavir, nefazodone, fluconazole, fluoxetine, grapefruit juice, fluvoxamine, zileuton, metronidazole, clotrimazole).
Nicotine	Nicotine potentiates vasoconstrictive action.
Propranolol	Propranolol potentiates vasoconstrictive action.
Sympathomimetics	Extreme BP elevation may occur with sympathomimetics.
Vasoconstrictors	Avoid vasoconstrictors.

Dihydroergotamine Mesylate (D.H.E. 45)

CYP3A4 inhibitors	Contraindicated with CYP3A4 inhibitors (eg, macrolides, protease inhibitors). Caution with less potent CYP3A4 inhibitors (eg, saquinavir, nefazodone, fluconazole, grapefruit juice, fluoxetine, fluvoxamine, zileuton, clotrimazole).
Macrolides	Increased plasma levels and peripheral vasoconstriction with macrolides.
Nicotine	Nicotine may potentiate the vasoconstrictive action.
Propranolol	Propranolol may potentiate the vasoconstrictive action.
Sumatriptan	Additive coronary vasospastic effect with sumatriptan; avoid within 24 hrs of each other.
Vasoconstrictors, central	Potentiated BP elevation with central vasoconstrictors.
Vasoconstrictors, peripheral	Potentiated BP elevation with peripheral vasoconstrictors.

Eletriptan Hydrobromide (Relpax)

5-HT$_1$ agonists	Avoid within 24 hours of other 5-HT$_1$ agonists.
CYP3A4 inhibitors, potent	Avoid within 72 hrs of potent CYP3A4 inhibitors (eg, ketoconazole, itraconazole, nefazodone, troleandomycin, clarithromycin, ritonavir, nelfinavir).
Ergot-containing drugs	Prolonged vasospastic reactions reported with ergot-containing drugs; avoid within 24 hours of each other.
Erythromycin	Erythromycin may increase levels.
Fluconazole	Fluconazole may increase levels.
Propranolol	Propranolol may increase levels.
Verapamil	Verapamil may increase levels.

Table 17.2: DRUG INTERACTIONS FOR NEUROLOGICAL AGENTS (cont.)

VASCULAR HEADACHE SUPPRESSANTS (cont.)

Frovatriptan Succinate (Frova)

5-HT$_{1B/1D}$ agonists	Avoid within 24 hours of other 5-HT$_{1B/1D}$ agonists.
Ergot-containing drugs	Prolonged vasospastic reactions reported with ergot-containing drugs; avoid within 24 hours of each other.
Selective serotonin reuptake inhibitors	Weakness, hyperreflexia, and incoordination reported with SSRIs (rare).

Naratriptan Hydrochloride (Amerge)

5-HT$_1$ agonists	Avoid other 5-HT$_1$ agonist drugs within 24 hr period due to additive effects.
Ergotamine-containing drugs	Ergotamine-containing drugs may cause prolonged vasospastic reactions.
Ergot-type drugs	Ergot-type (dihydroergotamine or methysergide) drugs may cause prolonged vasospastic reactions.
Selective serotonin reuptake inhibitors	SSRIs may cause weakness, hyperreflexia, and incoordination.

Rizatriptan Benzoate (Maxalt, Maxalt-MLT)

5-HT$_1$ agonists	Prolonged vasospastic reactions with other 5-HT$_1$ agonists.
Ergot-type agents	Prolonged vasospastic reactions with ergot-type agents.
MAOIs	Avoid MAOIs during or within 14 days.
Propranolol	Increased plasma levels with propranolol.
Selective serotonin reuptake inhibitors	SSRIs may cause weakness, hyperreflexia, and incoordination (rare).

Sumatriptan (Imitrex)

5-HT$_1$ agonists	Avoid other 5-HT$_1$ agonists.
Ergot-containing drugs	Prolonged vasospastic reactions with ergot-containing drugs; avoid use within 24 hrs.
MAOIs	Avoid MAOIs.
Selective Serotonin Reuptake Inhibitors	Weakness, hyperreflexia, and incoordination reported with SSRIs (rare).

Zolmitriptan (Zomig, Zomig-ZMT)

5-HT$_{1B/1D}$ agonists	Avoid 5-HT$_{1B/1D}$ agonists within 24 hrs.
Cimetidine	Half-life and AUC doubled with cimetidine.
Ergot-agents	Ergot-agents may prolong vasospastic reactions.
MAOIs	Avoid MAOIs, during or within 14 days of therapy.
Selective serotonin reuptake inhibitors	SSRIs may cause weakness, hyperreflexia, and incoordination.

Chapter 18

Psychoactive Drugs

Steven Ganzberg, D.M.D., M.S.

Approximately one of every three people will suffer from a mental illness at some point in his or her life. Many of these people will be placed on a regimen of psychoactive drugs, which may influence dental management. Psychiatric medications partially include antidepressant, antianxiety, antipsychotic, and antimanic drugs, drugs for attention deficit/hyper-activity disorders as well as sedatives and "sleeping pills."

When members of the dental team are treating a patient taking psychoactive medications, common sense dictates that they should take care in their personal interactions with the patient. Efforts to minimize anxiety, although routine in dental practice, should be given high priority.

General psychiatric drug information is provided in Tables 18.1 and 18.2, including adverse effects, precautions/contraindications, and interactions with other drugs.

Use of Psychoactive Drugs in Dental Practice

The prescription of psychoactive agents by dentists is indicated for a number of conditions, including acute anxiety associated with dental or oral surgery, management of bruxism and management of various orofacial pain conditions. These agents also have a place in dentistry for sedation (see Chapter 2) and general anesthesia (see Appendix N).

Anxiety Associated With Dental or Oral Surgery

The benzodiazepines are generally regarded as the drugs of choice for oral preoperative anxiolysis in dental practice. These drugs have a high margin of safety, especially when used as a single dose 30 minutes to 1 hour before a dental visit. Diazepam historically has been used in this regard, but with the advent of newer agents with different phamacokinetic properties, other agents may be preferred. Diazepam is an inexpensive drug, with a rapid onset of action and a long half-life with active metabolites. At a dose of 5-10 mg, 1 hour before a dental appointment, most adult patients will have some element of anxiolysis without significant sedation.

Another drug, triazolam, has a more rapid onset of action and the shortest half-life of any oral benzodiazepine, 1.5-5 hours without active metabolites. This agent may provide less postoperative sedation, which may be desirable. The typical adult oral preoperative anxiolytic dosage for triazolam would be 0.25-0.5 mg 1 hour before the dental appointment.

The intravenous drug midazolam has a similar pharmacokinetic profile to that of triazolam. This medication is FDA-approved for oral use in children.

With any of these agents, there should be minimal, if any, respiratory or cardiac depression when used alone. In elderly, medically compromised or smaller adult patients, the lower dose range should be prescribed initially. Some patients may experience significant sedation even at low doses. If oral premedication is prescribed, the patient must have a responsible adult escort present at all times until the effects of the sedative have worn off sufficiently. Patients who have taken an oral sedative before a dental appointment must not drive to or from the dental office. Patients should be cautioned about lingering sedative effects during the day and to avoid other central nervous system (CNS) depressants such as alcohol and opioids. Multiple dosing of oral sedative agents on the same treatment day, especially in doses exceeding the maximum recommended single home dose, can result in unpredictable levels of sedation beyond that which was intended.

Management of Nocturnal Bruxism

If an acute anxiety-producing circumstance leads to severe bruxism, a short course of a benzodiazepine at bedtime can be efficacious. Typically, diazepam 5-10 mg at bedtime has been used owing to its muscle-relaxing properties and anxiolytic effect. Other benzodiazepines are also effective. In general, this type of benzodiazepine use should be limited to no more than 2 weeks to avoid issues of dependence, rebound insomnia and alteration of sleep architecture. Benzodiazepines are relatively contraindicated in a depressed patient unless approved by the patient's psychiatrist in advance. Patients should be cautioned about lingering sedative effects during the day and to avoid other CNS depressants such as alcohol and opioids.

The tricyclic antidepressants have come into increasing use for the long-term management of nocturnal bruxism unresponsive to intraoral orthotic therapy. Although not fully understood, bruxism appears to occur during transitional stages of sleep or during rapid-eye-movement (REM) sleep. The tricyclic antidepressants decrease the number of awakenings, shorten time spent in transitional stages of sleep, increase stage III and IV sleep, and markedly decrease time spent in REM sleep. These effects may be beneficial for some patients with bruxism. Common agents used include amitriptyline, nortriptyline or doxepin. These drugs are usually started at 10 mg at bedtime and gradually titrated upward every few days. It is uncommon for most patients to require more than 50 mg at bedtime, which is substantially below the effective dose for use as an antidepressant.

These drugs are not benign. They have significant anticholinergic and antihistaminic side effects. They can cause cardiac dysrhythmias and may lower seizure threshold. In patients aged older than 40 years, pretreatment electrocardiogram evaluation may be appropriate. The dentist prescribing antidepressants for this use is presumed to have established a proper diagnosis and to be fully aware of the drug's interactions, adverse effects and contraindications. When used as antidepressants, these drugs should be prescribed only by clinicians who have had special training in the diagnosis and management of depression.

Management of Orofacial Pain

Psychotropic drugs have a long history of use for chronic pain conditions. A full listing of indications and prescribing information is not appropriate for this text. For the properly trained dentist, the use of psychoactive drugs is appropriate for the management of orofacial conditions such as primary headaches, neuropathic and musculoskeletal pains.

Antidepressants are commonly used for a variety of chronic pain conditions (including myofascial pain syndrome and migraine headache). Phenothiazines can be a useful adjunct for some types of neuropathic pains, and lithium is indicated for cluster headaches. The dentist using these drugs as therapeutic agents is presumed to be proficient in prescribing and managing these medications.

Antianxiety Agents

Anxiety is a state of uneasiness of mind that resembles fear, but usually has no identifiable source. Anxiety has both physiological and psychological components. The anxious patient may be tachycardic, nauseated, diaphoretic or light-headed. Although a patient may be diagnosed with a generalized anxiety disorder, at times clearly defined categories of anxiety apply. These categories include phobia, agoraphobia, panic attacks, obsessive-compulsive disorder, posttraumatic stress disorder and performance anxiety. Benzodiazepines, facilitators of gamma-aminobutyric acid-A ($GABA_A$) receptors, agonists, are commonly prescribed for these disorders. The development of dependence with these agents may limit the long-term use of these drugs in some patients. Oral overdose of benzodiazepines is rarely fatal unless combined with other central nervous system depressants such as opioids, barbiturates or alcohol. Another drug without dependence-producing characteristics, the selective serotonin agonist buspirone, may be effective for some generalized anxiety disorders. Antidepressants are frequently prescribed as primary therapy for anxiety or for those patients with coexisting anxiety and depression.

β-blockers more recently have been prescribed as an adjunct to benzodiazepine treatment and for control of performance anxiety. The antihistamine hydroxyzine is sometimes used for selected cases of anxiety disorders and combined with other agents for pediatric oral sedation.

See Tables 18.1 and 18.2 for general information on antianxiety agents. Other agents listed as sleep adjuncts, although not FDA-approved for treatment of anxiety, may be prescribed for these disorders. More information on sleep adjuncts appears later in this chapter.

Special Dental Considerations

These drugs may cause xerostomia and should be considered in the differential diagnosis of caries, periodontal disease or candidiasis.

These drugs may cause orthostatic hypotension. After supine positioning, the dentist should ask the patient to sit upright in the dental chair for a minute or two and then monitor the patient when standing.

If these drugs are used for oral preoperative anxiolysis for dental procedures, a competent adult should drive the patient to and from the dental office. Assistance to and from the dental chair may be needed, especially for elderly patients.

Drug Interactions of Dental Interest

Antianxiety agents may have an additive sedative effect with concomitantly administered CNS depressants.

Absorption of diazepam and chlordiazepoxide is delayed with antacids.

The metabolism of chlordiazepoxide, diazepam and triazolam is decreased if they are administered with cimetidine and erythromycin.

The clearance of diazepam is decreased if it is administered with some selective serotonin reuptake inhibitor (SSRI) antidepressants.

Special Patients

In elderly, medically compromised or smaller adult patients, the lower dose range should be prescribed initially. Some of these patients may experience significant sedation even at low doses.

Pharmacology

These agents are mainly benzodiazepines, which act at the $GABA_A$ receptor, a gated chloride-ion channel that has specific benzodiazepine and barbiturate receptor sites. Binding of benzodiazepines to the receptor complex opens the chloride channel to facilitate GABA receptor transmission. GABA is the main inhibitory neurotransmitter of the central nervous system. Activity of the GABA system provides antianxiety, sedative, anticonvulsant, amnestic and muscle-relaxing actions. Long-term use of benzodiazepines can lead to a withdrawal syndrome if abruptly discontinued. The sedative and antianxiety effects of these drugs are used to advantage in promoting short-term sleep improvement. These drugs are hepatically metabolized to active or inactive metabolites for excretion in the bile or urine.

Buspirone, a serotonin (5HT1$_A$) receptor partial agonist with weak dopamine receptor activity, has shown some utility in the management of generalized anxiety. Its onset of action is delayed, thus making this drug a poor choice for management of acute anxiety. Antidepressant pharmacology is discussed in the section below.

The antihistamines hydroxyzine and diphenhydramine are seldom-used older agents that have sedative and anticholinergic effects independent of GABA action.

Antidepressants

Depression is a common mental illness that will affect at least 5% of the population at some time in life. A great number of these patients will be placed on antidepressants. Antidepressants are classified as heterocyclic (tricyclic, tetracyclic), monoamine oxidase inhibitors (MAOIs), selective serotonin reuptake inhibitors (SSRIs), serotonin/norepinephrine reuptake inhibitors (SNRIs) and other miscellaneous agents. These drugs work by affecting neurotransmitter balance between serotonin, norepinephrine and, in some cases, dopamine in the CNS. Some of the SSRI antidepressants are also used for obsessive-compulsive disorder and are listed separately in the tables.

Implications in dental and oral surgery revolve around the use of vasoconstrictors in local anesthetics, medication side effects and issues of patient management.

See Tables 18.1 and 18.2 for basic information on antidepressants and for epinephrine/levonordefrin interaction information.

Special Dental Considerations

Most of these drugs cause decreased salivary flow. Consider this in the differential diagnosis of caries, periodontal disease or oral candidiasis.

The SSRIs (such as fluoxetine and sertraline) can initiate bruxism. The clinician should consider this in the differential diagnosis of bruxism-related signs and symptoms.

These drugs, in rare cases, cause blood dyscrasias and should be considered in the differential diagnosis of oral signs and symptoms.

Many of these drugs can cause orthostatic hypotension. The dentist should ask the patient to sit upright in the dental chair for a minute or two after being in a supine position and then monitor the patient when standing.

Amoxapine, and less commonly other antidepressants, can cause tardive dyskinesia or extrapyramidal symptoms, which are manifested as involuntary oral or facial movements. Management of bruxism, occlusal adjustments and bite registrations may be difficult to obtain. If newly diagnosed mouthing movements (involuntary mouth and tongue movements and/or drooling) are seen, which may indicate a serious medication side effect, consultation with the patient's physician may be appropriate.

Venlafaxine can, rarely, cause trismus.

Drug Interactions of Dental Interest

There has been much misunderstanding about the use of local anesthetics with epinephrine for patients taking antidepressants. Local anesthetics with epinephrine are not absolutely contraindicated for any patient taking any antidepressant—including tricyclic or MAOI agents, all of which increase the concentration of norepinephrine in the synaptic cleft. The potential concern is that these drug combinations might lead to a hypertensive/tachycardic crisis. Because a major route of metabolism of exogenously administered catecholamines (such as epinephrine) involves catechol-O-methyl transferase (COMT), use of epinephrine or levonordefrin in patients taking MAOIs is not likely to be of concern. Antidepressants that block norepinephrine reuptake (tricyclics, tetracyclics, venlafaxine, nefazodone) could cause unwanted cardiovascular effects when epinephrine-containing local anesthetics are administered. It is prudent, therefore, to monitor vital signs for dental patients taking antidepressants that affect norepinephrine reuptake blockade or monoamine oxidase A (MAO-A) activity.

For these agents, it is reasonable to administer no more than 40 µg of epinephrine in local anesthetic solutions (approximately one cartridge of local anesthetic with 1:50,000 epinephrine, two cartridges with 1:100,000 epinephrine, or four cartridges with 1:200,000 epinephrine) within a short period with careful aspiration technique. This may be particularly important in patients taking venlafaxine, which has been noted to produce a sustained increase in diastolic blood pressure and heart rate as a relatively common side effect. Additional anesthetic with vasoconstrictor may be administered if vital signs are acceptable. No vasoconstrictor contraindication exists for the SSRI antidepressants. Gingival retraction cord with epinephrine is contraindicated for all patients taking antidepressants other than SSRI and should be used with caution, if at all, in other patients.

Anticholinergics and antihistamines should be used cautiously due to additive xerostomia and CNS sedative effects.

CNS depressants (for example, alcohol, opioids and benzodiazepines) may potentiate sedative side effects.

Meperidine and dextromethorphan are specifically contraindicated in patients taking MAOIs. Hypermetabolic crisis may occur. Caution with other opioids may be warranted.

Tricyclic antidepressants (which might be used for bruxism) are contraindicated with MAOIs and should be used cautiously with SSRIs unless their use is cleared by a psychiatrist.

The anticoagulant effect of coumarin agents is increased when most antidepressants, including tricyclic agents, are administered concomitantly.

Antidepressants may lower the seizure threshold.

The therapeutic effect of tricyclic antidepressants may be decreased by concurrent administration of barbiturates, anticonvulsants or other hepatic-enzyme–inducing drugs.

With cimetidine, fluoxetine, methylphenidate and some estrogens (oral contraceptives), there is increased plasma concentration of tricyclic antidepressants.

Laboratory Value Alterations

- Blood glucose levels may increase or decrease.
- ECG changes are possible with tricyclic-antidepressants, especially with preexisting conduction abnormalities.

Special Patients

Side effects, such as xerostomia and orthostatic hypotension, are more pronounced in elderly patients.

Pharmacology

Antidepressants affect mood by altering the balance between serotonin, norepinephrine and dopamine in critical brain centers. Antidepressants, in general, increase the availability of neurotransmitters in the synaptic cleft, causing changes in the postsynaptic receptor. These changes take some time to develop, thus accounting for the delay in action of 2-4 weeks or longer for these drugs' mood-altering effects to become apparent. Due to the side-effect profile of many of the tricyclic and

MAOI agents, the SSRIs are frequently chosen as first-line therapy for depression. In pain management, both norepinephrine and serotonin reuptake blockade appear to be important for an analgesic effect, so the tricyclics and venlafaxine remain the preferred initial agents. Analgesia occurs well before the antidepressant effect and at lower doses that are not effective for management of depression in many patients with chronic pain.

The heterocyclic (tricyclic and tetracyclic) and selective serotonin reuptake inhibitor (SSRI) antidepressants block the reuptake of the neurotransmitters into the presynaptic neuron, a partial mechanism by which neurotransmitter activity is modulated. The SSRIs, as their name implies, are selective for serotonin reuptake blockade. Because of the receptor selectivity of these agents, they generally possess the fewest side effects of any antidepressant type. SNRIs inhibit the reuptake of serotonin and norepinephrine with few effects at other receptors. The heterocyclic (tricyclic, tetracyclic) antidepressants affect norepinephrine and serotonin, as well as a number of other important neurotransmitters, but to varying degrees. Amoxapine possesses strong dopamine reuptake blocking effects. The MAOIs block the action of MAO-A, an enzyme found in the presynaptic neuron, which degrades serotonin and norepinephrine after reuptake. Bupropion is a weak reuptake blocker of dopamine and, to a lesser extent, norepinephrine and serotonin. Mirtazapine is an α_2 antagonist affecting norepinephrine and, indirectly, serotonin.

Antimanic/Bipolar Disorder Drugs

Mania is a state of excessive excitement or enthusiasm and is frequently associated with hyperactivity or aggressive behavior. Approximately 90% of people who experience mania alternate these experiences with episodes of depression; this condition is termed "bipolar disorder" (manic-depression). Lithium carbonate has historically been the most prescribed agent, but now various anti-epileptic and antipsychotic agents are also being used as first-line treatments.

See Tables 18.1 and 18.2 for general information on antimanic/bipolar disorder drugs.

Special Dental Considerations: Lithium and Other Agents

Lithium can cause decreased salivary flow. Consider in the differential diagnosis of caries, periodontal disease or oral candidiasis.

Lithium can cause blood dyscrasias and should be considered in the differential diagnosis of oral signs and symptoms.

Lithium can cause orthostatic hypotension. The dentist should monitor vital signs and, after supine positioning, ask the patient to sit upright in the dental chair for a minute or two and then monitor the patient when standing.

Antipsychotic agents are discussed in the sections below. Anti-epileptic agents are discussed in Chapter 17, Neurological Drugs.

Drug Interactions of Dental Interest: Lithium and Other Agents

Vasoconstrictors in local anesthetics should be used with caution owing to lithium's hypotensive effects.

Opioids, alcohol and other hypotension-producing agents have additive hypotensive effects.

NSAIDs, except aspirin and sulindac, increase lithium's plasma concentration because of decreased renal clearance and should be prescribed, if at all, in consultations with the patient's psychiatrist.

Metronidazole increases plasma lithium concentration because of decreased renal clearance.

with or without psychotherapy, are frequently used for treatment. α_2 agonists, such as clonidine, are commonly used at bedtime to counteract the common adverse effect of insomnia. There is increasing recognition of this disorder in adults.

These drugs are also used for disorders of excessive somnolence, such as narcolepsy. Another drug for this indication is modafinil.

See Tables 18.1 and 18.2 for general information on drugs used for attention deficit/hyperactivity disorder.

Special Dental Considerations

Determine if the patient is taking any drug for attention deficit disorder or narcolepsy. Monitor vital signs because of possible sympathomimetic effects.

Many of these drugs can cause decreased salivary flow and should be considered in the differential diagnosis of caries, periodontal disease or oral candidiasis.

Amphetamines may cause gingival enlargement, which should be monitored by the dentist.

These drugs can, rarely, cause blood dyscrasias; the dentist should consider this in the differential diagnosis of oral signs and symptoms.

Drug Interactions of Dental Interest

Vasoconstrictors in local anesthetics have possible additive sympathomimetic effects. Depending on vital signs, it is reasonable to administer no more than 40 µg of epinephrine in local anesthetic solutions (approximately one cartridge of local anesthetic with 1:50,000 epinephrine, two cartridges with 1:100,000 epinephrine, or four cartridges with 1:200,000 epinephrine) within a short period with careful aspiration technique. If vital signs warrant, less vasoconstrictor should be used. Additional anesthetic with vasoconstrictor may be administered if vital signs are acceptable after a short period.

Tricyclic antidepressants (which may be used for bruxism) should be used with caution, because their metabolism is decreased by methylphenidate. Increased sympathomimetic effects are possible when tricyclic antidepressants are prescribed to patients taking dextroamphetamine because of norepinephrine reuptake blockade by tricyclics.

Anticholinergics have additive oral drying effects.

Pharmacology

Methylphenidate and pemoline appear to act by blocking dopamine reuptake. These drugs increase children's ability to pay attention and decrease their motor restlessness. Dextroamphetamine/amphetamine are sympathomimetic amines that block the reuptake of dopamine and norepinephrine, inhibits MAO and releases catecholamines. Atomoxepine selectively blocks the reuptake of norepinephrine. Because of the stimulant effects, use of these drugs may result in weight loss, insomnia and tachycardia. These effects are particularly prominent with dextroamphetamine. These drugs are also used to treat narcolepsy.

Obesity Agents

Obesity is defined as a Body-Mass Index, a measure of weight in respect to height, greater than 30. Obesity can lead to a number of medical complications including diabetes mellitus, hypertension, coronary artery disease, stroke, obstructive sleep apnea as well as many other conditions. While exercise and calorie reduction remain the mainstay of treatment, some patients require surgery and/or medication to help achieve weight reduction goals. Most medications are in the stimulant/amphetamine classification. Other antidepressant medications, particularly the SSRIs, may also be used in conjunction with stimulant medications.

Special Dental Considerations

Monitor vital signs because of possible sympathomimetic effects. Many of these drugs can cause decreased salivary flow and should be considered in the differential diagnosis of caries, periodontal disease or oral candidiasis. These drugs can, rarely, cause blood dyscrasias; the dentist should consider this in the differential diagnosis of oral signs and symptoms.

Drug Interactions of Dental Interest

Vasoconstrictors in local anesthetics have possible additive sympathomimetic effects. Depending on vital signs, it is reasonable to administer no more than 40 µg of epinephrine in local anesthetic solutions (approximately one cartridge of local anesthetic with 1:50,000 epinephrine, two cartridges with 1:100,000 epinephrine, or four cartridges with 1:200,000 epinephrine) within a short period with careful aspiration technique. If vital signs warrant, less vasoconstrictor should be used. Additional anesthetic with vasoconstrictor may be administered if vital signs are acceptable after a short period. Tricyclic antidepressants (which may be used for bruxism) should be used with caution, as increased sympathomimetic effects are possible. Anticholinergics have additive oral drying effects.

Pharmacology

Most drugs that help manage obesity are appetite suppressants of the amphetamine family. They block the reuptake of norepinephrine and dopamine and may also release these catecholamines from presynaptic nerves. Because of this, use of epinephrine in local anesthetic solutions may produce exaggerated cardiovascular effects.

Sleep Adjuncts

Sleep disorders include disorders in initiating or maintaining sleep, disorders of excessive somnolence, disorders of sleep-wake schedule and parasomnias (including nocturnal bruxism). Disorders of initiating and maintaining sleep are by far the most common complaints and will be addressed in this section.

The benzodiazepines, $GABA_A$ agonists, are the drugs most commonly prescribed for insomnia. Unfortunately, prolonged use can interfere with normal sleep architecture and be detrimental in the long term. The FDA indication for these drugs is for short-term use only, although they are frequently prescribed for many months or years. Dependence and rebound insomnia are frequently observed. Nevertheless, for short-term use, these agents are generally effective. The nonbenzodiazepine $GABA_A$ agonists—zolpidem, zaleplon, and eszopiclone—produce less disruption of sleep architecture and may have some effect in treating bruxism.

The more sedating tricyclic antidepressants and trazadone also have been used for some patients who require long-term treatment, as have sedating antihistamines. Clonidine is also used for some forms of insomnia. The older barbiturate drugs, such as secobarbital and pentobarbital, are rarely used today for insomnia.

See Tables 18.1 and 18.2 for general information on sleep adjuncts.

Special Dental Considerations

These drugs can cause xerostomia. The dentist should consider this in the differential diagnosis of caries, periodontal disease or candidiasis.

These drugs may cause orthostatic hypotension. The dentist should monitor vital signs, ask the patient to sit upright in the dental chair for 1-2 minutes after being in a supine position and then monitor the patient when standing.

If these drugs are used for preoperative anxiolysis for dental procedures, ensure that a competent adult drives the patient to and from the dental office. Assistance to and from the dental chair may be needed, especially for elderly patients.

Drug Interactions of Dental Interest

CNS depressants will have an additive effect with concomitantly administered CNS depressants.

Diazepam and chlordiazepoxide have delayed absorption with antacids.

The metabolism of chlordiazepoxide, diazepam and triazolam is decreased if they are administered with cimetidine and erythromycin.

The clearance of diazepam is decreased if it is administered with SSRI antidepressants.

Special Patients

In elderly, medically compromised or smaller adult patients, the lower dose range should be prescribed initially. Some of these patients may experience significant sedation even at low doses.

Pharmacology

See the description for antianxiety agents above.

Adverse Effects, Precautions and Contraindications

Table 18.1 provides adverse effects, precautions and contraindications of psychoactive drugs.

Suggested Readings

American Psychiatric Association. Diagnostic and statistical manual of mental disorders (DSM-IV). 4th ed. Washington, D.C.: American Psychiatric Association; 1994.

Brown RS, Bottomley WK. The utilization and mechanism of action of tricyclic antidepressants in the treatment of chronic facial pain: a review of the literature. Anes Prog 1990;37:223-9.

Eschalier A, Mestre C, Dubray C, Ardid D. Why are antidepressants effective as pain relief? CNS Drugs 1994;2:261-7.

Hasan AA, Ciancio S. Relationship between amphetamine ingestion and gingival enlargement. Pediatr Dent 2004 Sep-Oct;26(5):396-400.

Mortimer AM. Newer and older antipsychotics: a comparative review of appropriate use. CNS Drugs 1994;2:381-6.

Okeson JP, ed. Orofacial pain: guidelines for assessment, diagnosis and management. Lombard, Ill.: Quintessence; 1996.

Tucker GJ. Psychiatric disorders in medical practice. In: Wyngaarden JB, Smith LH Jr., Bennett JC, eds. Cecil textbook of medicine. 19th ed. Philadelphia: Saunders; 1992.

The United States Pharmacopeial Convention. Drug information for the health care professional. 23rd ed. Rockville, Md.: The United States Pharmacopeial Convention, Inc.; 2003.

Table 18.1: PRESCRIBING INFORMATION FOR PSYCHOACTIVE DRUGS

NAME	FORM/ STRENGTH	DOSAGE	WARNINGS/PRECAUTIONS & CONTRAINDICATIONS	ADVERSE EFFECTS†
ANTIANXIETY AGENTS				
BENZODIAZEPINES				
Alprazolam^{CIV} (Niravam, Xanax, Xanax XR)	**Tab, Orally Disintegrating: (Niravam)** 0.25mg*, 0.5mg*, 1mg*, 2mg*. **Tab: (Xanax)** 0.25mg*, 0.5mg*, 1mg*, 2mg*. **Tab, ER: (Xanax XR)** 0.5mg, 1mg, 2mg, 3mg	**Adults: (Niravam) Anxiety: Initial:** 0.25-0.5mg tid. **Titrate:** May increase every 3-4 days. **Max:** 4mg/day. **Panic Disorder: Initial:** 0.5mg tid. **Titrate:** Increase by no more than 1mg/day every 3-4 days; slower titration if ≥4mg/day. **Usual:** 1-10mg/day. Decrease dose slowly (no more than 0.5mg every 3 days). **Elderly/Advanced Liver Disease/Debilitated: Initial:** 0.25mg bid-tid. **Titrate:** Increase gradually as tolerated. **(Xanax) Anxiety: Initial:** 0.25-0.5mg tid. **Titrate:** May increase every 3-4 days. **Max:** 4mg/day. **Elderly/Advanced Liver Disease/Debilitated: Initial:** 0.25mg bid-tid. **Titrate:** Increase gradually as tolerated. **Panic Disorder: Initial:** 0.5mg tid. **Titrate:** Increase by no more than 1mg/day every 3-4 days; slower titration if ≥4mg/day. **Usual:** 1-10mg/day. Decrease dose slowly (no more than 0.5mg every 3 days). **(Xanax XR) Initial:** 0.5-1mg qd, preferably in am. **Titrate:** Increase by no more than 1mg/day every 3-4 days. **Maint:** 1-10mg/day. Usual: 3-6mg/day. Decrease dose slowly (no more than 0.5mg every 3 days). **Elderly/Advanced Liver Disease/Debilitated: Initial:** 0.5mg qd.	**W/P:** Risk of dependence. Withdrawal symptoms, including seizures, reported with dose reduction or abrupt discontinuation; avoid abrupt withdrawal. Caution with impaired renal, hepatic, or pulmonary function, severe depression, obesity, elderly, and debilitated. May cause fetal harm. Hypomania/mania reported with depression. Weak uricosuric effect. Periodically reassess usefulness. **Contra:** Acute narrow angle glaucoma, untreated open-angle glaucoma, concomitant ketoconazole or itraconazole. **P/N:** Category D, not for use in nursing	Drowsiness, lightheadedness, depression, headache, confusion, insomnia, **dry mouth**, constipation, diarrhea, nausea/vomiting, tachycardia/palpitations, blurred vision, nasal congestion, sedation, memory impairment, dysarthria, abnormal coordination, fatigue, mental impairment, decreased libido, increased/decreased appetite, irritability, cognitive disorder, dysarthria, hypotension, **increased salivation**.
Chlordiazepoxide Hydrochloride^{CIV} (Librium)	**Cap:** 5mg, 10mg, 25mg; **Inj:** 100mg	**Adults: Mild-Moderate Anxiety:** 5-10mg PO tid-qid. **Severe Anxiety:** 20-25mg PO tid-qid or 50-100mg IM/IV initially, then 25-50mg tid-qid as needed. **Alcohol Withdrawal:** 50-100mg IM/IV initially, may repeat in 2-4 hrs or 50-100mg PO, repeated until agitation is controlled. **Preoperative Anxiety:** 5-10mg PO tid-qid on days prior to surgery or 50-100mg IM 1 hr prior to surgery. **Max:** 300mg/q24h for above indications. **Elderly/Debilitated:** Reduce dose (25-50mg IM/IV) or 5mg PO bid-qid. **Pediatrics: PO: ≥6 yrs:** 5mg bid-qid. May increase to 10mg bid-tid for all conditions except acute alcohol withdrawal. **Acute Alcohol Withdrawal:** 50-100mg followed by repeated doses until agitation is controlled. **Max:** 300mg/day. **IM/IV: ≥12 yrs: Withdrawal Symptoms of Acute Alcoholism: Initial:** 25-50mg; repeat in 2 to 4hrs. prn. **Acute/Severe Anxiety: Initial:** 25-50mg, then 12.5-50mg tid-qid prn. **Preoperative Anxiety:** 25-50mg 1 hr prior to surgery.	**W/P:** Avoid in pregnancy. Paradoxical reactions reported in psychiatric patients and in hyperactive, aggressive pediatrics. Caution with porphyria, renal or hepatic dysfunction. Reduce dose in elderly, debilitated. Avoid abrupt withdrawal after extended therapy. Observe patients up to 3 hrs after IM/IV use. **P/N:** Not for use in pregnancy, safety in nursing not known.	Drowsiness, ataxia, confusion, skin eruptions, edema, nausea, constipation, extrapyramidal symptoms, libido changes, EEG changes.
Clorazepate Dipotassium^{CIV} (Tranxene-SD, Tranxene T-Tab)	**Tab: (Tranxene T-Tab)** 3.75mg*, 7.5mg*, 15mg*; **Tab, Extended Release: (Tranxene-SD)** 22.5mg,	**Adults: Anxiety: Initial:** (Tab) 15mg qhs. **Usual:** 30mg/day in divided doses. **Max:** 60mg/day. **Elderly/Debilitated: Initial:** 7.5-15mg/day. (Tab, Extended-Release) 22.5mg q24h, (may substitute for 7.5mg tid)	**W/P:** Avoid with depressive neuroses or psychotic reactions. Withdrawal symptoms with abrupt withdrawal; taper gradually. Caution with known drug dependency, renal/hepatic impairment. Suicidal tendencies reported; give	Drowsiness, dizziness, GI complaints, nervousness, blurred vision, dry mouth, headache, mental confusion.

*Scored.   †Bold entries denote special dental considerations.

NAME	FORM/ STRENGTH	DOSAGE	WARNINGS/PRECAUTIONS & CONTRAINDICATIONS	ADVERSE EFFECTS†
Clorazepate Dipotassium^{CIV} (cont.)	**(Tranxene-SD Half Strength)** 11.25mg*	or 11.25mg/day (may substitute for 3.75mg tid). Do not use Extended-Release for initial therapy. **Alcohol Withdrawal: Day 1:** (Tab) 30mg, then 30-60mg/day. **Day 2:** 45-90mg/day. **Day 3:** 22.5-45mg/day. **Day 4:** 15-30mg. Give in divided doses. Reduce dose and continue with 7.5-15mg/day; discontinue when stable. **Max:** 90mg/day. **Antiepileptic Adjunct: Initial:** (Tab) 7.5mg tid. **Titrate:** Increase by no more than 7.5mg/week. **Max:** 90mg/day. **Pediatrics: >9 yrs: Anxiety: Initial:** (Tab) 15mg qhs. **Usual:** 30mg/day in divided doses. **Max:** 60mg/day. (Tab, Extended-Release) 22.5mg q24h, (may substitute for 7.5mg tid) or 11.25mg q24h (may substitute for 3.75mg tid). Do not use Extended-Release for initial therapy. **>12 yrs: Antiepileptic Adjunct: Initial:** (Tab) 7.5 mg tid. **Titrate:** Increase by no more than 7.5mg/day. **Max:** 90mg/day. 9-12 yrs: **Initial:** 7.5mg bid. **Titrate:** Increase by no more than 7.5mg/week. **Max:** 60mg/day.	lowest effective dose. Monitor LFTs and blood counts periodically with long-term therapy. Use lowest effective dose in elderly. **Contra:** Acute narrow-angle glaucoma. **P/N:** Safety in pregnancy not known, not for use in nursing.	
Diazepam^{CIV} (Valium)	**Tab:** 2mg*, 5mg*, 10mg*	**Adults: Anxiety:** 2-10mg bid-qid. **Alcohol Withdrawal:** 10mg tid-qid for 24 hours. **Maint:** 5mg tid-qid prn. **Skeletal Muscle Spasm:** 2-10mg tid-qid. **Seizure Disorders:** 2-10mg bid-qid. **Elderly/Debilitated:** 2-2.5mg qd-bid initially; may increase gradually as needed and tolerated. **Pediatrics: ≥6 months:** 1-2.5mg tid-qid initially; may increase gradually as needed and tolerated. **Pediatrics: ≥6 months:** 1-2.5mg tid-qid initially; may increase gradually as needed and tolerated.	**W/P:** Monitor blood counts and LFTs in long-term use. Neutropenia and jaundice reported. Increase in grand mal seizures reported. Avoid abrupt withdrawal. Caution with kidney or hepatic dysfunction. **Contra:** Acute narrow angle glaucoma, untreated open angle glaucoma, patients <6 months. **P/N:** Not for use during pregnancy, safety in nursing not known.	Drowsiness, fatigue, ataxia, paradoxical reactions, minor EEG changes.
Lorazepam^{CIV} (Ativan, Ativan Injection)	**Inj:** 2mg/mL, 4mg/mL. **Tab:** 0.5mg, 1mg*, 2mg*	**Adults: (Inj) ≥18 yrs: Status Epilepticus:** 4mg IV (given slowly at 2mg/min); may repeat 1 dose after 10-15 minutes if seizures recur or fail to cease. **Preanesthetic Sedation: Usual:** 0.05mg/kg IM; 2mg or 0.044mg/kg IV (whichever is smaller). **Max:** 4mg IM/IV. **(Tab) Initial:** 2-3mg/day given bid-tid. Usual: 2-6mg/day in divided doses. **Insomnia:** 2-4mg qhs. **Elderly/Debilitated:** 1-2mg/day in divided doses. **Pediatrics: >12 yrs: Initial:** 2-3mg/day given bid-tid. **Usual:** 2-6mg/day in divided doses. **Insomnia:** 2-4mg qhs.	**W/P:** (Inj) Monitor all parameters to maintain vital function. Risk of respiratory depression or airway obstruction in heavily sedated patients. May cause fetal damage during pregnancy. Increased risk of CNS and respiratory depression in elderly. Avoid with hepatic/renal failure. Caution with mild to moderate hepatic/renal disease. Avoid outpatient endoscopic procedures. Possible propylene glycol toxicity in renal impairment. (Tab) Avoid with primary depression or psychosis. Withdrawal symptoms with abrupt discontinuation. Careful supervision if addiction-prone. Caution with elderly, and renal or hepatic dysfunction. Monitor for GI disease with prolonged therapy. Periodic blood counts and LFTs with long-term therapy. **Contra:** Acute narrow-angle glaucoma, sleep apnea syndrome, severe respiratory insufficiency. Not for intra-arterial injection. **P/N:** (Inj) Category D, not for use in nursing. (Tab) Not for use in pregnancy or nursing.	Sedation, dizziness, weakness, unsteadiness, transient amnesia, memory impairment, respiratory depression/ failure, hypotension, somnolence, headache, hypoventilation.

Table 18.1: PRESCRIBING INFORMATION FOR PSYCHOACTIVE DRUGS (cont.)

NAME	FORM/ STRENGTH	DOSAGE	WARNINGS/PRECAUTIONS & CONTRAINDICATIONS	ADVERSE EFFECTS†
ANTIANXIETY AGENTS (cont.)				
LorazepamCIV (Ativan Injection)	**Inj:** 2mg/mL, 4mg/mL	***Adults: ≥18 yrs: Status Epilepticus:*** 4mg IV (given slowly at 2mg/min); may repeat 1 dose after 10-15 minutes if seizures recur or fail to cease. **Preanesthetic Sedation: Usual:** 0.05mg/kg IM; 2mg or 0.044mg/kg IV (whichever is smaller). **Max:** 4mg IM/IV.	**W/P:** Monitor all parameters to maintain vital function. Risk of respiratory depression or airway obstruction in heavily sedated patients. May cause fetal damage during pregnancy. Increased risk of CNS and respiratory depression in elderly. Avoid with hepatic/renal failure. Caution with mild to moderate hepatic/renal disease. Avoid outpatient endoscopic procedures. Possible propylene glycol toxicity in renal impairment. **Contra:** Acute narrow-angle glaucoma, sleep apnea syndrome, severe respiratory insufficiency. **P/N:** Not for intra-arterial injection. Category D, not for use in nursing.	Respiratory depression/ failure, hypotension, somnolence, headache, hypoventilation.
OxazepamCIV (Serax)	**Cap:** 10mg, 15mg, 30mg; **Tab:** 15mg	***Adults: Anxiety: Mild-Moderate:*** 10-15mg tid-qid. **Severe:** 15-30mg tid-qid. **Elderly: Initial:** 10mg tid. **Titrate:** Increase to 15mg tid-qid. **Alcohol Withdrawal:** 15-30mg tid-qid.	**W/P:** May impair mental/physical abilities. Withdrawal symptoms with abrupt discontinuation. Caution in sensitivity to hypotension, elderly. Caution with tablets in tartrazine or ASA allergy. Risk of congenital malformations; avoid in pregnancy. **Contra:** Psychoses. **P/N:** Not for use in pregnancy or nursing.	Drowsiness, dizziness, vertigo, headache, paradoxical excitement, transient amnesia, memory impairment.
NONBENZODIAZEPINES				
Buspirone Hydrochloride (Buspar)	**Tab:** 5mg*, 10mg*, 15mg*, 30mg*	***Adults: Usual:*** 7.5mg bid. **Titrate:** May increase by 5mg/day every 2-3 days. **Usual:** 20-30mg/day. **Max:** 60mg/day. Use low dose with potent CYP450 3A4 inhibitors (eg, 2.5mg qd with nefazodone). Take consistently with or without food; bioavailabilty increased with food.	**W/P:** Avoid with hepatic or renal impairment. **P/N:** Category B, not for use in nursing.	Dizziness, nausea, headache, nervousness, lightheadedness, excitement.
Escitalopram Oxalate (Lexapro)	**Sol:** 5mg/5mL [240mL]; **Tab:** 5mg, 10mg*, 20mg*	***Adults: Initial:*** 10mg qd, in am or pm. **Titrate:** May increase to 20mg after a minimum of 1 week. **Elderly/Hepatic Impairment:** 10mg qd. Re-evaluate periodically.	**Antidepressants increased the risk of suicidal thinking and behavior (suicidality) in short-term studies in children and adolescents with major depressive disorder and other psychiatric disorders. Escitalopram is not approved for use in pediatric patients. W/P:** Avoid abrupt withdrawal. Activation of mania/hypomania, hyponatremia reported. SIADH reported with citalopram. Caution with history of mania or seizures, hepatic impairment, severe renal impairment, conditions that alter metabolism or hemodynamic responses, suicidal tendencies. May impair mental/physical abilities. Consider tapering dose during 3rd trimester of pregnancy. **Contra:** Concomitant MAOI therapy. **P/N:** Category C, not for use in nursing.	Nausea, insomnia, ejaculation disorder, increased sweating, somnolence, fatigue, diarrhea.
Fluoxetine Hydrochloride (Prozac, Sarafem)	**(Prozac) Cap:** 10mg, 20mg, 40mg; **Sol:** 20mg/5mL [120mL]; **Tab:** 10mg*; **(Sarafem) Cap:** 10mg, 20mg	**(Prozac)** ***Adults: Major Depressive Disorder: Daily Dosing: Initial:*** 20mg qam; increase dose if no improvement after several weeks. Doses >20mg/day, give qam or bid (am and noon). **Max:** 80mg/day. Obsessive-Compulsive Disorder: **Initial:** 20mg/day. **Maint:** 20-60mg/day given qd-bid, am and noon. **Max:** 80mg/day. **Bulimia**	**Antidepressants increased the risk of suicidal thinking and behavior (suicidality) in children and adolescents with Major Depressive Disorder and other psychiatric disorders. Fluoxetine is approved for use in pediatric patients with major depressive disorder and obsessive-compulsive disorder. Contra:** During or within 14 days	Nausea, diarrhea, insomnia, anxiety, nervousness, dizziness, somnolence, tremor, decreased libido, sweating, anorexia, asthenia, **dry mouth,** dyspepsia, headache.

*Scored.   †Bold entries denote special dental considerations.

NAME	FORM/STRENGTH	DOSAGE	WARNINGS/PRECAUTIONS & CONTRAINDICATIONS	ADVERSE EFFECTS†
Fluoxetine Hydrochloride *(cont.)*		**Nervosa:** 60mg qam. **Max:** 60mg/day. **Panic Disorder: Initial:** 10mg/day. May increase to 20mg/day after 1 week. May increase further after several weeks if no clinical improvement. **Max:** 60mg/day. **Hepatic Impairment/Elderly:** Use lower or less frequent dosage. *Pediatrics:* **Major Depressive Disorder:** ≥8 yrs: **Higher Weight Peds: Initial:** 10 or 20mg/day. After 1 week at 10mg/day, may increase to 20mg/day. **Lower Weight Peds: Initial:** 10mg/day. **Titrate:** May increase to 20mg/day after several weeks if clinical improvement not observed. **Obsessive-Compulsive Disorder:** ≥7 yrs: **Adolescents and Higher Weight Peds: Initial:** 10mg/day. **Titrate:** Increase to 20mg/day after 2 weeks. Consider additional dose increases after several more weeks if clinical improvement not observed. **Usual:** 20-60mg/day. **Lower Weight Peds: Initial:** 10mg/day. **Titrate:** Consider additional dose increases after several weeks if clinical improvement not observed. **Usual:** 20-30mg/day. **Max:** 60mg/day. **(Sarafem)** *Adults:* **Continuous: Initial:** 20mg qd. **Maint:** 20mg/day up to 6 months. **Max:** 60mg/day. **Intermittent: Initial:** 20mg qd; start 14 days before menses onset through 1st full day of menses. **Maint:** 20mg/day up to 3 months. **Max:** 60mg/day. **Hepatic Impairment/Concurrent Disease/Concomitant Medications:** Lower dose or less frequent dosing.	of MAOI therapy. Thioridazine within 5 weeks of discontinuation. **W/P:** Discontinue if unexplained allergic reaction occurs. Monitor for symptoms of mania/hypomania. Caution with diseases or conditions that could affect metabolism or hemodynamic responses, diabetes, history of seizures, suicidal tendencies. Altered platelet function, hyponatremia reported. Periodically monitor height and weight in pediatrics. Monitor for clinical worsening and/or suicidality, especially at initiation of therapy or dose changes. Avoid abrupt withdrawal. Monitor for discontinuation symptoms. Caution in third trimester of pregnancy due to risk of serious neonatal complications. **P/N:** Category C, not for use in nursing.	
Hydroxyzine Hydrochloride (Atarax)	**Inj:** 25mg/mL, 50mg/mL; **Syrup:** 10mg/5mL; **Tab:** 10mg, 25mg, 50mg, 100mg	*Adults:* **PO: Anxiety:** 50-100mg qid. **Pruritus:** 25mg tid-qid. **Sedation:** 50-100mg. **IM: Nausea/Vomiting:** 25-100mg. **Pre-/Postoperative and Pre-/Postpartum Adjunct:** 25-100mg. **Psychiatric/Emotional Emergencies:** 50-100mg q4-6h prn. *Pediatrics:* **PO: Anxiety/Pruritus:** <6 yrs: 50mg/day in divided doses. ≥6 yrs: 50-100mg in divided doses. **Sedation:** 0.6mg/kg. **IM: Nausea/Vomiting:** 0.5mg/lb. **Pre-/Postoperative Adjunct:** 0.5mg/lb.	**W/P:** Caution in elderly. May impair mental/physical abilities. Effectiveness as an antianxiety agent for long term use (>4 months) has not been established. **Contra:** Early pregnancy. Inj is intended only for IM administration and should not, under any circumstances, be injected subcutaneously, intra-arterially, or IV. **P/N:** Not for use in pregnancy or nursing.	**Dry mouth**, drowsiness, involuntary motor activity.
Hydroxyzine Pamoate (Vistaril)	**Cap:** 25mg, 50mg, 100mg; **Sus:** 25mg/5mL [120mL, 480mL]	*Adults:* **Anxiety:** 50-100mg qid. **Pruritus:** 25mg tid-qid. **Sedation:** 50-100mg. *Pediatrics:* **Anxiety/Pruritus:** >6 yrs: 50-100mg/day in divided doses. <6 yrs: 50mg/day in divided doses. **Sedation:** 0.6mg/kg.	**W/P:** Caution in elderly. May impair mental/physical abilities. Effectiveness as an antianxiety agent for long term use (>4 months) has not been established. **Contra:** Early pregnancy. **P/N:** Safety unknown in pregnancy and is contraindicated in early pregnancy, not for use in nursing.	**Dry mouth**, drowsiness, involuntary motor activity.
Paroxetine Hydrochloride (Paxil, Paxil CR)	**(Paxil) Sus:** 10mg/5mL [250mL]; **Tab:** 10mg*, 20mg*, 30mg, 40mg *scored; **(Paxil CR) Tab, Controlled Release:** 12.5mg, 25mg, 37.5mg	**(Paxil)** *Adults:* Give qd, usually in the AM. **MDD: Initial:** 20mg/day. **Max:** 50mg/day. **OCD: Initial:** 20mg qd. **Usual:** 40mg qd. **Max:** 60mg/day. **Panic Disorder: Initial:** 10mg qd. **Usual:** 40mg qd. **Max:** 60mg/day. **GAD: Initial:** 20mg/day. **Usual:** 20-50mg/day. **SAD: Initial/Usual:** 20mg/day. **PTSD: Initial:** 20mg/day. **Usual:** 20-50mg/day. To titrate, may increase weekly by 10mg/day. **Elderly/Debilitated/Severe Renal/**	**Antidepressants increased the risk of suicidal thinking and behavior (suicidality) in short-term studies in children and adolescents with major depressive disorder and other psychiatric disorders. Paroxetine is not approved for use in pediatric patients. W/P:** Caution with history of mania or seizures, conditions that affect metabolism or hemodynamic responses, narrow angle glaucoma. Discontinue if seizures occur.	Somnolence, insomnia, nausea, asthenia, abnormal ejaculation, **dry mouth**, constipation, dizziness, diarrhea, decreased libido, sweating.

Table 18.1: PRESCRIBING INFORMATION FOR PSYCHOACTIVE DRUGS (cont.)

NAME	FORM/STRENGTH	DOSAGE	WARNINGS/PRECAUTIONS & CONTRAINDICATIONS	ADVERSE EFFECTS†
ANTIANXIETY AGENTS (cont.)				
Paroxetine Hydrochloride (cont.)		**Hepatic Impairment: Initial:** 10mg qd. **Max:** 40mg/day. **(Paxil CR) Adults:** Give qd, usually in the AM. Swallow whole. **MDD: Initial:** 25mg/day. **Titrate:** May increase weekly by 12.5mg/day. **Max:** 62.5mg/day. **Panic Disorder: Initial:** 12.5mg/day. May increase weekly by 12.5mg/day. **Max:** 75mg/day. **SAD: Initial:** 12.5mg/day. May increase weekly by 12.5mg/day. **Max:** 37.5mg/day. **PMDD: Initial:** 12.5mg/day continuous or limited to luteal phase of cycle. May increase weekly by 12.5mg/day. **Elderly/Debilitated/Severe Renal/Hepatic Impairment: Initial:** 12.5mg/day. **Max:** 50mg/day.	Altered platelet function, hyponatremia, mydriasis reported. Avoid abrupt withdrawal. Re-evaluate periodically. Monitor for clinical worsening and/or suicidality, especially at initiation of therapy or dose changes. **Contra:** Concomitant MAOIs or thioridazine. **P/N:** (Paxil) Category D, caution in nursing. (Paxil CR) Category C, caution in nursing.	
Paroxetine Mesylate (Pexeva)	**Tab:** 10mg, 20mg, 30mg, 40mg	**Adult: MDD: Initial:** 20mg/day. **Max:** 50mg/day. **OCD: Initial:** 40mg/day. **Max:** 60mg/day. **Panic Disorder: Initial:** 10mg/day. **Titrate:** 10mg/day increments at intervals of at least 1 week. Max: 60mg/day. **Elderly/Debilitated/Severe Renal or Hepatic Impairment: Initial:** 10mg qd. **Max:** 40mg/day.	**Antidepressants increased the risk of suicidal thinking and behavior (suicidality) in short-term studies in children and adolescents with major depressive disorder (MDD) and other psychiatric disorders. Pexeva is not approved for use in pediatric patients. W/P:** Caution with history of mania or seizures, conditions that affect metabolism or hemodynamic responses, narrow angle glaucoma. Discontinue if seizures occur. Altered platelet function, hyponatremia, mydriasis reported. Avoid abrupt withdrawal. Re-evaluate periodically. Monitor for clinical worsening and/or suicidality, especially at initiation of therapy or dose changes. **P/N:** Category C, caution in nursing.	Asthenia, sweating, nausea, decreased appetite, somnolence, dizziness, insomnia, tremor, nervousness, abnormal ejaculation, **dry mouth**, constipation, decreased libido, impotence.
Sertraline Hydrochloride (Zoloft)	**Sol:** 20mg/mL [60mL]; **Tab:** 25mg*, 50mg*, 100mg*	**Adults: MDD/OCD:** 50mg qd. **Titrate:** Adjust dose at 1 week intervals. **Max:** 200mg/day. **Panic Disorder/PTSD/SAD: Initial:** 25mg qd. **Titrate:** Increase to 50mg qd after 1 week. Adjust dose at 1 week intervals. **Max:** 200mg/day. **PMDD: Initial:** 50mg qd continuous or limited to luteal phase of cycle. **Titrate:** Increase 50mg/cycle if needed up to 150mg/day for continuous or 100mg/day for luteal phase dosing. If 100mg/day is established for luteal phase dosing, a 50mg/day titration step for 3 days should take place at the beginning of each luteal phase dosing period. **Hepatic Impairment:** Use lower or less frequent doses. Dilute solution with 4oz of water, ginger ale, lemon/lime soda, lemonade or orange juice. Take immediately after mixing. **Pediatrics: OCD: Initial: 6-12 yrs:** 25mg qd. **13-17 yrs:** 50mg qd. **Titrate:** Adjust dose at 1 week intervals. **Max:** 200mg/day. **Hepatic Impairment:** Use lower or less frequent doses. Dilute solution with 4oz of water, ginger ale, lemon/lime soda, lemonade or orange juice. Take immediately after mixing.	**Antidepressants increased the risk of suicidal thinking and behavior (suicidality) in short-term studies in children and adolescents with major depressive disorder (MDD) and other psychiatric disorders. Sertraline HCl is not approved for use in pediatric patients except for patients with obsessive compulsive disorder. W/P:** Activation of mania/hypomania reported. Monitor weight loss. Caution with conditions that could affect metabolism or hemodynamic responses, seizure disorder. Dose adjust with liver dysfunction. Altered platelet function and hyponatremia reported. Weak uricosuric effects reported. Caution with latex sensitivity; solution dropper dispenser contains rubber. Monitor for clinical worsening and/or suicidality, especially at initiation of therapy or dose changes. Avoid abrupt withdrawal. Monitor for discontinuation symptoms. **Contra:** Concomitant use with MAOIs or pimozide. Concomitant disulfiram with solution. **P/N:** Category C, caution in nursing.	Ejaculation failure, **dry mouth**, increased sweating, somnolence, tremor, anorexia, dizziness, headache, vomiting, diarrhea, dyspepsia, nausea, agitation, insomnia, nervousness, abnormal vision.

*Scored.   †Bold entries denote special dental considerations.

NAME	FORM/ STRENGTH	DOSAGE	WARNINGS/PRECAUTIONS & CONTRAINDICATIONS	ADVERSE EFFECTS†
Venlafaxine Hydrochloride (Effexor, Effexor XR)	(Effexor) **Tab:** 25mg*, 37.5mg*, 50mg*, 75mg*, 100mg* *scored; **(Effexor-XR) Cap, Extended Release:** 37.5mg, 75mg, 150mg	(Effexor) *Adults:* ≥18 yrs: **Initial:** 75mg/day given bid-tid with food. **Titrate:** Increase by 75mg/day at no less than 4 day intervals. **Max:** 375mg/day. **Hepatic Impairment (moderate):** Reduce dose by 50%. **Renal Impairment (mild-to-moderate):** Reduce dose by 25%. **Hemodialysis:** Reduce dose by 50%. Withhold dose until after hemodialysis treatment completed. If drug used 6 weeks or longer, taper gradually (over 2 weeks or more) when discontinuing treatment. **(Effexor XR)** *Adults:* **MDD/ GAD/SAD: Initial:** 75mg qd, or 37.5mg qd increase to 75mg qd after 4-7 days. **Titrate:** May increase by 75mg/day at no less than 4 day intervals. **Max:** 225mg/day . **PD: Initial:** 37.5mg qd for 7 days. **Titrate:** May increase 75mg/day, as needed at no less than 7 day intervals. **Max:** 225mg/day. **Moderate Hepatic Impairment:** Reduce initial dose by 50%. **Renal Impairment:** Reduce total daily dose by 25-50%. **Hemodialysis:** Reduce total daily dose by 50%. Withhold dose until after hemodialysis treatment completed. If drug used 6 weeks or longer, taper gradually (over 2 weeks or more) when discontinuing treatment. Periodically reassess need for maintenance therapy. Take with food in the am or pm, the same time each day. May sprinkle on spoonful of applesauce. Do not divide, crush, chew or place in water.	**Antidepressants increased the risk of suicidal thinking and behavior (suicidality) in short-term studies in children and adolescents with major depressive disorder and other psychiatric disorders. Venlafaxine is not approved for use in pediatric patients. W/P:** May cause sustained increases in BP. Treatment-emergent anxiety, nervousness, insomnia, and anorexia reported. Caution with history of mania or seizures and conditions affecting hemodynamic responses. Monitor with increased IOP or if at risk of acute narrow angle glaucoma. Activation of mania/hypomania reported. Risk of hyponatremia, SIADH, skin and mucous membrane bleeding. Caution with hyperthyroidism, heart failure, recent MI, renal or hepatic impairment. **Contra:** Concomitant MAOI therapy. **P/N:** Category C, not for use in nursing.	Asthenia, sweating, nausea, constipation, anorexia, vomiting, insomnia, somnolence, **dry mouth**, dizziness, nervousness, anxiety, tremor, blurred vision, abnormal ejaculation/orgasm, impotence in men.

ANTIDEPRESSANTS

MONOAMINE OXIDASE INHIBITORS

Phenelzine Sulfate (Nardil)	**Tab:** 15mg	*Adults:* **Initial:** 15mg tid. **Titrate:** Increase to 60-90mg/day at a fairly rapid pace until maximum benefit. **Maint:** Reduce slowly over several weeks to 15mg qd or 15mg every other day.	**Antidepressants increased the risk of suicidal thinking and behavior (suicidality) in short-term studies in children and adolescents with major depressive disorder and other psychiatric disorders. Phenelzine is not approved for use in pediatric patients. W/P:** Hypertensive crisis, postural hypotension reported; monitor BP frequently. Caution with epilepsy, asthma, psychosis, DM. Discontinue if palpitations or headache occur. Excessive stimulation in schizophrenics. Discontinue 10 days prior to elective surgery. Avoid abrupt withdrawal. **Contra:** Pheochromocytoma, CHF, history of liver disease, abnormal LFTs, meperidine, MAOIs, dextromethorphan, CNS depressants, alcohol, certain narcotics, sympathomimetic drugs (eg, amphetamines, cocaine, methylphenidate, dopamine, epinephrine, norepinephrine),	Dizziness, headache, drowsiness, sleep disturbances, constipation, **dry mouth**, GI disturbances, elevated serum transaminases, weight gain, postural hypotension, edema, sexual disturbances.

Table 18.1: PRESCRIBING INFORMATION FOR PSYCHOACTIVE DRUGS (cont.)

NAME	FORM/ STRENGTH	DOSAGE	WARNINGS/PRECAUTIONS & CONTRAINDICATIONS	ADVERSE EFFECTS†
ANTIDEPRESSANTS (cont.)				
Phenelzine Sulfate (cont.)			or related compounds (eg, methyldopa, L-dopa, L-tryptophan, L-tyrosine, phenylalanine), high tyramine-containing food (eg, cheese, pickled herring, beer, wine, yeast extract, salami, yogurt), excessive caffeine and chocolate, dextromethorphan, CNS depressants, buspirone, serotoninergic agents (eg, dexfenfluramine, fluoxetine, fluvoxamine, paroxetine, sertraline, venlafaxine), bupropion, guanethidine. **P/N:** Safety in pregnancy and nursing not known.	
Tranylcypromine Sulfate (Parnate)	**Tab:** 10mg	**Adults: Usual:** 30mg/day in divided doses. **Titrate:** After 2 weeks, may increase by 10mg/day every 1-3 weeks depending on signs of improvement. **Max:** 60mg/day.	**Antidepressants increased the risk of suicidal thinking and behavior (suicidality) in short-term studies in children and adolescents with major depressive disorder and other psychiatric disorders. Tranylcypromine is not approved for use in pediatric patients. W/P:** Hypertensive crisis, postural hypotension reported; monitor BP frequently. Caution with epilepsy, asthma, psychosis, DM. Discontinue if palpitations or headache occur. Excessive stimulation in schizophrenics. Discontinue 10 days prior to elective surgery. Avoid abrupt withdrawal. **Contra:** Pheochromocytoma, CHF, history of liver disease, abnormal LFTs, meperidine, MAOIs, dextromethorphan, CNS depressants, alcohol, certain narcotics, sympathomimetic drugs (eg, amphetamines, cocaine, methylphenidate, dopamine, epinephrine, norepinephrine), or related compounds (eg, methyldopa, L-dopa, L-tryptophan, L-tyrosine, phenylalanine), high tyramine-containing food (eg, cheese, pickled herring, beer, wine, yeast extract, salami, yogurt), excessive caffeine and chocolate, dextromethorphan, CNS depressants, buspirone, serotoninergic agents (eg, dexfenfluramine, fluoxetine, fluvoxamine, paroxetine, sertraline, venlafaxine), bupropion, guanethidine. **P/N:** Safety in pregnancy and nursing not known.	Restlessness, insomnia, weakness, drowsiness, nausea, diarrhea, tachycardia, anorexia, edema, tinnitis, muscle spasm, overstimulation, dizziness, **dry mouth**, blood dyscrasias.
SELECTIVE SEROTONIN REUPTAKE INHIBITORS				
Citalopram Hydrobromide (Celexa)	**Sol:** 10mg/5mL [240mL]; **Tab:** 10mg, 20mg*, 40mg*	**Adults: Initial:** 20mg qd, in the am or pm. **Titrate:** Increase by 20mg at intervals of no less than 1 week. **Max:** 40mg/day (nonresponders may require 60mg/day). **Elderly/Hepatic Impairment:** 20mg/day; titrate to 40mg/day in nonresponders.	**Antidepressants increased the risk of suicidal thinking and behavior (suicidality) in short-term studies in children and adolescents with major depressive disorder and other psychiatric disorders. Citalopram is not approved for use in pediatric patients. Contra:** Concomitant MAOI therapy. **W/P:** Activation of mania/hypomania, SIADH, hyponatremia reported. Close supervision with high risk suicide patients. Caution with history of mania or seizures, hepatic impairment, severe renal impairment, conditions that alter metabolism or hemodynamic responses. May impair judgment, thinking, or motor skills. **P/N:** Category C, not for use in nursing.	Nausea, dyspepsia, vomiting, diarrhea, **dry mouth**, somnolence, insomnia, increased sweating, ejaculation disorder, rhinitis, anxiety, anorexia, skeletal pain, agitation.

*Scored.   †Bold entries denote special dental considerations.

NAME	FORM/STRENGTH	DOSAGE	WARNINGS/PRECAUTIONS & CONTRAINDICATIONS	ADVERSE EFFECTS†
Escitalopram Oxalate (Lexapro)	**Sol:** 5mg/5mL [240mL]; **Tab:** 5mg, 10mg*, 20mg*	**Adults: Initial:** 10mg qd, in am or pm. **Titrate:** May increase to 20mg after a minimum of 1 week. **Elderly/Hepatic Impairment:** 10mg qd. Re-evaluate periodically.	**Antidepressants increased the risk of suicidal thinking and behavior (suicidality) in short-term studies in children and adolescents with major depressive disorder and other psychiatric disorders. Escitalopram is not approved for use in pediatric patients. W/P:** Avoid abrupt withdrawal. Activation of mania/hypomania, hyponatremia reported. SIADH reported with citalopram. Caution with history of mania or seizures, hepatic impairment, severe renal impairment, conditions that alter metabolism or hemodynamic responses, suicidal tendencies. May impair mental/physical abilities. Consider tapering dose during 3rd trimester of pregnancy. **Contra:** Concomitant MAOI therapy. **P/N:** Category C, not for use in nursing.	Nausea, insomnia, ejaculation disorder, increased sweating, somnolence, fatigue, diarrhea.
Fluoxetine Hydrochloride (Prozac, Sarafem)	**(Prozac) Cap:** 10mg, 20mg, 40mg; **Sol:** 20mg/5mL [120mL]; **Tab:** 10mg*; **(Sarafem) Cap:** 10mg, 20mg	**(Prozac) Adults: MDD: Daily Dosing: Initial:** 20mg qam; increase dose if no improvement after several weeks. Doses >20mg/day, give qam or bid (am and noon). **Max:** 80mg/day. **OCD: Initial:** 20mg/day. **Maint:** 20-60mg/day given qd-bid, am and noon. **Max:** 80mg/day. **Bulimia Nervosa:** 60mg qam. **Max:** 60mg/day. **Panic Disorder: Initial:** 10mg/day. May increase to 20mg/day after 1 week. May increase further after several weeks if no clinical improvement. **Max:** 60mg/day. **Hepatic Impairment/Elderly:** Use lower or less frequent dosage. **Pediatrics: MDD: ≥8 yrs: Higher Weight Peds: Initial:** 10 or 20mg/day. After 1 week at 10mg/day, may increase to 20mg/day. **Lower Weight Peds: Initial:** 10mg/day. **Titrate:** May increase to 20mg/day after several weeks if clinical improvement not observed. **OCD: ≥7 yrs: Adolescents and Higher Weight Peds: Initial:** 10mg/day. **Titrate:** Increase to 20mg/day after 2 weeks. Consider additional dose increases after several more weeks if clinical improvement not observed. **Usual:** 20-60mg/day. **Lower Weight Peds: Initial:** 10mg/day. **Titrate:** Consider additional dose increases after several weeks if clinical improvement not observed. **Usual:** 20-30mg/day. **Max:** 60mg/day. **(Sarafem) Adults: Continuous: Initial:** 20mg qd. **Maint:** 20mg/day up to 6 months. **Max:** 60mg/day. **Intermittent: Initial:** 20mg qd; start 14 days before menses onset through 1st full day of menses. **Maint:** 20mg/day up to 3 months. **Max:** 60mg/day. **Hepatic Impairment/Concurrent Disease/Concomitant Medications:** Lower dose or less frequent dosing.	**Antidepressants increased the risk of suicidal thinking and behavior (suicidality) in short-term studies in children and adolescents with major depressive disorder and other psychiatric disorders. Fluoxetine is approved for use in pediatric patients with major depressive disorder and obsessive compulsive disorder. Contra:** During or within 14 days of MAOI therapy. Thioridazine within 5 weeks of discontinuation. **W/P:** Discontinue if unexplained allergic reaction occurs. Monitor for symptoms of mania/hypomania. Caution with diseases or conditions that could affect metabolism or hemodynamic responses, diabetes, history of seizures, suicidal tendencies. Altered platelet function, hyponatremia reported. Periodically monitor height and weight in pediatrics. Monitor for clinical worsening and/or suicidality, especially at initiation of therapy or dose changes. Avoid abrupt withdrawal. Monitor for discontinuation symptoms. Caution in third trimester of pregnancy due to risk of serious neonatal complications. **P/N:** Category C, not for use in nursing.	Nausea, diarrhea, insomnia, anxiety, nervousness, dizziness, somnolence, tremor, decreased libido, sweating, anorexia, asthenia, **dry mouth**, dyspepsia, headache.
Paroxetine Hydrochloride (Paxil, Paxil CR)	**(Paxil) Sus:** 10mg/5mL [250mL]; **Tab:** 10mg*, 20mg*, 30mg, 40mg *scored; **(Paxil**	**(Paxil) Adults:** Give qd, usually in the AM. **MDD: Initial:** 20mg/day. **Max:** 50mg/day. **OCD: Initial:** 20mg qd. **Usual:** 40mg qd. **Max:** 60mg/day. **Panic Disorder: Initial:** 10mg qd. **Usual:** 40mg/day. **Max:** 60mg/day.	**Antidepressants increased the risk of suicidal thinking and behavior (suicidality) in short-term studies in children and adolescents with major depressive disorder and other psychiatric disorders. Paroxetine is not**	Somnolence, insomnia, nausea, asthenia, abnormal ejaculation, **dry mouth**, constipation, dizziness, diarrhea, decreased

Table 18.1: PRESCRIBING INFORMATION FOR PSYCHOACTIVE DRUGS (cont.)

NAME	FORM/ STRENGTH	DOSAGE	WARNINGS/PRECAUTIONS & CONTRAINDICATIONS	ADVERSE EFFECTS†
ANTIDEPRESSANTS (cont.)				
Paroxetine Hydrochloride (cont.)	**CR) Tab, Controlled Release:** 12.5mg, 25mg, 37.5mg	**GAD: Initial:** 20mg/day. **Usual:** 20-50mg/day. **SAD: Initial/Usual:** 20mg/day. **PTSD: Initial:** 20mg/day. **Usual:** 20-50mg/day. To titrate, may increase weekly by 10mg/day. **Elderly/ Debilitated/Severe Renal/Hepatic Impairment: Initial:** 10mg qd. **Max: (Paxil CR) Adults:** Give qd, usually in the AM. Swallow whole. **MDD: Initial:** 25mg/day. **Titrate:** May increase weekly by 12.5mg/day. **Max:** 62.5mg/day. **Panic Disorder: Initial:** 12.5mg/day. May increase weekly by 12.5mg/day. **Max:** 75mg/day. **SAD: Initial:** 12.5mg/day. May increase weekly by 12.5mg/day. **Max:** 37.5mg/day. **PMDD: Initial:** 12.5mg/day continuous or limited to luteal phase of cycle. May increase weekly by 12.5mg/day. **Elderly/Debilitated/Severe Renal/Hepatic Impairment: Initial:** 12.5mg/day. **Max:** 50mg/day.	**approved for use in pediatric patients. W/P:** Caution with history of mania or seizures, conditions that affect metabolism or hemodynamic responses, narrow angle glaucoma. Discontinue if seizures occur. Altered platelet function, hyponatremia, mydriasis reported. Avoid abrupt withdrawal. Re-evaluate periodically. Monitor for clinical worsening and/or suicidality, especially at initiation of therapy or dose changes. **Contra:** Concomitant MAOIs or thioridazine. **P/N:** (Paxil) Category D, caution in nursing. (Paxil CR) Category C, caution in nursing.	libido, sweating.
Paroxetine Mesylate (Pexeva)	**Tab:** 10mg, 20mg, 30mg, 40mg	**Adult: MDD: Initial:** 20mg/day. **Max:** 50mg/day. **OCD: Initial:** 40mg/day. **Max:** 60mg/day. **Panic Disorder: Initial:** 10mg/day. **Titrate:** May increase in 10mg increments at intervals of at least 1 week. **Max:** 60mg/day. **Elderly/Debilitated/Severe Renal or Hepatic Impairment: Initial:** 10mg qd. **Max:** 40mg/day.	**Antidepressants increased the risk of suicidal thinking and behavior (suicidality) in short-term studies in children and adolescents with major depressive disorder and other psychiatric disorders. Pexeva is not approved for use in pediatric patients. W/P:** Caution with history of mania or seizures, conditions that affect metabolism or hemodynamic responses, narrow angle glaucoma. Discontinue if seizures occur. Altered platelet function, hyponatremia, mydriasis reported. Avoid abrupt withdrawal. Re-evaluate periodically. Monitor for clinical worsening and/or suicidality, especially at initiation of therapy or dose changes. **Contra:** Concomitant MAOIs or thioridazine. **P/N:** Category D, caution in nursing.	Asthenia, sweating, nausea, decreased appetite, somnolence, dizziness, insomnia, tremor, nervousness, abnormal ejaculation, dry mouth, constipation, decreased libido, impotence.
Sertraline Hydrochloride (Zoloft)	**Sol:** 20mg/mL [60mL]; **Tab:** 25mg*, 50mg*, 100mg* *scored	**Adults: MDD/OCD:** 50mg qd. **Titrate:** Adjust dose at 1 week intervals. **Max:** 200mg/day. **Panic Disorder/PTSD/SAD: Initial:** 25mg qd. **Titrate:** Increase to 50mg/day after 1 week. Adjust dose at 1 week intervals. **Max:** 200mg/day. **PMDD: Initial:** 50mg qd continuous or limited to luteal phase of cycle. **Titrate:** Increase 50mg/cycle if needed up to 150mg/day for continuous or 100mg/day for luteal phase dosing. If 100mg/day is established for luteal phase dosing, a 50mg/day titration step for 3 days should take place at the beginning of each luteal phase dosing period. **Hepatic Impairment:** Use lower or less frequent doses. Dilute solution with 4oz of water, ginger ale, lemon/ lime soda, lemonade **or orange juice. Take immediately after mixing.**	**Antidepressants increased the risk of suicidal thinking and behavior (suicidality) in short-term studies in children and adolescents with major depressive disorder and other psychiatric disorders. Sertraline HCl is not approved for use in pediatric patients except for patients with obsessive compulsive disorder. W/P:** Activation of mania/hypomania reported. Monitor weight loss. Caution with conditions that could affect metabolism or hemodynamic responses, seizure disorder. Dose adjust with liver dysfunction. Altered platelet function and hyponatremia reported. Weak uricosuric effects reported. Caution with latex sensitivity; solution dropper dispenser contains rubber. Monitor for clinical worsening and/or suicidality, especially at initiation of therapy or dose changes. Avoid abrupt withdrawal. Monitor for discontinuation symptoms. **Contra:** Concomitant use with MAOIs or pimozide. Concomitant disulfiram with solution.	Ejaculation failure, dry mouth, increased sweating, somnolence, tremor, anorexia, dizziness, headache, vomiting, diarrhea, dyspepsia, nausea, agitation, insomnia, nervousness, abnormal vision.

*Scored.   †Bold entries denote special dental considerations.

NAME	FORM/ STRENGTH	DOSAGE	WARNINGS/PRECAUTIONS & CONTRAINDICATIONS	ADVERSE EFFECTS†
Sertraline Hydrochloride *(cont.)*		***Pediatrics:*** **OCD: Initial: 6-12 yrs:** 25mg qd. **13-17 yrs:** 50mg qd. **Titrate:** Adjust dose at 1 week intervals. **Max:** 200mg/day. **Hepatic Impairment:** Use lower or less frequent doses. Dilute solution with 4oz of water, ginger ale, lemon/lime soda, lemonade or orange juice. Take immediately after mixing.	**P/N:** Category C, caution in nursing.	

SEROTONIN/NOREPINEPHRINE REUPTAKE INHIBITORS

NAME	FORM/ STRENGTH	DOSAGE	WARNINGS/PRECAUTIONS & CONTRAINDICATIONS	ADVERSE EFFECTS†
Duloxetine Hydrochloride (Cymbalta)	**Cap, Delayed-Release:** 20mg, 30mg, 60mg	***Adults:*** **MDD: Initial:** 40mg/day (given as 20mg bid) to 60mg/day (given once daily or as 30mg bid). Re-evaluate periodically. **Diabetic Peripheral Neuropathic Pain:** 60mg/day given once daily. May lower starting dose if tolerability is a concern. **Renal Impairment:** Consider lower starting dose with gradual increase. Do not chew or crush.	**Antidepressants increased the risk of suicidal thinking and behavior (suicidality) in short-term studies in children and adolescents with major depressive disorder and other psychiatric disorders. Duloxetine is not approved for use in pediatric patients. W/P:** Monitor for clinical worsening and/or suicidality. May increase risk of serum transaminase elevations. Avoid with chronic liver disease. May increase BP; obtain baseline and monitor periodically. Avoid abrupt cessation and in patients with severe renal impairment/ESRD or hepatic insufficiency. Caution with conditions that may slow gastric emptying, history of mania or seizures. May increase risk of mydriasis; caution in patients with controlled narrow-angle glaucoma. **Contra:** During or within 14 days of MAOI therapy, uncontrolled narrow-angle glaucoma. **P/N:** Category C, not for use in nursing.	Nausea, dry mouth, constipation, diarrhea, vomiting, decreased appetite, fatigue, dizziness, somnolence, increased sweating, blurred vision, insomnia, erectile dysfunction.
Nefazodone Hydrochloride	**Tab:** 50mg, 100mg*, 150mg*, 200mg, 250mg	***Adults:*** **Initial:** 100mg bid. **Usual:** 300-600mg/day. **Titrate:** May increase by 100-200mg/day at intervals of no less than 1 week. **Elderly/Debilitated: Initial:** 50mg bid.	**Antidepressants increased the risk of suicidal thinking and behavior (suicidality) in short-term studies in children and adolescents with major depressive disorder and other psychiatric disorders. Nefazodone is not approved for use in pediatric patients. Life-threatening hepatic failure reported. Avoid with active liver disease or elevated serum transaminases. Discontinue and do not retreat if symptoms of hepatic disease develop or if ALT/AST ≥3X ULN. W/P:** May cause postural hypotension. Caution with cardiovascular or cerebrovascular disease that could be exacerbated by hypotension and conditions with predisposition to hypotension (eg, dehydration, hypotension). May activate mania/hypomania. Priapism reported. Caution with history of MI, unstable heart disease, seizures, liver cirrhosis. Avoid with active liver disease. **Contra:** Coadministration of terfenadine, astemizole, cisapride, pimozide, carbamazepine, triazolam. Liver injury from previous treatment. **P/N:** Category C, caution in nursing.	Hepatic failure, somnolence, **dry mouth,** nausea, dizziness, insomnia, agitation, constipation, asthenia, lightheadedness, blurred vision, confusion, abnormal vision.
Venlafaxine Hydrochloride (Effexor, Effexor-XR)	**(Effexor) Tab:** 25mg*, 37.5mg*, 50mg*, 75mg*, 100mg*;	**(Effexor) *Adults:* ≥18 yrs: Initial:** 75mg/day given bid-tid with food. **Titrate:** Increase by 75mg/day at no less than 4-day intervals. **Max:** 375mg/day. **Hepatic Impairment (Moderate):**	**Antidepressants increased the risk of suicidal thinking and behavior in short-term studies in children and adolescents with major depressive disorder and other psychiatric**	Asthenia, sweating, nausea, constipation, anorexia, vomiting, insomnia, somnolence, **dry mouth,** dizziness,

Table 18.1: PRESCRIBING INFORMATION FOR PSYCHOACTIVE DRUGS (cont.)

NAME	FORM/ STRENGTH	DOSAGE	WARNINGS/PRECAUTIONS & CONTRAINDICATIONS	ADVERSE EFFECTS†
ANTIDEPRESSANTS (cont.)				
Venlafaxine Hydrochloride (cont.)	**(Effexor-XR) Cap, Extended Release:** 37.5mg, 75mg, 150mg	Reduce dose by 50%. **Renal Impairment (Mild-to-Moderate):** Reduce dose by 25%. **Hemodialysis:** Reduce dose by 50%. Withhold dose until after hemodialysis treatment completed. If drug used 6 weeks or longer, taper gradually (over 2 weeks or more) when discontinuing treatment. **(Effexor XR) Adults: MDD/GAD/SAD: Initial:** 75mg qd, or 37.5mg qd increase to 75mg qd after 4-7 days. **Titrate:** May increase by 75mg/day at no less than 4-day intervals. **Max:** 225mg/day. **PD: Initial:** 37.5mg qd for 7 days. **Titrate:** May increase 75mg/day, as needed at no less than 7-day intervals. **Max:** 225mg/day. **Moderate Hepatic Impairment:** Reduce initial dose by 50%. **Renal Impairment:** Reduce total daily dose by 25-50%. **Hemodialysis:** Reduce total daily dose by 50%. Withhold dose until after hemodialysis treatment completed. If drug used 6 weeks or longer, taper gradually (over 2 weeks or more) when discontinuing treatment. Periodically reassess need for maintenance therapy. Take with food in am or pm, the same time each day. May sprinkle on spoonful of applesauce. Do not divide, crush, chew or place in water.	**disorders. Venlafaxine is not approved for use in pediatric patients. W/P:** May cause sustained increases in BP. Treatment-emergent anxiety, nervousness, insomnia, and anorexia reported. Caution with history of mania or seizures and conditions affecting hemodynamic responses. Monitor with increased IOP or if at risk of acute narrow angle glaucoma. Activation of mania/hypomania reported. Risk of hyponatremia, SIADH, skin and mucous membrane bleeding. Caution with hyperthyroidism, heart failure, recent MI, renal or hepatic impairment. **Contra:** Concomitant MAOI therapy. **P/N:** Category C, not for use in nursing.	nervousness, anxiety, tremor, blurred vision, abnormal ejaculation/orgasm, impotence in men.
TETRACYCLIC AGENTS				
Maprotiline Hydrochloride	**Tab:** 25mg, 50mg, 75mg	**Adults: Outpatient: Initial:** 25-75mg qd for 2 weeks. **Maint:** Increase by 25mg. **Max:** 225mg/day. **Hospitalized: Initial:** 100-150mg qd. **Maint:** 150-225 mg/day. **Max:** 225mg/day.	**W/P:** Caution with bipolar disorder, cardiovascular disease, glaucoma, hepatic or renal damage, hypertensive patients receiving adrenergic blocking agents, hyperthyroidism, patients with history of myocardial infarction, patients with suicidal tendencies, pregnancy or lactation, prostatic hypertrophy, schizophrenia. Suicidal ideation and behavior or worsening depression; increased risk, particularly in children and adolescents, during the first few months of therapy. **Contra:** Acute recovery phase following myocardial infarction; coadministration with or within 2 weeks of treatment with monoamine oxidase inhibitors; seizure disorders. **P/N:** Category B, caution in nursing.	Hypotension, tachyarrhythmia, rash, weight gain, constipation, nausea, pancreatitis, **reduced salivation**, vomiting, **xerostomia**, asthenia, headache, myoclonus, somnolence, tremor, vertigo, blurred vision, agitation, anxiety, nervousness, micturition finding, delayed, urinary retention, fatigue.
Mirtazapine (Remeron, Remeron Soltab)	**Tab:** 15mg*, 30mg*, 45mg; **Tab, Disintegrating:** 15mg, 30mg, 45mg	**Adults: Initial:** 15mg qhs. **Titrate:** May increase every 1-2 weeks. **Max:** 45mg/day. Disintegrating tabs disintegrate rapidly on the tongue and can be swallowed with saliva; no water is needed. Do not cut tabs in half.	**Antidepressants increased the risk of suicidal thinking and behavior (suicidality) in short-term studies in children and adolescents with major depressive disorder and other psychiatric disorders. Mirtazapine is not approved for use in pediatric patients. W/P:** Risk of agranulocytosis. Discontinue if develop sore throat, fever, or stomatitis, along with low WBC count. May increase appetite, cholesterol, and triglycerides. Caution in history of seizures, mania/hypomania,	Somnolence, appetite increase, weight gain, dizziness, **dry mouth**, constipation, asthenia, flu syndrome, abnormal dreams.

*Scored.   †Bold entries denote special dental considerations.

NAME	FORM/ STRENGTH	DOSAGE	WARNINGS/PRECAUTIONS & CONTRAINDICATIONS	ADVERSE EFFECTS†
Mirtazapine *(cont.)*			hepatic or renal impairment, altered metabolic or hemodynamic conditions, elderly. Somnolence, dizziness reported. Close supervision with high risk suicide patients. May impair judgement, thinking, or motor skills. **P/N:** Category C, caution in nursing.	

TRICYCLIC AGENTS

NAME	FORM/ STRENGTH	DOSAGE	WARNINGS/PRECAUTIONS & CONTRAINDICATIONS	ADVERSE EFFECTS†
Amitriptyline Hydrochloride (Elavil)	**Inj:** 10mg/mL; **Tab:** 10mg, 25mg, 50mg, 75mg, 100mg, 150mg	***Adults:*** **PO: Initial: (Outpatient)** 75mg/day in divided doses or 50-100mg qhs. **(Inpatient)** 100mg/day. **Titrate: (Outpatient)** Increase by 25-50mg qhs. **(Inpatient)** Increase to 200mg/day. **Maint:** 50-100mg qhs. **Max: (Outpatient)** 150mg/day. **(Inpatient)** 300mg/day. **IM: Initial:** 20-30mg qid. **Elderly:** 10mg tid or 20mg qhs.	**Antidepressants increased the risk of suicidal thinking and behavior (suicidality) in short-term studies in children and adolescents with major depressive disorder and other psychiatric disorders. W/P:** Caution with history of seizures, urinary retention, angle-closure glaucoma, increased IOP, hyperthyroidism, cardiovascular disorders, liver dysfunction. Increases symptoms with schizophrenia and manic-depression. Discontinue several weeks before elective surgery. May alter blood glucose levels. **Contra:** MAOI use or within 14 days, acute recovery period following MI. **P/N:** Category C, not for use in nursing.	MI, stroke, seizure, paralytic ileus, urinary retention, constipation, blurred vision, **dry mouth**, hyperpyrexia, rash, bone marrow depression, testicular swelling, gynecomastia (male), breast enlargement (female), alopecia, edema.
Amitriptyline Hydrochloride/ Chlordiazepoxide[CIV] (Limbitrol, Limbitrol DS)	**(Chlordiazepoxide-Amitriptyline) Tab: (Limbitrol)** 5mg-12.5mg, **(Limbitrol DS)** 10mg-25mg	***Adults:*** **Initial:** 3-4 tabs/day in divided doses. **Max: (Limbitrol DS)** 6 tabs/day. **Elderly:** Start at low end of dosing range.	**Antidepressants increased the risk of suicidal thinking and behavior (suicidality) in children and adolescents with major depressive disorder and other psychiatric disorders. Chlordiazepoxide-Amitriptyline is not approved for use in pediatric patients. W/P:** Caution with urinary retention, angle-closure glaucoma, cardiovascular disorder, history of seizures, hyperthyroidism, renal or hepatic dysfunction. May produce arrhythmia, sinus tachycardia, and conduction time prolongation. May impair mental alertness. Caution in elderly. Avoid abrupt withdrawal. Monitor blood and LFT's periodically with long-term therapy. **Contra:** MAOI use during or within 14 days, acute recovery period following MI. **P/N:** Not for use in pregnancy or nursing.	Drowsiness, **dry mouth**, constipation, blurred vision, dizziness, bloating, anorexia, fatigue, weakness, restlessness, lethargy.
Amoxapine	**Tab:** 25mg*, 50mg*, 100mg*, 150mg*	***Adults:*** **Initial:** 50mg bid-tid. **Titrate:** May increase to 100mg bid-tid by end of first week. **Usual:** 200-300mg/day. **Max: Outpatients:** 400mg/day; **Inpatients:** 600mg/day. **Elderly: Initial:** 25mg bid-tid. **Titrate:** May increase to 50mg bid-tid by end of first week. **Max:** 300mg/day. Doses =300mg/day may be given as single dose at bedtime.	**Antidepressants increased the risk of suicidal thinking and behavior (suicidality) in short-term studies in children and adolescents with major depressive disorder and other psychiatric disorders. W/P:** Discontinue if NMS, tardive dyskinesia, rash and/or drug fever occur. Caution with history of urinary retention, angle-closure glaucoma, or increased IOP, suicidal tendencies. May induce sinus tachycardia, changes in conduction time, arrhythmias. MI, stroke reported. Extreme caution with history of seizure disorders. Activation of mania, increased psychosis reported. May impair mental/physical abilities. **Contra:** During or within 14 days of MAOIs, recent MI. **P/N:** Category C, caution in nursing.	Drowsiness, **dry mouth**, constipation, blurred vision.

Table 18.1: PRESCRIBING INFORMATION FOR PSYCHOACTIVE DRUGS *(cont.)*

ANTIDEPRESSANTS *(cont.)*

NAME	FORM/STRENGTH	DOSAGE	WARNINGS/PRECAUTIONS & CONTRAINDICATIONS	ADVERSE EFFECTS†
Clomipramine Hydrochloride (Anafranil)	**Cap:** 25mg, 50mg, 75mg	***Adults:* Initial:** 25mg/day with meals. **Titrate:** Increase within 2 weeks to 100mg/day. Increase further over several weeks. **Max:** 250mg/day. **Maint:** May give total daily dose at bedtime. ***Pediatrics:*** ≥10 yrs: **Initial:** 25mg/day with meals. **Titrate:** Increase within 2 weeks to 3mg/kg or 100mg/day, whichever is smaller. Increase further over several weeks. **Max:** 3mg/kg/day or 200mg/day. **Maint:** May give total daily dose at bedtime.	**Antidepressants increased the risk of suicidal thinking and behavior (suicidality) in short-term studies in children and adolescents with major depressive disorder and other psychiatric disorders. Clomipramine is not approved for use in pediatric patients except for patients with obsessive compulsive disorder. W/P:** Increased risks with electroconvulsive therapy. Discontinue prior to elective surgery. Avoid abrupt withdrawal. Caution with seizure disorder, conditions predisposing to seizures (eg, brain damage, alcoholism), urinary retention, narrow-angle glaucoma, adrenal medulla tumors, increased IOP, hyperthyroidism, cardiovascular disorders, liver dysfunction, significant renal dysfunction. Monitor hepatic enzymes with liver dysfunction. Weight changes, sexual dysfunction, blood dyscrasias, elevated liver enzymes reported. Hypomania/mania reported with affective disorder. Psychosis reported with schizophrenia. **Contra:** MAOI use within 14 days, acute recovery period following MI. **P/N:** Category C, not for use in nursing.	**Dry mouth**, constipation, nausea, dyspepsia, anorexia, weight gain, increased sweating, increased appetite, myoclonus, nervousness, libido change, dizziness, tremor, somnolence, impotence, visual changes.
Desipramine Hydrochloride (Norpramin)	**Tab:** 10mg, 25mg, 50mg, 75mg, 100mg, 150mg	***Adults:* Usual:** 100-200mg/day given qd or in divided doses. **Max:** 300mg/day. **Elderly/Adolescents: Usual:** 25-100mg/day given qd or in divided doses. **Max:** 150mg/day.	**Antidepressants increased the risk of suicidal thinking and behavior (suicidality) in short-term studies in children and adolescents with major depressive disorder and other psychiatric disorders. Desipramine is not approved for use in pediatric patients. W/P:** Hypomania with manic-depressive disease. Discontinue prior to elective surgery. Do not withdraw abruptly. Extreme caution with urinary retention, glaucoma, seizure disorders, cardiovascular disease, thyroid disease, alcohol abuse. May exacerbate psychosis; caution with schizophrenia. May impair mental or physical abilities. May alter blood glucose levels. **Contra:** MAOI use within 14 days, acute recovery period following MI. **P/N:** Safety in pregnancy and nursing not known.	Arrhythmias, hypotension, HTN, tachycardia, confusion, hallucination, dizziness, anxiety, numbness, tingling, ataxia, tremors, **dry mouth**, urinary retention, urticaria, photosensitivity, SIADH, altered libido.
Doxepin Hydrochloride (Sinequan)	**Cap:** 10mg, 25mg, 50mg, 75mg, 100mg, 150mg; **Sol, Concentrate:** 10mg/mL [120mL]	***Adults:* Very Mild Illness: Usual:** 25-50mg/day. **Mild-to-Moderate Severity: Initial:** 75mg/day. **Usual:** 75-150mg/day. **Severely Ill:** May increase up to 300mg/day. Dilute solution with 120mL of water, milk or juice. Give once daily or in divided doses. Divide dose if ≥150mg. **Elderly:** Use lower doses and monitor closely.	**Antidepressants increased the risk of suicidal thinking and behavior (suicidality) in short-term studies in children and adolescents with major depressive disorder and other psychiatric disorders. Doxepin is not approved for use in pediatric patients. W/P:** Monitor for suicidal tendencies and increased symptoms of psychosis. Avoid abrupt discontinuation. **Contra:** Glaucoma, urinary retention. **P/N:** Safety in pregnancy and nursing not known.	Drowsiness, **dry mouth**, blurred vision, constipation, urinary retention, hypotension, tachycardia, rash, edema, photosensitization, pruritus, eosinophilia, nausea, dizziness.
Imipramine Hydrochloride (Tofranil)	**Tab:** 10mg, 25mg, 50mg	***Adults:* Depression: Initial:** (Inpatient) 100mg/day in divided doses. **Titrate:** Increase to 200mg/day; up to 250-300mg/day after 2 weeks if needed.	**Antidepressants increased the risk of suicidal thinking and behavior (suicidality) in short-term studies in children and adolescents with major**	Orthostatic hypotension, HTN, confusion, hallucinations, numbness, tremors, **dry**

*Scored.   †Bold entries denote special dental considerations.

NAME	FORM/ STRENGTH	DOSAGE	WARNINGS/PRECAUTIONS & CONTRAINDICATIONS	ADVERSE EFFECTS†
Imipramine Hydrochloride *(cont.)*		**(Outpatient)** 75mg/day. **Titrate:** Increase to 150mg/day. **Maint:** 50-150mg/day. **Max:** 200mg/day.**Elderly/ Adolescents: Initial:** 30-40mg/day. **Max:** 100mg/day. *Pediatrics:* **Enuresis: ≥6 years old: Initial:** 25mg/day 1 hour before bedtime. **Titrate: 6-12 yrs:** If inadequate response in 1 week, increase to 50mg before bedtime. **≥12 yrs:** Increase to 75mg before bedtime after 1 week if needed. **Max:** 2.5mg/kg/day.	**depressive disorder and other psychiatric disorders. Imipramine HCl is not approved for use in pediatric patients except for patients with nocturnal enuresis. W/P:** Caution with elderly, serious depression, cardiovascular disease, hyperthyroidism, urinary retention, narrow-angle glaucoma, increased IOP, seizure disorders, renal and hepatic impairment. May activate psychosis in schizophrenia; reduce dose. Limit electroshock therapy. May alter blood glucose levels. Photosensitivity reported. Discontinue prior to elective surgery, or with hypomanic or manic episodes. Discontinue with pathological neutrophil depression. **Contra:** Within 14 days of MAOI therapy, or during acute recovery period following MI. **P/N:** Safety in pregnancy not known; not for use in nursing.	**mouth**, urticaria, nausea, vomiting, diarrhea, gynecomastia (male), breast enlargement (female), galactorrhea.
Imipramine Pamoate (Tofranil-PM)	**Cap:** 75mg, 100mg, 125mg, 150mg	*Adults:* **(Inpatient) Initial:** 100-150mg/day. **Titrate:** May increase to 200mg/day. After 2 weeks may increase up to 250-300mg/day if needed. **(Outpatient) Initial:** 75mg/day. **Titrate:** May increase to 150mg/day. **Max:** 200mg/day. **(Inpatient/Outpatient) Maint:** Following remission, maintain at lowest possible dose. **Usual:** 75-150mg/day. **Elderly/Adolescents:** Initiate with Tofranil 25-50mg/day. Switch to Tofranil-PM with doses ≥75mg. **Max:** 100mg/day.	**Antidepressants increased the risk of suicidal thinking and behavior (suicidality) in short-term studies in children and adolescents with major depressive disorder and other psychiatric disorders. Imipramine is not approved for use in pediatric patients. W/P:** Caution with elderly, serious depression, cardiovascular disease, hyperthyroidism, urinary retention, narrow-angle glaucoma, increased IOP, seizure disorders, renal and hepatic impairment. May activate psychosis in schizophrenia; reduce dose. Limit electroshock therapy. May alter blood glucose levels. Photosensitivity reported. Discontinue prior to elective surgery, or with hypomanic or manic episodes. Discontinue with pathological neutrophil depression. **Contra:** Within 14 days of MAOI therapy or during acute recovery period following MI. **P/N:** Safety in pregnancy not known; not for use in nursing.	Orthostatic hypotension, HTN, confusion, hallucinations, numbness, tremors, **dry mouth**, urticaria, nausea, vomiting, diarrhea, gynecomastia (male), breast enlargement (female), galactorrhea.
Nortriptyline Hydrochloride (Pamelor)	**Cap:** 10mg, 25mg, 50mg, 75mg; **Sol:** 10mg/5mL	*Adults:* 25mg tid-qid. **Max:** 150mg/day. Total daily dose may be given once a day. Monitor serum levels if dose >100mg/day. **Elderly/Adolescents:** 30-50mg/day in single or divided doses.	**Antidepressants increased the risk of suicidal thinking and behavior (suicidality) in short-term studies in children and adolescents with major depressive disorder and other psychiatric disorders. Nortriptyline is not approved for use in pediatric patients. W/P:** MI, arrhythmia, strokes have occurred. Caution with cardiovascular disease, glaucoma, history of urinary retention, hyperthyroidism. May lower seizure threshold, exacerbate psychosis or activate schizophrenia, cause symptoms of mania in bipolar disease, or alter glucose levels. Discontinue several days prior to elective surgery. **Contra:** MAOI use within 14 days, acute recovery period following MI. **P/N:** Safety during pregnancy and nursing not known.	Arrhythmias, hypotension, HTN, tachycardia, MI, heart block, stroke, confusion, hallucination, insomnia, tremors, ataxia, anxiety, **dry mouth**, blurred vision, skin rash, extrapyramidal symptoms, photosensitivity, SIADH, anorexia.

Table 18.1: PRESCRIBING INFORMATION FOR PSYCHOACTIVE DRUGS *(cont.)*

NAME	FORM/ STRENGTH	DOSAGE	WARNINGS/PRECAUTIONS & CONTRAINDICATIONS	ADVERSE EFFECTS†
ANTIDEPRESSANTS *(cont.)*				
Protriptyline Hydrochloride (Vivactil)	**Tab:** 5mg, 10mg	***Adults:*** **Usual:** 15-40mg/day taken tid-qid. **Titrate:** May increase to 60mg/day. **Max:** 60mg/day. **Elderly: Initial:** 5mg tid. **Titrate:** Increase gradually if needed. Monitor cardiovascular system with doses >20mg/day. ***Pediatrics: Adolescents: Initial:*** 5mg tid. **Titrate:** Increase gradually if needed.	**Antidepressants increased the risk of suicidal thinking and behavior (suicidality) in short-term studies in children and adolescents with major depressive disorder and other psychiatric disorders. Protriptyline is not approved for use in pediatric patients. W/P:** Caution with history of seizures, urinary retention, increased IOP, cardiovascular disorders, hyperthyroidism, elderly. May aggravate psychotic symptoms in schizophrenia, manic symptoms in manic-depressive psychosis, and anxiety/agitation in overactive/agitated patients. Discontinue several days before elective surgery. **Contra:** Within 14 days of MAOI therapy, cisapride, acute recovery period following MI. **P/N:** Safety in pregnancy and nursing not known.	Tachycardia, hypotension, confusion, anxiety, insomnia, nightmares, seizures, EPS, dizziness, headache, anticholinergic effects, rash, photosensitivity, blood dyscrasias, GI effects, impotence, decreased libido, flushing.
Trimipramine Maleate (Surmontil)	**Cap:** 25mg, 50mg, 100mg	***Adults:*** **Outpatient: Initial:** 75mg/day in divided doses. **Titrate:** Increase to 150mg/day. **Maint:** 50-150mg/day. **Max:** 200mg/day. **Hospitalized Patients: Initial:** 100mg/day in divided doses. **Titrate:** Increase gradually to 200mg/day. If no improvement after 2-3 weeks, may increase up to 250-300mg/day. **Elderly: Initial:** 50mg/day. **Titrate:** Increase gradually to 100mg/day. Take at bedtime for at least 3 months.	**Antidepressants increased the risk of suicidal thinking and behavior (suicidality) in short-term studies in children and adolescents with major depressive disorder and other psychiatric disorders. Trimipramine is not approved for use in pediatric patients. W/P:** Caution with cardiovascular disease, increased IOP, urinary retention, narrow-angle glaucoma, hyperthyroidism, seizure disorder, liver dysfunction. May impair ability to operate machinery. May alter glucose levels. May activate psychosis in schizophrenia. Manic or hypomanic episodes may occur. May increase hazards with electroshock therapy. **Contra:** Acute recovery period post-MI, within 14 days of MAOI therapy. **P/N:** Category C, safety in nursing not known.	Hypotension, HTN, arrhythmia, confusion, insomnia, incoordination, GI complaints, allergic reactions, gynecomastia, blood dyscrasias, **dry mouth**, blurred vision, urinary retention.
MISCELLANEOUS				
Bupropion Hydrochloride (Wellbutrin, Wellbutrin SR, Wellbutrin XL)	**(Wellbutrin) Tab:** 75mg, 100mg; **(Wellbutrin SR) Tab, Extended Release:** 100mg, 150mg, 200mg; **(Wellbutrin XL) Tab, Extended Release:** 150mg, 300mg	**(Wellbutrin/Wellbutrin SR)** ***Adults:*** **≥18 yrs: (Tab, Extended Release) Initial:** 150mg qd, may increase to 150mg bid after 3 days. **Usual:** 150mg bid. **Max:** 200mg bid. Separate doses by at least 8 hrs. **Severe Hepatic Cirrhosis:** 100mg/day or 150mg every other day. **Mild-Moderate Hepatic Cirrhosis/Renal Impairment:** Reduce frequency and/or dose. **Max:** 450mg/day, given in divided doses of not more than 150mg each. **Severe Hepatic Cirrhosis: Max:** 75mg qd. **(Wellbutrin XL)** ***Adults:*** **≥18 yrs:** Give qd in the AM. Swallow whole. **Initial:** 150mg qd, may increase to 300mg qd after 3 days. **Usual:** 300mg qd. **Max:** 450mg qd. **Mild-Moderate Hepatic Cirrhosis/Renal Impairment:** Reduce frequency and/or dose. **Severe Hepatic Cirrhosis: Max:** 150mg every other day.	**Antidepressants increased the risk of suicidal thinking and behavior (suicidality) in short-term studies in children and adolescents with major depressive disorder and other psychiatric disorders. Bupropion is not approved for use in pediatric patients. W/P:** Dose-related risk of seizures. Discontinue and do not restart if seizure occurs. **Initial:** (Tab) 100mg bid, may increase to 100mg tid after 3 days. **Usual:** 100mg tid. Extreme caution with history of seizure, cranial trauma, severe hepatic cirrhosis. Agitation, insomnia, psychosis, confusion and other neuropsychiatric signs reported. Caution with bipolar disorder, recent MI, unstable heart disease, renal impairment. Altered appetite/weight, allergic reactions, HTN reported. Monitor for clinical worsening and/or suicidality, especially at initiation of therapy or dose changes. **Contra:** Seizure disorder, bulimia or anorexia	Anorexia, **dry mouth**, rash, sweating, agitation, dizziness, insomnia, nausea, constipation, pharyngitis, abdominal pain, agitation, diarrhea, palpitations, myalgia, anxiety, tinnitus, sweating, urinary frequency.

*Scored.   †Bold entries denote special dental considerations.

NAME	FORM/ STRENGTH	DOSAGE	WARNINGS/PRECAUTIONS & CONTRAINDICATIONS	ADVERSE EFFECTS†
Bupropion Hydrochloride *(cont.)*			nervosa, within 14 days of MAOIs, other forms of bupropion, abrupt discontinuation of alcohol or sedatives. **P/N:** Category B, not for use in nursing.	
Trazodone Hydrochloride (Desyrel)	**Tab:** 50mg*, 100mg*, 150mg*, 300mg*	***Adults:*** **Initial:** 150mg/day in divided doses pc. **Titrate:** May increase by 50mg/day every 3-4 days. **Max: (Outpatient)** 400mg/day, **(Inpatient)** 600mg/day.	**Antidepressants increased the risk of suicidal thinking and behavior (suicidality) in short-term studies in children and adolescents with major depressive disorder and other psychiatric disorders. Trazodone is not approved for use in pediatric patients. W/P:** Avoid during initial recovery phase of MI. Caution in cardiac disease. Discontinue prior to elective surgery. **P/N:** Category C, caution in nursing.	**Dry mouth,** edema, constipation, blurred vision, fatigue, nervousness, drowsiness, dizziness, headache, insomnia, nausea, vomiting, musculoskeletal pain, hypotension, confusion, priaprism.

ANTIMANIC/BIPOLAR DISORDER AGENTS

ANTI-EPILEPTIC AGENTS

NAME	FORM/ STRENGTH	DOSAGE	WARNINGS/PRECAUTIONS & CONTRAINDICATIONS	ADVERSE EFFECTS†
Carbamazepine (Equetro)	**Cap, Extended Release:** 100mg, 200mg, 300mg	***Adults:*** **Initial:** 400mg/day, given in divided doses, bid. **Titrate:** 200mg qd. **Max:** 1600mg/day. Do not crush or chew.	**Aplastic anemia and agranulocytosis reported. Obtain complete pretreatment hematological testing as baseline. Discontinue if evidence of bone marrow depression develops. W/P:** Monitor blood levels. Avoid use with any other medication containing carbamazepine. May cause fetal harm during pregnancy. Severe dermatologic reactions, including toxic epidermal necrolysis (Lyell's syndrome) and Stevens-Johnson syndrome, reported with carbamazepine. Avoid abrupt discontinuation with seizure disorder. Carbamazepine has mild anticholinergic activity; observe closely with increased IOP. Caution in patients with a history of cardiac, hepatic, or renal damage; adverse hematologic reaction to other drugs; or interrupted courses of therapy with carbamazepine. Closely monitor patients at high-risk for suicide attempts. May cause activate latent psychosis. May cause confusion/agitation in elderly. Perform eye exam and monitor LFTs and renal function at baseline and periodically. **Contra:** Avoid in patients with a history of previous bone marrow depression, hypersensitivity to the drug, or known sensitivity to any of the tricyclic compounds. Use of MAOIs is not recommended and MAOIs should be discontinued for a minimum of 14 days prior to use. **P/N:** Category D, not for use in nursing.	Dizziness, somnolence, nausea, vomiting, ataxia, pruritus, **dry mouth,** headache, infection, pain, rash, diarrhea, dyspepsia, asthenia, amnesia.
Divalproex Sodium (Depakote, Depakote ER, Depakote Sprinkles)	**(Depakote/Depakote Sprinkles) Cap, Delayed Release: (Sprinkle)** 125mg; **Tab, Delayed Release:** 125mg, 250mg, 500mg; **(Depakote ER) Tab, Extended Release:** 250mg, 500mg	**(Depakote/Depakote Sprinkles)** ***Adults:*** **(Cap/Tab) Complex Partial Seizures:** **Initial:** 10-15mg/kg/day. **Titrate:** Increase by 5-10mg/kg/week. **Max:** 60mg/kg/day. **Absence Seizures: Initial:** 15mg/kg/day. **Titrate:** Increase weekly by 5-10mg/kg/day. **Max:** 60mg/kg/day. Give in divided doses if >250mg/day. **(Tab) Migraine: Initial:** ≥16 yrs: 250mg bid. **Max:** 1000mg/day. **Mania:** 750mg in divided doses. **Titrate:** Increase dose rapidly	**Fatal hepatic failure (<2 yrs at considerable risk), teratogenic effects (eg, neural tube defects), and life-threatening pancreatitis reported. W/P:** Hyperammonemic encephalopathy in elderly or debilitated patients; discontinue if this occurs. Prior to therapy, evaluate for urea cycle disorder in high risk patients (eg, history of unexplained encephalopathy, coma, etc). Measure ammonia levels if develop unexplained lethargy, vomiting, or mental status	Nausea, vomiting, diarrhea, somnolence, dyspepsia, thrombocytopenia, asthenia, abdominal pain, tremor, diplopia, blurred vision, weight gain, ataxia, nystagmus.Nausea, vomiting, diarrhea, somnolence, dyspepsia,

Table 18.1: PRESCRIBING INFORMATION FOR PSYCHOACTIVE DRUGS *(cont.)*

NAME	FORM/ STRENGTH	DOSAGE	WARNINGS/PRECAUTIONS & CONTRAINDICATIONS	ADVERSE EFFECTS†
ANTIMANIC/BIPOLAR DISORDER AGENTS *(cont.)*				
Divalproex Sodium *(cont.)*		to clinical effect. **Max:** 60mg/kg/day. **Elderly:** Reduce initial dose and titrate slowly. Decrease dose or discontinue if decreased food or fluid intake or if excessive somnolence occurs. ***Pediatrics:*** ≥ **10 yrs: (Cap/Tab) Complex Partial Seizures: Initial:** 10-15mg/Kg/day. **Titrate:** Incrase weekly by -mg/kg/day. **Max:** 60mg/kg/day. Give in divided does if > 250mg/day **(Depakote ER)** *Adults:* For qd dosing. **Migraine: Initial:** 500mg qd for 1 week. **Titrate:** Increase to 1000 kg qd ~~Max: 1000mg/day.~~ **Complex Partial Seizures: Monotherapy/Adjunct Therapy: Initial:** 10-15mg/kg/day. **Titrate:** Increase by 5-10mg/kg/week to optimal response. **Usual:** Less than 60mg/kg/day (accepted therapeutic range 50-100mcg/mL). When converting to monotherapy, reduce concomitant antiepilepsy drug by 25% every 2 weeks starting at initiation or delay 1-2 weeks after start of therapy. **Simple and Complex Absence Seizures: Initial:** 15mg/kg/day. **Titrate:** Increase weekly by 5-10mg/kg/day to optimal response. **Max:** 60mg/kg/day. **Mania: Initial:** 25mg/kg/day given once daily. **Titrate:** Increase dose rapidly to clinical effect. **Max:** 60mg/kg/day. **Conversion from Depakote:** Administer Depakote ER qd using a dose 8-20% higher than the total daily dose of Depakote. If cannot directly convert to Depakote ER, consider increasing to next higher Depakote total daily dose before converting to appropriate total daily Depakote ER dose. **Elderly:** Give lower initial dose and titrate slowly. Decrease dose or discontinue if decreased food or fluid intake or if excessive somnolence occurs. Swallow whole; do not crush or chew. *Pediatrics:* ≥ **10yrs:** For qd dosing. **Complex Partial Seizures: Monotherapy/Adjunct Therapy: Initial:** 10-15mg/kg/day.**Titrate:** Increase weekly by 5-10mg/kg/day to optimal response. **Max:** 60mg/kg/day. **Conversion from Depakote:** Administer Depakote ER qd using a dose 8-20% higher than the total daily dose of Depakote. If cannot directly convert to Depakote ER, consider increasing to next higher Depakote total daily dose before converting to appropriate total daily Depakote ER dose. Swallow whole; do not crush or chew.	changes. Caution with hepatic disease. Check LFTs prior to therapy, then frequently during first 6 months. Dose-related thrombocytopenia and elevated liver enzymes reported. Monitor platelet and coagulation tests prior to therapy, then periodically. Altered thyroid function tests and urine ketone test. May stimulate replication of HIV and CMV viruses. Avoid abrupt discontinuation. **Contra:** Hepatic disease, significant hepatic dysfunction, known urea cycle disorders. **P/N:** Category D, not for use in nursing.	asthenia, abdominal pain, tremor, headache, anorexia, diplopia, blurred vision, weight gain, ataxia, nystagmus.
Lamotrigine (Lamictal, Lamictal CD)	**Tab:** 25mg*, 100mg*, 150mg*, 200mg*; **Tab, Chewable: (Lamictal CD)**	*Adults:* **Epilepsy: Concomitant AEDs with valproate:** Weeks 1 and 2: 25mg every other day. Weeks 3 and 4: 25mg qd. **Titrate:** Increase every 1-2 weeks by 25-50mg/day. **Maint:** 100-400mg/day, given qd or bid; 100-200mg/day	**Serious life-threatening rash including Stevens-Johnson syndrome and toxic epidermal necrolysis reported. Occurs more often in pediatrics than adults. Discontinue at 1st sign of rash. W/P:** Risk of serious life-threatening rash;	Serious rash, dizziness, ataxia, somnolence, headache, diplopia, blurred vision, nausea, vomiting, insomnia, back/abdominal pain,

*Scored.   †Bold entries denote special dental considerations.

NAME	FORM/ STRENGTH	DOSAGE	WARNINGS/PRECAUTIONS & CONTRAINDICATIONS	ADVERSE EFFECTS†
Lamotrigine *(cont.)*	2mg, 5mg, 25mg	when added to valproate alone. **Concomitant EIAEDs without valproate: Weeks 1 and 2:** 50mg qd. **Weeks 3 and 4:** 50mg bid. **Titrate:** Increase every 1-2 weeks by 100mg/day. **Maint:** 150-250mg bid. **Conversion to Monotherapy From Single EIAED: ≥16 yrs: Weeks 1 and 2:** 50mg qd. **Weeks 3 and 4:** 50mg bid. **Titrate:** Increase every 1-2 weeks by 100mg/day. **Maint:** 250mg bid. Withdraw EIAED over 4 weeks. **Conversion to Monotherapy From valproate: ≥16 yrs: Step 1:** Follow Concomitant AEDs with valproate dosing regimen to achieve Lamictal dose of 200mg/day. Maintain previous valproate dose. **Step 2:** Maintain Lamictal 200mg/day. Decrease valproate to 500mg/day by decrements of ≥500mg/day per week. Maintain valproate 500mg/day for 1 week. **Step 3:** Increase to Lamictal 300mg/day for 1 week. Decrease valproate simultaneously to 250mg/day for 1 week. **Step 4:** Discontinue valproate. Increase Lamictal 100mg/day every week to maint dose of 500mg/day. **Bipolar Disorder: Patients not taking carbamazepine, other enzyme-inducing drugs or valproate: Weeks 1 and 2:** 25mg qd. **Weeks 3 and 4:** 50mg qd. **Week 5:** 100mg qd. **Weeks 6 and 7:** 200mg qd. **Patients taking valproate: Weeks 1 and 2:** 25mg every other day. **Weeks 3 and 4:** 25mg qd. **Week 5:** 50mg qd. **Weeks 6 and 7:** 100mg qd. **Patients taking carbamazepine (or other enzyme-inducing drugs) and not taking valproate: Weeks 1 and 2:** 50mg qd. **Weeks 3 and 4:** 100mg qd (divided doses). **Week 5:** 200mg qd (divided doses). **Week 6:** 300mg qd (divided doses). **Week 7:** up to 400mg qd (divided doses). **After discontinuation of psychotropic drugs excluding valproate carbamazepine, or other enzyme-inducing drugs:** Maintain current dose. **After discontinuation of valproate and current lamotrigine dose of 100mg qd: Week 1:** 150mg qd. **Week 2 and onward:** 200mg qd. **After discontinuation of carbamazepine or other enzyme-inducing drugs and current lamotrigine dose of 400mg qd: Week 1:** 400mg qd. **Week 2:** 300mg qd. **Week 3 and onward:** 200mg qd. **Hepatic Impairment: Initial/Titrate/ Maint:** Reduce by 50% for moderate (Child-Pugh Grade B) and 75% for severe (Child-Pugh Grade C) impairment. **Significant Renal Impairment: Maint:** Reduce dose. **Elderly:** Start at low end of dosing range. ***Pediatrics:*** Round dose down to nearest whole tab. **2-12 yrs: ≥6.7kg: Lennox-Gastaut/Partial Seizures: Concomitant AEDs with valproate: Weeks 1 and 2:** 0.15mg/kg/day given qd-bid. **Weeks 3 and 4:** 0.3mg/kg/day	discontinue if rash occurs. Multiorgan failure, sudden unexplained death, hypersensitivity reactions, and pure red cell aplasia reported. Avoid abrupt withdrawal. Caution with renal, hepatic, or cardiac functional impairment. May cause ophthalmic toxicity. Do not exceed recommended initial dose and dose escalations. Caution in elderly. Chewable tabs may be swallowed whole, chewed with water/diluted fruit juice or dissolved in water/diluted fruit juice; do administer partial quantities. **P/N:** Category C, not for use in nursing.	fatigue, **xerostomia,** rhinitis.

Table 18.1: PRESCRIBING INFORMATION FOR PSYCHOACTIVE DRUGS (cont.)

NAME	FORM/ STRENGTH	DOSAGE	WARNINGS/PRECAUTIONS & CONTRAINDICATIONS	ADVERSE EFFECTS†
ANTIMANIC/BIPOLAR DISORDER AGENTS (cont.)				
Lamotrigine (cont.)		given qd or bid. **Titrate:** Increase every 1-2 weeks by 0.3mg/kg/day. **Maint:** 1-5mg/kg/day given qd or bid; 1-3mg/kg/day when added to valproate alone. Max: 200mg/day. Concomitant EIAEDs without valproate: Weeks 1 and 2: 0.3mg/kg bid. **Weeks 3 and 4:** 0.6mg/kg bid. **Titrate:** Increase every 1-2 weeks by 1.2mg/kg/day. **Maint:** 2.5-7.5mg/kg bid. **Max:** 400mg/day. **>12 yrs: Concomitant AEDs with valproate: Weeks 1 and 2:** 25mg every other day. **Weeks 3 and 4:** 25mg qd. Titrate: Increase every 1-2 weeks by 25-50mg/day. **Maint:** 100-400mg/day, given qd or bid; 100-200mg/day when added to valproate alone. **Concomitant EIAEDs without valproate: Weeks 1 and 2:** 50mg qd. **Weeks 3 and 4:** 50mg bid. **Titrate:** Increase every 1-2 weeks by 100mg/day. **Maint:** 150-250mg bid. **Hepatic Impairment: Initial/Titrate/ Maint:** Reduce by 50% for moderate (Child-Pugh Grade B) and 75% for se- vere (Child-Pugh Grade C) impairment. **Significant renal Impairment: Maint:** Reduce dose.		
LITHIUM				
Lithium Carbonate (Eskalith, Eskalith-CR)	**Cap: (Eskalith)** 300mg; **Tab, Ex- tended Release: (Eskalith CR)** 450mg*	*Adults:* **(Cap)** 300mg tid-qid. **(Tab, Extended Release)** 450mg q12h. Monitor every 1-2 weeks and adjust dose if needed. When stable, monitor every 2 months to achieve levels of 0.6- 1.2mEq/L. **Maint:** 900-1200mg/day. **Acute Mania:** 1800mg/day in divided doses. Monitor levels twice weekly to achieve 1-1.5mEq/L. When switching to extended-release tabs, give same total daily dose when possible. *Pediatrics:* ≥12 yrs: **(Cap)** 300mg tid-qid. **(Tab, Extended Release)** 450mg q12h. Monitor every 1-2 weeks and adjust dose if needed. When stable, monitor every 2 months to achieve levels of 0.6- 1.2 mEq/L. **Maint:** 900-1200mg/day. **Acute Mania:** 1800mg/day in divided doses. Monitor levels twice weekly to achieve 1-1.5mEq/L. When switching to extended-release tabs, give same total daily dose when possible.	**Lithium toxicity is related to serum levels, and can occur at doses close to therapeutic levels. W/P:** Avoid with significant renal or cardiovas- cular disease, severe debilitation, dehydration, or sodium depletion. Risk of encephalopathic syndrome (eg, weak- ness, lethargy, fever, tremulousness, confusion, EPS); discontinue therapy. Maintain normal diet, adequate salt/fluid intake. Reduce dose or discontinue with sweating, diarrhea, infection with elevated temperatures. Caution with hypothyroidism; may need supplemental therapy. Chronic therapy associated with diminution of renal concentrat- ing ability, glomerular and interstitial fibrosis, and nephron atrophy. **P/N:** Safety in pregnancy not known, not for use in nursing.	Fine hand tremor, polyuria, **mild thirst**, nausea, general discomfort, diarrhea, vomiting, drowsiness, muscular weakness.
ANTIPSYCHOTIC AGENTS				
Aripiprazole (Abilify)	**Tab:** 5mg, 10mg, 15mg, 20mg, 30mg; **Sol:** 1mg/mL [50mL, 150mL, 480mL]	*Adults:* **Schizophrenia: Initial/Target:** 10 to 15mg qd. **Titrate:** Should not increase before 2 weeks. **Bipolar mania: Initial:** 30mg qd. **Titrate:** May decrease to 15mg qd based on assess- ment and tolerability. Oral solution can be given on a mg-per-mg basis up to 25mg. Patients receiving 30mg tablets should receive 25mg of the solution. **Concomitant CYP3A4 Inhibitors (eg, ketoconazole):** Reduce usual	**Elderly patients with dementia-related psychosis treated with atypical anti- psychotic drugs are at an increased risk of death; most appeared to be cardiovascular (eg, heart failure, sudden death) or infectious (eg, pneu- monia) in nature. Aripiprazole is not approved for the treatment of patients with dementia-related psychosis. W/P:** May develop tardive dyskinesia, NMS. Monitor for hyperglycemia, worsening	Headache, asthenia, rash, blurred vision, rhinitis, cough, tremor, anxiety, insomnia, nausea, vomiting, lightheadedness, som- nolence, constipation, akathisia.

*Scored.   †Bold entries denote special dental considerations.

NAME	FORM/ STRENGTH	DOSAGE	WARNINGS/PRECAUTIONS & CONTRAINDICATIONS	ADVERSE EFFECTS†
Aripiprazole *(cont.)*		aripiprazole dose by 50%. **Concomitant CYP2D6 Inhibitors (eg, quinidine, fluoxetine, paroxetine):** Reduce usual aripiprazole dose by 50%. **Concomitant CYP3A4 Inducers (eg, carbamazepine):** Double aripiprazole dose (to 20mg or 30mg). Periodically reassess for maintenance therapy.	of glucose control with DM, FBG levels with diabetes risk. Increased incidence of cerebrovascular adverse events (stroke) in elderly dementia patients. Not approved for treatment of patients with dementia related psychosis. Orthostatic hypotension reported; caution with cardiovascular disease, conditions predisposed to hypotension (eg, dehydration, hypovolemia). May lower seizure threshold. Potential for cognitive and motor impairment. May disrupt body's temperature regulation. Possible esophageal dysmotility and aspiration; caution in patients at risk for aspiration pneumonia. Observe vigilance in treating psychosis associated with Alzheimer's. **P/N:** Category C, not for use in nursing.	
Olanzapine (Zyprexa)	**Inj:** 10mg; **Tab:** 2.5mg, 5mg, 7.5mg, 10mg, 15mg, 20mg; **Tab, Disintegrating:** (Zydis) 5mg, 10mg, 15mg, 20mg	***Adults:*** **(Tab) Schizophrenia: Initial/ Usual:** 5-10mg qd. **Titrate:** Adjust by 5mg daily at weekly intervals. **Max:** 20mg/day. **Bipolar Mania: Initial:** 10-15mg qd. **Titrate:** Increase by 5mg daily. **Max:** 20mg/day. **With Lithium or Valproate: Initial/Usual:** 10mg qd. **Max:** 20mg/day. **Debilitated/Hypotension Risk/Slow metabolizers/Sensitivity to olanzapine effects: Initial:** 5mg qd. **Titrate:** Increase cautiously. **(IM) Agitation: Initial:** 10mg IM. **Usual:** 2.5-10mg IM. **Max:** 3 doses of 10mg q 2-4h. **Elderly:** 5mg IM. **Debilitated/Hypotension Risk/Sensitivity to olanzapine effects:** 2.5mg IM. May initiate PO therapy when clinically appropriate.	**Elderly patients with dementia-related psychosis treated with atypical antipsychotic drugs are at an increased risk of death; most appeared to be cardiovascular (eg, heart failure, sudden death) or infectious (eg, pneumonia) in nature. Olanzapine is not approved for the treatment of patients with dementia-related psychosis. W/P:** Monitor for hyperglycemia, worsening of glucose control with DM, FBG levels with diabetes risk. Risk of NMS, tardive dyskinesia, orthostatic hypotension, seizures. Caution in hepatic impairment, prostatic hypertrophy, narrow-angle glaucoma, history of paralytic ileus, elderly patients with dementia or Parkinson's disease, cardio- or cerebrovascular disease, hypotension risk (eg, hypovolemia, dehydration), risk for aspiration pneumonia, suicidal tendencies. Elevated transaminases, hyperprolactinemia reported. May cause disruption of body temperature regulation. Re-evaluate periodically. **P/N:** Category C, not for use in nursing.	Postural hypotension, constipation, dry mouth, weight gain, somnolence, dizziness, akathisia, asthenia, dyspepsia, tremor, increased appetite.
Olanzapine/ Fluoxetine Hydrochloride (Symbyax)	**Cap:** (Olanzapine-Fluoxetine): 6-25mg, 6-50mg, 12-25mg, 12-50mg	***Adults:*** **≥18yrs: Initial:** 6-25mg cap qpm. **Titrate:** Adjust dose based on efficacy and tolerability. **Max:** 18mg/75mg. **Hypotension Risk/Hepatic Impairment/Slow Metabolizers: Initial:** 6-25mg cap qpm. **Titrate:** Increase cautiously. Re-evaluate periodically.	**Antidepressants increased the risk of suicidal thinking and behavior (suicidality) in short-term studies in children and adolescents with major depressive disorder and other psychiatric disorders. Fluoxetine is not approved for use in pediatric patients. Elderly patients with BB: dementia-related psychosis treated with atypical antipsychotic drugs are at an increased risk of death; most appeared to be cardiovascular (eg, heart failure, sudden death) or infectious (eg, pneumonia) in nature. Olanzapine is not approved for the treatment of patients with dementia-related psychosis. W/P:** Monitor for hyperglycemia, worsening of glucose control with DM, FBG levels with diabetes risk. Not for use with dementia-related psychosis. Risk of orthostatic hypotension, NMS, tardive dyskinesia, hyperprolactinemia, hyponatremia, seizures. Caution with	Asthenia, somnolence, weight gain, edema, increased appetite, peripheral edema, **pharyngitis**, abnormal thinking, tremors.

Table 18.1: PRESCRIBING INFORMATION FOR PSYCHOACTIVE DRUGS *(cont.)*

NAME	FORM/ STRENGTH	DOSAGE	WARNINGS/PRECAUTIONS & CONTRAINDICATIONS	ADVERSE EFFECTS†
ANTIMANIC/BIPOLAR DISORDER AGENTS *(cont.)*				
Olanzapine/ Fluoxetine Hydrochloride *(cont.)*			cardio- or cerebrovascular disease, hypotension risk (eg, dehydration, hypovolemia), history of seizures or conditions that lower the seizure threshold, elderly (especially with dementia), hepatic impairment, risk of aspiration pneumonia, conditions that affect metabolism or hemodynamic responses, prostatic hypertrophy, narrow-angle glaucoma, history of paralytic ileus, suicidal tendencies. Discontinue if unexplained allergic reaction occurs. Elevated transaminases, bleeding episodes reported. Monitor for symptoms of mania/hypomania. May cause disruption of body temperature regulation. **Contra:** During or within 14 days of MAOIs, thioridazine within 5 weeks of discontinuation. **P/N:** Category C, not for use in nursing.	
Quetiapine Fumarate (Seroquel)	**Tab:** 25mg, 100mg, 200mg, 300mg	***Adults: Acute Bipolar Mania: Monotherapy/Adjunctive:*** Give bid. Initial: 100mg/day. **Titrate:** Increase to 400mg/day on Day 4 in increments of up to 100mg/day. Adjust doses up to 800mg/day by Day 6 in increments ≤200mg/day. **Max:** 800mg/day. **Schizophrenia: Initial:** 25mg bid. **Titrate:** Increase by 25-50mg bid-tid on the 2nd and 3rd day to 300-400mg/day given bid-tid by the 4th day. Adjust doses by 25-50mg bid at intervals of at least 2 days. **Maint:** Lowest effective dose. Max: 800mg/day. **Hepatic Impairment: Initial:** 25mg/day. **Titrate:** Increase by 25-50mg/day to effective dose. **Elderly/Debilitated/Predisposition to hypotension: Initial:** 25mg bid. **Titrate:** Increase cautiously.	**Elderly patients with dementia-related psychosis treated with atypical antipsychotic drugs are at an increased risk of death; most appeared to be cardiovascular (eg, heart failure, sudden death) or infectious (eg, pneumonia) in nature. Quetiapine is not approved for the treatment of patients with dementia-related psychosis. W/P:** NMS reported. May develop tardive dyskinesia. May induce orthostatic hypotension. Caution with cardiovascular disease, cerebrovascular disease, conditions which predispose to hypotension (eg, dehydration, hypovolemia), history of seizures. Monitor for cataracts at initiation, then every 6 months. Possible hypothyroidism. Hepatic enzyme, cholesterol and triglyceride elevations reported. May impair judgment, thinking and motor skills. Priapism reported. May disrupt body's ability to reduce core temperature. Caution in patients at risk for aspiration, elderly, debilitated. **P/N:** Category C, not for use in nursing.	Headache, dizziness, postural hypotension, **dry mouth**, dyspepsia, tachycardia, somnolence, constipation.
Risperidone (Risperdal, Risperdal Consta, Risperdal M-Tab)	**Inj: (Consta)** 25mg, 37.5mg, 50mg. **Sol:** 1mg/ mL [30mL]; **Tab:** 0.25mg, 0.5mg, 1mg, 2mg, 3mg, 4mg; **Tab, Disintegrating: (M-Tab)** 0.5mg, 1mg, 2mg	***Adults: Schizophrenia: (Inj)*** 25mg IM every 2 weeks. **Max:** 50mg/dose. Give 1st injection with oral dosage form or other oral antipsychotic. Continue for 3 weeks, then discontinue oral. **Titrate:** Increase at intervals of no more than every 4 weeks. **(Sol, Tab) Initial:** 1mg bid. **Titrate:** Increase by 1mg bid on the 2nd and 3rd day until target dose of 3mg bid by third day. Adjust further at intervals of at least 1 week. **Usual:** 4-8mg/day. **Max:** 16mg/day. Doses up to 8mg can be taken once daily. **Bipolar Mania: (Sol, Tab): Initial:** 2-3mg qd. **Titrate:** Increase/Decrease by 1mg qd. **Usual:** 1-6mg/day. **Max:** 6mg/day. **Elderly/Debilitated/Hypotension/Severe Renal or Hepatic Impairment: Initial:** 0.5mg bid. **Titrate:** Increase by no more than 0.5mg bid. Increase at	**Elderly patients with dementia-related psychosis treated with atypical antipsychotic drugs are at an increased risk of death; most appeared to be cardiovascular (eg, heart failure, sudden death) or infectious (eg, pneumonia) in nature. Risperidone is not approved for the treatment of patients with dementia-related psychosis. W/P:** NMS, tardive dyskinesia may occur. Monitor for hyperglycemia; perform FBG testing if symptoms develop or with risk factors for DM. Cerebrovascular events (eg, stroke, TIA) reported in elderly with dementia-related psychosis. Not approved for the treatment of dementia-related psychosis. May induce orthostatic hypotension, elevate prolactin levels, have an antiemetic effect. Caution in elderly, severe renal/hepatic impairment,	Insomnia, agitation, anxiety, somnolence, extrapyramidal symptoms, hyperkinesia, headache, dizziness, constipation, dyspepsia, rhinitis, rash, akathisia, dystonia, parkinsonism.

*Scored.   †Bold entries denote special dental considerations.

NAME	FORM/ STRENGTH	DOSAGE	WARNINGS/PRECAUTIONS & CONTRAINDICATIONS	ADVERSE EFFECTS†
Risperidone *(cont.)*		intervals of at least 1 week for dosage >1.5mg bid.	history of seizures, cardio- or cerebro-vascular disease, suicidal tendencies, risk of aspiration pneumonia, conditions predisposing to hypotension (eg, hypovolemia, dehydration) or affecting metabolism or hemodynamic responses. May disrupt body temperature regulation; caution in patients exposed to temperature extremes. Re-evaluate periodically. **P/N:** Category C, not for use in nursing.	
Ziprasidone (Geodon)	**Cap:** (HCl) 20mg, 40mg, 60mg, 80mg; **Inj:** (Mesylate) 20mg/mL	**Adults: Schizophrenia: (Cap) Initial:** 20mg bid with food. **Titrate:** May increase up to 80mg bid; adjust dose at intervals of not less than 2 days. **Maint:** 20-80mg bid for up to 52 weeks. **(Inj)** 10-20mg IM up to max 40mg/day. May give 10mg q2h or 20mg q4h up to 40mg/day for 3 days. **Bipolar Mania: (Cap) Initial:** 40mg bid with food. **Titrate:** Increase to 60-80mg bid on 2nd day of treatment. **Maint:** 40-80mg bid.	**Elderly patients with dementia-related psychosis treated with atypical antipsychotic drugs are at an increased risk of death; most appeared to be cardiovascular (eg, heart failure, sudden death) or infectious (eg, pneumonia) in nature. Ziprasidone is not approved for the treatment of patients with dementia-related psychosis. W/P:** Discontinue if persistent QTc measurements >500 msec, NMS, tardive dyskinesia occurs. Monitor for hyperglycemia in patients with DM or at risk for DM. Avoid with congenital long QT syndrome, history of arrhythmia. Caution in history of seizures. Esophageal dysmotility and aspiration reported. May elevate prolactin levels. Orthostatic hypotension reported; caution with cardiovascular or cerebrovascular disease, conditions predisposed to hypotension (eg, dehydration, hypovolemia). Caution with IM use in renal dysfunction. **Contra:** Concomitant dofetilide, sotalol, quinidine, Class Ia/III antiarrhythmics, mesoridazine, thioridazine, chlorpromazine, droperidol, pimozide, sparfloxacin, gatifloxacin, moxifloxacin, halofantrine, mefloquine, pentamidine, arsenic trioxide, levomethadyl acetate, dolasetron, probucol, tacrolimus, and drugs that prolong QT interval. History of QT prolongation, recent acute MI, uncompensated heart failure. **P/N:** Category C, not for use in nursing.	Asthenia, nausea, constipation, dyspepsia, diarrhea, dry mouth, rash, somnolence, akathisia, dizziness, EPS, dystonia, hypertonia, respiratory disorder, upper respiratory infection, vomiting, headache, injection site pain.

ANTIPSYCHOTIC AGENTS

NAME	FORM/ STRENGTH	DOSAGE	WARNINGS/PRECAUTIONS & CONTRAINDICATIONS	ADVERSE EFFECTS†
Aripiprazole (Abilify)	**Tab:** 5mg, 10mg, 15mg, 20mg, 30mg; **Sol:** 1mg/mL [50mL, 150mL, 480mL]	**Adults: Schizophrenia: Initial/Target:** 10 to 15mg qd. **Titrate:** Should not increase before 2 weeks. **Bipolar Mania: Initial:** 30mg qd. Titrate: May decrease to 15mg qd based on assessment and tolerability. Oral solution can be given on a mg-per-mg basis up to 25mg. Patients receiving 30mg tablets should receive 25mg of the solution. **Concomitant CYP3A4 Inhibitors (eg, ketoconazole):** Reduce usual aripiprazole dose by 50%. **Concomitant CYP2D6 Inhibitors (eg, quinidine, fluoxetine, paroxetine):** Reduce usual aripiprazole dose by 50%. **Concomitant CYP3A4 Inducers (eg, carbamazepine):** Double aripiprazole dose (to 20mg or 30mg). Periodically reassess for maintenance therapy.	**Elderly patients with dementia-related psychosis treated with atypical antipsychotic drugs are at an increased risk of death; most appeared to be cardiovascular (eg, heart failure, sudden death) or infectious (eg, pneumonia) in nature. Aripiprazole is not approved for the treatment of patients with dementia-related psychosis. W/P:** May develop tardive dyskinesia, NMS. Monitor for hyperglycemia, worsening of glucose control with DM, FBG levels with diabetes risk. Increased incidence of cerebrovascular adverse events (stroke) in elderly dementia patients. Not approved for treatment of patients with dementia related psychosis. Orthostatic hypotension reported; caution with cardiovascular disease, conditions	Headache, asthenia, rash, blurred vision, rhinitis, cough, tremors, anxiety, insomnia, nausea, vomiting, lightheadedness, somnolence, constipation, akathisia.

Table 18.1: PRESCRIBING INFORMATION FOR PSYCHOACTIVE DRUGS (cont.)

NAME	FORM/ STRENGTH	DOSAGE	WARNINGS/PRECAUTIONS & CONTRAINDICATIONS	ADVERSE EFFECTS†
ANTIPSYCHOTIC AGENTS (cont.)				
Aripiprazole (cont.)			predisposed to hypotension (eg, dehydration, hypovolemia). May lower seizure threshold. Potential for cognitive and motor impairment. May disrupt body's temperature regulation. Possible esophageal dysmotility and aspiration; caution in patients at risk for aspiration pneumonia. Observe vigilance in treating psychosis associated with Alzheimer's. **P/N:** Category C, not for use in nursing.	
Chlorpromazine Hydrochloride (Thorazine)	**Cap, Extended Release:** 30mg, 75mg, 150mg; **Inj:** 25mg/mL; **Sup:** 25mg, 100mg; **Syrup:** 10mg/5mL [120mL]; **Tab:** 10mg, 25mg, 50mg, 100mg, 200mg	**Adults: Severe Behavioral Problems: Inpatient: Acute Schizophrenic/Manic State:** 25mg IM, then 25-50mg IM in 1 hr if needed. **Titrate:** Increase over several days up to 400mg q4-6h until controlled then switch to PO. **Usual:** 500mg/day PO. **Max:** 1000mg/day PO. **Less Acutely Disturbed:** 25mg PO tid. **Titrate:** Increase gradually to 400mg/day. **Outpatient:** 10mg PO tid-qid or 25mg PO bid-tid. **More Severe:** 25mg PO tid. **Titrate:** After 1-2 days, increase by 20-50mg twice weekly until calm. **Prompt Control of Severe Symptoms:** 25mg IM, may repeat in 1 hr then 25-50mg PO tid. **Nausea/Vomiting: Usual:** 10-25mg PO q4-6h prn; 25mg IM then, if no hypotension, 25-50mg q3-4h prn until vomiting stops then switch to PO; 100mg rectally q6-8h prn. **Nausea/Vomiting in Surgery:** 12.5mg IM, may repeat in 1/2 hr; 2mg IV per fractional injection at 2 minute intervals. **Max:** 25mg. **Presurgical Apprehension:** 25-50mg PO 2-3 hrs pre-op; 12.5-25mg IM 1-2 hrs pre-op. **Intractable Hiccups:** 25-50mg PO tid-qid; if symptoms persist after 2-3 days, give 25-50mg IM; if symptoms still persist, give 25-50mg slow IV. **Porphyria:** 25-50mg PO tid-qid; 25mg IM tid-qid until PO therapy. **Tetanus:** 25-50mg IM tid-qid; 25-50mg IV. **Elderly:** Use lower doses, increase dose more gradually, monitor closely. **Pediatrics: 6 months-12 yrs: Severe Behavioral Problems: Outpatient:** 0.25mg/lb PO q4-6h prn; 0.5mg/lb sup rectally q6-8h prn; 0.25mg/lb IM q6-8h prn. **Inpatient:** Start low and increase gradually to 50-100mg/day; ≤200mg/day in older children. **Max:** 500mg/day. **<5 yrs (<50lbs): Max:** ≥40mg/day IM. **5-12 yrs (50-100lbs): Max:** ≥75mg/day IM. **Nausea/Vomiting:** 0.25mg/lb PO q4-6h; 0.5mg/lb sup rectally q6-8 prn. 0.25mg/lb IM q6-8h prn. **Max: 6 months-5 yrs (or 50 lbs):** <40mg/day. **5-12 yrs (or 50-100lbs):** <75mg/day except in severe cases. **During Surgery:** 0.125mg/lb IM repeat in 1/2 hr if needed; 1mg IV per fractional injection at 2-minute intervals and not exceeding recommended IM dosage.	**W/P:** Tardive dyskinesia, NMS may occur. Caution with chronic respiratory disorders, acute respiratory infections (especially in children), glaucoma, cardiovascular, hepatic, or renal disease, history of hepatic encephalopathy due to cirrhosis. Suppresses cough reflex; aspiration of vomitus possible. Caution if exposed to extreme heat or organophosphates. Avoid in children/adolescents with signs of Reye's syndrome. Lowers seizure threshold. Reduce dose gradually to prevent side effects. May mask signs of overdoses to other drugs and obscure diagnosis of other conditions (eg, intestinal obstruction, brain tumor, Reye's syndrome). May produce false-positive PKU test. May elevate prolactin levels. Injection contains sulfites. **Contra:** Comatose states, or with large amounts of CNS depressants. Hypersensitivity to phenothiazines. **P/N:** Safety in pregnancy not known. Not for use in nursing.	Drowsiness, jaundice, agranulocytosis, hypotensive effects, EKG changes, dystonias, motor restlessness, pseudo-parkinsonism, tardive dyskinesia, anticholinergic effects, NMS, ocular changes.

*Scored.   †Bold entries denote special dental considerations.

NAME	FORM/ STRENGTH	DOSAGE	WARNINGS/PRECAUTIONS & CONTRAINDICATIONS	ADVERSE EFFECTS†
Chlorpromazine Hydrochloride *(cont.)*		**Presurgical Apprehension:** 0.25mg/lb PO 2-3 hrs (or IM 1-2 hrs) before operation. **Tetanus:** 0.25mg/lb IM/IV q6-8h. **<50lbs: Max:** ≤40mg/day; **50-100lbs: Max:** ≤75mg/day.		
Clozapine (Clozaril, Fazaclo)	**Tab: (Clozapine)** 12.5mg, 25mg, 100mg; **(Clozaril)** 25mg*, 100mg*	*Adults:* **Initial:** 12.5mg qd-bid. **Titrate:** Increase by 25-50mg/day, up to 300-450mg/day by end of 2nd week, then increase weekly or bi-weekly by up to 100mg. **Usual:** 100-900mg/day given tid. **Max:** 900mg/day. If at risk of suicidal behavior then treat for at least 2 yrs then assess; reassess thereafter at regular intervals. To discontinue, gradually reduce dose over 1-2 weeks. Monitor for psychotic symptoms if abrupt discontinuation warranted (eg, leukopenia).	**Risk of agranulocytosis, seizures, myocarditis, and other cardiovascular and respiratory effects. Conduct baseline WBC and differential before therapy, then regularly, and 4 weeks after discontinuation. Elderly patients with dementia-related psychosis treated with atypical antipsychotic drugs are at an increased risk of death; most appeared to be cardio-vascular (eg, heart failure, sudden death) or infectious (eg, pneumonia) in nature. Clozapine is not approved for the treatment of patients with dementia-related psychosis. W/P:** Re-serve treatment for severely ill patients unresponsive to other schizophrenia therapies. Monitor for hyperglycemia, worsening of glucose control with DM, FBG levels with diabetes risk. Significant risk of orthostatic hypotension, and tachycardia. May impair alertness with initial doses. May cause high fever, hyperglycemia, or pulmonary embolism. Cardiomyopathy reported; discontinue unless benefit outweighs risk. Caution with prostatic enlargement, narrow angle glaucoma, and renal, hepatic, or cardiac/pulmonary disease. NMS and tardive dyskinesia reported. Acquire WBC and ANC at baseline, then weekly for 1st 6 months of therapy, then every 2 weeks for 6 months, and then every 4 weeks thereafter if WBCs and ANC are acceptable. Avoid initiation of treatment if WBCs <3500/mm³, ANC <2000/mm³, history of myeloproliferative disorder, previous clozapine-induced agranulocy-tosis or granulocytopenia. Discontinue treatment if WBCs <3000/mm³, ANC <1500/mm³, eosinophils >4000/mm³, or if myocarditis develops. Discontinue over 1-2 weeks. Varying degrees of intestinal peristalsis impairment (eg, constipation, intestinal obstruction, paralytic ileus), ECG changes reported. **Contra:** Myeloproliferative disorders, uncontrolled epilepsy, paralytic ileus, history of clozapine-induced agranulocy-tosis or severe granulocytopenia, severe CNS depression, coma, with agents with potential to cause agranulocytosis or suppress bone marrow function. **P/N:** Category B, not for use in nursing.	Drowsiness, vertigo, headache, tremor, salivation, sweating, **dry mouth**, visual dis-turbances, tachycardia, hypotension, syncope, constipation, nausea, blood dyscrasias, fever.
Fluphenazine	**(HCl) Inj:** 2.5mg/mL; **Elixir:** 2.5mg/5mL; **Sol, Concentrate:** 5mg/mL; **Tab:** 1mg, 5mg, 10mg; **(Decanoate) Inj:** 25mg/mL.	*Adults:* **(PO) Initial:** 2.5-10mg/day in divided doses q6-8h. **Titrate:** May in-crease up to 40mg/day. **Maint:** 1-5mg qd. **Elderly: Initial:** 1-2.5mg/day. **(Inj, HCl) Initial:** 1.25mg IM q6-8h. **Max:** 10mg/day. **(Decanoate) Initial:** 12.5-25mg IM/SC every 4-6 weeks. **Max:** 100mg/dose. For doses >50mg,	**W/P:** May develop tardive dyskinesia, NMS. Caution with history of choles-tatic jaundice, dermatoses or allergic reactions to phenothiazine derivatives. Elevated prolactin levels reported. Avoid abrupt withdrawal. Caution if exposed to extreme heat or phosphorous insecti-cides, seizure disorder, cardiovascular	Extrapyramidal symptoms, tardive dyskinesia, HTN, hypotension, allergic reactions, nausea, loss of appetite, **dry mouth**, headache, constipa-tion, perspiration,

Table 18.1: PRESCRIBING INFORMATION FOR PSYCHOACTIVE DRUGS (cont.)

NAME	FORM/ STRENGTH	DOSAGE	WARNINGS/PRECAUTIONS & CONTRAINDICATIONS	ADVERSE EFFECTS†

ANTIPSYCHOTIC AGENTS (cont.)

NAME	FORM/ STRENGTH	DOSAGE	WARNINGS/PRECAUTIONS & CONTRAINDICATIONS	ADVERSE EFFECTS†
Fluphenazine (cont.)		succeeding doses should be increased in increments of 12.5mg.	disease, pheochromocytoma. May develop liver damage, pigmentary retinopathy, lenticular and corneal dyskinesias with prolonged therapy. Monitor for hypotension in patients on large doses undergoing surgery. **Contra:** Comatose state, severe depression, concomitant large dose hypnotics, blood dyscrasia, hepatic impairment, subcortical brain damage, cross-sensitivity to phenothiazine derivatives. **P/N:** Safety in pregnancy or nursing not known.	**salivation**, polyuria, hepatic dysfunction.
Haloperidol (Haldol)	**Inj:** 5mg/mL; **Inj:** (Decanoate) 50mg/mL, 100mg/mL; **Sol:** 2mg/mL; **Tab:** 0.5mg*, 1mg*, 2mg*, 5mg*, 10mg*, 20mg*	**Adults: Psychosis: (Immediate Release) PO: Moderate Symptoms/Elderly/Debilitated:** 0.5-2mg bid-tid. **Severe Symptoms/Resistant Patients:** 3-5mg bid-tid. **Max:** 100mg/day. **IM: Acute Agitation:** 2-5mg every 4-8 hrs or hourly as needed for moderately severe to very severe symptoms. **Max:** 100mg/day. **(Decanoate)** Give every 4 weeks or monthly. **Initial:** 10-20 times daily oral dose up to 100mg. Give remainder of dose 3-7 days later if initial dose >100mg. **Usual:** 10-15 times daily oral dose. **Max:** 450mg/month. **Elderly/Debilitated: Initial:** 10-15 times daily oral dose. **Pediatrics: 3-12 yrs (15-40 kg): PO: Psychosis:** 0.05-0.15mg/kg/day given bid-tid. **Nonpsychotic Disorder/Tourette's:** 0.05-0.075mg/kg/day given bid-tid. **Max:** 6mg/day.	**W/P:** Risk of tardive dyskinesia, especially in elderly. NMS, hyperpyrexia, heat stroke, bronchopneumonia reported. Decreased cholesterol, cutaneous and/or ocular changes may occur. Neurotoxicity may occur with thyrotoxicosis. Caution with cardiovascular disease, seizures, EEG abnormalities, elderly. **Contra:** Comatose states, severe toxic CNS depression, Parkinson's disease. **P/N:** Category C, not for use in nursing.	Extrapyramidal symptoms, tardive dyskinesia, tardive dystonia, ECG changes, gynecomastia, insomnia, drowsiness, skin reactions, anorexia, anticholinergic effects, **laryngospasm**, cataracts.
Loxapine Succinate (Loxitane)	**Cap:** 5mg, 10mg, 25mg, 50mg; **Inj:** 50mg/mL; **Sol: Concentrate: (Loxitane C)** 25mg/mL [120mL]	**Adults: (PO) Initial:** 10mg bid, up to 50mg/day for severely disturbed. **Titrate:** Increase rapidly over 7-10 days. **Maint:** 60-100mg/day. **Max:** 250mg/day. Mix concentrate with orange or grapefruit juice; use dropper to dose. **(IM)** 12.5-50mg q4-6h. Individualize dose.	**W/P:** Extrapyramidal symptoms, tardive dyskinesia, NMS can occur. May lower seizure threshold. May mask symptoms of overdose of other drugs. May obscure diagnosis of intestinal obstruction, brain tumor. Ocular toxicity reported. Caution in cardiovascular disease, glaucoma, urinary retention. Elevates prolactin levels. Caution with activities requiring alertness. **Contra:** Comatose states, severe drug-induced depressed states (eg, alcohol, barbiturates, narcotics). **P/N:** Safety in pregnancy not known. Not for use in nursing.	Drowsiness, weakness, NMS, tachycardia, hypotension, HTN, syncope, edema, **dry mouth**, constipation, blurred vision.
Molindone Hydrochloride (Moban)	**Tab:** 5mg, 10mg, 25mg*, 50mg*	**Adults: Initial:** 50-75mg/day. **Titrate:** Increase to 100mg/day in 3-4 days; adjust to patient response. **Maint: Mild:** 5-15mg tid-qid. **Moderate:** 10-25mg tid-qid. **Severe:** 225mg/day. **Pediatrics: ≥12 yrs: Initial:** 50-75mg/day. **Titrate:** Increase to 100mg/day in 3-4 days; adjust to patient response. **Maint: Mild:** 5-15mg tid-qid. **Moderate:** 10-25mg tid-qid. **Severe:** 225mg/day.	**W/P:** Tardive dyskinesia, NMS may occur. Concentrate contains sulfites. Caution with activities requiring alertness. Convulsions, increased activity reported. May obscure signs of intestinal obstruction or brain tumor. May elevate prolactin levels. **Contra:** Severe CNS depression (alcohol, barbiturates, narcotics), comatose states. **P/N:** Safety in pregnancy and nursing not known.	Drowsiness, depression, hyperactivity, euphoria, extrapyramidal reactions, akathisia, Parkinson's syndrome, blurred vision, nausea, **dry mouth**.
Olanzapine (Zyprexa)	**Inj:** 10mg; **Tab:** 2.5mg, 5mg, 7.5mg, 10mg, 15mg, 20mg; **Tab, Disintegrating: (Zydis)** 5mg,	**Adults: (Tab) Schizophrenia: Initial/Usual:** 5-10mg qd. **Titrate:** Adjust by 5mg daily at weekly intervals. **Max:** 20mg/day. **Bipolar Mania: Initial:** 10-15mg qd. **Titrate:** Increase by 5mg daily. **Max:** 20mg/day. **With Lithium**	Elderly patients with dementia-related psychosis treated with atypical antipsychotic drugs are at an increased risk of death; most appeared to be cardiovascular (eg, heart failure, sudden death) or infectious (eg, pneumonia) in nature. Olanzapine is not	Postural hypotension, constipation, **dry mouth**, weight gain, somnolence, dizziness, personality disorder, akathisia, asthenia, dyspepsia, tremor,

*Scored.   †Bold entries denote special dental considerations.

NAME	FORM/ STRENGTH	DOSAGE	WARNINGS/PRECAUTIONS & CONTRAINDICATIONS	ADVERSE EFFECTS†
Olanzapine *(cont.)*	10mg, 15mg, 20mg	**or Valproate: Initial/Usual:** 10mg qd. Max: 20mg/day. **Debilitated/Hypotension Risk/Slow metabolizers/Sensitivity to olanzapine effects: Initial:** 5mg qd. **Titrate:** Increase cautiously. (IM) **Agitation: Initial:** 10mg IM. **Usual:** 2.5-10mg IM. **Max:** 3 doses of 10mg q 2-4h. **Elderly:** 5mg IM. **Debilitated/Hypotension Risk/Sensitivity to olanzapine effects:** 2.5mg IM. May initiate PO therapy when clinically appropriate.	approved for the treatment of patients with dementia-related psychosis. W/P: Monitor for hyperglycemia, worsening of glucose control with DM, FBG levels with diabetes risk. Risk of NMS, tardive dyskinesia, orthostatic hypotension, seizures. Caution in hepatic impairment, prostatic hypertrophy, narrow-angle glaucoma, history of paralytic ileus, elderly patients with dementia or Parkinson's disease, cardio- or cerebrovascular disease, hypotension risk (eg, hypovolemia, dehydration), risk for aspiration pneumonia, suicidal tendencies. Elevated transaminases, hyperprolactinemia reported. May cause disruption of body temperature regulation. Re-evaluate periodically. **P/N:** Category C, not for use in nursing.	increased appetite.
Perphenazine	**Tab:** 2mg, 4mg, 8mg, 16mg	*Adults:* **Moderately Disturbed Non-Hospitalized With Schizophrenia: Initial:** 4-8mg tid. **Maint:** Reduce to minimum effective dose. **Hospitalized Psychotic Patients With Schizophrenia:** 8-16mg bid-qid. **Max:** 64mg/day. **Severe Nausea/Vomiting:** 8-16mg/day in divided doses. **Max:** 24mg/day. **Elderly:** Lower dosages recommended. *Pediatrics:* **≥12 yrs:** Use lowest limits of adult dose.	**W/P:** Tardive dyskinesia may develop. NMS, photosensitivity reported. May lower convulsive threshold; caution with alcohol withdrawal. Caution with psychic depression, renal impairment, respiratory impairment. May impair mental/physical abilities. May mask signs of overdosage to other drugs. May obscure diagnosis of intestinal obstruction, brain tumor. Severe hypotension may occur in surgery. May elevate prolactin levels. Monitor hepatic/renal functions, blood counts. Increased risk of liver damage, jaundice, corneal and lenticular deposits, and irreversible dyskinesias with long-term use. **Contra:** Comatose or greatly obtunded patients, large doses of CNS depressants (eg, barbiturates, alcohol, narcotics, analgesics, or antihistamines), blood dyscrasias, bone marrow depression, liver damage, subcortical brain damage with or without hypothalamic involvement. **P/N:** Safety in pregnancy and nursing not known.	Aching/numbness of the limbs, motor restlessness, cerebral edema, seizures, drowsiness, dry mouth, salivation, nausea, vomiting, diarrhea, lactation, postural hypotension, tachycardia.
Risperidone (Risperdal, Risperdal Consta, Risperdal M-Tab)	**Inj: (Consta)** 25mg, 37.5mg, 50mg. **Sol:** 1mg/mL [30mL]; **Tab:** 0.25mg, 0.5mg, 1mg, 2mg, 3mg, 4mg; **Tab, Disintegrating: (M-Tab)** 0.5mg, 1mg, 2mg	*Adults:* **Schizophrenia: (Inj)** 25mg IM every 2 weeks. **Max:** 50mg/dose. Give 1st injection with oral dosage form or other oral antipsychotic. Continue for 3 weeks, then discontinue oral. **Titrate:** Increase at intervals of no more than every 4 weeks. **(Sol, Tab) Initial:** 1mg bid. **Titrate:** Increase by 1mg bid on the 2nd and 3rd day until target dose of 3mg bid by third day. Adjust further at intervals of at least 1 week. **Usual:** 4-8mg/day. **Max:** 16mg/day. Doses up to 8mg can be taken once daily. **Bipolar Mania: (Sol, Tab): Initial:** 2-3mg qd. **Titrate:** Increase/Decrease by 1mg qd. **Usual:** 1-6mg/day. **Max:** 6mg/day. **Elderly/Debilitated/Hypotension/Severe Renal or Hepatic Impairment: Initial:** 0.5mg bid. **Titrate:** Increase by no more than 0.5mg bid. Increase at intervals of at least 1 week for dosage >1.5mg bid.	**Elderly patients with dementia-related psychosis treated with atypical antipsychotic drugs are at an increased risk of death; most appeared to be cardiovascular (eg, heart failure, sudden death) or infectious (eg, pneumonia) in nature. Risperidone is not approved for the treatment of patients with dementia-related psychosis. W/P:** NMS, tardive dyskinesia may occur. Monitor for hyperglycemia; perform fasting blood glucose testing if symptoms develop or with risk factors for DM. Cerebrovascular events (eg, stroke, TIA) reported in elderly with dementia-related psychosis. Not approved for the treatment of dementia-related psychosis. May induce orthostatic hypotension, elevate prolactin levels, have an antiemetic effect. Caution in elderly, severe renal/hepatic impairment, history of seizures, cardio- or cerebrovascular disease, suicidal tendencies, risk of aspiration pneumonia,	Insomnia, agitation, anxiety, somnolence, extrapyramidal symptoms, hyperkinesia, headache, dizziness, constipation, dyspepsia, rhinitis, rash, akathisia, dystonia, parkinsonism.

Table 18.1: PRESCRIBING INFORMATION FOR PSYCHOACTIVE DRUGS *(cont.)*

NAME	FORM/ STRENGTH	DOSAGE	WARNINGS/PRECAUTIONS & CONTRAINDICATIONS	ADVERSE EFFECTS†
ANTIPSYCHOTIC AGENTS *(cont.)*				
Risperidone *(cont.)*			conditions predisposing to hypotension (eg, hypovolemia, dehydration) or affecting metabolism or hemodynamic responses. May disrupt body temperature regulation; caution in patients exposed to temperature extremes. Re-evaluate periodically. **P/N:** Category C, not for use in nursing.	
Thioridazine Hydrochloride (Mellaril)	**Sol, Concentrate:** 30mg/mL, 100mg/mL [120mL]; **Tab:** 10mg, 15mg, 25mg, 50mg, 100mg, 150mg, 200mg	***Adults:*** **Initial:** 50-100mg tid. **Titrate:** Increase gradually. **Usual:** 200-800mg/ day given bid-qid. **Max:** 800mg/day. Dilute concentrate in juice, distilled or acidified tap water. ***Pediatrics:*** **Initial:** 0.5mg/kg/day given in divided doses. **Titrate:** Increase gradually. **Max:** 3mg/kg/day. Dilute concentrate in juice, distilled or acidified tap water.	**Prolongation of QTc interval reported in a dose related manner. Associated with torsade de pointes and sudden death; reserve for patients not responding to or cannot tolerate other antipsychotics.** **W/P:** Perform baseline ECG and measure baseline potassium level; monitor periodically thereafter. May develop tardive dyskinesia. NMS, seizures, leukopenia, agranulocytosis reported. Caution with activities requiring alertness. May elevate prolactin levels. **Contra:** Severe CNS depression, comatose states, severe hypo- or hypertensive heart disease. Drugs that prolong QTc interval, congenital long QT syndrome, cardiac arrhythmias, drugs that inhibit CYP450 2D6 (eg, fluoxetine, paroxetine), patients with reduced activity of CYP450 2D6. **P/N:** Safety in pregnancy and nursing not known.	Tardive dyskinesia, ECG changes, drowsiness, **dry mouth,** blurred vision, peripheral edema, galactorrhea, nausea, vomiting, gynecomastia, impotence, constipation, diarrhea.
Thiothixene (Navane)	**Cap:** 2mg, 5mg, 10mg, 20mg	***Adults:*** **Mild Condition: Initial:** 2mg tid. **Titrate:** May increase to 15mg/day. **Severe Condition: Initial:** 5mg bid. **Usual:** 20-30mg/day. **Max:** 60mg/day.	**W/P:** May develop tardive dyskinesia, NMS. May mask symptoms of overdose of toxic drugs. May obscure conditions such as intestinal obstruction and brain tumor. May lower seizure threshold. Monitor for pigmentary retinopathy and lenticular pigmentation. Caution with cardiovascular disease, extreme heat exposure, activities requiring alertness. May elevate prolactin levels. **Contra:** Circulatory collapse, comatose states, CNS depression, blood dyscrasias. **P/N:** Safety in pregnancy and nursing not known.	Tachycardia, hypotension, lightheadedness, syncope, drowsiness, agitation, insomnia, hyperreflexia, cerebral edema, pseudoparkinsonism, LFT elevation, blood dyscrasias, rash, photosensitivity, **dry mouth,** blurred vision.
Trifluoperazine Hydrochloride	**Tab:** 1mg, 2mg, 5mg, 10mg	***Adults:*** **Psychotic Disorders: Initial:** 2-5mg PO bid. **Usual:** 15-20mg/day. **Max:** 40mg/day or more if needed. **Non-Psychotic Anxiety:** 1-2mg bid. **Max:** 6mg/day or >12 weeks. **Elderly:** Lower dose and increase more gradually. ***Pediatrics:*** **Psychotic Disorders: 6-12 yrs: Initial:** 1mg PO qd-bid. **Titrate:** Increase gradually until symptoms controlled. **Usual:** 15mg/day.	**W/P:** May develop tardive dyskinesia, NMS. May elevate prolactin levels; caution with prolactin-dependent tumors. May mask drug toxicity and drug overdose due to antiemetic effects. May obscure diagnosis and treatment of intestinal obstruction, brain tumor, and Reye's syndrome. Risk of hypotension; avoid large doses and IV use with cardiovascular disease. Caution with glaucoma, angina, and elderly. May cause retinopathy; discontinue if retinal changes occur. Evaluate therapy periodically with prolonged use. May interfere with thermoregulatory mechanism; caution in extreme heat. Solution contains sodium bisulfite. Jaundice, hepatic damage reported. May cause false-positive PKU test. **Contra:** Comatose or greatly depressed states due to CNS depressants, bone marrow depression, blood dyscrasias, hepatic damage. **P/N:** Safety in pregnancy not known. Not for use in nursing.	EPS, motor restlessness, dystonias, pseudo-parkinsonism, tardive dyskinesia, convulsions, **dry mouth,** headache, nausea, blood dycrasias.

*Scored.   †Bold entries denote special dental considerations.

NAME	FORM/ STRENGTH	DOSAGE	WARNINGS/PRECAUTIONS & CONTRAINDICATIONS	ADVERSE EFFECTS†
Ziprasidone (Geodon)	**Cap:** (HCl) 20mg, 40mg, 60mg, 80mg; **Inj:** (Mesylate) 20mg/mL	*Adults:* **Schizophrenia: (Cap) Initial:** 20mg bid with food. **Titrate:** May increase up to 80mg bid; adjust dose at intervals of not less than 2 days. **Maint:** 20-80mg bid for up to 52 weeks. **(Inj)** 10-20mg IM up to max 40mg/day. May give 10mg q2h or 20mg q4h up to 40mg/day for 3 days. **Bipolar Mania: (Cap) Initial:** 40mg bid with food. **Titrate:** Increase to 60-80mg bid on 2nd day of treatment. **Maint:** 40-80mg bid.	**Elderly patients with dementia-related psychosis treated with atypical antipsychotic drugs are at an increased risk of death; most appeared to be cardiovascular (eg, heart failure, sudden death) or infectious (eg, pneumonia) in nature. Ziprasidone is not approved for the treatment of patients with dementia-related psychosis. W/P:** Discontinue if persistent QTc measurements >500 msec, NMS, tardive dyskinesia occurs. Monitor for hyperglycemia in patients with DM or at risk for DM. Avoid with congenital long QT syndrome, history of arrhythmia. Caution in history of seizures. Esophageal dysmotility and aspiration reported. May elevate prolactin levels. Orthostatic hypotension reported; caution with cardiovascular or cerebrovascular disease, conditions predisposed to hypotension (eg, dehydration, hypovolemia). Caution with IM use in renal dysfunction. **Contra:** Concomitant dofetilide, sotalol, quinidine, Class Ia/III antiarrhythmics, mesoridazine, thioridazine, chlorpromazine, droperidol, pimozide, sparfloxacin, gatifloxacin, moxifloxacin, halofantrine, mefloquine, pentamidine, arsenic trioxide, levomethadyl acetate, dolasetron, probucol, tacrolimus, and drugs that prolong QT interval. History of QT prolongation, recent acute MI, uncompensated heart failure. **P/N:** Category C, not for use in nursing.	Asthenia, nausea, constipation, dyspepsia, diarrhea, dry mouth, rash, somnolence, akathisia, dizziness, EPS, dystonia, hypertonia, respiratory disorder, upper respiratory infection, vomiting, headache, injection site pain.

ATTENTION DEFICIT/HYPERACTIVITY DISORDER AGENTS

NAME	FORM/ STRENGTH	DOSAGE	WARNINGS/PRECAUTIONS & CONTRAINDICATIONS	ADVERSE EFFECTS†
Amphetamine Aspartate/Amphetamine Sulfate/Dextroamphetamine Saccharate/Dextroamphetamine Sulfate CII (Adderall, Adderall XR)	**Tab:** 5mg*, 7.5mg*, 10mg*, 12.5mg*, 15mg*, 20mg*, 30mg*; **Cap, Extended Release:** 5mg, 10mg, 15mg, 20mg, 25mg, 30mg	**(Adderall)** *Adults:* **Narcolepsy: Initial:** 10mg/day. **Titrate:** May increase by 10mg/day every week. **Usual:** 5-60mg/day. Give 1st dose upon awakening, additional doses every 4-6 hrs. *Pediatrics:* **ADHD: 3-5 yrs: Initial:** 2.5mg qd. **Titrate:** May increase by 2.5mg weekly. **≥6 yrs:** 5mg qd-bid. May increase by 5mg weekly. **Max (usual):** 40mg/day. **Narcolepsy: 6-12 yrs: Initial:** 5mg/day. May increase by 5mg weekly. **≥12 yrs: Initial:** 10mg/day. **Titrate:** May increase by 10mg/day every week. **Usual:** 5-60mg/day. Give 1st dose upon awakening, and additional doses q4-6h. **(Adderall XR)** *Adults:* **Initial:** 20mg qam. **Currently Using Adderall:** Switch to Adderall XR at the same total daily dose, taken once daily. Titrate at weekly intervals as needed. Swallow cap whole or open cap and sprinkle contents on applesauce; do not chew beads. *Pediatrics:* **≥6 yrs: Initial:** 10mg qam. **Titrate:** May increase weekly by 5-10mg/day. **Max:** 30mg/day. **13 to 17 yrs: Initial:** 10mg/day. **Titrate:** May increase to 20mg/day after one week. **Currently Using Adderall:** Switch to Adderall XR at the same total daily dose, taken once daily. Titrate at weekly intervals as	**High potential for abuse; avoid prolonged use. Misuse of amphetamine may cause sudden death and serious cardiovascular adverse events. W/P:** Exacerbation of Tourette's syndrome and phonic or motor tics. Caution with HTN. May exacerbate symptoms of behavior disturbance and thought disorder in psychotic children. Monitor growth in children. Interrupt occasionally to determine if patient requires continued therapy. Sudden death reported in children with structural cardiac abnormalities; avoid use in children or adults with structural cardiac abnormalities. **Contra:** Advanced arteriosclerosis, symptomatic cardiovascular disease, moderate to severe HTN, hyperthyroidism, glaucoma, agitated states, history of drug abuse, during or within 14 days of MAOI use. **P/N:** Category C, not for use in nursing.	HTN, tachycardia, palpitations, CNS over-stimulation, **dry mouth, gingival enlargement,** GI disorders, anorexia, impotence, urticaria, abdominal pain, asthenia, fever, loss of appetite, diarrhea, nausea, vomiting, emotional lability, insomnia, nervousness, weight loss, headache.

Table 18.1: PRESCRIBING INFORMATION FOR PSYCHOACTIVE DRUGS *(cont.)*

NAME	FORM/ STRENGTH	DOSAGE	WARNINGS/PRECAUTIONS & CONTRAINDICATIONS	ADVERSE EFFECTS†
ATTENTION DEFICIT/HYPERACTIVITY DISORDER AGENTS *(cont.)*				
Amphetamine Aspartate/ Amphetamine Sulfate/ Dextro-amphetamine Saccharate/ Dextroamphet-amine Sulfate^{CII} *(cont.)*		needed. Swallow cap whole or open cap and sprinkle contents on apple-sauce; do not chew beads.		
Atomoxetine Hydrochloride (Strattera)	**Cap:** 10mg, 18mg, 25mg, 40mg, 60mg	***Adults:* Initial:** 40mg/day given qam or evenly divided doses in the am and late afternoon/early evening. **Titrate:** Increase after minimum of 3 days to target dose of about 80mg/day. After 2-4 weeks, may increase to max of 100mg/day. **Max:** 100mg/day. **Hepatic Insufficiency: Moderate (Child-Pugh Class B):** Reduce initial and target doses to 50% of normal dose. **Severe (Child-Pugh Class C):** Reduce initial and target doses to 25% of normal dose. **Concomitant CYP450 2D6 inhibitor (eg, paroxetine, fluoxetine, quinidine): Initial:** 40mg/day. **Titrate:** Only increase to 80mg/day if symptoms fail to improve after 4 weeks. ***Pediatrics:* ≥6yrs: ≤70kg: Initial:** 0.5mg/kg/day given qam or evenly divided doses in the am and late afternoon or early evening. **Titrate:** Increase after minimum of 3 days to target dose of about 1.2mg/kg/day. **Max:** 1.4mg/kg/day or 100mg, whichever is less. **>70kg: Initial:** 40mg/day given qam or evenly divided doses in the am and late afternoon/early evening. **Titrate:** Increase after minimum of 3 days to target dose of about 80mg/day. After 2-4 weeks, may increase to max of 100mg/day. **Max:** 100mg/day. **Hepatic Insufficiency: Moderate (Child-Pugh Class B):** Reduce initial and target doses to 50% of the normal dose. **Severe (Child-Pugh Class C):** Reduce initial and target doses to 25% of normal dose. **Concomitant CYP450 2D6 inhibitor (eg, paroxetine, fluoxetine, quinidine): ≥6yrs: ≤70kg: Initial:** 0.5mg/kg/day. **Titrate:** Only increase to 1.2mg/kg/day if symptoms fail to improve after 4 weeks. **>70kg: Initial:** 40mg/day. **Titrate:** Only increase to 80mg/day if symptoms fail to improve after 4 weeks.	**Increased risk of suicidal ideation in short-term studies in children or adolescents with ADHD. Closely monitor for suicidality, clinical worsening, or unusual changes in behavior. Close observation/communication with prescriber by families and caregivers is advised. W/P:** Allergic reactions and orthostatic hypotension reported. Monitor growth. May increase blood pressure and heart rate; caution with HTN, tachycardia, or cardiovascular or cerebrovascular disease. May increase urinary retention and urinary hesitation. May cause severe liver injury in rare cases; monitor liver enzymes and discontinue with jaundice or liver injury. **Contra:** During or within 14 days of MAOI use; narrow angle glaucoma. **P/N:** Category C, caution in nursing.	(Pediatrics) Upper abdominal pain, headache, vomiting, decreased appetite, cough, irritability, dizziness, somnolence. (Adults) **Dry mouth,** headache, insomnia, nausea, decreased appetite, constipation, dysmenorrhea, ejaculation failure/disorder.
Dexmethylphe-nidate Hydrochloride^{CII} (Focalin, Focalin XR)	**(Focalin) Tab:** 2.5mg, 5mg, 10mg; **(Focalin XR) Cap, Extended Release:** 5mg, 10mg, 20mg	**(Focalin)** *Adults:* Take bid at least 4 hrs apart. **Methylphenidate Naive: Initial:** 2.5mg bid. **Titrate:** Increase weekly by 2.5-5mg/day. **Max:** 20mg/day. **Currently on Methylphenidate: Initial:** Take 1/2 of methylphenidate dose. **Max:** 20mg/day. Reduce or discontinue if paradoxical aggravation of symptoms. Discontinue if no improvement after appropriate dosage adjustments	**W/P:** Caution in drug dependence or alcoholism. Psychotic episodes can occur with parenteral abuse. Not for management of severe depression or normal fatigue states. Monitor growth, CBC, differential, and platelets with prolonged therapy. May exacerbate behavior disturbance and thought disorder in psychotic children. Discontinue in the presence of seizures. Caution in HTN.	Abdominal pain, fever, anorexia, nausea, nervousness, insomnia. (Adults) **Dry mouth, pharyngolaryngeal pain,** feeling jittery, dizziness. (Children) Loss of appetite, weight loss, tachycardia.

*Scored.   †Bold entries denote special dental considerations.

NAME	FORM/ STRENGTH	DOSAGE	WARNINGS/PRECAUTIONS & CONTRAINDICATIONS	ADVERSE EFFECTS†
Dexmethylphe- nidate HydrochlorideCII *(cont.)*		over 1 month. *Pediatrics:* ≥6 yrs: Take bid at least 4 hrs apart. **Methylpheni- date Naive: Initial:** 2.5mg bid. **Titrate:** Increase weekly by 2.5-5mg/day. **Max:** 20mg/day. **Currently on Methylpheni- date: Initial:** Take 1/2 of methylpheni- date dose. **Max:** 20mg/day. Reduce or discontinue if paradoxical aggravation of symptoms. Discontinue if no improvement after appropriate dosage adjustments over 1 month. **(Focalin XR)** *Adults:* **Methylphenidate Naive: Initial:** 10mg/day. **Titrate:** May adjust weekly by 10mg/day. **Max:** 20mg/day. **Currently on Methylphenidate: Initial:** Take 1/2 of methylphenidate dose. **Max:** 20mg/day. Reduce or discontinue if paradoxical aggravation of symptoms. Swallow capsule whole or sprinkle contents on applesauce; contents should not be crushed, chewed or divided. Discontinue if no improvement after appropriate dosage adjustments over 1 month. *Pediatrics:* **≥6 yrs: Methylphenidate Naive: Initial:** 5mg/day. **Titrate:** May adjust weekly by 5mg/day. **Max:** 20mg/day. **Currently on Methylphenidate: Initial:** Take 1/2 of methylphenidate dose. **Max:** 20mg/day. Reduce or discontinue if paradoxical aggravation of symptoms. Swallow capsule whole or sprinkle contents on applesauce; contents should not be crushed, chewed or divided. Discontinue if no improvement after appropriate dosage adjustments over 1 month.	Visual disturbances reported. **Contra:** Marked anxiety, tension, and agitation; glaucoma; motor tics or family history or diagnosis of Tourette's syndrome; during or within 14 days of MAOI use. **P/N:** Category C, caution in nursing.	
Dextroamphet- amine SulfateCII (Dexedrine, Dexedrine Spansules)	**Cap, Extended Release:** (Span- sules) 5mg, 10mg, 15mg; **Tab:** 5mg*	*Adults:* **Narcolepsy: Initial:** 10mg/day. **Titrate:** May increase by 10mg/day every week. **Usual:** 5-60mg/day. For tabs, give 1st dose upon awakening and additional every 4-6 hrs. May give caps once daily. *Pediatrics:* **Narcolepsy: 6-12 yrs: Initial:** 5mg/day. **Titrate:** Increase weekly by 5mg/day. **≥12 yrs: Initial:** 10mg qd. **Titrate:** Increase weekly by 10mg/day. **Usual:** 5-60mg/day in divided doses. **ADHD: Initial: 3-5 yrs:** 2.5mg qd. **Titrate:** Increase weekly by 2.5mg/day. **≥6 yrs:** 5mg qd-bid. **Titrate:** Increase weekly by 5mg/day. **Max:** 40mg/day. For tabs, give 1st dose upon awakening and additional every 4-6 hrs. May give caps once daily.	**High potential for abuse. Avoid prolonged use. W/P:** Caution with HTN. Tablets contain tartrazine; may cause allergy reactions. Exacerbation of motor and phonic tics and Tourette's syn- drome. May exacerbate behavior distur- bance and thought disorder in psychotic pediatrics. Interrupt occasionally to determine if patient requires continued therapy. Monitor growth in children. **Contra:** Advanced arteriosclerosis, symptomatic cardiovascular disease, moderate to severe HTN, hyperthyroid- ism, glaucoma, agitated states, history of drug abuse, during or within 14 days of MAOI use. **P/N:** Category C, not for use in nursing.	Palpitations, tachy- cardia, BP elevation, CNS overstimulation, restlessness, insomnia, **dry mouth, gingival enlargement,** GI disturbances, anorexia, urticaria, impotence.
Methamphet- amine HydrochlorideCII (Desoxyn)	**Tab:** 5mg	*Adults:* **Obesity:** 5mg, 1/2 hr before each meal. Do not exceed a few weeks of treatment. *Pediatrics:* **ADHD:** ≥6 yrs: **Initial:** 5mg/day. **Titrate:** Increase weekly by 5mg/day until optimum response. **Usual:** 20-25mg/day given bid. **Obesity:** ≥12 yrs: 5mg, 1/2 hr before each meal. Do not exceed a few weeks of treatment.	**High potential for abuse. Avoid prolonged therapy in obesity. W/P:** Tolerance to anorectic effect develops within a few weeks, do not exceed recommended dose to increase effect. Monitor growth in children. Caution with HTN. Do not use to combat fatigue or replace rest. Exacerbation of motor and phonic tics and Tourette's syndrome. May exacerbate behavior disturbance and thought disorder in psychotic	BP elevation, tachycar- dia, palpitation, dizzi- ness, insomnia, tremor, diarrhea, constipation, **dry mouth,** urticaria, impotence, changes in libido.

Table 18.1: PRESCRIBING INFORMATION FOR PSYCHOACTIVE DRUGS (cont.)

NAME	FORM/STRENGTH	DOSAGE	WARNINGS/PRECAUTIONS & CONTRAINDICATIONS	ADVERSE EFFECTS†
ATTENTION DEFICIT/HYPERACTIVITY DISORDER AGENTS (cont.)				
Methamphet-amine Hydrochloride^{CII} (cont.)			pediatrics. Interrupt occasionally to determine if patient requires continued therapy. **Contra:** Advanced arterio-sclerosis, symptomatic cardiovascular disease, moderate to severe HTN, hyper-thyroidism, glaucoma, agitated states, history of drug abuse, during or within 14 days of MAOI use. **P/N:** Category C, not for use in nursing.	
Methylphenidate Hydrochloride^{CII} (Concerta, Metadate CD, Metadate ER, Methylin, Ritalin, Ritalin LA, Rit-alin-SR)	**(Concerta) Tab, Extended Release:** 18mg, 27mg, 36mg, 54mg; **(Metadate CD) Cap, Extended Release:** 10mg, 20mg, 30mg; **(Metadate ER) Tab, Extended Release:** 10mg, 20mg; **(Methylin) Sol:** 5mg/5mL [500mL], 10mg/5mL [500mL]; **Tab:** 5mg, 10mg, 20mg; **Tab, Chewable:** 2.5mg, 5mg, 10mg; **Tab, Extended Release:** 10mg, 20mg; **(Ritalin) Cap, ER (Ritalin LA):** 10mg, 20mg, 30mg, 40mg; **Tab (Ritalin):** 5mg, 10mg*, 20mg*; **Tab, ER (Ritalin-SR):** 20mg	**(Concerta) Adults: Methylphenidate-Naive or Receiving Other Stimulant: Initial:** 18mg qam. **Titrate:** Adjust dose at weekly intervals. **Previous Methylphenidate Use: Initial:** 18mg qam if previous dose 10-15mg/day; 36mg qam if previous dose 20-30mg/day; 54mg qam if previous dose 30-45mg/day. Initial conversion should not exceed 54mg/day. **Titrate:** Adjust dose at weekly intervals. **Max:** 72mg/day. Reduce dose or discontinue if paradoxical aggravation of symptoms occurs. Discontinue if no improvement after appropriate dosage adjustments over 1 month. Swallow whole with liquids. Do not crush, chew, or divide. *Pediatrics:* **≥6 yrs: Methylphenidate Naive or Receiving Other Stimulant: Initial:** 18mg qam. **Titrate:** Adjust dose at weekly intervals. **Max: 6-12 yrs:** 54mg/day. **13-17 yrs:** 72mg/day not to exceed 2mg/kg/day. **Previous Methylphenidate Use: Initial:** 18mg qam if previous dose 10-15mg/day; 36mg qam if previous dose 20-30mg/day; 54mg qam if previous dose 30-45mg/day. Initial conversion should not exceed 54mg/day. **Titrate:** Adjust dose at weekly intervals. **Max:** 72mg/day. Reduce dose or discontinue if paradoxical aggravation of symptoms occurs. Discontinue if no improvement after appropriate dosage adjustments over 1 month. Swallow whole with liquids. Do not crush, chew, or divide. **(Metadate CD)** *Pediatrics:* **≥6 yrs: Usual:** 20mg qam before breakfast. **Titrate:** Increase weekly by 20mg depending on tolerability/effi-cacy. **Max:** 60mg/day. Reduce dose or discontinue if paradoxical aggravation of symptoms occur. Discontinue if no improvement after appropriate dose adjustments over 1 month. Swallow whole with liquids or open and sprinkle on 1 tbs applesauce followed by water. Do not crush, chew, or divide. **(Metadate ER)** *Adults:* **(Immediate-Release Methylphenidate)** 10-60mg/day given bid-tid 30-45 minutes ac. Take last dose before 6 pm if insomnia occurs. **(Tab, Extended Release)** May use in place of immediate release tabs when the 8 hr dose corresponds to the	**W/P:** Monitor growth during treatment in children. Not for severe depression or fatigue. May exacerbate symptoms of behavior disturbance and thought dis-order in psychotic patients. Avoid with severe GI narrowing (eg, esophageal motility disorders, small bowel inflam-matory disease, short-gut syndrome). May lower seizure threshold, especially in known EEG abnormalities. Caution with HTN, conditions affected by BP or heart rate elevation, history of drug abuse or alcoholism. Monitor during withdrawal from abusive use. Visual disturbances may occur (rare). Monitor CBC, differential, and platelets with prolonged use. **Contra:** Marked anxiety, tension, and agitation; glaucoma; motor tics or family history or diagnosis of Tourette's syndrome, during or within 14 days of MAOI use. **P/N:** Category C, caution in nursing. (Methylin/Rit-alin/Ritalin SR) Safety in pregnancy and nursing not known.	Headache, abdominal pain, anorexia, insom-nia, upper respiratory tract infection, nervous-ness, hypersensitiv-ity reactions, nausea, dizziness, palpitations, dyskinesia, drowsiness, BP and pulse changes, tachycardia, angina, arrhythmia.

*Scored.   †Bold entries denote special dental considerations.

NAME	FORM/ STRENGTH	DOSAGE	WARNINGS/PRECAUTIONS & CONTRAINDICATIONS	ADVERSE EFFECTS†
Methylphenidate HydrochlorideCII *(cont.)*		titrated 8 hr immediate release dose. Swallow whole; do not chew or crush. *Pediatrics:* ≥6 yrs: **(Immediate-Release Methylphenidate) Initial:** 5mg bid before breakfast and lunch. **Titrate:** Increase gradually by 5-10mg weekly. **Max:** 60mg/day. **(Tab, Extended Release)** May use in place of immediate release tabs when the 8 hr dose corresponds to the titrated 8 hr immediate release dose. Swallow whole; do not chew or crush. Reduce dose or discontinue if paradoxical aggravation of symptoms occur. Discontinue if no improvement after appropriate dose adjustment over 1 month. **(Methylin)** *Adults:* **(Sol/Tab/Tab, Chewable)** 10-60mg/day given bid-tid 30-45 minutes ac. Take last dose before 6 pm if insomnia occurs. **(Tab, Extended Release)** May use in place of immediate release tabs when the 8 hr dose corresponds to the titrated 8 hr immediate release dose. Swallow whole; do not chew or crush. *Pediatrics:* ≥6 yrs: **(Sol/Tab/Tab, Chewable) Initial:** 5mg bid before breakfast and lunch. **Titrate:** Increase gradually by 5-10mg weekly. **Max:** 60mg/day. **(Tab, Extended Release)** May be used in place of immediate release tabs when the 8 hr dose corresponds to the titrated 8 hr immediate release dose. Swallow whole; do not chew or crush. Reduce dose or discontinue if paradoxical aggravation of symptoms occur. Discontinue if no improvement after appropriate dose adjustment over 1 month. **(Ritalin)** *Adults:* **(Tab)** 10-60mg/day given bid-tid 30-45 minutes ac. Take last dose before 6 pm if insomnia occurs. **(Tab, ER)** May use in place of immediate release (IR) when the 8 hr dose corresponds to the titrated 8 hr IR dose. Swallow whole; do not chew or crush. *Pediatrics:* ≥6 yrs: **(Tab) Initial:** 5mg bid before breakfast and lunch. **Titrate:** Increase gradually by 5-10mg weekly. **Max:** 60mg/day. **(Tab, ER)** May use in place of immediate release (IR) when the 8 hr dose corresponds to the titrated 8 hr IR dose. Swallow whole; do not chew or crush. **(Cap, ER) Initial:** 10-20mg qam. **Titrate:** Adjust weekly by 10mg. **Max:** 60mg qam. **Previous Methylphenidate Use:** May use as qd in place of IR dosed bid or daily dose of methylphenidate-SR. Swallow whole or sprinkle over spoonful of applesauce. Do not crush, chew, or divide. Reduce dose or discontinue if paradoxical aggravation of symptoms occurs. Discontinue if no improvement after appropriate dose adjustment over 1 month.		

Table 18.1: PRESCRIBING INFORMATION FOR PSYCHOACTIVE DRUGS *(cont.)*

NAME	FORM/ STRENGTH	DOSAGE	WARNINGS/PRECAUTIONS & CONTRAINDICATIONS	ADVERSE EFFECTS†
ATTENTION DEFICIT/HYPERACTIVITY DISORDER AGENTS *(cont.)*				
Modafinil^{CIV} (Provigil)	Tab: 100mg, 200mg*	**Adults:** 200mg qd. **Narcolepsy/OSAHS:** Take in am. **SWSD:** Take 1 hr prior to start of work shift. **Hepatic Dysfunction:** 100mg qd. **Elderly:** Consider dose reduction. **Pediatrics:** ≥16 yrs: 200mg qd. **Narcolepsy/OSAHS:** Take in am. **SWSD:** Take 1 hr prior to start of work shift. **Hepatic Dysfunction:** 100mg qd.	**W/P:** Avoid in history of left ventricular hypertrophy, ischemic ECG changes, chest pain, arrhythmia or other manifestations of mitral valve prolapse with CNS stimulants. Caution if recent MI, unstable angina, history of psychosis. Monitor hypertensive patients. **P/N:** Category C, caution in nursing.	Headache, infection, nausea, nervousness, anxiety, insomnia.
SLEEP ADJUNCTS				
BENZODIAZEPINES				
Alprazolam^{CIV} (Niravam, Xanax, Xanax XR)	Tab, Orally Disintegrating: (Niravam) 0.25mg*, 0.5mg*, 1mg*, 2mg*; Tab: (Xanax) 0.25mg*, 0.5mg*, 1mg*, 2mg*; Tab, ER: (Xanax XR) 0.5mg, 1mg, 2mg, 3mg	**Adults:** (Niravam) **Anxiety: Initial:** 0.25-0.5mg tid. **Titrate:** May increase every 3-4 days. **Max:** 4mg/day. **Panic Disorder: Initial:** 0.5mg tid. **Titrate:** Increase by no more than 1mg/day every 3-4 days; slower titration if ≥4mg/day. **Usual:** 1-10mg/day. Decrease dose slowly (no more than 0.5mg every 3 days). **Elderly/Advanced Liver Disease/Debilitated: Initial:** 0.25mg bid-tid. **Titrate:** Increase gradually as tolerated. **(Xanax) Anxiety: Initial:** 0.25-0.5mg tid. **Titrate:** May increase every 3-4 days. **Max:** 4mg/day. **Elderly/Advanced Liver Disease/Debilitated: Initial:** 0.25mg bid-tid. **Titrate:** Increase gradually as tolerated. **Panic Disorder: Initial:** 0.5mg tid. **Titrate:** Increase by no more than 1mg/day every 3-4 days; slower titration if ≥4mg/day. **Usual:** 1-10mg/day. Decrease dose slowly (no more than 0.5mg every 3 days). **(Xanax XR) Initial:** 0.5-1mg qd, preferably in am. **Titrate:** Increase by no more than 1mg/day every 3-4 days. **Maint:** 1-10mg/day. Usual: 3-6mg/day. Decrease dose slowly (no more than 0.5mg every 3 days). **Elderly/Advanced Liver Disease/Debilitated: Initial:** 0.5mg qd.	**W/P:** Risk of dependence. Withdrawal symptoms, including seizures, reported with dose reduction or abrupt discontinuation; avoid abrupt withdrawal. Caution with impaired renal, hepatic, or pulmonary function, severe depression, obesity, elderly, and debilitated. May cause fetal harm. Hypomania/mania reported with depression. Weak uricosuric effect. Periodically reassess usefulness. **Contra:** Acute narrow angle glaucoma, untreated open angle glaucoma, concomitant ketoconazole or itraconazole. **P/N:** Category D, not for use in nursing	Drowsiness, light-headedness, depression, headache, confusion, insomnia, **dry mouth**, constipation, diarrhea, nausea/vomiting, tachycardia/palpitations, blurred vision, nasal congestion, sedation, somnolence, memory impairment, dysarthria, abnormal coordination, fatigue, mental impairment, ataxia, decreased libido, increased/decreased appetite, irritability cognitive disorder, dysarthria, decreased libido, confusional state, hypotension, **increased salivation**.
Diazepam^{CIV} (Valium)	Tab: 2mg*, 5mg*, 10mg*	**Adults: Anxiety:** 2-10mg bid-qid. **Alcohol Withdrawal:** 10mg tid-qid for 24 hours. **Maint:** 5mg tid-qid prn. **Skeletal Muscle Spasm:** 2-10mg tid-qid: **Seizure Disorders:** 2-10mg bid-qid. **Elderly/Debilitated:** 2-2.5mg qd-bid initially; may increase gradually as needed and tolerated. **Pediatrics:** ≥6 months: 1-2.5mg tid-qid initially; may increase gradually as needed and tolerated.	**W/P:** Monitor blood counts and LFTs in long-term use. Neutropenia and jaundice reported. Increase in grand mal seizures reported. Avoid abrupt withdrawal. Caution with kidney or hepatic dysfunction. **Contra:** Acute narrow angle glaucoma, untreated open angle glaucoma, patients <6 months. **P/N:** Not for use during pregnancy, safety in nursing not known.	Drowsiness, fatigue, ataxia, paradoxical reactions, minor EEG changes.
Estazolam^{CIV} (ProSom)	Tab: 1mg*, 2mg*	**Adults: Initial:** 1mg qhs. May increase to 2mg qhs. **Small/Debilitated/Elderly: Initial:** 0.5mg qhs.	**W/P:** Avoid abrupt withdrawal after prolonged use. Caution with depression, elderly/debilitated, renal/hepatic impairment. May cause respiratory depression. **Contra:** Pregnancy. **P/N:** Category X, not for use in nursing.	Somnolence, hypokinesia, dizziness, abnormal coordination, constipation, **dry mouth**, amnesia, paradoxical reactions.

*Scored.   †Bold entries denote special dental considerations.

NAME	FORM/ STRENGTH	DOSAGE	WARNINGS/PRECAUTIONS & CONTRAINDICATIONS	ADVERSE EFFECTS†
Flurazepam HydrochlorideCIV (Dalmane)	**Cap:** 15mg, 30mg	***Adults:* Usual:** 15-30mg at bedtime. **Elderly/Debilitated: Initial:** 15mg at bedtime. ***Pediatrics:* ≥15 yrs: Usual:** 15-30mg at bedtime.	**W/P:** Caution in elderly, debilitated, severely depressed, those with suicidal tendencies, hepatic/renal impairment, respiratory disease. Ataxia and falls reported in elderly and debilitated. Withdrawal symptoms after discontinuation; avoid abrupt discontinuation. **Contra:** Pregnancy. **P/N:** Not for use in pregnancy or nursing.	Confusion, dizziness, drowsiness, lightheadedness, ataxia.
LorazepamCIV (Ativan, Ativan Injection)	**Inj:** 2mg/mL, 4mg/mL; **Tab:** 0.5mg, 1mg*, 2mg*	***Adults:* (Inj) ≥18 yrs: Status Epilepticus:** 4mg IV (given slowly at 2mg/min); may repeat 1 dose after 10-15 minutes if seizures recur or fail to cease. **Preanesthetic Sedation: Usual:** 0.05mg/kg IM; 2mg or 0.044mg/kg IV (whichever is smaller). **Max:** 4mg IM/IV. **(Tab) Initial:** 2-3mg/day given bid-tid. **Usual:** 2-6mg/day in divided doses. **Insomnia:** 2-4mg qhs. **Elderly/Debilitated:** 1-2mg/day in divided doses. ***Pediatrics:* >12 yrs: Initial:** 2-3mg/day given bid-tid. **Usual:** 2-6mg/day in divided doses. **Insomnia:** 2-4mg qhs.	**W/P:** (Inj) Monitor all parameters to maintain vital function. Risk of respiratory depression or airway obstruction in heavily sedated patients. May cause fetal damage during pregnancy. Increased risk of CNS and respiratory depression in elderly. Avoid with hepatic/renal failure. Caution with mild to moderate hepatic/renal disease. Avoid outpatient endoscopic procedures. Possible propylene glycol toxicity in renal impairment. (Tab) Avoid with primary depression or psychosis. Withdrawal symptoms with abrupt discontinuation. Careful supervision if addiction-prone. Caution with elderly, and renal or hepatic dysfunction. Monitor for GI disease with prolonged therapy. Periodic blood counts and LFTs with long-term therapy. **Contra:** Acute narrow-angle glaucoma, sleep apnea syndrome, severe respiratory insufficiency. Not for intra-arterial injection. **P/N:** (Inj) Category D, not for use in nursing. (Tab) Not for use in pregnancy or nursing.	Sedation, dizziness, weakness, unsteadiness, transient amnesia, memory impairment, respiratory depression/ failure, hypotension, somnolence, headache, hypoventilation.
Midazolam HydrochlorideCIV (Versed)	**Inj:** 1mg/mL, 5mg/mL **Syrup:** 2mg/mL	***Adults:* IV: Sedation/Anxiolysis/Amnesia Induction: <60 yrs: Initial:** 1-2.5mg IV over 2 min. **Max:** 5mg. **Titrate:** In small increments at 2 min intervals if needed. **Concomitant Narcotics/Other CNS Depressants:** Reduce by 30%. **≥60 yrs/Debilitated/ Chronically Ill: Initial:** 1-1.5mg IV over 2 min. **Max:** 3.5mg. **Titrate:** In small increments at 2 min intervals if needed. **Concomitant Narcotics/Other CNS Depressants:** Reduce by 50%. **Maint:** 25% of sedation dose by slow titration. **IM: Preoperative Sedation/Anxiolysis/Amnesia: <60 yrs:** 0.07-0.08mg/kg IM up to 1 hr before surgery. **≥60 yrs/Debilitated:** 1-3mg IM. **Anesthesia Induction: Unpremedicated: <55 yrs: Initially:** 0.3-0.35mg/kg IV over 20-30 seconds. May give additional doses of 25% of initial dose to complete induction. **≥55 yrs: Initial:** 0.3mg/kg IV. **Debilitated: Initial:** 0.15-0.25mg/kg IV. **Premedicated: <55 yrs: Initial:** 0.25mg/kg IV over 20-30 seconds. **≥55 yrs: Initial:** 0.2mg/kg IV. **Debilitated: Initial:** 0.15mg/kg IV. **Maintenance Sedation: LD:** 0.01-0.05mg/kg IV. May repeat dose at 10-15 min intervals until adequate sedation. **Maint:** 0.02-0.1mg/kg/hr.	**Associated with respiratory depression and respiratory arrest especially when used for sedation in noncritical care settings. Do not administer by rapid injection to neonates. Continuous monitoring required. W/P:** Agitation, involuntary movements, hyperactivity, and combativeness reported. Caution with CHF, chronic renal failure, pulmonary disease, uncompensated acute illnesses (eg, severe fluid or electrolyte disturbances), elderly or debilitated. Avoid use with shock or coma, or in acute alcohol intoxication with depression of vital signs. Contains benzyl alcohol. **Contra:** Acute narrow-angle glaucoma, untreated open-angle glaucoma, intrathecal or epidural use. **P/N:** Category D, caution in nursing.	Decreased tidal volume and/or respiratory rate, BP/HR variations, apnea, hypotension, pain and local reactions at injection site, **hiccups,** nausea, vomiting, **desaturation.**

Table 18.1: PRESCRIBING INFORMATION FOR PSYCHOACTIVE DRUGS *(cont.)*

NAME	FORM/ STRENGTH	DOSAGE	WARNINGS/PRECAUTIONS & CONTRAINDICATIONS	ADVERSE EFFECTS†
SLEEP ADJUNCTS *(cont.)*				
Midazolam HydrochlorideCIV *(cont.)*		Titrate to desired level of sedation using 25-50% adjustments. Infusion rate should be decreased 10-25% every few hrs to find minimum effective infusion rate. *Pediatrics:* 0.25-1mg/kg single dose. **Max:** 20mg.		
TemazepamCIV (Restoril)	**Cap:** 7.5mg, 15mg, 22.5mg, 30mg	**Adults:** Usual: 7.5-30mg qhs. **Transient Insomnia:** 7.5mg qhs. **Elderly/ Debilitated: Initial:** 7.5mg qhs.	**W/P:** Caution in elderly, debilitated, severely depressed, those with suicidal tendencies, hepati 'renal impairment, pulmonary insufficiency. Avoid abrupt discontinuation. If no improvement after 7-10 days, may indicate primary psychiatric and/or medical condition. **Contra:** Pregnancy. **P/N:** Category X, caution in nursing.	Headache, dizziness, drowsiness, fatigue, nervousness, nausea, lethargy, hangover.
TriazolamCIV (Halcion)	**Tab:** 0.125mg, 0.25mg*	**Adults:** 0.25mg qhs. **Max:** 0.5mg. **Elderly/Debilitated: Initial:** 0.125mg. **Max:** 0.25mg.	**W/P:** Worsening or failure of response after 7-10 days may indicate other medical conditions. Increased daytime anxiety, abnormal thinking and behavioral changes have occurred. May impair mental/physical abilities. Anterograde amnesia reported with therapeutic doses. Caution with baseline depression, suicidal tendencies, history of drug dependence, elderly/debilitated, renal/hepatic impairment, chronic pulmonary insufficiency, and sleep apnea. Withdrawal symptoms after discontinuation; avoid abrupt withdrawal. **Contra:** Pregnancy. With ketoconazole, itraconazole, nefazodone, medications that impair CYP3A. **P/N:** Category X, not for use in nursing.	Drowsiness, dizziness, lightheadedness, headache, nausea, vomiting, coordination disorders, ataxia.
NONBENZODIAZEPINES				
EszopicloneCIV (Lunesta)	**Tab:** 1mg, 2mg, 3mg	**Adults:Initial:** 2mg qhs. **Max:** 3mg qhs. **Elderly: Difficulty Falling Asleep: Initial:** 1mg qhs. **Max:** 2mg qhs. **Difficulty Staying Asleep: Initial/Max:** 2mg qhs. Avoid high-fat meal.	**W/P:** A variety of abnormal thinking and behavior changes have been reported to occur in association with the use of sedative/hypnotics. Some of these changes may be characterized by decreased inhibition, similar to effects produced by alcohol and other CNS depressants. Other reported behavioral changes have included bizarre behavior, agitation, hallucinations, and depersonalization. Amnesia and other neuropsychiatric symptoms may occur unpredictably. In primarily depressed patients, worsening of depression, including suicidal thinking, has been reported in association with the use of sedative/hypnotics. Rapid dose decrease or abrupt discontinuation of use of sedative/hypnotics can result in signs and symptoms similar to those associated with withdrawal from other CNS-depressant drugs. Eszopiclone, like other hypnotics, has CNS-depressant effects and because of rapid onset of action eszopiclone should only be taken immediately prior to going to bed or after the patient has gone to bed and has experienced difficulty falling asleep.	Headache, **unpleasant taste**, somnolence, **dry mouth**, dizziness, infection, rash, chest pain, peripheral edema, migraine.

*Scored.   †Bold entries denote special dental considerations.

NAME	FORM/ STRENGTH	DOSAGE	WARNINGS/PRECAUTIONS & CONTRAINDICATIONS	ADVERSE EFFECTS†
EszopicloneCIV *(cont.)*			Patients should be cautioned against engaging in hazardous occupations requiring complete mental alertness or motor coordination after taking eszopiclone. Eszopiclone should be used with caution in patients with diseases or conditions that could affect metabolism or hemodynamic responses. Reduced dose should be given in patients with severe hepatic impairment or in patients who are taking potent inhibitors of CYP3A4. Eszopiclone should be used with caution in patients exhibiting signs and symptoms of depression, suicidal tendencies may present in such patients and protective measures may be required. **P/N:** Category C, caution in nursing.	
Ramelteon (Rozerem)	**Tab:** 8mg	***Adults:*** 8mg within 30 minutes of bedtime. Do not take with or after high fat meal.	**W/P:** Sleep disturbances may be presenting manifestations of a physical and/or psychiatric disorder, initiate therapy only after careful evaluation. Do not use in severe hepatic impairment. A variety of abnormal thinking and behavior changes have been reported to occur in association with the use of hypnotics. In primarily depressed patients, worsening of depression, including suicidal ideation, has been reported in association with the use of hypnotics. May impair physical/mental abilities. Not recommended in patients with severe sleep apnea or severe COPD. Caution with alcohol. May affect reproductive hormones. **P/N:** Category C, not for use in nursing	Headache, somnolence, fatigue, dizziness, nausea, exacerbated insomnia, upper respiratory tract infection.
ZaleplonCIV (Sonata)	**Cap:** 5mg, 10mg	***Adults:*** **Insomnia:** 10mg qhs. **Low Weight Patients:** Start with 5mg hs. **Max:** 20mg/day. **Elderly/Debilitated/ Concomitant Cimetidine:** 5mg qhs. **Max:** 10mg/day. **Mild to Moderate Hepatic Dysfunction:** 5mg qhs. Take immediately prior to bedtime.	**W/P:** Monitor elderly/debilitated closely. Abnormal thinking and behavioral changes reported. Avoid abrupt withdrawal. Abuse potential exist. Caution in respiratory disorders, depression, conditions affecting metabolism or hemodynamic responses, and mild-to-moderate hepatic insufficiency. Not for use in severe hepatic impairment. May cause impaired coordination even the following day. Re-evaluate if no improvement of insomnia after 7-10 days of therapy. Contains tartrazine. **P/N:** Category C, not for use in nursing.	Headache, asthenia, nausea, dizziness, amnesia, somnolence, eye pain, dysmenorrhea, abdominal pain.
Zolpidem TartrateCIV (Ambien, Ambien-CR)	**Tab: (Ambien)** 5mg, 10mg; **Tab, Extended-Release: (Ambien-CR)** 6.25mg, 12.5mg	***Adults:*** **Tab:** **Usual:** 10mg qhs. **Elderly/ Debilitated/Hepatic Insufficiency: Initial:** 5mg. Decrease dose with other CNS-depressants. **Max:** 10mg qd. Use should be limited to 7-10 days. Revaluate if patient needs to take for more than 2-3 weeks. **(Tab, ER)** 12.5mg qhs. **Elderly/Debilitated/Hepatic Insufficiency:** 6.25mg qhs. Swallow whole; do not divide, crush, or chew.	**W/P:** (Tab) Monitor elderly and debilitated patients for impaired motor performance. Caution with depression and conditions that could affect metabolism or hemodynamic responses. (Tab, ER) Use smallest possible effective dose, especially in the elderly. Abnormal thinking and behavior changes have been reported with the use of sedative/hypnotics. Caution with depression and conditions that could affect metabolism or hemodynamic responses. Signs and symptoms of withdrawal reported with abrupt discontinuation of sedative/hypnotics. Monitor elderly and debilitated patients for impaired motor and/or cognitive performance. **P/N:** (Tab) Category B; not for use in nursing. (Tab, ER) Category C, not for use in nursing.	Drowsiness, dizziness, headache, nausea, drugged feeling, dyspepsia, myalgia, confusion, dependence, somnolence, hallucinations, back pain, fatigue.

Table 18.1: PRESCRIBING INFORMATION FOR PSYCHOACTIVE DRUGS *(cont.)*

NAME	FORM/STRENGTH	DOSAGE	WARNINGS/PRECAUTIONS & CONTRAINDICATIONS	ADVERSE EFFECTS†
OBESITY AGENTS (Centrally Acting)				
Benzphetamine Hydrochloride^{CIII} (Didrex)	**Tab:** 50mg*	*Adults:* **Initial:** 25-50mg qd. **Usual:** 25-50mg qd-tid. *Pediatrics:* ≥12 yrs: **Initial:** 25-50mg qd. **Usual:** 25-50mg qd-tid.	**W/P:** Caution with mild HTN. Discontinue if tolerance develops. Psychological disturbances reported when used with restrictive dietary regimen. **Contra:** Advanced arteriosclerosis, symptomatic cardiovascular disease, moderate to severe HTN, agitated states, hyperthyroidism, glaucoma, history of drug abuse, concomitant CNS stimulants, MAOI use within 14 days, pregnancy. **P/N:** Category X, not for use in nursing.	Palpitations, tachycardia, BP elevation, restlessness, dizziness, insomnia, headache, tremor, sweating, **dry mouth**, nausea, diarrhea, **unpleasant tastes**, urticaria, altered libido.
Diethylpropion Hydrochloride^{CIV} (Tenuate)	**Tab:** (Tenuate) 25mg; **Tab, Extended Release:** (Tenuate Dospan) 75mg	*Adults:* ~~(Tab)~~ 25mg tid 1 hour before meals, and mid-evening if needed for night hunger. **(Tab, ER):** 75mg at qd in mid-morning, swallowed whole. *Pediatrics:* ≥16 yrs: **(Tab)** 25mg tid 1 hour before meals, and mid-evening if needed for night hunger. **(Tab, ER):** 75mg at qd in mid-morning, swallowed whole.	**W/P:** Possible risk of pulmonary hypertension and valvular heart disease. Caution in HTN, symptomatic cardiovascular disease. Avoid with heart murmur, valvular heart disease, severe HTN. May increase convulsions with epilepsy. Prolonged use may induce dependence with withdrawal symptoms. Discontinue if tolerance develops or if insignificant weight loss after 4 weeks of therapy. **Contra:** Advanced arteriosclerosis, hyperthyroidism, glaucoma, pulmonary HTN, severe HTN, within 14 days of MAOI use, agitated states, history of drug abuse, other concomitant anorectics. **P/N:** Category B, caution in nursing.	Palpitations, tachycardia, arrhythmias, blurred vision, dizziness, anxiety, insomnia, depression, urticaria, gynecomastia, nausea, vomiting, GI disturbances, bone marrow depression, impotence.
Phendimetrazine Tartrate^{CIII} (Bontril PDM, Bontril Slow-Release)	**Cap, Extended Release:** (Slow-Release) 105mg; **Tab:** (PDM) 35mg*	*Adults:* **(Slow-Release)** 105mg qam, 30-60 minutes before breakfast. **(PDM)** 35mg bid-tid, 1 hr before meals; may reduce to 17.5mg/dose. **Max:** 70mg tid. *Pediatrics:* ≥12 yrs: **(Slow-Release)** 105mg qam, 30-60 minutes before breakfast. **(PDM)** 35mg bid-tid, 1 hr before meals; may reduce to 17.5mg/dose. **Max:** 70mg tabs tid.	**W/P:** Tolerance to anorectic effect develops within a few weeks, discontinue if this occurs. Fatigue and depression with abrupt withdrawal after prolonged high dose therapy. Caution in mild HTN. **Contra:** Advanced arteriosclerosis, symptomatic cardiovascular disease, moderate and severe HTN, hyperthyroidism, glaucoma, agitated states, history of drug abuse, concomitant CNS stimulants including MAOIs. **P/N:** Not for use in pregnancy, safety in nursing not known.	Palpitation, tachycardia, BP elevation, overstimulation, restlessness, dizziness, **dry mouth**, diarrhea, constipation, nausea, libido changes, dysuria, insomnia.
Phentermine Hydrochloride^{CIV} (Adipex-P)	**Cap:** 37.5mg; **Tab:** 37.5mg*	*Adults:* **Usual:** 37.5mg before breakfast or 1-2 hrs after breakfast. **Alternate Schedule:** 18.75mg qd-bid. Avoid late evening dosing. *Pediatrics:* >16 yrs: **Usual:** 37.5mg before breakfast or 1-2 hrs after breakfast. **Alternate Schedule:** 18.75mg qd-bid. Avoid late evening dosing.	**W/P:** Only for short-term therapy. Primary pulmonary HTN and valvular heart disease reported. Abuse potential. Caution with mild HTN. Tolerance may develop. **Contra:** Advanced arteriosclerosis, cardiovascular disease, moderate to severe HTN, hyperthyroidism, glaucoma, agitated states, history of drug abuse, within 14 days of MAOI use. **P/N:** Category C, not for use in nursing.	Primary pulmonary hypertension, regurgitant valvular heart disease, palpitation, tachycardia, blood pressure elevation, CNS overstimulation, **dry mouth**, impotence, urticaria.
Phentermine Resin^{CIV} (Ionamin)	**Cap:** 15mg, 30mg	*Adults:* 15-30mg before breakfast or 10-14 hrs before bedtime. Swallow caps whole.	**W/P:** Primary pulmonary HTN and valvular heart disease reported. Discontinue if tolerance occurs. Abuse potential. Caution with mild HTN. **Contra:** Advanced arteriosclerosis, CVD, moderate to severe HTN, hyperthyroidism, glaucoma, agitated states, history of drug abuse, within 14 days of MAOI use. **P/N:** Safety in pregnancy and nursing not known.	Primary pulmonary HTN, palpitations, tachycardia, BP elevation, restlessness, dizziness, insomnia, headache, diarrhea, constipation, impotence.

*Scored.   †Bold entries denote special dental considerations.

NAME	FORM/ STRENGTH	DOSAGE	WARNINGS/PRECAUTIONS & CONTRAINDICATIONS	ADVERSE EFFECTS†
Sibutramine Hydrochloride^{CIV} (Meridia)	Cap: 5mg, 10mg, 15mg	*Adults:* Initial: 10mg qd. Titrate: May increase after 4 weeks to 15mg qd. Max: 15mg/day. Use 5mg/day in patients unable to tolerate 10mg/day. May continue for up to 2 yrs. *Pediatrics:* ≥16 yrs: Initial: 10mg qd. Titrate: May increase after 4 weeks to 15mg qd. Use 5mg/day in patients unable to tolerate 10mg/day. Max: 15mg/day. May continue for up to 2 yrs.	W/P: May increase BP and/or pulse. Avoid with uncontrolled or poorly controlled HTN, coronary artery disease, CHF, arrhythmias, stroke, severe hepatic or renal dysfunction. Monitor BP and pulse before therapy and regularly thereafter. Caution with narrow angle glaucoma, mild to moderate renal impairment, seizures and in patients predisposed to bleeding. Exclude organic causes of obesity. Gallstones precipitated with weight loss. Contra: Concomitant MAOIs or centrally acting appetite suppressants, anorexia nervosa. P/N: Category C, not for use in nursing.	Anorexia, constipation, increased appetite, nausea, dyspepsia, dry mouth, insomnia, dizziness, nervousness, HTN, tachycardia, dysmenorrhea, headache.

OBSESSIVE-COMPULSIVE DISORDER AGENTS

NAME	FORM/ STRENGTH	DOSAGE	WARNINGS/PRECAUTIONS & CONTRAINDICATIONS	ADVERSE EFFECTS†
Fluoxetine Hydrochloride (Prozac)	Cap: 10mg, 20mg, 40mg; Sol: 20mg/5mL [120mL]; Tab: 10mg*	*Adults:* MDD: Daily Dosing: Initial: 20mg qam; increase dose if no improvement after several weeks. Doses >20mg/ day, give qam or bid (am and noon). Max: 80mg/day. OCD: Initial: 20mg/day. Maint: 20-60mg/day given qd-bid, am and noon. Max: 80mg/day. Bulimia Nervosa: 60mg q am. Max: 60mg/day. Panic Disorder: Initial: 10mg/day. May increase to 20mg/day after 1 week. May increase further after several weeks if no clinical improvement. Max: 60mg/day. Hepatic Impairment/Elderly: Use lower or less frequent dosage. *Pediatrics:* MDD: ≥8 yrs: Higher Weight Peds: Initial: 10 or 20mg/day. After 1 week at 10mg/day, may increase to 20mg/day. Lower Weight Peds: Initial: 10mg/day. Titrate: May increase to 20mg/day after several weeks if clinical improvement not observed. OCD: ≥7 yrs: Adolescents and Higher Weight Peds: Initial: 10mg/day. Titrate: Increase to 20mg/day after 2 weeks. Consider additional dose increases after several more weeks if clinical improvement not observed. Usual: 20-60mg/day. Lower Weight Peds: Initial: 10mg/day. Titrate: Consider additional dose increases after several weeks if clinical improvement not observed. Usual: 20-30mg/day. Max: 60mg/day.	Antidepressants increased the risk of suicidal thinking and behavior (suicidality) in short-term studies in children and adolescents with major depressive disorder and other psychiatric disorders. Fluoxetine is approved for use in pediatric patients with major depressive disorder and obsessive compulsive disorder. W/P: Discontinue if unexplained allergic reaction occurs. Monitor for symptoms of mania/hypomania. Caution with diseases or conditions that could affect metabolism or hemodynamic responses, diabetes, history of seizures, suicidal tendencies. Altered platelet function, hyponatremia reported. Periodically monitor height and weight in pediatrics. Monitor for clinical worsening and/or suicidality, especially at initiation of therapy or dose changes. Avoid abrupt withdrawal. Monitor for discontinuation symptoms. Caution in third trimester of pregnancy due to risk of serious neonatal complications. Contra: During or within 14 days of MAOI therapy. Thioridazine within 5 weeks of discontinuation. P/N: Category C, not for use in nursing.	Nausea, diarrhea, insomnia, anxiety, nervousness, dizziness, somnolence, tremor, decreased libido, sweating, anorexia, asthenia, dry mouth, dyspepsia, headache.
Fluvoxamine Maleate	Tab: 25mg, 50mg*, 100mg*	*Adults:* Initial: 50mg qhs. Titrate: Increase by 50mg every 4-7 days. Maint: 100-300mg/day. Give bid if total dose >100mg daily. Max: 300mg/day. Elderly/Hepatic Impairment: Modify initial dose and titration. *Pediatrics:* 8-17 yrs: Initial: 25mg qhs. Titrate: Increase by 25mg every 4-7 days. Maint: 50-200mg/day. Max: 8-11 yrs: 200mg/day. Adolescents: 300mg/day. Give bid if total dose >50mg daily.	Antidepressants increased the risk of suicidal thinking and behavior (suicidality) in short-term studies in children and adolescents with major depressive disorder and other psychiatric disorders. Fluvoxamine is not approved for use in pediatric patients except for patients with obsessive compulsive disorder. W/P: Activation of mania/hypomania, SIADH, and hyponatremia reported. Close supervision with high risk suicide patients. Caution with history of seizures, hepatic dysfunction, with conditions altering metabolism or hemodynamic responses. Smoking increases metabolism. Contra: Co-administration of thioridazine, terfenadine, astemizole, cisapride, pimozide, alosetron, tizanidine. P/N: Category C, not for use in nursing.	Headache, asthenia, nausea, diarrhea, vomiting, anorexia, dyspepsia, insomnia, somnolence, nervousness, agitation, dizziness, anxiety, dry mouth, sweating, tremor, abnormal ejaculation.

Table 18.1: PRESCRIBING INFORMATION FOR PSYCHOACTIVE DRUGS (cont.)

NAME	FORM/STRENGTH	DOSAGE	WARNINGS/PRECAUTIONS & CONTRAINDICATIONS	ADVERSE EFFECTS†

OBSESSIVE-COMPULSIVE DISORDER AGENTS (cont.)

NAME	FORM/STRENGTH	DOSAGE	WARNINGS/PRECAUTIONS & CONTRAINDICATIONS	ADVERSE EFFECTS†
Paroxetine Hydrochloride (Paxil)	**Sus:** 10mg/5mL [250mL]; **Tab:** 10mg*, 20mg*, 30mg, 40mg	**Adults:** Give qd, usually in the AM. **Major Depressive Disorder: Initial:** 20mg/day. **Max:** 50mg/day. **Obsessive-Compulsive Disorder: Initial:** 20mg qd. **Usual:** 40mg qd. **Max:** 60mg/day. **Panic Disorder: Initial:** 10mg qd. **Usual:** 40mg/day. **Max:** 60mg/day. **Generalized Anxiety Disorder: Initial:** 20mg/day. **Usual:** 20-50mg/day. **Seasonal Affective Disoder: Initial/Usual:** 20mg/day. **Post-Traumatic Stress Disorder: Initial:** 20mg/day. **Usual:** 20-50mg/day. To titrate, may increase weekly by 10mg/day. **Elderly/Debilitated/Severe Renal/Hepatic Impairment: Initial:** 10mg qd. **Max:** 40mg/day.	**Antidepressants increased the risk of suicidal thinking and behavior (suicidality) in short-term studies in children and adolescents with major depressive disorder and other psychiatric disorders. Paroxetine is not approved for use in pediatric patients. W/P:** Caution with history of mania or seizures, conditions that affect metabolism or hemodynamic responses, narrow angle glaucoma. Discontinue if seizures occur. Altered platelet function, hyponatremia, mydriasis reported. Avoid abrupt withdrawal. Re-evaluate periodically. Monitor for clinical worsening and/or suicidality, especially at initiation of therapy or dose changes. **Contra:** Concomitant MAOIs or thioridazine. **P/N:** Category D, caution in nursing.	Somnolence, insomnia, nausea, asthenia, abnormal ejaculation, **dry mouth**, constipation, dizziness, diarrhea, decreased libido, sweating.
Paroxetine Mesylate (Pexeva)	**Tab:** 10mg, 20mg, 30mg, 40mg	**Adult: Major Depressive Disorder: Initial:** 20mg/day. **Max:** 50mg/day. **Obsessive-Compulsive Disorder: Initial:** 40mg/day. **Max:** 60mg/day. **Panic Disorder: Initial:** 10mg/day. **Titrate:** 10mg/day increments at intervals of at least 1 week. Max: 60mg/day. **Elderly/Debilitated/Severe Renal or Hepatic Impairment: Initial:** 10mg qd. **Max:** 40mg/day.	**Antidepressants increased the risk of suicidal thinking and behavior (suicidality) in short-term studies in children and adolescents with major depressive disorder and other psychiatric disorders. Pexeva is not approved for use in pediatric patients. W/P:** Caution with history of mania or seizures, conditions that affect metabolism or hemodynamic responses, narrow angle glaucoma. Discontinue if seizures occur. Altered platelet function, hyponatremia, mydriasis reported. Avoid abrupt withdrawal. Re-evaluate periodically. Monitor for clinical worsening and/or suicidality, especially at initiation of therapy or dose changes. **P/N:** Category D, caution in nursing.	Asthenia, sweating, nausea, decreased appetite, somnolence, dizziness, insomnia, tremor, nervousness, abnormal ejaculation, **dry mouth**, constipation, decreased libido, impotence.
Sertraline Hydrochloride (Zoloft)	**Sol:** 20mg/mL [60mL]; **Tab:** 25mg*, 50mg*, 100mg*	**Adults: Major Depressive Disorder/Obsessive-Compulsive Disorder:** 50mg qd. **Titrate:** Adjust dose at 1 week intervals. **Max:** 200mg/day. **Panic Disorder/Post-Traumatic Stress Disoder/Seasonal Affective Disorder: Initial:** 25mg qd. **Titrate:** Increase to 50mg qd after 1 week. Adjust dose at 1 week intervals. **Max:** 200mg/day. **Premenstrual Dysphoric Disorder: Initial:** 50mg qd continuous or limited to luteal phase of cycle. **Titrate:** Increase 50mg/cycle if needed up to 150mg/day for continuous or 100mg/day for luteal phase dosing. If 100mg/day is established for luteal phase dosing, a 50mg/day titration step for 3 days should take place at the beginning of each luteal phase dosing period. **Hepatic Impairment:** Use lower or less frequent doses. Dilute solution with 4oz of water, ginger ale, lemon/lime soda, lemonade or orange	**Antidepressants increased the risk of suicidal thinking and behavior (suicidality) in short-term studies in children and adolescents with major depressive disorder and other psychiatric disorders. Sertraline HCl is not approved for use in pediatric patients except for patients with obsessive-compulsive disorder. W/P:** Activation of mania/hypomania reported. Monitor weight loss. Caution with conditions that could affect metabolism or hemodynamic responses, seizure disorder. Dose adjust with liver dysfunction. Altered platelet function and hyponatremia reported. Weak uricosuric effects reported. Caution with latex sensitivity; solution dropper dispenser contains rubber. Monitor for clinical worsening and/or suicidality, especially at initiation of therapy or dose changes. Avoid abrupt withdrawal. Monitor for discontinuation symptoms.	Ejaculation failure, **dry mouth**, increased sweating, somnolence, tremor, anorexia, dizziness, headache, vomiting, diarrhea, dyspepsia, nausea, agitation, insomnia, nervousness, abnormal vision.

*Scored.   †Bold entries denote special dental considerations.

NAME	FORM/ STRENGTH	DOSAGE	WARNINGS/PRECAUTIONS & CONTRAINDICATIONS	ADVERSE EFFECTS†
Sertraline Hydrochloride *(cont.)*		juice. Take immediately after mixing. ***Pediatrics:* Obsessive-Compulsive Disorder: Initial: 6-12 yrs:** 25mg qd. **13-17 yrs:** 50mg qd. **Titrate:** Adjust dose at 1 week intervals. **Max:** 200mg/day. **Hepatic Impairment:** Use lower or less frequent doses. Dilute solution with 4oz of water, ginger ale, lemon/lime soda, lemonade or orange juice. Take immediately after mixing.	**Contra:** Concomitant use with MAOIs or pimozide. Concomitant disulfiram with solution. **P/N:** Category C, caution in nursing.	

Table 18.2: DRUG INTERACTIONS FOR PSYCHOACTIVE DRUGS

ANTIANXIETY AGENTS

BENZODIAZEPINES

Alprazolam[CIV] (Niravam, Xanax, Xanax XR)

Amiodarone	Caution with amiodarone.
Anticonvulsants	Additive CNS depressant effects with anticonvulsants.
Antihistamines	Additive CNS depressant effects with antihistamines.
Azole antifungals	Avoid azole antifungals.
Carbamazepine	Decreased plasma levels with carbamazepine.
Cimetidine	Potentiated by cimetidine.
Contraceptives, oral	Potentiated by oral contraceptives.
Cyclosporine	Caution with cyclosporine.
CYP3A inducers	Decreased levels with CYP3A inducers (eg, carbamazepine).
CYP3A inhibitors	Avoid with potent CYP3A inhibitors (eg, azole antifungals). Caution with other CYP3A inhibitors.
Desipramine	Increases levels of desipramine.
Diltiazem	Caution with diltiazem.
Ergotamine	Caution with ergotamine.
Ethanol	Additive CNS depressant effects with ethanol.
Fluoxetine	Potentiated by fluoxetine.
Fluvoxamine	Potentiated by fluvoxamine.
Grapefruit juice	Caution with grapefruit juice.
Imipramine	Increases levels of imipramine.
Isoniazid	Caution with isoniazid.
Itraconazole	Contraindicated with concomitant itraconazole.
Ketoconazole	Contraindicated with concomitant ketoconazole.
Macrolids	Caution with macrolides.
Nefazodone	Potentiated by nefazodone.
Nicardipine	Caution with nicardipine.
Nifedipine	Caution with nifedipine.
Paroxetine	Caution with paroxetine.
Propoxyphene	Decreased plasma levels with propoxyphene.
Psychotropic agents	Additive CNS depressant effects with psychotropic agents.

ANTIANXIETY AGENTS *(cont.)*

Alprazolam^{CIV} (Niravam, Xanax, Xanax XR) *(cont.)*

Sertraline	Caution with sertraline.

Chlordiazepoxide Hydrochloride^{CIV} (Librium)

Alcohol	Additive effects with alcohol.
CNS depressants	Additive effects with CNS depressants.
Psychotropic agents	Avoid other psychotropic agents.

Clorazepate Dipotassium^{CIV} (Tranxene T-Tab, Tranxene-SD)

Alcohol	Additive CNS depression with alcohol.
Antidepressants	Potentiated by other antidepressants.
Barbiturates	Potentiated by barbiturates.
CNS depressants	Additive CNS depression with CNS depressants.
Hypnotics	Increased sedation with hypnotics.
MAOIs	Potentiated by MAOIs.
Narcotics	Potentiated by narcotics.
Phenothiazines	Potentiated by phenothiazines.

Diazepam^{CIV} (Valium)

Alcohol	Avoid alcohol.
Antidepressants	Other antidepressants may potentiate effects.
Barbiturates	Barbiturates may potentiate effects.
Cimetidine	Delayed clearance with cimetidine.
CNS depressants	Avoid other CNS-depressants.
Flumazenil	Risk of seizure with flumazenil.
MAOIs	MAOIs may potentiate effects.
Narcotics	Narcotics may potentiate effects.
Phenothiazines	Phenothiazines may potentiate effects.

Lorazepam^{CIV} (Ativan)

Alcohol	CNS-depressant effects with alcohol. Diminished tolerance to alcohol.
Barbiturates	CNS-depressant effects with barbiturates.
CNS depressants	Diminished tolerance to other CNS depressants.

Oxazepam^{CIV}

Alcohol	Additive effects with alcohol and other CNS depressants.
CNS depressants	Additive effects with alcohol and other CNS depressants.

Table 18.2: DRUG INTERACTIONS FOR PSYCHOACTIVE DRUGS *(cont.)*

ANTIANXIETY AGENTS *(cont.)*

NONBENZODIAZEPINES

Buspirone Hydrochloride (Buspar)

Alcohol	Avoid alcohol.
Cimetidine	Cimetidine increases plasma levels.
CNS depressants	Withdraw other CNS depressants gradually before therapy.
CYP3A4 inducers	CYP3A4 inducers may increase metabolism of buspirone; may need dose adjustment.
CYP3A4 inhibitors	CYP3A4 inhibitors may increase plasma levels; may need dose adjustment.
Digoxin	May displace digoxin.
Diltiazem	Diltiazem increases plasma levels.
Erythromycin	Erythromycin increases plasma levels.
Food	Presystemic clearance may be decreased with food.
Grapefruit juice	Grapefruit juice increases plasma levels.
Haloperidol	Increases haloperidol levels.
Itraconazole	Itraconazole increases plasma levels.
MAOIs	Avoid MAOIs.
Nefazodone	Nefazodone increases plasma levels. May increase levels of both drugs with nefazodone; decrease dose of buspirone.
Psychotropics	Caution with psychotropics.
Rifampin	Decreased plasma levels and effects with rifampin; may need to adjust buspirone dose.
Trazodone	Elevated liver transaminases reported with trazodone.
Verapamil	Verapamil increases plasma levels.

Fluoxetine Hydrochloride (Prozac, Sarafem)

Alcohol	Avoid alcohol.
Antidepressants	May potentiate other antidepressants.
Antidiabetic	Antidiabetic drugs may need adjustment.
Antipsychotics	May potentiate antipsychotics (eg, haloperidol, clozapine).
Benzodiazepine	May increase benzodiazepine levels.
Carbamazepine	May increase carbamazepine levels.
Clozapine	May increase clozapine levels.
CNS drugs	Caution with CNS drugs.
CYP2D6 metabolized drugs	May potentiate drugs metabolized by CYP2D6.

ANTIANXIETY AGENTS *(cont.)*

Fluoxetine Hydrochloride (Prozac, Sarafem)

Haloperidol	May increase haloperidol levels.
Hemostasis-interfering drugs	Caution with drugs that interfere with hemostasis (eg, nonselective NSAIDs, aspirin, warfarin) due to increased risk of bleeding.
Lithium	Lithium levels may increase/decrease; monitor lithium levels.
MAOIs	Do not use with or within 14 days of MAOIs.
Phenytoin	May increase phenytoin levels.
Plasma-bound drugs	May shift concentrations with plasma-bound drugs (eg, coumadin, digitoxin).
Thioridazine	May increase thioridazine levels.
Tricyclic antidepressants	May increase TCAs levels.
Tryptophan	Increased adverse effects with tryptophan.
Warfarin	May alter warfarin effects.

Hydroxyzine Hydrochloride (Atarax)

Alcohol	May increase alcohol effects.
CNS depressants	Potentiates CNS depression with other CNS depressants (eg, narcotics, non-narcotic analgesics, barbiturates, alcohol).

Hydroxyzine Pamoate (Vistaril)

CNS depressants	Potentiated by CNS depressants (eg, narcotics, non-narcotic analgesics, barbiturates); reduce dose.

Paroxetine Hydrochloride (Paxil, Paxil CR)

Alcohol	Avoid alcohol.
Anticoagulants, oral	Increased risk of bleeding with oral anticoagulants.
Aspirin	Increased risk of bleeding with aspirin.
Atomoxetine	May increase levels of atomoxetine; dosage adjustment of atomoxetine may be necessary and initiate atomoxetine at reduced dose.
Cimetidine	Caution with cimetidine.
CYP2D6 inhibitors	Caution with drugs that inhibit CYP2D6 (eg, quinidine).
CYP2D6 metabolized drugs	Caution with drugs metabolized by CYP2D6 (eg, antidepressants, phenothiazines, Type 1C antiarrhythmics).
Digoxin	Caution with digoxin.
Diuretics	Caution with diuretics.

Table 18.2: DRUG INTERACTIONS FOR PSYCHOACTIVE DRUGS *(cont.)*

ANTIANXIETY AGENTS *(cont.)*

Paroxetine Hydrochloride (Paxil, Paxil CR) *(cont.)*

Lithium	Caution with lithium.
NSAIDs	Increased risk of bleeding with NSAIDs.
Phenobarbital	Caution with phenobarbital.
Phenytoin	Caution with phenytoin.
Plasma-bound drugs	May shift concentrations with plasma-bound drugs.
Procyclidine	Reduce procyclidine dose if anticholinergic effects occur.
Risperidone	May increase levels of risperidone.
Sumatriptan	Rare reports of weakness, hyperreflexia, incoordination with an SSRI and sumatriptan.
Theophylline	Monitor theophylline.
Tricyclic antidepressants	May inhibit metabolism of TCAs. Caution with TCAs.
Tryptophan	Avoid tryptophan.
Warfarin	Caution with warfarin.

Paroxetine Mesylate (Pexeva)

Alcohol	Avoid alcohol.
Anticoagulants, oral	Increased risk of bleeding with oral anticoagulants.
Aspirin	Increased risk of bleeding with aspirin.
Cimetidine	Caution with cimetidine.
CYP2D6 metabolized drugs	Caution with drugs metabolized by CYP2D6 (eg, antidepressants, phenothiazines, Type 1C antiarrhythmics).
Digoxin	Caution with digoxin.
Diuretics	Caution with diuretics.
Lithium	Caution with lithium.
MAOI therapy	Avoid within 14 days of MAOI therapy.
NSAIDs	Increased risk of bleeding with NSAIDs.
Phenobarbital	Caution with phenobarbital.
Phenytoin	Caution with phenytoin.
Plasma-bound drugs	May shift concentrations with plasma-bound drugs.
Procyclidine	Reduce procyclidine dose if anticholinergic effects occur.

ANTIANXIETY AGENTS *(cont.)*

Paroxetine Mesylate (Pexeva) *(cont.)*

Quinidine	Caution with quinidine.
Sumatriptan	Rare reports of weakness, hyperreflexia, incoordination with an SSRI and sumatriptan.
Theophylline	Monitor theophylline.
Thioridazine	Avoid thioridazine.
Tricyclic antidepressants	May inhibit metabolism of TCAs.
Tryptophan	Avoid tryptophan.
Warfarin	Caution with warfarin.

Sertraline Hydrochloride (Zoloft)

Alcohol	Avoid with alcohol.
Cimetidine	Increased levels with cimetidine.
Cisapride	May induce metabolism of cisapride.
CNS drugs	Caution with CNS drugs (eg, diazepam).
CYP2D6 metabolized drugs	May potentiate drugs metabolized by CYP2D6 (eg, TCAs, Type 1C antiarrhythmics).
Hemostasis-interfering drugs	Caution with drugs that interfere with hemostasis (eg, nonselective NSAIDs, aspirin, warfarin) due to increased risk of bleeding.
Lithium	Monitor lithium.
MAOIs	Avoid with MAOIs.
OTC products	Caution with OTC products.
Pimozide	Avoid with pimozide.
Plasma protein-bound-drugs	May shift concentrations with plasma protein-bound drugs (eg, warfarin, digitoxin).
Sumatriptan	Rare reports of weakness, hyperreflexia, incoordination with an SSRI and sumatriptan.
Tolbutamide	Decreases clearance of tolbutamide.
Tricyclic antidepressants	Caution with TCAs; may need dose adjustment.
Warfarin	Monitor PT with warfarin.

Venlafaxine Hydrochloride (Effexor, Effexor-XR)

Alcohol	Avoid alcohol.
Cimetidine	Caution with cimetidine in elderly, HTN, hepatic dysfunction
CNS-active drugs	Caution with CNS-active drugs (eg, triptans, SSRIs, lithium).

Table 18.2: DRUG INTERACTIONS FOR PSYCHOACTIVE DRUGS *(cont.)*

ANTIANXIETY AGENTS *(cont.)*

Venlafaxine Hydrochloride (Effexor, Effexor-XR) *(cont.)*

CYP2D6 inhibitors, potent	Caution with potent inhibitors of CYP2D6.
CYP3A4 inhibitors, potent	Caution with potent inhibitors of CYP3A4.
Desipramine	Increases desipramine plasma levels.
Diuretics	Caution with diuretics.
Haloperidol	Decreases clearance of haloperidol.
Indinavir	Decreases indinavir plasma levels.
MAOI therapy	Avoid within 14 days of MAOI therapy. Upon discontinuation, wait at least 7 days before starting MAOI therapy.
Risperidone	Increases risperidone plasma levels.

ANTIDEPRESSANTS

Monoamine Oxidase Inhibitors

Phenelzine Sulfate (Nardil)

Anesthesia	Avoid general/local/spinal anesthesia.
Antidepressant	Allow 10 days between starting another antidepressant.
Antihypertensives	Exaggerated hypotensive effects with antihypertensives.
Barbiturates	Reduce dose of barbiturates.
Bupropion	Allow 2 weeks after discontinuing therapy before starting bupropion.
Buspirone	Allow 10 days before starting buspirone.
Cocaine	Avoid cocaine.
Fluoxetine	Allow 5 weeks after discontinuing fluoxetine before starting therapy.
MAOIs	Hypertensive crisis with other MAOIs. Allow 10 days between starting another MAOI.
Meperidine	Excitation, seizures, delirium, hyperpyrexia, circulatory collapse, coma, and death have been reported with meperidine.
Rauwolfia alkaloids	Caution with rauwolfia alkaloids.
Serotoninergic agents	Serious reactions reported with serotoninergic agents.
Sympathomimetics	Hypertensive crisis with sympathomimetics.

ANTIDEPRESSANTS *(cont.)*

Phenelzine Sulfate (Nardil) *(cont.)*

Tyramine-containing foods	Hypertensive crisis with high tyramine-containing foods.

Tranylcypromine Sulfate (Parnate)

Disulfiram	Caution with disulfiram.
Metrizamide	Avoid metrizamide; discontinue 48hrs before myelography and may resume 24hrs post-procedure.
Phenothiazines	Additive hypotensive effects with phenothiazines.
Tryptophan	Tryptophan may precipitate disorientation, memory impairment and other neurological and behavioral signs.

Selective Serotonin Reuptake Inhibitors

Citalopram Hydrobromide (Celexa)

Alcohol	Avoid alcohol.
Aspirin	Increased risk of bleeding with aspirin.
Carbamazepine	Caution with carbamazepine.
Cimetidine	Caution with cimetidine.
CNS drugs	Caution with other CNS drugs.
CYP2C19 inhibitors, potent	Clearance may be decreased with potent CYP2C19 (eg, omeprazole) inhibitors.
CYP3A4 inhibitors, potent	Clearance may be decreased with potent CYP3A4 (eg, ketoconazole, itraconazole, fluconazole, erythromycin) inhibitors.
Lithium	Caution with lithium.
Metoprolol	May increase metoprolol levels which leads to decreased cardioselectivity.
NSAIDs	Increased risk of bleeding with NSAIDs.
Sumatriptan	Rare reports of weakness, hyperreflexia, incoordination with an SSRI and sumatriptan.
Tricyclic antidepressants	Caution with TCAs.
Warfarin	Increased risk of bleeding with warfarin.

Escitalopram Oxalate (Lexapro)

Alcohol	Avoid alcohol within 14 days of MAOI therapy.
Aspirin	Increased risk of bleeding with aspirin.
Carbamazepine	Caution with carbamazepine.

Table 18.2: DRUG INTERACTIONS FOR PSYCHOACTIVE DRUGS *(cont.)*

ANTIDEPRESSANTS *(cont.)*

Escitalopram Oxalate (Lexapro) *(cont.)*

Cimetidine	Caution with cimetidine.
Citalopram	Avoid citalopram within 14 days of MAOI therapy.
CNS drugs	Caution with other CNS drugs.
CYP2D6 metabolized drugs	Avoid drugs metabolized by CYP2D6 (eg, desipramine).
Linezolid	Serotonin syndrome reported with linezolid.
Lithium	Caution with lithium.
Metoprolol	May increase metoprolol levels which leads to decreased cardioselectivity.
NSAIDs	Increased risk of bleeding with NSAIDs.
Sumatriptan	Rare reports of weakness, hyperreflexia, incoordination with an SSRI and sumatriptan.
Warfarin	Increased risk of bleeding with warfarin.

Fluoxetine Hydrochloride (Prozac, Sarafem)

Alcohol	Avoid alcohol.
Antidepressants	May potentiate other antidepressants.
Antidiabetic	Antidiabetic drugs may need adjustment.
Antipsychotics	May potentiate antipsychotics (eg, haloperidol, clozapine).
Benzodiazepine	May increase benzodiazepine levels.
Carbamazepine	May increase carbamazepine levels.
Clozapine	May increase clozapine levels.
CNS drugs	Caution with CNS drugs.
CYP2D6 metabolized drugs	May potentiate drugs metabolized by CYP2D6.
Haloperidol	May increase haloperidol levels.
Hemostasis-interfering drugs	Caution with drugs that interfere with hemostasis (eg, nonselective NSAIDs, aspirin, warfarin) due to increased risk of bleeding.
Lithium	Lithium levels may increase/decrease; monitor lithium levels.
MAOIs	Do not use with or within 14 days of MAOIs.
Phenytoin	May increase phenytoin levels.
Plasma-bound drugs	May shift concentrations with plasma-bound drugs (eg, coumadin, digitoxin).
Thioridazine	May increase thioridazine levels.
Tricyclic antidepressants	May increase TCAs levels.

ANTIDEPRESSANTS *(cont.)*

Fluoxetine Hydrochloride (Prozac, Sarafem) *(cont.)*

Tryptophan	Increased adverse effects with tryptophan.
Warfarin	May alter warfarin effects.

Paroxetine Hydrochloride (Paxil, Paxil CR)

Alcohol	Avoid alcohol.
Anticoagulants, oral	Increased risk of bleeding with oral anticoagulants.
Aspirin	Increased risk of bleeding with aspirin.
Atomoxetine	May increase levels of atomoxetine; dosage adjustment of atomoxetine may be necessary and initiate atomoxetine at reduced dose.
Cimetidine	Caution with cimetidine.
CYP2D6 inhibitors	Caution with drugs that inhibit CYP2D6 (eg, quinidine).
CYP2D6 metabolized drugs	Caution with drugs metabolized by CYP2D6 (eg, antidepressants, phenothiazines, Type 1C antiarrhythmics).
Digoxin	Caution with digoxin.
Diuretics	Caution with diuretics.
Lithium	Caution with lithium.
NSAIDs	Increased risk of bleeding with NSAIDs.
Phenobarbital	Caution with phenobarbital.
Phenytoin	Caution with phenytoin.
Plasma-bound drugs	May shift concentrations with plasma-bound drugs.
Procyclidine	Reduce procyclidine dose if anticholinergic effects occur.
Risperidone	May increase levels of risperidone.
Sumatriptan	Rare reports of weakness, hyperreflexia, incoordination with an SSRI and sumatriptan.
Theophylline	Monitor theophylline.
Tricyclic antidepressants	May inhibit metabolism of TCAs. Caution with TCAs.
Tryptophan	Avoid tryptophan.
Warfarin	Caution with warfarin.

Paroxetine Mesylate (Pexeva)

Alcohol	Avoid alcohol.
Anticoagulants, oral	Increased risk of bleeding with oral anticoagulants.

Table 18.2: DRUG INTERACTIONS FOR PSYCHOACTIVE DRUGS (cont.)

ANTIDEPRESSANTS (cont.)

Paroxetine Mesylate (Pexeva) (cont.)

Aspirin	Increased risk of bleeding with aspirin.
Cimetidine	Caution with cimetidine.
CYP2D6 metabolized drugs	Caution with drugs metabolized by CYP2D6 (eg, antidepressants, phenothiazines, Type 1C antiarrhythmics).
Digoxin	Caution with digoxin.
Diuretics	Caution with diuretics.
Lithium	Caution with lithium.
MAOI therapy	Avoid within 14 days of MAOI therapy.
NSAIDs	Increased risk of bleeding with NSAIDs.
Phenobarbital	Caution with phenobarbital.
Phenytoin	Caution with phenytoin.
Plasma-bound drugs	May shift concentrations with plasma-bound drugs.
Procyclidine	Reduce procyclidine dose if anticholinergic effects occur.
Quinidine	Caution with quinidine.
Sumatriptan	Rare reports of weakness, hyperreflexia, incoordination with an SSRI and sumatriptan.
Theophylline	Monitor theophylline.
Thioridazine	Avoid thioridazine.
Tricyclic antidepressants	May inhibit metabolism of TCAs.
Tryptophan	Avoid tryptophan.
Warfarin	Caution with warfarin.

Sertraline Hydrochloride (Zoloft)

Alcohol	Avoid with alcohol.
Cimetidine	Increased levels with cimetidine.
Cisapride	May induce metabolism of cisapride.
CNS drugs	Caution with CNS drugs (eg, diazepam).
CYP2D6 metabolized drugs	May potentiate drugs metabolized by CYP2D6 (eg, tricyclic antidepressants, Type 1C antiarrhythmics).
Hemostasis-interfering drugs	Caution with drugs that interfere with hemostasis (eg, nonselective NSAIDs, aspirin, warfarin) due to increased risk of bleeding.
Lithium	Monitor lithium.

ANTIDEPRESSANTS *(cont.)*

Sertraline Hydrochloride (Zoloft) *(cont.)*

MAOIs	Avoid with MAOIs.
OTC products	Caution with OTC products.
Pimozide	Avoid with pimozide.
Plasma protein-bound drugs	May shift concentrations with plasma protein-bound drugs (eg, warfarin, digitoxin).
Sumatriptan	Rare reports of weakness, hyperreflexia, incoordination with an SSRI and sumatriptan.
Tolbutamide	Decreases clearance of tolbutamide.
Tricyclic antidepressants	Caution with TCAs; may need dose adjustment.
Warfarin	Monitor PT with warfarin.

SEROTONIN/NOREPINEPHRINE REUPTAKE INHIBITORS

Duloxetine Hydrochloride (Cymbalta)

Alcohol	Avoid substantial alcohol use.
CNS-active drugs	Caution with CNS-active drugs.
CYP1A2 inhibitors	Avoid CYP1A2 inhibitors (eg, fluvoxamine, some quinolone antibiotics).
CYP2D6 inhibitors	Increased levels with potent CYP2D6 inhibitors (eg, paroxetine, fluoxetine, quinidine).
CYP2D6 metabolized drugs	Caution with drugs metabolized by CYP2D6 having a narrow therapeutic index (eg, tricyclic antidepressants, phenothiazines, Type 1C antiarrhythmics).
Gastric acidity, drugs affecting	Potential for interaction with drugs that affect gastric acidity.
MAOI therapy	Avoid within 14 days of MAOI therapy. Upon discontinuation, wait at least 5 days before starting MAOI therapy.
Protein-bound drugs (highly)	May increase free concentration levels of highly protein-bound drugs.
Thioridazine	Avoid thioridazine.

Nefazodone Hydrochloride

Alcohol	Avoid alcohol.
Astemizole	Avoid astemizole.
Buspirone	May increase buspirone levels; decrease buspirone dose to 2.5mg qd.
Carbamazepine	Effects antagonized by carbamazepine.
Cisapride	Avoid cisapride.
CNS-active drugs	Caution with CNS-active drugs.
Cyclosporine	Increases plasma levels of cyclosporine.

Table 18.2: DRUG INTERACTIONS FOR PSYCHOACTIVE DRUGS *(cont.)*

ANTIDEPRESSANTS *(cont.)*

Nefazodone Hydrochloride *(cont.)*

CYP3A4 metabolized drugs	Caution with drugs metabolized by CYP3A4.
Digoxin	Monitor digoxin.
Epinephrine	Administer no more than 40µg epinephrine in local anesthetic solutions (two cartridges of 2% liodocaine with 1:100,000 epinephrine or its equivalent) within short period with careful aspiration technique; additional anesthetic with vasoconstrictor may be given if vital signs are acceptable.
Fluoxetine	Institute a wash-out period and lower doses if used after fluoxetine therapy.
General anesthesia	Discontinue prior to general anesthesia.
Haloperidol	Haloperidol may need dose adjustment.
Lovastatin	Rhabdomyolysis (rare) reported with lovastatin.
MAOIs	Avoid MAOIs within 14 days of use.
Pimozide	Avoid pimozide.
Protein-bound drugs (highly)	Caution with highly protein bound drugs.
Simvastatin	Rhabdomyolysis (rare) reported with simvastatin.
Tacrolimus	Increases plasma levels of tacrolimus.
Terfenadine	Avoid terfenadine.
Triazolam	Reduce triazolam dose by 75% and avoid in elderly.

Venlafaxine Hydrochloride (Effexor, Effexor-XR)

Alcohol	Avoid alcohol.
Cimetidine	Caution with cimetidine in elderly, HTN, hepatic dysfunction.
CNS-active drugs	Caution with CNS-active drugs (eg, triptans, SSRIs, lithium).
CYP2D6 inhibitors, potent	Caution with potent inhibitors of CYP2D6.
CYP3A4 inhibitors, potent	Caution with potent inhibitors of CYP3A4.
Desipramine	Increases desipramine plasma levels.
Diuretics	Caution with diuretics.
Epinephrine	Administer no more than 40µg epinephrine in local anesthetic solutions (two cartridges of 2% liodocaine with 1:100,000 epinephrine or its equivalent) within short period with careful aspiration technique; additional anesthetic with vasoconstrictor may be given if vital signs are acceptable.
Haloperidol	Decreases clearance of haloperidol.

ANTIDEPRESSANTS *(cont.)*

Venlafaxine Hydrochloride (Effexor, Effexor-XR) *(cont.)*

Indinavir	Decreases indinavir plasma levels.
MAOI therapy	Avoid within 14 days of MAOI therapy. Upon discontinuation, wait at least 7 days before starting MAOI therapy.
Risperidone	Increases risperidone plasma levels.

TETRACYCLIC AGENTS

Maprotiline Hydrochloride

Cisapride	Use with cisapride can cause cardiotoxicity (QT prolongation, torsades de pointes, cardiac arrest).
Epinephrine	Administer no more than 40µg epinephrine in local anesthetic solutions (two cartridges of 2% liodocaine with 1:100,000 epinephrine or its equivalent) within short period with careful aspiration technique; additional anesthetic with vasoconstrictor may be given if vital signs are acceptable.
Fluvoxamine	Increased risk of maprotiline toxicity (dry mouth, urinary retention, sedation).
MAOIs	Concurrent use with monoamine oxidase inhibitors is contraindicated.

Mirtazapine (Remeron, Remeron Soltab)

Alcohol	Alcohol increases cognitive and motor skill impairment.
Diazepam	Diazepam increase cognitive and motor skill impairment.
Epinephrine	Administer no more than 40µg epinephrine in local anesthetic solutions (two cartridges of 2% liodocaine with 1:100,000 epinephrine or its equivalent) within short period with careful aspiration technique; additional anesthetic with vasoconstrictor may be given if vital signs are acceptable.
MAOIs	Avoid MAOIs within 14 days of use.

TRICYCLIC AGENTS

Amitriptyline Hydrochloride (Elavil)

Alcohol	Potentiates alcohol.
Anticholinergics	Paralytic ileus and hyperpyrexia with anticholinergics.
Barbiturates	Potentiates barbiturates.
CNS depressants	Potentiates other CNS depressants.
CYP2D6 inhibitors	Increased levels with CYP2D6 inhibitors (eg, quinidine, cimetidine, SSRIs).
Disulfiram	Delirium reported with disulfiram.
Enzyme substrates	Increased levels with enzyme substrates (eg, phenothiazines, propafenone, flecainide).
Epinephrine	Administer no more than 40µg epinephrine in local anesthetic solutions (two cartridges of 2% liodocaine with 1:100,000 epinephrine or its equivalent) within short period with careful aspiration technique; additional anesthetic with vasoconstrictor may be given if vital signs are acceptable.

Table 18.2: DRUG INTERACTIONS FOR PSYCHOACTIVE DRUGS *(cont.)*

ANTIDEPRESSANTS *(cont.)*

Amitriptyline Hydrochloride (Elavil) *(cont.)*

Ethchlorvynol	Delirium reported with ethchlorvynol.
Fluoxetine	Avoid within 5 weeks of fluoxetine use.
Guanethidine	May block antihypertensive effects of guanethidine.
Neuroleptics	Monitor with neuroleptics.
Sympathomimet-ics	Monitor with sympathomimetics.
Thyroid drugs	Caution with thyroid drugs.

Amitriptyline Hydrochloride/Chlordiazepoxide (Limbitrol, Limbitrol DS)

Alcohol	Additive sedative effects with alcohol.
Anticholinergics	Severe constipation with anticholinergics.
Antihypertensives	May antagonize antihypertensives (eg, guanethidine).
CNS depressants	Additive sedative effects with CNS depressants.
CYP2D6 inhibitors	Increased levels with CYP2D6 inhibitors (eg, quinidine, cimetidine, SSRIs).
Enzyme substrates	Increased levels with enzyme substrates (eg, phenothiazines, propafenone, flecainide).
Fluoxetine	Avoid within 5 weeks of fluoxetine use.
Psychotropics	Additive effects may occur with psychotropics.
Thyroid drugs	Caution with thyroid agents.

Amoxapine

Alcohol	Additive effects with alcohol.
Antidepressants	Increased levels in other antidepressants.
Barbiturates	Additive effects with barbiturates.
Cimetidine	Increased levels in cimetidine.
CNS depressants	Additive effects with other CNS depressants.
CYP2D6, poor metabolizers	Increased levels in poor metabolizers of CYP2D6.
Flecainide	Increased levels in flecainide.
MAOIs	Avoid MAOIs (during or within 14 days of therapy).
Phenothiazines	Increased levels in phenothiazines.
Propafenone	Increased levels in propafenone.
Quinidine	Increased levels in quinidine.
Selective serotonin reuptake inhibitors	Caution with SSRIs.

ANTIDEPRESSANTS *(cont.)*

Clomipramine Hydrochloride (Anafranil)

Alcohol	Additive effects with alcohol.
Anticholinergics	Caution with anticholinergics.
Barbiturates	Additive effects with barbiturates.
Clonidine	Blocks effects of clonidine.
CNS depressants	Additive effects with CNS depressants.
CNS drugs	Caution with CNS drugs.
CYP2D6 inhibitors	Increased levels with CYP2D6 inhibitors (eg, quinidine, cimetidine, SSRIs).
Enzyme inducers	Decreased levels with enzyme inducers (eg, barbiturates, phenytoin).
Enzyme substrates	Increased levels with enzyme substrates (eg, phenothiazines, propafenone, flecainide).
Fluoxetine	At least 5 weeks must elapse before starting tricyclic antidepressants therapy after fluoxetine discontinuation.
Guanethidine	Blocks effects of guanethidine.
Haloperidol	Increased levels with haloperidol.
Protein bound drugs (highly)	Increased levels with highly protein bound drugs. Increases highly protein bound drugs (eg, warfarin, digoxin) plasma levels.
Methyphenidate	Increased levels with methyphenidate.
Neuroleptics	NMS reported with neuroleptics.
Phenobarbital	Increases phenobarbital plasma levels.
Sympathomimet-ics	Caution with sympathomimetics.
Thyroid drugs	Caution with thyroid drugs.

Doxepin Hydrochloride (Sinequan)

Alcohol	Increased danger of overdose with alcohol.
Anticholinergics	Increased side effects with anticholinergics.
CYP2D6 inhibitors	Potentiated by inhibitors (eg, cimetidine, quinidine, SSRIs) of CYP2D6.
CYP2D6 substrates	Potentiated by substrates (other antidepressants, phenothiazines, propafenone, flecainide) of CYP2D6.
CYP2D6 metabolized drugs	Caution with drugs metabolized by CYP2D6.
MAOI therapy	Avoid within 2 weeks of MAOI therapy.
Selective serotonin reuptake inhibitors	Caution when switching from tricyclic antidepressants to SSRIs ($\geq$5 weeks may be needed before initiating tricyclic antidepressant treatment after withdrawal from fluoxetine).
Tolazamide	Hypoglycemia reported with tolazamide.

Table 18.2: DRUG INTERACTIONS FOR PSYCHOACTIVE DRUGS (cont.)

ANTIDEPRESSANTS (cont.)

Imipramine Hydrochloride (Tofranil)

Alcohol	Additive effects with alcohol.
Anticholinergics	Additive effects with anticholinergics. Paralytic ileus with anticholinergics.
Blood pressure lowering drugs	Caution with drugs that lower BP.
Clonidine	Blocks effects of clonidine.
CNS depressants	Additive effects with CNS depressants.
CYP2D6 inhibitors	Increased levels with CYP2D6 inhibitors (eg, quinidine, cimetidine, SSRIs).
Enzyme inducers	Decreased levels with enzyme inducers (eg, barbiturates, phenytoin).
Enzyme substrates	Increased levels with enzyme substrates (eg, phenothiazines, other antidepressants, propafenone, flecainide).
Guanethidine	Blocks effects of guanethidine.
Methyphenidate	Increased levels with methyphenidate.
Selective serotonin reuptake inhibitors	Wait 5 weeks after discontinuing SSRIs before initiating tricyclic antidepressants.
Sympathomimetic amines	Avoid preparations that contain a sympathomimetic amine (eg, epinephrine, norepinephrine); may potentiate catecholamine effect.
Thyroid drugs	Caution with thyroid drugs.

Imipramine Pamoate (Tofranil-PM)

Alcohol	Additive effects with alcohol.
Anticholinergics	Additive effects with anticholinergics. Paralytic ileus with anticholinergics.
Blood pressure lowering drugs	Caution with drugs that lower BP.
Clonidine	Blocks effects of clonidine.
CNS depressants	Additive effects with CNS depressants.
CYP2D6 inhibitors	Increased levels with CYP2D6 inhibitors (eg, quinidine, cimetidine, SSRIs).
Enzyme inducers	Decreased levels with enzyme inducers (eg, barbiturates, phenytoin).
Enzyme substrates	Increased levels with enzyme substrates (eg, phenothiazines, other antidepressants, propafenone, flecainide).
Guanethidine	Blocks effects of guanethidine.
Methyphenidate	Increased levels with methyphenidate.
Selective serotonin reuptake inhibitors	Wait 5 weeks after discontinuing SSRIs before initiating TCAs.

ANTIDEPRESSANTS *(cont.)*

Imipramine Pamoate (Tofranil-PM) *(cont.)*

Sympathomimetic amines	Avoid preparations that contain a sympathomimetic amine (eg, epinephrine, norepinephrine); may potentiate catecholamine effect.
Thyroid drugs	Caution with thyroid drugs.

Nortriptyline Hydrochloride (Pamelor)

Alcohol	Alcohol may potentiate effects.
Anticholinergics	Monitor with anticholinergic drugs.
Antidepressants	Antidepressants may potentiate effects.
Chlorpropamide	Hypoglycemia reported with chlorpropamide.
Cimetidine	Increased plasma levels with cimetidine.
CYP2D6 inhibitors	CYP2D6 inhibitors (eg, quinidine) may potentiate effects.
Fecainide	Flecainide may potentiate effects.
Guanethidine	May block guanethidine effects.
Phenothiazines	Phenothiazines may potentiate effects.
Propafenone	Propafenone may potentiate effects.
Quinidine	Decreased clearance with quinidine.
Selective serotonin reuptake inhibitors	Tricyclic antidepressants may potentiate effects.
Sympathomimetics	Monitor with sympathomimetic drugs.
Thyroid agents	Arrhythmia risk with thyroid agents.

Protriptyline Hydrochloride (Vivactil)

Alcohol	Enhanced response to alcohol.
Anticholinergics	Risk of hyperpyrexia with anticholinergics.
Barbiturates	Enhanced response to barbiturates.
Cimetidine	Reduced hepatic metabolism with cimetidine.
CNS depressants	Enhanced response to other CNS depressants.
CYP2D6 enzyme inhibitors	Use with CYP2D6 enzyme inhibitors (eg, quinidine, cimetidine, other antidepressants, phenothiazines, propafenone, flecainide, SSRIs) require lower doses for either tricyclic antidepressants or other drugs.
Guanethidine (or similarly acting compounds)	May block antihypertensive effect of guanethidine, or similarly acting compounds.

Table 18.2: DRUG INTERACTIONS FOR PSYCHOACTIVE DRUGS *(cont.)*

ANTIDEPRESSANTS *(cont.)*

Protriptyline Hydrochloride (Vivactil) *(cont.)*

MAOIs	Hyperpyretic crises, severe convulsions, and deaths reported with MAOIs.
Neuroleptics	Risk of hyperpyrexia with neuroleptics.
Tramadol	Enhanced seizure risk with tramadol.

Trimipramine Maleate (Surmontil)

Alcohol	Alcohol may exaggerate effects.
Anticholinergics	May potentiate anticholinergic effects.
Catecholamine	May potentiate catecholamine.
Cimetidine	Cimetidine inhibits elimination.
CYP2D6 inhibitors	Potentiated by CYP2D6 inhibitors (eg, quinidine).
CYP2D6 substrates	Potentiated by CYP2D6 substrates (eg, other antidepressants, phenothiazines, propafenone, fleccainide).
MAOIs	Avoid MAOIs.
Selective serotonin reuptake inhibitors	Caution with SSRIs; wait 5 weeks after fluoxetine withdrawal before initiating therapy.

MISCELLANEOUS

Bupropion Hydrochloride (Wellbutrin, Wellbutrin SR, Wellbutrin XL, Zyban)

Alcohol	Increased seizure risk with excessive use or abrupt discontinuation of alcohol. Minimize or avoid alcohol.
Amantadine	Caution with amantadine; use low initial dose and gradually titrate.
Bupropion-containing drugs	Avoid other bupropion-containing drugs.
Carbamazepine	Carbamazepine may induce metabolism of bupropion.
Cimetidine	Cimetidine may induce metabolism of bupropion.
Cocaine	Increased seizure risk with cocaine addiction.
CYP2B6 inhibitors	Caution with CYP2B6 inhibitors (eg, orphenadrine, cyclophosphamide, thiotepa).
CYP2B6 substrates	Caution with CYP2B6 substrates.
CYP2D6 metabolized drugs	Caution with drugs that are metabolized by CYP2D6 (eg, SSRIs, tricyclic antidepressants, antipsychotics, beta-blockers, type 1C antiarrhythmics); use low initial dose and gradually titrate.
Hypoglycemics, oral	Increased seizure risk with oral hypoglycemics.
Insulin	Increased seizure risk with insulin.

ANTIDEPRESSANTS *(cont.)*

Bupropion Hydrochloride (Wellbutrin, Wellbutrin SR, Wellbutrin XL, Zyban) *(cont.)*

Levodopa	Caution with levodopa; use low initial dose and gradually titrate.
Opioids	Increased seizure risk with opioid addiction.
OTC anorectics	Increased seizure risk with OTC anorectics.
OTC stimulants	Increased seizure risk with OTC stimulants.
Phenobarbital	Phenobarbital may induce metabolism of bupropion.
Phenytoin	Phenytoin may induce metabolism of bupropion.
Sedatives	Increased seizure risk with excessive use or abrupt discontinuation of sedatives.
Seizure-threshold-lowering drugs	Extreme caution with drugs that lower seizure threshold (eg, antidepressants, antipsychotics, theophylline, systemic steroids).
Stimulants	Increased seizure risk with stimulant addiction.
Transdermal nicotine	Monitor HTN with transdermal nicotine.

Trazodone Hydrochloride (Desyrel)

Alcohol	May enhance response to alcohol.
Antihypertensives	Caution with antihypertensives.
Barbiturates	May enhance response to barbiturates.
Carbamazepine	Carbamazepine decreases levels.
CNS depressants	May enhance response to other CNS depressants.
CYP3A4 inhibitors	Potent CYP3A4 inhibitors (eg, ritonavir, ketoconazole, indinavir, itraconazole, nefazodone) may increase levels.
Digoxin	Increases digoxin serum levels.
MAOIs	Caution with MAOIs.
Phenytoin	Increases phenytoin serum levels.
Warfarin	May affect PT in patients on warfarin.

ANTIMANIC/BIPOLAR DISORDER AGENTS

Aripiprazole (Abilify)

2D6 inhibitors	2D6 inhibitors (eg, quinidine, fluoxetine, paroxetine) can increase blood levels.
Alcohol	Avoid alcohol.
Anticholinergics	Caution with anticholinergic agents.
Antihypertensives	May potentiate effect of antihypertensives.
Centrally acting drugs	Caution with other centrally acting drugs.

Table 18.2: DRUG INTERACTIONS FOR PSYCHOACTIVE DRUGS *(cont.)*

ANTIMANIC/BIPOLAR DISORDER AGENTS *(cont.)*

Aripiprazole (Abilify) *(cont.)*

CYP3A4 inducers	CYP3A4 inducers (eg, carbamazepine) may lower blood levels.
CYP3A4 inhibitors	CYP3A4 inhibitors (eg, ketoconazole, itraconazole) can increase blood levels.

Carbamazepine (Equetro)

Alcohol	Caution with alcohol.
Anti-malarial drugs	Anti-malarial drugs may antagonize the activity of carbamazepine.
Centrally acting drugs	Caution with other centrally acting drugs.
Clomipramine	May increase plasma levels of clomipramine.
CYP1A2 metabolized drugs	May induce CYP1A2; may interact with any agent metabolized by this enzyme.
CYP3A4 inducers	CYP3A4 inducers may decrease plasma levels.
CYP3A4 inhibitors	CYP3A4 inhibitors may increase plasma levels.
CYP3A4 metabolized drugs	May induce CYP3A4; may interact with any agent metabolized by this enzyme.
Delavirdine	Co-administration with delavirdine may lead to loss of virologic response and possible resistance to non-nucleoside reverse transcriptase inhibitors.
Lithium	May increase risk of neurotoxic side effects of lithium.
Phenytoin	May increase plasma levels of phenytoin.
Primidone	May increase plasma levels of primidone.

Divalproex Sodium (Depakote)

Alcohol	CNS depression with alcohol.
Amitriptyline	Potentiates amitriptyline.
ASA	Efficacy potentiated by ASA.
Carbamazepine	Potentiates carbamazepine. Efficacy reduced by carbamazepine.
Clonazepam	Clonazepam may induce absence status in patients with absence type seizures.
CNS depressants	CNS depression with other CNS depressants.
Diazepam	Potentiates diazepam.
Ethosuximide	Potentiates ethosuximide.
Felbamate	Efficacy potentiated by felbamate.
Lamotrigine	Potentiates lamotrigine.
Lorazepam	Potentiates lorazepam.
Nortriptyline	Potentiates nortriptyline.

ANTIMANIC/BIPOLAR DISORDER AGENTS *(cont.)*

Divalproex Sodium (Depakote) *(cont.)*

Phenobarbital	Potentiates phenobarbital. Efficacy reduced by phenobarbital.
Phenytoin	Potentiates phenytoin. Efficacy reduced by phenytoin.
Primidone	Potentiates primidone. Efficacy reduced by primidone.
Rifampin	Efficacy reduced by rifampin.
Tolbutamide	Potentiates tolbutamide.
Warfarin	Monitor PT/INR with warfarin.
Zidovudine	Potentiates zidovudine.

Lamotrigine (Lamictal, Lamictal CD)

Carbamazepine	Decreased levels with carbamazepine.
Folate inhibitors	May potentiate folate inhibitors.
Phenobarbital	Decreased levels with phenobarbital.
Phenytoin	Decreased levels with phenytoin.
Primidone	Decreased levels with primidone.
Valproic acid	Risk of life-threatening rash with valproic acid. Lamotrigine decreases valproic acid levels; valproic acid increases lamotrigine levels.

Lithium Carbonate (Eskalith, Eskalith-CR)

ACE inhibitors	Increased plasma levels with ACE inhibitors.
Acetazolamide	Decreased levels with acetazolamide.
Alkalinizing agents	Decreased levels with alkalinizing agents.
Angiotensin II receptor antagonists	Increased plasma levels with angiotensin II receptor antagonists.
Calcium channel blockers	Increased risk of neurotoxicity with calcium channel blockers.
Carbamazepine	Interacts with carbamazepine.
COX-2 inhibitors	Increased plasma levels with COX-2 inhibitors.
Diuretics	Increased risk of toxicity with diuretics.
Indomethacin	Increased plasma levels with indomethacin.
Methyldopa	Interacts with methyldopa.
Metronidazole	Increased risk of toxicity with metronidazole.
Neuromuscular blockers	May prolong effects of neuromuscular blockers.

Table 18.2: DRUG INTERACTIONS FOR PSYCHOACTIVE DRUGS *(cont.)*

ANTIMANIC/BIPOLAR DISORDER AGENTS *(cont.)*

Lithium Carbonate (Eskalith, Eskalith-CR) *(cont.)*

NSAIDs	Increased plasma levels with other NSAIDs.
Phenytoin	Interacts with phenytoin.
Piroxicam	Increased plasma levels with piroxicam.
Selective serotonin reuptake inhibitors	Caution with SSRIs.
Urea	Decreased levels with urea.
Xanthine agents	Decreased levels with xanthine agents.

Olanzapine (Zyprexa)

Activated charcoal	Decreased levels with activated charcoal.
Alcohol	Caution with alcohol.
Antihypertensives	May potentiate antihypertensives.
Carbamazepine	Increased clearance with carbamazepine.
CNS drugs	Caution with other CNS drugs.
CYP1A2 inducers	Inducers of CYP1A2 may increase clearance.
CYP1A2 inhibitors	Inhibitors of CYP1A2 may decrease clearance.
Dopamine agonists	May antagonize dopamine agonists.
Fluvoxamine	Increased levels with fluvoxamine; lower olanzapine dose.
Glucuronyl transferase	Glucuronyl transferase (eg, omeprazole, rifampin) may increase clearance.
Levodopa	May antagonize levodopa agonists.

Olanzapine/Fluoxetine Hydrochloride (Symbyax)

Alcohol	Risk of orthostatic hypotension with alcohol.
Antihypertensives	Risk of orthostatic hypotension with antihypertensives.
Aspirin	Increased risk of bleeding with aspirin.
Benzodiazepines	Risk of orthostatic hypotension with benzodiazepines.
Carbamazepine	Increased clearance with carbamazepine.
Clozapine	Increase in clozapine levels.
CNS-drugs	Caution with other CNS drugs.
CYP1A2 inducers	Increased clearance with other inducers of CYP1A2.
CYP1A2 inhibitors	Decreased clearance with other CYP1A2 inhibitors.
CYP2D6 metabolized drugs	Inhibits drugs metabolized by CYP2D6 (eg, flecainide, vinblastine, tricyclic antidepressants); initiate at lower end of dosage range.

ANTIMANIC/BIPOLAR DISORDER AGENTS *(cont.)*

Olanzapine/Fluoxetine Hydrochloride (Symbyax) *(cont.)*

Dopamine agonists	May antagonize dopamine agonists.
Fluoroquinolones	Decreased clearance with fluoroquinolones.
Fluoxetine-containing products	Caution with other fluoxetine-containing products.
Fluvoxamine	Decreased clearance with fluvoxamine.
Glucuronyl transferase	Increased clearance with glucuronyl transferase.
Haloperidol	Increase in haloperidol levels.
Hepatotoxic drugs	Caution with hepatotoxic drugs.
Protein-bound drugs (highly)	Caution with other highly protein bound drugs (eg, warfarin, digitoxin).
Levodopa	May antagonize levodopa agonists.
Lithium	Monitor lithium levels.
NSAIDs	Increased risk of bleeding with NSAIDs.
Olanzapine-containing products	Caution with other olanzapine-containing products.
Omeprazole	Increased clearance with omeprazole.
Phenytoin	Increase in phenytoin levels.
Rifampin	Increased clearance with carbamazepine.
Sumatriptan	Caution with other sumatriptan.
Tricyclic antidepressants	May increase TCA levels; may require reduction in TCA dose.
Tryptophan	Caution with other tryptophan.
Warfarin	Increased risk of bleeding with warfarin.

Quetiapine Fumarate (Seroquel)

Alcohol	Increased cognitive and motor effects of alcohol.
Antihypertensives	May enhance effects of antihypertensives.
CNS drugs	Caution with other CNS drugs.
CYP3A inhibitors	Caution with inhibitors of CYP3A (eg, itraconazole, ketoconazole, fluconazole, erythromycin).
Dopamine agonists	May antagonize dopamine agonists.
Hepatic enzyme inducers	Other hepatic enzyme inducers (eg, carbamazepine, barbiturates, glucocorticoids) may reduce levels.

Table 18.2: DRUG INTERACTIONS FOR PSYCHOACTIVE DRUGS (cont.)

ANTIMANIC/BIPOLAR DISORDER AGENTS (cont.)

Quetiapine Fumarate (Seroquel) (cont.)

Levodopa	May antagonize levodopa agonists.
Lorazepam	May reduce oral clearance of lorazepam.
Phenytoin	Phenytoin may reduce levels.
Thioridazine	Increased clearance with thioridazine.

Risperidone (Risperdal, Risperdal Consta, Risperdal M-Tab)

Alcohol	Caution with alcohol.
Antihypertensives	May potentiate antihypertensives.
Clozapine	Increased levels with clozapine.
CNS-drugs	Caution with other CNS drugs.
Dopamine agonists	May antagonize dopamine agonists.
Enzyme inducers	Enzyme inducers (eg, carbamazepine, phenytoin, rifampin, phenobarbital) may decrease levels.
Fluoxetine	Increased levels with fluoxetine.
Furosemide	Increased mortality with furosemide in elderly patients.
Levodopa	May antagonize levodopa agonists.
Paroxetine	Increased levels with paroxetine.
Valproate	May increase valproate levels.

Ziprasidone (Geodon)

Antihypertensives	May enhance effects of antihypertensives.
Carbamazepine	Carbamazepine may decrease levels.
Centrally acting drugs	Caution with centrally acting drugs.
CYP3A4 inhibitors	CYP3A4 inhibitors may increase levels.
Dopamine agonists	May antagonize effects of dopamine agonists.
Levodopa	May antagonize effects of levodopa agonists.

ANTIPSYCHOTIC AGENTS

Aripiprazole (Abilify)

2D6 inhibitors	2D6 inhibitors (eg, quinidine, fluoxetine, paroxetine) can increase blood levels.
Alcohol	Avoid alcohol.
Anticholinergics	Caution with anticholinergic agents.

ANTIPSYCHOTIC AGENTS *(cont.)*

Aripiprazole (Abilify) *(cont.)*

Antihypertensives	May potentiate effect of antihypertensives.
Centrally acting drugs	Caution with other centrally acting drugs.
CYP3A4 inducers	CYP3A4 inducers (eg, carbamazepine) may lower blood levels.
CYP3A4 inhibitors	CYP3A4 inhibitors (eg, ketoconazole, itraconazole) can increase blood levels.

Chlorpromazine Hydrochloride (Thorazine)

Amipaque	Do not use with Amipaque; discontinue at least 48hrs before myelography and resume at least 24hrs after. Can cause α-adrenergic blockade.
Anticoagulants, oral	May decrease effects of oral anticoagulants.
Anticonvulsants	Anticonvulsants may need adjustment; phenytoin toxicity reported.
Atropine or related drugs	Caution with atropine or related drugs.
CNS depressants	Potentiates effects of CNS depressants (eg, anesthetic, barbiturates, narcotics); reduce doses of these drugs by 1/4 to 1/2.
Guanethidine	May decrease effects of guanethidine.
Lithium	Encephalopathic syndrome reported with lithium.
Propranolol	Propranolol increases plasma levels of both agents.
Thiazide diuretics	Thiazide diuretics may potentiate orthostatic hypotension.

Clozapine (Clozaril, Fazaclo)

2D6 inhibitors	Caution with 2D6 inhibitors.
2D6 inducers	Caution with 2D6 inducers.
3A4 inhibitors	Caution with 3A4 inhibitors.
3A4 inducers	Caution with 3A4 inducers.
Alcohol	Caution with alcohol.
Anesthesia, general	Caution with general anesthesia.
Benzodiazepines	Caution with benzodiazepines.
Bone marrow suppressants	Avoid with bone marrow suppressants.
Carbamazepine	Avoid with carbamazepine.
CNS-active drugs	Caution with CNS-active drugs.
CYP1A2 inhibitors	Caution with CYP1A2 inhibitors.

Table 18.2: DRUG INTERACTIONS FOR PSYCHOACTIVE DRUGS *(cont.)*

ANTIPSYCHOTIC AGENTS *(cont.)*

Clozapine (Clozaril, Fazaclo) *(cont.)*

CYP1A2 inducers	Caution with CYP1A2 inducers.
CYP450 inducers	CYP450 inducers (eg, phenytoin, nicotine, rifampin) decrease plasma levels.
CYP450 inhibitors	CYP450 inhibitors (eg, cimetidine, caffeine, erythromycin, citalopram) increase plasma levels.
Epinephrine	Avoid with epinephrine.
Fluvoxamine	Caution with fluvoxamine.
Paroxetine	Caution with paroxetine.
Psychotropics	Caution with other psychotropics.
Sertraline	Caution with sertraline.

Fluphenazine

Alcohol	Potentiates alcohol effects.
Anesthetics	Reduce dose of anesthetics prior to surgery.
Anticholinergics	May potentiate anticholinergics.
CNS depressants	Reduce dose of CNS depressants prior to surgery.

Haloperidol (Haldol)

Alcohol	May potentiate CNS depression with alcohol.
Anesthetics	May potentiate CNS depression with anesthetics.
Anticholinergics	Caution with anticholinergics.
Anticoagulants	Caution with anticoagulants.
Anticonvulsants	Caution with anticonvulsants.
Antiparkinson agents	Caution with antiparkinson agents.
CNS depressants	May potentiate CNS depression with other CNS depressants.
Epinephrine	Antagonizes epinephrine.
Lithium	Monitor for neurological toxicity with lithium.
Opiates	May potentiate CNS depression with opiates.
Rifampin	Caution with rifampin.

Loxapine Succinate (Loxitane)

CNS-active drugs	Caution with CNS-active drugs, including alcohol.
Epinephrine	Antagonizes epinephrine.
Lorazepam	Significant respiratory depression and hypotension reported with lorazepam (rare).

ANTIPSYCHOTIC AGENTS *(cont.)*

Molindone Hydrochloride (Moban)

Calcium sulfate	Tabs contain calcium sulfate; may interfere with phenytoin sodium and tetracycline absorption.

Olanzapine (Zyprexa)

Activated charcoal	Decreased levels with activated charcoal.
Alcohol	Caution with alcohol.
Antihypertensives	May potentiate antihypertensives.
Carbamazepine	Increased clearance with carbamazepine.
CNS drugs	Caution with other CNS drugs.
CYP1A2 inducers	Inducers of CYP1A2 may increase clearance.
CYP1A2 inhibitors	Inhibitors of CYP1A2 may decrease clearance.
Dopamine agonists	May antagonize dopamine agonists.
Fluvoxamine	Increased levels with fluvoxamine; lower olanzapine dose.
Glucuronyl transferase	Glucuronyl transferase (eg, omeprazole, rifampin) may increase clearance.
Levodopa	May antagonize levodopa agonists.

Perphenazine

Alcohol	Additive effects and hypotension may occur with alcohol.
Atropine/atropine-like drugs	Additive anticholinergic effects with atropine/atropine-like drugs.
CNS depressants	Additive effects with CNS depressants; use reduced amount of added drug.
Cytochrome P450 2D6 inhibitors	Cytochrome P450 2D6 inhibitors (tricyclic antidepressants, SSRIs) may increase levels; lower doses may be required.
Phenothiazine	Additive effects with phenothiazine; use reduced amount of added drug.
Phosphorous insecticide	Additive anticholinergic effects with exposure to phosphorous insecticide.

Quetiapine Fumarate (Seroquel)

Alcohol	Increased cognitive and motor effects of alcohol.
Antihypertensives	May enhance effects of antihypertensives.
CNS drugs	Caution with other CNS drugs.
CYP3A inhibitors	Caution with inhibitors of CYP3A (eg, itraconazole, ketoconazole, fluconazole, erythromycin).
Dopamine agonists	May antagonize dopamine agonists.

Table 18.2: DRUG INTERACTIONS FOR PSYCHOACTIVE DRUGS *(cont.)*

ANTIPSYCHOTIC AGENTS *(cont.)*

Quetiapine Fumarate (Seroquel) *(cont.)*

Hepatic enzyme inducers	Other hepatic enzyme inducers (eg, carbamazepine, barbiturates, glucocorticoids) may reduce levels.
Levodopa	May antagonize levodopa agonists.
Lorazepam	May reduce oral clearance of lorazepam.
Phenytoin	Phenytoin may reduce levels.
Thioridazine	Increased clearance with thioridazine.

Risperidone (Risperdal, Risperdal Consta, Risperdal M-Tab)

Alcohol	Caution with alcohol.
Antihypertensives	May potentiate antihypertensives.
Clozapine	Increased levels with clozapine.
CNS drugs	Caution with other CNS drugs.
Dopamine agonists	May antagonize dopamine agonists.
Enzyme inducers	Enzyme inducers (eg, carbamazepine, phenytoin, rifampin, phenobarbital) may decrease levels.
Fluoxetine	Increased levels with fluoxetine.
Furosemide	Increased mortality with furosemide in elderly patients.
Levodopa	May antagonize levodopa agonists.
Paroxetine	Increased levels with paroxetine.
Valproate	May increase valproate levels.

Thioridazine Hydrochloride

Alcohol	May potentiate alcohol.
Atropine	May potentiate atropine.
CNS depressants	May potentiate CNS depressants.
CYP2D6 inhibitors	Avoid CYP2D6 inhibitors (eg, fluoxetine, paroxetine); increased risk of arrhythmias.
Fluvoxamine	Fluvoxamine increases thioridazine plasma levels; avoid concomitant use.
Phosphorus insecticides	May potentiate phosphorus insecticides.
Pindolol	Pindolol increases thioridazine plasma levels; avoid concomitant use.
Propranolol	Propranolol increases thioridazine plasma levels; avoid concomitant use.

Thiothixene (Navane)

Alcohol	Possible additive effects including hypotension with alcohol.

ANTIPSYCHOTIC AGENTS *(cont.)*

Thiothixene (Navane) *(cont.)*

Atropine or related drugs	Caution with atropine or related drugs.
CNS depressants	Possible additive effects including hypotension with CNS depressants.
Pressor agents	Paradoxical effects with pressor agents.

Trifluoperazine Hydrochloride

Alpha-adrenergic blockade	May potentiate alpha-adrenergic blockade.
Amipaque	Discontinue 48 hrs before myelography, resume 24 hrs post procedure.
Anticoagulants, oral	May decrease effects of oral anticoagulants.
Anticonvulsants	May lower seizure threshold; adjust anticonvulsants.
CNS depressants	Additive CNS depression with other CNS depressants (eg, sedatives, narcotics, anesthetics, tranquilizers, alcohol).
Guanethidine	May decrease effects of guanethidine.
Lithium	Risk of encephalopathic syndrome with lithium.
Phenytoin	May cause phenytoin toxicity.
Propranolol	Propranolol may increase levels of both drugs.
Thiazide diuretics	Thiazide diuretics may potentiate orthostatic hypotension.

Ziprasidone (Geodon)

Antihypertensives	May enhance effects of antihypertensives.
Carbamazepine	Carbamazepine may decrease levels.
Centrally acting drugs	Caution with centrally acting drugs.
CYP3A4 inhibitors	CYP3A4 inhibitors may increase levels.
Dopamine agonists	May antagonize effects of dopamine agonists.
Levodopa	May antagonize effects of levodopa agonists.

ATTENTION DEFICIT/HYPERACTIVITY DISORDER AGENTS

Amphetamine Aspartate/Amphetamine Sulfate/Dextroamphetamine Saccharate/ Dextroamphetamine Sulfate (Adderall, Adderall XR)

Adrenergic blockers	Antagonizes adrenergic blockers.
Antihistamines	Antagonizes antihistamines.

Table 18.2: DRUG INTERACTIONS FOR PSYCHOACTIVE DRUGS *(cont.)*

ATTENTION DEFICIT/HYPERACTIVITY DISORDER AGENTS *(cont.)*

Amphetamine Aspartate/Amphetamine Sulfate/Dextroamphetamine Saccharate/Dextroamphetamine Sulfate (Adderall, Adderall XR) *(cont.)*

Antihypertensives	Antagonizes antihypertensives.
Chlorpromazine	Antagonized by chlorpromazine.
Ethosuximide	May delay absorption of ethosuximide.
GI acidifying agents	GI acidifying agents (guanethidine, reserpine, glutamic acid, etc.) decrease efficacy.
GI alkalinizers	Potentiated by GI alkalinizers.
Haloperidol	Antagonized by haloperidol.
Lithium	Antagonized by lithium.
MAOIs	MAOIs may cause hypertensive crisis.
Meperidine	Potentiates meperidine.
Norepinephrine	Potentiates norepinephrine.
Phenobarbital	May delay absorption of phenobarbital. Potentiates phenobarbital.
Phenytoin	May delay absorption of phenytoin. Potentiates phenytoin.
Propoxyphene	Potentiated by propoxyphene overdose.
Tricyclic antidepressants	Potentiated effects of both agents with TCAs.
Urinary acidifying agents	Urinary acidifying agents (ammonium chloride, etc.) decrease efficacy.
Urinary alkalinizers	Potentiated by urinary alkalinizers.
Veratrum alkaloids	Antagonizes veratrum alkaloids (antihypertensive).

Atomoxetine Hydrochloride (Strattera)

Albuterol	May potentiate the cardiovascular effects of albuterol.
β_2-agonists	May potentiate the cardiovascular effects of other β_2-agonists.
CYP2D6 inhibitors	Increased levels in extensive metabolizers with CYP2D6 inhibitors (eg, paroxetine, fluoxetine, quinidine); atomoxetine may need dose adjustment.
Pressor agents	Caution with pressor agents.

Dexmethylphenidate Hydrochloride (Focalin, Focalin XR)

Acid supressants	Acid supressants could alter the release of dexmethylphenidate.
Antacids	Antacids could alter the release of dexmethylphenidate.
Anticonvulsants	May inhibit metabolism of anticonvulsants; adjust dose.
Antidepressants	May inhibit metabolism of some antidepressants; adjust dose.
Antihypertensives	May decrease the effectiveness of antihypertensives.

ATTENTION DEFICIT/HYPERACTIVITY DISORDER AGENTS *(cont.)*

Dexmethylphenidate Hydrochloride (Focalin, Focalin XR) *(cont.)*

Clonidine	Adverse events reported with clonidine.
Coumarin anticoagulants	May inhibit metabolism of coumarin anticoagulants; adjust dose.
Pressor agents	Caution with pressor agents.
Tricyclic drugs	May inhibit metabolism of tricyclic drugs; adjust dose.

Dextroamphetamine Sulfate (Dexedrine, Dexedrine Spansules)

Antihistamines	Antagonizes antihistamines.
Antihypertensives	Antagonizes antihypertensives.
Chlorpromazine	Antagonized by chlorpromazine.
Ethosuximide	May delay absorption of ethosuximide.
GI acidifying agents	GI acidifying agents (guanethidine, reserpine, glutamic acid, etc.) decrease efficacy.
GI alkalinizers	Potentiated by GI alkalinizers.
Haloperidol	Antagonized by haloperidol.
Lithium	Antagonized by lithium.
MAOIs	MAOIs may cause hypertensive crisis.
Meperidine	Potentiates meperidine.
Norepinephrine	Potentiates norepinephrine.
Phenobarbital	May delay absorption of phenobarbital. Potentiates phenobarbital.
Phenytoin	May delay absorption of phenytoin. Potentiates phenytoin.
Propoxyphene	Potentiated by propoxyphene overdose.
Tricyclic antidepressants	Potentiated effects of both agents with TCAs.
Urinary acidifying agents	Urinary acidifying agents (ammonium chloride, etc.) decrease efficacy.
Urinary alkalinizers	Potentiated by urinary alkalinizers.
Veratrum alkaloids	Antagonizes veratrum alkaloids (antihypertensive).

Methamphetamine Hydrochloride (Desoxyn)

Guanethidine	May decrease hypotensive effect of guanethidine.
Insulin	May alter insulin requirements.
MAOIs	Avoid MAOIs.
Phenothiazines	Antagonized by phenothiazines.

Table 18.2: DRUG INTERACTIONS FOR PSYCHOACTIVE DRUGS (cont.)

ATTENTION DEFICIT/HYPERACTIVITY DISORDER AGENTS (cont.)

Methamphetamine Hydrochloride (Desoxyn) (cont.)

Sympathomimetic amines, indirect acting	Caution with indirect acting sympathomimetic amines.
Tricyclic antidepressants	Caution with TCAs.

Methylphenidate Hydrochloride (Concerta, Metadate CD, Metadate ER, Methylin, Ritalin, Ritalin LA, Ritalin-SR)

α_2-agonist	Caution with α_2-agonist (eg, clonidine).
Acid suppressants, (Cap, Extended-Release)	Acid suppressants may alter release characteristics of capsule.
Antacids, (Cap, Extended-Release)	Antacids may alter release characteristics of capsule.
Anticoagulants	Potentiates anticoagulants; monitor plasma drug levels or PT/INR.
Anticonvulsants	Potentiates anticonvulsants (eg, phenobarbital, phenytoin, primidone); monitor plasma drug levels or PT/INR.
Guanethidine	May decrease hypotensive effect of guanethidine.
MAOIs	Avoid during or within 14 days of MAOI use.
Phenylbutazone	Potentiates phenylbutazone; monitor plasma drug levels or PT/INR.
Pressor agents	Caution with pressor agents.
Selective serotonin reuptake inhibitors	Potentiates SSRIs.
Tricyclic antidepressants	Potentiates TCAs (eg, imipramine, clomipramine, desipramine); monitor plasma drug levels or PT/INR.

Modafinil (Provigil)

Alcohol	Avoid alcohol.
Clomipramine	May increase levels of clomipramine.
CYP2C19 metabolized drugs	May increase levels of drugs metabolized by CYP2C19 (eg, diazepam, propranolol, phenytoin) .
CYP2C9 metabolized drugs	May increase levels of drugs metabolized by CYP2C9 (eg, warfarin).
CYP3A4 inducers	CYP3A4 inducers (eg, carbamazepine, phenobarbital, rifampin) may decrease levels.
CYP3A4 inhibitors	CYP3A4 inhibitors (eg, ketoconazole, itraconazole) may increase levels.
CYP3A4 metabolized drugs	May decrease levels of drugs metabolized by CYP3A4 (eg, cyclosporine, steroidal contraceptives, theophylline).

ATTENTION DEFICIT/HYPERACTIVITY DISORDER AGENTS *(cont.)*

Modafinil (Provigil) *(cont.)*

Desipramine	May increase levels of desipramine.
MAOIs	Caution with MAOIs.
Methylphenidate	Methylphenidate may delay absorption.
Phenytoin	Monitor for toxicity with phenytoin.
Steroidal contraceptives	May reduce efficacy of steroidal contraceptives up to 1 month after discontinuation.
Warfarin	Monitor PT with warfarin.

SLEEP ADJUNCTS

Alprazolam[CIV] (Niravam, Xanax, Xanax XR)

Amiodarone	Caution with amiodarone.
Anticonvulsants	Additive CNS depressant effects with anticonvulsants.
Antihistamines	Additive CNS depressant effects with antihistamines.
Azole antifungals	Avoid azole antifungals.
Carbamazepine	Decreased plasma levels with carbamazepine.
Cimetidine	Potentiated by cimetidine.
Contraceptives, oral	Potentiated by oral contraceptives.
Cyclosporine	Caution with cyclosporine.
CYP3A inducers	Decreased levels with CYP3A inducers (eg, carbamazepine).
CYP3A inhibitors	Avoid with potent CYP3A inhibitors (eg, azole antifungals). Caution with other CYP3A inhibitors.
Desipramine	Increases levels of desipramine.
Diltiazem	Caution with diltiazem.
Ergotamine	Caution with ergotamine.
Ethanol	Additive CNS depressant effects with ethanol.
Fluoxetine	Potentiated by fluoxetine.
Fluvoxamine	Potentiated by fluvoxamine.
Grapefruit juice	Caution with grapefruit juice.
Imipramine	Increases levels of imipramine.
Isoniazid	Caution with isoniazid.
Itraconazole	Contraindicated with concomitant itraconazole.
Ketoconazole	Contraindicated with concomitant ketoconazole.

Table 18.2: DRUG INTERACTIONS FOR PSYCHOACTIVE DRUGS *(cont.)*

SLEEP ADJUNCTS *(cont.)*

Alprazolam[CIV] (Niravam, Xanax, Xanax XR) *(cont.)*

Macrolids	Caution with macrolides.
Nefazodone	Potentiated by nefazodone.
Nicardipine	Caution with nicardipine.
Nifedipine	Caution with nifedipine.
Paroxetine	Caution with paroxetine.
Propoxyphene	Decreased plasma levels with propoxyphene.
Psychotropic agents	Additive CNS depressant effects with psychotropic agents.
Sertraline	Caution with sertraline.

Diazepam[CIV] (Valium)

Alcohol	Avoid alcohol.
Antidepressants	Other antidepressants may potentiate effects.
Barbiturates	Barbiturates may potentiate effects.
Cimetidine	Delayed clearance with cimetidine.
CNS depressants	Avoid other CNS depressants.
Flumazenil	Risk of seizure with flumazenil.
MAOIs	MAOIs may potentiate effects.
Narcotics	Narcotics may potentiate effects.
Phenothiazines	Phenothiazines may potentiate effects.

Estazolam[CIV] (ProSom)

Alcohol	Potentiated effects with alcohol.
Anticonvulsants	Potentiated effects with anticonvulsants.
Antihistamines	Potentiated effects with antihistamines.
Barbiturates	Potentiated effects with barbiturates.
CNS depressants	Potentiated effects with other CNS depressants
MAOIs	Potentiated effects with MAOIs.
Narcotics	Potentiated effects with narcotics.
Phenothiazines	Potentiated effects with phenothiazines.
Psychotropic medications	Potentiated effects with psychotropic medications.
Smoking	Smoking may increase clearance.

SLEEP ADJUNCTS *(cont.)*

Flurazepam Hydrochloride^{CIV} (Dalmane)

Alcohol	Additive effects with alcohol.
CNS depressants	Additive effects with other CNS depressants.

Lorazepam^{CIV} (Ativan)

Alcohol	CNS-depressant effects with alcohol. Diminished tolerance to alcohol.
Barbiturates	CNS-depressant effects with barbiturates.
CNS depressants	Diminished tolerance to other CNS depressants.

Midazolam Hydrochloride^{CIV} (Versed)

Alcohol	Avoid use with acute alcohol intoxication.
CNS depressants	Increased sedative effects with other CNS depressants.
CYP450 3A4 inhibitors	Prolonged sedation with CYP450 3A4 inhibitors (eg, erythromycin, diltiazem, verapamil, ketoconazole, itraconazole, saquinavir, cimetidine).
Droperidol	Increased sedative effects with droperidol.
Fentanyl	Increased sedative effects with fentanyl. May cause severe hypotension with concomitant use of fentanyl in neonates.
Halothane	Decreases concentration of halothane required for anesthesia.
Meperidine	Increased sedative effects with meperidine.
Morphine	Increased sedative effects with morphine.
Secobarbital	Increased sedative effects with secobarbital.
Thiopental	Decreases concentration of thiopental required for anesthesia.

Temazepam^{CIV} (Restoril)

Alcohol	Additive CNS depressant effects with alcohol.
CNS depressants	Additive CNS depressant effects with CNS depressants.
Diphenhydramine	May be synergistic with diphenhydramine.

Triazolam^{CIV} (Halcion)

Alcohol	Additive CNS depression with alcohol.
Amiodarone	Caution with famiodarone.
Anticonvulsants	Additive CNS depression with anticonvulsants.
Antihistamines	Additive CNS depression with antihistamines.
Cimetidine	Caution with cimetidine.
Contraceptives, oral	Potentiated by the coadministration of oral contraceptives.
Cyclosporine	Caution with cyclosporine.

Table 18.2: DRUG INTERACTIONS FOR PSYCHOACTIVE DRUGS *(cont.)*

SLEEP ADJUNCTS *(cont.)*

Triazolam^CIV (Halcion) *(cont.)*

CYP3A, medications that impair	Contraindicated with medications that impair CYP3A.
CYP3A inhibitors	Avoid the concomitant use with inhibitors of the CYP3A (eg, ketoconazole, itraconazole, all azole-type antifungals, nefazodone).
Diltiazem	Caution with diltiazem.
Ergotamine	Caution with ergotamine.
Fluvoxamine	Caution with fluvoxamine.
Grapefruit juice	Potentiated by the coadministration of grapefruit juice.
Intraconazole	Contraindicated with itraconazole.
Isoniazid	Potentiated by the coadministration of isoniazid.
Ketoconazole	Contraindicated with ketoconazole.
Marcrolides	Caution with macrolides.
Nefazodone	Contraindicated with nefazodone.
Nicardipine	Caution with nicardipine
Paroxetine	Caution with paroxetine.
Psychotropics	Additive CNS depression with psychotropics.
Ranitidine	Potentiated by the coadministration of ranitidine.
Sertraline	Caution with sertraline.
Verapamil	Caution with verapamil.

Eszopiclone^CIV (Lunesta)

CYP3A4	Strong inhibitors of CYP3A4 may significantly increase the AUC of eszopiclone.
Ethanol	Possible additive effect on psychomotor performance with ethanol.
Olanzapine	Coadministration with olanzapine produced a decrease in DSST score.

Ramelteon (Rozerem)

Alcohol	Additive effect with alcohol.
CYP inducers	Decreased efficacy with strong CYP inducers (rifampin).
CYP1A2 inhibitors	Do not use with strong CYP1A2 inhibitors (fluvoxamine). Caution with less strong CYP1A2 inhibitors.
CYP2C9 inhibitors	Caution with strong CYP2C9 inhibitors (fluconazole).
CYP3A4 inhibitors	Caution with strong CYP3A4 inhibitors (ketoconazole).

Zaleplon^CIV (Sonata)

Alcohol	Potentiates CNS depression with alcohol.

SLEEP ADJUNCTS *(cont.)*

Zaleplon[CIV] (Sonata) *(cont.)*

Anticonvulsants	Potentiates CNS depression with anticonvulsants.
Antihistamines	Potentiates CNS depression with antihistamines.
Cimetidine	Potentiated by cimetidine.
CNS depressants	Potentiates CNS depression with other CNS depressants.
CYP3A4 inducers	CYP3A4 inducers (eg, rifampin, phenytoin, carbamazepine and phenobarbital) decreases levels.
Psychotropic medications	Potentiates CNS depression with psychotropics (eg, thioridazine, imipramine).

Ramelteon (Rozerem)

Alcohol	Additive effect with alcohol.
CYP inducers	Decreased efficacy with strong CYP inducers (rifampin).
CYP1A2 inhibitors	Do not use with strong CYP1A2 inhibitors (fluvoxamine). Caution with less strong CYP1A2 inhibitors.
CYP2C9 inhibitors	Caution with strong CYP2C9 inhibitors (fluconazole).
CYP3A4 inhibitors	Caution with strong CYP3A4 inhibitors (ketoconazole).

Zaleplon[CIV] (Sonata)

Alcohol	Potentiates CNS depression with alcohol.
Anticonvulsants	Potentiates CNS depression with anticonvulsants.
Antihistamines	Potentiates CNS depression with antihistamines.
Cimetidine	Potentiated by cimetidine.
CNS depressants	Potentiates CNS depression with other CNS depressants.
CYP3A4 inducers	CYP3A4 inducers (eg, rifampin, phenytoin, carbamazepine and phenobarbital) decreases levels.
Psychotropic medications	Potentiates CNS depression with psychotropics (eg, thioridazine, imipramine).

Zolpidem Tartrate[CIV] (Ambien, Ambien-CR)

Alcohol	Increased effect with alcohol.
CNS depressants	Increased effect with other CNS depressants.
Flumazenil	Flumazenil reverses effect.
Rifampin	Rifampin may decrease effects.

OBESITY AGENTS

Benzphetamine Hydrochloride (Didrex)

Antihypertensives	Decreases effects of antihypertensives.

Table 18.2: DRUG INTERACTIONS FOR PSYCHOACTIVE DRUGS *(cont.)*

OBESITY AGENTS *(cont.)*

Benzphetamine Hydrochloride (Didrex) *(cont.)*

CNS stimulants	Avoid with other CNS stimulants.
Insulin	May alter insulin requirements.
MAOIs	Hypertensive crisis risk if used within 14 days of MAOIs.
Tricyclic antidepressants	Potentiates TCAs.
Urinary acidifying agents	Reduced effect with urinary acidifying agents.
Urinary alkalinizing agents	Potentiated by urinary alkalinizing agents.

Diethylpropion Hydrochloride (Tenuate)

Alcohol	Adverse reactions with alcohol.
Anesthetics, general	Potential for arrhythmias with general anesthetics.
Anorectic agents	Avoid with other anorectic agents (prescription, OTC, herbal products) or if used within prior year.
Antidiabetics	Antidiabetic drug requirements may be altered.
Antihypertensives	May interfere with antihypertensives (eg, guanethidine, methyldopa).
Dexfenfluramine	Valvular heart disease reported with dexfenfluramine.
Fenfluramine	Valvular heart disease reported with fenfluramine.
MAOIs	MAOIs may cause hypertensive crisis.
Phenothiazines	Phenothiazines may antagonize anorectic effects.

Phendimetrazine Tartrate (Bontril PDM, Bontril Slow-Release)

Guanethidine	May decrease hypotensive effects of guanethidine.
Insulin	May alter insulin requirements.
MAOIs	Hypertensive crisis risk if used within 14 days of MAOIs.

Phentermine Hydrochloride (Adipex-P)

Alcohol	Avoid alcohol.
Dexfenfluramine	Valvular heart disease and primary pulmonary hypertension reported with dexfenfluramine.
Fenfluramine	Valvular heart disease and primary pulmonary hypertension reported with fenfluramine.
Guanethidine	May decrease effects of guanethidine.
Insulin	May alter insulin requirements.
Selective serotonin reuptake inhibitors	Avoid SSRIs.

OBESITY AGENTS *(cont.)*

Phentermine Hydrochloride (Adipex-P) *(cont.)*

Weight loss products	Avoid other weight loss products.

Phentermine Resin (Ionamin)

Dexfenfluramine	Valvular heart disease and primary pulmonary hypertension reported with dexfenfluramine.
Fenfluramine	Valvular heart disease and primary pulmonary hypertension reported with fenfluramine.
Insulin	May alter insulin requirements.
Neuron blocking agents	May decrease effects of adrenergic neuron blocking agents.
Selective serotonin reuptake inhibitors	Avoid SSRIs.
Weight loss products	Avoid with weight loss products.

Sibutramine Hydrochloride (Meridia)

Alcohol	Avoid excess alcohol within 14 days of MAOI use.
Blood pressor, agents that increase	Caution with other agents that increase BP.
CNS-active drugs	Avoid CNS-active drugs within 14 days of MAOI use.
Ephedrine	Caution with ephedrine.
Erythromycin	Possible decreased metabolism with erythromycin.
Heart rate, agents that increase	Caution with other agents that increase BP, heart rate.
Hemostasis, drugs affecting	Caution with drugs affecting hemostasis.
Ketoconazole	Possible decreased metabolism with ketoconazole.
Platelet function, drugs affecting	Caution with drugs affecting platelet function.
Pseudoephedrine	Caution with pseudoephedrine.
Serotonergic agents	Avoid other serotonergic agents (eg, SSRIs, migraine therapy agents, certain opioids), within 14 days of MAOI use.

OBSESSIVE-COMPULSIVE DISORDER AGENTS

Fluoxetine Hydrochloride (Prozac, Sarafem)

Alcohol	Avoid alcohol.
Antidepressants	May potentiate other antidepressants.

Table 18.2: DRUG INTERACTIONS FOR PSYCHOACTIVE DRUGS *(cont.)*

OBSESSIVE-COMPULSIVE DISORDER AGENTS *(cont.)*

Fluoxetine Hydrochloride (Prozac, Sarafem) *(cont.)*

Antidiabetic	Antidiabetic drugs may need adjustment.
Antipsychotics	May potentiate antipsychotics (eg, haloperidol, clozapine).
Benzodiazepine	May increase benzodiazepine levels.
Carbamazepine	May increase carbamazepine levels.
Clozapine	May increase clozapine levels.
CNS drugs	Caution with CNS drugs.
CYP2D6 metabolized drugs	May potentiate drugs metabolized by CYP2D6.
Haloperidol	May increase haloperidol levels.
Hemostasis-interfering drugs	Caution with drugs that interfere with hemostasis (eg, nonselective NSAIDs, aspirin, warfarin) due to increased risk of bleeding.
Lithium	Lithium levels may increase/decrease; monitor lithium levels.
MAOIs	Do not use with or within 14 days of MAOIs.
Phenytoin	May increase phenytoin levels.
Plasma-bound drugs	May shift concentrations with plasma-bound drugs (eg, coumadin, digitoxin).
Thioridazine	May increase thioridazine levels.
Tricyclic antidepressants	May increase TCAs levels.
Tryptophan	Increased adverse effects with tryptophan.
Warfarin	May alter warfarin effects.

Fluvoxamine Maleate

Alcohol	Avoid alcohol.
Astemizole	Avoid astemizole.
Benzodiazepines	Reduces clearance of benzodiazepines metabolized by hepatic oxidation (eg, alprazolam, midazolam, triazolam).
Carbamazepine	Increases serum levels of carbamazepine.
Cisapride	Avoid cisapride.
Clozapine	Increases serum levels of clozapine.
Diazepam	Avoid diazepam.
Diltiazem	Bradycardia with diltiazem.
Lithium	Lithium may increase serotonergic effects.
MAOIs	Potential for serious, fatal interactions with MAOIs.

OBSESSIVE-COMPULSIVE DISORDER AGENTS *(cont.)*

Fluvoxamine Maleate *(cont.)*

Methadone	Increases serum levels of methadone.
Metoprolol	May potentiate metoprolol.
Mexiletine	Reduces clearance of mexiletine metabolized by hepatic oxidation (eg, alprazolam, midazolam, triazolam).
Primozide	Avoid primozide.
Propranolol	May potentiate propranolol.
Sumatriptan	Caution with sumatriptan.
Tacrine	Increases tacrine serum levels.
Terfenadine	Avoid terfenadine.
Theophylline	Increases serum levels of theophylline.
Thioridazine	Avoid thioridazine; produces dose-related QTc interval prolongation.
Tricyclic antidepressants	Caution with TCAs.
Tryptophan	Caution with tryptophan.
Warfarin	Increases serum levels of warfarin.

Paroxetine Hydrochloride (Paxil, Paxil CR)

Alcohol	Avoid alcohol.
Anticoagulants, oral	Increased risk of bleeding with oral anticoagulants.
Aspirin	Increased risk of bleeding with aspirin.
Atomoxetine	May increase levels of atomoxetine; dosage adjustment of atomoxetine may be necessary and initiate atomoxetine at reduced dose.
Cimetidine	Caution with cimetidine.
CYP2D6 inhibitors	Caution with drugs that inhibit CYP2D6 (eg, quinidine).
CYP2D6 metabolized drugs	Caution with drugs metabolized by CYP2D6 (eg, antidepressants, phenothiazines, Type 1C antiarrhythmics).
Digoxin	Caution with digoxin.
Diuretics	Caution with diuretics.
Lithium	Caution with lithium.
NSAIDs	Increased risk of bleeding with NSAIDs.
Phenobarbital	Caution with phenobarbital.
Phenytoin	Caution with phenytoin.
Plasma-bound drugs	May shift concentrations with plasma-bound drugs.

Table 18.2: DRUG INTERACTIONS FOR PSYCHOACTIVE DRUGS *(cont.)*

OBSESSIVE-COMPULSIVE DISORDER AGENTS *(cont.)*

Paroxetine Hydrochloride (Paxil, Paxil CR) *(cont.)*

Procyclidine	Reduce procyclidine dose if anticholinergic effects occur.
Risperidone	May increase levels of risperidone.
Sumatriptan	Rare reports of weakness, hyperreflexia, incoordination with an SSRI and sumatriptan.
Tricyclic antidepressants	May inhibit metabolism of TCAs. Caution with TCAs.
Theophylline	Monitor theophylline.
Tryptophan	Avoid tryptophan.
Warfarin	Caution with warfarin.

Paroxetine Mesylate (Pexeva)

Alcohol	Avoid alcohol.
Anticoagulants, oral	Increased risk of bleeding with oral anticoagulants.
Aspirin	Increased risk of bleeding with aspirin.
Cimetidine	Caution with cimetidine.
CYP2D6 metabolized drugs	Caution with drugs metabolized by CYP2D6 (eg, antidepressants, phenothiazines, Type 1C antiarrhythmics).
Digoxin	Caution with digoxin.
Diuretics	Caution with diuretics.
Lithium	Caution with lithium.
MAOI therapy	Avoid within 14 days of MAOI therapy.
NSAIDs	Increased risk of bleeding with NSAIDs.
Phenobarbital	Caution with phenobarbital.
Phenytoin	Caution with phenytoin.
Plasma-bound drugs	May shift concentrations with plasma-bound drugs.
Procyclidine	Reduce procyclidine dose if anticholinergic effects occur.
Quinidine	Caution with quinidine.
Sumatriptan	Rare reports of weakness, hyperreflexia, incoordination with an SSRI and sumatriptan.
Theophylline	Monitor theophylline.
Thioridazine	Avoid thioridazine.
Tricyclic antidepressants	May inhibit metabolism of TCAs.

OBSESSIVE-COMPULSIVE DISORDER AGENTS *(cont.)*

Paroxetine Mesylate (Pexeva) *(cont.)*

Tryptophan	Avoid tryptophan.
Warfarin	Caution with warfarin.

Sertraline Hydrochloride (Zoloft)

Alcohol	Avoid with alcohol.
Cimetidine	Increased levels with cimetidine.
Cisapride	May induce metabolism of cisapride.
CNS drugs	Caution with CNS drugs (eg, diazepam).
CYP2D6 metabolized drugs	May potentiate drugs metabolized by CYP2D6 (eg, tricyclic antidepressants, Type 1C antiarrhythmics).
Hemostasis-interfering drugs	Caution with drugs that interfere with hemostasis (eg, nonselective NSAIDs, aspirin, warfarin) due to increased risk of bleeding.
Lithium	Monitor lithium.
MAOIs	Avoid with MAOIs.
OTC products	Caution with OTC products.
Pimozide	Avoid with pimozide.
Plasma protein-bound drugs	May shift concentrations with plasma protein-bound drugs (eg, warfarin, digitoxin).
Sumatriptan	Rare reports of weakness, hyperreflexia, incoordination with an SSRI and sumatriptan.
Tolbutamide	Decreases clearance of tolbutamide.
Tricyclic antidepressants	Caution with TCAs; may need dose adjustment.
Warfarin	Monitor PT with warfarin.

Chapter 19

Hematologic Drugs

Angelo J. Mariotti, D.D.S., Ph.D.

Hematologic disturbances involve a wide variety of diseases that affect erythrocyte production (anemia or erythrocytosis), leukocytes (leukopenia or leukocytosis), platelets (thrombocytopenia or thrombocytosis), homeostasis (hemorrhage) and normal growth of the lymphoreticular system. Because various drugs, including hormones, growth factors, vitamins and minerals, can directly or indirectly influence the blood as well as blood-forming organs, the treatment of hematologic disorders should always be directed to the specific cause of the disorder; accordingly, proper testing is an important factor in diagnosing the hematologic disturbance.

range of hemoglobin is 14 mg/dL-18 mg/dL and the normal hematocrit is 42%-52%. For adult females, the normal range of hemoglobin is 12 mg/dL-16 mg/dL and the normal hematocrit range is 37%-47%. Laboratory values falling below these ranges may indicate anemia.

See Tables 19.1 and 19.2 for general information on antianemic agents.

Pharmacology

Iron supplements provide adequate amounts of iron necessary for erythropoeisis and increased oxygen transport capacity in the blood. Epoetin alfa induces erythropoeisis by stimulating erythroid progenitor cells to divide and differentiate into mature red blood cells.

Antianemic Agents

Special Dental Considerations

Clinical signs of iron toxicity sometimes include bluish-colored lips, fingernails or palms of hands.

Drug Interactions of Dental Interest

Use of iron supplements reduces the absorption of tetracyclines.

Laboratory Value Alterations

The normal daily recommended intake of elemental iron for adolescent and adult males is 10 mg; for nonpregnant adolescent and adult females, the amount ranges from 10 to 15 mg. Common methods to ascertain iron levels in the human body usually measure iron indirectly via hemoglobin levels or hematocrits. For adult males, the normal

Anticoagulant Agents

Special Dental Considerations

Early signs of overdose include bleeding from noninflamed gingivae on brushing or unexplained bruising on skin or in the mouth. In addition, the patient may exhibit purplish areas on the skin, unprovoked nosebleeds, prolonged and intense bleeding from minor cuts or wounds, or all of these. There is some controversy about whether patients receiving therapeutic levels of continuous anticoagulant therapy need to be removed from drug therapy before undergoing dental treatment (such as root planing or extractions). Although sound reasons exist to continue anticoagulation therapy during dental treatment, there also is a risk of hemorrhage in patients who are at therapeutic levels of anticoagulation. Generally, a patient who is taking anticoagulants and has an international normalized ratio (INR) of less than 3.0 is considered safe in undergoing scaling and root planing. Nonetheless, as the risk of localized bleeding after dental procedures (such as scaling, root planing and surgical procedures) can increase in a patient who is taking anticoagulants, the dentist must consult with the patient's physician to determine whether temporary reduction or withdrawal of the drug is advisable.

Drug Interactions of Dental Interest

All drug interactions affecting anticoagulants have not been identified; therefore, monitoring INR is recommended when any drug is added to or withdrawn from a patient's regimen.

Special Patients

Women of childbearing age should take additional nonhormonal precautions to prevent pregnancy when using anticoagulant agents. Anticoagulant use is not recommended during pregnancy or labor and delivery.

See Tables 19.1 and 19.2 for general information on anticoagulant agents.

Pharmacology

These agents inhibit vitamin K γ-carboxylation of procoagulation factors II, VII, IX and X in the liver. Heparin potentiates the effects of antithrombin III and neutralizes thrombin.

Antidotes

Special Dental Considerations

In most cases, patients who receive folinic acid are suffering from toxicity (symptoms such as gastrointestinal bleeding and thrombocytopenia) owing to methotrexate, pyrimethamine or trimethoprim therapy for a neoplasm.

See Tables 19.1 and 19.2 for general information on the antidote leucovorin.

Pharmacology

The principal use of leucovorin is to circumvent the actions of dihydrofolate reductase inhibitors.

Antifibrinolytic Agent

Special Dental Considerations

Aminocaproic acid has been used for postsurgical hemorrhage after oral surgical procedures. See Chapter 4 for further discussion of this and other agents that modify blood coagulation.

Drug Interactions of Dental Interest

Aminocaproic acid and drugs containing estrogen may increase thrombus formation.

Special Patients

In women using oral contraceptives, concurrent use of aminocaproic acid increases the chance of thrombus formation.

See Tables 19.1 and 19.2 for general information on the antifibrinolytic agent aminocaproic acid.

Pharmacology

This agent inhibits the activation of plasminogen.

Antithrombotic Agents

Special Dental Considerations

As increased risk of localized bleeding can occur after dental procedures (such as scaling, root planing and surgical procedures), the dentist should consider consulting the patient's physician to determine whether temporary reduction or withdrawal of the drug is advisable. It is recommended that these drugs be discontinued 10-14 days before any dental surgery. Ticlopidine also may induce neutropenia, leading to microbial infections, delayed healing and gingival bleeding. Dental work should be delayed if severe neutropenia occurs.

Drug Interactions of Dental Interest
There are additive effects of dipyridamole with aspirin on platelet aggregation. Therefore, there is a risk of increased bleeding when these agents are used with aspirin or nonsteroidal anti-inflammatory drugs (NSAIDs).

Laboratory Value Alterations
Blood pressure and bleeding times should be monitored. Normal bleeding times range between 3 and 10 minutes, depending on the method used to determine bleeding times. Normal neutrophil levels are 3,000-7,000/cm³.

See Tables 19.1 and 19.2 for general information on antithrombotic agents.

Pharmacology
These agents either decrease or increase platelet aggregation.

Nutritional Supplements

Special Dental Considerations
Anemic patients may exhibit pallor in the mouth. Cyanocobalamin and folic acid are dietary supplements used to treat anemia.

Drug Interactions of Dental Interest
Antibiotics can interfere with the assay of serum vitamin B_{12} concentrations or serum folic acid concentrations. Sulfonamides will inhibit the absorption of folate.

See Tables 19.1 and 19.2 for general information on nutritional supplements.

Pharmacology
These supplements provide adequate amounts of vitamin K or folic acid to prevent anemia.

Thrombolytic Agents

Special Dental Considerations
These agents are used intensively for short periods in a hospital setting; therefore, drug interactions are not normally observed in a dental office.

Drug Interactions of Dental Interest
Antibiotics (cefamandole, cefoperazone, cefotetan), aspirin and NSAIDs may increase the risk of bleeding when used in conjunction with thrombolytic agents.

See Tables 19.1 and 19.2 for general information on thrombolytic agents.

Pharmacology
These agents activate the endogenous fibrinolytic system by converting plasminogen to plasmin.

Adverse Effects, Precautions and Contraindications

Dental care professionals should be aware of the possible adverse effects of hematologic drugs, as well as precautions and contraindications for their use (Table 19.1).

Suggested Readings

Johnson BS. Antianemic and hematopoietic stimulating drugs. In: Pharmacology and Therapeutics for Dentistry. 5th ed. Yagiela JA, Dowd FJ, Neidle EA (eds). Elsevier Mosby, St. Louis, 2004, pp. 483-502.

Johnson BS. Procoagulant, anticoagulant and thrombolytic drugs. In: Pharmacology and Therapeutics for Dentistry. 5th ed. Yagiela JA, Dowd FJ, Neidle EA (eds). Elsevier Mosby, St. Louis, 2004, pp. 503-27.

Mariotti A. Laboratory testing of patients for systemic conditions in periodontal practice. Periodontol 2000. 2004;34:84-108.

O'Donnell M, Kearon C. Perioperative management of oral coagulation. Clin Geriatr Med 2006;22:199-213.

Stern R, Karlis V, Kinney L, Glickman R. Using the international normalized ratio to standardize prothrombin time. JADA 1997;128:1121-2.

Wahl MJ. Myths of dental surgery in patients receiving anticoagulant therapy. JADA 2000;131:77-81.

Table 19.1: PRESCRIBING INFORMATION FOR HEMATOLOGIC DRUGS

NAME	FORM/ STRENGTH	DOSAGE	WARNINGS/PRECAUTIONS & CONTRAINDICATIONS	ADVERSE EFFECTS†
ANTIANEMIC AGENTS				
Darbepoetin Alfa (Aranesp)	**Inj: Syringe:** 0.025mg/0.42mL, 0.04mg/0.4mL, 0.06mg/0.3mL, 0.1mg/0.5mL, 0.15mg/0.3mL, 0.2mg/0.4mL, 0.3mg/0.6mL, 0.5mg/mL; **SDV:** 0.025mg/mL, 0.04mg/mL, 0.06mg/mL, 0.1mg/ mL, 0.15mg/ 0.75mL, 0.2mg/mL, 0.3mg/mL	***Adults:* CRF: Initial:** 0.45mcg/kg IV/SC weekly. **Conversion from Epoetin Alfa:** Base dose on weekly epoetin dose. Give once weekly if receiving epoetin 2-3x/week. Give every 2 weeks if receiving epoetin once weekly. (See labeling for more informatioln). **Titrate:** Adjust to target Hgb <12g/dL. If Hgb increases >1g/dL in a 2-week period or is approaching 12g/dL, decrease dose by 25%. If Hgb continues to increase, hold dose until Hgb begins to decrease, and reinitiate at 25% below previous dose. Do not increase dose more than once monthly. **Malignancy: Initial:** 2.25mcg/kg SC weekly. **Titrate:** Increase to 4.5mcg/kg if Hgb increases <1g/dL after 6 weeks of therapy. If Hgb increases by more than 1g/dL in a 2-week period or if Hgb >12g/dL, decrease dose by 25%. If Hgb >13g/dL, hold dose until Hgb falls to 12g/dL and reinitiate at 25% below previous dose.	**W/P:** Pure red cell aplasia and severe anemia (with or without other cytopenias) may occur. Due to increased Hgb, increased risk of cardiovascular events including death may occur. Control BP before therapy. Seizures reported. Increased risk of thrombotic events. Pure red cell aplasia reported; discontinue if this occurs. Evaluate etiology if lac k/loss of response occurs. Permanently discontinue if serious allergic reaction occurs. Monitor renal function, fluid, and electrolytes. Albumin solution carries risk of transmission of viral diseases. May need interval of 2-6 weeks between dose adjustment and response. Monitor Hgb weekly until stabilized and maintenance dose is established, and for at least 4 weeks after dosage change. Monitor iron status before and during therapy. Increases RBCs and decreases plasma volume. **Contra:** Uncontrolled HTN. **P/N:** Category C, caution in nursing.	Thrombic events, infection, myalgia, HTN, hypotension, headache, diarrhea, fatigue, edema, nausea, vomiting, fever, dyspnea.
Epoetin Alfa (Epogen, Procrit)	**(Epogen) Inj:** 2000U/mL, 3000U/ mL, 4000U/mL, 10,000U/mL, 20,000U/mL, 40,000U/mL; **(Procrit) Inj:** 2000U/mL, 3000U/ mL, 4000U/mL, 10,000U/mL, 20,000U/mL, 40,000U/mL	**(Epogen) *Adults:* CRF: Initial:** 50-100U/kg IV/SC 3x/week. IV is preferred route in dialysis patients. Reduce dose when Hct approaches 36% or increase by >4 points in any 2 week period. Increase dose if Hct does not increase by 5-6 points after 8 weeks of therapy and Hct is below target range. **Maint:** Individually titrate. **Zidovudine-Treated HIV Patients:** Serum erythropoietin ≤500mU/mL and zidovudine dose ≤4200mg/week: 100U/kg IV/SC 3x/week for 8 weeks. **Max:** 300U/kg 3x/week. **Maint:** Individualize dose to maintain Hct within 30%-36%. **Chemotherapy-Induced Anemia: Initial:** 150U/kg SC 3x/week. **Titrate:** May increase to 300U/kg 3x/week after 8 weeks of therapy. **Surgery:** 300U/kg/day SC for 10 days before, on day of, and 4 days after surgery; or 600U/kg SC once weekly on 21, 14, and 7 days before surgery, and a 4th dose on day of surgery. ***Pediatrics:* CRF: Initial:** 50U/kg 3x/week IV/SC. Reduce dose when Hct approaches 36% or increase by >4 points in any 2 week period. Increase dose if Hct does not increase by 5-6 points after 8 weeks of therapy and Hct is below target range. **Maint:** Individually titrate. **(Procrit) *Adults:* CRF: Initial:** 50-100U/kg IV/SC 3x/week. IV is preferred route in dialysis patients. **Titrate:** Reduce if Hgb approaches 12g/dL or if Hgb increases >1g/dL in any 2-week period. Increase when Hgb does not increase by 2g/dL after 8 weeks of therapy and Hgb is below	**W/P:** Pure red cell aplasia and severe anemia (without or without other cytopenias) may occur. Caution with porphyria, HTN, or history of seizures. Evaluate iron stores before and during therapy; most patients need iron supplementation. Monitor Hgb, BP, iron levels, serum chemistry, and CBC. Menses may resume. Multidose formulation contains benzyl alcohol. **Contra:** Uncontrolled HTN. Hypersensitivity to mammalian cell-derived products and albumin (human). **P/N:** Category C, caution in nursing.	HTN, headache, fatigue, arthralgias, nausea, vomiting, diarrhea, edema, rash, pyrexia, clotted vascular access, respiratory congestion, dyspnea, asthenia, dizziness, seizures, thrombotic events.

*Scored.   †Bold entries denote special dental considerations.

NAME	FORM/ STRENGTH	DOSAGE	WARNINGS/PRECAUTIONS & CONTRAINDICATIONS	ADVERSE EFFECTS†
Epoetin Alfa *(cont.)*		target range (10-12g/dL). **Maint:** Individually titrate. **Zidovudine-Treated HIV Patients:** If serum erythropoietin levels ≤500mU/mL and zidovudine ≤4200mg/week give 100U/kg IV/SC 3x/week for 8 weeks. **Titrate:** Increase by 50-100U/kg 3x/week after 8 weeks if necessary. **Maint:** If Hgb >13g/dL, discontinue until Hgb <12g/dL, then reduce dose by 25% when resume therapy. **Max:** 300U/kg 3x/week. **Chemotherapy Induced Anemia: Initial:** 150U/kg SC 3x/week. **Titrate:** Reduce by 25% when Hgb approaches 12g/dL or Hgb increases >1g/dL in any 2-week period. If Hgb >13g/dL, withhold until Hgb <12g/dL then restart at 25% below previous dose. May increase to 300U/kg 3x/week if no response after 8 weeks of therapy. **Max:** 300U/kg 3x/week. **Weekly Dosing:** 40,000U SC weekly. **Titrate:** If Hgb not increased by ≥1g/dL after 4 weeks, increase to 60,000U weekly. If Hgb >13g/dL, withhold until Hgb <12g/dL then restart with 25% dose reduction. Reduce dose by 25% if very rapid Hgb response (eg, increase >1g/dL in any 2-week period. **Max:** 60,000U weekly. **Surgery:** 300U/kg/day SC for 10 days before surgery, on surgery day, and 4 days post-op or 600U/kg SC once weekly on 21, 14, and 7 days before surgery and a 4th dose on surgery day, with adequate iron supplement. ***Pediatrics:*** **CRF: Initial:** 50U/kg 3x/week IV/SC. **Titrate:** Reduce if Hgb approaches 12g/dL or if Hgb increases by >1g/dL in any 2-week period. Increase if Hgb does not increase by 2g/dL after 8 weeks of therapy and Hgb is below target range (10-12g/dL). **Maint:** Individually titrate.		
Oprelvekin (Neumega)	**Inj:** 5mg	***Adults:*** 50mcg/kg qd SC. Initiate 6-24 hrs after chemotherapy completion. Monitor platelets to assess optimal duration of therapy. Continue therapy until post-nadir platelets ≥50,000 cells/mcL. Discontinue at least 2 days before next chemotherapy cycle. **Max:** 21 days of therapy.	**W/P:** Fluid retention reported; caution in CHF, pleural or pericardial effusions, and patients receiving aggressive hydration. Monitor fluid and electrolyte balance with chronic diuretic therapy, renal dysfunction. Permanently discontinue if significant allergic reactions occur. Moderate decreases in Hgb, Hct, and RBCs; transient, mild visual disturbances; papilledema; and rash reported. Caution with history of atrial arrhythmias. May develop antibodies to therapy. Obtain CBC before therapy, then regularly. Monitor platelets during expected nadir time, and until adequate recovery. **P/N:** Category C, not for use in nursing.	Edema, atrial fibrillation/ flutter, **oral moniliasis**, tachycardia, palpitations, dyspnea, pleural effusion, conjunctival injection, asthenia, pain, chills, abdominal pain, infection, anorexia, constipation, alopecia, myalgia, dyspepsia, ecchymosis.

ANTICOAGULANT AGENTS

NAME	FORM/ STRENGTH	DOSAGE	WARNINGS/PRECAUTIONS & CONTRAINDICATIONS	ADVERSE EFFECTS†
Dalteparin Sodium (Fragmin)	**Inj: Syringe:** 2500 IU/0.2mL, 5000 IU/0.2mL, 7500 IU/0.3mL, 10,000 IU/mL; **Multidose:**	***Adults:*** Administer SC. **Unstable Angina/Non-Q-Wave MI:** 120 IU/kg up to 10,000 IU q12h with ASA (75-165mg/day) for 5-8 days. **Hip Surgery: Initial (if start 2 hrs pre-op):** 2500 IU	**Risk of paralysis by spinal/epidural hematoma with neuraxial anesthesia or spinal puncture. Increased risk with indwelling epidural catheters for analgesia, drugs affecting hemostasis**	Hemorrhage, injection site pain, allergic reactions, thrombocytopenia.

Table 19.1: PRESCRIBING INFORMATION FOR HEMATOLOGIC DRUGS *(cont.)*

NAME	FORM/ STRENGTH	DOSAGE	WARNINGS/PRECAUTIONS & CONTRAINDICATIONS	ADVERSE EFFECTS†
ANTICOAGULANT AGENTS *(cont.)*				
Dalteparin Sodium *(cont.)*	25,000 IU/mL [3.8mL], 10,000 IU/mL [9.5mL]	pre-op, then 2500 IU 4-8 hrs post-op. **Initial (if start 10-14 hrs pre-op):** 5000 IU 10-14 hrs pre-op, then 5000 IU 4-8 hrs post-op. **Maint (for either initial dose):** 5000 IU SC qd for 5-10 days post-op (up to 14 days). **Abdominal Surgery:** 2500 IU 1-2 hrs pre-op, then 2500 IU qd for 5-10 days post-op. **Abdominal Surgery with High Risk:** 5000 IU the evening before surgery, then 5000 IU qd for 5-10 days post-op. **Abdominal Surgery with Malignancy: Initial:** 2500 IU 1-2 hrs pre-op, then 2500 IU 12 hrs later. **Maint:** 5000 IU qd for 5-10 days post-op. **Severely Restricted Mobility During Acute Illness:** 5000 IU qd for 12-14 days.	**(eg, NSAIDs, platelet inhibitors, anticoagulants), and traumatic or repeated epidural or spinal puncture. W/P:** Not for IM injection. Cannot use interchangeably unit for unit with heparin or other low molecular weight heparins. Extreme caution with HIT, conditions with increased risk of hemorrhage (eg, bacterial endocarditis, hemorrhagic stroke, etc). Hemorrhage, thrombocytopenia, HIT may occur. Caution with bleeding diathesis, platelet defects, severe hepatic/kidney dysfunction, hypertensive or diabetic retinopathy, recent GI bleeding or in elderly with low body weight (<45kg) and predisposed to decreased renal function. Discontinue if thromboembolic event occurs. Perform periodic CBC, platelets, stool occult blood test. Multiple dose vial contains benzyl alcohol. **Contra:** Heparin or pork allergy, regional anesthesia with unstable angina or non-Q-wave MI, active major bleeding, thrombocytopenia with a positive in vitro test for anti-platelet antibody. **P/N:** Category B, caution in nursing.	
Enoxaparin Sodium (Lovenox)	**Inj: Multi-Dose Vial:** 300mg/3mL; **Syringe:** 30mg/0.3mL, 40mg/0.4mL, 60mg/0.6mL, 80mg/0.8mL, 100mg/mL, 120mg/0.8mL, 150mg/mL	*Adults:* **Hip/Knee Surgery:** 30mg SC q12h, starting 12-24 hrs post-op, for 7-10 days (up to 14 days) or 40mg SC qd for hip surgery for 3 weeks. **Abdominal Surgery:** 40mg SC qd, starting 2 hrs pre-op, for 7-10 days (up to 14 days). **DVT with or without PE treatment: (inpatient/outpatient)** 1mg/kg SC q12h or (inpatient) 1.5mg/kg qd with warfarin (start within 72 hrs) for 7 days (up to 17 days). **Acute Illness:** 40mg SC qd for 6-11 days (up to 14 days). **Unstable Angina/Non-Q-Wave MI:** 1mg/kg SC q12h with 100-325mg/day of ASA for 2-8 days (up to 12.5 days). **CrCl <30mL/min: Surgery/Acute Illness:** 30mg SC qd. **DVT with or without PE treatment (inpatient/outpatient)/ Unstable Angina/Non-Q-Wave MI:** 1mg/kg SC qd.	**Risk of paralysis by spinal/epidural hematoma with neuraxial anesthesia or spinal puncture. Increased risk with indwelling epidural catheters for analgesia, drugs affecting hemostasis (eg, NSAIDs, platelet inhibitors, anticoagulants), and traumatic or repeated epidural or spinal puncture. W/P:** Not for IM injection. Cannot use interchangeably unit for unit with heparin or other low molecular weight heparins. Extreme caution with HIT, conditions with an increased risk of hemorrhage (eg, bacterial endocarditis, hemorrhagic stroke, etc). Major hemorrhages (eg, retroperitoneal, intracranial), thrombocytopenia reported. Discontinue if platelets <100,000/mm³. Perform periodic CBC, platelets, and stool occult blood test. Caution with bleeding diathesis, uncontrolled arterial HTN, recent GI ulceration, diabetic retinopathy, hemorrhage. Delayed elimination with elderly or in renal dysfunction. Monitor elderly with low body weight (<45 kg) and predisposition to decreased renal function. Higher risk of thromboembolism in pregnant women with prosthetic heart valves. Not for thromboprophylaxis in prosthetic heart valve patients. **Contra:** Heparin or pork allergy, active major bleeding, thrombocytopenia with a positive *in vitro* test for anti-platelet antibody. Hypersensitivity to benzyl alcohol (multi-dose formulation). **P/N:** Category B, caution in nursing.	Hemorrhage, thrombocytopenia, local reactions (ecchymosis, erythema), anemia.

*Scored.   †Bold entries denote special dental considerations.

NAME	FORM/ STRENGTH	DOSAGE	WARNINGS/PRECAUTIONS & CONTRAINDICATIONS	ADVERSE EFFECTS†
Heparin Sodium	**Inj:** 1000U/mL, 2500U/mL, 5000U/ mL, 7500U/mL, 10,000U/mL	***Adults:*** Based on 68kg: **Initial:** 5000U IV, then 10,000-20,000U SC. **Maint:** 8000-10,000U q8h or 15,000-20,000U q12h. **Intermittent IV Injection: Initial:** 10,000U. **Maint:** 5000-10,000U q4-6h. **Continuous IV Infusion: Initial:** 5000U. **Maint:** 20,000-40,000U/24 hours. Adjust to coagulation test results. See labeling for details in specific disease states. ***Pediatrics:*** **Initial:** 50U/kg IV drip. **Maint:** 100U/kg IV drip q4h or 20,000U/m²/24 hrs continuously.	**W/P:** Not for IM use. Hemorrhage can occur at any site; caution with increased danger of hemorrhage (severe HTN, bacterial endocarditis, surgery, etc.). Monitor blood coagulation tests frequently. Thrombocytopenia reported; discontinue if platelets <100,000mm³ or if recurrent thrombosis develops. Contains benzyl alcohol. White-clot syndrome reported. Monitor platelets, Hct, and occult blood in the stool. Increased heparin resistance with fever, thrombosis, thrombophlebitis, infections with thrombosing tendencies, MI, cancer, and post-op. Higher bleeding incidence in women >60 yrs. **Contra:** Severe thrombocytopenia, if cannot perform appropriate blood-coagulation tests (with full-dose heparin), uncontrollable active bleeding state (except in DIC). **P/N:** Category C, safe in nursing.	Hemorrhage, local irritation, erythema, mild pain, hematoma, chills, fever, urticaria.
Tinzaparin Sodium (Innohep)	**Inj:** 20,000 anti-Xa IU/mL	***Adults:*** 175 anti-Xa IU/kg SC qd for at least 6 days and until anticoagulated with warfarin (INR is at least 2 for 2 days). Begin warfarin within 1-3 days of therapy.	**Risk of paralysis by spinal/epidural hematoma with neuraxial anesthesia or spinal puncture. Increased risk with indwelling epidural catheters for analgesia, drugs affecting hemostasis (eg, NSAIDs, platelet inhibitors, anticoagulants), and traumatic or repeated epidural or spinal puncture. W/P:** Not for IM injection. Cannot use interchangeably unit for unit with heparin or other low molecular weight heparins. Extreme caution in conditions with an increased risk of hemorrhage (eg, bacterial endocarditis, hemorrhagic stroke, etc). Bleeding can occur at any site during therapy. Discontinue if severe hemorrhage occurs. Perform periodic CBC, platelets, and stool occult blood test. Asymptomatic increase in AST and ALT. Priapism reported (rare). Thrombocytopenia can occur; discontinue if platelets <100,000/mm³. Multiple dose vial contains benzyl alcohol. Contains sodium metabisulfite. Caution with bleeding diathesis, uncontrolled arterial HTN, recent GI ulceration, diabetic retinopathy, hemorrhage. Reduced elimination with elderly or in renal dysfunction; use with caution. **Contra:** Heparin, sulfite, benzoyl alcohol, or pork allergy. Active major bleeding, with or history of heparin-induced thrombocytopenia (HIT). **P/N:** Category B, caution use in nursing.	Hemorrhage, thrombocytopenia, elevated LFTs, local reactions (ecchymosis, hematoma), hypersensitivity reactions.
Warfarin Sodium (Coumadin)	**Inj:** 5mg; **Tab:** 1mg*, 2mg*, 2.5mg*, 3mg*, 4mg*, 5mg*, 6mg*, 7.5mg*, 10mg*	***Adults:*** ≥18 yrs: Adjust dose based on PT/INR. Give IV as alternate to PO. **Initial:** 2-5mg qd. **Usual:** 2-10mg qd. **Venous Thromboembolism (including pulmonary embolism):** INR 2-3. **Atrial Fibrillation:** INR 2-3. **Post-MI:** Initiate 2-4 weeks post-infarct and maintain INR 2.5-3.5. **Mechanical/Bioprosthetic Heart Valve:** INR 2-3 for 12	**W/P:** Monitor PT/INR; many endogenous and exogenous factors affect the PT/INR. Weigh benefits/risks with severe-moderate hepatic or renal insufficiency, infectious disease, intestinal flora disturbance, lactation, surgery, trauma, severe-moderate HTN, protein C deficiency, polycythemia vera, vasculitis, severe DM, indwelling catheters.	Tissue or organ hemorrhage/necrosis, paresthesia, vasculitis, fever, rash, abdominal pain, hepatic disorders, fatigue, headache, alopecia.

Table 19.1: PRESCRIBING INFORMATION FOR HEMATOLOGIC DRUGS (cont.)

NAME	FORM/ STRENGTH	DOSAGE	WARNINGS/PRECAUTIONS & CONTRAINDICATIONS	ADVERSE EFFECTS†
ANTICOAGULANT AGENTS (cont.)				
Warfarin Sodium (cont.)		weeks after valve insertion, then INR 2.5-3.5 long term.	Discontinue if tissue necrosis, systemic cholesterol microemboliza- tion ("purple toe syndrome") occurs. Caution with HIT, DVT, elderly. Warfarin resistance, allergic reactions reported. **Contra:** Hemorrhagic tendencies, blood dyscrasias, CNS surgery, ophthalmic or traumatic surgery, inadequate lab facility, threatened abortion, eclampsia, preeclampsia, major regional lumbar block anesthesia, malignant HTN, pregnancy and unsupervised senile, alcoholic or psychotic patients. Bleed- ing of GI, GU or respiratory tract, aneurysms, pericarditis and pericar- dial effusion, bacterial endocarditis, cerebrovascular hemorrhage, spinal puncture, procedures with potential for uncontrollable bleeding. **P/N:** Category X, weigh benefits/risks with nursing.	
ANTIFIBRINOLYTIC AGENT				
Aminocaproic Acid (Amicar)	**Inj:** 250mg/mL; **Syr:** 1.25g/5mL; **Tab:** 500mg*, 1000mg*	**Adults: IV:** 16-20mL (4-5g) in 250mL diluent during 1st hr, then 4mL/hr (1g) in 50mL of diluent. **PO:** 5g during 1st hr, then 5mL (syr) or 1g (tabs) per hr. Continue therapy for 8 hrs or until bleeding is controlled.	**W/P:** Avoid in hematuria of upper uri- nary tract origin due to risk of intrarenal obstruction from glomerular capillary thrombosis or clots in renal pelvis and ureters. Skeletal muscle weakness with necrosis of muscle fibers reported after prolonged therapy. Consider cardiac muscle damage with skeletal myopathy. Avoid rapid IV infusion. Thrombo- phlebitis may occur. Contains benzyl alcohol; do not administer to neonates due to risk of fatal gasping syndrome. Do not administer without a definite diagnosis of hyperfibrinolysis. **Contra:** Active intravascular clotting process, disseminated intravascular coagulation without concomitant heparin. **P/N:** Category C, caution in nursing.	Edema, headache, ana- phylactoid reactions, injection site reactions, pain, bradycardia, hypotension, abdominal pain, diarrhea, nausea, vomiting, agranulocy- tosis, increased CPK, confusion, dyspnea, pruritus, tinnitus.
ANTIHEMOPHILIC FACTOR				
Antihemo- philic Factor (Recombinant) Plasma/ Albumin-Free (Advate)		**Adults: Hemophilia A: Treatment and Prophylaxis:** Body weight (kg) X 0.5 IU/kg X factor VIII activity increase desired (%). **Mild Hemorrhage:** 10-15 IU/kg IV for one dose (20% to 30% cor- rection); may be repeated every 12-24 hours if needed. **Moderate Hemorrhage:** 15-25 IU/kg IV for one dose (30% to 50% correction); may continue with 10-15 IU/kg IV (20% to 30% correction) every 8-24 hours if needed. **Serious Hemorrhage:** 40-50 IU/kg IV (80% to 100% correction) given once; followed by 20-25 IU/kg IV (40% to 50% correc- tion) every 8-12 hours. **Surgery:** 25-50 IU/kg IV preoperatively (50% to 100% correction), postoperatively maintain Factor VIII levels at or above 30% for 2 weeks. **Dental Procedures:** 30-40 IU/kg IV (60% to 80% correction)	**W/P:** Formation of inhibitor antibodies may occur. Hemolysis may occur with administration of large doses of concentrate to patients with blood groups A, B, or AB. Reactivation of viral infections (eg, cytomegalovirus, Ep- stein-Barr) or seroconversion (hepatitis A virus, parvovirus) have occurred in a small number of patients treated with recombinant factor VIII. Transmission of viral agents (hepatitis B, hepatitis C, HIV); risk reduced with newer purification methods and minimal with recombinant formulations. **Contra:** Hypersensitivity to mouse (murine) protein (for antihemophilic factor concentrates purified via monoclonal antibody affinity chromatography); hypersensitivity to mouse, hamster, or bovine proteins (for antihemophilic	Angina, cold extremi- ties, hypotension, nau- sea, vomiting, **unusual taste**, rash, hemolytic anemia, thrombocy- topenia

*Scored.   †Bold entries denote special dental considerations.

NAME	FORM/ STRENGTH	DOSAGE	WARNINGS/PRECAUTIONS & CONTRAINDICATIONS	ADVERSE EFFECTS[†]
Antihemo- philic Factor (Recombinant) Plasma/ Albumin-Free *(cont.)*		immediately prior to procedure, readminister if necessary. **Prophylactic administration:** 7.5 IU/kg IV (15% correction) once daily or every other day. **von Willebrand disease type 1: Mild: Major Hemorrhage:** Loading dose of 40-60 IU (vWF:Rcof)/kg IV, then 40-50 IU/kg every 8-12 hours for 3 days to keep the nadir level of vWF:Rcof greater than 50%, then 40-50 IU/kg daily for a total of up to 7 days of treatment. **Moderate or Severe: Minor Hemorrhage:** 40-50 IU (vWF:RCof)/kg IV (1 or 2 doses). **Major Hemorrhage:** Loading dose of 50-75 IU (vWF:RCof)/kg, then 40-60 IU/kg every 8-12 hours for 3 days to keep the nadir level of vWF:Rcof greater than 50%, then 40-60 IU/kg daily for a total of up to 7 days of treatment. **von Willebrand Disease Type 2: Minor Hemorrhage:** 40-50 IU (vWF:RCof)/kg IV (1 or 2 doses). **Major Hemorrhage:** Loading dose of 60-80 IU (vWF:RCof)/kg, then 40-60 IU/kg every 8-12 hours for 3 days to keep the nadir level of vWF:Rcof greater than 50%, then 40-60 IU/kg daily for a total of up to 7 days of treatment. von Willebrand disease type 3: **Minor Hemorrhage:** 40-50 IU (vWF:RCof)/kg IV (1 or 2 doses). **Major Hemorrhage:** loading dose of 60-80 IU (vWF:RCof)/kg, then 40-60 international units/kg every 8-12 hours for 3 days to keep the nadir level of vWF:Rcof greater than 50%, then 40-60 international units/kg daily for a total of up to 7 days of treatment. *Pediatric:* **von Willebrand Disease Type 1: Mild: Major Hemorrhage:** Loading dose of 40-60 IU (vWF:Rcof)/kg IV, then 40-50 international units/kg every 8-12 hours for 3 days to keep the nadir level of vWF:Rcof greater than 50%, then 40-50 IU/kg daily for a total of up to 7 days of treatment. **von Willebrand Disease Type 1: Moderate or Severe: Minor Hemorrhage:** 40-50 IU (vWF:RCof)/kg IV (1 or 2 doses). **Major Hemorrhage:** loading dose of 50-75 IU (vWF:RCof)/kg, then 40-60 IU/kg every 8-12 hours for 3 days to keep the nadir level of vWF:Rcof greater than 50%, then 40-60 IU/kg daily for a total of up to 7 days of treatment. **von Willebrand Disease Type 2: Minor Hemorrhage:** 40-50 IU (vWF:RCof)/kg IV (1 or 2 doses). **Major Hemorrhage:** Loading dose of 60-80 IU (vWF:RCof)/kg, then 40-60 IU/kg every 8-12 hours for 3 days to keep the nadir level of vWF:Rcof greater than 50%, then 40-60 IU/kg daily for a total of up to 7 days of treatment. **von Willebrand Disease Type 3: Minor Hemorrhage:** 40-50 IU (vWF:RCof)/kg IV (1 or 2 doses). **Major Hemorrhage:** Loading dose of 60-80 IU (vWF:RCof)/kg, then 40-60 IU/kg every 8-12 hours	factor concentrates derived from re- combinant technology); hypersensitivity to antihemophilic factor. **P/N:** Category C, caution with nursing.	

Table 19.1: PRESCRIBING INFORMATION FOR HEMATOLOGIC DRUGS *(cont.)*

NAME	FORM/ STRENGTH	DOSAGE	WARNINGS/PRECAUTIONS & CONTRAINDICATIONS	ADVERSE EFFECTS†
ANTIHEMOPHILIC FACTOR *(cont.)*				
Antihemo-philic Factor (Recombinant) Plasma/ Albumin-Free *(cont.)*		for 3 days to keep the nadir level of vWF:Rcof greater than 50%, then 40-60 IU/kg daily for a total of up to 7 days of treatment.		
Antihemophilic Factor VIII (Recombinant) Sucrose Formulated (Helixate FS, Kogenate FS)	**Inj:** 250 IU, 500 IU, 1000 IU	***Adults:*** **Minor Hemorrhage:** 10-20 IU/kg IV; repeat if evidence of further bleeding. **Moderate-To-Major Hemorrhage/surgery (minor):** 15-30 IU/kg IV; repeat one dose at 12-24 hrs if needed. **Major to life-Threatening Hemorrhage/fractures/head Trauma: Surgery (major): Preoperative dose:** 50 IU/kg IV (verify 100% FVIII activity prior to surgery); repeat as necessary after 6-12 hrs initially, and for 10-14 days until healing is complete.	**W/P:** Development of circulating neutralizing antibodies to FVIII may occur; monitor by appropriate clinical observation and laboratory tests. Hypotension, urticaria, and chest tightness in association with hypersensitivity reported. **Contra:** Known hypersensitivity to mouse or hamster protein. **Initial:** 40-50 IU/kg IV; repeat dose 20-25 IU/kg IV q 8-12 hrs. **P/N:** Category C, safety not known in nursing.	Local injection site reactions, dizziness, rash, **unusual taste**, mild increase in BP, pruritus, depersonalization, nausea, rhinitis.
Antihemophilic Factor VIII [Recombinant] (Recombinate, Refacto)	**Inj: (Recombinate)** 250 IU, 500 IU, 1000 IU; **(Refacto)** 250 IU, 500 IU, 1000 IU, 2000 IU	***Adults:*** **Hemophilia A: Treatment and Prophylaxis:** dosage calculation, body weight (kg) X 0.5 IU/kg X factor VIII activity increase desired (%) = dose required. **Mild Hemorrhage:** 10-15 IU/kg IV for one dose (20% to 30% correction); may be repeated every 12-24 hours if needed. **Moderate Hemorrhage:** 15-25 IU/kg IV for one dose (30% to 50% correction); may continue with 10-15 IU/kg IV (20% to 30% correction) every 8-24 hours if needed. **Serious Hemorrhage:** 40-50 IU/kg IV (80% to 100% correction) given once; followed by 20-25 IU/kg IV (40% to 50% correction) every 8-12 hours. **Surgery:** 25-50 IU/kg IV preoperatively (50% to 100% correction), postoperatively maintain Factor VIII levels at or above 30% for 2 weeks. **Dental Procedures:** 30-40 IU/kg IV (60% to 80% correction) immediately prior to procedure, readminister if necessary. **Prophylactic Administration:** 7.5 international unit/kg IV (15% correction) once daily or every other day. **von Willebrand Disease Type 1: Mild: Major Hemorrhage:** Loading dose of 40-60 IU (vWF:Rcof)/kg IV, then 40-50 IU/kg every 8-12 hours for 3 days to keep the nadir level of vWF:Rcof greater than 50%, then 40-50 IU/kg daily for a total of up to 7 days of treatment. **Moderate or Severe: Minor Hemorrhage:** 40-50 IU (vWF:RCof)/kg IV (1 or 2 doses). **Major Hemorrhage:** Loading dose of 50-75 IU (vWF:RCof)/kg, then 40-60 IU/kg every 8-12 hours for 3 days to keep the nadir level of vWF:Rcof greater than 50%, then 40-60 IU/kg daily for a total of up to 7 days of treatment.	**W/P:** Hypersensitivity reactions are possible. **Contra:** Known hypersensitivity to mouse, hamster or bovine protein may be a contraindication to the use of Antihemophilic Factor (Recombinant). **P/N:** Category C, safety not known in nursing.	Headache, fever, chills, flushing, nausea, vomiting, lethargy.

*Scored.   †Bold entries denote special dental considerations.

NAME	FORM/ STRENGTH	DOSAGE	WARNINGS/PRECAUTIONS & CONTRAINDICATIONS	ADVERSE EFFECTS†
Antihemophilic Factor VIII [Recombinant] *(cont.)*		**von Willebr and Disease Type 2: Minor Hemorrhage:** 40-50 IU (vWF:RCof)/kg IV (1 or 2 doses). **Major Hemorrhage:** Loading dose of 60-80 IU (vWF: RCof)/kg, then 40-60 IU/kg every 8-12 hours for 3 days to keep the nadir level of vWF:Rcof greater than 50%, then 40-60 IU/kg daily for a total of up to 7 days of treatment. **von Willebrand Disease Type 3: Minor Hemorrhage:** 40-50 IU (vWF:RCof)/kg IV (1 or 2 doses). **Major Hemorrhage:** Loading dose of 60-80 IU (vWF:RCof)/kg, then 40-60 IU/kg every 8-12 hours for 3 days to keep the nadir level of vWF: Rcof greater than 50%, then 40-60 IU/kg daily for a total of up to 7 days of treatment. ***Pediatric:* von Willebrand Disease Type 1: Mild: Major Hemorrhage:** Loading dose of 40-60 IU (vWF:Rcof)/kg IV, then 40-50 IU/kg every 8-12 hours for 3 days to keep the nadir level of vWF:Rcof greater than 50%, then 40-50 IU/kg daily for a total of up to 7 days of treatment. **Moderate or Severe: Minor Hemorrhage:** 40-50 IU (vWF:RCof)/kg IV (1 or 2 doses). **Major Hemorrhage:** Loading dose of 50-75 IU (vWF:RCof)/kg, then 40-60 IU/kg every 8-12 hours for 3 days to keep the nadir level of vWF: Rcof greater than 50%, then 40-60 IU/kg daily for a total of up to 7 days of treatment. **von Willebrand Disease Type 2: Minor Hemorrhage:** 40-50 IU (vWF:RCof)/kg IV (1 or 2 doses) **Major Hemorrhage:** Loading dose of 60-80 IU (vWF:RCof)/kg, then 40-60 IU/kg every 8-12 hours for 3 days to keep the nadir level of vWF:Rcof greater than 50%, then 40-60 IU/kg daily for a total of up to 7 days of treatment. **von Willebrand Disease Type 3: Minor Hemorrhage:** 40-50 IU (vWF:RCof)/kg IV (1 or 2 doses). **Major Hemorrhage:** Loading dose of 60-80 IU (vWF: RCof)/kg, then 40-60 IU/kg every 8-12 hours for 3 days to keep the nadir level of vWF: Rcof greater than 50%, then 40-60 IU/kg daily for a total of up to 7 days of treatment.		
Antihemo- philic Factor VIII: C Human (Hemofil-M, Monarc-M)		***Adults:* Hemophilia A: Treatment and Prophylaxis:** dosage calculation, body weight (kg) X 0.5 IU/kg X factor VIII activity increase desired (%) = dose required. **Mild Hemorrhage:** 10-15 IU/kg IV for one dose (20% to 30% correction); may be repeated every 12-24 hours if needed. **Moderate Hemorrhage:** 15-25 IU/kg IV for one dose (30% to 50% correction); may continue with 10-15 IU/kg IV (20% to 30% correction) every 8-24 hours if needed. **Serious Hemorrhage:** 40-50 IU/kg IV (80% to 100% correction)	**W/P:** Hypersensitivity reactions are possible. **Contra:** Known hypersensitiv- ity to mouse protein. **P/N:** Category C, safety not known in nursing.	Nausea, fever, chills, urticaria, **disorder of taste**.

Table 19.1: PRESCRIBING INFORMATION FOR HEMATOLOGIC DRUGS *(cont.)*

NAME	FORM/STRENGTH	DOSAGE	WARNINGS/PRECAUTIONS & CONTRAINDICATIONS	ADVERSE EFFECTS†
ANTIHEMOPHILIC FACTOR *(cont.)*				
Antihemo-philic Factor VIII:C Human *(cont.)*		given once; followed by 20-25 IU/kg IV (40% to 50% correction) every 8-12 hours. **Surgery:** 25-50 IU/kg IV preoperatively (50% to 100% correction), postoperatively maintain Factor VIII levels at or above 30% for 2 weeks. **Dental Procedures:** 30-40 IU/kg IV (60% to 80% correction) immediately prior to procedure, readminister if necessary. **Prophylactic Administration:** 7.5 IU/kg IV (15% correction) once daily or every other day. **von Willebrand Disease Type 1: Mild: Major Hemorrhage:** Loading dose of 40-60 IU (vWF:Rcof)/kg IV, then 40-50 IU/kg every 8-12 hours for Rcof greater than 50%, then 40-50 IU/kg daily for a total of up to 7 days of treatment. **Moderate or Severe: Minor Hemorrhage:** 40-50 IU (vWF:RCof)/kg IV (1 or 2 doses). **Major Hemorrhage:** Loading dose of 50-75 IU (vWF:RCof)/kg, then 40-60 IU/kg every 8-12 hours for 3 days to keep the nadir level of vWF:Rcof greater than 50%, then 40-60 IU/kg daily for a total of up to 7 days of treatment. **von Willebrand Disease Type 2: Minor Hemorrhage:** 40-50 IU (vWF:RCof)/kg IV (1 or 2 doses) **Major Hemorrhage:** Loading dose of 60-80 IU (vWF:RCof)/kg, then 40-60 IU/kg every 8-12 hours for 3 days to keep the nadir level of vWF:Rcof greater than 50%, then 40-60 IU/kg daily for a total of up to 7 days of treatment. **von Willebrand Disease Type 3: Minor Hemorrhage:** 40-50 IU (vWF:RCof)/kg IV (1 or 2 doses). **Major Hemorrhage:** Loading dose of 60-80 IU (vWF:RCof)/kg, then 40-60 IU/kg every 8-12 hours for 3 days to keep the nadir level of vWF.Rcof greater than 50%, then 40-60 IU/kg daily for a total of up to 7 days of treatment. 3 days to keep the nadir level of vWF. *Pediatric:* **von Willebrand Disease Type 1: Mild:** Major Hemorrhage: Loading dose of 40-60 IU (vWF: Rcof)/kg IV, then 40-50 IU/kg every 8-12 hours for 3 days to keep the nadir level of vWF:Rcof greater than 50%, then 40-50 IU/kg daily for a total of up to 7 days of treatment. **Moderate or Severe: Minor Hemorrhage:** 40-50 IU (vWF:RCof)/kg IV (1 or 2 doses). **Major Hemorrhage:** Loading dose of 50-75 IU (vWF:RCof)/kg, then 40-60 IU/kg every 8-12 hours for 3 days to keep the nadir level of vWF:Rcof greater than 50%, then 40-60 IU/kg daily for a total of up to 7 days of treatment. **von Willebrand Disease Type 2: Minor Hemorrhage:** 40-50 IU (vWF: RCof)/kg IV (1 or 2 doses). **Major Hemorrhage:** Loading dose of 60-80 IU (vWF:RCof)/kg, then 40-60 IU/kg every 8-12 hours for 3 days to keep the		

*Scored.   †Bold entries denote special dental considerations.

NAME	FORM/ STRENGTH	DOSAGE	WARNINGS/PRECAUTIONS & CONTRAINDICATIONS	ADVERSE EFFECTS†
Antihemo- philic Factor VIII:C Human *(cont.)*		nadir level of vWF:Rcof greater than 50%, then 40-60 IU/kg daily for a total of up to 7 days of treatment. **von Willebrand Disease Type 3: Minor Hemorrhage:** 40-50 IU (vWF:RCof)/kg IV (1 or 2 doses). **Major Hemorrhage:** Loading dose of 60-80 international units (vWF:RCof)/kg, then 40-60 IU/kg every 8-12 hours for 3 days to keep the nadir level of vWF:Rcof greater than 50%, then 40-60 IU/kg daily for a total of up to 7 days of treatment.		
Antihemophilic Factor VIII: C Human/Von Willebrand Factor Complex [Human] (Humate-P)		***Adults:* Hemophilia A: Treatment and Prophylaxis:** Dosage calculation, body weight (kg) X 0.5 IU/kg X factor VIII activity increase desired (%) = dose required. **Mild Hemorrhage:** 10-15 IU/kg IV for one dose (20% to 30% correction); may be repeated every 12-24 hours if needed. **Moderate Hemorrhage:** 15-25 IU/kg IV for one dose (30% to 50% correction); may continue with 10-15 IU/kg IV (20% to 30% correction) every 8-24 hours if needed. **Serious Hemorrhage:** 40-50 IU/kg IV (80% to 100% correction) given once; followed by 20-25 IU/kg IV (40% to 50% correction) every 8-12 hours. **Surgery:** 25-50 IU/kg IV preoperatively (50% to 100% correction), postoperatively maintain Factor VIII levels at or above 30% for 2 weeks. **Dental Procedures:** 30-40 IU/kg IV (60% to 80% correction) immediately prior to procedure, readminister if necessary. **Prophylactic Administration:** 7.5 IU/kg IV (15% correction) once daily or every other day. **von Willebrand disease type 1: Mild: Major Hemorrhage:** Loading dose of 40-60 IU (vWF:Rcof)/kg IV, then 40-50 IU/kg every 8-12 hours for 3 days to keep the nadir level of vWF: Rcof greater than 50%, then 40-50 IU/kg daily for a total of up to 7 days of treatment. **Moderate or Severe: Minor Hemorrhage:** 40-50 IU (vWF:RCof)/kg IV (1 or 2 doses). **Major Hemorrhage:** Loading dose of 50-75 IU (vWF: RCof)/kg, then 40-60 IU/kg every 8-12 hours for 3 days to keep the nadir level of vWF:Rcof greater than 50%, then 40-60 IU/kg daily for a total of up to 7 days of treatment. **von Willebrand Disease Type 2: Minor Hemorrhage:** 40-50 IU (vWF:RCof)/kg IV (1 or 2 doses) **Major Hemorrhage:** Loading dose of 60-80 IU (vWF:RCof)/kg, then 40-60 IU/kg every 8-12 hours for 3 days to keep the nadir level of vWF:Rcof greater than 50%, then 40-60 IU/kg daily for a total of up to 7 days of treatment. **von Willebrand Disease Type 3: Minor Hemorrhage:** 40-50 IU (vWF:RCof)/kg IV (1 or 2 doses). **Major Hemorrhage:** Loading dose of 60-80 IU (vWF:RCof)/kg, then 40-60 IU/kg every 8-12 hours for 3 days to keep the nadir level of	**W/P:** Hypersensitivity reactions are possible. **Contra:** Known hypersensitivity to mouse protein. **P/N:** Category C, safety not known in nursing.	Nausea, fever, chills, urticaria, **disorder of taste**.

Table 19.1: PRESCRIBING INFORMATION FOR HEMATOLOGIC DRUGS (cont.)

NAME	FORM/ STRENGTH	DOSAGE	WARNINGS/PRECAUTIONS & CONTRAINDICATIONS	ADVERSE EFFECTS†
ANTIHEMOPHILIC FACTOR (cont.)				
Antihemophilic Factor VIII: C Human/Von Willebrand Factor Complex [Human] (cont.)		vWF:Rcof greater than 50%, then 40-60 IU/kg daily for a total of up to 7 days of treatment. **Pediatric: von Willebrand Disease Type 1: Mild: Major Hemorrhage:** Loading dose of 40-60 IU (vWF:Rcof)/kg IV, then 40-50 IU/kg every 8-12 hours for 3 days to keep the nadir level of vWF:Rcof greater than 50%, then 40-50 IU/kg daily for a total of up to 7 days of treatment. **Moderate or Severe: Minor Hemorrhage:** 40-50 IU (vWF:RCof)/kg IV (1 or 2 doses). **Major Hemorrhage:** Loading dose of 50-75 IU (vWF:RCof)/kg, then 40-60 IU/kg every 8-12 hours for 3 days to keep the nadir level of vWF:Rcof greater than 50%, then 40-60 IU/kg daily for a total of up to 7 days of treatment. **von Willebrand Disease Type 2: Minor Hemorrhage:** 40-50 IU (vWF:RCof)/kg IV (1 or 2 doses) **Major Hemorrhage:** Loading dose of 60-80 IU (vWF:RCof)/kg, then 40-60 IU/kg every 8-12 hours for 3 days to keep the nadir level of vWF:Rcof greater than 50%, then 40-60 IU/kg daily for a total of up to 7 days of treatment. **von Willebrand Disease Type 3: Minor Hemorrhage:** 40-50 IU (vWF:RCof)/kg IV (1 or 2 doses). **Major Hemorrhage:** Loading dose of 60-80 IU (vWF:RCof)/kg, then 40-60 IU/kg every 8-12 hours for 3 days to keep the nadir level of vWF: Rcof greater than 50%, then 40-60 IU/kg daily for a total of up to 7 days of treatment.		
Factor IX Complex Recombinant (Benefix)	**Inj:** 250 IU, 500 IU, 1000 IU	**Adults: Hemophilia B - Hemorrhage:** Number of Factor IX international units required = body weight (kg) times desired Factor IX increase (%) times 1 IU/kg. **Mild Hemorrhage:** (20% to 30% of normal Factor IX level), 20-30 IU/kg IV twice daily until hemorrhage stops and healing is achieved (1 to 2 days). **Moderate Hemorrhage:** (25% to 50% of normal Factor IX level), 25-50 IU/kg IV twice a day until healing is achieved (2-7 days). **Major Hemorrhage:** (50% of normal Factor IX level), 30-50 IU/kilogram IV twice a day for at least 3 to 5 days. Followed by 20 IU/kg IV (20% of normal Factor IX level) twice a day. Treatment may need to be continued for up to 10 days. Surgery (50% to 100% of normal Factor IX level), 50-100 IU/kg IV twice daily for 7 to 10 days. **Dental Procedures:** (50% of normal Factor IX level), 50 IU/kilogram IV prior to the procedure, repeat if bleeding recurs. **Pediatrics: Hemophilia B - Hemorrhage:** Dose required = body weight (kg) times desired Factor IX increase (%) times 1 IU/kg.	**W/P:** Hypersensitivity reactions are possible. **Contra:** Contraindicated in patients with a known history of hypersensitivity to hamster protein. **P/N:** Category C, safety not known in nursing.	Headache, fever, chills, flushing, nausea, vomiting, lethargy, taste perversion.

*Scored.   †Bold entries denote special dental considerations.

NAME	FORM/STRENGTH	DOSAGE	WARNINGS/PRECAUTIONS & CONTRAINDICATIONS	ADVERSE EFFECTS†
Factor IX Human, Purified (Alphanine SD, Mononine)	**Inj:** 500 IU, 1000 IU	*Adults*: **Hemophilia B - Hemorrhage:** Number of factor IX international units required = body weight (kg) times desired Factor IX increase (%) times 1 IU/kg. **Mild Hemorrhage:** (20% to 30% of normal factor IX level), 20-30 IU/kg IV twice daily until hemorrhage stops and healing is achieved (1 to 2 days). **Moderate Hemorrhage:** (25% to 50% of normal Factor IX level), 25-50 IU/kg IV twice a day until healing is achieved (2-7 days). **Major Hemorrhage:** (50% of normal Factor IX level), 30-50 IU/kilogram IV twice a day for at least 3 to 5 days. Followed by 20 IU/kg IV (20% of normal Factor IX level) twice a day. Treatment may need to be continued for up to 10 days. Surgery (50% to 100% of normal Factor IX level), 50-100 IU/kg IV twice daily for 7 to 10 days. **Dental Procedures:** (50% of normal Factor IX level), 50 IU/kilogram IV prior to the procedure, repeat if bleeding recurs. *Pediatrics*: **Hemophilia B - Hemorrhage:** dose required = body weight (kg) times desired Factor IX increase (%) times 1 IU/kg.	**W/P:** Hypersensitivity reactions are possible. **Contra:** Contraindicated in patients with a known history of hypersensitivity to hamster protein. **P/N:** Category C, safety not known in nursing.	Headache, fever, chills, flushing, nausea, vomiting, lethargy, taste perversion.

ANTIPLATELET AGENTS

NAME	FORM/STRENGTH	DOSAGE	WARNINGS/PRECAUTIONS & CONTRAINDICATIONS	ADVERSE EFFECTS†
Abciximab (Reopro)	**Inj:** 2mg/mL	*Adults*: **PCI:** 0.25mg/kg IV bolus given 10-60 minutes before start PCI, followed by 0.125 mcg/kg/min IV infusion (**Max:** 10mcg/min) for 12 hrs. **Angina:** 0.25mg/kg IV bolus followed by 10mcg/min infusion for 18-24 hrs, concluding 1 hr after PCI.	**W/P:** Increased risk of bleeding. Monitor all potential bleeding sites (eg, catheter insertion sites, arterial and venous puncture sites, cutdown sites). Minimize vascular and other trauma. Discontinue if serious, uncontrollable bleeding, thrombocytopenia, or emergency surgery occurs. Anaphylaxis may occur. Antibody (HACA) formation may occur; risk of hypersensitivity, thrombocytopenia, decreased benefit with readministration. Monitor platelets, PT, aPTT, ACT before infusion. **Contra:** Active internal bleeding, recent (within 6 weeks) significant GI or GU bleeding, CVA within 2 years, CVA with significant residual neurological deficit, bleeding diathesis, oral anticoagulants within 7 days (unless PT =1.2x control), thrombocytopenia, recent (within 6 weeks) major surgery or trauma, intracranial neoplasm, arteriovenous malformation, aneurysm, severe uncontrolled HTN, history of vasculitis, IV dextran use before PCI or during an intervention. **P/N:** Category C, caution in nursing.	Bleeding, thrombocytopenia, hypotension, bradycardia, nausea, vomiting, back/chest pain, headache.
Anagrelide Hydrochloride (Agrylin)	**Cap:** 0.5mg, 1mg	*Adults*: **Initial:** 0.5mg qid or 1mg bid for at least 1 week. **Moderate Hepatic Impairment: Initial:** 0.5mg qd for at least 1 week. **Titrate:** Increase by no more than 0.5mg/day per week. **Max:** 10mg/day or 2.5mg/dose. Adjust lowest effective dose to reduce and maintain platelets <600,000/mcL. Monitor platelets every 2 days during first week, then weekly thereafter until reach maintenance dose.	**W/P:** Caution with heart disease, renal or hepatic dysfunction. Perform pre-treatment cardiovascular exam and monitor during treatment; may cause cardiovascular effects (eg, vasodilation, tachycardia, palpitations, CHF). Monitor closely for renal toxicity if creatinine ≥2mg/dL or hepatic toxicity if bilirubin, SGOT, or LFTs >1.5X ULN). Monitor blood counts, renal and hepatic function while platelets are lowered. Increase	Headache, palpitations, asthenia, edema, GI effects, dizziness, pain, dyspnea, fever, chest pain, rash, tachycardia, malaise, **pharyngitis**, cough, paresthesia.

Table 19.1: PRESCRIBING INFORMATION FOR HEMATOLOGIC DRUGS *(cont.)*

NAME	FORM/ STRENGTH	DOSAGE	WARNINGS/PRECAUTIONS & CONTRAINDICATIONS	ADVERSE EFFECTS†
ANTIPLATELET AGENTS *(cont.)*				
Anagrelide Hydrochloride *(cont.)*			in platelets after therapy interruption. Reduce dose in moderate hepatic impairment. **Contra:** Severe hepatic impairment. **P/N:** Category C, not for use in nursing.	
Aspirin/ Dipyridamole (Aggrenox)	**Cap:** (Dipyridamole Extended Release-ASA) 200mg-25mg	***Adults:*** 1 cap bid (am and pm).	**W/P:** Increased risk of bleeding with chronic, heavy alcohol use. Caution with inherited or acquired bleeding disorders, severe CAD, and hypotension. Monitor for signs of GI ulcers and bleeding. Avoid with history of peptic ulcer disease, severe renal failure (CrCl <10mL/min). Risk of hepatic dysfunction. Not interchangeable with individual components of aspirin and Persantine® Tablets. Avoid in 3rd trimester of pregnancy. **Contra:** NSAID allergy, children or teenagers with viral infections, syndrome of asthma, rhinitis, nasal polyps. **P/N:** Category B (dipyridamole), Category D (aspirin), caution in nursing.	Headache, dyspepsia, abdominal pain, nausea, diarrhea, vomiting, fatigue, arthralgia, pain, hemorrhage.
Cilostazol (Pletal)	**Tab:** 50mg, 100mg	***Adults:*** 100mg bid, 1/2 hr before or 2 hrs after breakfast and dinner. **Concomitant CYP3A4 and CYP2C19 Inhibitors:** Consider 50mg bid.	**Contraindicated with CHF of any severity due to possible decrease in survival. W/P:** Risks not known in patients with severe underlying heart disease, moderate or severe hepatic impairment, or with long-term use. Rare cases of thrombocytopenia or leukopenia reported. **Contra:** CHF of any severity. **P/N:** Category C, not for use in nursing.	Headache, palpitation, tachycardia, abnormal stool, diarrhea, peripheral edema, dizziness, infection.
Clopidogrel Hydrogen Sulfate (Plavix)	**Tab:** 75mg	***Adults:*** **MI/Stroke/PAD:** 75mg qd. **Acute Coronary Syndrome:** Take with 75-325mg ASA qd. **LD:** 300mg. **Maint:** 75mg qd.	**W/P:** Caution with risk of increased bleeding, ulcers or lesions with a propensity to bleed, severe hepatic or renal impairment. Discontinue 5 days before surgery if antiplatelet effect is not desired. Monitor blood cell count and other appropriate tests if symptoms of bleeding or undesirable hematological effects arise. Thrombotic thrombocytopenic purpura (TTP) reported (rare). **Contra:** Active pathological bleeding (eg, peptic ulcer, intracranial hemorrhage). **P/N:** Category B, not for use in nursing.	Chest pain, influenza-like symptoms, pain, edema, HTN, headache, dizziness, abdominal pain, dyspepsia, diarrhea, arthralgia, purpura, upper respiratory tract infection, back pain, dyspnea.
Dipyridamole (Persantine)	**Tab:** 25mg, 50mg, 75mg	***Adults:*** 75-100mg qid.	**W/P:** Caution with hypotension or severe coronary artery disease (eg, unstable angina or recent MI); may aggravate chest pain. Elevated hepatic enzymes and hepatic failure reported. **P/N:** Category B, caution in nursing.	Dizziness, abdominal distress.
Eptifibatide (Integrilin)	**Sol:** 0.75mg/mL, 2mg/mL	***Adults:*** **ACS: SCr <2mg/dL:** 180mcg/kg IV bolus, then 2mcg/kg/min IV infusion until discharge, initiation of CABG, or up to 72 hrs. If undergoing PCI, continue until discharge or 18-24 hrs post-PCI. **SCr 2-4 mg/dL:** 180mcg/kg IV bolus, then 1mcg/kg/min IV infusion. **PCI: SCr <2mg/dL:** 180mcg/kg IV bolus immediately before PCI, then 2mcg/kg/min IV	**W/P:** Bleeding reported. Caution with renal dysfunction, platelets ≤100,000mm³, femeral access site in PCI. Minimize vascular and other trauma. Discontinue if thrombocytopenia occurs. Monitor Hct, Hgb, platelets, serum creatinine (SCr), and PT/aPTT before therapy (and activated clotting time before PCI). Discontinue before	Bleeding, thrombocytopenia, hypotension.

*Scored.   †Bold entries denote special dental considerations.

NAME	FORM/ STRENGTH	DOSAGE	WARNINGS/PRECAUTIONS & CONTRAINDICATIONS	ADVERSE EFFECTS†
Eptifibatide *(cont.)*		infusion. Give 2nd bolus of 180mcg/kg 10 minutes after 1st bolus. Continue until discharge or 18-24 hrs post-PCI. **SCr: 2-4 mg/dL:** 180mcg/kg IV bolus immediately before PCI, then 1mcg/ kg/min IV infusion. Give 2nd bolus of 180mcg/kg 10 minutes after 1st bolus. **ACS/PCI: >121kg: SCr <2mg/dL: Max:** 22.6mg IV bolus, then 15mg/hr IV infusion. **SCr 2-4mg/dL: Max:** 22.6mg IV bolus, then 7.5mg/hr IV infusion. See labeling for concomitant ASA and heparin doses.	CABG surgery. **Contra:** Active abnormal bleeding, history of bleeding diathesis, or stroke within past 30 days. Severe HTN uncontrolled with antihyperten- sives, major surgery within preceding 6 weeks, history of hemorrhagic stroke, concomitant parenteral glycopro- tein IIb/IIIa inhibitor, renal dialysis dependency. **P/N:** Category B, caution in nursing.	
Ticlopidine Hydrochloride (Ticlid)	**Tab:** 250mg	**Adults:** Take with food. **Stroke:** 250mg bid. **Coronary Artery Stenting:** 250mg bid with ASA up to 30 days after stent implant.	**Can cause life-threatening hematological adverse reactions, including neutropenia/agranulocy- tosis, thrombotic thrombocytopenic purpura (TTP), and aplastic anemia.** **W/P:** Monitor for hematologic toxicity before treatment, then every 2 weeks for 1st 3 months, and 2 weeks after discontinuation. Monitor more frequently if signs of hematological adverse reactions; discontinue if neu- trophils <1200/mm^3, aplastic anemia or TTP occurs. Discontinue 10-14 days before surgery. Caution in trauma, surgery, bleeding disorders. May need dose adjustment with renal or hepatic impairment. May elevate LFTs, TG, and cholesterol. **Contra:** Hematopoietic disorders (eg, neutropenia, thrombo- cytopenia), history of TTP or aplastic anemia, hemostatic disorders, active pathological bleeding, severe liver impairment. **P/N:** Category B, not for use in nursing.	Diarrhea, rash, nausea, GI pain, rash, dyspep- sia, neutropenia.
Tirofiban Hydrochloride (Aggrastat)	**Inj:** 0.05mg/mL, 0.25mg/mL	**Adults: Initial:** 0.4mcg/kg/min IV for 30 minutes. **Maint:** 0.1mcg/kg/min IV. Continue through angiography and for 12-24 hrs after angioplasty or atherec- tomy. **CrCl <30mL/min:** Administer half of the usual rate of infusion.	**W/P:** Bleeding reported. Monitor platelets, Hgb, Hct before treatment, within 6 hrs after loading infusion, and daily during therapy. Monitor platelets earlier if previous GP IIb/IIIa inhibitor use. Determine APTT before and during therapy with heparin. Caution with platelets <150,000/mm^3, hemorrhagic retinopathy, chronic hemodialysis patients, femoral ac- cess site in percutaneous coronary intervention. Minimize vascular and other trauma. Discontinue if throm- bocytopenia confirmed or if bleeding cannot be controlled by pressure. **Contra:** Active internal bleeding, acute pericarditis, severe HTN, concomitant parenteral GP IIb/IIIa inhibitor, hemorrhagic stroke, aortic dissec- tion, thrombocytopenia with prior exposure. Bleeding diathesis, stroke, major surgical procedure, or severe physical trauma within past 30 days. History of intracranial hemorrhage or neoplasm, arteriovenous malforma- tion, aneurysm. **P/N:** Category B, not for use in nursing.	Bleeding, nausea, fever, headache, edema, anaphylaxis.

Table 19.1: PRESCRIBING INFORMATION FOR HEMATOLOGIC DRUGS *(cont.)*

NAME	FORM/STRENGTH	DOSAGE	WARNINGS/PRECAUTIONS & CONTRAINDICATIONS	ADVERSE EFFECTS†
NUTRITIONAL SUPPLEMENTS				
Ascorbic Acid/Calcium Carbonate/ Cyanoco- balamin/Folic Acid/Iron/ Niacinamide/ Pyridoxine/ Riboflavin/ Thiamine/ Vitamin A/Vitamin D (Nu-Iron-V)	**Tab:** Iron (Elemental) 60 mg; Folic Acid 1 mg; Ascorbic Acid 50 mg; Cyanocobalamin 3 mcg; Vitamin A 4,000 IU; Vitamin D 2 400 IU; Thiamine Mononitrate 3 mg; Riboflavin 3 mg; Pyridoxine Hydrochloride 2 mg; Niacinamide 10 mg; Calcium Carbonate 312 mg	*Adults:* 1 tab qd.	**W/P:** Accidental overdose of iron-containing products is a leading cause of fatal poisoning in children under 6 years of age. May cause darkening of stool. **P/N:** Safety in pregnancy and nursing not known.	Nausea, constipation, diarrhea, or stomach painrash, itching, vomiting, stomach pain, black or green bowel movements.
Ascorbic Acid/Calcium Pantothenate/ Cyanocobala- min/ Ferrous Sulfate/Folic Acid/Niacin/ Pyrido xine/Riboflavin/Thiamine (Iberet-Folic-500)	**Tab, Extended Release:** Ferrous Sulfate 105mg-Folic Acid 0.8mg-Vitamin B_1 6mg-Vitamin B_2 6mg-Vitamin B_3 30mg-Vitamin B_5 10mg-Vitamin B_6 5mg-Vitamin B_{12} 25mcg-Vitamin C 500mg	*Adults:* 1 tab qd on empty stomach.	**W/P:** May mask pernicious anemia. **Contra:** Pernicious anemia. **P/N:** Category A, caution in nursing.	Allergic sensitization.
Ascorbic Acid/ Cyanocobala- min/Ferrous Bisglycinate Chelate/Folic Acid/Iron Polysaccharide (Niferex-150 Forte)	**Cap:** (Folic Acid-Iron-Vitamin B_{12}-Vitamin C) 1mg-150mg-25mcg-60mg	*Adults:* 1 cap qd.	**W/P:** Fatal poisoning reported in children <6 yrs with accidental overdose of iron-containing products. Determination of type, cause of anemia is recommended before starting therapy. Folic acid >0.1mg/day may obscure pernicious anemia. **Contra:** Hemochromatosis, hemosiderosis. **P/N:** Safety in pregnancy and nursing not known.	Constipation, diarrhea, nausea, vomiting, dark stools, abdominal pain.
Ascorbic Acid/Ferrous Bisglycinate Chelate/Iron Polysaccharide (Niferex-150)	**Cap:** (Iron-Vitamin C) 150mg-50mg	*Adults:* 1-2 caps qd.	**W/P:** Fatal poisoning reported in children <6 yrs with accidental overdose of iron-containing products. **P/N:** Safety in pregnancy and nursing not known.	
Ascorbic Acid/Ferrous Fumarate (Fero-Grad-500, Vitron-C, Vitron-C Plus)	**Tab, Extended Release:** Ferrous Sulfate 105mg-Vitamin C 500mg	*Adults:* 1 tab qd. *Pediatrics:* ≥4 yrs: 1 tab qd.		
Ascorbic Acid/Ferrous Sulfate/ Folic Acid (Fero-Folic 500)	**(Ferrous Sulfate-Folic Acid-Vitamin C) Tab, ER:** 525mg-0.8mg-500mg	*Adults:* 1 tab qd.	**W/P:** May mask pernicious anemia. **Contra:** Pernicious anemia. **P/N:** Category A, safety in nursing not known.	Gastric intolerance, allergic sensitization.
Cyanocobalamin	**Lozenge/Troche:** 100mcg, 250mcg, 500mcg, 2000mcg; **Nasal Gel/Jelly:** 500mcg/0.1mL; **Nasal Spray:**	*Adults:* Cobalamin Deficiency: Normal Absorption: 1000mcg/day PO. Cobalamin Deficiency: Malabsorption: 100mcg IM or deep SC injection daily for 6 or 7 days; if clinical improvement and reticulocyte	**W/P:** Caution with Leber's disease (hereditary optic nerve atrophy). Some brands contain benzyl alcohol, associated with fatal gasping syndrome in premature infants. All hematological parameters should be normal before	Diarrhea, injection site pain, headache.

*Scored.   †Bold entries denote special dental considerations.

NAME	FORM/ STRENGTH	DOSAGE	WARNINGS/PRECAUTIONS & CONTRAINDICATIONS	ADVERSE EFFECTS†
Cyanocobalamin *(cont.)*	500mcg/0.1mL; **Sol:** 2mcg/mL, 100mcg/mL, 1000mcg/mL; **Tab:** 25mcg, 50mcg, 100mcg, 250mcg, 500mcg, 1000mcg, 2000mcg; **Tab, Extended Release:** 1000mcg, 1500mcg; **Tab, Sublingual:** 1000mcg, 2500mcg, 5000mcg	response, give same amount on alternate days for 7 doses; then every 3-4 days for another 2-3 wk; then 100mcg monthly for life. **Prophylaxis:** 500mcg gel or spray intranasally into one nostril once weekly. **Homocystinemia:** 400mcg/day PO with folic acid. **Malabsorption of Cyanocobalamin: Diagnosis - Schilling Test:** Flushing dose, 1000mcg IM. **Pernicious Anemia:** 100mcg IM or deep SC injection daily for 6 or 7 days; if clinical improvement and reticulocyte response, give same amount on alternate days for 7 doses; then every 3-4 days for another 2-3 wk; then 100mcg monthly for life. **Maintenance:** 1000mcg/day PO. **Recommended Dietary Allowance: Men:** 2.4mcg/day. **Women:** 2.4mcg/day. **Pregnancy:** 2.6mcg/day. **Lactation:** 2.8mcg/day. **Schilling Test:** 18.5-37 kBq (0.5-1 mCi) cyanocobalamin Co 57 PO, followed by 1000mcg cyanocobalamin IM 2hr later. *Pediatrics:* **Cobalamin Deficiency:** 1000mcg/day PO, IM route is preferred; 30-50mcg IM daily for 2 or more wk; then 100mcg monthly to sustain remission. **Malabsorption of Cyanocobalamin: Diagnosis - Schilling Test:** flushing dose, 1000mcg IM. **Pernicious Anemia:** 30-50mcg IM daily for 2 or more wk; then 100mcg monthly to sustain remission. **Recommended Dietary Allowance: (up to 6 months)** 0.4mcg/day; **(6 months-1 yr)** 0.5mcg/day; **(1-3 yr)** 0.9mcg/day; **(4-8 yr)** 1.2mcg/day; **(9-13 yr)** 1.8mcg/day; **(14 yr and older)** 2.4mcg/day. **Transcobalamin Deficiency, Congenital:** 1000mcg IM twice weekly.	beginning treatment with cyanocobalamin nasal gel. **P/N:** Category C, safe in nursing.	
Cyanocobalamin/ Folic Acid/Iron Polysaccharide (Hemocyte-F)	**Tab:** (Ferrous Fumarate-Folic Acid) 324mg-1mg	***Adults:*** 1 tab qd. **Elderly:** Start at low end of dosing range.	**W/P:** Toxic when overdoses are ingested by children. Not for the treatment of pernicious anemia and other megaloblastic anemias where vitamin B_{12} is deficient. Folic acid >0.1mg-0.4mg/day may obscure pernicious anemia. Caution with peptic ulcer, regional enteritis, ulcerative colitis. **Contra:** Hemochromatosis, hemosiderosis, pernicious anemia.	GI disturbances, abdominal cramps, diarrhea, constipation, heartburn, nausea, vomiting, black stools, allergic sensitization.
Cyanocobalamin/Folic Acid/Pyridoxine (Folgard RX 2.2)	**Tab:** Folic Acid 2.2mg-Vitamin B_6 25mg-Vitamin B_{12} 0.5mg*	***Adults:*** 1 tab qd.	**W/P:** Folic acid >0.1mg/day may obscure pernicious anemia. **P/N:** Safety in pregnancy and nursing is not known.	Allergic sensitization.
Ferrous Bisglycinate Chelate/Iron Polysaccharide (Niferex)	**Cap:** 60mg; **Sol:** 100mg/5mL	***Adults:*** 1-2 tabs bid or 5-10mL qd. ***Pediatrics:*** **≥6 yrs:** 1-2 tabs qd or 5mL qd. **<6 yrs: (Sol)** Individualize dose.	**W/P:** Fatal poisoning reported in children <6 yrs with accidental overdose of iron-containing products. **P/N:** Safety in pregnancy and nursing not known.	
Ferrous Fumarate (Feostat, Ferretts, Ferrocite, Hemocyte, Ircon)	**Tab:** 324mg (106mg elemental iron)	***Adults:*** 1 tab up to bid, between meals.	**W/P:** May aggravate existing GI disorders. Ineffective with steatorrhea, partial gastrectomy. **Contra:** Hemochromatosis, hemosiderosis, hemolytic anemia.	

Table 19.1: PRESCRIBING INFORMATION FOR HEMATOLOGIC DRUGS (cont.)

NAME	FORM/STRENGTH	DOSAGE	WARNINGS/PRECAUTIONS & CONTRAINDICATIONS	ADVERSE EFFECTS†
NUTRITIONAL SUPPLEMENTS (cont.)				
Ferrous Fumarate/Docusate Sodium (Ferro-Sequels)	Tab, ER: (Ferrous Fumarate-Docusate Sodium) 50mg-40mg	*Adults:* 1 tab qd.	**W/P:** Fatal poisoning reported in children <6 yrs with accidental overdose of iron-containing products. **P/N:** Safety in pregnancy and nursing not known.	
Ferrous Fumarate/Folic Acid (Hemocyte-F, Ircon-FA)	Tab: (Ferrous Fumarate-Folic Acid) 324mg-1mg	*Adults:* 1 tab qd. **Elderly:** Start at low end of dosing range.	**W/P:** Toxic when overdoses are ingested by children. Not for the treatment of pernicious anemia and other megaloblastic anemias where vitamin B_{12} is deficient. Folic acid >0.1mg-0.4mg/day may obscure pernicious anemia. Caution with peptic ulcer, regional enteritis, ulcerative colitis. **Contra:** Hemochromatosis, hemosiderosis, pernicious anemia.	GI disturbances, abdominal cramps, diarrhea, constipation, heartburn, nausea, vomiting, black stools, allergic sensitization.
Ferrous Gluconate (Fergon, Feronate)	Tab: 240mg (27mg elemental iron)	*Adults:* 1 tab qd with food.	**W/P:** Accidental overdose of iron-containing products is a leading cause of fatal poisoning in children under 6. **P/N:** Safety in pregnancy and nursing not known.	Nausea, GI disturbance, constipation, diarrhea.
Ferrous Sulfate (Feosol, Slow FE)	Tab: (Feosol Tablet) 200mg (65mg elemental iron); (Slow-FE) 160 mg (50mg elemental iron)	*Adults:* 1 tab qd with food. *Pediatrics:* ≥12 yrs: 1 tab qd with food.	**W/P:** Keep product out of reach of children. Accidental overdose of iron-containing products is a leading cause of fatal poisoning in children <6 yrs. **P/N:** Safety in pregnancy and nursing not known.	Nausea, GI disturbance, constipation, diarrhea.
Ferrous Sulfate/Folic Acid (Slow FE w/Folic Acid)	Tab: (elemental iron-folic acid) 47.5mg-350mg	*Adults:* 1-2 tabs qd with food. *Pediatrics:* ≥12 yrs: 1-2 tab qd with food.	**W/P:** Accidental overdose of iron-containing products is a leading cause of fatal poisoning in children under 6. Keep this product out of reach of children. **P/N:** Safety in pregnancy and nursing not known.	
Folic Acid	Inj: 5mg/mL; Tab: (OTC) 0.4mg, 0.8mg, (Rx) 1mg	*Adults:* **Usual:** Up to 1mg/day. **Maint:** 0.4mg qd. **Pregnancy/Nursing: Maint:** 0.8mg qd. **Max:** 1mg/day. Increase maintenance dose with alcoholism, hemolytic anemia, anticonvulsant therapy, chronic infection. *Pediatrics:* **Usual:** Up to 1mg/day. **Maint: Infants:** 0.1mg qd. **<4 yrs:** 0.3mg qd. **≥4 yrs:** 0.4mg qd.	**W/P:** Not for monotherapy in pernicious anemia and other megaloblastic anemias with B_{12} deficiency. May obscure pernicious anemia in dosage >0.1 mg/day. Decreased B_{12} serum levels with prolonged therapy. **P/N:** Category A, requirement increases during nursing.	Allergic sensitization.
Folic Acid/Iron Polysaccharide (Irofol)	(Folic Acid-Polysaccharide Iron Complex) Liquid: 1mg-100mg/5mL; Tab: 1mg-150mg	*Adults:* 1-2 tabs or 5-10mL qd. *Pediatrics:* >12 yrs: 1-2 tabs or 5-10mL qd.	**W/P:** Not for the treatment of pernicious anemia and other megaloblastic anemias. Folic acid >0.1mg/day may obscure pernicious anemia. **P/N:** Safety in pregnancy and nursing not known.	Gastric intolerance, allergic sensitization.
Iron Dextran (Infed)	Inj: 50mg/mL	*Adults:* **Iron Deficiency Anemia:** Dose (mL)=0.0442 (desired Hgb-observed Hgb) x LBW + (0.26 x LBW); LBW=lean body weight (kg). See labeling for more details. **Blood Loss:** Replace equivalent amount of iron in blood loss. *Pediatrics:* ≥4 months: >15kg: **Iron Deficiency Anemia:** Dose (mL)=0.0442 (desired Hgb-observed Hgb) x LBW + (0.26 x LBW); LBW=lean body weight (kg). **5-15kg:** Dose (mL)=0.0442 (desired Hgb-observed Hgb) x weight + (0.26 x weight). See labeling for more details. **Blood Loss:**	**Anaphylactic-type reactions and death possible. Only use when indication clearly established and lab investigations confirm iron deficient state not amenable to oral therapy. W/P:** Large IV doses associated with increased incidence of adverse effects. Caution with serious hepatic impairment, significant allergies, asthma. Avoid during acute phase of infectious kidney disease. May exacerbate cardiovascular complications in pre-existing cardiovascular disease and joint pain or swelling in rheumatoid arthritis. Hypersensitivity	Anaphylactic reactions, chest pain/tightness, urticaria, pruritus, abdominal pain, nausea, arthralgia, convulsions, respiratory arrest, hematuria, febrile episodes.

*Scored.   †Bold entries denote special dental considerations.

NAME	FORM/ STRENGTH	DOSAGE	WARNINGS/PRECAUTIONS & CONTRAINDICATIONS	ADVERSE EFFECTS†
Iron Dextran *(cont.)*		Replace equivalent amount of iron in blood loss.	reactions reported after uneventful test doses. Unwarranted therapy can cause exogenous hemosiderosis. Have epinephrine (1:1000) available. Risk of carcinogenesis with IM use. Give 0.5mL test dose before IM/IV administration. **Contra:** Anemia not associated with iron deficiency. **P/N:** Category C, caution in nursing.	
Iron Sucrose (Venofer)	**Inj:** 20mg/mL	***Adults:*** **HDD-CKD:** 100mg IV injection over 2 to 5 minutes or 100mg infusion over at least 15 minutes per consecutive hemodialysis session for a total cumulative dose of 1000mg. **NDD-CKD:** 1000mg over a 14 day period as a 200mg slow IV injection undiluted over 2 to 5 minutes on 5 different occasions within the 14 day period.	**W/P:** Fatal hypersensitivity reactions characterized by anaphylactic shock, collapse, hypotension, and dyspnea reported. Caution with administration; hypotension may occur. Monitor hematologic and hematinic parameters periodically. **Contra:** Iron overload, anemia not caused by iron deficiency. **P/N:** Category B, caution in nursing.	Headache, fever, pain, asthenia, malaise, hypotension, chest pain, HTN, hypervolemia, nausea, vomiting, cramps, musculoskeletal pain, dyspnea, cough, pruritus, application site reaction.
Sodium Ferric Gluconate Complex (Ferrlecit)	**Inj:** 62.5mg elemental iron/5mL	***Adults:*** 10mL (125mg) as IV infusion (diluted in 100mL NS) over 1 hr or undiluted as a slow IV injection (at a rate of up to 12.5mg/min). **Min:** 1g elemental iron over 8 sequential dialysis sessions.	**W/P:** Hypersensitivity reactions reported. **Contra:** Anemia not associated with iron deficiency. Iron overload. **P/N:** Category B, caution in nursing.	Injection site reactions, nausea, vomiting, diarrhea, hypotension, cramps, HTN, dizziness, dyspnea, abnormal erythrocytes, leg cramps, pain, chest pain.

THROMBOLYTIC/ANTITHROMBIN AGENTS

NAME	FORM/ STRENGTH	DOSAGE	WARNINGS/PRECAUTIONS & CONTRAINDICATIONS	ADVERSE EFFECTS†
Alteplase, Recombinant (Activase)	**Inj:** 50mg, 100mg	***Adults:*** **AMI: Accelerated Infusion:** **>67kg:** 15mg IV bolus, then 50mg over next 30 minutes, and then 35mg over next 60 minutes. **≥67kg:** 15mg IV bolus, then 0.75mg/kg (max 50mg) over next 30 minutes, then 0.5mg/kg (max 35mg) over next 60 minutes. **Max:** 100mg total dose. **3-Hr Infusion:** **≥65kg:** 60mg in 1st hr (give 6-10mg as IV bolus), then 20mg over 2nd hr, then 20mg over 3rd hr. **< 65kg:** 1.25mg/kg over 3 hrs as described above. **Stroke:** 0.9mg/kg IV over 1 hr (max 90mg total dose). Administer 10% of total dose as IV bolus over 1 minute. **PE:** 100mg IV over 2 hrs. Start heparin at end or immediately after infusion when PTT or PT ≤2x normal.	**W/P:** Weigh benefits/risks with recent major surgery, cerebrovascular disease, recent GI or GU bleeding, recent trauma, HTN, left heart thrombus, acute pericarditis, subacute bacterial endocarditis, hemostatic defects, severe hepatic dysfunction, pregnancy, diabetic hemorrhagic retinopathy or other hemorrhagic ophthalmic conditions, septic thrombophlebitis or occluded AV cannula at a seriously infected site, elderly, any other bleeding condition that is difficult to manage. For stroke, also weigh benefits/risks with severe neurological deficit or major early infarct signs on CT. Cholesterol embolism and internal/superficial bleeding reported. Arrhythmias may occur with reperfusion. Avoid IM injection, noncompressible arterial puncture, and internal jugular or subclavian venous puncture. Caution with readministration. **Contra:** (AMI, PE) Active internal bleeding, history of CVA, recent intracranial/intraspinal surgery or trauma, intracranial neoplasm, arteriovenous (AV) malformation, aneurysm, bleeding diathesis, severe uncontrolled HTN. (Stroke) Active internal bleeding, AV malformation, intracranial neoplasm or hemorrhage, aneurysm, bleeding diathesis, uncontrolled HTN, SAH, seizure at on stroke onset. Recent intracranial or intraspinal surgery, serious head trauma, previous stroke. **P/N:** Category C, caution in nursing.	Bleeding.

Table 19.1: PRESCRIBING INFORMATION FOR HEMATOLOGIC DRUGS *(cont.)*

NAME	FORM/ STRENGTH	DOSAGE	WARNINGS/PRECAUTIONS & CONTRAINDICATIONS	ADVERSE EFFECTS†
THROMBOLYTIC/ANTITHROMBIN AGENTS *(cont.)*				
Antithrombin III Human (Thrombate III)	**Intravenous Powder for Solution:** 1 IU, 500 IU	***Adults:*** **Antithrombin III deficiency, Acquired - Thromboembolic disorder: Initial:** Dose calculation = (desired minus current antithrombin III level as % of normal level) times weight (kg) divided by 1.4, up to 6000 units IV daily; initial target plasma AT-III peak level (20 min postinfusion) is 120% of normal activity. **Maint:** Administered every 24 hr to maintain plasma AT-III levels greater than 80% of normal activity. **Treatment and Prophylaxis: Initial:** dose calculation = (desired minus current antithrombin III level as % of normal level) times weight (kg) divided by 1.4, up to 6000 units IV daily; initial target plasma AT-III peak level (20 min postinfusion) is 120% of normal activity. **Maint:** Administered every 24 hr to maintain plasma AT-III levels greater than 80% of normal activity. ***Pediatrics:*** **Disseminated Intravascular Coagulation:** 40-60 units/kg/day to achieve AT-III levels of 30-80% of average adult levels; administer with heparin initial dose of 50-100 units/kg/day.	**W/P:** Reduce heparin dose during concurrent therapy. **P/N:** Category B, caution in nursing.	**Bad taste in mouth,** nausea, dizziness, fever.
Argatroban	**Inj:** 100mg/mL	***Adults:*** **Thrombosis:** Discontinue heparin and obtain baseline aPTT. **Initial:** 2mcg/kg/min IV. Check aPTT after 2 hrs. **Titrate:** Increase dose until aPTT is 1.5-3x the initial baseline. **Max:** 10mcg/kg/min. **Moderate Hepatic Impairment: Initial:** 0.5mcg/kg/min. **PCI: Initial:** 350mcg/kg bolus with 25mcg/kg/min IV. Check activated clotting time (ACT) 5-10 minutes after bolus. Proceed with PCI if ACT >300 seconds. If ACT <300 seconds, give additional 150mcg/kg bolus and increase infusion to 30mcg/kg/min. Check ACT 5-10 minutes later. If ACT >450 seconds, decrease to 15mcg/kg/min and check ACT 5-10 minutes later. Continue infusion dose at therapeutic ACT (300-450 seconds) during procedure. May give additional 150mcg/kg bolus and increase infusion to 40mcg/kg/min if dissection, impending abrupt closure, thrombus formation, or inability to achieve/maintain ACT >300 seconds. After PCI, may use lower infusion rate if anticoagulation is needed.	**W/P:** Discontinue all parenteral anticoagulants before administering. Extreme caution in conditions associated with an increased danger of hemorrhage (eg, severe HTN, immediately following lumbar puncture, bleeding disorder, GI lesions, spinal anesthesia, major surgery, etc). Caution in hepatic impairment. Avoid high doses in PCI patients with significant hepatic disease or AST/ALT ≥3X ULN. Monitor aPTT. For PCI, obtain ACT before dose, 5-10 minutes after dose, and infusion rate change, at the end of PCI, and every 20-30 minutes during prolonged procedures. **Contra:** Overt major bleeding. **P/N:** Category B, not for use in nursing.	GI bleed, GU bleed, Hct/Hgb decrease, hypotension, fever, diarrhea, nausea, ventricular tachycardia, vomiting, allergic reactions, chest pain (in PCI).
Bivalirudin (Angiomax)	**Inj:** 250mg	***Adults:*** **Initial:** 0.75mg/kg IV bolus, then 1.75mg/kg/hr for duration of PCI procedure. Additional bolus of 0.3mg/kg can be given if needed based on ACT. Continuation of infusion for up to 4 hrs post-procedure is optional. After 4 hrs, if needed, an additional 0.2mg/kg/hr IV for up to 20 hrs may be initiated. **Renal Impairment: CrCl <30mL/min:** 1mg/kg/hr infusion. **Hemodialysis:** 0.25mg/kg/hr infusion. Reduction in bolus dose not necessary; monitor anticoagulation.	**W/P:** Not for IM administration. Hemorrhage can occur at any site. Discontinue with unexplained symptom, fall in BP or Hct. There is no known antidote to treatment, but can be hemodialyzable. **Contra:** Active major bleeding. **P/N:** Category B, caution in nursing.	Bleeding, back pain, pain, nausea, vomiting, headache, hypotension, HTN, bradycardia, dyspepsia, urinary retention, insomnia, anxiety, abdominal pain, fever, nervousness.

*Scored.   †Bold entries denote special dental considerations.

NAME	FORM/ STRENGTH	DOSAGE	WARNINGS/PRECAUTIONS & CONTRAINDICATIONS	ADVERSE EFFECTS†
Fondaparinux Sodium (Arixtra)	**Inj: Syringe:** 2.5mg/0.5mL, 5mg/0.4mL, 7.5mg/0.6mL, 10mg/0.8mL	***Adults:* DVT Prophylaxis:** 2.5mg SC qd, starting 6-8 hrs post-op for 5-9 days (up to 11 days). **Hip Fracture Surgery:** Extended prophylaxis up to 24 additional days is recommended. **DVT/PE Treatment: <50kg:** 5mg SC qd. **50-100kg:** 7.5mg SC qd. **>100kg:** 10mg SC qd. Add concomitant warfarin ASAP (usually within 72 hrs) and continue for 5-9 days (up to 26 days) until INR=2-3.	**Risk of paralysis by spinal/epidural hematoma with neuraxial anesthesia or spinal puncture. Increased risk with indwelling epidural catheters for analgesia, drugs affecting hemostasis (eg, NSAIDs, platelet inhibitors, anticoagulants), and traumatic or repeated epidural or spinal puncture. W/P:** Not for IM injection. Cannot use interchangeably unit for unit with heparin or other low molecular weight heparins. Risk of hemorrhage increases with renal impairment. Caution with moderate renal dysfunction, elderly, history of HIT, bleeding diathesis, uncontrolled arterial HTN, recent GI ulceration, diabetic retinopathy, hemorrhage. Monitor renal function periodically. Extreme caution in conditions with an increased risk of hemorrhage (eg, bleeding disorders, hemorrhagic stroke, etc). Perform routine CBC, SCr, stool occult blood tests. Discontinue if platelets <100,000/mm^3. Thrombocytopenia reported. Major bleeding with abdominal surgery reported. **Contra:** Severe renal impairment (CrCl <30mL/min), body weight <50kg undergoing hip fracture, hip/knee replacement or abdominal surgery, bacterial endocarditis, active major bleeding, thrombocytopenia with a positive in vitro test for anti-platelet antibody. **P/N:** Category B, caution in nursing.	Hemorrhage, thrombocytopenia, local reactions (eg, rash, pruritus), AST/ALT elevations, anemia, fever, nausea, edema, constipation, vomiting.
Lepirudin (Refludan)	**Inj:** 50mg	***Adults:* LD:** 0.4mg/kg (**Max:** 44mg) IV over 15-20 seconds. **Initial:** 0.15mg/kg/hr (max 16.5mg/hr) continuous infusion for 2-10 days. Adjust dose based on aPTT. If aPTT is above target range, stop infusion for 2 hrs and restart at 50% of previous rate. Check aPTT 4 hrs later. If aPTT is below target range, increase rate in steps of 20% and check aPTT 4 hrs later. Do not exceed 0.21mg/kg/hr. **Renal Impairment: LD:** 0.2mg/kg. **Initial: CrCl 45-60 mL/min:** 0.075mg/kg/hr. **CrCl 30-44mL/min:** 0.045mg/kg/hr. **CrCl 15-29 mL/min:** 0.0225mg/kg/hr. **CrCl <15mL/min/Hemodialysis:** Avoid or stop infusion. **Concomitant Thrombolytic Therapy: LD:** 0.2mg/kg. **Initial:** 0.1mg/kg/hr.	**W/P:** Risk of bleeding. Weigh risks/benefits with recent puncture of large vessels or organ biopsy, anomaly of vessels or organs, recent CVA, stroke, intracerebral surgery or other neuraxial procedures, severe uncontrolled HTN, bacterial endocarditis, advanced renal impairment, hemorrhagic diathesis, recent major surgery or bleeding. Avoid with baseline aPTT ≥2.5. Monitor aPTT 4 hrs after initiate infusion and at least once daily. Liver injury may enhance anticoagulant effects. Antihirudin antibodies reported; may increase anticoagulant effects. **P/N:** Category B, not for use in nursing.	Hemorrhagic events (eg, bleeding, anemia, hematoma, hematuria, epistaxis, hemothorax), fever, liver dysfunction, pneumonia, sepsis, allergic skin reactions, multiorgan failure.
Reteplase, Recombinant (Retavase)	**Inj:** 10.4 U	***Adults:*** 10 U IV over 2 minutes. Repeat in 30 minutes.	**W/P:** Weigh benefits/risks with recent major surgery, previous puncture of noncompressible vessels, cerebrovascular disease, recent GI or GU bleeding, recent trauma, HTN, left heart thrombus, acute pericarditis, subacute bacterial endocarditis, hemostatic defects, severe hepatic or renal dysfunction, pregnancy, diabetic hemorrhagic retinopathy or other hemorrhagic ophthalmic conditions, septic thrombophlebitis or occluded AV cannula at a seriously infected site,	Bleeding, allergic reactions, dyspnea, hypotension.

Table 19.1: PRESCRIBING INFORMATION FOR HEMATOLOGIC DRUGS *(cont.)*

THROMBOLYTIC/ANTITHROMBIN AGENTS *(cont.)*

NAME	FORM/ STRENGTH	DOSAGE	WARNINGS/PRECAUTIONS & CONTRAINDICATIONS	ADVERSE EFFECTS†
Reteplase, Recombinant *(cont.)*			elderly, any other bleeding condition that is difficult to manage. Cholesterol embolism and internal/superficial bleeding reported. Arrhythmias may occur with reperfusion. Avoid IM injection, noncompressible arterial puncture, and internal jugular or subclavian venous puncture. **Contra:** Active internal bleeding, history of CVA, recent intracranial or intraspinal surgery or trauma, intracranial neoplasm, arteriovenous malformation, aneurysm, bleeding diathesis, severe uncontrolled HTN. **P/N:** Category C, caution in nursing.	
Streptokinase (Streptase)	**Inj:** 250,000 IU, 750,000 IU, 1.5 MIU	***Adults*: AMI: IV:** 1.5 MIU within 60 minutes. **Intracoronary:** 20,000 IU infusion bolus, then 2000 IU/min for 60 minutes for total 140,000U. **PE:** LD: 250,000 IU over 30 minutes. **IV Infusion:** 100,000 IU/hr for 24 hrs (72 hrs if concurrent DVT). **DVT:** LD: 250,000 IU over 30 minutes. **IV Infusion:** 100,000 IU/hr for 72 hrs. **Arterial Thrombosis or Embolism: LD:** 250,000 IU over 30 minutes. **IV Infusion:** 100,000 IU/hr for 24-72 hrs. **AV Cannulae Occlusion:** Instill 250,000 IU in 2mL of solution into occluded limb of cannula; clamp off cannula limb for 2 hrs. Aspirate contents after therapy, flush with saline, and reconnect cannula.	**W/P:** Weigh benefits/risks with recent major surgery, previous puncture of noncompressible vessels, cerebrovascular disease, recent serious GI bleeding or trauma, HTN, left heart thrombus, subacute bacterial endocarditis, hemostatic defects, pregnancy, diabetic hemorrhagic retinopathy, septic thrombophlebitis or occluded AV cannula at a seriously infected site, >75 yrs, any other bleeding condition that is difficult to manage. Cholesterol embolism, non-cardiogenic pulmonary edema, hypotension, and bleeding reported. Arrhythmias may occur with reperfusion. Increased resistance due to antistreptokinase antibody. **Contra:** Active internal bleeding, recent CVA, recent intracranial or intraspinal surgery, intracranial neoplasm, severe uncontrolled HTN. **P/N:** Category C, safety not known in nursing.	Bleeding, allergic reactions (eg, fever, shivering), respiratory depression.
Tenecteplase (TNKase)	**Inj:** 50mg	***Adults*:** Administer as single IV bolus over 5 seconds. **<60kg:** 30mg. **60 to <70kg:** 35mg. **70 to <80kg:** 40mg. **80 to <90kg:** 45mg. **≥90kg:** 50mg. **Max:** 50mg/dose.	**W/P:** Weigh benefits/risks with recent major surgery, cerebrovascular disease, recent GI or GU bleeding, recent trauma, HTN, left heart thrombus, acute pericarditis, subacute bacterial endocarditis, hemostatic defects, severe hepatic dysfunction, pregnancy, diabetic hemorrhagic retinopathy or other hemorrhagic ophthalmic conditions, septic thrombophlebitis or occluded AV cannula at a seriously infected site, elderly, any other bleeding condition that is difficult to manage. Cholesterol embolism and internal/superficial bleeding reported. Arrhythmias may occur with reperfusion. Avoid IM injection, noncompressible arterial puncture, and internal jugular or subclavian venous puncture. Caution with readmission. **Contra:** Active internal bleeding, history of CVA, intracranial or intraspinal surgery or trauma within 2 months, intracranial neoplasm, arteriovenous malformation, aneurysm, bleeding diathesis, severe uncontrolled HTN. **P/N:** Category C, caution in nursing.	Bleeding.

*Scored.   †Bold entries denote special dental considerations.

NAME	FORM/ STRENGTH	DOSAGE	WARNINGS/PRECAUTIONS & CONTRAINDICATIONS	ADVERSE EFFECTS†
Urokinase (Abbokinase)	**Inj:** 250,000IU	**Adults: LD:** 4400 IU/kg IV at 90 mL/hr over 10 minutes. **Maint:** 4400 IU/kg/hr IV at 15mL/hr for 12 hrs. Flush line after each cycle.	**W/P:** Prior to use obtain Hct, platelet count, and aPTT. Increased risk of bleeding; fatalities due to hemorrhage, including intracranial and retroperitoneal, reported. Avoid IM injections, nonessential patient handling, frequent venipunctures. Use upper extremity vessels when performing arterial punctures. Increased risk of bleeding with recent (within 10 days) major surgery, obstetrical delivery, organ biopsy, previous puncture of noncompressible vessels, serious GI bleeding, high likelihood of left heart thrombus, subacute bacterial endocarditis, hemostatic defects including those secondary to severe hepatic or renal disease, pregnancy, cerebrovascular disease, diabetic hemorrhagic retinopathy, and any other condition in which bleeding may be a significant hazard or difficult to manage. May carry risk of transmitting infectious agents. **Contra:** Active internal bleeding, intracranial neoplasm, arteriovenous malformation, aneurysm, bleeding diathesis, severe uncontrolled arterial HTN. Recent (within 2 months) CVA, intracranial or intraspinal surgery, trauma including resuscitation. **P/N:** Category B, caution with nursing.	Bleeding, fatal hemorrhage, anaphylaxis, allergic-type or infusion reactions.

MISCELLANEOUS

NAME	FORM/ STRENGTH	DOSAGE	WARNINGS/PRECAUTIONS & CONTRAINDICATIONS	ADVERSE EFFECTS†
Aprotinin (Trasylol)	**Inj:** 10,000 KIU/mL	**Adults: IV:** Administer through central line. Do not administer other drugs in the same line. **Test Dose:** 1mL 10 minutes before LD. **Regimen A: LD:** 200mL IV over 20-30 minutes. **Pump Prime Dose:** Add 200mL to recirculating priming fluid. **Constant Infusion Dose:** 50mL/hr. **Regimen B:** Give 1/2 doses of Regimen A.	**Possible anaphylactic or anaphylactoid reactions; increased risk if re-exposed to aprotinin-containing products. Weigh benefit against risks in primary CABG surgery if second exposure to aprotinin is required. W/P:** Discontinue if hypersensitivity reactions occur. Take precautions with re-exposure to aprotinin: have emergency anaphylactic treatment available; give test dose and LD only when conditions for rapid cannulation present; delay aprotinin addition into pump prime solution until after LD safely given. Consider giving H_1 and H_2 blockers 15 minutes before test dose. Greater risk of hypersensitivity to aprotinin if history of allergic reactions to other agents. Administer test dose 10 minutes before LD. Administer LD in supine position over 20-30 minutes. Rapid IV administration may cause hypotension. **P/N:** Category B, safety in nursing not known.	Fever, infection, arrhythmia, hypotension, MI, CHF, pericarditis, peripheral edema, GI effects, confusion, insomnia, lung disorder, pleural effusion, atelectasis, dyspnea, pneumothorax, abnormal LFTs and renal function, urinary retention.
Drotrecogin Alfa (Xigris)	**Inj:** 5mg, 20mg	**Adults:** 24mcg/kg/hr IV for 96 hrs.	**W/P:** Increased risk of bleed with platelets <30,000 x 10^6/L (even if platelets increased by transfusions), PT-INR >3, GI bleed within 6 weeks, ischemic stroke within 3 months, intracranial arteriovenous malformation or aneurysm,	Bleeding.

Table 19.1: PRESCRIBING INFORMATION FOR HEMATOLOGIC DRUGS *(cont.)*

NAME	FORM/ STRENGTH	DOSAGE	WARNINGS/PRECAUTIONS & CONTRAINDICATIONS	ADVERSE EFFECTS†
MISCELLANEOUS *(cont.)*				
Drotrecogin Alfa *(cont.)*			known bleeding diathesis, chronic severe hepatic disease, or condition where bleeding is a significant hazard or difficult to manage due to location. If bleeding occurs, stop infusion. Discontinue 2 hrs before invasive surgical procedures or procedures with risk of bleeding. Patients with single organ dysfunction and recent surgery may not be at high risk of death irrespective of APACHE II score and therefore may not be among the indicated population; use in these patients only after careful consideration. **Contra:** Active internal bleeding, hemorrhagic stroke within 3 months, intracranial or intraspinal surgery or severe head trauma within 2 months, trauma with an increased risk of life-threatening bleeding, epidural catheter, intracranial neoplasm or mass lesion, evidence of cerebral herniation. **P/N:** Category C, not for use in nursing.	
Filgrastim (Neupogen)	**Inj:** 300mcg/0.5mL, 300mcg/mL, 480mcg/0.8mL, 480mcg/1.6mL [10^s]	**Adults: Myelosuppressive Chemotherapy: Initial:** 5mcg/kg qd SC bolus, short IV infusion, or continuous SC/IV infusion. Monitor CBCs and platelets before therapy, twice weekly during therapy. **Titrate:** Increase 5mcg/kg for each chemotherapy cycle according to duration and severity of ANC nadir. Avoid 24 hours before through 24 hours after cytotoxic chemotherapy. Perform CBC twice weekly during therapy. Continue therapy after chemotherapy until the post nadir ANC =10,000/mm^3. BMT: Following BMT, 10mcg/kg/day by IV infusion of 4 or 24 hrs, or by continuous 24-hr SC infusion. First dose at least 24 hrs after chemotherapy and at least 24 hrs after bone marrow infusion. **Dose Adjustment:** If ANC >1000/mm^3 for 3 days, 5mcg/kg/day; increase to 10mcg/kg/day if ANC <1000/mm$_3$. If ANC >1000/mm^3 for 3 more days, stop therapy. If ANC drops to <1000/mm^3, resume 5mcg/kg/day. **PBPC:** 10mcg/kg/day bolus or continuous SC 4 days before and for 6-7 days with leukapheresis on days 5, 6 and 7. Monitor neutrophils after 4 days and adjust if WBC >100,000/mm^3. **Chronic Neutropenia: Congenital Neutropenia: Initial:** 6mcg/kg SC bid. **Idiopathic or Cyclic Neutropenia: Initial:** 5mcg/kg SC qd. Adjust dose based on clinical course and ANC.	**W/P:** Allergic-type reactions may occur. Rare cases of splenic rupture reported, some fatal. Evaluate for enlarged spleen or splenic rupture if complaints of left upper abdominal and/or shoulder tip pain. Adult respiratory distress syndrome reported with sepsis; discontinue until resolved. Sickle cell crisis reported with sickle cell disease; keep patient well hydrated. Potential for immunogenicity. **Contra:** Hypersensitivity to *E.coli*-derived proteins. **P/N:** Category C, caution in nursing.	Bone pain, nausea, vomiting, HTN, rash.
Pegfilgrastim (Neulasta)	**Inj:** 6mg/0.6mL	**Adults:** 6mg SC, once per chemotherapy cycle. Do not administer in the period 14 days before and 24 hrs after chemotherapy.	**W/P:** Rare cases of splenic rupture reported, some fatal. Evaluate for enlarged spleen or splenic rupture if complaints of upper abdominal and/or shoulder tip pain. ARDS, allergic reactions (eg, anaphylaxis, rash) reported with filgrastim. Caution with sickle cell disease; monitor for sickle cell crises. Obtain CBC, platelets before chemotherapy.	Medullary bone pain, nausea, fatigue, alopecia, diarrhea, vomiting, constipation, fever, anorexia, headache.

*Scored.   †Bold entries denote special dental considerations.

NAME	FORM/ STRENGTH	DOSAGE	WARNINGS/PRECAUTIONS & CONTRAINDICATIONS	ADVERSE EFFECTS†
Pegfilgrastim *(cont.)*			Monitor Hct, platelets regularly. Do not use in infants, children, and smaller adolescents <45kg. **Contra:** Hypersensitivity to *E.coli*-derived proteins. **P/N:** Category C, caution in nursing.	
Pentoxifylline (Trental)	**Tab, Extended Release:** 400mg	***Adults:*** 400mg tid with meals for at least 8 weeks. Reduce to 400mg bid if digestive and GI side effects occur; discontinue if side effects persist.	**W/P:** Monitor Hgb and Hct with risk factors complicated by hemorrhage (eg, recent surgery, peptic ulceration, cerebral/retinal bleeding). **Contra:** Recent cerebral and/or retinal hemorrhage, intolerance to methylxanthines (eg, caffeine, theophylline, theobromine). **P/N:** Category C, not for use in nursing.	Bloating, dyspepsia, nausea, vomiting, dizziness, headache.
Phytonadione	**Sol:** 1mg/0.5mL, 10mg/mL; **Tab:** 0.1mg, 5mg, 100mcg	***Adults:*** Anticoagulant therapy, Oral - Drug Action Reversal: 2.5-25mg SC/IM/IV/PO (rarely up to 50mg); oral is preferred over subcutaneous. **Factor II Deficiency:** 2.5-25mg SC/IM/IV/PO (rarely up to 50 mg); may repeat dose in 6-8 hr if there is inadequate response. ***Pediatrics:*** **Hemorrhage of Newborn:** 1mg SC or IM. **Prophylaxis:** 0.5-1 mg IM/SC within 1 hr of birth.	**Severe reactions, including fatalities, have occurred during and immediately after intravenous injection of phytonadione, even when precautions have been taken to dilute the phytonadione and to avoid rapid infusion. Severe reactions, including fatalities, have also been reported following intramuscular administration. Typically these severe reactions have resembled hypersensitivity or anaphylaxis, including shock and cardiac and/or respiratory arrest. Some patients have exhibited these severe reactions on receiving phytonadione for the first time. Therefore the intravenous and intramuscular routes should be restricted to those situations where the subcutaneous route is not feasible and the serious risk involved is considered justified. W/P:** Caution with liver disease. Severe reactions, including fatalities, have occurred with IV and IM administration. **P/N:** Category C, safe in nursing.	Skin reaction.
Protamine Sulfate	**Inj:** 10mg/mL	***Adults:*** Administer as slow IV infusion over 10 minutes, at doses not to exceed 50mg. Determine dose by blood coagulation studies. Each mg neutralizes about 90U heparin derived from lung tissue or 115U heparin derived from intestinal mucosa.	**W/P:** May cause allergic reactions with fish hypersensitivity. Rapid administration may cause severe hypotensive and anaphylactoid-like reactions. Caution in cardiac surgeries; hyperheparinemia or bleeding reported. Previous exposure to protamine/protamine-containing insulin may induce humoral immune response; severe hypersensitivity reaction, including life-threatening anaphylaxis reported. Increased risk of antiprotamine antibodies in infertile or vasectomized men. **P/N:** Category C, caution in nursing.	Hypotension, bradycardia, transitory flushing/ feeling of warmth, lassitude, dyspnea, nausea, vomiting, back pain, anaphylaxis that causes severe respiratory distress, circulatory collapse, noncardiogenic pulmonary edema, acute pulmonary HTN.
Sargramostim (Leukine)	**Inj:** 250mcg/vial, 500mcg/mL	***Adults:*** **Myeloid Reconstitution After BMT:** 250mcg/m²/day IV over 2 hrs 2-4 hrs post bone marrow infusion and not less than 24 hrs after last dose of chemo- or radiotherapy. Do not give until ANC <500 cells/mm³. Continue until ANC >1500 cells/mm³ for 3 consecutive days. May reduce dose by 50% or temporarily discontinue if severe adverse reaction occurs. Discontinue immediately if blast cells appear or disease progression occurs.	**W/P:** Contains benzyl alcohol; avoid use in neonates. Caution with pre-existing fluid retention, pulmonary infiltrate, CHF, hypoxia, cardiac disease, renal/hepatic dysfunction, or myeloid malignancies. Monitor CBC twice weekly and renal/hepatic function every other week with pre-existing dysfunction. **Contra:** Excessive leukemic myeloid blasts in bone marrow or peripheral blood (≥10%), concomitant chemotherapy or radiotherapy. **P/N:** Category C, caution in nursing.	Fever, nausea, diarrhea, vomiting, alopecia, rash, headache, **stomatitis**, anorexia, mucous membrane disorder, asthenia, malaise, abdominal pain, edema, HTN.

NAME	FORM/STRENGTH	DOSAGE	WARNINGS/PRECAUTIONS & CONTRAINDICATIONS	ADVERSE EFFECTS[†]
MISCELLANEOUS *(cont.)*				
Sargramostim *(cont.)*		**BMT Failure/Engraftment Delay:** 250mcg/m^2/day IV over 2 hrs for 14 days. May repeat after 7 days if needed. Give third course after another 7 days of 500mcg/m^2/day IV for 14 days if needed. May reduce dose by 50% or temporarily discontinue if severe adverse reaction occurs. Discontinue immediately if blast cells appear or disease progression occurs. Reduce dose by 50% or interrupt treatment if ANC >20,000 cells/mm^3. **Post Peripheral Blood Progenitor Cell Transplant:** 250mcg/m^2/day IV over 24 hrs or SC once daily. Begin immediately after infusion of progenitor cells and continue until ANC >1500 cells/mm^3 for 3 consecutive days. **Mobilization of Peripheral Blood Progenitor Cells (PBPC):** 250mcg/m^2/day IV over 24 hrs or SC once daily. Continue through PBPC collection period. Reduce dose by 50% if WBC >50,000 cells/mm^3. **Neutrophil Recovery Post-Chemo in AML: ≥55 yrs: Hypoplastic Bone Marrow With <5% Blasts:** 250mcg/m^2/day IV over 4 hrs starting on day 11 or 4 days after completion of induction chemo. If 2nd cycle of induction chemo is needed, give 4 days after completion of chemo. Continue until ANC >1500 cells/mm^3 for 3 consecutive days or max of 42 days. Discontinue immediately if leukemic regrowth occurs. May reduce dose by 50% or temporarily discontinue if severe adverse reaction occurs.		
MISCELLANEOUS–ANTIDOTE				
Leucovorin Calcium	**Inj:** 10mg/mL, 50mg, 100mg, 200mg, 350mg, 500mg; **Tab:** 5mg, 10mg, 15mg, 25mg	***Adults:* Colorectal Cancer:** 200mg/m^2 slow IV push over 3 min. followed by 5-FU 370mg/m^2 IV qd for 5 days, or 20mg/m^2 IV qd followed by 5-FU 425mg/m^2 IV qd for 5 days. May repeat at 4-wk intervals for 2 courses then at 4-to 5-wk intervals.May increase 5-FU dose by 10% if no toxicity. Reduce 5-FU dose by 20% with moderate GI/hematologic toxicity and by 30% with severe toxicity. **Leucovorin Rescue:** 15mg q6h for 10 doses starting 24 hrs after start of MTX until serum MTX is <5x10-8M. Give IV/IM with GI toxicity. See labeling for leucovorin adjustments and extended therapy. **Impaired MTX Elimination/Overdose:** 10mg/m^2 IV/IM/PO q6h until serum MTX is <10-8M. Increase to 100mg/m^2 q3h if 24-hr serum creatinine is 50% over baseline, or if 24-hr serum MTX is >5x10-6M, or the 48-hr level is >9x10-7M. Give IV/IM wvith GI toxicity. Start ASAP after overdose and within 24 hrs of MTX with delayed excretion. **Megaloblastic Anemia:** Up to 1mg/day. **Elderly:** Caution with dose selection.	**W/P:** Do not administer >160mg/min. Do not give intrathecally. Monitor serum MTX. Higher than recommended PO doses must be given IV. Increased risk of severe toxicity in elderly/debilitated colorectal cancer patients taking 5-FU with leucovorin. Monitor renal function in elderly. **Contra:** Improper therapy for pernicious anemia and other megaloblastic anemias secondary to lack of vitamin B$_{12}$. **P/N:** Category C, caution in nursing.	Allergic sensitization.

*Scored.   †Bold entries denote special dental considerations.

Table 19.2: DRUG INTERACTIONS FOR HEMATOLOGIC DRUGS

ANTIANEMIC AGENTS

Epoetin Alfa (Epogen, Procrit)

Anticoagulant	Adjust anticoagulant dose in dialysis patients.

ANTICOAGULANT AGENTS

Dalteparin Sodium (Fragmin)

Anticoagulants, oral	Caution with oral anticoagulants due to increased risk of bleeding.
Platelet inhibitors	Caution with platelet inhibitors due to increased risk of bleeding.
Thrombolytic agents	Caution with thrombolytic agents due to increased risk of bleeding.

Enoxaparin Sodium (Lovenox)

Hemorrhage inducers	Discontinue agents that increase risk of hemorrhage (eg, anticoagulants, acetylsalicylic acid, salicylates, NSAIDs, dipyridamole, sulfinpyrazone), unless really needed; monitor closely if co-administered.

Heparin Sodium

Antihistamines	Antihistamines may counteract anticoagulant action.
Dicumarol	Wait ≥5 hrs after last IV dose or 24 hrs after last SQ dose before measure PT for dicumarol.
Digitalis	Digitalis may counteract anticoagulant action.
Nicotine	Nicotine may counteract anticoagulant action.
Platelet inhibitors	Platelet inhibitors (eg, acetylsalicylic acid, dextran, phenylbutazone, ibuprofen, indomethacin, dipyridamole, hydroxychloroquine) may induce bleeding.
Tetracyclines	Tetracyclines may counteract anticoagulant action.
Warfarin	Wait ≥5 hrs after last IV dose or 24 hrs after last SQ dose before measure PT for dicumarol.

Tinzaparin Sodium (Innohep)

Anticoagulants	Increased risk of bleeding with anticoagulants; monitor closely if co-administered.
Platelet inhibitors	Increased risk of bleeding with platelet inhibitors (eg, salicylates, dipyridamole, sulfinpyrazone, dextran, NSAIDs, ticlopidine, clopidogrel); monitor closely if co-administered.
Thrombolytics	Increased risk of bleeding with thrombolytics; monitor closely if co-administered.

Warfarin Sodium (Coumadin)

Anticonvulsant drugs	Potentiates anticonvulsant drugs.
Hemorrhage inducers	Caution with drugs that may cause hemorrhage (eg, NSAIDs, ASA).
Hepatic enzyme inducers	Interacts with hepatic enzyme inducers.

Table 19.2: DRUG INTERACTIONS FOR HEMATOLGIC DRUGS *(cont.)*

ANTICOAGULANT AGENTS *(cont.)*

Warfarin Sodium (Coumadin) *(cont.)*

Hepatic enzyme inhibitors	Interacts with hepatic enzyme inhibitors.
Hypoglycemic drugs	Potentiates hypoglycemic drugs.
Protein bound drugs	Interacts with protein bound drugs.

ANTIFIBRINOLYTIC AGENT

Aminocaproic Acid (Amicar)

Anti-inhibitor coagulant concentrates	Increase risk of thrombosis with anti-inhibitor coagulant concentrates.
Factor IX complex concentrates	Increase risk of thrombosis with factor IX complex concentrates.

ANTIPLATELET AGENTS

Abciximab (Reopro)

Anticoagulants	Increased risk of bleeding with anticoagulants.
Antiplatelets	Increased risk of bleeding with antiplatelets.
Hemostasis affecting drugs	Caution with other drugs that affect hemostasis (eg, thrombolytics, heparin, oral anticoagulants, NSAIDs, dipyridamole, ticlopidine).
Monoclonal antibody agents	If have HACA titers, possible allergic reactions with monoclonal antibody agents.
Thrombolytics	Increased risk of bleeding with thrombolytics.

Anagrelide Hydrochloride (Agrylin)

Cyclic AMP PDE III inhibitors	Exacerbated effects of products that inhibit cyclic AMP PDE III (inotropes: milrinone, enoximone, amrinone, olparinone, cilostazol).
Sucralfate	Sucralfate may interfere with absorption.

Aspirin/Dipyridamole (Aggrenox)

ACE inhibitors	May decrease effects of ACE inhibitors.
Acetazolamide	Potentiates acetazolamide.
Adenosine	Potentiates adenosine.
Anticoagulants	Anticoagulants increase risk of bleeding.
β-blockers	May decrease effects of beta-blockers.
Cholinesterase inhibitors	May decrease effects of cholinesterase inhibitors.
Diuretics	Decreased effects of diuretics in renal or cardiovascular disease.
Hypoglycemics, oral	Potentiates oral hypoglycemics.

ANTIPLATELET AGENTS *(cont.)*

Aspirin/Dipyridamole (Aggrenox) *(cont.)*

Methotrexate	Potentiates methotrexate.
NSAIDs	NSAIDs may increase risk of bleeding and decrease renal function.
Phenytoin	May decrease effects of phenytoin.
Uricosuric agents	May antagonize uricosuric agents.
Valproic acid	Potentiates valproic acid.

Cilostazol (Pletal)

CYP3A4 inhibitors	Caution with CYP3A4 inhibitors (eg, ketoconazole, diltiazem, erythromycin); may increase cilostazol levels.
CYP2C19 inhibitors	Caution with CYP2C19 inhibitors (eg, omeprazole); may increase cilostazol levels.
Grapefruit juice	Avoid grapefruit juice.

Clopidogrel Hydrogen Sulfate (Plavix)

Aspirin	Potentiates effect of aspirin on collagen-induced platelet aggregation.
CYP2C9	Inhibits CYP2C9.
Fluvastatin	Caution with fluvastatin.
NSAIDs	Increased occult GI loss with NSAIDs. Caution with many NSAIDs.
Phenytoin	Caution with phenytoin.
Tamoxifen	Caution with tamoxifen.
Tolbutamide	Caution with tolbutamide
Torsemide	Caution with torsemide.
Warfarin	Caution with warfarin.

Dipyridamole (Persantine)

Adenosine	Increases levels of adenosine.
Cholinesterase inhibitors	May counteract effects of cholinesterase inhibitors.

Eptifibatide (Integrilin)

ASA	Cerebral, pulmonary, GI hemorrhage reported with ASA.
Glycoprotein IIb/IIIa inhibitors	Avoid other glycoprotein IIb/IIIa inhibitors.
Hemostasis affecting drugs	Caution with other drugs that affect hemostasis (eg, thrombolytics, anticoagulants, NSAIDs, dipyridamole).
Heparin	Cerebral, pulmonary, GI hemorrhage reported with heparin.

Ticlopidine Hydrochloride (Ticlid)

Antacids	Antacids reduce plasma levels.

Table 19.2: DRUG INTERACTIONS FOR HEMATOLGIC DRUGS *(cont.)*

ANTIPLATELET AGENTS *(cont.)*

Ticlopidine Hydrochloride (Ticlid) *(cont.)*

Anticoagulants	Discontinue anticoagulants.
ASA	Potentiates ASA effect on platelet aggregation.
Cimetidine	Cimetidine reduces clearance.
CYP450, drugs metabolized by	Adjust dose with drugs metabolized by CYP450 with low therapeutic ratios or with hepatic impairment.
Digoxin	Decreases digoxin plasma levels.
Fibrinolytics	Discontinue fibrinolytics.
Food	Increased bioavailability with food.
NSAIDs	Potentiates NSAIDs effect on platelet aggregation.
Phenytoin	Caution with phenytoin.
Propranolol	Caution with propranolol.
Theophylline	Significant decrease of theophylline plasma clearance.

Tirofiban Hydrochloride (Aggrastat)

ASA	Increased bleeding with ASA.
GP IIb/IIIa inhibitors, parenteral	Avoid other parenteral GP IIb/IIIa inhibitors.
Hemostasis affecting drugs	Caution with other drugs that affect hemostasis (eg, warfarin).
Heparin	Increased bleeding with heparin.
Levothyroxine	Increased clearance with levothyroxine.
Omeprazole	Increased clearance with omeprazole.

NUTRITIONAL SUPPLEMENTS

Ascorbic Acid/Calcium Carbonate/Cyanocobalamin/Folic Acid/Iron/Niacinamide/Pyridoxine/Riboflavin/Thiamine/Vitamin A/Vitamin D (Nu-Iron-V)

Antacids containing carbonates	Iron absorption is inhibited by antacids containg carbonates.
Magnesium trisilicate	Iron absorption is inhibited by magnesium trisilicate.
Levodopa	Pyridoxine may reverse antiparkinsonism effects of levodopa.
Tetracyclines	May interfere with absorption of tetracyclines.

Ascorbic Acid/Calcium Pantothenate/Cyanocobalamin/Ferrous Sulfate/Folic Acid/Niacin/Pyridoxine/ Riboflavin/Thiamine (Iberet-Folic-500)

Antacids containing carbonates	Iron absorption is inhibited by antacids containg carbonates.

NUTRITIONAL SUPPLEMENTS *(cont.)*

Ascorbic Acid/Calcium Pantothenate/Cyanocobalamin/Ferrous Sulfate/Folic Acid/ Niacin/Pyridoxine/ Riboflavin/Thiamine (Iberet-Folic-500) *(cont.)*

Magnesium trisilicate	Iron absorption is inhibited by magnesium trisilicate.
Levodopa	Pyridoxine may reverse antiparkinsonism effects of levodopa.
Tetracyclines	May interfere with absorption of tetracyclines.

Ascorbic Acid/Cyanocobalamin/Ferrous Bisglycinate Chelate/Folic Acid/Iron Polysaccharide (Niferex-150 Forte)

Antacids containing carbonates	Iron absorption is inhibited by antacids containing carbonates.
Magnesium trisilicate	Iron absorption is inhibited by magnesium trisilicate.
Tetracyclines	May interfere with absorption of tetracyclines.

Ascorbic Acid/Ferrous Bisglycinate Chelate/Iron Polysaccharide (Niferex-150)

Antacids containing carbonates	Iron absorption is inhibited by antacids containing carbonates.
Magnesium trisilicate	Iron absorption is inhibited by magnesium trisilicate.
Tetracyclines	May interfere with absorption of tetracyclines.

Ascorbic Acid/Ferrous Fumarate (Fero-Grad-500, Vitron-C, Vitron-C Plus)

Antacids containing carbonates	Absorption may be inhibited by antacids containing carbonates.
Magnesium trisilicate	Absorption may be inhibited by magnesium trisilicate.
Tetracyclines	May interfere with the absorption of tetracyclines.

Ascorbic Acid/Ferrous Sulfate/Folic Acid (Fero-Folic 500)

Antacids containing carbonates	Absorption may be inhibited by antacids containing carbonates.
Magnesium trisilicate	Absorption may be inhibited by magnesium trisilicate.
Tetracyclines	May interfere with the absorption of tetracyclines.

Cyanocobalamin/Folic Acid/Iron Polysaccharide (Hemocyte-F)

Antacids containing carbonates	Absorption may be inhibited by antacids containing carbonates.
Magnesium trisilicate	Absorption may be inhibited by magnesium trisilicate.
Tetracyclines	May interfere with the absorption of tetracyclines.

Cyanocobalamin/Folic Acid/Iron Polysaccharide (Poly-Iron 150 Forte)

Antacids containing carbonates	Absorption may be inhibited by antacids containing carbonates.
Magnesium trisilicate	Absorption may be inhibited by magnesium trisilicate.
Tetracyclines	May interfere with the absorption of tetracyclines.

Table 19.2: DRUG INTERACTIONS FOR HEMATOLGIC DRUGS *(cont.)*

NUTRITIONAL SUPPLEMENTS *(cont.)*

Ferrous Bisglycinate Chelate/Iron Polysaccharide (Niferex)

Antacids containing carbonates	Absorption may be inhibited by antacids containing carbonates.
Magnesium trisilicate	Absorption may be inhibited by magnesium trisilicate.
Tetracyclines	May interfere with the absorption of tetracyclines.

Ferrous Fumarate (Feostat, Ferretts, Ferrocite, Hemocyte, Ircon)

Antacids containing carbonates	Absorption may be inhibited by antacids containing carbonates.
Magnesium trisilicate	Absorption may be inhibited by magnesium trisilicate.
Tetracyclines	May interfere with the absorption of tetracyclines.

Ferrous Fumarate/Folic Acid (Hemocyte-F, Ircon-FA)

Antacids containing carbonates	Absorption may be inhibited by antacids containing carbonates.
Magnesium trisilicate	Absorption may be inhibited by magnesium trisilicate.
Tetracyclines	May interfere with the absorption of tetracyclines.

Ferrous Gluconate (Fergon, Feronate)

Antacids containing carbonates	Absorption may be inhibited by antacids containing carbonates.
Magnesium trisilicate	Absorption may be inhibited by magnesium trisilicate.
Tetracyclines	May interfere with the absorption of tetracyclines.

Ferrous Sulfate (Feosol, Feratab, Fer-in-sol, Ferrousal, Slow Fe)

Antacids containing carbonates	Absorption may be inhibited by antacids containing carbonates.
Magnesium trisilicate	Absorption may be inhibited by magnesium trisilicate.
Tetracyclines	May interfere with the absorption of tetracyclines.

Ferrous Sulfate/Folic Acid (Slow Fe w/Folic Acid)

Antacids containing carbonates	Absorption may be inhibited by antacids containing carbonates.
Magnesium trisilicate	Absorption may be inhibited by magnesium trisilicate.
Tetracyclines	May interfere with the absorption of tetracyclines.

Folic Acid

Alcohol	Alcohol increases loss of folate.
Alcoholic cirrhosis	Alcoholic cirrhosis increases loss of folate.
Barbiturates	Barbiturates increases loss of folate.

NUTRITIONAL SUPPLEMENTS *(cont.)*

Folic Acid *(cont.)*

Methotrexate	Methotrexate increases loss of folate.
Nitrofurantoin	Nitrofurantoin increases loss of folate.
Phenobarbital	Increased seizures with phenobarbital reported.
Phenytoin	Antagonizes phenytoin effects. Phenytoin increases loss of folate. Increased seizures with phenytoin reported.
Primidone	Primidone increases loss of folate. Increased seizures with primidone reported.
Pyrimethamine	Pyrimethamine increases loss of folate.
Tetracycline	Tetracycline may cause false low serum and red cell folate due to suppression of *Lactobacillus casei*.

Folic Acid/Iron Polysaccharide (Irofol)

Antacids containing carbonates	Absorption may be inhibited by antacids containing carbonates.
Magnesium trisilicate	Absorption may be inhibited by magnesium trisilicate.
Trisilicate	May interfere with the absorption of tetracyclines.

Iron Dextran (Infed)

Iron, oral	Discontinue oral iron before use.

Iron Sucrose (Venofer)

Iron, oral	Avoid oral iron preparations.

THROMBOLYTIC/ANTITHROMBIN AGENTS

Alteplase, Recombinant (Activase)

Heparin	Increased risk of bleeding with heparin given before, during, or after alteplase therapy.
Platelet, altering drugs	Increased risk of bleeding with drugs altering platelets (eg, ASA, dipyridamole, abciximab) given before, during, or after alteplase therapy.
Vitamin K antagonists	Increased risk of bleeding with vitamin K antagonists given before, during, or after alteplase therapy.

Antithrombin III Human (Thrombate III)

Heparin	The anticoagulant effect of heparin is enhanced.

Argatroban

Anticoagulants	Other anticoagulants may increase risk of bleeding. Discontinue all anticoagulants before argatroban administration.
Antiplatelets	Antiplatelets may increase risk of bleeding.
Heparin	Initiate after cessation of heparin therapy; allow time for heparin's effect on the aPTT to decrease.

Table 19.2: DRUG INTERACTIONS FOR HEMATOLGIC DRUGS *(cont.)*

THROMBOLYTIC/ANTITHROMBIN AGENTS *(cont.)*

Alteplase, Recombinant (Activase)

Thrombolytics	Thrombolytics may increase risk of bleeding.
Warfarin	Prolongation of PT and INR with warfarin.

Bivalirudin (Angiomax)

Heparin	Increased risk of major bleeding with heparin.
Warfarin	Increased risk of major bleeding with warfarin.
Thrombolytics	Increased risk of major bleeding with thrombolytics.

Fondaparinux Sodium (Arixtra)

Hemorrhage inducers	Discontinue agents that may enhance risk of hemorrhage (eg, platelet inhibitors); monitor closely if co-administered.

Lepirudin (Refludan)

Coumarin	Increased risk of bleeding with coumarin derivatives.
Platelet inhibitors	Increased risk of bleeding with other drugs that affect platelet function.
Thrombolytics	Thrombolytics increase risk of life-threatening intracranial bleeding or other bleeding complications and may enhance the effect on a PTT prolongation.

Reteplase, Recombinant (Retavase)

Anticoagulants	Weigh benefits/risks with oral anticoagulants.
Heparin	Increased risk of bleeding with heparin before or after therapy.
Platelet inhibitors	Increased risk of bleeding with drugs that alter platelet function (eg, ASA, NSAIDs, dipyridamole, abciximab) before or after therapy.
Vitamin K antagonists	Increased risk of bleeding with vitamin K antagonists before or after therapy.

Streptokinase (Streptase)

Anticoagulants	Anticoagulants may cause bleeding problems.
Antiplatelets	Antiplatelets may cause bleeding problems.

Tenecteplase (TNKase)

Anticoagulants, oral	Weigh benefits/risks with oral anticoagulants.
GP IIb/IIIa inhibitors	Weigh benefits/risks with GP IIb/IIIa inhibitors.
Heparin	Increased risk of bleeding with heparin before or after therapy.
Platelet inhibitors	Increased risk of bleeding with drugs that alter platelet function (eg, ASA, NSAIDs, dipyridamole, GP IIb/IIIa inhibitors) before or after therapy.
Vitamin K antagonists	Increased risk of bleeding with vitamin K antagonists before or after therapy.

Urokinase (Abbokinase)

Anticoagulants	Increased risk of serious bleeding with anticoagulants.

THROMBOLYTIC/ANTITHROMBIN AGENTS *(cont.)*

Urokinase (Abbokinase) *(cont.)*

Platelet inhibitors	Increased risk of serious bleeding with agents inhibiting platelet function (eg, ASA, other NSAIDs, dipyridamole, GP IIb/IIIa inhibitors).
Thrombolytics	Increased risk of serious bleeding with other thrombolytic agents.

MISCELLANEOUS

Aprotinin (Trasylol)

Captopril	May block acute hypotensive effect of captopril.
Fibrinolytic agents	May inhibit effects of fibrinolytic agents.
Heparin	Concomitant heparin may prolong activated clotting time.
Anticoagulants, oral	Increased risk of bleed with oral anticoagulants.
ASA	Increased risk of bleed with ASA > 650mg.
Glycoprotein IIb/IIIa inhibitors	Increased risk of bleed with glycoprotein IIb/IIIa inhibitors within 7 days.
Hemostasis affecting drugs	Caution with drugs that affect hemostasis.
Heparin	Increased risk of bleed with therapeutic heparin.
Platelet inhibitors	Increased risk of bleed with platelet inhibitors.
Thrombolytic therapy	Increased risk of bleed with therapeutic thrombolytic therapy within 3 days.

Filgrastim (Neupogen)

Neutrophils enhancers	Caution with drugs that may potentiate the release of neutrophils (eg, lithium).

Pegfilgrastim (Neulasta)

Lithium	Lithium may potentiate release of neutrophils; monitor neutrophil counts.

Pentoxifylline (Trental)

Antihypertensives	May increase effect of antihypertensives.
Theophylline	May increase in theophylline levels; risk of theophylline toxicity.
Warfarin	Increase risk of bleeding with warfarin; monitor PT/INR more frequently.

Protamine Sulfate

Antibiotics	Incompatible with certain antibiotics, such as cephalosporins and penicillins.

Sargramostim (Leukine)

Myeloproliferative enhancers	Caution with drugs that may potentiate myeloproliferative effects (eg, lithium, corticosteroids).

Table 19.2: DRUG INTERACTIONS FOR HEMATOLGIC DRUGS *(cont.)*

MISCELLANEOUS–ANTIDOTE

Leucovorin Calcium

5-FU	May enhance 5-FU toxicity.
Folic acid	Folic acid in large amounts may antagonize phenobarbital, phenytoin, and primidone, and increase seizure frequency in children.
MTX	May reduce MTX efficacy.
TMP-SMZ	Increased treatment failure and morbidity in TMP-SMZ-treated HIV patients with PCP.

Chapter 20

Endocrine/Hormonal and Bone Metabolism Drugs

Angelo J. Mariotti, D.D.S., Ph.D.

Hormones are chemical substances that are secreted from various organs into the blood stream and have specific regulatory effects on target tissues. The general functions of hormones can be divided into reproduction; growth and development; homeostasis of the internal environment; and energy production, use and storage.

Although the effects of hormones are diverse and complex, hormones can be divided into two broad categories according to their chemical structure: polypeptides and steroids. The polypeptides or amino acid derivates represent a majority of hormones. This category comprises hormones that are secreted from a variety of organs (such as brain, pancreas, thyroid and adrenal glands) and include large polypeptides (such as luteinizing hormone), medium-sized peptides (such as insulin), small peptides (such as thyrotropin-releasing hormone), dipeptides (such as thyroxine) and single amino acid byproducts (such as histamine).

The remaining hormones are derivatives of cholesterol and are called steroid hormones. Similarly to the polypeptide hormones, steroid hormones are secreted from a variety of organs (such as adrenal glands, testis and ovary). But unlike the polypeptide hormones, they are more uniform in their chemical structure, because each steroid hormone must contain a cyclopentanoperhydrophenanthrene ring system (for example, estradiol).

Hormones, regardless of their chemical structure, have common characteristics. First, hormones are found in low concentrations in the blood circulation. Most polypeptide hormone concentrations in the blood range from 1 to 100 femtomolar, while thyroid and steroid hormone concentrations range between picomolar and micromolar concentrations. Second, hormones must be directed to their sites of action, and this is most commonly accomplished by special protein molecules (receptors) that recognize specific hormones. Polypeptide hormone receptors are proteins that are fixed on the cell membrane; thyroid and steroid hormone receptors are proteins located inside the cell.

Although most drugs are considered to be substances foreign to the body, naturally occurring hormones, analogs of hormones and hormone antagonists can be used as drugs and can exert important effects on the body. For example, endocrine drugs can be used to treat osteoporosis. Although the theories regarding the pathogenesis of osteoporosis are diverse, it is known that estrogen deficiency in women is an important factor in bone loss. A variety of endocrine drugs have been used to help treat osteoporosis. Drugs such as androgens, estrogens, oral contraceptives, serum estrogen receptor modulators and calcitonin have been used.

In addition to these endocrine drugs, other important medications for treating osteoporosis are bone metabolism agents such as bisphosphonates.

Androgens

Special Dental Considerations
Androgens can exacerbate patients' inflammatory status, causing erythema and an increased tendency toward gingival bleeding. A controlled oral hygiene program that combines professional cleanings and plaque control will minimize androgen-induced sequelae.

Drug Interactions of Dental Interest
Androgens are responsible for the growth and development of male sex organs and for the maintenance of secondary sexual characteristics in males. Androgens can be used for replacement therapy in androgen-deficient men or for treatment of certain neoplasms. Androgens may enhance the actions of oral anticoagulants, oral hypoglycemic agents and glucocorticoids.

See Tables 20.1 and 20.2 for general information on androgens.

Pharmacology
Androgens bind to intracellular androgen receptors that regulate RNA and DNA in target tissues.

Estrogens

Special Dental Considerations
Estrogens can exacerbate patients' inflammatory status, causing erythema and an increased tendency toward gingival bleeding. In some instances, estrogens have been reported to induce gingival enlargements. A controlled

oral hygiene program that combines professional cleanings and plaque control will minimize estrogen-induced sequelae.

Drug Interactions of Dental Interest
Estrogens are responsible for the growth and development of female sex organs and for the maintenance of secondary sexual characteristics in women. Estrogens can be used to treat a variety of estrogen-deficiency states, as well as for certain neoplasms. Estrogen may change the requirements for oral anticoagulants, oral hypoglycemics, insulin or barbiturates.

See Tables 20.1 and 20.2 for general information on estrogens.

Pharmacology
Estrogens bind to intracellular estrogen receptors that regulate RNA and DNA in target tissues.

Serum Estrogen Receptor Modulators

Special Dental Considerations
The effects of serum estrogen receptor modulators (SERMs) on the oral cavity are largely unknown. SERMs can have variable effects depending on the type of estrogen receptor found in the oral cavity. Patients taking raloxifene will have lowered bone mineral density and, as a result, also may be more susceptible to periodontitis.

See Tables 20.1 and 20.2 for general information on SERMs.

Drug Interactions of Dental Interest
Caution should be used when prescribing diazepam, ibuprofen or naproxen with raloxifene, as these drugs can affect the binding of raloxifene to plasma proteins.

Pharmacology
Depending on the subtype of estrogen receptor found in a tissue, SERMs (such as

raloxifene and tamoxifen) may act as either estrogen receptor agonists or estrogen receptor antagonists.

Oral Contraceptives

Special Dental Considerations

Most studies recording changes in gingival tissues associated with oral contraceptives were completed when contraceptive concentrations were at much higher levels than are available today. These investigations reported an exacerbation of the gingival inflammatory response sometimes leading to a gingival enlargement. A recent clinical study evaluating the effects of current oral contraceptives on gingival inflammation in young women found these hormonal agents to have no effect on gingival tissues. From these data, it appears that current compositions of oral contraceptives probably are not as harmful to the periodontium as were the early formulations. Nonetheless, a controlled oral hygiene program that includes regular oral examinations, professional cleanings and plaque control will minimize the effects of oral contraceptives. These drugs also may increase the incidence of local alveolar osteitis after extraction of teeth.

Drug Interactions of Dental Interest

Oral contraceptives are used primarily to prevent ovulation. The effectiveness of oral contraceptives may be decreased by penicillin, chloramphenicol, oral neomycin, sulfonamides, barbiturates, glucocorticoids, griseofulvin and tetracyclines.

See Tables 20.1 and 20.2 for general information on oral contraceptives.

Pharmacology

Oral contraceptives prevent conception by suppressing ovulation, preventing nidation or slowing migration of sperm to the ovum.

Progestins

Special Dental Considerations

Progestins can exacerbate patients' inflammatory status, causing erythema and an increased tendency toward gingival bleeding. In some instances, progestins have been reported to induce gingival enlargement. A controlled oral hygiene program that includes regular oral examinations, professional cleanings and plaque control will minimize the effects of progestins.

Drug Interactions of Dental Interest

Progestins are responsible for maintenance of the female reproductive system in pregnant and nonpregnant women. Progestins are used for the treatment of certain female hormone imbalances as well as for the treatment of some neoplasms. Drug interactions with progestins are limited and involve drugs not normally prescribed by dentists.

See Tables 20.1 and 20.2 for general information on progestins.

Pharmacology

Progestins bind to intracellular progesterone receptors that regulate RNA and DNA in target tissues.

Insulin

Special Dental Considerations

Patients with diabetes mellitus are at risk of developing periodontal disease. A thorough evaluation of the mouth followed by a controlled oral hygiene program—including regular oral examinations, professional cleanings and plaque control—are recommended. Because diabetics have an increased risk of developing leukopenia and thrombocytopenia, an increased frequency of infection, altered wound healing and gingival bleeding are possible. Dental treatment should be delayed if leukopenia or cytopenia occurs.

People who have either type 1 or type 2 diabetes mellitus can experience untoward effects in the dental office. These can occur when a patient's insulin dose is not correctly titrated and blood glucose levels are either too low or too high. In patients whose diabetes is well-controlled by insulin (or other hypoglycemic agents), these concerns are minimized by proper medication in conjunction with proper diet. Signs of hypo- and hyperglycemia are listed in Table 20.3.

Drug Interactions of Dental Interest

Insulin can be used for the treatment of patients with either type 1 or type 2 diabetes mellitus. Corticosteroids may enhance blood glucose levels, and large doses of salicylates and nonsteroidal anti-inflammatory drugs may increase the hypoglycemic effect of insulin.

Laboratory Value Alterations

- Values for leukocytes in leukopenia: less than 4,000 cells per cubic millimeter as opposed to the normal values, 5,000-10,000 cells/mm^3.
- Values for platelets in thrombocytopenia: less than 20,000 platelets/mm^3 as opposed to the normal values of 150,000-350,000 platelets/mm^3.
See Tables 20.1 and 20.2 for general information on insulin.

Pharmacology

Insulin binds to fixed receptors on the cell membrane to control the storage and metabolism of carbohydrates, proteins and lipids.

Oral Hypoglycemic Agents

Special Dental Considerations

Patients with diabetes mellitus are at risk of developing periodontal disease. In patients whose diabetes is well-controlled by hypoglycemic agents, concerns are minimized with proper medication, proper diet and proper oral hygiene. It is recommended that these patients receive a thorough evaluation of the mouth followed by a controlled oral hygiene program that includes regular oral examinations, professional cleanings and plaque control. Owing to an increased risk of leukopenia and thrombocytopenia in diabetic patients, an increased frequency of infection, altered wound healing and gingival bleeding is possible. Dental treatment should be delayed if leukopenia or cytopenia occurs.

Drug Interactions of Dental Interest

Oral hypoglycemic agents can be used only for the treatment of type 2 diabetes mellitus. Glucocorticoids may decrease the effectiveness of oral hypoglycemic agents. Nonsteroidal anti-inflammatory drugs and salicylates may increase the risk of hypoglycemia. See the box on page 430 for a listing of signs of hypoglycemia.

Laboratory Value Alterations

- Values for leukocytes in leukopenia: less than 4,000 cells/mm^3 as opposed to the normal values of 5,000-10,000 cells/mm^3.
- Values for platelets in thrombocytopenia: less than 20,000 platelets/mm^3 as opposed to the normal values of 150,000-350,000 platelets/mm^3.
See Tables 20.1 and 20.2 for general information on oral hypoglycemic agents.

Pharmacology

Oral hypoglycemics lower blood glucose levels by stimulating the functioning of β cells of the pancreatic islets to secrete insulin.

Calcitonin

Special Dental Considerations

Calcitonin is administered primarily intranasally to treat Paget's disease, osteoporosis or hypercalcemia. As a result of the nasal administration, a variety of oral-facial sequelae (such as skin rash, urticaria, flushing, redness and swelling) can occur. Except for allergic reactions, these signs and symptoms should not be considered for medical attention unless they continue or are bothersome.

See Tables 20.1 and 20.2 for general information on calcitonin.

Drug Interactions of Dental Interest
When calcitonin is delivered via a nasal route, it can cause nasal symptoms that include the development of crusts, dryness, epistaxis, inflammation, rhinitis and itching.

Pharmacology
Calcitonin is a polypeptide hormone that is secreted from the C cells of the thyroid gland. Calcitonin binds to the cell surface receptor and inhibits osteoclastic bone resorption while promoting the renal excretion of calcium, phosphate, sodium, magnesium and potassium. Calcitonin ultimately acts to lower calcium in the bloodstream.

Thyroid Hormones

Special Dental Considerations
Patients with well-controlled hypothyroidism can receive any dental treatment. Dental treatment should be delayed in patients whose thyroid symptoms are not appropriately controlled pharmacologically.

Drug Interactions of Dental Interest
Thyroid hormones, a mixture of liothyroxin and levothyroxine, are necessary for the homeostasis of the human body. Liothyroxin and/or levothyroxine are used for replacement therapy in patients with diminished thyroid function. Glucocorticoids and sym-

pathomimetic agents may interfere with the actions of the drugs.

See Tables 20.1 and 20.2 for general information on thyroid hormones.

Pharmacology
Thyroid hormones bind to nuclear thyroid hormone receptors that regulate catabolic and anabolic effects necessary for homeostasis.

Antithyroid Agents

Special Dental Considerations
Dental treatment should be delayed in patients with hyperthyroidism whose symptoms are not appropriately controlled pharmacologically or surgically. Antithyroid hormones are a group of drugs used to decrease the production of thyroid hormones. Because these agents have the potential to depress cells in the bone marrow, the incidence of microbial infections can increase, resulting in delayed healing and gingival bleeding. A patient who is using antithyroid drugs may exhibit leukopenia, thrombocytopenia or both, and any dental work should be deferred until blood counts return to normal.

Drug Interactions of Dental Interest
Methimazole and propylthiouracil are used in the treatment of patients with hyperthyroidism before surgery or radiotherapy. These drugs can cause mouth sores, sialadenopathy, loss of taste, gingival bleeding and delayed wound healing.

See Tables 20.1 and 20.2 for general information on antithyroid hormones.

Pharmacology
Antithyroid hormones inhibit the synthesis of thyroid hormones by interfering with the oxidation of iodide to iodine, thereby blocking the synthesis of thyroxine.

Bisphosphonates

Special Dental Considerations

Drugs that are used to treat osteoporosis may be very important to the dentist, since initial studies have suggested that there might be an association between periodontitis and osteoporosis. Additional studies are needed to demonstrate if a causative relationship exists between osteoporosis and tooth loss. Initial short-term studies in patients with periodontitis who are using bisphosphonates have suggested that these agents may play an important role in the maintenance of alveolar bone. Concomitant use of salicylates or salicylate-containing compounds with bisphosphonates is not recommended since an increased incidence of upper gastrointestinal adverse events can occur.

One of the more important considerations with bisphosphonates for the dentist are the reports of osteonecrosis of the jaw associated with the use of these drugs. The majority of cases of bisphosphonate-associated osteonecrosis (BON) have been associated with the intravenous administration of these agents; however, BON has been reported (at a significantly lower prevalence) with the enteral administration of bisphosphonates. Currently, data are limited regarding the incidence and prevalence of this condition and in identifying the risk factors that may influence BON in patients taking these drugs orally. See Appendix P for ADA recommendations on the dental management of patients on oral bisphosphonate therapy.

Pharmacology

Bisphosphonates work to inhibit osteoclast activity and help to preserve bone mass.

Adverse Effects, Precautions and Contraindications

Table 20.1 presents contraindications, precautions and adverse effects of endocrine/hormonal and bone metabolism drugs.

Suggested Readings

Galasko GT. Pituitary, thyroid and parathyroid pharmacology. In: Pharmacology and Therapeutics for Dentistry. 5th ed. Yagiela JA, Dowd FJ, Neidle EA (eds). St. Louis: Elsevier Mosby; 2004:555-64.

Galasko GT. Insulin, oral hypoglycemics, and glucagon. In: Pharmacology and Therapeutics for Dentistry. 5th ed. Yagiela JA, Dowd FJ, Neidle EA (eds). St. Louis: Elsevier Mosby; 2004:573-82.

Mariotti A. Sex steroid hormones and cell dynamics in the periodontium. Crit Rev Oral Biol Med 1994;5:27-53.

Mariotti AJ. Steroid hormones of reproduction and sexual development. In: Pharmacology and Therapeutics for Dentistry. 5th ed. Yagiela JA, Dowd FJ, Neidle EA (eds). St. Louis: Elsevier Mosby; 2004:583-94.

Preshaw PM, Knutsen M, Mariotti A. Experimental gingivitis in women using oral contraceptives. J Dent Res 2001;80:2011-15.

Table 20.1: PRESCRIBING INFORMATION FOR ENDOCRINE/HORMONAL AND BONE METABOLISM DRUGS

NAME	FORM/ STRENGTH	DOSAGE	WARNINGS/PRECAUTIONS & CONTRAINDICATIONS	ADVERSE EFFECTS†
ANDROGENS				
Methyltestos-teroneCIII (Testred)	**Cap:** 10mg	***Adults:*** Dose based on age, sex, and diagnosis. Adjust dose according to clinical response and adverse events. **Male Replacement Therapy:** 10-50mg/day. **Breast Carcinoma:** 50-200mg/day. ***Pediatrics:*** Dose based on age, sex, and diagnosis. Adjust dose according to clinical response and adverse events. **Delayed Puberty:** Use lower range of 10-50mg/day for 4-6 months. Caution in pediatrics.	**W/P:** Discontinue if hypercalcemia occurs in breast cancer; monitor calcium levels. Monitor for virilization in females. Risk of compromised stature in pediatrics; monitor bone growth every 6 months. Risk of hepatic damage with long-term use. Discontinue if jaundice or cholestatic hepatitis occurs. Risk of edema; caution with pre-existing cardiac, renal, or hepatic disease. Caution in the elderly; increased risk of prostatic hypertrophy and prostatic carcinoma. Should not be used for enhancement of athletic performance. Monitor LFTs, Hct, and Hgb periodically. **Contra:** Pregnancy. Males with breast or prostate carcinoma. **P/N:** Category X, not for use in nursing.	Amenorrhea, virilization, menstrual irregularities, gynecomastia, excessive frequency/duration of penile erections, male pattern baldness, increased/decreased libido, oligospermia, hirsutism, acne, fluid and electrolyte disturbances, nausea, hypercholesterolemia, clotting factor suppression, polycythemia, altered LFTs, priapism, anxiety, and depression.
OxandroloneCIII (Oxandrin)	**Tab:** 2.5mg*, 10mg	***Adults:*** Usual: 2.5-20mg/day given bid-qid for 2-4 weeks. May repeat course intermittently as indicated. **Elderly:** 5mg bid. ***Pediatrics:*** ≤0.1mg/kg/day. May repeat intermittently as indicated.	**W/P:** Discontinue if peliosis hepatis, liver cell tumors, cholestatic hepatitis, jaundice, LFT abnormalities, hypercalcemia, or signs of virilization (females) occur. Edema with or without CHF may occur with pre-existing cardiac, renal, or hepatic disease. Monitor bone growth in children every 6 months. Increased risk of prostatic hypertrophy/carcinoma in the elderly. May decrease levels of thyroxine-binding globulin, suppress clotting factors II, V, VII, and X, and increase PT. Caution with CAD and history of MI. Lower dose recommended in elderly. **Contra:** Carcinoma of the prostate or breast, carcinoma of the breast in females with hypercalcemia, pregnancy, nephrosis, hypercalcemia. **P/N:** Category X, not for use in nursing.	Cholestatic jaundice, gynecomastia, edema, CNS effects, acne, phallic enlargement, increased frequency/persistence of erections, inhibition of testicular function, chronic priapism, epididymitis, impotence, testicular atrophy, oligospermia, bladder irritability, menstrual irregularities, and virilization.
Testosterone (Androderm, Androgel, Testim)	**Patch: (Androderm)** 2.5mg/24hrs [60s], 5mg/24 hrs [30s] **Gel: (Androgel)** 1% [2.5g, 5g packets, 75g pump] **Gel: (Testim)** 1% [5g (50mg)/tube 30s]	***Adults:*** **Androderm: Initial:** 5mg/day. **Maint:** 2.5mg-7.5mg/day. Apply patch nightly to intact skin of the back, abdomen, upper arm, or thigh. Rotate sites; avoid same site for 7 days. Do not apply to scrotum or oily, damaged, irritated areas. May apply 2 patches at same time. **Androgel:** Apply 5g qd to clean, dry, intact skin of shoulders and upper arms and/or abdomen. Allow to dry prior to dressing. **Titrate:** May increase to 7.5g qd, then 10g qd if response not achieved. Do not apply to scrotum/genitals. **Testim:** Apply 5g qd, preferably in the am, to clean, dry, intact skin of shoulders and/or upper arms. Allow to dry prior to dressing. **Titrate:** May increase to 10g qd if response not achieved or serum concentration is below normal range. Do not apply to genitals or abdomen. To maintain serum testosterone levels, do not wash site of application for at least 2 hrs.	**W/P:** Prolonged use is associated with serious hepatic effects. Increased risk for prostatic hyperplasia/carcinoma in elderly. Risk of edema with pre-existing cardiac, renal, or hepatic disease; discontinue if edema occurs. Risk of virilization of female sex partner. Monitor LFTs, Hgb, Hct, PSA, cholesterol, and lipids. May potentiate sleep apnea. Transfer of testosterone can occur with skin-to-skin contact. Gels are flammable; avoid fire, flame, or smoking during use. **Contra:** Breast or prostate carcinoma in men. Pregnant women should avoid skin contact with application sites in men. **P/N:** Category X, not for use in nursing.	Gynecomastia, pruritus/ erythema/vesicles/blister at application site, prostate abnormalities, headache, and depression.

*Scored.   †Bold entries denote special dental considerations.

Table 20.1: PRESCRIBING INFORMATION FOR ENDOCRINE/HORMONAL AND BONE METABOLISM DRUGS (cont.)

NAME	FORM/ STRENGTH	DOSAGE	WARNINGS/PRECAUTIONS & CONTRAINDICATIONS	ADVERSE EFFECTS†
ANDROGENS (cont.)				
Testosterone Cypionate^{CIII} (Depo-Testosterone)	**Inj:** 100mg/mL, 200mg/mL	**Adults: Male Hypogonadism:** 50-400mg IM every 2-4 weeks. Dose based on age, sex, and diagnosis. Adjust dose according to response and adverse reactions. **Pediatrics:** ≥12 yrs: Male Hypogonadism: 50-400mg IM every 2-4 weeks. Dose based on age, sex, and diagnosis. Adjust dose according to response and adverse reactions.	**W/P:** May accelerate bone maturation without linear growth; monitor bone growth every 6 months. Risk of hepatic damage with long-term use. Discontinue if hypercalcemia occurs in immobilized patients. Discontinue with acute urethral obstruction, priapism, excessive sexual stimulation, or oligospermia; restart at lower doses. Risk of edema; caution with pre-existing cardiac, renal, or hepatic disease. Caution in the elderly; increased risk of prostatic hypertrophy and prostatic carcinoma. Caution with BPH. Should not be used for enhancement of athletic performance. Do not administer IV. Monitor Hct, Hgb, and cholesterol periodically. **Contra:** Severe renal, hepatic, and cardiac disease. Males with carcinoma of the breast or prostate gland. Pregnancy. **P/N:** Category X, not for use in nursing.	Gynecomastia, excessive frequency/duration of penile erections, male pattern baldness, increased/decreased libido, oligospermia, hirsutism, acne, fluid and electrolyte disturbances, nausea, hypercholesterolemia, clotting factor suppression, polycythemia, altered LFTs, priapism, anxiety, and depression.
CONTRACEPTIVES (Oral)				
Desogestrel/ Ethinyl Estradiol (Cyclessa, Desogen, Mircette, Orthocept); **Drospirenone/ Ethinyl Estradiol** (Yasmin, YAZ); **Ethinyl Estradiol/Ethynodiol Diacetate** (Demulen 1/35-28, Demulen 1/50-21, Demulen 1/50-28); **Ethinyl Estradiol/Etonogestrel** (Nuvaring); **Ethinyl Estradiol/ Ferrous Fumarate/ Norethindrone Acetate** (Estrostep FE, Loestrin FE 1.5/30, Loestrin FE 1/20); **Ethinyl Estradiol/ Levonorgestrel** (Alesse 28, Levlen, Levlite 28, Nordette-28, Seasonale, Tri-Levlen, Triphasil-21, Triphasil-28); **Ethinyl Estradiol/ Norelgestromin** (Ortho Evra);	See manufacturer's package insert for specific brand information.	See manufacturer's package insert for specific brand information.	**W/P: [ALL]** Cigarette smoking increases risk of serious cardiovascular side effects. Risk increases with age (especially >35 yrs) and heavy smoking. Increased risk of MI, vascular disease, thromboembolism, stroke, and gallbladder disease. Retinal thrombosis, hepatic neoplasia, carcinoma of breast and reproductive organs reported. May cause glucose intolerance. May increase BP, elevate LDL levels or cause other lipid changes, fluid retention, breakthrough bleeding, and spotting. May cause or exacerbate migraine. May develop visual changes with contact lens. Increased risk of MI with HTN, hyperlipidemia, obesity or diabetes. Discontinue if jaundice, significant depression or ophthalmic irregularities develop. Not for use before menarche or with uncontrolled HTN. Alternate method recommended with history of HTN or renal disease. Perform annual physical exam. May affect certain endocrine, LFTs, and blood components. **[Seasonale]** Weigh benefit of fewer planned menses against inconvenience of increased intermenstrual bleeding or spotting. **[Yasmin, YAZ]** Monitor K+ levels during 1st cycle with conditions predisposing to hyperkalemia. **Contra: [ALL]** Thrombophlebitis, deep-vein thrombosis or thromboembolic disorders, pregnancy, cerebrovascular or coronary artery disease, undiagnosed abnormal genital bleeding, cholestatic jaundice of pregnancy or jaundice with prior pill use, hepatic adenomas or carcinomas, breast cancer, endometrium carcinoma or other estrogen-dependent	Nausea, vomiting, breakthrough bleeding, spotting, amenorrhea, migraine, depression, vaginal candidiasis, edema, weight changes.

*Scored.   †Bold entries denote special dental considerations.

NAME	FORM/ STRENGTH	DOSAGE	WARNINGS/PRECAUTIONS & CONTRAINDICATIONS	ADVERSE EFFECTS†

CONTRACEPTIVES (Oral) *(cont.)*

Ethinyl Estradiol/ Norethindrone (Loestrin 21 1.5/30, Loestrin 21 1/20, Modicon, Ortho-Novum 1/35, Ortho-Novum 10/11, Ortho-Novum 7/7/7, Ovcon 35, Ovcon 50, Tri-Norinyl); **Ethinyl Estradiol/ Norgestimate** (Ortho-cyclen, Ortho Tri-cyclen, Ortho Tri-cyclen LO); **Ethinyl Estradiol/Norg-estrel** (Lo/Ovral-28); **Mestranol/ Norethindrone** (Ortho-Novum 1/50); **Norethindrone** (Nor-QD)			neoplasia. **[Alesse, Triphasil, Lo/Ovral]** Thrombogenic valvulopathies, thrombogenic rhythm disorders, diabetes with vascular involvement, uncontrolled HTN, active liver disease (as long as liver function has not returned to normal). **[Ortho-Cyclen, Ortho Tri-Cyclen]** Migraine with focal aura, acute or chronic hepatocellular disease. **[Ortho Tri-Cyclen Lo]** Valvular heart disease with complications, severe HTN, diabetes with vascular involvement, headaches with focal neurological symptoms, major surgery with prolonged immobilization. **[Yasmin, YAZ]** Renal or adrenal insufficiency, hepatic dysfunction, liver tumor, active liver disease, heavy smoking (≥15 cigarettes daily) and >35 yrs old.	

ESTROGENS

Conjugated Estrogens (Premarin, Premarin Intravenous); **Conjugated Estrogens Synthetic A** (Cenestin); **Esterified Estrogens** (Menest); **Estradiol** (Alora, Climara, Es **Conjugated Estrogens** (Premarin, Premarin Intravenous); **Conjugated Estrogens Synthetic A** (Cenestin); **Esterified Estrogens** (Menest); **Estradiol** (Alora, Climara, Esclim, Estrace, Estraderm, Menostar, Vivelle, Vivelle-Dot); **Estradiol Cypionate** (Depo-Estradiol); **Estradiol Valerate** (Delestrogen); **Estropipate** (Ogen)	See manufacturer's package insert for specific brand information.	See manufacturer's package insert for specific brand information.	**Estrogens increase the risk of endometrial cancer. Estrogens, with or without progestins, should not be used for the prevention of CVD or dementia. Increased risks of MI, stroke, invasive breast cancer, pulmonary embolism, and deep-vein thrombosis in postmenopausal women (50-79 yrs) reported. Increased risk of developing probable dementia in postmenopausal women ≥65 yrs reported. W/P:** May increase risk of CV events (eg, MI, stroke), venous thrombosis, and pulmonary embolism; discontinue immediately if any of these events occur or are suspected. May increase risk of breast/endometrial cancer and gallbladder disease. May lead to severe hypercalcemia with breast cancer and bone metastases; monitor and discontinue if hypercalcemia occurs. Retinal vascular thrombosis reported; monitor and discontinue if papilledema or retinal vascular lesions occur. Consider addition of a progestin if no hysterectomy. May elevate BP; monitor at regular intervals. May cause elevations of plasma triglycerides with pre-existing hypertriglyceridemia. Caution with history of cholestatic jaundice associated with past estrogen use or with pregnancy; discontinue with recurrence. May lead to increased thyroid-binding globulin levels; monitor thyroid function. May cause fluid retention;	Altered vaginal bleeding, vaginal candidiasis, breast tenderness/enlargement, GI effects, melasma, CNS effects, weight changes, edema, and altered libido.

Table 20.1: PRESCRIBING INFORMATION FOR ENDOCRINE/HORMONAL AND BONE METABOLISM DRUGS *(cont.)*

NAME	FORM/ STRENGTH	DOSAGE	WARNINGS/PRECAUTIONS & CONTRAINDICATIONS	ADVERSE EFFECTS†
ESTROGENS *(cont.)*				
			caution with cardiac/renal dysfunction. Caution with severe hypocalcemia. May increase risk of ovarian cancer. May exacerbate endometriosis, asthma, diabetes, epilepsy, migraine, porphyria, lupus, and hepatic hemangiomas; use with caution. **Contra:** Pregnancy, undiagnosed abnormal genital bleeding, breast cancer unless being treated for metastatic disease, estrogen-dependent neoplasia, deep-vein thrombosis/pulmonary embolism, active or recent (eg, within past year) arterial thromboembolic disease (eg, stroke, MI), liver dysfunction or disease. **P/N:** Category X, caution in nursing.	
ESTROGEN COMBINATIONS				
Conjugated Estrogens/ Medroxyprogesterone Acetate (Premphase, Prempro); **Esterified Estrogens/ Methyltestosterone** (Estratest, Estratest HS); **Estradiol/Levonorgestrel** (Climara Pro); **Estradiol/ Norethindrone Acetate** (Activella, Combipatch); **Estradiol/Norgestimate** (Prefest); **Ethinyl Estradiol/ Norethindrone Acetate** (Femhrt 1/5, Femhrt LO)	See manufacturer's package insert for specific brand information.	See manufacturer's package insert for specific brand information.	**Estrogens and progestins should not be used for prevention of CVD or dementia. Increased risk of MI, stroke, invasive breast cancer, pulmonary embolism, and deep-vein thrombosis in postmenopausal women (50-79 yrs) reported. Increased risk of developing probable dementia in postmenopausal women ≥65 yrs reported.** **W/P:** May increase risk of cardiovascular events (eg, MI, stroke), venous thrombosis, and pulmonary embolism; discontinue immediately if any of these events occur or are suspected. May increase risk of breast/endometrial cancer and gallbladder disease. May lead to severe hypercalcemia with breast cancer and bone metastases; monitor and discontinue if hypercalcemia occurs. Retinal vascular thrombosis reported; monitor and discontinue if papilledema or retinal vascular lesions occur. May elevate BP; monitor at regular intervals. May cause elevations of plasma triglycerides with pre-existing hypertriglyceridemia. Caution with history of cholestatic jaundice associated with past estrogen use or with pregnancy; discontinue with recurrence. May lead to increased thyroid-binding globulin levels; monitor thyroid function. May cause fluid retention; caution with cardiac/renal dysfunction. Caution with severe hypocalcemia. May increase risk of ovarian cancer. May exacerbate endometriosis, asthma, diabetes, epilepsy, migraine, porphyria, lupus, and hepatic hemangiomas; use with caution. **Contra:** Pregnancy, undiagnosed abnormal genital bleeding, breast cancer, estrogen dependent neoplasia, deep-vein thrombosis/pulmonary embolism, active or recent (eg, within past year) arterial thromboembolic disease (eg, stroke, MI), and liver dysfunction or disease. **P/N:** Category X, caution in nursing.	Abdominal pain, dysmenorrhea, vaginal moniliasis, breast pain, nausea, arthralgia, headache, depression, back pain, infection, pain, vaginal hemorrhage, and vaginitis.

*Scored.   †Bold entries denote special dental considerations.

PROGESTINS

NAME	FORM/STRENGTH	DOSAGE	WARNINGS/PRECAUTIONS & CONTRAINDICATIONS	ADVERSE EFFECTS[†]
Medroxyprogesterone Acetate (Depo-provera, Depo-provera contraceptive Depo-SubQ-provera 104, Provera)	**Inj:** (Depo-provera) 400mg/mL; (Depo-provera contraceptive) 150mg/mL; (Depo-SubQ-provera 104) 104mg/0.65mL; **Tab:** (Provera) 2.5mg*, 5mg*, 10mg*	***Adults:*** (Depo-provera) **Initial:** 400-1000mg IM weekly. **Maint:** 400mg/month if disease stabilizes and/or improves within a few weeks or months. **(Depo-provera contraceptive)** 150mg IM every 3 months (13 weeks) in gluteal or deltoid muscle. Give 1st injection during 1st 5 days of menses; within 1st 5 days postpartum if not nursing; or 6 weeks postpartum if nursing. **(Depo-SubQ-provera)** 104mg SC once every 3 months in the anterior thigh or abdomen. Give 1st injection during 1st 5 days of menses or 6 weeks postpartum if nursing. **(Provera) Secondary Amenorrhea:** 5-10mg qd for 5-10 days. **Abnormal Uterine Bleeding:** 5-10mg qd for 5-10 days beginning on day 16 or day 21 of cycle. **Endometrial Hyperplasia:** 5-10mg qd for 12-14 consecutive days per month beginning on day 1 or day 16 of cycle.	(Depo-provera contraceptive/Depo-SubQ-provera) **May cause significant loss of BMD; greater with increasing duration of use and may not be completely reversible. Should be used as long-term birth control (>2 yrs) only if other birth control methods are inadequate. Unknown if use during adolescence or early adulthood will reduce peak bone mass and increase risk of osteoporotic fractures in later life. W/P:** (Depo-provera) Avoid during 1st 4 months of pregnancy. May cause thromboembolic disorders, ocular disorders, and fluid retention. Caution with depression, family history of breast cancer, or patients with breast nodules. May mask the onset of climacteric. (Depo-provera contraceptive/Depo-SubQ-provera) Loss of BMD; may cause bleeding irregularities, cancer risk, thromboembolic disorders, ocular disorders, unexpected pregnancies, ectopic pregnancy, anaphylaxis and anaphylactoid reaction, fluid retention, return of fertility, or decrease in glucose metabolism. Caution with CNS or convulsive disorders. Discontinue if jaundice develops. (Provera) Discontinue if develop thrombotic disorders, papilledema, or retinal vascular lesions. Discontinue pending exam if sudden onset of proptosis, sudden partial or complete loss of vision, diplopia, or migraine. Include pap smear in pre-treatment exam. Caution with depression, DM, and conditions aggravated by fluid retention (eg, epilepsy, migraine, asthma, cardiac, or renal dysfunction). **Contra:** Pregnancy, undiagnosed vaginal bleeding, breast malignancy, thrombophlebitis, thromboembolic disorders, cerebral vascular disease, and liver dysfunction. **P/N:** (Depo-provera/Depo SubQ-provera) Safety in pregnancy and nursing not known. (Depo-provera contraceptive/Provera) Category X, caution in nursing.	Menstrual irregularities, nervousness, dizziness, edema, weight changes, cholestatic jaundice, breast tenderness, galactorrhea, rash, acne, alopecia, hirsutism, depression, pyrexia, fatigue, insomnia, nausea, urticaria, pruritus, thromboembolic phenomena, insomnia, and somnolence.
Norethindrone Acetate (Aygestin)	**Tab:** 5mg*	***Adults:*** Assume interval between menses is 28 days. **Secondary Amenorrhea/Abnormal Uterine Bleeding:** 2.5-10mg qd for 5-10 days during second half of menstrual cycle. **Endometriosis: Initial:** 5mg qd for 2 weeks. **Titrate:** Increase by 2.5mg qd every 2 weeks until 15mg/day. Continue for 6-9 months or until breakthrough bleeding demands temporary termination.	**W/P:** Discontinue with migraine, vision loss, proptosis, diplopia, papilledema, or retinal vascular lesions. May cause thrombophlebitis, pulmonary embolism, and fluid retention. Caution with epilepsy, migraine, psychic depression, asthma, cardiac or renal dysfunction, DM, and hyperlipidemia. May mask onset of climacteric. Not for use during the first trimester of pregnancy; risk to the fetus. **Contra:** Pregnancy, thrombophlebitis, thromboembolic disorders, cerebral apoplexy, liver impairment, breast carcinoma, undiagnosed vaginal bleeding, missed abortion, use as a pregnancy diagnostic test. **P/N:** Category X, safety in nursing is not known.	Breakthrough bleeding, spotting, change in menstrual flow, amenorrhea, edema, weight changes, cervical changes, cholestatic jaundice, rash, melasma, chloasma, and depression.

Table 20.1: PRESCRIBING INFORMATION FOR ENDOCRINE/HORMONAL AND BONE METABOLISM DRUGS (cont.)

NAME	FORM/ STRENGTH	DOSAGE	WARNINGS/PRECAUTIONS & CONTRAINDICATIONS	ADVERSE EFFECTS†
PROGESTINS (cont.)				
Progesterone (Prometrium)	**Cap:** 100mg, 200mg	**Adults: Prevention of Endometrial Hyperplasia:** 200mg qpm for 12 days sequentially per 28-day cycle. **Secondary Amenorrhea:** 400mg qhs for 10 days.	**Progestins and estrogens should not be used for the prevention of CVD. Increased risk of MI, stroke, invasive breast cancer, pulmonary emboli, DVT, and development of probable dementia in postmenopausal women. W/P:** Discontinue if develop thrombotic disorders, papilledema, or retinal vascular lesions. Discontinue pending exam if sudden onset of proptosis, sudden partial or complete loss of vision, diplopia, or migraine. Include pap smear in pretreatment exam. Caution with depression, DM, and conditions aggravated by fluid retention (eg, epilepsy, migraine, asthma, cardiac dysfunction, or renal dysfunction). **Contra:** Peanut allergy, undiagnosed abnormal genital bleeding, breast cancer, DVT, PE, thromboembolic disorders (stroke or myocardial infarction), liver dysfunction or disease, or pregnancy. **P/N:** Category B, caution in nursing.	Dizziness, headache, breast pain, nausea, diarrhea, dizziness, abdominal pain and distension, emotional lability, and upper respiratory infection.
SERUM ESTROGEN RECEPTOR MODULATOR				
Raloxifene Hydrochloride (Evista)	**Tab:** 60mg	**Adults:** 60mg qd with or without meals.	**W/P:** Increases risk of venous thromboembolism. Discontinue 72 hrs prior to and during prolonged immobilization. Lowers total and LDL cholesterol. Not for use in premenopausal women. Serum levels increase with hepatic dysfunction. Not for use with systemic estrogens. **Contra:** Nursing, pregnancy, venous thromboembolic events (eg, DVT, pulmonary embolism or retinal vein thrombosis). **P/N:** Category X, contraindicated in nursing.	Hot flashes, leg cramps, abdominal pain, vaginal bleeding, arthralgia, rhinitis, and headache.
HYPOGLYCEMIC AGENTS				
INSULIN				
Insulin Aspart Protamine, Recombinant/ Insulin Aspart, Recombinant (Novolog 70/30)	(Insulin Aspart Protamine-Insulin Aspart) **Inj:** 70U-30U/mL; **PenFill:** 70U-30U/mL; **Prefilled:** 70U-30U/mL	**Adults:** Individualize dose. For SC injection only. Inject SC bid within 15 min before breakfast and dinner. Do not mix with other insulins or use in insulin pumps.	**W/P:** Any change of insulin should be made cautiously. Changes in strength, manufacturer, and type or method of manufacture may result in the need for a change in dosage. Hypoglycemia and hypokalemia may occur; caution with fasting and autonomic neuropathy. Illness, stress, change in meals, and exercise may change insulin requirements. Smoking, temperature, and exercise affect insulin absorption. Caution with liver or kidney disease. Administration of insulin SC can result in lipoatrophy. **Contra:** Hypoglycemia. **P/N:** Category C, safety in nursing not known.	Hypoglycemia, hypokalemia, lipodystrophy, hypersensitivity reaction, injection site reactions, pruritus, and rash.
Insulin Aspart, Recombinant (Novolog)	**Inj:** 100U/mL; **PenFill:** 100U/ mL; **Prefilled:** 100U/mL	**Adults:** Individualize dose. Inject SC within 5-10 min before a meal. Draw first when mixing with NPH human insulin; inject immediately. Do not mix with crystalline zinc	**W/P:** Any change of insulin should be made cautiously. Changes in strength, manufacturer, type, or method of manufacture may result in the need for a change in dosage. Hypoglycemia may	Hypoglycemia, hypokalemia, lipodystrophy, hypersensitivity reaction, injection site reactions, pruritus, and rash.

*Scored.   †Bold entries denote special dental considerations.

NAME	FORM/ STRENGTH	DOSAGE	WARNINGS/PRECAUTIONS & CONTRAINDICATIONS	ADVERSE EFFECTS†
Insulin Aspart, Recombinant *(cont.)*		insulins, animal source insulins, or other manufacturer insulins. **External Insulin Pump:** Do not dilute or mix with other insulins. *Pediatrics:* Individualize dose. Inject SC within 5-10 min before a meal. Draw first when mixing with NPH human insulin; inject immediately. Do not mix with crystalline zinc insulins, animal source insulins, or other manufacturer insulins. **External Insulin Pump:** Do not dilute or mix with other insulins.	occur from taking too much insulin; missing or delaying meals; exercising or working more than usual; diseases of adrenal, pituitary, or thyroid glands; or progression of kidney or liver disease. Dosage adjustments may be needed with hepatic or renal dysfunction, during any infection, illness (especially with diarrhea or vomiting), or pregnancy. A longer-acting insulin is usually required to maintain adequate glucose control. Infusion sets and the insulin in the infusion sets should be changed q48h or sooner. Do not use in quick-release infusion sets or cartridge adapters. **Contra:** Hypoglycemia. **P/N:** Category C, caution in nursing.	
Insulin Glargine, Recombinant (Lantus)	**Inj:** 100U/mL; **OptiPen:** 100U/mL	*Adults:* Individualize dose. For SC injection only. Administer qd at same time each day. Insulin-naive patients on oral antidiabetic drugs, start with 10U qd. Switching from once-daily NPH or Ultralente does not require initial dose change. Switching from bid NPH, reduce initial dose by 20%. **Maint:** 2-100U/day. *Pediatrics:* ≥6 yrs: Individualize dose. For SC injection only. Administer qd at same time each day. Insulin-naive patients on oral antidiabetic drugs, start with 10U qd. Switching from once-daily NPH or Ultralente does not require initial dose change. Switching from bid NPH, reduce initial dose by 20%. **Maint:** 2-100U/day.	**W/P:** Human insulin differs from animal-source insulin. Any change of insulin should be made cautiously. Changes in strength, manufacturer, type, or method of manufacture may result in the need for a change in dosage. Hypoglycemia may occur with taking too much insulin, missing or delaying meals, or exercising or working more than usual. An infection or illness (especially with diarrhea or vomiting) may change insulin requirements. Administration of insulin SC can result in lipodystrophy. Not for IV use. Do not mix with other insulins. May cause sodium retention and edema. **P/N:** Category C, caution in nursing.	Hypoglycemia, allergic reactions, injection site reactions, lipodystrophy, pruritus, and rash.
Insulin Human Isophane [NPH] (Humulin N, Novolin N)	**Inj:** 100U/mL **Pen:** 100U/mL	*Adults/Pediatrics:* Individualize dose.	**W/P:** Human insulin differs from animal-source insulin. Any change of insulin should be made cautiously. Changes in strength, manufacturer, type, or method of manufacture may result in the need for a change in dosage. Hypoglycemia may occur with taking too much insulin, missing or delaying meals, or exercising or working more than usual. An infection or illness (especially with diarrhea or vomiting) may change insulin requirements. Administration of insulin SC can result in lipoatrophy. **P/N:** Pregnancy category is not known.	Hypoglycemia, sweating, dizziness, palpitation, tremor, hunger, restlessness, lightheadedness, inability to concentrate, headache, injection site reaction, and allergic reaction.
Insulin Human Regular (Humulin R, Novolin R)	**Inj:** 100U/mL, 500U/mL	*Adults/Pediatrics:* Individualize dose.	**W/P:** Human insulin differs from animal-source insulin. Any change of insulin should be made cautiously. Changes in strength, manufacturer, type, or method of manufacture may result in the need for a change in dosage. Hypoglycemia may occur with taking too much insulin, missing or delaying meals, or exercising or working more than usual. An infection or illness (especially with diarrhea or vomiting) may change insulin requirements. Administration of insulin SC can result in lipoatrophy. **P/N:** Pregnancy category is not known.	Hypoglycemia, sweating, dizziness, palpitation, tremor, hunger, restlessness, lightheadedness, inability to concentrate, headache, injection site reaction, and allergic reaction.

NAME	FORM/ STRENGTH	DOSAGE	WARNINGS/PRECAUTIONS & CONTRAINDICATIONS	ADVERSE EFFECTS†
HYPOGLYCEMIC AGENTS (cont.)				
Insulin Human Zinc [Lente] (Humulin L)	**Inj:** 100U/mL	***Adults/Pediatrics:*** Individualize dose.	**W/P:** Human insulin differs from animal source insulin. Any change of insulin should be made cautiously. Changes in strength, manufacturer, type, or method of manufacture may result in the need for a change in dosage. Hypoglycemia may occur with taking too much insulin, missing or delaying meals, or exercising or working more than usual. An infection or illness (especially with diarrhea or vomiting) may change insulin requirements. Administration of insulin SC can result in lipoatrophy. **P/N:** Pregnancy category is not known.	Hypoglycemia, sweating, dizziness, palpitation, tremor, hunger, restlessness, lightheadedness, inability to concentrate, headache, injection site reaction, and allergic reaction.
Insulin Human Zinc, Extended [Ultralente] (Humulin U)	**Inj:** 100U/mL	***Adults/Pediatrics:*** Individualize dose.	**W/P:** Human insulin differs from animal source insulin. Any change of insulin should be made cautiously. Changes in strength, manufacturer, type, or method of manufacture may result in the need for a change in dosage. Hypoglycemia may occur with taking too much insulin, missing or delaying meals, or exercising or working more than usual. An infection or illness (especially with diarrhea or vomiting) may change insulin requirements. Administration of insulin SC can result in lipoatrophy. **P/N:** Pregnancy category is not known.	Hypoglycemia, sweating, dizziness, palpitation, tremor, hunger, restlessness, lightheadedness, inability to concentrate, headache, injection site reaction, and allergic reaction.
Insulin Lispro Protamine, Recombinant/ Insulin Lispro, Recombinant (Humalog Mix 75/25)	**Inj:** 75U-25U/mL; **Pen:** 75U-25U/mL	***Adults:*** Individualize dose. Inject SC within 15 min before a meal. May need to reduce/adjust dose with renal or hepatic impairment.	**W/P:** Any change of insulin should be made cautiously. Changes in strength, manufacturer, type, or method of manufacture may result in the need for a change in dosage. Hypoglycemia may occur with taking too much insulin, missing or delaying meals, or exercising or working more than usual. An infection or illness (especially with diarrhea or vomiting) may change insulin requirements. **Contra:** Hypoglycemia. **P/N:** Category B, caution in nursing.	Hypoglycemia, hypokalemia, allergic reaction, injection site reaction, lipodystrophy, pruritus, and rash.
Insulin Lispro, Recombinant (Humalog)	**Cartridge:** 100U/mL; **Inj:** 100U/mL; **Pen:** 100U/mL	***Adults:*** Individualize dose. Inject SC within 15 min before or immediately after a meal. May use with external insulin pump; do not dilute or mix with other insulin when used with pump. ***Pediatrics:*** ≥3 yrs: Individualize dose. Inject SC within 15 min before or immediately after a meal. May use with external insulin pump; do not dilute or mix with other insulin when used with pump.	**W/P:** Any change of insulin should be made cautiously. Changes in strength, manufacturer, type, or method of manufacture may result in the need for a change in dosage. Hypoglycemia may occur with taking too much insulin, missing or delaying meals, or exercising or working more than usual. An infection or illness (especially with diarrhea or vomiting) may change insulin requirements. With type 1 DM a longer-acting insulin is usually required to maintain glucose control; not required with type 2 DM if regimen includes sulfonylureas. May be diluted with sterile diluent. **Contra:** Hypoglycemia. **P/N:** Category B, caution in nursing.	Hypoglycemia, hypokalemia, allergic reaction, injection site reaction, lipodystrophy, pruritus, and rash.

*Scored.   †Bold entries denote special dental considerations.

NAME	FORM/ STRENGTH	DOSAGE	WARNINGS/PRECAUTIONS & CONTRAINDICATIONS	ADVERSE EFFECTS†
Insulin Pork Isophane [NPH] (Iletin II NPH Pork)	**Inj:** 100U/mL	***Adults:*** Individualize dose. ***Pediatrics:*** Individualize dose.	**W/P:** Make any change of insulin cautiously. Changes in strength, manufacturer, type, or method of manufacture may result in the need to change dosage. Hypoglycemia may occur with too much insulin, missing or delaying meals, or exercising or working more than usual. An infection or illness (especially with diarrhea or vomiting) may change insulin requirements. **P/N:** Pregnancy category is not known.	Hypoglycemia, sweating, dizziness, palpitation, tremor, hunger, restlessness, lightheadedness, inability to concentrate, headache, injection site reaction, and allergic reaction.
Insulin Pork Regular (Iletin II Regular Pork)	**Inj:** 100U/mL	***Adults:*** Individualize dose. ***Pediatrics:*** Individualize dose.	**W/P:** Make any change of insulin cautiously. Changes in strength, manufacturer, type, or method of manufacture may result in the need to change dosage. Hypoglycemia may occur with too much insulin, missing or delaying meals, or exercising or working more than usual. An infection or illness (especially with diarrhea or vomiting) may change insulin requirements. **P/N:** Pregnancy category is not known.	Hypoglycemia, sweating, dizziness, palpitation, tremor, hunger, restlessness, lightheadedness, inability to concentrate, headache, injection site reaction, and allergic reaction.
Insulin Pork Zinc [Lente] (Iletin II Lente Pork)	**Inj:** 100U/mL	***Adults:*** Individualize dose. ***Pediatrics:*** Individualize dose.	**W/P:** Make any change of insulin cautiously. Changes in strength, manufacturer, type, or method of manufacture may result in the need to change dosage. Hypoglycemia may occur with too much insulin, missing or delaying meals, or exercising or working more than usual. An infection or illness (especially with diarrhea or vomiting) may change insulin requirements. **P/N:** Pregnancy category is not known.	Hypoglycemia, sweating, dizziness, palpitation, tremor, hunger, restlessness, lightheadedness, inability to concentrate, headache, injection site reaction, and allergic reaction.

ORAL AGENTS

NAME	FORM/ STRENGTH	DOSAGE	WARNINGS/PRECAUTIONS & CONTRAINDICATIONS	ADVERSE EFFECTS†
Acarbose (Precose)	**Tab:** 25mg, 50mg, 100mg	***Adults:*** **Initial:** 25mg tid with first bite of each main meal. **To Minimize GI Effects:** 25mg qd, increase gradually to 25mg tid. **Titrate:** After reaching 25mg tid, may increase at 4-8-week intervals. **Maint:** 50-100mg tid. **Max:** **≥60kg:** 50mg tid. >60kg: 100mg tid. If no further reduction in postprandial glucose level or HbA$_{1c}$ occurs with 100mg tid, consider reducing dose.	**W/P:** Avoid with significant renal dysfunction (SCr >2mg/dL). May need to discontinue and give insulin with stress (eg, fever or trauma). Dose-related elevated serum transaminase levels reported. Monitor serum transaminases every 3 months for the first year, then periodically. Reduce dose or discontinue if elevated serum transaminases persist. Use glucose (dextrose) instead of sucrose (sugar cane) to treat mild to moderate hypoglycemia. **Contra:** Diabetic ketoacidosis, cirrhosis, inflammatory bowel disease, colonic ulceration, partial or predisposition to intestinal obstruction, chronic intestinal disease with marked disorders of digestion or absorption, and conditions that may deteriorate from increased intestinal gas formation. **P/N:** Category B, not for use in nursing.	Transient flatulence, diarrhea, and abdominal pain.
Chlorpropamide (Diabinese)	**Tab:** 100mg*, 250mg*	***Adults:*** **Initial:** 250mg qd. **Titrate:** After 5-7 days, adjust by 50-125mg/day every 3-5 days for control. **Maint:** 100-500 qd. **Max:** 750mg qd.	**W/P:** Increased risk of cardiovascular mortality. Hypoglycemia risk especially with renal/hepatic insufficiency, elderly, debilitated, malnourished, and	Hypoglycemia, cholestatic jaundice, diarrhea, nausea, vomiting, anorexia, pruritus, photosensitivity

Table 20.1: PRESCRIBING INFORMATION FOR ENDOCRINE/HORMONAL AND BONE METABOLISM DRUGS (cont.)

NAME	FORM/ STRENGTH	DOSAGE	WARNINGS/PRECAUTIONS & CONTRAINDICATIONS	ADVERSE EFFECTS[†]
HYPOGLYCEMIC AGENTS (cont.)				
Chlorpropamide (cont.)		**Elderly, Debilitated, Malnourished, or Renal or Hepatic Dysfunction: Initial:** 100-125mg qd. **Maint:** Conservative dosing. Take with breakfast. Divide dose with GI intolerance. If <40U/day insulin, discontinue therapy. If ≥40U/day insulin, decrease dose by 50% and start chlorpropamide therapy. Adjust insulin dose depending on response.	adrenal/pituitary insufficiency. Loss of blood glucose control when exposed to stress (fever, trauma, infection, or surgery); discontinue therapy and start insulin. Secondary failure can occur over a period of time. **Contra:** Diabetic ketoacidosis. **P/N:** Category C, not for use in nursing.	reactions, skin eruptions, blood dyscrasias, hepatic porphyria, and disulfiram-like reactions.
Glimepiride (Amaryl)	**Tab:** 1mg*, 2mg*, 4mg*	**Adults: Initial:** 1-2mg qd with breakfast or 1st main meal. **Titrate:** After 2mg, may increase by up to 2mg every 1-2 weeks. **Maint:** 1-4mg qd. **Max:** 8mg qd. **Amaryl/Metformin:** Add Metformin to 8mg qd for better glucose control. **Amaryl/Insulin Therapy:** If FBG >150mg/dL on 8mg qd, add low-dose insulin; increase insulin weekly as needed. **Renal Insufficiency: Initial:** 1mg qd. **Elderly, Debilitated, Malnourished, or Hepatic Insufficiency:** Dose conservatively to avoid hypoglycemia.	**W/P:** Increased cardiovascular mortality. Hypoglycemia risk if debilitated, malnourished, or with adrenal, pituitary, renal, or hepatic insufficiency. Hypoglycemia may be masked in elderly. May lose blood-glucose control with stress. Secondary failure may occur. Discontinue if skin reactions persist or worsen. **Contra:** Diabetic ketoacidosis. **P/N:** Category C, not for use in nursing.	Dizziness, nausea, asthenia, headache, hypoglycemia.
Glipizide (Glucotrol, Glucotrol XL)	**Tab:** (Glucotrol) 5mg*, 10mg*; **Tab, Extended Release:** (XL) 2.5mg, 5mg, 10mg	**Adults: (Glucotrol XL)** Do not chew, divide, or crush. **Initial:** 5mg qd with breakfast. Use lower doses if sensitive to hypoglycemics. **Usual:** 5-10mg qd. **Max:** 20mg/day. **Combination Therapy: Initial:** 5mg qd. **(Glucotrol): Initial:** 5mg qd 30 min before breakfast. **Geriatric/Hepatic Impairment: Initial:** 2.5mg qd. **Titrate:** Increase by 2.5-5mg after several days. **Max:** 40mg/day. Divide doses >15mg and give 30 min before a meal. **(Glucotrol XL, Glucotrol) Switch From Insulin:** If on ≤20U/day: Stop insulin; start Glucotrol XL or Glucotrol 5mg qd. If on >20U/day: Reduce insulin dose by 50% and add Glucotrol XL or Glucotrol 5mg qd. Further insulin reductions depend on response.	**W/P:** Increased risk of hypoglycemia with elderly, debilitated, malnourished, renal or hepatic disease, or adrenal or pituitary insufficiency. Increased risk of CV mortality. Loss of blood glucose control when exposed to stress (fever, trauma, infection, or surgery); discontinue therapy and start insulin. Secondary failure can occur over a period of time. (XL) GI disease will reduce retention time of the drug. Caution with pre-existing severe GI narrowing. **Contra:** Diabetic ketoacidosis. **P/N:** Category C, not for use in nursing.	Hypoglycemia, nausea, diarrhea, allergic skin reactions, disulfiram-like reactions, dizziness, drowsiness, asthenia, and headache.
Glipizide/ Metformin Hydrochloride (Metaglip)	**Tab:** (Glipizide-Metformin) 2.5mg-250mg, 2.5mg-500mg, 5mg-500mg	**Adults: Initial:** 2.5mg-250mg qd. If FBG 280-320mg/dL, give 2.5mg-500mg bid. **Titrate:** Increase by 1 tab/day every 2 weeks. **Max:** 10mg-1g/day or 10mg-2g/day given in divided doses. **Second-Line Therapy: Initial:** 2.5mg-500mg or 5mg-500mg bid (with morning and evening meals). Starting dose should not exceed daily dose of metformin or glipizide already being taken. **Titrate:** Increase by no more than 5mg-500mg/day. **Max:** 20mg-2g/day. **Elderly/Debilitated/Malnourished:** Do not titrate to max dose. Take with meals.	**W/P:** Lactic acidosis reported (rare); increased risk with renal dysfunction, increased age, DM, CHF, and other conditions with risk of hypoperfusion and hypoxemia. Avoid use in patients ≥80 yrs unless renal function is normal. Increased risk of cardiovascular mortality. Increased risk of hypoglycemia in elderly, debilitated/malnourished, adrenal or pituitary insufficiency, or alcohol intoxication. Discontinue in hypoxic states (eg, CHF, shock, acute MI) and prior to surgical procedures (due to restricted food intake). Avoid in renal/hepatic impairment. May decrease serum vitamin B_{12} levels.	Upper respiratory tract infection, HTN, headache, diarrhea, dizziness, musculoskeletal pain, nausea, vomiting, and abdominal pain.

*Scored.   †Bold entries denote special dental considerations.

NAME	FORM/ STRENGTH	DOSAGE	WARNINGS/PRECAUTIONS & CONTRAINDICATIONS	ADVERSE EFFECTS†
Glipizide/ Metformin Hydrochloride *(cont.)*			Impaired renal and/or hepatic function may slow glipizide excretion. With-hold treatment with any condition associated with dehydration or sepsis. Monitor renal function. **Contra:** Renal disease/dysfunction (SCr ≥1.5mg/dL [males], ≥1.4mg/dL [females], abnor-mal CrCl), CHF, metabolic acidosis, and diabetic ketoacidosis. Discontinue temporarily (48hrs) for radiologic studies with intravascular iodinated contrast materials. **P/N:** Category C, not for use in nursing.	
Glyburide (Diabeta, Micronase)	**Tab:** 1.25mg*, 2.5mg*, 5mg*	***Adults:*** **Initial:** 2.5-5mg qd with breakfast or first main meal; give 1.25mg if sensitive to hypoglycemia. **Titrate:** Increase by no more than 2.5mg/day at weekly intervals. **Maint:** 1.25-20mg given qd or in divided doses. **Max:** 20mg/day. May give bid with >10mg/day. **Renal/Hepatic Disease, Elderly, Debilitated, Malnourished, or Adrenal or Pituitary Insufficiency: Initial:** 1.25mg qd. **Transfer From Other Oral Antidiabetic Agents: Initial:** 2.5-5mg/day. **Switch From Insulin:** If >40U/day, decrease dose by 50% and give 5mg qd. **Titrate:** Progressive withdrawal of insulin, and increase by 1.25-2.5mg/day every 2-10 days.	**W/P:** Increased risk of CV mortality. Risk of hypoglycemia, especially with renal or hepatic disease, or elderly, debilitated, or malnourished patients, and those with adrenal or pituitary insufficiency. May need to discontinue and give insulin with stress (eg, fever or trauma). Secondary failure may oc-cur. Discontinue if jaundice, hepatitis, or persistent skin reaction occurs. He-matologic reactions and hyponatremia reported. **Contra:** Diabetic ketoacidosis. **P/N:** (Diabeta) Category C, not for use in nursing. (Micronase) Category B, not for use in nursing.	Hypoglycemia, nausea, epigastric fullness, heartburn, allergic skin reactions, disulfiram-like reactions (rarely), hypo-natremia, liver function abnormalities, and photo-sensitivity reactions.
Glyburide, Micronized (Glynase Pres-Tab)	**Tab:** 1.5mg*, 3mg*, 6mg*	***Adults:*** **Initial:** 1.5-3mg qd with breakfast or first main meal. **Renal or Hepatic Disease, Elderly, Debili-tated, Malnourished, or Adrenal or Pituitary Insufficiency: Initial:** 0.75mg qd. **Titrate:** Increase by no more than 1.5mg/day at weekly intervals. **Maint:** 0.75-12mg qd or in divided doses. **Max:** 12mg/day given qd or bid. **Transfer from Other Sulfonylureas:** Starting dose should not exceed 3mg/day. **Switch from Insulin:** If <20U/day, substitute with 1.5-3mg qd. If 20-40U/day, give 3mg qd. If >40U/day, decrease insulin dose by 50% and give 3mg qd. **Titrate:** Progressive withdrawal of insulin and increase by 0.75-1.5mg every 2-10 days.	**W/P:** Increased risk of CV mortality. Risk of hypoglycemia, especially with renal or hepatic disease, elderly, debilitated, malnourished, or adrenal or pituitary insufficiency. Loss of blood glucose control when exposed to stress (eg, fever, trauma, infection, or surgery); discontinue therapy and start insulin. Secondary failure can occur over a period of time. Discontinue if cholestatic jaundice or hepatitis occur. Retitrate when transferring from other glyburide products. **Contra:** Diabetic ketoacidosis and as sole therapy of type 1 DM. **P/N:** Category B, not for use in nursing.	Hypoglycemia, nausea, epigastric fullness, heartburn, allergic skin reactions, disulfiram-like reactions (rarely), hypona-tremia, blood dyscrasias, LFT abnormalities, and photosensitivity reactions.
Glyburide/ Metformin Hydrochloride (Glucovance)	**Tab:** (Glyburide-Metformin) 1.25mg-250mg, 2.5mg-500mg, 5mg-500mg	***Adults:*** Take with meals. **Initial:** 1.25mg-250mg qd. If HbA$_{1c}$ >9% or FPG >200mg/dL, give 1.25mg-250mg bid. **Titrate:** Increase by 1.25mg-250mg/day every 2 weeks. Do not use 50mg-500mg tab for initial therapy. **Second-Line Therapy: Initial:** 2.5mg-500mg or 5mg-500mg bid. Starting dose should not exceed daily doses of glyburide (or sulfonyl-urea equivalent) or metformin	**W/P:** Lactic acidosis reported (rare); increased risk with renal dysfunction, increased age, DM, CHF, and other con-ditions with risk of hypoperfusion and hypoxemia. Avoid use in patients ≥80 yrs unless renal function is normal. Increased risk of cardiovascular mortal-ity. Increased risk of hypoglycemia in elderly, debilitated/malnourished, adre-nal or pituitary insufficiency, or alcohol intoxication. Discontinue in hypoxic	Hypoglycemia, nausea, vomiting, abdominal pain, upper respiratory infec-tion, headache, dizziness, and diarrhea.

Table 20.1: PRESCRIBING INFORMATION FOR ENDOCRINE/HORMONAL AND BONE METABOLISM DRUGS (cont.)

NAME	FORM/STRENGTH	DOSAGE	WARNINGS/PRECAUTIONS & CONTRAINDICATIONS	ADVERSE EFFECTS†

HYPOGLYCEMIC AGENTS (cont.)

NAME	FORM/STRENGTH	DOSAGE	WARNINGS/PRECAUTIONS & CONTRAINDICATIONS	ADVERSE EFFECTS†
Glyburide/ Metformin Hydrochloride (cont.)		already being taken. **Titrate:** Increase by no more than 5mg-500mg/day. **Max:** 20mg-2000mg/day. **With Concomitant Thiazolidinedion:** Initiate and titrate thiazolidinedion as recommended. If hypoglycemia occurs, reduce glyburide component. **Elderly, Debilitated, or Malnourished:** Conservative dosing; do not titrate to max.	states (eg, CHF, shock, acute MI), loss of blood glucose control due to stress (give insulin), acidosis, and prior to surgical procedures (due to restricted food intake). Monitor renal function and for ketoacidosis and metabolic acidosis. Avoid in renal/hepatic impairment. May decrease serum vitamin B_{12} levels. When used with a thiazolidinedion, monitor LFTs and weight gain. Withhold treatment with any condition associated with hypoxemia, dehydration, or sepsis. **Contra:** Renal disease/dysfunction (SCr ≥1.5mg/dL [males], ≥1.4mg/dL [females], abnormal CrCl), CHF, metabolic acidosis, and diabetic ketoacidosis. Discontinue temporarily (48hrs) for radiologic studies with IV iodinated contrast materials. **P/N:** Category B, not for use in nursing.	
Metformin Hydrochloride (Fortamet, Glucophage, Glucophage XR, Riomet)	**Tab, Extended Release: (Fortamet)** 500mg, 1000mg **Sol: (Riomet)** 500mg/5mL; **Tab:** (Glucophage) 500mg, 850mg, 1000mg*; **Tab, Extended Release: (Glucophage XR)** 500mg, 750mg; **(Fortamet)** 500mg, 1000mg	**Adults:** **(Sol, Tab) Initial:** 500mg bid or 850mg qd with meals. **Titrate:** Increase by 500mg/week, or 850mg every 2 weeks, or may increase from 500mg bid to 850mg bid after 2 weeks. **Max:** 2550mg/day. Give in 3 divided doses with meals if dose is >2g/day. **(Tab, Extended Release) Initial: ≥17 yrs:** 500mg qd with evening meal. **Titrate:** Increase by 500mg/week. **Max:** 2000mg/day. **With Insulin: Initial:** 500mg qd. **Titrate:** Increase by 500mg/week. **Max:** 2500mg/day and 2000mg/day (XR). Decrease insulin dose by 10-25% when FPG <120mg/dL. Swallow whole; do not crush or chew. **Elderly, Debilitated, or Malnourished:** Conservative dosing; do not titrate to max.	**W/P:** Lactic acidosis reported (rare); increased risk with renal dysfunction, increased age, DM, CHF, and other conditions with risk of hypoperfusion and hypoxemia. Avoid use in patients ≥80 yrs unless renal function is normal. Monitor renal function and for ketoacidosis and metabolic acidosis. Avoid in renal/hepatic impairment. Discontinue in hypoxic states (eg, CHF, shock, and acute MI), loss of blood glucose control due to stress (give insulin), acidosis, dehydration, or sepsis. Temporarily discontinue prior to surgery (due to restricted food intake) and procedures requiring intravascular iodinated contrast materials. May decrease serum vitamin B_{12} levels. Increased risk of hypoglycemia in elderly, debilitated, malnourished, adrenal or pituitary insufficiency, or alcohol intoxication. **Contra:** Renal disease or dysfunction (SCr ≥1.5mg/dL [males], ≥1.4mg/dL [females], abnormal CrCl), CHF, metabolic acidosis, or diabetic ketoacidosis. Discontinue temporarily (48hrs) for radiologic studies with intravascular iodinated contrast materials. **P/N:** Category B, not for use in nursing.	Diarrhea, nausea, dyspepsia, flatulence, and abdominal pain.
Metformin Hydrochloride/ Rosiglitazone Maleate (Avandamet)	**Tab:** (Rosiglitazone-Metformin) 1mg-500mg, 2mg-500mg, 4mg-500mg, 2mg-1g, 4mg-1g	**Adults:** **Prior Metformin Therapy of 1g/day: Initial:** 2mg-500mg tab bid. **Prior Metformin Therapy of 2g/day: Initial:** 2mg-1g tab bid. **Prior Rosiglitazone Therapy of 4mg/day: Initial:** 2mg-500mg tab bid. **Prior Rosiglitazone Therapy of 8mg/day: Initial:** 4mg-500mg tab bid. **Titrate:** May increase by increments of 4mg rosiglitazone and/or 500mg metformin. **Max:** 8mg-2g/day. **Elderly, Debilitated, or Malnourished:** Conservative dosing; do not titrate to max dose. Take with meals.	**W/P:** Lactic acidosis reported (rare); increased risk with renal dysfunction, increased age, DM, CHF, and other conditions with risk of hypoperfusion and hypoxemia. Avoid use in patients ≥80 years unless renal function is normal. Monitor renal function and for ketoacidosis and metabolic acidosis. Discontinue in hypoxic states (eg, CHF, shock, and acute MI), loss of blood glucose control due to stress, acidosis, and prior to surgical procedures (due to restricted food intake). May decrease serum vitamin B_{12} levels. Increased risk	Upper respiratory tract infection, headache, back pain, fatigue, sinusitis, diarrhea, viral infection, arthralgia, and anemia.

*Scored.   †Bold entries denote special dental considerations.

NAME	FORM/ STRENGTH	DOSAGE	WARNINGS/PRECAUTIONS & CONTRAINDICATIONS	ADVERSE EFFECTS†
Metformin Hydrochloride/ Rosiglitazone Maleate *(cont.)*			of hypoglycemia in elderly, debilitated, malnourished, adrenal or pituitary insufficiency, or alcohol intoxication. May cause fluid retention and exacerbation or initiation of heart failure; discontinue if cardiac status deteriorates. Avoid if NYHA Class III or IV cardiac status. Not for use in type 1 diabetes or for diabetic ketoacidosis treatment. Caution with edema. Dose-related weight gain reported. Ovulation in premenopausal anovulatory patients may occur; risk of pregnancy with inadequate contraception. May decrease Hgb and Hct. Avoid with active liver disease, if ALT levels >2.5X ULN, or if jaundice occurred with troglitazone. Check LFTs before therapy, every 2 months for 1 year, and periodically thereafter, or if hepatic-dysfunction symptoms occur. Discontinue if ALT >3X ULN on therapy. Not for use with insulin. **Contra:** Renal disease/dysfunction (SCr ≥1.5mg/dL [males], ≥1.4mg/dL [females], abnormal CrCl), CHF, metabolic acidosis, or diabetic ketoacidosis. Discontinue temporarily (48hrs) for radiologic studies with intravascular iodinated contrast materials. **P/N:** Category C, not for use in nursing.	
Miglitol (Glyset)	**Tab:** 25mg, 50mg, 100mg	***Adults:* Initial:** 25mg tid. May give 25mg qd (to minimize GI side effects) and gradually increase to tid. **Titrate:** After 4-8 weeks, increase to 50mg tid. **Maint:** 50mg tid. After 3 months may increase to 100mg tid if needed. **Max:** 100mg tid. Take with first bite of each main meal.	**W/P:** Use glucose (dextrose) not sucrose (cane sugar) to treat mild-to-moderate hypoglycemia. Temporary insulin therapy may be necessary at times of stress such as fever, trauma, infection, or surgery. Not recommended with renal impairment (SCr >2mg/dL). **Contra:** Ketoacidosis, inflammatory bowel disease, colonic ulceration, or partial intestinal obstruction, or if predisposed to intestinal obstruction. Chronic intestinal diseases with digestion or absorption disorders or conditions may deteriorate with increased gas formation in the intestine. **P/N:** Category B, not for use in nursing.	Flatulence, diarrhea, abdominal pain, skin rash, and decreased serum iron.
Nateglinide (Starlix)	**Tab:** 60mg, 120mg	***Adults:* Initial/Maint:** 120mg tid before meals (with or without metformin or thiazolidinedion). Take 1-30 minutes before meals. May use 60mg tid (with or without metformin or thiazolidinedion) in patients near goal HbA₁ᴄ. Skip dose if meal is skipped.	**W/P:** Caution in moderate to severe hepatic impairment. Transient loss of glucose control with trauma, surgery, fever, and infection; may need insulin therapy. Secondary failure may occur in prolonged therapy. Hypoglycemia risk in elderly, debilitated, or malnourished, with strenuous exercise, or with adrenal or pituitary insufficiency. Autonomic neuropathy may mask hypoglycemia. **Contra:** Type 1 diabetes, and diabetic ketoacidosis. **P/N:** Category C, not for use in nursing.	Upper respiratory infection, flu symptoms, dizziness, arthropathy, diarrhea, hypoglycemia, and back pain.
Pioglitazone Hydrochloride (Actos)	**Tab:** 15mg, 30mg, 45mg	***Adults:* Monotherapy: Initial:** 15-30mg qd. **Max:** 45mg/day. **Combination Therapy: Initial:** 15-30mg qd. **Max:** 30mg/day. Decrease insulin dose by 10-25% if hypoglycemia occurs or if plasma glucose	**W/P:** May cause fluid retention and exacerbation or initiation of heart failure; discontinue if cardiac status deteriorates. Avoid if NYHA Class III or IV cardiac status. Use lowest approved dose if systolic heart failure (NYHA	Upper respiratory tract infection, myalgia, **tooth disorder**, headache, sinusitis, **pharyngitis**, transient CPK level elevations, CHF, weight gain, aggravated DM, edema, and dyspnea.

Table 20.1: PRESCRIBING INFORMATION FOR ENDOCRINE/HORMONAL AND BONE METABOLISM DRUGS *(cont.)*

NAME	FORM/ STRENGTH	DOSAGE	WARNINGS/PRECAUTIONS & CONTRAINDICATIONS	ADVERSE EFFECTS[†]

HYPOGLYCEMIC AGENTS *(cont.)*

NAME	FORM/ STRENGTH	DOSAGE	WARNINGS/PRECAUTIONS & CONTRAINDICATIONS	ADVERSE EFFECTS[†]
Pioglitazone Hydrochloride *(cont.)*		is <100mg/dL. Decrease sulfonyl-urea dose with hypoglycemia.	Class II). Not for use in type 1 diabetes or for diabetic ketoacidosis treatment. Caution with edema. Dose-related weight gain reported. Ovulation in pre-menopausal anovulatory patients may occur; risk of pregnancy with inade-quate contraception. May decrease Hgb and Hct. Avoid with active liver disease, if ALT levels >2.5X ULN, or if jaundice occurred with troglitazone. Check LFTs before therapy, every 2 months for 1 year, and periodically thereafter, or if hepatic dysfunction symptoms occur. Discontinue if jaundice occurs or ALT >3X ULN on therapy. **P/N:** Category C, not for use in nursing.	
Repaglinide (Prandin)	**Tab:** 0.5mg, 1mg, 2mg	***Adults:*** Take within 15-30 min before meals. Skip dose if skipping meal; add dose if adding meal. **Initial: Treatment-Naive or HbA$_{1c}$ <8%:** 0.5mg with each meal. **Previous Oral Therapy/Combination Therapy and HbA1c ≥8%:** 1-2mg with each meal. **Titrate:** May double preprandial dose up to 4mg (bid-qid) at no less than 1-week intervals. **Maint:** 0.5-4mg with meals. **Max:** 16mg/day. If hypoglycemia with combination metformin or thiazolidinedion oc-curs, reduce repaglinide dose. **Renal Dysfunction: CrCl 20-40mg/dL: Initial:** 0.5mg with each meal; titrate carefully. **Hepatic Dysfunction:** Increase intervals between dose adjustments.	**W/P:** Hypoglycemia risk especially with renal or hepatic insufficiency, elderly, malnourished, or adrenal/pituitary insufficiency. Loss of blood glucose control when exposed to stress (fever, trauma, infection, or surgery); discontinue therapy and start insulin. Secondary failure can occur over a period of time. Caution with hepatic and renal dysfunction. Not indicated for use in combination with NPH insulin. **Contra:** Diabetic ketoacidosis and type 1 diabetes. **P/N:** Category C, not for use in nursing.	Hypoglycemia, cardiovas-cular effects, respiratory infections, UTI, bronchitis, sinusitis, rhinitis, pares-thesia, nausea, diarrhea, constipation, vomiting, dyspepsia, arthralgia, back pain, headache, and chest pain.
Rosiglitazone Maleate (Avandia)	**Tab:** 2mg, 4mg, 8mg	***Adults:* ≥18 yrs: Initial:** 2mg bid or 4mg qd. **Titrate:** May increase after 8-12 weeks to 4mg bid or 8mg qd. **Max:** 8mg/day as monotherapy or with metformin; 4mg/day in combination with sulfonylureas or insulin. Decrease insulin by 10-25% if hypoglycemic or FPG <100mg/dL; individualize further adjustments based on glucose lowering response.	**W/P:** May cause fluid retention and exacerbation or initiation of heart failure; discontinue if cardiac status deteriorates. Avoid if NYHA Class III or IV cardiac status. Not for use in type 1 Dm or for diabetic ketoacidosis treatment. Caution with edema. Dose-related weight gain reported. Ovulation in premenopausal anovulatory patients may occur; risk of pregnancy with in-adequate contraception. May decrease Hgb and Hct. Avoid with active liver disease, if ALT levels >2.5X ULN, or if jaundice occurred with troglitazone. Check LFTs before therapy, every 2 months for 1 year, and periodically thereafter, or if hepatic dysfunction symptoms occur. Discontinue if ALT >3X ULN on therapy. **Contra:** Combina-tion use with metformin with renal impairment. **P/N:** Category C, not for use in nursing.	Upper respiratory tract infection, injury, headache, back pain, hyperglycemia, fatigue, sinusitis, anemia, and edema.
Tolazamide (Tolinase)	**Tab:** 100mg, 250mg, 500mg	***Adults:* Initial:** 100-250mg qd w/breakfast. **Titrate:** May increase by 100-250mg/week. **Maint:** 100-1000mg/day. **Max:** 1000mg/day. Divide dose if >500.	**W/P:** Hypoglycemia; loss of glycemic control due to secondary failure; stress due to infection, fever, trauma, or surgery. **Contra:** Diabetic ketoaci-dosis. **P/N:** Category C, not for use in nursing.	Heartburn, nausea, and hypoglycemia.

*Scored.   †Bold entries denote special dental considerations.

NAME	FORM/ STRENGTH	DOSAGE	WARNINGS/PRECAUTIONS & CONTRAINDICATIONS	ADVERSE EFFECTS†
Tolbutamide (Tol-Tab)	**Tab:** 500mg	***Adults:*** **Usual/Initial:** 1-2g qd 30 min ac. **Maint:** 0.25-3g/day. **Max:** 3g/day.	**W/P:** Hypoglycemia; loss of glycemic control due to secondary failure; stress due to infection, fever, trauma, or surgery. **Contra:** Diabetic ketoacidosis. **P/N:** Category C, not for use in nursing.	Heartburn, nausea, and hypoglycemia.

MISCELLANEOUS

NAME	FORM/ STRENGTH	DOSAGE	WARNINGS/PRECAUTIONS & CONTRAINDICATIONS	ADVERSE EFFECTS†
Exenatide (Byetta)	**Inj:** 5µg/dose, 10µg/dose [60-dose Prefilled Pen]	***Adults:*** 5µg SC bid, 60 min before morning and evening meals. **Titrate:** May increase to 10µg bid after 1 month. Reduction of sulfonylurea dose may be considered to reduce risk of hypoglycemia.	**W/P:** Not a substitute for insulin. Do not use with type 1 DM, for treatment of diabetic ketoacidosis, end-stage renal disease, severe renal impairment (CrCl <30mL/min), or severe GI disease. Increased incidence of hypoglycemia with sulfonylurea. **P/N:** Category C, caution in nursing.	Nausea, vomiting, diarrhea, feeling jittery, dizziness, headache, and dyspepsia.

THYROID HORMONES

NAME	FORM/ STRENGTH	DOSAGE	WARNINGS/PRECAUTIONS & CONTRAINDICATIONS	ADVERSE EFFECTS†
Calcitonin-Salmon (Miacalcin)	**Inj:** 200 IU/mL; **Nasal Spray:** 200 IU/inh [2mL 2s]	***Adults:*** **(Inj) Paget's Disease: Usual:** 100 IU IM/SQ qd. **Hypercalcemia: Initial:** 4 IU/kg IM/SQ q12h. **Titrate:** May increase to 8 IU/kg q12h after 1-2 days, then to 8 IU/kg q6h after 2 days if unsatisfactory response. **Osteoporosis: (Inj)** 100 IU IM/SQ every other day. If >2mL, use IM injection. **(Spray)** 200 IU qd intranasally. Alternate nostrils daily. Take with supplemental calcium and vitamin D for postmenopausal osteoporosis.	**W/P:** Possibility of systemic allergic reactions. Monitor urine sediment periodically with chronic use. If nasal mucosa ulceration occurs, discontinue until healed. Discontinue if severe ulceration of the nasal mucosa occurs. Perform periodic nasal exams. Monitor drug effects. **P/N:** Category C, not for use in nursing.	(Inj) Nausea, vomiting, injection site inflammation, flushing of face or hands, nocturia, ear lobe pruritus, poor appetite, abdominal pain. (Spray) Nasal symptoms, back pain, headache, arthralgia.
Calcitonin-Salmon (rDNA origin) (Fortical)	**Nasal Spray:** 200 IU/inh	***Adults:*** 200 IU qd intranasally. Alternate nostrils daily.	**W/P:** Possibility of systemic allergic reactions. Consider skin testing if sensitivity suspected. If nasal mucosa ulceration occurs, discontinue until healed. Discontinue if severe ulceration of the nasal mucosa occurs. Perform periodic nasal exams. **Contra:** Clinical allergy to calcitonin-salmon. **P/N:** Category C, not for use in nursing.	Rhinitis, nasal symptoms, back pain, arthralgia, epistaxis, headache.
Levothyroxine Sodium (Levoxyl, Synthroid)	**Tab:** 25µg*, 50µg*, 75µg*, 88µg*, 100µg*, 112µg*, 125µg*, 137µg*, 150µg*, 175µg*, 200µg*, 300µg*	***Adults:*** Take in am at least one-half hour before food. **Hypothyroid: Usual:** 1.7µg/kg/day. >200µg/day (seldom). **>50 yrs or <50 yrs with CVD: Initial:** 25-50µg/day. **Titrate:** Increase by 12.5-25µg/day every 6-8 weeks until euthyroid. **Elderly with CVD: Initial:** 12.5-25µg/day. **Titrate:** Increase by 12.5-25µg/day every 4-6 weeks until euthyroid. **Severe Hypothyroidism: Initial:** 12.5-25µg/day. **Titrate:** Increase by 25µg/day every 2-4 weeks until euthyroid. **Pregnancy:** May increase dose requirements. **Subclinical Hypothyroidism:** Lower doses required. ***Pediatrics:*** Take in am at least 30 min before food. **Hypothyroidism: 0-3 months:** 10-15µg/kg/day. **3-6 months:** 8-10µg/kg/day. **6-12 months:** 6-8µg/kg/day. **1-5 yrs:** 5-6µg/kg/day. **6-12 yrs:** 4-5µg/kg/day. **>12 yrs:** 2-3µg/kg/day. **Growth/Puberty Complete:** 1.7µg/kg/day. **Cardiac Risk: Initial:** Use lower dose. **Titrate:** Increase	**W/P:** Do not use in the treatment of obesity; larger doses in euthyroid patients can cause serious or even life-threatening toxicity. Caution with CVD, CAD, adrenal insufficiency, and elderly with risk of occult CVD. Carefully titrate dose to avoid over or under treatment. Decreased bone mineral density with long-term use. Caution with non-toxic diffuse goiter or nodular thyroid disease. With adrenal insufficiency, supplement with glucocorticoids before therapy. **Contra:** Untreated thyrotoxicosis, acute MI, and uncorrected adrenal insufficiency. **P/N:** Category A, caution in nursing.	Pseudotumor cerebri in children reported. Seizures (rare), hypersensitivity reactions, dysphagia, choking, gagging, and hyperthyroidism (increased appetite, weight loss, heat intolerance, hyperactivity, tremors, palpitations, tachycardia, diarrhea, vomiting, or hair loss).

Table 20.1: PRESCRIBING INFORMATION FOR ENDOCRINE/HORMONAL AND BONE METABOLISM DRUGS (cont.)

NAME	FORM/ STRENGTH	DOSAGE	WARNINGS/PRECAUTIONS & CONTRAINDICATIONS	ADVERSE EFFECTS†
THYROID HORMONES (cont.)				
Levothyroxine Sodium (cont.)		dose every 4-6 weeks until euthyroid. **Infants with Serum T4 <5µg/dL: Initial:** 50µg/day. **Chronic/Severe Hypothyroidism: Children: Initial:** 25µg/day. **Titrate:** Increase by 25µg/day every 2-4 weeks until desired effect. **Minimize Hyperactivity in Older Children: Initial:** Give 25% of full replacement dose. **Titrate:** Increase by same amount weekly until full dose achieved. May crush tab and mix with 5-10mL water.		
Levothyroxine Sodium/ Liothyronine Sodium (Thyrolar)	(T3-T4) **Tab:** (1/4) 3.1µg-12.5µg, (1/2) 6.25µg-25µg, (1) 12.5µg-50µg, (2) 25µg-100µg, (3) 37.5µg-150µg	**Adults: Hypothyroidism: Usual:** 12.5µg-50µg to 25µg-100µg qd. **Elderly/Coronary Artery Disease: Initial:** 6.25µg-25µg qd. **Chronic Myxedema:** 3.1µg-12.5µg qd. **Titrate:** Increase by 3.1µg-12.5µg/d q 2-3 weeks. Reduce dose if angina occurs. **Myxedema Coma:** 400µg IV levothyroxine sodium (100µg/mL rapidly) followed by 100-200µg/day IV. Switch to PO when stable. **Thyroid Suppression:** 1.56mg/kg/d levothyroxine (T₄) for 7-10 days. **Pediatrics: Hypothyroidism: >12 years:** 18.75µg-75µg qd. **6-12 years:** 12.5µg-50µg to 18.75µg-75µg qd. **1-5 years:** 9.35µg-37.5µg to 12.5µg-50µg qd. **6-12 months:** 6.25µg-25µg to 9.35µg-37.5µg qd. **0-6 months:** 3.1µg-12.5µg to 6.25µg-25µg qd.	**W/P:** Do not use in the treatment of obesity; larger doses in euthyroid patients can cause serious or even life-threatening toxicity. Caution with angina pectoris and elderly; use lower doses. May aggravate DM or insipidus and adrenal cortical insufficiency. Excessive doses may cause craniosynostosis. Extreme caution with long-standing myxedema especially with CV impairment. **Contra:** Untreated thyrotoxicosis or uncorrected adrenal cortical insufficiency. **P/N:** Category A, caution in nursing.	
Liothyronine Sodium (Cytomel)	**Tab:** 5µg, 25µg*, 50µg*	**Adults: Mild Hypothyroidism: Initial:** 25µg qd. **Titrate:** May increase by up to 25µg qd every 1-2 weeks. **Maint:** 25-75µg qd. **Myxedema: Initial:** 5µg qd. **Titrate:** May increase by 5-10µg qd every 1-2 weeks up to 25µg qd, then increase by 5-25µg qd every 1-2 weeks. **Maint:** 50-100µg/day. **Goiter: Initial:** 5µg/day. **Titrate:** May increase by 5-10µg qd every 1-2 weeks up to 25µg qd, then by 12.5-25µg qd every 1-2 weeks. **Maint:** 75µg qd. **Elderly/CAD: Initial:** 5µg qd. **Titrate:** Increase by no more than 5µg qd every 2 weeks. **Thyroid Suppression Therapy:** 75-100µg qd for 7 days. Radioactive iodine uptake is determined before and after administration of hormone. **Pediatrics: Congenital Hypothyroidism: Initial:** 5µg qd. **Titrate:** Increase by 5µg qd every 3-4 days until desired response. **Maint: <1 year:** 20µg qd. **1-3 years:** 50µg qd. **>3 years:** 25-75µg/day.	**W/P:** Do not use in the treatment of obesity; larger doses in euthyroid patients can cause serious or even life-threatening toxicity. Caution with angina pectoris and elderly; use lower doses. Rule out hypogonadism and nephrosis prior to therapy. With prolonged and severe hypothyroidism supplement with adrenocortical steroids. May aggravate DM or diabetes insipidus and adrenal cortical insufficiency. Add glucocorticoid with myxedema coma. Excessive doses may cause craniosynostosis in infants. **Contra:** Uncorrected adrenal cortical insufficiency and untreated thyrotoxicosis. **P/N:** Category A, caution in nursing.	Allergic skin reactions (rare).
Thyroid (Armour Thyroid)	**Tab:** 15mg, 30mg, 60mg, 90mg, 120mg, 180mg, 240mg, 300mg	**Adults: Hypothyroidism: Initial:** 30mg qd. **Titrate:** Increase by 15mg q2-3 weeks. **Myxedema with CVD:** 15mg qd. **Maint:** 60-120mg/day. **Thyroid Cancer:** Higher doses then replacement therapy is required. **Myxedema Coma: Levothyroxine Sodium: Initial:** 400µg IV then 100-200µg/day IV.	**W/P:** Do not use in the treatment of obesity; larger doses in euthyroid patients can cause serious or even life-threatening toxicity. Caution with CVD, DM, diabetes insipidus, elderly, and adrenal cortical insufficiency. **Contra:** Untreated thyrotoxicosis or uncorrected adrenal cortical insufficiency.	

*Scored.   †Bold entries denote special dental considerations.

NAME	FORM/ STRENGTH	DOSAGE	WARNINGS/PRECAUTIONS & CONTRAINDICATIONS	ADVERSE EFFECTS†
Thyroid *(cont.)*		Continue with oral therapy when stabilized. **Thyroid Suppression:** 1.56mg/kg/day for 7-10 days. **Elderly: Initial:** Use lower dose (eg, 15-30mg qd). *Pediatrics:* **Hypothyroidism: 0-6months:** 4.8-6mg/kg/day; **6-12 months:** 3.6-4.8mg/kg/day; **1-5 years:** 3-3.6mg/kg/day; **6-12 years:** 2.4-3mg/kg/day; **>12 yrs:** 1.2-1.8mg/kg/day.	**P/N:** Category A, caution in nursing.	

ANTITHYROID HORMONES

NAME	FORM/ STRENGTH	DOSAGE	WARNINGS/PRECAUTIONS & CONTRAINDICATIONS	ADVERSE EFFECTS†
Methimazole (Tapazole)	**Tab:** 5mg*, 10mg*	*Adults:* **Initial: Mild Hyperthyroidism:** 5mg q8h. **Moderately Severe Hyperthyroidism:** 30-40mg/day, in divided doses q8h. **Severe Hyperthyroidism:** 20mg q8h. **Maint:** 5-15mg/day. *Pediatrics:* **Initial:** 0.4mg/kg/day in divided doses q8h. **Maint:** 1/2 of initial dose.	**W/P:** Can cause fetal harm. Agranulocytosis, leukopenia, thrombocytopenia, or aplastic anemia may occur; monitor bone marrow function. Discontinue with agranulocytosis, aplastic anemia, or exfoliative dermatitis. Discontinue with liver abnormality (eg, hepatitis), including transaminases ≥3X ULN. Monitor thyroid function periodically. May cause hypoprothrombinemia and bleeding; monitor PT. **Contra:** Nursing mothers. **P/N:** Category D, contraindicated in nursing.	Rash, urticaria, nausea, vomiting, arthralgia, paresthesia, myalgia, neuritis, vertigo, edema, **altered taste,** hair loss, lymphadenopathy, lupus-like syndrome, and insulin autoimmune syndrome.
Propylthiouracil	**Tab:** 50mg	*Adults:* **Initial:** 300mg/day in 3 divided doses q8h. **Severe Hyperthyroidism/Very Large Goiters: Initial:** 400mg/day in 3 divided doses; may give up to 600-900mg/day if needed. **Maint:** 100-150mg/day. *Pediatrics:* **6-10 years: Initial:** 50-150mg/day. **≥10 years: Initial:** 150-300mg/day. **Maint:** Determine by patient response.	**W/P:** Discontinue with agranulocytosis, aplastic anemia, hepatitis, fever, or exfoliative dermatitis. Rare reports of severe hepatic reactions exist. Discontinue with significant hepatic abnormality, including transaminases >3X ULN. Caution with pregnancy, may cause fetal harm. Monitor PT and TFTs. **Contra:** Nursing mothers. **P/N:** Category D, contraindicated in nursing.	Agranulocytosis, skin rash, urticaria, nausea, vomiting, epigastric distress, arthralgia, paresthesias, **loss of taste,** myalgia, headache, pruritus, drowsiness, neuritis, edema, vertigo, and jaundice.

BONE METABOLISM DRUGS

BISPHOSPHONATES

NAME	FORM/ STRENGTH	DOSAGE	WARNINGS/PRECAUTIONS & CONTRAINDICATIONS	ADVERSE EFFECTS†
Alendronate sodium (Fosamax)	**Sol:** 70mg [75mL]; **Tab:** 5mg, 10mg, 35mg, 40mg, 70mg	*Adults:* **Osteoporosis: Treatment:** 70mg once weekly or 10mg qd. **Prevention:** 35mg once weekly or 5mg qd. **Glucocorticoid-Induced:** 5mg qd; 10mg qd for postmenopausal women not on estrogen. **Paget's Disease:** 40mg qd for 6 months. Take at least 30 minutes before the first food, beverage (other than water), or medication. Take tabs with 6-8 oz plain water or 2 oz with oral solution. Do not lie down for at least 30 minutes and until after the first food of the day.	**W/P:** Caution with active upper GI problems. May cause local irritation of the upper GI mucosa. Correct hypocalcemia or other mineral metabolism disturbances before initiating therapy. Supplement calcium and vitamin D if needed. Not recommended with renal insufficiency (CrCl <35mL/min). Discontinue if symptoms of esophageal disease develop. When combined with glucocorticoids perform BMD test at initiation and 6-12 months later. Rare reports of osteonecrosis, primarily in the jaw, and severe, incapacitating bone, joint, and/or muscle pain. **Contra:** Esophagus abnormalities which delay esophageal emptying such as stricture or achalasia; inability to stand or sit upright for at least 30 minutes; hypocalcemia. **P/N:** Category C, caution in nursing.	Abdominal pain, nausea, dyspepsia, constipation, diarrhea, flatulence, acid regurgitation, musculoskeletal pain, gastric ulcers, **jaw osteonecrosis (rare).**
Etidronate disodium (Didronel)	**Tab:** 200mg, 400mg*	*Adults:* Give as single dose (preferred) or in divided doses. **Paget's Disease: Initial:** 5-10mg/kg/day up to 6 months or 11-20mg/kg/day up to 3 months. May re-treat after drug-free period of 90 days only if	**W/P:** Therapy response in Paget's Disease may be of slow onset and continue for months after stopping. Maintain adequate dietary intake of calcium and vitamin D. Diarrhea reported with enterocolitis. Monitor	Diarrhea, nausea, increased bone pain in Paget's, alopecia, arthropathy, esophagitis, hypersensitivity reactions, osteomalacia, amnesia,

Table 20.1: PRESCRIBING INFORMATION FOR ENDOCRINE/HORMONAL AND BONE METABOLISM DRUGS (cont.)

NAME	FORM/ STRENGTH	DOSAGE	WARNINGS/PRECAUTIONS & CONTRAINDICATIONS	ADVERSE EFFECTS†
BONE METABOLISM DRUGS (cont.)				
Etidronate disodium (cont.)		evidence of active disease process. **Heterotopic Ossification: Hip Replacement:** 20mg/kg/day 1 month before and 3 months after surgery. **Spinal Cord:** 20mg/kg/day for 2 weeks, followed by 10mg/kg/day for 10 weeks.	with renal impairment. Reduce dose with decreased GFR. Max dose (20mg/day) or long-term therapy (>6 months) may increase fracture risk. Rachitic syndrome reported in children at doses of 10mg/kg/day for prolonged periods (approaching or exceeding 1 year). Rare reports of osteonecrosis, primarily in the jaw, and severe, incapacitating bone, joint, and/or muscle pain have been reported with other bisphosphonates, although not with etidronate specifically. **Contra:** Overt osteomalacia. **P/N:** Category C, caution with nursing.	confusion; **rare reports of jaw osteonecrosis with other bisphosphonates**.
Ibandronate sodium (Boniva)	**Tab:** 2.5mg, 150mg	**Adults:** 2.5mg qd or 150mg once monthly. Swallow whole with 6-8 oz. of water. Do not lie down for 60 minutes after dose. Take at least 60 minutes before first food, drink (other than water), medication, or supplements.	**W/P:** May cause upper GI disorders (eg, dysphagia, esophagitis, esophageal or gastric ulcer). Not recommended in severe renal impairment (CrCl <30mL/min). Rare reports of osteonecrosis, primarily in the jaw, and severe, incapacitating bone, joint, and/ or muscle pain. **Contra:** Hypocalcemia; inability to stand or sit upright for at least 60 minutes. **P/N:** Category C, caution in nursing.	HTN, dyspepsia, nausea, back pain, arthralgia, abdominal pain, diarrhea, constipation, influenza, nasopharyngitis, headache, bronchitis, **jaw osteonecrosis (rare)**.
Pamidronate disodium (Aredia)	**Inj:** 30mg, 90mg	**Adults: Moderate Hypercalcemia:** 60-90mg IV single dose over 2-24 hrs. **Severe Hypercalcemia:** 90mg IV single dose over 2-24 hrs. **Retreatment:** May repeat after 7 days. **Paget's Disease:** 30mg IV over 4 hrs for 3 consecutive days. **Osteolytic Bone Lesions of Multiple Myeloma:** 90mg IV over 4 hrs once a month. **Osteolytic Bone Metastases of Breast Cancer:** 90mg IV over 2 hrs every 3-4 weeks. **Max:** 90mg/single dose for all indications. **Renal Dysfunction With Bone Metastases:** Withhold dose if SrCr increases by 0.5mg/dL (normal baseline) or by 1mg/dL (abnormal baseline). Resume when SrCr returns to within 10% of baseline.	**W/P:** Associated with renal toxicity; monitor serum creatinine prior to each treatment. Monitor serum calcium, electrolytes, phosphate, magnesium, CBC with differential, Hct/Hgb closely. Monitor for 2 weeks post-treatment if pre-existing anemia, leukopenia, thrombocytopenia. Increased risk of renal adverse reactions with renal impairment; monitor renal function. Avoid treatment of bone metastases in severe renal impairment. Reports of osteonecrosis of the jaw in cancer patients treated with IV bisphosphonates; avoid invasive dental procedures. Rare reports of severe, incapacitating bone, joint, and/or muscle pain with bisphosphonate therapy. **P/N:** Category D, caution in nursing.	Malaise, fever, convulsions, hypomagnesemia, hypocalcemia, hypokalemia, fluid overload, hypophosphatemia, nausea, diarrhea, constipation, anorexia, abnormal hepatic function, bone pain, dyspnea, **jaw osteonecrosis (rare)**.
Risedronate sodium (Actonel)	**Tab:** 5mg, 30mg, 35mg	**Adults: Paget's Disease:** 30mg qd for 2 months. May retreat after 2 months. **Postmenopausal Osteoporosis:** 5mg qd or 35mg once weekly. **Glucocorticoid-Induced Osteoporosis:** 5mg qd. Take at least 30 minutes before the 1st food or drink of the day other than water. Swallow tab in upright position with 6-8 oz of plain water. Do not lie down for 30 minutes after dose.	**W/P:** May cause upper GI disorders (eg, dysphagia, esophagitis, esophageal or gastric ulcer). Treat hypocalcemia and other disturbances of bone and mineral metabolism before therapy. Give supplemental calcium and vitamin D if dietary intake is inadequate. Avoid with severe renal impairment (CrCl <30mL/min). Rare reports of osteonecrosis, primarily in the jaw, and severe, incapacitating bone, joint, and/or muscle pain. **Contra:** Hypocalcemia; inability to stand or sit upright for at least 30 minutes. **P/N:** Category C, not for use in nursing.	Asthenia, diarrhea, abdominal pain, nausea, constipation, peripheral edema, arthralgia, leg cramps, headache, dizziness, sinusitis, rash, tinnitus, **jaw osteonecrosis (rare)**.

*Scored.   †Bold entries denote special dental considerations.

NAME	FORM/ STRENGTH	DOSAGE	WARNINGS/PRECAUTIONS & CONTRAINDICATIONS	ADVERSE EFFECTS[†]
Tiluronate disodium (Skelid)	**Tab:** 200mg	***Adults:*** 400mg qd for 3 months. After therapy, wait 3 months to assess response. Take with 6-8 oz of water. Take 2 hrs after food.	**W/P:** May cause GI disorders (eg, dysphagia, esophagitis, esophageal or gastric ulcers). Maintain adequate Vitamin D and calcium intake. Avoid in severe renal failure. Rare reports of osteonecrosis, primarily in the jaw, and severe, incapacitating bone, joint, and/or muscle pain have been reported with other bisphosphonates, although not with tiluronate specifically. **P/N:** Category C, caution in nursing.	Pain, headache, dizziness, paresthesia, diarrhea, nausea, dyspepsia, vomiting, rhinitis, upper respiratory infection; **rare reports of jaw osteonecrosis with other bisphosphonates**.
Zoledronic acid (Zometa)	**Inj:** 4mg/5mL	***Adults:* Hypercalcemia of Malignancy: Max:** 4mg IV over no less than 15 minutes. **Retreatment (if necessary):** Wait at least 7 days from initial dose. **Multiple Myeloma/Bone Metastases:** 4mg IV over 15 minutes every 3-4 weeks. CrCl 50-60mL/min: 3.5mg; CrCl 40-49mL/min: 3.3mg; CrCl 30-39mL/min: 3.0mg. Measure serum creatinine prior to each dose. Withhold dose with renal deterioration; resume when serum creatinine returns to within 10% of baseline. Take with oral calcium 500mg/day and Vitamin D 400 IU/day.	**W/P:** Caution with hepatic insufficiency, aspirin-sensitive asthma, and the elderly. Risk of renal toxicity/failure. In severe renal impairment, avoid with bone metastases and use caution with hypercalcemia of malignancy. Rehydrate before use with hypercalcemia of malignancy. Monitor serum creatinine before each dose, and serum calcium, electrolytes, phosphate, magnesium, and Hct/Hgb regularly. May cause fetal harm during pregnancy. Osteonecrosis of the jaw reported in cancer patients treated with IV bisphosphonates; avoid invasive dental procedures. Rare reports of severe, incapacitating bone, joint, and/or muscle pain with bisphosphonate therapy. **P/N:** Category D, not for use in nursing.	Fever, chills, bone pain, arthralgia, myalgia, nausea, vomiting, diarrhea, constipation, injection site reactions, conjunctivitis, hypomagnesemia, abnormal serum creatinine, hypophosphatemia, hypocalcemia, **jaw osteonecrosis (rare)**.

BISPHOSPHONATE COMBINATIONS

NAME	FORM/ STRENGTH	DOSAGE	WARNINGS/PRECAUTIONS & CONTRAINDICATIONS	ADVERSE EFFECTS[†]
Alendronate Sodium/ Cholecalciferol (Fosamax Plus D)	**Tab:** (Alendronate Sodium-Cholecalciferol) 70mg-2800 IU	***Adults:*** 1 tab (70mg/2800 IU) once weekly. Take at least 30 minutes before the first food, beverage (other than water), or medication. Do not lie down for at least 30 minutes and until after first food of the day.	**W/P:** Caution with active upper GI problems. May cause local irritation of the upper GI mucosa. Correct hypocalcemia and other mineral metabolism disturbances before initiating therapy. Do not use to treat vitamin D deficiency. May worsen hypercalcemia and/or hypercalciuria. Supplement calcium if needed. Not recommended with renal insufficiency (CrCl <35mL/min). Discontinue if symptoms of esophageal disease develop. Rare reports of osteonecrosis, primarily in the jaw, and severe, incapacitating bone, joint, and/or muscle pain. **Contra:** Esophagus abnormalities which delay esophageal emptying such as stricture or achalasia; inability to stand or sit upright for at least 30 minutes; hypocalcemia. **P/N:** Category C, caution in nursing.	Abdominal pain, nausea, dyspepsia, constipation, diarrhea, flatulence, acid regurgitation, musculoskeletal pain, gastric ulcers, **jaw osteonecrosis (rare)**.
Risedronate Sodium/ Calcium Carbonate (Actonel with Calcium)	**Tab:** (Risedronate Sodium) 35mg; **Tab:** (Calcium Carbonate) 1250mg	***Adults:* Risedronate:** 35mg once weekly (Day 1 of the 7-day treatment cycle). Take at least 30 minutes before 1st food or drink of the day other than water. Swallow tab in upright position with 6-8 oz of plain water. Do not lie down for 30 minutes after dose. **Calcium:** 1250mg qd with food on each of the remaining 6 days (Days 2-7 of the 7-day treatment cycle).	**W/P:** Risedronate: May cause upper GI disorders (eg, dysphagia, esophagitis, esophageal or gastric ulcer). Treat hypocalcemia and other disturbances of bone and mineral metabolism before therapy. May cause osteonecrosis, primarily in the jaw. Avoid with severe renal impairment (CrCl <30mL/min). Calcium: Should not be used to treat hypocalcemia. Daily intake above	(Risedronate) Infection, pain, flu syndrome, abdominal pain, headache, asthenia, hypertension, constipation, dyspepsia, nausea, arthralgia, diarrhea, dizziness, myalgia, **jaw osteonecrosis (rare)**. (Calcium) Constipation, flatulence, nausea,

Table 20.1: PRESCRIBING INFORMATION FOR ENDOCRINE/HORMONAL AND BONE METABOLISM DRUGS *(cont.)*

NAME	FORM/ STRENGTH	DOSAGE	WARNINGS/PRECAUTIONS & CONTRAINDICATIONS	ADVERSE EFFECTS†
BONE METABOLISM DRUGS *(cont.)*				
Risedronate Sodium/ Calcium Carbonate *(cont.)*			2000mg has been associated with increased risk of adverse effects, including hypercalcemia and kidney stones. Patients with achlorhydria may have decreased absorption of calcium. Rare reports of osteonecrosis, primarily in the jaw, and severe, incapacitating bone, joint, and/or muscle pain. **Contra:** Risedronate: Hypocalcemia; inability to stand or sit upright for at least 30 minutes. Calcium: Hypercalcemia from any cause (eg, hyperparathyroidism, hypercalcemia of malignancy, or sarcoidosis). **P/N:** Category C, not for use in nursing.	abdominal pain, bloating.
MISCELLANEOUS BONE METABOLISM DRUG				
Teriparatide (Forteo)	**Inj:** 250mcg/mL [3mL pen]	***Adults:*** 20mcg qd SC into thigh or abdominal wall. Administer initially under circumstances where patient can sit or lie down if symptoms of orthostatic hypotension occur. Discard pen after 28 days. Use for >2 yrs is not recommended.	**Increased incidence of osteosarcoma seen in rats. Only prescribe when benefits outweigh risks. Not for those at increased baseline risk for osteosarcoma, including Paget's disease or unexplained alkaline phosphatase elevations, open epiphyses, or prior radiation therapy involving the skeleton. W/P:** Avoid in pediatrics, or with bone metastases, or history of skeletal malignancies, metabolic bone diseases other than osteoporosis, or pre-existing hypercalcemia (eg, primary hyperparathyroidism). Potential exacerbation of active or recent urolithiasis. Transient episodes of symptomatic orthostatic hypotension observed infrequently. Increases serum uric acid levels. Transient calcium increases. **P/N:** Category C; not for use in nursing.	Pain, arthralgia, asthenia, nausea, rhinitis, dizziness, headache, HTN, increased cough, pharyngitis, constipation, diarrhea, dyspepsia.

*Scored.   †Bold entries denote special dental considerations.

Table 20.2: DRUG INTERACTIONS FOR ENDOCRINE/HORMONAL AND BONE METABOLISM DRUGS

ANDROGENS

Methyltestosterone[CIII] (Testred)

Anticoagulants	Potentiates oral anticoagulants and oxyphenbutazone.
Insulin	May decrease blood glucose and insulin requirements in diabetics.
Oxyphenbutazone	Potentiates oral anticoagulants and oxyphenbutazone.

Oxandrolone[CIII] (Oxandrin)

ACTH	May increase edema.
Adrenal cortical steroids	May increase edema.
Anticoagulants	Increased sensitivity to oral anticoagulants (eg, warfarin).
Hypoglycemics	May inhibit metabolism of oral hypoglycemics.

Oxymetholone (Anadrol-50)

Anticoagulants	Increased sensitivity to oral anticoagulants (eg, warfarin); anticoagulant dosages may need to be decreased.
Hypoglycemics	Dosage of insulin and oral hypoglycemic medications may need to be adjusted because of oxymetholone's potential to increase plasma blood glucose.
Insulin	Dosage of insulin and oral hypoglycemic medications may need to be adjusted because of oxymetholone's potential to increase plasma blood glucose.

Testosterone (Androderm, Androgel, Testim)

Anticoagulants	May potentiate effects of anticoagulants.
Corticosteroids	May enhance edema; caution with cardiac or hepatic disease.
Insulin	May decrease blood glucose and insulin requirements in diabetics.
Oxyphenbutazone	May elevate oxyphenbutazone levels.
Propranolol	May increase clearance of propranolol.

Testosterone Cypionate[CIII] (Depo-Testosterone)

Anticoagulants	Potentiates oral anticoagulants (eg, warfarin).
Insulin	May decrease blood glucose and insulin requirements in diabetics.
Oxyphenbutazone	Potentiates oxyphenbutazone.

Table 20.2: DRUG INTERACTIONS FOR ENDOCRINE/HORMONAL AND BONE METABOLISM DRUGS *(cont.)*

CONTRACEPTIVES (Oral)

Desogestrel/Ethinyl Estradiol (Cyclessa, Desogen, Mircette, Orthocept); **Drospirenone/Ethinyl Estradiol** (Yasmin, YAZ); **Ethinyl Estradiol/Ethynodiol Diacetate** (Demulen 1/35-28, Demulen 1/50-21, Demulen 1/50-28); **Ethinyl Estradiol/Etonogestrel** (Nuvaring); **Ethinyl Estradiol/Ferrous Fumarate/Norethindrone Acetate** (Estrostep FE, Loestrin FE 1.5/30, Loestrin FE 1/20); **Ethinyl Estradiol/Levonorgestrel** (Alesse 28, Levlen, Levlite 28, Nordette-28, Seasonale, Tri-Levlen, Triphasil-21, Triphasil-28); **Ethinyl Estradiol/Norelgestromin** (Ortho Evra); **Ethinyl Estradiol/Norethindrone** (Loestrin 21 1.5/30, Loestrin 21 1/20, Modicon, Ortho-Novum 1/35, Ortho-Novum 10/11, Ortho-Novum 7/7/7, Ovcon 35, Ovcon 50, Tri-Norinyl); **Ethinyl Estradiol/Norgestimate** (Ortho-cyclen, Ortho Tri-cyclen, Ortho Tri-cyclen LO); **Ethinyl Estradiol/Norgestrel** (Lo/Ovral-28); Mestranol/Norethindrone (Ortho-Novum 1/50); **Norethindrone** (Nor-QD)

ACE inhibitors	Risk of hyperkalemia with ACE inhibitors.
Acetaminophen	May increase plasma levels of ethinyl estradiol; acetaminophen levels may decrease.
Aldosterone antagonists	Risk of hyperkalemia with aldosterone antagonists.
Angiotensin II receptor antagonists	Risk of hyperkalemia with ACE inhibitors, angiotensin II receptor antagonists.
Antibiotics	Reduced effects, increased breakthrough bleeding, and menstrual irregularities with some antibiotics.
Anticonvulsants	Reduced effects, increased breakthrough bleeding, and menstrual irregularities with some anticonvulsants.
Antifungals	Reduced effects, increased breakthrough bleeding, and menstrual irregularities with some antifungals.
Ascorbic acid	May increase plasma levels of oral contraceptives.
Barbiturates	Reduced effects, increased breakthrough bleeding, and menstrual irregularities with barbiturates.
Carbamazepine	Reduced effects, increased breakthrough bleeding, and menstrual irregularities with carbamazepine.
Corticosteroids	May affect corticosteroid levels.
Cyclosporine	Increased plasma concentrations of cyclosporine.
CYP450 inducers	Reduced effects with hepatic enzyme inducers (eg, rifampin, phenytoin, carbamazepine, barbiturates).
CYP3A4 inhibitors	Increased levels of ethinyl estradiol with CYP3A4 inhibitors (eg, ketoconazole, itraconazole).
Griseofulvin	Possible reduced effects, increased breakthrough bleeding, and menstrual irregularities with with griseofulvin.
Phenylbutazone	Reduced effects, increased breakthrough bleeding, and menstrual irregularities with phenylbutazone.
Phenytoin	Reduced effects, increased breakthrough bleeding, and menstrual irregularities with phenytoin.
Potassium-sparing diuretics	Risk of hyperkalemia with potassium-sparing diuretics.
Prednisolone	Increased plasma concentrations of prednisolone.

CONTRACEPTIVES (Oral) *(cont.)*

Protease inhibitors	May increase/decrease levels. Reduced effects, increased breakthrough bleeding, and menstrual irregularities with some protease inhibitors.
Rifampin	Reduced effects, increased breakthrough bleeding, and menstrual irregularities with rifampin.
Salicylic acid	May increase clearance of salicylic acid.
St. John's wort	May induce hepatic enzymes and reduce effectiveness.
Temazepam	May increase clearance of temazepam.
Tetracyclines	Possible reduced effects, increased breakthrough bleeding, and menstrual irregularities with tetracyclines.
Theophylline	Increased plasma concentrations of theophylline.
Topiramate	Reduced effects, increased breakthrough bleeding, and menstrual irregularities with topiramate.

ESTROGENS

Conjugated Estrogens (Premarin, Premarin Intravenous); **Conjugated Estrogens Synthetic A** (Cenestin); **Esterified Estrogens** (Menest); **Estradiol** (Alora, Climara, Esclim, Estrace, Estraderm, Menostar, Vivelle, Vivelle-Dot); **Estradiol Cypionate** (Depo-Estradiol); **Estradiol Valerate** (Delestrogen); **Estropipate** (Ogen)

CYP3A4 inducers	CYP3A4 inducers (eg, St. John's wort, phenobarbital, carbamazepine, rifampin) may decrease levels, possibly decreasing therapeutic effects and/or changing uterine bleeding profile.
CYP3A4 inhibitors	CYP3A4 inhibitors (eg, erythromycin, clarithromycin, ketoconazole, itraconazole, ritonavir, grapefruit juice) may increase levels, possibly resulting in side effects.

ESTROGEN COMBINATIONS

Conjugated Estrogens/Medroxyprogesterone Acetate (Premphase, Prempro); **Esterified Estrogens/Methyltestosterone** (Estratest, Estratest HS); **Estradiol/Levonorgestrel** (Climara Pro); **Estradiol/Norethindrone Acetate** (Activella, Combipatch); **Estradiol/Norgestimate** (Prefest); **Ethinyl Estradiol/Norethindrone Acetate** (Femhrt 1/5, Femhrt LO)

Acetaminophen	May increase levels of ethinyl estradiol; acetaminophen levels may decrease.
Anticoagulants	May increase anticoagulant requirements.
Clofibric acid	May increase clearance of clofibric acid.
Cyclosporine	Increases plasma levels of cyclosporine.
CYP3A4 inducers	CYP3A4 inducers (eg, St. John's wort, phenobarbital, carbamazepine, rifampin) may decrease levels, possibly decreasing therapeutic effects and/or changing uterine bleeding profile.
CYP3A4 inhibitors	CYP3A4 inhibitors (eg, erythromycin, clarithromycin, ketoconazole, itraconazole, ritonavir, grapefruit juice) may increase levels, possibly resulting in side effects.
Insulin	May decrease insulin requirements.

Table 20.2: DRUG INTERACTIONS FOR ENDOCRINE/HORMONAL AND BONE METABOLISM DRUGS *(cont.)*

ESTROGEN COMBINATIONS *(cont.)*

Morphine	May increase clearance of morphine.
Oxyphenbutazone	May increase levels of oxyphenbutazone.
Prednisolone	Increases plasma levels of prednisolone.
Salicylic acid	May increase clearance of salicylic acid.
Temazapam	May increase clearance of temazapam.
Theophylline	Increases plasma levels of theophylline.

PROGESTINS

Medroxyprogesterone Acetate (Depo-provera, Depo-SubQ-provera 104, Provera)

Aminoglutethimide	May decrease serum levels.
Estrogen	Caution with estrogen.

Progesterone (Prometrium)

CYP3A4 inhibitors	CYP3A4 inhibitors (eg, ketoconazole) may increase bioavailability of progesterone.

SERUM ESTROGEN RECEPTOR MODULATOR

Raloxifene Hydrochloride (Evista)

Anion exchange resins	Avoid concomitant use with anion exchange resins.
Cholestyramine	Cholestyramine decreases absorption.
Protein-bound drugs	Caution with other highly protein-bound drugs (eg, diazepam, diazoxide, lidocaine).
Warfarin/ anticoagulants	Monitor PT/INR with warfarin and other anticoagulants.

HYPOGLYCEMIC AGENTS

INSULIN

Insulin Aspart Protamine, Recombinant/Insulin Aspart, Recombinant (Novolog 70/30)

ACE inhibitors	Increased glucose-lowering effects with ACE inhibitors.
Alcohol	May potentiate or weaken glucose-lowering effect.
Antidiabetics	Increased glucose-lowering effects with oral antidiabetics.
β-blockers	β-blockers may potentiate or weaken glucose-lowering effect and may reduce or mask signs of hypoglycemia.
Clonidine	May potentiate or weaken glucose-lowering effect and may reduce or mask signs of hypoglycemia.

HYPOGLYCEMIC AGENTS *(cont.)*

Insulin Aspart Protamine, Recombinant/Insulin Aspart, Recombinant (Novolog 70/30) *(cont.)*

Corticosteroids	Decreased blood glucose-lowering effects with corticosteroids.
Danazol	Decreased blood glucose-lowering effects with danazol.
Disopyramide	Increased glucose-lowering effects with disopyramide.
Diuretics	Decreased blood glucose-lowering effects with diuretics.
Estrogens	Decreased blood glucose-lowering effects with estrogens.
Fibrates	Increased glucose-lowering effects with fibrates.
Fluoxetine	Increased glucose-lowering effects with fluoxetine.
Guanethidine	May reduce or mask signs of hypoglycemia.
Insulin	Do not mix with other insulin products.
Isoniazid	Decreased blood glucose-lowering effects with isoniazid.
Lithium salts	May potentiate or weaken glucose-lowering effects.
MAOIs	Increased glucose-lowering effects with MAOIs.
Niacin	Decreased blood glucose-lowering effects with niacin.
Pentamidine	May cause hypoglycemia, followed by hyperglycemia.
Phenothiazine derivatives	Decreased blood glucose-lowering effects with phenothiazine derivatives.
Potassium-lowering drugs	Caution with potassium-lowering drugs and drugs sensitive to serum potassium levels.
Progesterones	Decreased blood glucose-lowering effects with progesterones.
Propoxyphene	Increased glucose-lowering effects with propoxyphene.
Reserpine	May reduce or mask signs of hypoglycemia.
Salicylates	Increased glucose-lowering effects with salicylates.
Somatostatin analog	Increased glucose-lowering effects with somatostatin analog.
Somatropin	Decreased blood glucose-lowering effects with somatropin.
Sulfonamide antibiotics	Increased glucose-lowering effects with sulfonamide antibiotics.
Sympathomimetics	Decreased blood glucose-lowering effects with sympathomimetics.
Thyroid hormones	Decreased blood glucose-lowering effects with thyroid hormones.

Insulin Aspart, Recombinant (Novolog)

ACE inhibitors	Increased glucose-lowering effects with ACE inhibitors.

Table 20.2: DRUG INTERACTIONS FOR ENDOCRINE/HORMONAL AND BONE METABOLISM DRUGS *(cont.)*

HYPOGLYCEMIC AGENTS *(cont.)*

Insulin Aspart, Recombinant (Novolog) *(cont.)*

Alcohol	May potentiate or weaken glucose-lowering effect.
β-blockers	May potentiate or weaken glucose-lowering effect. Masked or reduced hypoglycemic symptoms with β-blockers.
Clonidine	May potentiate or weaken glucose-lowering effect and may reduce or mask signs of hypoglycemia.
Corticosteroids	Decreased blood glucose-lowering effects with corticosteroids.
Danazol	Decreased blood blood glucose-lowering effects with danazol.
Disopyramide	Increased blood glucose-lowering effects with disopyramide.
Diuretics	Decreased blood glucose-lowering effects with diuretics.
Estrogens	Decreased blood glucose-lowering effects with estrogens.
Fibrates	Increased blood glucose-lowering effects with fibrates.
Fluoxetine	Increased blood glucose-lowering effects with fluoxetine.
Guanethidine	Masked or reduced hypoglycemic symptoms with guanethidine.
Isoniazid	Decreased blood glucose-lowering effects with isoniazid.
Lithium salts	May potentiate or weaken glucose-lowering effect.
MAOIs	Increased blood glucose-lowering effects with MAOIs.
Niacin	Decreased blood glucose-lowering effects with niacin.
Pentamidine	May cause hypoglycemia followed by hyperglycemia.
Phenothiazine derivatives	Decreased blood glucose-lowering effects with phenothiazine derivatives.
Progesterones	Decreased blood glucose-lowering effects with progesterones.
Propoxyphene	Increased blood glucose-lowering effects with propoxyphene.
Reserpine	Masked or reduced hypoglycemic symptoms with reserpine.
Salicylates	Increased blood glucose-lowering effects with salicylates.
Somatostatin analog	Increased blood glucose-lowering effects with somatostatin analog.
Somatropin	Decreased blood glucose-lowering effects with somatropin.
Sulfonamide antibiotics	Increased blood glucose-lowering effects with sulfonamide antibiotics and other antidiabetic agents.
Sympathomimetic agents	Decreased blood glucose-lowering effects with sympathomimetic agents.
Thyroid hormones	Decreased blood glucose-lowering effects with thyroid hormones.

HYPOGLYCEMIC AGENTS *(cont.)*

Insulin Glargine, Recombinant (Lantus)

ACE inhibitors	Increased blood glucose-lowering effects with ACE inhibitors.
Alcohol	May potentiate or weaken blood glucose-lowering effect.
Antidiabetic agents	Increased blood glucose-lowering effects with sulfonamide antibiotics and other antidiabetic agents.
β-blockers	May potentiate or weaken blood glucose-lowering effect and may reduce or mask signs of hypoglycemia.
Clonidine	May potentiate or weaken blood glucose-lowering effect and may reduce or mask signs of hypoglycemia.
Corticosteroids	Decreased blood glucose-lowering effects with corticosteroids.
Danazol	Decreased blood glucose-lowering effects with danazol.
Diuretics	Decreased blood glucose-lowering effects with diuretics.
Estrogens	Decreased blood glucose-lowering effects with estrogens.
Fibrates	Increased blood glucose-lowering effects with fibrates.
Fluoxetine	Increased blood glucose-lowering effects with fluoxetine.
Guanethidine	May reduce or mask signs of hypoglycemia.
Isoniazid	Decreased blood glucose-lowering effects with isoniazid.
Isopyramide	Increased blood glucose-lowering effects with disopyramide.
Lithium salts	May potentiate or weaken blood glucose-lowering effect.
MAOIs	Increased blood glucose-lowering effects with MAOIs.
Pentamidine	May cause hypoglycemia, followed by hyperglycemia.
Phenothiazine derivatives	Decreased blood glucose-lowering effects with phenothiazine derivatives.
Progestogens	Decreased blood glucose-lowering effects with progestogens.
Propoxyphene	Increased blood glucose-lowering effects with propoxyphene.
Reserpine	May reduce or mask signs of hypoglycemia.
Salicylates	Increased blood glucose-lowering effects with salicylates.
Somatostatin analog	Increased blood glucose-lowering effects with somatostatin analog.
Somatropin	Decreased blood glucose-lowering effects with somatropin.
Sulfonamide antibiotics	Increased blood glucose-lowering effects with sulfonamide antibiotics and other antidiabetic agents.

Table 20.2: DRUG INTERACTIONS FOR ENDOCRINE/HORMONAL AND BONE METABOLISM DRUGS *(cont.)*

HYPOGLYCEMIC AGENTS *(cont.)*

Insulin Glargine, Recombinant (Lantus) *(cont.)*

Sympathomimetic amines	Decreased blood glucose-lowering effects with sympathomimetic amines.
Thyroid hormones	Decreased blood glucose-lowering effects with thyroid hormones.

Insulin Human Isophane [NPH] (Humulin N, Novolin N)

Alcohol	May change insulin requirements.
Antidepressants	Reduced insulin requirements with certain antidepressants.
β-blockers	May mask symptoms of hypoglycemia.
Contraceptives	Increased insulin requirements with oral contraceptives.
Corticosteroids	Increased insulin requirements with corticosteroids.
Hypoglycemics	Reduced insulin requirements with oral hypoglycemics.
Salicylates	Reduced insulin requirements with salicylates.
Sulfa antibiotics	Reduced insulin requirements with sulfa antibiotics.
Thyroid replacement therapy	Increased insulin requirements with thyroid replacement therapy.

Insulin Human Regular (Humulin R, Novolin R)

Alcohol	May change insulin requirements.
Antidepressants	Reduced insulin requirements with certain antidepressants.
β-blockers	May mask symptoms of hypoglycemia.
Contraceptives	Increased insulin requirements with oral contraceptives.
Corticosteroids	Increased insulin requirements with corticosteroids.
Hypoglycemics	Reduced insulin requirements with oral hypoglycemics.
Salicylates	Reduced insulin requirements with salicylates.
Sulfa antibiotics	Reduced insulin requirements with sulfa antibiotics.
Thyroid replacement therapy	Increased insulin requirements with thyroid replacement therapy.

Insulin Human Zinc [Lente] (Humulin L)

Alcohol	May change insulin requirements.
Antidepressants	Reduced insulin requirements with certain antidepressants.
β-blockers	May mask symptoms of hypoglycemia.
Contraceptives	Increased insulin requirements with oral contraceptives.
Corticosteroids	Increased insulin requirements with corticosteroids.

HYPOGLYCEMIC AGENTS *(cont.)*

Insulin Human Zinc [Lente] (Humulin L) *(cont.)*

Hypoglycemics	Reduced insulin requirements with oral hypoglycemics.
Salicylates	Reduced insulin requirements with salicylates.
Sulfa antibiotics	Reduced insulin requirements with sulfa antibiotics.
Thyroid replacement therapy	Increased insulin requirements with thyroid replacement therapy.

Insulin Human Zinc, Extended [Ultralente] (Humulin U)

Alcohol	May change insulin requirements.
Antidepressants	Reduced insulin requirements with certain antidepressants.
β-blockers	May mask symptoms of hypoglycemia.
Contraceptives	Increased insulin requirements with oral contraceptives.
Corticosteroids	Increased insulin requirements with corticosteroids.
Hypoglycemics	Reduced insulin requirements with oral hypoglycemics.
Salicylates	Reduced insulin requirements with salicylates.
Sulfa antibiotics	Reduced insulin requirements with sulfa antibiotics.
Thyroid replacement therapy	Increased insulin requirements with thyroid replacement therapy.

Insulin Lispro Protamine, Recombinant/Insulin Lispro, Recombinant (Humalog Mix 75/25)

ACE inhibitors	Decreased insulin requirements with ACE inhibitors.
Alcohol	Decreased insulin requirements with alcohol.
β-blockers	Decreased insulin requirements with β-blockers and may mask symptoms of hypoglycemia.
Contraceptives	Increased insulin requirements with oral contraceptives.
Corticosteroids	Increased insulin requirements with corticosteroids.
Estrogens	Increased insulin requirements with estrogens.
Hypoglycemics	Decreased insulin requirements with oral hypoglycemics.
Isoniazid	Increased insulin requirements with isoniazid.
MAOIs	Decreased insulin requirements with MAOIs.
Niacin	Increased insulin requirements with niacin.
Octreotide	Decreased insulin requirements with octreotide.
Phenothiazines	Increased insulin requirements with phenothiazines.
Salicylates	Decreased insulin requirements with salicylates.
Sulfa antibiotics	Decreased insulin requirements with sulfa antibiotics.

Table 20.2: DRUG INTERACTIONS FOR ENDOCRINE/HORMONAL AND BONE METABOLISM DRUGS (cont.)

HYPOGLYCEMIC AGENTS (cont.)

Insulin Lispro Protamine, Recombinant/Insulin Lispro, Recombinant (Humalog Mix 75/25) (cont.)

Thyroid replacement therapy	Increased insulin requirements with thyroid replacement therapy.

Insulin Lispro, Recombinant (Humalog)

ACE inhibitors	Decreased insulin requirements with ACE inhibitors.
Alcohol	Decreased insulin requirements with alcohol.
β-blockers	Decreased insulin requirements with β-blockers and may mask symptoms of hypoglycemia.
Contraceptives	Increased insulin requirements with oral contraceptives.
Corticosteroids	Increased insulin requirements with corticosteroids.
Estrogens	Increased insulin requirements with estrogens.
Hypoglycemics	Decreased insulin requirements with oral hypoglycemics.
Isoniazid	Increased insulin requirements with isoniazid.
MAOIs	Decreased insulin requirements with MAOIs.
Niacin	Increased insulin requirements with niacin.
Octreotide	Decreased insulin requirements with octreotide.
Phenothiazines	Increased insulin requirements with phenothiazines.
Potassium-lowering drugs	Caution with potassium-lowering drugs and with drugs sensitive to serum potassium levels.
Salicylates	Decreased insulin requirements with salicylates.
Sulfa antibiotics	Decreased insulin requirements with sulfa antibiotics.
Thyroid replacement therapy	Increased insulin requirements with thyroid replacement therapy.

Insulin Pork Isophane [NPH] (Iletin II NPH Pork)

Alcohol	May change insulin requirements.
Antidepressants	Insulin requirements may be reduced with certain antidepressants.
β-blockers	May mask symptoms of hypoglycemia.
Contraceptives	Insulin requirements may be increased with oral contraceptives.
Corticosteroids	Insulin requirements may be increased with corticosteroids.
Hypoglycemics	Insulin requirements may be reduced with oral hypoglycemics.
Salicylates	Insulin requirements may be reduced with salicylates.
Sulfa antibiotics	Insulin requirements may be reduced with sulfa antibiotics.
Thyroid replacement therapy	Insulin requirements may be increased with thyroid replacement therapy.

HYPOGLYCEMIC AGENTS *(cont.)*

Insulin Pork Regular (Iletin II Regular Pork) *(cont.)*

Alcohol	May change insulin requirements.
Antidepressants	Insulin requirements may be reduced with certain antidepressants.
β-blockers	May mask symptoms of hypoglycemia.
Contraceptives	Insulin requirements may be increased with oral contraceptives.
Corticosteroids	Insulin requirements may be increased with corticosteroids.
Hypoglycemics	Insulin requirements may be reduced with oral hypoglycemics.
Salicylates	Insulin requirements may be reduced with salicylates.
Sulfa antibiotics	Insulin requirements may be reduced with sulfa antibiotics.
Thyroid replacement therapy	Insulin requirements may be increased with thyroid replacement therapy.

Insulin Pork Zinc [Lente] (Iletin II Lente Pork)

Alcohol	May change insulin requirements.
Antidepressants	Insulin requirements may be reduced with certain antidepressants.
β-blockers	May mask symptoms of hypoglycemia.
Contraceptives	Insulin requirements may be increased with oral contraceptives.
Corticosteroids	Insulin requirements may be increased with corticosteroids.
Hypoglycemics	Insulin requirements may be reduced with oral hypoglycemics.
Salicylates	Insulin requirements may be reduced with salicylates.
Sulfa antibiotics	Insulin requirements may be reduced with sulfa antibiotics.
Thyroid replacement therapy	Insulin requirements may be increased with thyroid replacement therapy.

ORAL DIABETIC AGENTS

Acarbose (Precose)

Calcium channel blockers	Risk of hyperglycemia with calcium channel blockers.
Carbohydrate-splitting enzymes	Reduced effect with digestive enzymes containing carbohydrate-splitting enzymes (eg, amylase, pancreatin); avoid concomitant use.
Charcoal	Reduced effect with intestinal adsorbents (eg, charcoal); avoid concomitant use.
Corticosteroids	Risk of hyperglycemia with corticosteroids.
Digoxin	May affect digoxin bioavailability; may require dose adjustment of digoxin.
Diuretics	Risk of hyperglycemia with diuretics.
Estrogens	Risk of hyperglycemia with estrogens.

Table 20.2: DRUG INTERACTIONS FOR ENDOCRINE/HORMONAL AND BONE METABOLISM DRUGS *(cont.)*

HYPOGLYCEMIC AGENTS *(cont.)*

Acarbose (Precose) *(cont.)*

Insulin	Monitor for hypoglycemia with insulin.
Intestinal adsorbents	Reduced effect with intestinal adsorbents (eg, charcoal); avoid concomitant use.
Isoniazid	Risk of hyperglycemia with isoniazid.
Nicotinic acid	Risk of hyperglycemia with nicotinic acid.
Oral contraceptives	Risk of hyperglycemia with oral contraceptives.
Phenothiazines	Risk of hyperglycemia with phenothiazines.
Phenytoin	Risk of hyperglycemia with phenytoin.
Sulfonylureas	Monitor for hypoglycemia with sulfonylureas.
Sympathomimetics	Risk of hyperglycemia with sympathomimetics.
Thyroid products	Risk of hyperglycemia with thyroid products.

Chlorpropamide (Diabinese)

Alcohol	May produce disulfiram-like reaction.
β-blockers	Potentiated hypoglycemia with β-blockers, may mask signs of hypoglycemia.
Barbiturates	Caution with barbiturates.
Calcium channel blockers	Risk of hyperglycemia with calcium channel blockers.
Chloramphenicol	Potentiated hypoglycemia with chloramphenicol.
Contraceptives	Risk of hyperglycemia with oral contraceptives.
Corticosteroids	Risk of hyperglycemia corticosteroids.
Coumarins	Potentiated hypoglycemia with coumarins.
Diuretics	Risk of hyperglycemia with diuretics.
Estrogens	Risk of hyperglycemia with estrogens.
Isoniazid	Risk of hyperglycemia with isoniazid.
MAOIs	Potentiated hypoglycemia with MAOIs.
Miconazole	Caution with miconazole.
Nicotinic acid	Risk of hyperglycemia with nicotinic acid.
NSAIDs	Potentiated hypoglycemia with NSAIDs.
Phenothiazines	Risk of hyperglycemia with phenothiazines.
Phenytoin	Risk of hyperglycemia with phenytoin.
Probenecid	Potentiated hypoglycemia with probenecid.
Protein-bound drugs	Potentiated hypoglycemia with highly protein-bound drugs.

HYPOGLYCEMIC AGENTS *(cont.)*

Chlorpropamide (Diabinese) *(cont.)*

Salicylates	Potentiated hypoglycemia with salicylates.
Sulfonamides	Potentiated hypoglycemia with sulfonamides.
Sympathomimetics	Risk of hyperglycemia with sympathomimetics.
Thyroid products	Risk of hyperglycemia with thyroid products.

Glimepiride (Amaryl)

Alcohol	Potentiated hypoglycemia with alcohol.
β-blockers/ sympatholytic agents	Hypoglycemia may be masked with β-blockers/sympatholytic agents.
Contraceptives	Risk of hyperglycemia with oral contraceptives.
Corticosteroids	Risk of hyperglycemia with corticosteroids.
Diuretics	Risk of hyperglycemia with diuretics.
Estrogens	Risk of hyperglycemia with estrogens.
Insulin/metformin	Monitor for hypoglycemia with combination therapy with insulin and metformin.
Isoniazid	Risk of hyperglycemia with isoniazid.
Nicotinic acid	Risk of hyperglycemia with nicotinic acid.
NSAIDs	Potentiated hypoglycemia with NSAIDs.
Phenothiazines	Risk of hyperglycemia with phenothiazines.
Phenytoin	Risk of hyperglycemia with phenytoin.
Protein-bound drugs	Potentiated hypoglycemia with highly protein-bound drugs(eg,.salicylates, sulfonamides, chloramphenicol, coumarins, probenecid, MAOIs, miconazole, and β-blockers).
Sulfonylurea	Monitor for hypoglycemia when switching from long-acting sulfonylurea.
Sympathomimetics	Risk of hyperglycemia with sympathomimetics.
Thyroid products	Risk of hyperglycemia with thyroid products.

Glipizide (Glucotrol, Glucotrol XL)

Alcohol	Potentiated hypoglycemia with alcohol.
Azoles	Potentiated hypoglycemia with some azoles (eg, miconazole, fluconazole).
β-blockers	Potentiated hypoglycemia with β-blockers and may mask signs of hypoglycemia.
Calcium channel blockers	Risk of hyperglycemia with calcium channel blockers.
Chloramphenicol	Potentiated hypoglycemia with chloramphenicol.
Contraceptives	Risk of hyperglycemia with oral contraceptives.

Table 20.2: DRUG INTERACTIONS FOR ENDOCRINE/HORMONAL AND BONE METABOLISM DRUGS *(cont.)*

HYPOGLYCEMIC AGENTS *(cont.)*

Glipizide (Glucotrol, Glucotrol XL) *(cont.)*

Corticosteroids	Risk of hyperglycemia with diuretics, corticosteroids.
Coumarins	Potentiated hypoglycemia with courmarins.
Diuretics	Risk of hyperglycemia with diuretics.
Estrogens	Risk of hyperglycemia with estrogens.
Isoniazid	Risk of hyperglycemia with isoniazid.
MAOIs	Potentiated hypoglycemia with MAOIs.
Nicotinic acid	Risk of hyperglycemia with nicotinic acid.
NSAIDs	Potentiated hypoglycemia with NSAIDs.
Phenothiazines	Risk of hyperglycemia with diuretics, corticosteroids, phenothiazines.
Phenytoin	Risk of hyperglycemia with phenytoin.
Probenecid	Potentiated hypoglycemia with probenecid.
Protein-bound drugs	Potentiated hypoglycemia with highly protein-bound drugs.
Salicylates	Potentiated hypoglycemia with salicylates.
Sulfonamides	Potentiated hypoglycemia with sulfonamides.
Sympathomimetics	Risk of hyperglycemia with sympathomimetics.
Thyroid products	Risk of hyperglycemia with thyroid products.

Glipizide/Metformin Hydrochloride (Metaglip)

Alcohol	Potentiated hypoglycemia with alcohol and potentiates effect of metformin on lactate metabolism.
Azoles	Potentiated hypoglycemia with some azoles and other highly protein-bound drugs.
β-blockers	Potentiated hypoglycemia with β-blockers.
Calcium channel blockers	May cause hyperglycemia.
Cationic drugs (eg, digoxin, amiloride, procainamide, quinidine, quinine, ranitidine, trimethoprim, vancomycin, triamterene, morphine)	May increase metformin levels.
Chloramphenicol	Potentiated hypoglycemia with chloramphenicol.
Cimetidine	May increase metformin levels.

HYPOGLYCEMIC AGENTS *(cont.)*

Glipizide/Metformin Hydrochloride (Metaglip) *(cont.)*

Contraceptives	May cause hyperglycemia.
Corticosteroids	May cause hyperglycemia.
Coumarins	Potentiated hypoglycemia with coumarins.
Estrogens	May cause hyperglycemia.
Furosemide	May increase metformin levels and may decrease furosemide levels.
Isoniazid	May cause hyperglycemia.
MAOIs	Potentiated hypoglycemia with MAOIs.
Nicotinic acid	May cause hyperglycemia.
Nifedipine	May increase metformin levels.
NSAIDs	Potentiated hypoglycemia with NSAIDs.
Miconazole	Severe hypoglycemia reported with concomitant oral miconazole.
Phenothiazines	May cause hyperglycemia.
Phenytoin	May cause hyperglycemia.
Probenecid	Potentiated hypoglycemia with probenecid.
Salicylates	Potentiated hypoglycemia with salicylates.
Sulfonamides	Potentiated hypoglycemia with sulfonamides.
Sympathomimetics	May cause hyperglycemia.
Thiazides and other diuretics	May cause hyperglycemia.
Thyroid products	May cause hyperglycemia.

Glyburide (Diabeta, Micronase)

Alcohol	Potentiated hypoglycemia and disulfiram-like reactions (rarely) with alcohol.
β-blockers	Potentiated hypoglycemia with β-blockers and may mask hypoglycemia.
Calcium channel blockers	Risk of hyperglycemia with calcium channel blockers.
Chloramphenicol	Potentiated hypoglycemia with chloramphenicol.
Contraceptives	Risk of hyperglycemia with oral contraceptives.
Corticosteroids	Risk of hyperglycemia with corticosteroids.
Coumarins	Potentiated hypoglycemia with coumarins and increased or decreased coumarin effects.
Diuretics	Risk of hyperglycemia with diuretics.
Estrogens	Risk of hyperglycemia with estrogens.
Fluoroquinolones	Potentiated hypoglycemia with fluoroquinolones.

Table 20.2: DRUG INTERACTIONS FOR ENDOCRINE/HORMONAL AND BONE METABOLISM DRUGS *(cont.)*

HYPOGLYCEMIC AGENTS *(cont.)*

Glyburide (Diabeta, Micronase) *(cont.)*

INH	Risk of hyperglycemia with INH.
MAOIs	Potentiated hypoglycemia with MAOIs.
Miconazole	Potentiated hypoglycemia with miconazole.
Nicotinic acid	Risk of hyperglycemia with nicotinic acid.
NSAIDs	Potentiated hypoglycemia with NSAIDs.
Phenothiazines	Risk of hyperglycemia with phenothiazines.
Phenytoin	Risk of hyperglycemia with phenytoin.
Probenecid	Potentiated hypoglycemia with probenecid.
Protein-bound drugs	Potentiated hypoglycemia with highly protein-bound drugs.
Salicylates	Potentiated hypoglycemia with salicylates.
Sulfonamides	Potentiated hypoglycemia with sulfonamides.
Sympathomimetics	Risk of hyperglycemia with sympathomimetics.
Thyroid products	Risk of hyperglycemia with thyroid products.

Glyburide, Micronized (Glynase Pres-Tab)

Alcohol	Hypoglycemia potentiated by alcohol.
β-blockers	Hypoglycemia potentiated by β-blockers and may mask hypoglycemia.
Calcium channel blockers	Risk of hyperglycemia with calcium channel blockers.
Chloramphenicol	Hypoglycemia potentiated by chloramphenicol.
Ciprofloxacin	Hypoglycemia potentiated by ciprofloxacin.
Contraceptives	Risk of hyperglycemia with oral contraceptives.
Corticosteroids	Risk of hyperglycemia with corticosteroids.
Coumarins	Hypoglycemia potentiated by coumarins.
Diuretics	Risk of hyperglycemia with diuretics.
Estrogens	Risk of hyperglycemia with estrogens.
Isoniazid	Risk of hyperglycemia with isoniazid.
MAOIs	Hypoglycemia potentiated by MAOIs.
Miconazole	Hypoglycemia potentiated by miconazole.
Nicotinic acid	Risk of hyperglycemia with nicotinic acid.
NSAIDs	Hypoglycemia potentiated by NSAIDs.
Phenothiazines	Risk of hyperglycemia with phenothiazines.

HYPOGLYCEMIC AGENTS *(cont.)*

Glyburide, Micronized (Glynase Pres-Tab) *(cont.)*

Phenytoin	Risk of hyperglycemia with phenytoin.
Probenecid	Hypoglycemia potentiated by probenecid.
Protein-bound drugs	Hypoglycemia potentiated by highly protein-bound drugs.
Salicylates	Hypoglycemia potentiated by salicylates.
Sulfonamides	Hypoglycemia potentiated by sulfonamides.
Sympathomimetics	Risk of hyperglycemia with sympathomimetics.
Thyroid products	Risk of hyperglycemia with thyroid products.

Glyburide/Metformin Hydrochloride (Glucovance)

Alcohol	Potentiated hypoglycemia with alcohol and excess alcohol may increase potential for lactic acidosis.
β-blockers	Potentiated hypoglycemia with β-blockers.
Calcium channel blockers	May cause hyperglycemia.
Cationic drugs (eg, digoxin, amiloride, procainamide, quinidine, quinine, ranitidine, trimethoprim, vancomycin, triamterene, morphine)	May increase metformin levels.
Chloramphenicol	Potentiated hypoglycemia with chloramphenicol.
Cimetidine	May increase metformin levels.
Ciprofloxacin	Potentiated hypoglycemia with ciprofloxacin.
Contraceptives	May cause hyperglycemia.
Corticosteroids	May cause hyperglycemia.
Coumarins	Potentiated hypoglycemia with coumarins.
Estrogens	May cause hyperglycemia.
Furosemide	May increase metformin levels and metformin may decrease furosemide levels.
Isoniazid	May cause hyperglycemia.
MAOIs	Potentiated hypoglycemia with MAOIs.
Miconazole	Potentiated hypoglycemia with miconazole.
Nicotinic acid	May cause hyperglycemia.
Nifedipine	May increase metformin levels.

Table 20.2: DRUG INTERACTIONS FOR ENDOCRINE/HORMONAL AND BONE METABOLISM DRUGS (cont.)

HYPOGLYCEMIC AGENTS (cont.)

Glyburide/Metformin Hydrochloride (Glucovance) (cont.)

NSAIDs	Potentiated hypoglycemia with NSAIDs.
Phenothiazines	May cause hyperglycemia.
Phenytoin	May cause hyperglycemia.
Probenecid	Potentiated hypoglycemia with probenecid.
Salicylates	Potentiated hypoglycemia with salicylates.
Sulfonamides	Potentiated hypoglycemia with sulfonamides.
Sympathomimetics	May cause hyperglycemia.
Thiazides and other diuretics	May cause hyperglycemia.
Thyroid products	May cause hyperglycemia.
TZDs	Potentiated hypoglycemia with TZDs (eg, rosiglitazone).

Metformin Hydrochloride (Fortamet, Glucophage, Glucophage XR, Riomet)

Alcohol	Risk of hypoglycemia with alcohol and excess alcohol may increase potential for lactic acidosis.
Calcium channel blockers	May cause hyperglycemia.
Cationic drugs (eg, digoxin, amiloride, procainamide, quinidine, quinine, ranitidine, trimethoprim, vancomycin, triamterene, morphine)	May increase metformin levels.
Cimetidine	May increase metformin levels.
Contraceptives	May cause hyperglycemia.
Corticosteroids	May cause hyperglycemia.
Estrogens	May cause hyperglycemia.
Furosemide	May increase metformin levels and metformin may decrease furosemide levels.
Isoniazid	May cause hyperglycemia.
Nicotinic acid	May cause hyperglycemia.
Nifedipine	May increase metformin levels.
Phenothiazines	May cause hyperglycemia.
Phenytoin	May cause hyperglycemia.

Metformin Hydrochloride (Fortamet, Glucophage, Glucophage XR, Riomet) *(cont.)*

Sympathomimetics	May cause hyperglycemia.
Thiazides and other diuretics	May cause hyperglycemia.
Thyroid products	May cause hyperglycemia.

Metformin Hydrochloride/Rosiglitazone Maleate (Avandamet)

Alcohol	Risk of hypoglycemia with alcohol and excess alcohol may increase potential for lactic acidosis.
Calcium channel blockers	May cause hyperglycemia.
Cationic drugs (eg, digoxin, amiloride, procainamide, quinidine, quinine, ranitidine, trimethoprim, vancomycin, triamterene, morphine)	May increase metformin levels.
Cimetidine	May increase metformin levels.
Contraceptives	May cause hyperglycemia.
Corticosteroids	May cause hyperglycemia.
CYP2C8 inhibitors	Inhibitors of CYP2C8 (eg, gemfibrozil) may increase rosiglitazone AUC and inducers of CYP2C8 (eg, rifampin) may decrease rosiglitazone AUC.
Estrogens	May cause hyperglycemia.
Furosemide	May increase metformin levels and metformin may decrease furosemide levels.
Isoniazid	May cause hyperglycemia.
Nicotinic acid	May cause hyperglycemia.
Nifedipine	May increase metformin levels.
Phenothiazines	May cause hyperglycemia.
Phenytoin	May cause hyperglycemia.
Sympathomimetics	May cause hyperglycemia.
Thiazides and other diuretics	May cause hyperglycemia.
Thyroid products	May cause hyperglycemia.

Table 20.2: DRUG INTERACTIONS FOR ENDOCRINE/HORMONAL AND BONE METABOLISM DRUGS *(cont.)*

HYPOGLYCEMIC AGENTS *(cont.)*

Miglitol (Glyset)

Charcoal	Intestinal absorbents (eg, charcoal) may reduce effects.
Digestive enzyme	Digestive enzyme preparations (eg, amylase, pancreatin) May reduce effects.
Digoxin	May interact with digoxin.
Glyburide	May interact with glyburide.
Metformin	May interact with metformin.
Propranolol	May reduce bioavailability of propranolol.
Ranitidine	May reduce bioavailability of ranitidine.

Nateglinide (Starlix)

Alcohol	Potentiated hypoglycemia with alcohol.
β-blockers	Potentiated hypoglycemia with nonselective β-blockers, which may also mask hypoglycemic effects.
Corticosteroids	Risk of hyperglycemia with corticosteroids.
Liquid meals	Peak plasma levels reduced with liquid meals.
MAOIs	Potentiated hypoglycemia with MAOIs.
NSAIDs	Potentiated hypoglycemia with NSAIDs.
Protein-bound drugs	Caution with highly protein-bound drugs.
Salicylates	Potentiated hypoglycemia with salicylates.
Sympathomimetics	Risk of hyperglycemia with sympathomimetics.
Thiazides	Risk of hyperglycemia with thiazides.
Thyroid products	Risk of hyperglycemia with thyroid products.
Tolbutamide	May potentiate tolbutamide.

Pioglitazone Hydrochloride (Actos)

Ethinyl estradiol	Possible loss of contraception with ethinyl estradiol; caution when co-administering.
Hypoglycemic agents	Risk for hypoglycemia with insulin or oral hypoglycemic agents.
Insulin	Risk for hypoglycemia with insulin.
Ketoconazole	May inhibit pioglitazone metabolism; evaluate glycemic control more frequently.
Midazolam	May cause reduction of midazolam levels.
Norethindrone	Possible loss of contraception with norethindrone; caution when co-administering.

Repaglinide (Prandin)

Alcohol	Potentiated hypoglycemia with alcohol.

HYPOGLYCEMIC AGENTS *(cont.)*

Repaglinide (Prandin) *(cont.)*

β-blockers	Potentiated hypoglycemia with β-blockers and may mask hypoglycemia.
Calcium channel blockers	Risk of hyperglycemia with calcium channel blockers.
Chloramphenicol	Potentiated hypoglycemia with chloramphenicol.
Corticosteroids	Risk of hyperglycemia with corticosteroids.
Coumarins	Potentiated hypoglycemia with coumarins.
CYP3A4 inducers	Increased metabolism with CYP3A4 inducers (eg, rifampin, barbiturates, carbamazepine).
Diuretics	Risk of hyperglycemia with diuretics.
CYP3A4 inhibitors	CYP3A4 inhibitors (eg, erythromycin) may inhibit metabolism.
Estrogens	Potentiated hypoglycemia with estrogens.
Ethinyl estradiol	Increased levels with ethinyl estradiol and increases ethinyl estradiol levels.
Gemfibrozil	Increased levels with gemfibrozil; use caution and monitor levels if already on both drugs, avoid initiation of concurrent use.
Isoniazid	Risk of hyperglycemia with isoniazid.
Itraconazole	Avoid itraconazole if already on gemfibrozil and repaglinide; synergistic effect may occur.
Ketoconazole	May inhibit metabolism.
Levonorgestrel	Increased levels with levonorgestrel and increases levonorgestrel levels.
MAOIs	Potentiated hypoglycemia with MAOIs.
Miconazole	May inhibit metabolism.
Nicotinic acid	Risk of hyperglycemia with nicotinic acid.
NSAIDs	Potentiated hypoglycemia with NSAIDs and other highly protein-bound drugs.
Phenothiazines	Potentiated hypoglycemia with phenothiazines.
Phenytoin	Risk of hyperglycemia with phenytoin.
Probenecid	Potentiated hypoglycemia with probenecid.
Salicylates	Potentiated hypoglycemia with salicylates.
Simvastatin	Increased levels with simvastatin.
Sulfonamides	Potentiated hypoglycemia with sulfonamides.
Sympathomimetics	Risk of hyperglycemia with sympathomimetics.
Thyroid products	Potentiated hypoglycemia with thyroid products.

Rosiglitazone Maleate (Avandia)

Hypoglycemic agents	Risk of hypoglycemia when used in combination with other hypoglycemic agents.

Table 20.2: DRUG INTERACTIONS FOR ENDOCRINE/HORMONAL AND BONE METABOLISM DRUGS (cont.)

HYPOGLYCEMIC AGENTS (cont.)

Tolazamide

Alcohol	Potentiated hypoglycemia with alcohol.
β-blockers	Potentiated hypoglycemia with β-blockers, may mask signs of hypoglycemia.
Calcium channel blockers	Risk of hyperglycemia with calcium channel blockers.
Chloramphenicol	Potentiated hypoglycemia with chloramphenicol.
Contraceptives	Risk of hyperglycemia with oral contraceptives.
Corticosteroids	Risk of hyperglycemia with corticosteroids.
Coumarins	Potentiated hypoglycemia with coumarins.
Diuretics	Risk of hyperglycemia with diuretics.
Estrogens	Risk of hyperglycemia with estrogens.
Isoniazid	Risk of hyperglycemia with isoniazid.
MAOIs	Potentiated hypoglycemia with MAOIs.
Miconazole	Caution with miconazole; severe hypoglycemia reported.
Nicotinic acid	Risk of hyperglycemia with nicotinic acid.
NSAIDs	Potentiated hypoglycemia with NSAIDs.
Phenothiazines	Risk of hyperglycemia with phenothiazines.
Phenytoin	Risk of hyperglycemia with phenytoin.
Probenecid	Potentiated hypoglycemia with probenecid.
Protein bound drugs	Potentiated hypoglycemia with highly protein bound drugs.
Salicylates	Potentiated hypoglycemia with salicylates.
Sulfonamides	Potentiated hypoglycemia with sulfonamides.
Sympathomimetics	Risk of hyperglycemia with sympathomimetics.
Thyroid products	Risk of hyperglycemia with thyroid products.

MISCELLANEOUS DIABETIC AGENT

Exenatide (Byetta)

Antibiotics	Drugs that are dependent on threshold concentrations for efficacy (eg, contraceptives, antibiotics) should be taken 1 hour before.
Contraceptives	Drugs that are dependent on threshold concentrations for efficacy (eg, contraceptives, antibiotics) should be taken 1 hour before.
Gastrointestinal absorption	Caution with drugs that require rapid gastrointestinal absorption.

THYROID HORMONES

Levothyroxine Sodium (Levoxyl, Synthroid)

5-FU	Increased serum TBG concentration with 5-FU.
6-mercaptopurine	Altered levels of thyroid hormone and/or TSH level with 6-mercaptopurine.
Aluminum hydroxide	May decrease absorption.
Aminoglutethimide	Decreased thyroid hormone secretion with aminoglutethimide.
Amiodarone	Decreased conversion of T_4 to T_3 levels with amiodarone, decreased thyroid hormone secretion with amiodarone.
Androgens/ anabolic steroids	Decreased serum TBG concentration with androgens/anabolic steroids.
Antacids	Decreased T_4 absorption with antacids (aluminum and magnesium hydroxides).
Anticoagulants	May potentiate oral anticoagulant effects; adjust dose and monitor PT/INR.
Antidepressants	Additive effects of both agents with antidepressants.
Asparaginase	Decreased serum TBG concentration with asparaginase.
β-adrenergic antagonists	Decreased conversion of T_4 to T_3 levels with β-adrenergic antagonists (propranolol >160mg/day).
Bile acid sequestrants	Decreased T_4 absorption with bile acid sequestrants (cholestyramine, colestipol).
Calcium carbonate	Decreased T_4 absorption with calcium carbonate.
Cation exchange resins	Decreased T_4 absorption with cation exchange resins (kayexalate).
Cholestyramine	May decrease absorption.
Choral hydrate	Altered levels of thyroid hormone and/or TSH level with choral hydrate.
Clofibrate	Increased serum TBG concentration with clofibrate.
Colestipol	May decrease absorption.
Cottonseed meal	Decreased absorption with cottonseed meal.
Diazepam	Altered levels of thyroid hormone and/or TSH level with diazepam.
Digitalis glycosides	May decrease levels and effects of digitalis glycosides.
Dopamine/ dopamine agonists	Reduced TSH secretion with dopamine/dopamine agonists.
Estrogens	Increased serum TBG concentration with estrogens.
Ethionamide	Altered levels of thyroid hormone and/or TSH level with ethionamide.
Ferrous sulfate	Decreased T_4 absorption with ferrous sulfate.
Fiber	Decreased absorption with fiber.

Table 20.2: DRUG INTERACTIONS FOR ENDOCRINE/HORMONAL AND BONE METABOLISM DRUGS *(cont.)*

THYROID HORMONES *(cont.)*

Levothyroxine Sodium (Levoxyl, Synthroid) *(cont.)*

Furosemide	Protein-binding site displacement with furosemide.
Glucocorticoids	Decreased conversion of T_4 to T_3 levels with glucocorticoids (dexamethasone >4mg/day). Decreased serum TBG concentration.
Glucocorticoids	Reduced TSH secretion with glucocorticoids.
Growth hormones	Excessive use with growth hormones may accelerate epiphyseal closure.
Heparin	Protein-binding site displacement with heparin.
Heroin/methadone	Increased serum TBG concentration with heroin/methadone.
Hydantoins	Protein-binding site displacement with hydantoins.
Hypoglycemic agents	Upward dose adjustments needed for oral hypoglycemic agents.
Insulin	Upward dose adjustments needed for insulin.
Interferon-α	May cause development of antithyroid microsomal antibodies causing transient hypothyroidism, hyperthyroidism, or both.
Interleukin-2	Associated with transient painless thyroiditis.
Iodine	Decreased thyroid hormone secretion with iodine (including iodine-containing radiographic contrast agents). May reduce uptake of iodine-containing radiographic contrast agents.
Ketamine	May produce marked HTN and tachycardia.
Lithium	Reduced TSH secretion with lithium.
Lovastatin	Altered levels of thyroid hormone and/or TSH level with lovastatin.
Methimazole	Reduced TSH secretion with methimazole.
Metoclopramide	Altered levels of thyroid hormone and/or TSH level with metoclopramide.
Mitotane	Increased serum TBG concentration with mitotane.
Nicotinic acid (slow-release)	Decreased serum TBG concentration with nicotinic acid (slow-release).
Nitroprusside	Altered levels of thyroid hormone and/or TSH level with nitroprusside.
Octreotide	Reduced TSH secretion with octreotide.
Para-aminosalicylate sodium	Altered levels of thyroid hormone and/or TSH level with para-aminosalicylate sodium.
Perphenazine	Altered levels of thyroid hormone and/or TSH level with perphenazine.
Phenobarbital	Protein-binding site displacement with phenobarbital.
PTU	Reduced TSH secretion, decreased conversion of T_4 to T_3 levels with PTU.
Resorcinol	Altered levels of thyroid hormone and/or TSH level with resorcinol (excessive topical use).
Rifampin	Protein-binding site displacement with rifampin.

THYROID HORMONES *(cont.)*

Levothyroxine Sodium (Levoxyl, Synthroid) *(cont.)*

Simethicone	Decreased T$_4$ absorption with simethicone.
Sodium polystyrene	May decrease absorption.
Soybean flour (infant formula)	Decreased absorption with soybean flour (infant formula).
Sucralfate	Decreased T$_4$ absorption with sucralfate.
Sulfonamides	Reduced TSH secretion with sulfonamides.
Sympathomimetics	May increase risk of coronary insufficiency with CAD.
Tamoxifen	Increased serum TBG concentration with clofibrate, estrogens, heroin/methadone, 5-FU, mitotane, tamoxifen.
Thiazide diuretics	Altered levels of thyroid hormone and/or TSH level with thiazide diuretics.
Tolbutamide	Decreased thyroid hormone secretion with tolbutamide.
Walnuts	Decreased absorption with walnuts.

Levothyroxine Sodium/Liothyronine Sodium (Thyrolar)

Androgens	May interfere with thyroid lab tests.
Cholestyramine	Decreased absorption with cholestyramine; space dosing by 4-5hrs.
Colestipol	Decreased absorption with colestipol; space dosing by 4-5hrs.
Corticosteroids	May interfere with thyroid lab tests.
Estrogens	Estrogens increase thyroxine-binding globulin; increase in thyroid dose may be needed. May interfere with thyroid lab tests.
Insulin	May increase insulin requirements.
Iodine-containing preparations	May interfere with thyroid lab tests.
Anticoagulants	Altered effect of oral anticoagulants; monitor PT/INR.
Hypoglycemic drugs	May increase oral hypoglycemic drug requirements.
Salicylates	May interfere with thyroid lab tests.
Sympathomimetic amines	Serious or life-threatening side effects can occur with sympathomimetic amines.

Liothyronine Sodium (Cytomel)

Anticoagulants	Hypothyroidism decreases and hyperthyroidism increases sensitivity to oral anticoagulants; monitor PT/INR.
Catecholamines	Increased adrenergic effects of catecholamines; caution with CAD.
Cholestyramine	Decreased absorption with cholestyramine; space dosing by 4-5 hrs.

Table 20.2: DRUG INTERACTIONS FOR ENDOCRINE/HORMONAL AND BONE METABOLISM DRUGS *(cont.)*

THYROID HORMONES *(cont.)*

Liothyronine Sodium (Cytomel) *(cont.)*

Digitalis	May potentiate digitalis toxicity.
Estrogens	Estrogens increase thyroxine-binding globulin; increase in thyroid dose may be needed.
Hypoglycemic drugs	Monitor oral hypoglycemic drug requirements.
Insulin	Monitor insulin requirements.
Ketamine	HTN and tachycardia with ketamine.
Sympathomimetic amines	Large dose may cause life-threatening toxicities with sympathomimetic amines.
TCAs	Additive effects of both agents with TCAs.

Thyroid (Armour Thyroid)

Androgens	May interfere with thyroid lab tests.
Anticoagulants	Altered effect of oral anticoagulants; monitor PT/INR.
Cholestyramine	Reduced absorption with cholestyramine; space dosing by 4-5 hrs.
Colestipol	Reduced absorption with colestipol; space dosing by 4-5 hrs.
Corticosteroids	May interfere with thyroid lab tests.
Estrogens	Estrogens increase thyroxine-binding globulin; increase in thyroid dose may be needed. May interfere with thyroid lab tests.
Hypoglycemic drugs	May increase oral hypoglycemic requirements.
Insulin	May increase insulin requirements.
Iodine-containing preparations	May interfere with thyroid lab tests.
Salicylates	May interfere with thyroid lab tests.
Sympathomimetic amines	Serious or life-threatening side effects can occur with sympathomimetic amines.

ANTITHYROID HORMONES

Methimazole (Tapazole)

Anticoagulants	May potentiate anticoagulants.
β-blockers	May need dose reduction when patient becomes euthyroid.
Digitalis	May need dose reduction when patient becomes euthyroid.
Theophylline	May need dose reduction when patient becomes euthyroid.

Propylthiouracil

Anticoagulants	May potentiate anticoagulant effects.

ANTITHYROID HORMONES *(cont.)*

Propylthiouracil *(cont.)*

β-blockers	Hyperthyroidism increases clearance of β-blockers; reduce β-blocker dose when patient becomes euthyroid.
Digitalis	Increased digitalis glycoside levels when patient becomes euthyroid; reduce digitalis dose.
Theophylline	Decreased theophylline clearance when patient becomes euthyroid; reduce theophylline dose.

BONE METABOLISM DRUGS

BISPHOSPHONATES

Alendronate sodium (Fosamax)

Antacids	Antacids may interfere with absorption; dose at least one-half hour after alendronate.
Aspirin	Increased GI irritation with aspirin and alendronate >10mg.
Calcium supplements	Calcium supplements and other oral medications may interfere with absorption; dose at least one-half hour after alendronate.
NSAIDs	Caution with NSAIDs, other GI irritants.

Etidronate disodium (Didronel)

Antacids	Antacids that contain calcium, iron, aluminum, or magnesium reduce absorption; space dosing by 2 hrs.
Vitamins	Vitamins with mineral supplements reduce absorption; space dosing by 2 hrs.
Warfarin	Monitor PT with warfarin.

Ibandronate sodium (Boniva)

Calcium	Calcium and other multivalent cations cations may interfere with absorption.

Risedronate sodium (Actonel)

Aluminum	Aluminum-containing agents may interfere with absorption; space dosing by 2 hrs.
Calcium supplements	Calcium supplements may interfere with absorption; space dosing by 2 hrs.
Magnesium	Magnesium-containing agents may interfere with absorption; space dosing by 2 hrs.

Tiluronate disodium (Skelid)

Antacids, aluminum-containing	Decreased bioavailability with aluminum-containing antacids; space dosing by 2 hrs.
Antacids, magnesium-containing	Decreased bioavailability with magnesium-containing antacids; space dosing by 2 hrs.
Aspirin	Decreased bioavailability with aspirin; space dosing by 2 hrs.
Calcium supplements	Decreased bioavailability with calcium supplements; space dosing by 2 hrs.
Indomethacin	Increased bioavailability with indomethacin; space dosing by 2 hrs.

Table 20.2: DRUG INTERACTIONS FOR ENDOCRINE/HORMONAL AND BONE METABOLISM DRUGS (cont.)

BONE METABOLISM DRUGS (cont.)

Zoledronic acid (Zometa)

Aminoglycosides	Additive effect/risk of hypocalcemia with aminoglycosides.
Loop diuretics	Additive effect/risk of hypocalcemia with loop diuretics.
Nephrotoxic drugs	Caution with other nephrotoxic drugs.
Thalidomide	Increased risk of renal dysfunction with thalidomide in multiple myeloma patients.

BISPHOSPHONATE COMBINATIONS

Alendronate Sodium-Cholecalciferol (Fosamax Plus D)

Antacids	Antacids may interfere with absorption; dose at least one-half hour after alendronate.
Anticonvulsants	Anticonvulsants may increase catabolism.
Bile acid sequestrants	Bile acid sequestrants may impair absorption.
Calcium supplements	Calcium supplements and other oral medications may interfere with absorption; dose at least one-half hour after alendronate.
Cimetidine	Cimetidine may increase catabolism.
Mineral oils	Mineral oils may impair absorption.
NSAIDs	Caution with NSAIDs, other GI irritants.
Olestra	Olestra may impair absorption.
Orlistat	Orlistat may impair absorption.
Thiazides	Thiazides may increase catabolism.

Risedronate Sodium/Calcium Carbonate (Actonel with Calcium)

Calcium supplements	Calcium supplements may interfere with absorption; space dosing by 2 hrs.
Aluminum	Aluminum-containing agents may interfere with absorption; space dosing by 2 hrs.
Fluoroquinolones	Calcium may reduce absorption of fluoroquinolones.
Glucocorticoids, systemic	Calcium absorption reduced when taken with systemic glucocorticoids.
Iron	May interfere with absorption of iron; take iron and calcium at different times of the day.
Levothyroxine	Calcium may reduce absorption of levothyroxine.
Magnesium	Magnesium-containing agents may interfere with absorption; space dosing by 2 hrs.
Tetracycline	Calcium may reduce absorption of tetracycline.
Thiazide diuretics	Reduced urinary excretion of calcium with use of thiazide diuretics.
Vitamin D	Absorption of calcium increased with use of vitamin D and analogues.

MISCELLANEOUS BONE METABOLISM DRUG

Teriparatide (Forteo)

Digitalis	Hypercalcemia may predispose to digitalis toxicity; caution with concomitant use.

Table 20.3: SIGNS OF HYPO- AND HYPERGLYCEMIA

HYPOGLYCEMIA	HYPERGLYCEMIA
Anxiety	Xerostomia
Blood pressure normal or increased	Blood pressure normal or decreased
Breath normal in odor	Smell of acetone on breath
Breathing may be stertorous but at normal depth and rate	Breathing is deep and fast
Confusion, inability to concentrate	Warm and dry skin
Cool and moist skin	Loss of appetite
Hunger	Normal or depressed reflexes
Hyperactive reflexes	Lethargy
Lethargy	Gradual onset of symptoms
Rapid onset of symptoms	Rapid, normal or thready pulse
Rapid pulse	
Tired, weak	
Unsteadiness	
Vision problems	

Chapter 21

Drugs Used for Connective Tissue Disorders and Oral Mucosal Diseases

Eric T. Stoopler, D.M.D., Martin S. Greenberg, D.D.S.

This chapter describes the major drugs used to manage connective tissue diseases as well as the drugs used to treat diseases of the oral mucosa. Dentists have a major responsibility for the diagnosis and management of diseases affecting the oral mucosa; therefore, this chapter emphasizes the clinical application of these drugs. The section devoted to connective tissue disorders highlights the effect of this group of drugs on oral health and the precautions necessary when providing dental treatment for patients receiving drug therapy for this group of diseases.

Connective Tissue Disorder Drugs

The connective tissue diseases are a group of disorders with a prominent feature of tissue damage caused by the patient's own immune system. These diseases are often classified as autoimmune and the cause of tissue damage is complex and multifactorial. The major connective tissue diseases include lupus erythematosus, rheumatoid arthritis, scleroderma (systemic sclerosis), dermatomyositis, mixed connective tissue disease and Sjögren's syndrome.

See Tables 21.1 and 21.2 for general information on connective tissue disorder drugs.

Lupus Erythematosus Drugs

Lupus erythematosus is caused by the formation of autoantibodies to nuclear components, particularly DNA. Tissue damage may result directly from autoantibodies or more commonly from immune complexes composed of antigen, antibody, and complement, which cause an inflammatory reaction involving skin, mucosa, internal organs (particularly the kidneys and brain) or joints.

Discoid lupus is confined to the skin and mucosa and causes skin lesions with scales that project into hair follicles (follicular plugging). Typical oral lesions of discoid lupus appear as a mixture of inflammation, atrophy, ulceration and keratosis. The lesions easily may be confused with lichen planus or, occasionally, leukoplakia. Systemic lupus is a multisystem disease with a strong genetic component that most commonly affects women in their childbearing years. Patients with systemic lupus have skin and mucosal lesions, as well as renal, central nervous, cardiovascular and hematologic systemic manifestations. Patients with systemic lupus may have discoid lupus-type oral lesions or nonspecific ulcers caused by vasculitis. Dentists should be suspicious of the possibility of systemic lupus when a woman between the ages of 20 and 40 years develops oral lesions with associated symptoms, such as joint pains or skin lesions.

The lesions of discoid lupus often respond to use of topical and intralesional glucocorticoids (see Chapter 5 for a discussion-of-those drugs). Patients with discoid lupus that does not respond to this therapy may be placed on systemic therapy with antimalarial agents such as hydroxychloroquine (Plaquenil). Patients with mild-to-moderate manifestations of lupus are treated symptomatically for joint pains and skin or mucosal lesions. Patients with serious organ involvement such as kidney or central nervous system manifestations are treated with systemic glucocorticoids alone or glucocorticoids in combination with immunosuppressive drugs such as azathioprine or cyclophosphamide. Mycophenolate mofetil, a newer immunosuppressive agent, is being used in combination with glucocorticoids to treat discoid lupus lesions that are refractory to conventional therapies.

Rheumatoid Arthritis Drugs

Rheumatoid arthritis (RA) is a systemic inflammatory disease whose chief manifestation is destruction of the synovial membrane that spreads to the joint cartilage. Susceptibility to the disease has a strong hereditary basis, and an infectious etiology is suspected but not proven. RA chiefly manifests itself as symmetrical swelling and pain of the joints in people between the ages of 30 and 50 years. RA is a systemic disease; therefore, generalized manifestations such as weakness, fatigue and subcutaneous nodules are also common.

A form of RA, Felty's syndrome, affects the blood, causing anemia and a decrease in white blood cells and platelets. Dentists treating patients who have this syndrome must be aware of the potential for infection and bleeding. Involvement of the temporomandibular joints is common, but it is a major problem for only a small percentage of patients.

Dentists treating patients with RA must be aware of the drugs prescribed and their possible effect on dental treatment. The major classes of drugs used to treat RA include the following:

- nonsteroidal anti-inflammatory drugs (NSAIDs), which can increase bleeding after surgery;
- gold sodium thiomalate, which can cause oral ulcers, decreased white blood cells and decreased platelets; patients receiving systemic gold should receive periodic hematologic evaluations, and dentists performing surgical procedures on such patients should obtain the results of recent laboratory tests;
- penicillamine D, which may cause decreased white blood cells and platelets, drug-induced pemphigus with oral lesions or nephrotic syndrome; patients must have periodic hematologic evaluation; loss of taste has also been reported;
- systemic glucocorticoids (see Chapter 5);
- immunosuppressive drugs (see Chapter 23);
- tumor necrosis factor (TNF) inhibitors may increase the risk of infection when used in combination with immunosuppressive agents and may cause reactivation of latent tuberculosis (TB); patients must have periodic hematologic evaluations; status of TB must be determined prior to dental treatment and elective treatment should be deferred if active; patients should be monitored for TB-associated oral lesions.

Scleroderma Drugs

Patients with scleroderma (systemic sclerosis) develop fibrosis of the skin and internal organs owing to the overproduction of collagen. Tightening of the skin, especially around the face and hands, is a characteristic of the disease. Raynaud's phenomenon, ischemia and blanching of the fingers caused by vasoconstriction are common. Patients with this form of scleroderma may develop fibrosis of the heart, kidney or lung, and dentists treating these patients should consult with the managing physician regarding the extent of organ involvement before performing dental treatment.

Drugs frequently used to treat scleroderma include the following:

- penicillamine D (see RA on previous page);
- systemic glucocorticoids (see Chapter 5);
- immunosuppressive drugs (see Chapter 23).

Calcium channel blockers such as nifedipine are used to manage Raynaud's phenomenon. These drugs may cause gingival enlargement that can be minimized by good oral hygiene.

Dermatomyositis Drugs

Patients with dermatomyositis have skin lesions and muscle weakness. The term "polymyositis" is used when patients have only muscle involvement. The disease may occur alone or in association with an underlying malignancy or another connective-tissue disease. Oral involvement may include weakness of the palatal muscles and oral mucosal lesions.

Treatment of dermatomyositis includes use of high doses of systemic glucocorticoids (Chapter 5) and cytotoxic immunosuppressive drugs (Chapter 23).

Mixed Connective Tissue Disease Drugs

Patients with mixed connective tissue disease (MCTD) have signs and symptoms that overlap more than one connective tissue disease. MCTD is considered a separate disorder as patients have a distinct laboratory finding of high levels of autoantibodies to nuclear ribonucleoprotein. The drugs taken by patients with MCTD are determined by the particular overlap syndrome. They take the same drugs described above

for use with lupus, RA, scleroderma and dermatomyositis.

Sjögren's Syndrome Agents

Sjögren's syndrome (SS) is an autoimmune disease that primarily affects the lacrimal and salivary glands, but also may be associated with other connective tissue diseases or lymphoma. Primary SS, which occurs primarily in women (at a 9:1 ratio), causes destruction of salivary and lacrimal gland tissue and leads to severe xerostomia and dry eyes. Oral manifestations include an increased incidence of dental caries and candidiasis owing to a decrease in both the detergent and the antibacterial properties of saliva. Patients with SS also have difficulty wearing dentures. People with secondary SS have dry eyes and mouth in association with any one of the connective tissue diseases described above, most frequently RA. A major concern of clinicians managing patients who have SS is the high incidence of lymphoma in people with this condition. The diagnosis of SS is made by testing for salivary and lacrimal gland function and abnormal serologic findings and detection of inflammatory foci in biopsy specimens of minor salivary glands.

The medical management of xerostomia in patients with SS includes use of topical rinses, such as artificial saliva substitutes, and use of systemic medications to increase salivary flow. Pilocarpine 5 mg taken three times daily 30 minutes before meals increases salivary flow for patients who still have functional salivary gland tissue. The most common side effects of pilocarpine include sweating and gastrointestinal symptoms. Pilocarpine should not be used for patients with asthma, chronic bronchitis, narrow-angle glaucoma or chronic obstructive pulmonary disease. It should also be used with caution in patients with severe cardiovascular disease. Cevimeline 30 mg three times a day has been shown to increase salivary output in patients with SS. The most common side effects of cevimeline include nausea and sweating; however, these symptoms are mild compared to similar adverse reactions induced by pilocarpine. See Chapter 8 for further information on xerostomia and agents used to treat it.

Special Dental Considerations

Drug Interactions of Dental Interest

Many of the drugs taken by patients receiving treatment for a connective tissue disease may have a profound effect on both oral disease and the safety of dental treatment. Dentists treating a patient with a connective tissue disease must take a careful drug history and understand the potential side effects of the drugs the patient is taking and how they may affect the safety of dental treatment. Many of the drugs described in this chapter affect the hematologic and immune systems and, therefore, increase the risk of both infection and bleeding. Long-term glucocorticoid or immunosuppressive drug therapy, for example, may require significant modification of the dental treatment plan. Dentists may be consulted to treat oral and dental complications of connective tissue diseases, such as oral mucosal lesions in patients who have lupus or xerostomia in patients who have SS. Knowledge of the use of topical and intralesional glucocorticoids for patients with lupus and systemic medications for patients with SS, such as pilocarpine and cevimeline, can be an important component of good medical therapy.

Lupus. Dentists should be aware of a disorder called "drug-induced lupus," which occurs when patients develop symptoms and signs of lupus triggered by drug therapy. Drugs most frequently associated with drug-induced lupus include hydralazine, procainamide, penicillamine D and oral contraceptives. Dentists should also be aware that drug therapy may exacerbate systemic lupus. Antibiotics such as penicillin and sulfonamides as well as NSAIDs have been reported to cause lupus flare-ups. Dentists should check with the treating medical specialist before prescribing these drugs for patients with lupus.

Scleroderma. Scleroderma of the face results in a progressive decrease in oral opening that leads to difficulty with both oral home care and dental treatment. Difficulty with proper oral hygiene increases the risk of dental caries, especially when scleroderma is complicated by xerostomia as a result of secondary SS.

Sjögren's syndrome. Patients with SS systemic manifestations may be receiving therapy from their internist with antimalarial drugs such as hydroxychloroquine, particularly when there is joint involvement. Systemic glucocorticoids and/or immunosuppressive drugs also are used to manage severe systemic manifestations of SS. Patients receiving antimalarial therapy should be closely monitored for the development of blood dyscrasias, including neutropenia and agranulocytosis. Patients receiving antimalarials may develop dark pigmentation of the skin and mucosa and may ask their dentist about the cause of a pigmented area discovered on the oral mucosa.

Laboratory Value Alterations

Many drugs used to treat connective tissue diseases—such as immunosuppressive drugs, gold sodium thiomalate and penicillamine—may cause bone marrow suppression. Patients taking these drugs should have a hematologic evaluation, including a white blood cell and platelet count, before undergoing dental and oral surgical procedures.

Adverse Effects, Precautions and Contraindications

Table 21.1 lists adverse effects related to connective tissue disorder drugs.

Pharmacology

Cevimeline. Cevimeline is a parasympathetic agonist that is specific for M3 muscarinic receptors, the major receptor subtype found on salivary gland tissue. As compared to pilocarpine, onset of increased salivation may be later; however, duration of action is generally longer and the adverse effects are milder.

Gold sodium thiomalate. The mechanism that makes this drug an effective anti-inflammatory agent for patients with rheumatoid arthritis is unknown. It is effective in reducing synovitis in patients with active joint inflammation.

Hydroxychloroquine. This is an antimalarial drug that also is effective in the treatment of discoid and systemic lupus erythematosus. The mechanism of action in patients with lupus is not understood.

Immunosuppressive drugs. Azathioprine is an immunosuppressive drug used to prevent graft rejection in organ transplant patients. It also is effective for the management of some autoimmune and connective tissue diseases owing to its effect on lymphocyte response and delayed hypersensitivity.

Cyclophosphamide is used in cancer chemotherapy, which also suppresses the immune response and therefore is useful in the management of autoimmune and connective tissue diseases such as pemphigus and lupus erythematosus.

Mycophenolate mofetil is a potent immunosuppressive agent and was originally approved to prevent rejection of kidney transplants. Currently, mycophenolate mofetil is also being used to treat discoid lupus erythematosus, pemphigus, and mucous membrane pemphigoid.

Tumor necrosis factor (TNF) inhibitors decrease the amount of circulating TNF-α, an inflammatory cytokine that is present in increased concentrations in patients with RA. Etanercept is a receptor protein that prevents TNF-α from attaching to its cellular receptors and neutralizes its inflammatory behavior. Infliximab is a monoclonal antibody that binds to TNF-α, rendering it inactive. It may also promote lysis of TNF-producing cells. Both medications have demonstrated efficacy in managing symptoms associated with RA.

Nonsteroidal anti-inflammatory drugs. Pharmacological information on these drugs is provided in Chapter 3.

Penicillamine D. This drug decreases the level of rheumatoid factor related to immunoglobulin M. It also depresses the activity of T-lymphocytes.

Oral Mucosal Disease Drugs

This portion of the chapter will discuss the therapy for the major oral mucosal diseases not covered in other chapters.

Erythema Multiforme Drugs

Erythema multiforme (EM) is an acute inflammatory disease that may affect the mucosa, the skin or both. EM that involves multiple sites—including the mouth, conjunctiva, skin and genitals—is called Stevens-Johnson syndrome. Toxic epidermal necrolysis is a severe, life-threatening form of EM in which large areas of skin peel away, leaving the patient susceptible to fluid and electrolyte imbalance as well as secondary infection. EM may be caused by drug reactions or reactions to microorganisms. Drugs that most commonly cause EM include sulfonamides, oxicam NSAIDs (such as piroxicam), allopurinol and anticonvulsant drugs such as phenytoin and carbamazepine. Herpes simplex virus is the microorganism most commonly responsible for triggering episodes of EM, and recurrent herpes infections are believed to be the most common cause of recurrent episodes of EM. Mycoplasma infections also trigger cases of EM.

The oral lesions associated with EM can be extensive and cause severe ulceration of the lips and intraoral mucosa. Patients may have oral lesions as the sole or chief manifestation of EM. Extensive oral lesions are frequently present as part of generalized EM.

The management of mild cases of oral EM includes supportive care with topical anesthetic agents, such as viscous lidocaine. Severe cases of EM in adults frequently are treated with a short course of systemic glucocorticoids. The use of glucocorticoids to treat EM has been controversial, but studies have demonstrated both relief of symptoms and shortened healing times with few significant side effects when the drug is administered to adults. Children treated with glucocorticoids for EM have a higher incidence of side effects, particularly gastrointestinal bleeding or secondary infection. Patients with recurrent episodes of EM caused by herpes simplex virus benefit from prophylaxis with antiherpes drugs such as acyclovir or valacyclovir. Patients with severe stomatitis resulting from EM or other causes may obtain temporary relief with the use of topical anesthetic agents such as viscous lidocaine.

Lichen Planus Drugs

Lichen planus (LP) is a chronic mucocutaneous disease that affects the skin, mucosal surfaces or both. The oral mucosa is a common site of involvement, and LP oral lesions can present as reticular white lines, white plaques, areas of desquamation or ulcers. LP is also the most common cause of desquamative gingivitis. When LP is characterized by ulceration, desquamation or blisters, it is called "erosive LP." The etiology of the disease is unknown, but LP is divided into idiopathic and lichenoid reactions. Patients with idiopathic LP have no identifiable underlying trigger for the disease, whereas patients with lichenoid reactions have an underlying cause such as drug therapy, contact allergy or a systemic disease such as hepatitis C.

The lesions of idiopathic LP and lichenoid reactions cannot be reliably distinguished either clinically or histologically; therefore, dentists or dental specialists who manage patients with oral LP should obtain a thorough history to rule out a possible underlying cause, particularly in severe cases of erosive LP. The drugs most commonly associated with LP include angiotensin-converting enzyme (ACE) inhibitors such as captopril, β-blockers and NSAIDs. Allergic reactions to dental materials (such as amalgam or gold) that are directly in contact with the lesions also have been reported as a cause of LP.

Proper management of oral LP includes an attempt to identify an underlying cause, such as a lichenoid drug reaction, and then to control symptomatic lesions with topical or, occasionally, systemic agents. Topical glucocorticoids are the most effective agents for a majority of patients with lesions symptomatic of erosive LP. The effectiveness of topical glucocorticoids when managing desquamative gingival lesions can be improved by fabrication of a soft splint or mouthguard that covers the gingiva and holds the glucocorticoid in place more effectively. In severe cases, the topical glucocorticoid may be supplemented with intralesional glucocorticoid injections. Plaque-like lesions of LP, which require therapy, have been successfully managed with the use of topical retinoids such as tretinoin. Cyclosporine, an immunosuppressive drug used to prevent graft rejection in organ transplant patients, has been used topically to treat oral LP. The usefulness of this therapy is limited because it is significantly more expensive than the use of topical glucocorticoids. Tacrolimus is a nonsteroidal topical immunomodulator that inhibits production of inflammatory cytokines and is effective in the treatment of erosive LP that is refractory to topical glucocorticoid treatment. Patients should be informed that LP is a chronic disease that may last for many years and that treatment is designed to control the lesions, not cure the disease. Data strongly suggest that patients with oral LP have an increased risk of developing oral cancer; therefore, patients with LP should be evaluated periodically for the presence of suspicious lesions.

Mucous Membrane Pemphigoid Drugs

Mucous membrane pemphigoid (MMP), also called "cicatricial pemphigoid," is a chronic, blistering autoimmune disease caused by antibodies that destroy proteins in the basement membrane of the epithelium, thus causing separation of the epidermis from the dermis. The oral mucosa is the most common site of involvement in MMP, and desquamation of the gingiva is the most common oral manifestation. Involvement of the conjunctiva may lead to blindness, and in some cases the genital, tracheal and esophageal mucosa also may be affected. Diagnosis is made by biopsy of lesions that should be studied by means of both routine histology and direct immunofluorescence.

Oral lesions of MMP initially are treated with potent topical glucocorticoids, which can be more effective when held in place with occlusive dental splints if gingival or palatal lesions are involved. Intralesional glucocorticoids can be used when extensive localized lesions do not respond to topical glucocorticoids alone. Systemic therapy may be necessary to control severe cases of MMP. Systemic therapy found effective in some cases includes dapsone, tetracycline, immunosuppressive drugs (such as azathioprine and mycophenolate mofetil) and systemic glucocorticoids. These drugs can have serious side effects and should be prescribed only by a dental or medical specialist trained in managing patients who are taking these drugs.

Pemphigus Vulgaris Drugs

Pemphigus vulgaris (PV) is an autoimmune disease caused by antibodies that destroy the attachment between epithelial cells and cause separation of the cells (called "acantholysis") and blister formation. PV may occur alone or in association with other autoimmune diseases, such as myasthenia gravis. The blistering and peeling of the skin and mucosa are potentially fatal if not treated. The oral mucosa is often the initial site of involvement, and PV is frequently diagnosed by biopsy of oral lesions using both routine histology and direct immunofluorescence. Most cases of PV are of unknown origin, but a minority of cases are caused by a reaction to drugs, particularly penicillamine or captopril. Paraneoplastic pemphigus is a form of PV triggered by neoplasms, such as lymphomas.

Systemic glucocorticoid therapy is the mainstay of treatment of PV. Adjuvant therapy with immunosuppressive drugs such as azathioprine allows the clinician to use lower doses of systemic glucocorticoids, which reduces the risk of serious side effects. Mycophenolate mofetil, described earlier in this chapter, has a lower incidence of hepatotoxicity and nephrotoxicity compared to other immunosuppressive agents, and is used in the treatment of PV.

Recurrent Aphthous Stomatitis Drugs

Recurrent aphthous stomatitis (RAS) is a disease of unknown etiology, but it is clear that the tendency to develop RAS is inherited. RAS affects approximately 15% of the population and is commonly seen in dental patients. The disease is characterized by recurring oral ulcers with no other signs or symptoms of disease on other mucosal or skin surfaces and no evidence of involvement of other organ systems. Dentists managing patients with recurring oral ulcers should eliminate the possibility of other serious disorders that can cause recurring oral ulcers, such as connective tissue disease, blood dyscrasias or human immunodeficiency virus

(HIV) infection, by obtaining a thorough history and performing a careful examination. In severe or unusual cases, laboratory tests may be necessary to eliminate the possibility of underlying systemic disease. RAS is divided into minor and major forms. Patients with the minor form experience ulcers that are less than 1 cm in diameter and heal in 10 to 14 days. The major form of RAS is less common and causes ulcers that are greater than 1 cm in diameter, take weeks to months to heal and cause scarring.

The mainstay of treatment for RAS is the use of topical glucocorticoids. High-potency glucocorticoids such as fluocinonide placed directly on the lesion shorten the healing time of the lesion and increase patient comfort in a majority of cases, but do not prevent the formation of new lesions. Less potent glucocorticoids appear to have little effect. Other topical preparations that can decrease the healing time of RAS include amlexanox paste (Aphthasol) and topical tetracycline mouthrinses. The latter therapy may cause candidiasis or allergic reactions.

Patients with severe major aphthae may not experience adequate relief from topical preparations. Drugs that have been reported effective in reducing the number of ulcers in some cases of major RAS include colchicine, pentoxifylline and dapsone. Pentoxifylline is a methylxanthine related to caffeine, which is used chiefly to treat peripheral vascular disease because of its effect on the flexibility of red blood cells. Because it also has an effect on leukocytes, it appears useful for a number of inflammatory diseases. There have been several reports and uncontrolled trials of the successful use of pentoxifylline for the treatment of severe aphthous stomatitis.

Thalidomide has been shown to reduce the incidence and severity of RAS in both HIV and non-HIV patients, but it must be used with extreme caution in women of childbearing years owing to its potential for causing severe life-threatening and deforming birth defects. Clinicians prescribing thalidomide must be registered with the System for Thalidomide Education and Prescribing Safety Prescriber Registry, and patients receiving the drug must be carefully counseled regarding proper use of birth control methods during treatment with this drug. Other side effects of thalidomide include peripheral neuropathy, drowsiness and gastrointestinal disturbances.

See Tables 21.1 and 21.2 for general information on oral mucosal disease drugs.

Special Dental Considerations

Topical glucocorticoids. Treatment with topical glucocorticoids is common for patients with inflammatory diseases involving the oral mucosa. Topical glucocorticoids are largely synthetic derivatives of hydrocortisone with an 11-β-hydroxyl group required for anti-inflammatory action. The topical glucocorticoids are effective anti-inflammatory agents; these agents' effectiveness results from a combination of activities, including increased vasoconstriction, decreased migration of leukocytes, decreased complement activity and decreased fibroblast proliferation.

Long-term repeated use of topical glucocorticoids may cause resistance to the anti-inflammatory effects owing to tachyphylaxis, which primarily results from a decreased ability to cause vasoconstriction. Discontinuing the use of the drug for 3-4 days restores the normal response. Vasoconstriction is an important part of the action of topical glucocorticoids, and the potency of these drugs is established by an assay that measures vasoconstriction.

Topical glucocorticoids are grouped according to their potency. Examples of drugs in each group are as follows:
- Group 1: ultra high potency—betamethasone dipropionate 0.05%, clobetasol 0.05%;

- Group 2: high potency—fluocinonide 0.05%, desoximetasone 0.25%, 0.05%;
- Group 3: medium potency—betamethasone dipropionate 0.05%, triamcinolone acetonide 0.5%;
- Group 4: lower potency—triamcinolone acetonide, fluocinolone acetonide.

The effect of topical glucocorticoids on the desquamative lesions of LP may be enhanced by the use of soft occlusive dental splints that fit over the teeth and hold the glucocorticoid onto the attached gingiva, increasing contact of the glucocorticoid and preventing the medication from being washed away by saliva. The most frequent complication of the long-term use of topical glucocorticoids when treating chronic oral mucosal lesions such as LP or MMP is oral candidiasis. The incidence of candidiasis can be decreased by the concomitant use of topical antifungal agents such as nystatin suspension or clotrimazole troches. Dentists prescribing prolonged use of topical glucocorticoids must carefully instruct patients regarding safe use in the mouth, warn about overuse, and periodically monitor patients who are using these medications for extensive oral lesions.

Intralesional glucocorticoids. Patients with chronic, severe lesions of LP, MMP or major RAS that do not respond to topical glucocorticoids may be helped by the use of intralesional glucocorticoids. Glucocorticoids developed for intralesional use such as triamcinolone hexacetonide 5 mg/cc are useful in managing resistant lesions in patients with major aphthae, LP or MMP.

Systemic glucocorticoids. Many clinicians recommend a short course of systemic glucocorticoids for the management of EM. Use of systemic glucocorticoids in the management of chronic oral mucosal disease should be rare and for short periods to manage acute, severe exacerbations of diseases such as LP that are not life-threatening.

Topical immunomodulators. Tacrolimus is a calcineurin inhibitor, a type of drug that prevents the formation of numerous cytokines, which are critical in the development of various inflammatory skin disorders. Originally developed to prevent transplant rejection, the topical formulation of tacrolimus is primarily used for treatment of atopic dermatitis (eczema). It is also effective for treatment of erosive LP that is refractory to topical glucocorticoid therapy. Topical tacrolimus ointment is currently available in concentrations of 0.03% and 0.1%, with the latter formulation demonstrating greater clinical results when used to treat erosive LP.

Retinoids. Retinoids include vitamin A and its synthetic analogues. Systemic retinoids such as isotretinoin (13-cis-retinoic acid) and etretinate have been shown to promote healing of premalignant oral leukoplakias in a significant number of cases and to reduce the incidence of second cancers in patients with a history of head and neck malignancies. Systemic retinoids have the potential for inducing serious side effects, such as severe birth defects; benign intracranial hypertension (pseudotumor cerebri); an increase in plasma triglycerides, high-density lipoproteins and cholesterol; and liver toxicity. Patients taking systemic retinoids may also develop mucocutaneous signs such as cheilitis and conjunctivitis. Topical retinoids have been used to treat oral mucosal leukoplakia and LP. The white plaques or reticulated lesions of LP have been reversed with the use of topical tretinoin. Mucosal irritation may result from use of topical retinoids.

Dapsone. Dapsone, a synthetic sulfone, was used initially to treat leprosy and malaria. In the 1950s, the drug's anti-inflammatory properties became known, and it was used to successfully treat a number of inflammatory disorders, particularly those with neutrophil-rich infiltrates such as dermatitis herpetiformis. In oral medicine, dapsone is used most frequently to treat mucous membrane pemphigoid; however, according to some controlled studies, it also has been used in severe refractory cases of major aphthous ulcers, pemphigus and LP. Side effects of dapsone are common, and the drug should be prescribed by a clinician experienced in its use. The most common side effects are hemolytic anemia and methemoglobinemia, and most patients receiving the drug will demonstrate a decrease in hemoglobin. Anemia can be minimized by concurrent use of cimetidine and vitamin E. The use of dapsone is contraindicated in patients with glucose-6-phosphate dehydrogenase (G6PD) deficiency. Before prescribing dapsone, the clinician must screen the patient for this deficiency.

Thalidomide. This drug, which originally was prescribed for the treatment of nausea in pregnant women, was banned in the United States because it causes severe birth defects and fetal death. The drug was approved for limited use in 1998 for the treatment of erythema nodosum leprosum, but it also has been shown to be beneficial in the management of severe minor and major recurrent aphthous ulcers in some patients, including some patients with HIV infection. The drug may be prescribed to pregnant women only by specially registered physicians or dentists who have received formal education on the risk of fetal abnormalities. Use of thalidomide for recurrent aphthous stomatitis should be reserved for patients with severe intractable forms of the disease who have not responded to other less toxic forms of therapy. In addition to birth efects, the side effects of thalidomide include eripheral neuropathy, constipation, drowsiness and neutropenia.

Adverse Effects, Precautions and Contraindications
Table 21.1 lists adverse effects related to oral mucosal disease drugs.

Pharmacology
Colchicine. Colchicine suppresses white blood cell function by interfering on the cellular level with microtubule formation, inhibiting lysosomal degranulation and increasing the level of cyclic AMP. This decreases both the chemotactic and the phagocytic activity of neutrophils.

Cyclosporine. Cyclosporine is an immunosuppressive drug used to prevent graft rejection in organ transplant patients. It has a potent effect on the response of T-lymphocytes and cell-mediated immunity. It also has been used to treat connective tissue and autoimmune diseases.

Dapsone. Dapsone is a sulfone that has been used for its antibacterial properties for more than 50 years. It continues to be used to treat leprosy, malaria and *Pneumocystis carinii* infections in people with HIV. The anti-inflammatory properties of dapsone are unrelated to its antibacterial actions, but diseases that respond favorably to the drug are associated with significant neutrophil infiltration. There is evidence that dapsone suppresses neutrophil function by interfering with the myeloperoxidase-H_2O_2-halide cytotoxic function of neutrophils, as well as inhibiting the synthesis of prostaglandins by neutrophils.

Retinoids. This class of drugs has a major effect on cellular growth and cell differentiation. The use of these drugs can reverse keratinization and premalignant changes. There also is evidence that retinoids have anti-inflammatory properties.

Tacrolimus. The major adverse reaction associated with topical tacrolimus ointment is burning at the site of application. Recently, the U.S. Food and Drug Administration (FDA) issued an alert that use of topical tacrolimus ointment for treatment of atopic dermatitis in pediatric patients may increase the risk of developing cancer; further clinical studies are needed to substantiate this advisory.

Thalidomide. This drug was marketed as a nonaddictive sedative until its severe teratogenic properties became known and its use was discontinued. More recently, it has been used for its immune-modulating effects and its angiogenesis-inhibiting properties, which are believed to result from suppression of tumor necrosis factor α and inhibition of leukocyte migration.

Viscous lidocaine. Pharmacological information on this drug is provided in Chapter 1.

Suggested Readings

Akintoye SO, Greenberg MS. Recurrent aphthous stomatitis. Dent Clin North Am 2005;49:31-47.

Beck LA. The efficacy and safety of tacrolimus ointment: A clinical review. J Am Acad Dermatol 2005;53: S165-70.

Ciarrocca KN, Greenberg MS. Immunologic diseases. In: Greenberg MS, Glick M, eds. Burket's oral medicine: Diagnosis and treatment. 10th ed. Ontario: BC Decker; 2003:478-502.

Hartmann M, Enk A. Mycophenolate mofetil and skin diseases. Lupus 2005;14:S58-63.

Greenberg MS: Ulcerative, vesicular, and bullous lesions. In Greenberg MS, Glick M, editors. Burket's oral medicine: Diagnosis and treatment. 10th ed. Ontario: BC Decker; 2003:50-84.

Rindfleisch JA, Muller D. Diagnosis and management of rheumatoid arthritis. Am Fam Physician 2005;72: 1037-47, 1049-50.

Williams PM, Conklin RJ. Erythema multiforme: A review and contrast from Stevens-Johnson syndrome/toxic epidermal necrolysis. Dent Clin North Am 2005;49:67-76.

Table 21.1: PRESCRIBING INFORMATION FOR AGENTS USED TO TREAT CONNECTIVE TISSUE DISORDERS AND ORAL MUCOSAL DISEASES

NAME	FORM/ STRENGTH	DOSAGE	WARNINGS/PRECAUTIONS & CONTRAINDICATIONS	ADVERSE EFFECTS†
ANTI-INFLAMMATORY AGENT				
Amlexanox (Aphthasol)	**Paste:** 5% [5g]	**Adults:** Begin at 1st sign of aphthous ulcer. Apply 1/4 inch qid, pc and qhs, following oral hygiene. Use until ulcer heals. Re-evaluate if healing or pain reduction has not occurred after 10 days of use.	**W/P:** Wash hands immediately after applying paste. Discontinue if rash or contact mucositis occurs. Avoid eyes. **P/N:** Category B, caution in nursing.	Transient pain, stinging, burning.
ANTIMALARIAL AGENT				
Hydroxychloro- quine Sulfate (Plaquenil)	**Tab:** 200mg (200mg tab = 155mg base)	**Adults: Malaria Suppression:** 400mg weekly. Begin 2 weeks before exposure and continue for 8 weeks after leaving endemic area. Give 400mg q6h for 2 doses if therapy is not begun before exposure. **Acute Attack:** 800mg, then 400mg 6-8 hrs later, then 400mg for 2 more days. **RA: Initial:** 400-600mg qd with food or milk; increase until optimum response. **Maint:** After 4-12 weeks, 200-400mg qd with food or milk. **Lupus Erythematosus: Initial:** 400mg qd-bid for several weeks depending on response. **Maint:** 200-400mg/day. **Pediatrics: Malaria Suppression:** 5mg/kg (base) weekly. **Max:** 400mg/dose. Begin 2 weeks before exposure and continue for 8 weeks after leaving endemic area. q6h for 2 doses if therapy is not begun before exposure. **Acute Attack:** 10mg base/kg (**Max:** 800mg/dose) then 5mg base/kg (**Max:** 400mg/dose) at 6, 24 and 48 hrs after 1st dose.	**Be familiar with complete prescrib- ing information before prescribing hydroxychloroquine. W/P:** Caution with hepatic disease, G6PD deficiency, alcoholism, psoriasis, and porphyria. Perform baseline and periodic (3 months) ophthalmo- logic exams and blood cell counts with prolonged therapy. Test periodically for muscle weakness. Discontinue if blood disorders occur. Avoid if possible in pregnancy. Discontinue after 6 months if no improvement in rheumatoid arthritis. **Contra:** Long term therapy in children or if retinal/visual field changes due to 4-aminoquinoline compounds. **P/N:** Safety in pregnancy and nursing not known.	Headache, dizziness, diarrhea, loss of appe- tite, muscle weakness, nausea, abdominal cramps, bleaching of hair, dermatitis, ocular toxicity, visual field defects.
GOLD COMPOUND				
Gold Sodium Thiomalate (Myochrysine)	**Inj:** 50mg/mL	**Adults: RA: Initial:** 10mg IM 1st week, 25mg IM 2nd week, then 25-50mg IM weekly until response, toxicity or 1g cumulative dose. **Maint:** 25-50mg every other week, then every third week, then every forth week as tolerated. **Pediatrics:** 10mg IM, then 1mg/ kg (maximum 50mg/day) IM weekly for 20 weeks; maintenance, 1mg/kg IM (maximum 50mg/dose) every 2-4 weeks.	**W/P:** Caution with compromised cardio- vascular circulation, compromised cere- bral circulation, concurrent penicillamine, history of blood dyscrasias, previous hepatic insufficiency, previous renal insuf- ficiency, severe hypertension, skin rash. **Contra:** Moderate to severe renal failure, systemic lupus erythematosus, severe debilitation, toxicity to gold/heavy metals. **P/N:** Category C, caution with nursing.	Pruritis, rash, **stomatitis**.
IMMUNOSUPPRESSIVE DRUGS				
Azathioprine (Imuran)	**Tab:** 50mg*	**Adults: Renal Homo Transplantation: Initial:** 3-5mg/kg/day, start at time of transplant. **Maint:** 1-3mg/kg/day. **Rheumatoid Arthritis: Initial:** 1mg/kg/day given qd-bid. **Titrate:** Increase by 0.5mg/kg/day after 6-8 weeks, then at 4 week intervals. **Max:** 2.5mg/kg/day. **Maint:** Lowest effective dose. Decrease by 0.5mg/kg/day or 25mg/day every 4 weeks. If no response by Week 12, then considered refractory. **Renal Dysfunction:** Lower dose.	**Increased risk of neoplasia with chronic therapy. Mutagenic potential and possible hematological tox- icities. W/P:** Dose-related leukopenia, thrombocytopenia, macrocytic anemia, pancytopenia and severe bone marrow suppression may occur. Monitor CBCs, including platelets, weekly during the 1st month, twice monthly for the 2nd and 3rd months, then monthly or more fre- quently if dose/therapy changes. Monitor for infections. **Contra:** Pregnancy in RA treatment. Previous treatment of RA with alkylating agents (eg, cyclophospha- mide, chlorambucil, melphalan) may increase risk of neoplasia. **P/N:** Category D, not for use in nursing.	Leukopenia, thrombo- cytopenia, infections, nausea, vomiting, hepatotoxicity.

*Scored.   †Bold entries denote special dental considerations.

NAME	FORM/ STRENGTH	DOSAGE	WARNINGS/PRECAUTIONS & CONTRAINDICATIONS	ADVERSE EFFECTS[†]
Cyclophospha- mide (Cytoxan)	Inj (Ly- ophilized): 100mg, 200mg, 500mg, 1g, 2g; Tab: 25mg, 50mg	**Adults: Malignant Diseases (Without Hematologic Deficiency): Monotherapy: Initial:** 40-50mg/kg IV in divided doses over 2-5 days, or 10-15mg/kg IV given every 7-10 days, or 3-5mg/kg twice weekly. **Oral Dosing: Initial/Maint:** 1-5mg/kg/day PO. Adjust dose according to antitumor activity and/or leukopenia. May need to reduce dose when combined with other cytotoxic drugs. **Pediatrics: Malignant Diseases (Without Hematologic Deficiency): Monotherapy: Initial:** 40-50mg/kg IV in divided doses over 2-5 days, or 10-15mg/kg IV given every 7-10 days, or 3-5mg/kg twice weekly. **Oral Dosing: Initial/Maint:** 1-5mg/kg/day PO. Adjust dose according to antitumor activity and/or leukopenia. May need to reduce dose when combined with other cytotoxic drugs. **Nephrotic Syndrome:** 2.5-3mg/kg/day PO for 60-90 days.	**W/P:** Second malignancies, cardiac dysfunction, and hemorrhagic cystitis reported. May cause fetal harm in pregnancy. Serious, fatal infections may develop if severely immunosuppressed. Monitor for toxicity with leukopenia, thrombocytopenia, tumor cell infiltration of bone marrow, previous x-ray therapy or cytotoxic therapy, and impaired hepatic and/or renal function. Monitor hematologic profile for hematopoietic suppression. Examine urine for red blood cells. Anaphylactic reactions reported. Possible cross-sensitivity with other alkylating agents. May cause ste- rility. May interfere with normal wound healing. Consider dose adjustment with adrenalectomy. **Contra:** Severely depressed bone mar- row function. **P/N:** Category D, not for use in nursing.	Impairment of fertility, amenorrhea, nausea, vomiting, anorexia, abdominal discomfort, diarrhea, alopecia, leukopenia, thrombo- cytopenia, hemorrhagic ureteritis, interstitial pneumonitis, malaise, asthenia, renal tubular necrosis.
Cyclosporine (Sandimmune)	Cap: 25mg, 100mg; Inj: 50mg/mL; Sol: 100mg/ mL [50mL]	**Adults: Initial: PO:** 15mg/kg single dose 4-12 hrs before transplant; continue same dose qd for 1-2 weeks. **Usual:** Taper by 5% per week until 5-10mg/ kg/day. May mix oral solution with milk, chocolate milk, or orange juice. **IV:** 1/3 PO dose. **Initial:** 5-6mg/kg/day single dose; begin 4 to 12 hrs prior to transplantation. **Maint:** Continue single daily dose until PO forms are tolerated. Due to risk of anaphylaxis, only use injection if unable to take oral agents. **Pediatrics: Initial: PO:** 15mg/kg single dose 4-12 hrs before transplant; continue same dose qd for 1-2 weeks. **Usual:** Taper by 5% per week until 5-10mg/ kg/day. May mix oral solution with milk, chocolate milk, or orange juice. **IV:** 1/3 PO dose. **Initial:** 5-6mg/kg/day single dose; begin 4 to 12 hrs prior to transplantation. **Maint:** Continue single daily dose until PO forms are tolerated. Due to risk of anaphylaxis, only use injection if unable to take oral agents.	**Give with adrenal corticosteroids but not with other immunosuppressives. Increased susceptibility to infection and development of lymphoma. Sandimmune and Neoral are not bioequivalent. Monitor blood levels to avoid toxicity. W/P:** May cause hepatotoxic- ity and nephrotoxicity. Convulsions, elevated serum creatinine, and BUN levels reported. Thrombocytopenia and microangiopathic hemolytic anemia may develop. Monitor for hyperkalemia. Increases risk for development of lymphomas and other malignancies. Observe for 30 minutes after the start of infusion and frequently thereafter. Caution with malabsorption. **Contra:** Hypersensitivity to Cremophor EL (polyoxyethylated castor oil). **P/N:** Category C, not for use in nursing.	Renal dysfunction, tremor, hirsutism, HTN, **gum hyperplasia,** HTN, glomerular capillary thrombosis, cramps, acne, convulsions, headache, diarrhea, hepatotoxity, abdominal discomfort, paresthesia, flushing.
Cyclosporine, Modified (Neoral)	Cap: 25mg, 100mg; Sol: 100mg/ mL [50mL]	**Adults: Transplant:** Give initial oral dose 4-12 hrs before transplant or post-op. Dose bid. **Initial: Renal Transplant:** 9±3mg/kg/day. **Liver Transplant:** 8±4mg/kg/day. **Heart Transplant:** 7±3mg/kg/day. Give with corticosteroids initially. **Conversion from Sandimmune:** 1:1 dose conversion. Adjust to trough levels. Monitor every 4-7 days. **RA: Initial:** 1.25mg/kg bid. **Titrate:** May increase by 0.5-0.75mg/kg/ day after 8 weeks, again after 12 weeks. **Max:** 4mg/kg/day. Discontinue if no benefit by week 16. **Psoriasis: Initial:** 1.25mg/kg bid for 4 weeks.	**Increased susceptibility to infection, and development of neoplasia, HTN, nephrotoxicity. Monitor blood levels to avoid toxicity. Neoral is not bioequivalent to Sandimmune. Risk of skin malignancies if previously treated with PUVA, UVB, coal tar, radiation, MTX, or other immunosup- pressives. W/P:** Risk of hepatotoxic- ity and nephrotoxicity. Caution in elderly. Hyperkalemia, hyperuricemia, thrombocytopenia, microangiopathic hemolytic anemia, and encephalopathy reported in transplant patients. Monitor CBC and LFTs monthly with MTX. Monitor BP and renal function before therapy, every 2 weeks during 1st 3 months, then monthly if stable with RA or psoriasis.	Renal dysfunction, HTN, hirsutism, muscle cramps, acne, tremor, headache, **gingival hyperplasia,** diarrhea, nausea, vomiting, paresthesia, flushing, dyspepsia, hypertri- chosis, **stomatitis,** hypomagnesemia.

Table 21.1: PRESCRIBING INFORMATION FOR AGENTS USED TO TREAT CONNECTIVE TISSUE DISORDERS AND ORAL MUCOSAL DISEASES *(cont.)*

NAME	FORM/ STRENGTH	DOSAGE	WARNINGS/PRECAUTIONS & CONTRAINDICATIONS	ADVERSE EFFECTS†
IMMUNOSUPPRESSIVE DRUGS *(cont.)*				
Cyclosporine, Modified *(cont.)*		**Titrate:** May increase by 0.5mg/kg/day every 2 weeks. **Max:** 4mg/kg/day. Decrease dose by 25-50% to control adverse events. Take at the same time every day. Dilute sol in orange or apple juice that is room temp.	Monitor SCr after initiate or increase NSAID dose in RA. Monitor CBC, uric acid, K⁺, lipids, and magnesium every 2 weeks during 1st 3 months, then monthly if stable in RA. Monitor LFTs repeatedly. Monitor CBC, SCr with transplants. **Contra:** Abnormal renal function, uncontrolled HTN, malignancies. PUVA or UVB therapy, MTX, other immuno-suppressants, coal tar, or radiation in psoriasis patients. **P/N:** Category C, not for use in nursing.	
Mycophenolate mofetil (Cellcept)	**Cap:** 250mg; **Inj:** 500mg; **Sus:** 200mg/ mL [175mL]; **Tab:** 500mg	*Adults:* **Renal Transplant:** 1g IV/PO bid. **Cardiac Transplant:** 1.5g IV/PO bid. **Hepatic Transplant:** 1g IV bid or 1.5g PO bid. Start PO as soon as possible after transplant. Start IV within 24 hrs after transplant; can continue for up to 14 days. Switch to oral when tolerated. Give on an empty stomach. *Pediatrics:* **Renal Transplant:** (Sus) 600mg/m² PO bid. **Max:** 2g/day (10 mL/day). **(Cap) BSA 1.25m² to 1.5m²:** 750mg PO bid. **(Cap/Tab) BSA >1.5m²:** 1g bid.	**Increased susceptibility to infection. May develop lymphoma.** **W/P:** Risk of lymphomas and other malignancies, especially of the skin. Avoid sunlight to decrease risk of skin cancer. May cause fetal harm during pregnancy. Must have negative serum/urine pregnancy test within 1 week before therapy. Two reliable forms of contraception required before and during therapy, and 6 weeks following discontinuation. Monitor for bone marrow suppression. Risk of GI ulceration, hemorrhage, and perforation; caution with active digestive system disease. Caution with delayed renal graft function post-transplant. Oral suspension contains phenylalanine; caution with phenylketonurics. Monitor CBC weekly during the 1st month, twice monthly for the 2nd and 3rd months, and then monthly through 1st year. Avoid with rare hereditary deficiency of hypoxanthine-guanine phosphoribo-syl-transferase (eg, Lesch-Nyhan and Kelley-Seegmiller syndrome). **Contra:** (Inj) Hypersensitivity to Poly-sorbate 80 (TWEEN). **P/N:** Category C, not for use in nursing.	Infections, diarrhea, leukopenia, sepsis, vomiting, GI bleeding, pain, abdominal pain, fever, headache, asthenia, chest pain, back pain, anemia, leukopenia, thrombocytopenia.
Penicillamine (Cuprimine)	**Cap:** (Cuprimine): 125mg, 250mg; **Tab:** (Depen) 250mg*	*Adults:* **Wilson's Disease:** Determine dosage by 24-hr urinary copper excretion. **Maint:** 0.75-1.5g/day for 3 months. **Max:** Up to 2g/day, based on serum free copper. **Cystinuria: Initial:** 250mg qd. **Usual:** 250mg-1g qid. **RA: Initial:** 125-250mg qid. **Titrate:** May increase by 125mg or 250mg/ day every 1-3 months. If needed after 2-3 months, increase by 250mg/day every 2-3 months. Discontinue if no improvement after 3-4 months at dose of 1-1.5g/day. **Maint:** 500-750mg/day. **Max:** 1.5g/day. Give on an empty stomach, 1 hr before or 2 hrs after meals, and 1 hr apart from any other drug, food or milk. Supplemental pyridoxine 25mg/day recommended. *Pediatrics:* **Cystinuria:** 30mg/kg/day given qid.	**Supervise closely due to toxicity, special dosage considerations, and therapeutic benefits.** **W/P:** Aplastic anemia, agranulocy-tosis, drug fever, thrombocytopenia, Goodpasture's syndrome, myasthenia gravis, pemphigus foliaceus/vulgaris, obliterative bronchiolitis, proteinuria and hematuria reported. Routine urinalysis, CBC with differentials, Hgb and platelet count every 2 weeks for 6 months, then monthly. **Contra:** Pregnancy (except for treatment of Wilson's disease or certain cases of cystinuria), nursing, RA patients with renal insufficiency, history of penicillamine-related aplastic anemia or agranulocytosis. **P/N:** Category D, not for use in nursing.	Rash, urticaria, anorexia, epigastric pain, nausea, vomiting, diarrhea, leukopenia, thrombocytopenia, proteinuria.

*Scored.   †Bold entries denote special dental considerations.

NAME	FORM/ STRENGTH	DOSAGE	WARNINGS/PRECAUTIONS & CONTRAINDICATIONS	ADVERSE EFFECTS†

LOCAL ANESTHETIC

NAME	FORM/ STRENGTH	DOSAGE	WARNINGS/PRECAUTIONS & CONTRAINDICATIONS	ADVERSE EFFECTS†
Lidocaine Hydrochloride (Xylocaine)	**Inj:** 0.5%, 1%, 2%; (MPF) 0.5%, 1%, 1.5%, 2%; **Jelly:** 2% [Tube: 5mL, 30mL; Syringe: 10mL, 20mL]; **Sol:** 2% [100mL, 450mL]	**(Inj)** *Adults:* Dosage varies depending on procedure, depth and duration of anesthesia, degree of muscular relaxation, and patient physical condition. **Max:** 4.5mg/kg or total dose of 300mg. **Epidural/Caudal Anesthesia: Max:** Intervals not less than 90 minutes. **Paracervical Block: Max:** 200mg/90 minutes. **Regional Anesthesia: IV: Max:** 4mg/kg. **Children/Elderly/Debilitated/Cardiac or Liver Disease:** Reduce dose. *Pediatrics:* **>3 yrs: Max:** 1.5-2mg/lb. **Regional Anesthesia: IV: Max:** 3mg/kg. **(Jelly)** *Adults:* **Max:** 600mg/12 hrs. **Surface Anesthesia of Male Urethra:** Instill about 15mL (300mg). Instill an additional dose of not more than 15mL if needed. **Prior to Sounding or Cystoscopy:** A total dose of 30mL (600mg) is usually required. **Prior to Catheterization:** 5-10mL usually adequate. **Surface Anesthesia of Female Urethra:** Instill 3-5mL. **Elderly/Debilitated:** Reduce dose. *Pediatrics:* Determine dose by age and weight. **Max:** 4.5mg/kg. **(Sol)** *Adults:* **Irritated/Inflamed Mucous Membranes: Usual:** 15mL undiluted. (Mouth) Swish and spit out. (Pharynx) Gargle and may swallow. Do not administer in <3 hr intervals. **Max:** 8 doses/24hr; (Single Dose) 4.5mg/kg or total of 300mg. *Pediatrics:* **>3 yrs: Max:** Determine by age and weight. **Infants <3 yrs:** Apply 1.25mL with cotton-tipped applicator to immediate area. Do not administer in <3 hour intervals. **Max:** 8 doses/24hr.	**W/P:** (Inj) Acidosis, cardiac arrest, death reported from delay in toxicity management. Local anesthetic solutions containing antimicrobial preservatives should not be used for epidural or spinal anesthesia. Use lowest effective dose. During epidural anesthesia, administer initial test dose and monitor for CNS and cardiovascular toxicity as well as for signs of unintended intrathecal administration. Reduce dose with debilitated, elderly, acutely ill, and children. Extreme caution when using lumbar and caudal epidural anesthesia with existing neurological disease, spinal deformities, septicemia, and severe HTN. Monitor cardiovascular and respiratory vital signs and state of consciousness after each injection. Caution with hepatic disease, cardiovascular disorders. Monitor circulation and respiration with injections into head and neck area. (Jelly) Avoid excessive dosage or frequent administration; may result in serious adverse effects requiring resuscitative measures. Caution with heart block and severe shock. Extreme caution if mucosa traumatized or sepsis is present in the area of application; risk of rapid systemic absorption. **P/N:** Category B, caution in nursing. (Sol) Reduce dose in elderly, debilitated, acutely ill and children. Caution with heart block and severe shock. Excessive dosage or too frequent administration may result in high plasma levels and serious adverse effects requiring resuscitative measures. Extreme caution if mucosa traumatized; risk of rapid systemic absorption. Overdose reported in pediatrics due to inappropriate dosing.	Lightheadedness, nervousness, euphoria, confusion, dizziness, drowsiness, tinnitus, blurred vision, vomiting, heat/cold sensations, twitching, tremors, convulsions, respiratory depression, bradycardia, hypotension, urticaria, edema, anaphylactoid reactions.

RECURRENT APHTHOUS STOMATITIS DRUGS

NAME	FORM/ STRENGTH	DOSAGE	WARNINGS/PRECAUTIONS & CONTRAINDICATIONS	ADVERSE EFFECTS†
Colchicine	**Tab:** 0.5mg, 0.6mg	*Adults:* **Acute Treatment: Initial:** 1-1.2mg, followed by 0.5-0.6mg q1h, or 1-1.2mg q2h or 0.5-0.6mg q2-3h until pain relief, GI discomfort or diarrhea ensues. **Usual:** 4-8mg/attack. Wait 3 days before retreatment. **Prophylaxis: <1attack/yr:** 0.5-0.6mg/day given 3-4 times/week. **>1attack/yr:** 0.5-0.6mg qd. **Severe Cases:** 2-3 tabs of 0.5mg or 0.6mg daily. **Surgical Gout Prophylaxis:** 0.5-0.6mg tid 3 days before and 3 days after surgery.	**W/P:** Caution in elderly and debilitated, or those with GI, renal, hepatic, cardiac and hematologic disorders. Discontinue if nausea, vomiting or diarrhea occurs. Monitor blood counts periodically with long-term therapy. May adversely affect spermatogenesis. Elevates SGOT and alkaline phosphatase. May cause false (+) for urine RBC and Hgb. **Contra:** Serious GI, renal, hepatic or cardiac disorders and blood dyscrasias. **P/N:** Category C, caution in nursing.	Bone marrow depression, peripheral neuritis, purpura, myopathy, alopecia, dermatoses, reversible azoospermia, nausea, vomiting, diarrhea.
Pentoxifylline (Trental)	**Tab, Extended Release:** 400mg	*Adults:* 400mg tid with meals for at least 8 weeks. Reduce to 400mg bid if digestive and GI side effects occur; discontinue if side effects persist.	**W/P:** Monitor Hgb and Hct with risk factors complicated by hemorrhage (eg, recent surgery, peptic ulceration, cerebral/retinal bleeding). **Contra:** Recent cerebral and/or retinal hemorrhage, intolerance to methylxanthines (eg, caffeine, theophylline, theobromine). **P/N:** Category C, not for use in nursing.	Bloating, dyspepsia, nausea, vomiting, dizziness, headache.

Table 21.1: PRESCRIBING INFORMATION FOR AGENTS USED TO TREAT CONNECTIVE TISSUE DISORDERS AND ORAL MUCOSAL DISEASES (cont.)

NAME	FORM/STRENGTH	DOSAGE	WARNINGS/PRECAUTIONS & CONTRAINDICATIONS	ADVERSE EFFECTS†
RETINOID				
Isotretinoin (Accutane)	**Cap:** 10mg, 20mg, 40mg	***Adults:* Initial/Usual:** 0.5-1mg/kg/day given bid for 15-20 weeks. **Max:** 2mg/kg/day (for very serious cases). Adjust for side effects and disease response. May discontinue if nodule count reduced by >70% prior to completion. Repeat only if necessary after 2 months off drug. Take with food.	**Not for use by females who are or may become pregnant, or if breast feeding. Birth defects have been documented. Approved for marketing only under special restricted distribution program called iPLEDGE. Must have 2 (-) pregnancy tests. Repeat pregnancy test monthly. Use 2 forms of contraception at least 1 month prior, during, and 1 month following discontinuation. Must fill written prescriptions within 7 days; refills require new prescriptions. May dispense maximum of 1 month supply. Prescriber and patient must be registered with iPLEDGE.** **W/P:** Acute pancreatitis, impaired hearing, anaphylactic reactions, inflammatory bowel disease, elevated TG and LFTs, hepatotoxicity, premature epiphyseal closure, and hyperostosis reported. May cause depression, psychosis, aggressive and/or violent behaviors, rarely suicidal ideation/attempts and suicide; may need further evaluation after discontinuation. May cause decreased night vision, and corneal opacities. Associated with pseudotumor cerebri. Check lipids before therapy, and then at intervals until response established (within 4 weeks). Discontinue if significant decrease in WBC, hearing or visual impairment, abdominal pain, rectal bleeding, or severe diarrhea occurs. Monitor LFTs before therapy, weekly or biweekly until response established. May develop musculoskeletal symptoms. Avoid prolonged UV rays or sunlight, and donating blood up to 1 month after discontinuing therapy. Caution with genetic predisposition for age-related osteoporosis, history of childhood osteoporosis, osteomalacia, other bone metabolism disorders (eg, anorexia nervosa). Spontaneous osteoporosis, osteopenia, bone fractures, and delayed fracture healing reported; caution in sports with repetitive impact. **Contra:** Pregnancy, paraben sensitivity (preservative in gelatin cap). **P/N:** Category X, not for use in nursing.	Cheilitis, dry skin and mucous membranes, conjunctivitis, blood dyscrasias, epistaxis, decreased HDL, elevated cholesterol and TG, elevated blood sugar, arthralgias, back pain, hearing/vision impairment, rash, photosensitivity reactions, psychiatric disorders.
SEDATIVE-HYPNOTIC AGENT				
Thalidomide (Thalomid)	**Cap:** 50mg, 100mg, 200mg	***Adults:* Acute ENL: Initial:** 100-300mg qhs with water at least 1 hr after evening meal. **<50kg:** Start therapy at lower end of dosing range. **Severe Cutaneous ENL: Initial:** 400mg qhs with water at least 1 hour after evening meal. Use with corticosteroids in moderate to severe neuritis with severe ENL. Taper steroid where neuritis is ameliorated. Duration of therapy is usually 2 weeks. **Taper Dose:** Decrease by 50mg every 2-4 weeks.	**Severe, life-threatening human birth defects if taken during pregnancy. Women of childbearing potential should have a pregnancy test before starting therapy, then weekly for 1st month, and monthly thereafter. Males must use latex condoms in sexual intercourse with females of childbearing potential. Only prescribers and pharmacists registered with the S.T.E.P.S.® distribution program can prescribe and dispense.**	Drowsiness, somnolence, peripheral neuropathy, dizziness, orthostatic hypotension, neutropenia, increased HIV viral load, rash.

*Scored.   †Bold entries denote special dental considerations.

NAME	FORM/ STRENGTH	DOSAGE	WARNINGS/PRECAUTIONS & CONTRAINDICATIONS	ADVERSE EFFECTS†
Thalidomide (cont.)		**Maintenance Therapy for Prevention/Suppression of ENL Recurrence:** Use minimum dose to control reaction. **Taper Dose:** Every 3-6 months, attempt to decrease dose by 50mg every 2-4 weeks. *Pediatrics:* **≥12 yrs: Acute ENL: Initial:** 100-300mg qhs with water at least 1 hr after evening meal. **<50kg:** Start therapy at lower end of dosing range. **Severe Cutaneous ENL: Initial:** 400mg qhs with water at least 1 hour after evening meal. Use with corticosteroids in moderate to severe neuritis with severe ENL. Taper steroid where neuritis is ameliorated. Duration of therapy is usually 2 weeks. **Taper Dose:** Decrease by 50mg every 2-4 weeks. **Maintenance Therapy for Prevention/Suppression of ENL Recurrence:** Use minimum dose to control reaction. **Taper Dose:** Every 3-6 months, attempt to decrease dose by 50mg every 2-4 weeks.	**W/P:** If hypersensitivity reaction occurs such as rash, fever, tachycardia, discontinue drug. Stevens-Johnson syndrome and toxic epidermal necrolysis reported. Can cause severe birth defects. Drowsiness and somnolence reported, caution when operating machinery. May cause neuropathy, monitor for symptoms. If symptoms of neuropathy arise, discontinue immediately. Do not initiate if ANC <750/mm³. Measure viral load of HIV patients after 1st and 3rd month of therapy and every 3 months thereafter. **Contra:** Women of childbearing potential unless alternative therapies are considered inappropriate and if precautions are taken to avoid pregnancy. Sexually mature males unless they comply with the S.T.E.P.S.® program and mandatory contraceptive measures. **P/N:** Category X, not for use in nursing.	

SULFONE

NAME	FORM/ STRENGTH	DOSAGE	WARNINGS/PRECAUTIONS & CONTRAINDICATIONS	ADVERSE EFFECTS†
Dapsone	**Tab:** 25mg*, 100mg*	*Adults:* **Dermatitis Herpetiformis: Initial:** 50mg/day. **Usual:** 50-300mg/day, may increase dose if needed. Reduce to minimum maintenance dose. **Leprosy:** Give with 1 or more anti-leprosy drugs. **Maint:** 100mg/day. *Pediatrics:* Same schedule as adults but with correspondingly smaller doses.	**W/P:** Agranulocytosis, aplastic anemia and other blood dyscrasias reported. CBC weekly for the 1st month, monthly for 6 months and semi-annually thereafter. Discontinue if a significant reduction in leukocytes, platelets or hemopoiesis occurs. Treat severe anemia prior to therapy. Discontinue if sensitivity occurs. Caution in those with G6PD deficiency, methemoglobin reductase deficiency, or hemoglobin M. Toxic hepatitis and cholestatic jaundice reported. Monitor LFT's. **P/N:** Category C, not for use in nursing.	Hemolysis, peripheral neuropathy, nausea, vomiting, abdominal pain, pancreatitis, vertigo, blurred vision, tinnitus, insomnia, fever, headache, psychosis, phototoxicity, pulmonary eosinophilia, tachycardia, albuminuria, renal papillary necrosis, male infertility.

MISCELLANEOUS

NAME	FORM/ STRENGTH	DOSAGE	WARNINGS/PRECAUTIONS & CONTRAINDICATIONS	ADVERSE EFFECTS†
Etanercept (Enbrel)	**Inj:** 25mg [vial], 50mg/ mL [syringe]	*Adults:* **≥18 yrs: RA/Psoriatic Arthritis/AS:** 50mg SC per week, given as one SC injection. May continue MTX, glucocorticoids, salicylates, NSAIDs, or analgesics. **Psoriasis: Initial:** 50mg SC twice weekly given 3 or 4 days apart for 3 months. May begin with 25-50mg/week. **Maint:** 50mg/week. *Pediatrics:* **4-17 yrs: JRA:** 0.8mg/kg SC per week. **Max:** 50mg/week. **Max per injection site:** 25mg. **≤31kg:** One SC injection once weekly. **>31kg:** Two SC injections on same day or 3 or 4 days apart. May continue glucocorticoids, NSAIDs, or analgesics.	**W/P:** Discontinue if severe allergic reaction or infection (eg, sepsis) occurs. May cause autoimmune antibodies. Serious, fatal infections including sepsis reported. Avoid with active infections. Monitor closely if develop new infection. JRA patients should be brought up to date with current immunization guidelines prior to initiating therapy. Discontinue temporarily with significant varicella virus exposure and consider prophylaxis. Avoid with Wegener's granulomatosis. **Contra:** Sepsis. **P/N:** Category B, not for use in nursing.	(Adults, pediatrics) Injection site reactions, infections, headache. (Pediatrics) Varicella, gastroenteritis, depression, cutaneous ulcer, esophagitis.
Infliximab (Remicade)	**Inj:** 100mg	*Adults:* **RA (Combo with MTX):** 3mg/kg IV, repeat at 2 and 6 weeks. **Maint:** 3mg/kg every 8 weeks. **Incomplete Response:** Increase to 10mg/kg or give every 4 weeks. **Crohn's Disease/Fistulizing Crohn's Disease: Induction Regimen:** 5mg/kg IV at 0, 2, and 6 weeks. **Maint:** 5mg/kg every 8 weeks. For patients who respond then lose	**Reports of TB, invasive fungal infections, and other opportunistic infections. Evaluate for latent TB and treat if necessary prior to initiation of therapy. W/P:** Leukopenia, neutropenia, thrombocytopenia, and pancytopenia reported. Serious infections, including sepsis and pneumonia, reported.	Nausea, infections, infusion reactions, headache, sinusitis, **pharyngitis**, coughing, abdominal pain, diarrhea, bronchitis, dyspepsia, fatigue, rhinitis, pain, arthralgia.

Table 21.1: PRESCRIBING INFORMATION FOR AGENTS USED TO TREAT CONNECTIVE TISSUE DISORDERS AND ORAL MUCOSAL DISEASES *(cont.)*

NAME	FORM/ STRENGTH	DOSAGE	WARNINGS/PRECAUTIONS & CONTRAINDICATIONS	ADVERSE EFFECTS†
MISCELLANEOUS *(cont.)*				
Infliximab *(cont.)*		their response, may increase to 10mg/kg. Consider discontinuing therapy if no response to therapy by week 14. **Ankylosing Spondylitis:** 5mg/kg IV, repeat at 2 and 6 weeks. **Maint:** 5mg/kg every 6 weeks. **Psoriatic Arthritis:** 5mg/kg IV, repeat at 2 and 6 weeks. **Maint:** 5mg/kg every 8 weeks. May be used with or without MTX. **Ulcerative Colitis:** 5mg/kg at 0, 2, and 6 weeks. **Maint:** 5mg/kg every 8 weeks.	Avoid with active infection. Monitor for signs of infection during and after therapy; discontinue if serious infection develops. Caution in patients who have resided in areas where histoplasmosis or coccidioidomycosis are endemic. Hypersensitivity reactions reported. Caution with optic neuritis, chronic and recurrent infections, CNS demyelinating disease (eg, MS) and seizure disorder. May result in autoantibody formation; discontinue if lupus-like syndrome develops. Monitor closely and discontinue if new or worsening symptoms of heart failure appear. Lymphoma reported; caution with malignancies. Severe hepatic reactions, including acute liver failure, jaundice, hepatitis and cholestasis have been reported rarely. Caution in elderly. **Contra:** Hypersensitivity to murine proteins. Moderate or severe CHF (NYHA Class III/IV) with doses >5mg/kg. **P/N:** Category B, not for use in nursing.	
Cevimeline (Evoxac)	**Cap:** 30mg	**Adults:** 30mg tid.	**W/P:** May alter cardiac conduction and/or heart rate; caution with angina or MI. Potential to increase airway resistance, bronchial smooth muscle tone, and bronchial secretions; caution with controlled asthma, chronic bronchitis, or COPD. Toxicity characterized by exaggerated parasympathomimetic effects (eg, headache, visual disturbance, lacrimation, sweating, respiratory distress, GI spasm, nausea, vomiting, cardiac abnormalities, mental confusion, tremors). Caution with history of nephrolithiasis, cholelithiasis. Ophthalmic formulations decrease visual acuity; caution while night driving or hazardous activities in reduced lighting. **Contra:** Uncontrolled asthma, when miosis in undesirable (eg, acute iritis, narrow-angle glaucoma). **P/N:** Category C, not for use in nursing.	Excessive sweating, nausea, rhinitis, diarrhea, cough, sinusitis, upper respiratory infection.
Tacrolimus (Protopic)	**Oint:** 0.03%, 0.1% [30g, 60g, 100g]	**Adults:** (0.03% or 0.1%) Apply thin layer bid. Rub in gently. Continue for 1 week after symptoms clear. **Pediatrics: ≥16 yrs:** (0.03% or 0.1%) Apply thin layer bid. Rub in gently. Continue for 1 week after symptoms clear. **2-15 yrs:** (0.03%) Apply thin layer bid. Rub in gently. Continue for 1 week after symptoms clear.	**W/P:** Do not use with occlusive dressings. Increased risk of varicella zoster, herpes simplex, or eczema herpeticum. Lymphadenopathy reported; monitor closely. Discontinue if unknown etiology of lymphadenopathy or presence of acute infectious mononucleosis. Avoid in Netherton's syndrome. Minimize or avoid exposure to natural or artificial sunlight. **P/N:** Category C, not for use in nursing.	Skin burning, pruritus, flu-like symptoms, allergic reaction, skin erythema, headache, skin infection, fever, herpes simplex, rhinitis.

*Scored.   †Bold entries denote special dental considerations.

Table 21.2: DRUG INTERACTIONS FOR AGENTS USED TO TREAT CONNECTIVE TISSUE DISORDERS AND ORAL MUCOSAL DISEASES

ANTIMALARIAL AGENT

Hydroxychloroquine Sulfate (Plaquenil)

Hepatotoxic drugs	Caution with hepatotoxic drugs.

GOLD COMPOUND

Gold Sodium Thiomalate (Myochrysine)

Penicillamine	May cause bone marrow depression and rash.

IMMUNOSUPPRESSIVE DRUGS

Azathioprine (Imuran)

ACE inhibitors	May induce anemia, leukopenia.
Allopurinol	Reduce dose by one third to one fourth.
Cotrimazole	May exaggerate leukopenia.
Warfarin	Inhibited anticoagulant effects of warfarin.

Cyclophosphamide (Cytoxan)

Doxorubicin	Potentiates doxorubicin induced cardiotoxicity.
Phenobarbital	High doses increase metabolism and leukopenic activity.
Succinylcholine-chloride	Potentiates effects of succinylcholine.

Cyclosporine (Sandimmune, Neoral)

ACE inhibitors	Caution with ACE inhibitors.
Allopurinol	May increase levels.
Amiodarone	May increase levels.
Amphotericin B	May potentiate renal dysfunction.
Angiotensin II blockers	Caution with angiotensin II blockers.
Azaporpazon	May potentiate renal dysfunction.
Azithromycin	May increase levels.
Bezafirate	May potentiate renal dysfunction.
Bromocriptine	May increase levels.
Carbamazepine	May decrease levels.
Cimetidine	May potentiate renal dysfunction.
Ciprofloxacin	May potentiate renal dysfunction.
Clarithromycin	May increase levels.

Table 21.2: DRUG INTERACTIONS FOR AGENTS USED TO TREAT CONNECTIVE TISSUE DISORDERS AND ORAL MUCOSAL DISEASES *(cont.)*

IMMUNOSUPPRESSIVE DRUGS *(cont.)*

Cyclosporine (Sandimmune, Neoral) *(cont.)*

Colchicine	May potentiate renal dysfunction; may increase levels.
Danazol	May increase levels.
Diclofenac	May potenetiate renal dysfunction.
Diltiazem	May increase levels.
Erythromycin	May increase levels.
Fenofibrate	May potentiate renal dysfunction.
Fluconazole	May increase levels.
Gentamicin	May potentiate renal dysfunction.
Grapefruit juice	May decrease levels.
Imatinib	May increase levels.
Itraconazole	May increase levels.
Ketoconazole	May potentiate renal dysfunction; may increase levels.
Live vaccines	Avoid live vaccines.
Melphalan	May potentiate renal dysfunction.
Methylprednisolone	Convulsion reported with high dose.
Metoclopramide	May increase levels.
Naficillin	May decrease levels.
Naproxen	May potentiate renal dysfunction.
Nicardipine	May increase levels.
Nifedipine	Frequent gingival hyperplasia.
NSAIDs	Caution with NSAIDs.
Octreotide	May decrease levels.
Oral contraceptives	May increase levels.
Orlistat	May decrease levels.
Phenobarbital	May decrease levels.
Phenytoin	May decrease levels.
Potassium-sparing diuretics	Avoid with potassium-sparing diuretics.
Protease inhibitors	May increase levels.
Quinupristin	May increase levels.

IMMUNOSUPPRESSIVE DRUGS *(cont.)*

Cyclosporine (Sandimmune, Neoral) *(cont.)*

Ranitidine	May potentiate renal dysfunction.
Rifampin	May decrease levels.
Sirolimus	Increased levels of sirolimus; give 4 hrs after cyclosporine.
SMZ/TMP	May potentiate renal dysfunction.
Statins	Myotoxicity with statins.
St. John's wort	May decrease levels.
Sulfinpyrazone	May decrease levels.
Sulindac	May potentiate renal dysfunction.
Tacrolimus	May potentiate renal dysfunction.
Terbinafine	May decrease levels.
Ticlopidine	May decrease levels.
Tobramycin	May potentiate renal dysfunction.
Vancomycin	May potentiate renal dysfunction.
Verapamil	May increase levels.

Mycophenolate Mofetil (Cellcept)

Acyclovir	May increase levels.
Antacids (magnesium- and aluminum-containing)	Decreases levels; space dosing.
Azithioprine	Additive bone marrow suppression; avoid use.
Cholestyramine	Reduced efficacy with drugs that interfere with enterohepatic recirculation.
Ganciclovir	May increase levels.
Live attenuated vaccines	Avoid live attenuated vaccines.
Oral contraceptives	Decreased effects of oral contraceptives.
Probenecid	May increase levels.

Penicillamine (Cupramine)

Antimalarial drugs	Hematologic and renal adverse reactions increased.
Cytotoxic drugs	Hematologic and renal adverse reactions increased.
Gold therapy	Hematologic and adverse renal reactions increased.

Table 21.2: DRUG INTERACTIONS FOR AGENTS USED TO TREAT CONNECTIVE TISSUE DISORDERS AND ORAL MUCOSAL DISEASES *(cont.)*

IMMUNOSUPPRESSIVE DRUGS *(cont.)*

Penicillamine (Cupramine) *(cont.)*

Iron	Systemic levels lowered by iron; separate doses by 2 hrs.
Oxyphenbutazole	Hematologic and renal adverse reactions increased.
Phenylbutazone	Hematologic and renal adverse reactions increased.

RECURRENT APHTHOUS STOMATITIS DRUGS

Colchicine

Acidifying agents	Inhibited by acidifying agents.
Alkalinizing agents	Potentiated by alkalinizing agents.
CNS depressants	Potentiates CNS depressants.
Sympathomimetics	Potentiates sympathomimetic agents.

Pentoxifylline (Trental)

Antihypertensives	May increase effect of antihypertensives.
Theophylline	May increase theophylline levels; risk of theophylline toxicity.
Warfarin	Increased risk of bleeding; monitor PT/INR more frequently.

RETINOID

Isotretinoin (Accutane)

Alcohol	Limit alcohol consumption.
Corticosteroids	Caution with drugs that cause drug-induced osteoporosis/osteomalacia and affect vitamin D metabolism.
Tetracyclines	Increased incidence of pseudotumor cerebri.
Oral contraceptives	Pregnancy reported with oral and injectable/implantable contraceptives; may cause break-through bleeding with oral contraceptives.
St. John's wort	Avoid St. John's wort.
Vitamin A	Avoid vitamin A.

SEDATIVE-HYPNOTIC AGENT

Thaliomide (Thalomid)

Alcohol	Enhanced sedation.
Barbiturates	Enhanced sedation.
Chlorpromazine	Enhanced sedation.
Reserpine	Enhanced sedation.

SULFONE

Dapsone

Folic acid antagonists (eg, pyrimethamine)	May increase hematologic reactions.
Rifampin	Lowers plasma levels.
Trimethoprim	Raises the level of each other.

MISCELLANEOUS

Etanercept (Enbrel)

Live vaccines	Do not give live vaccines.
Cyclophosphamide	Avoid with cyclophosphamide.

Infliximab (Remicade)

Anakinra	May increase risk of serious infections and neutropenia.
Live vaccines	Do not give live vaccines.

Cevimeline (Evoxac)

β-antagonists	Possible conduction disturbances.
CYP450 2D6 deficiency	Caution with deficiency.
CYP450 2D6 inhibitors	Inhibit the metabolism of cevimeline.
CYP450 3A3/4 inhibitors	Inhibit the metabolism of cevimeline.
Parasympathomimetics	Additive effects with parasympathomimetics.

Tacrolimus (Protopic)

CYP450 3A4 inhibitors	Caution with CYP 3A4 inhibitors in widespread and/or erythrodermic disease.
Immunosuppressive therapy	Increased risk of lymphomas in transplant patients receiving other immunosuppresive therapy.

Chapter 22

Skeletal Muscle Relaxants

Lida Radfar D.D.S., M.S.; Lakshmanan Suresh, D.D.S., M.S.

Skeletal muscle relaxants have a myriad of indications in dentistry. They may be used to reduce facial pain from muscle spasms associated with temporomandibular disorders and trismus after dental or oral surgical procedures. In addition, centrally acting muscle relaxants such as benzodiazepines are commonly used as antianxiety agents for patients undergoing dental procedures.

Muscle relaxants are divided into two major therapeutic groups: neuromuscular blockers and spasmolytics. Neuromuscular blockers are peripherally acting agents used primarily in combination with general anesthetics to induce muscle relaxation and, thus, provide an optimal surgical working condition. Spasmolytics are centrally acting agents used to reduce spasticity in a variety of neurologic conditions such as cerebral palsy, inflammation and multiple sclerosis. Drugs within this class of muscle relaxants also are commonly used for antianxiety effects and to induce amnesia. The skeletal muscles are innervated by large myelinated nerve fibers that originate in the large motor neurons of the spinal cord. The nerve ending joins the muscle at the neuromuscular junction. When the action potential in the nerve reaches the nerve terminal, a neurotransmitter is released. In the case of skeletal muscle, the neurotransmitter is acetylcholine. Acetylcholine is released into the synaptic cleft, which allows it to bind to its receptor on the muscle membrane. This binding results in a conformational change that increases the permeability of the muscle terminal to potassium and sodium ions, leading to skeletal muscle contraction. The released acetylcholine is removed from the end plate by diffusion and rapid enzymatic destruction by acetylcholinesterase.

Neuromuscular Blockers

Neuromuscular blocking agents are used to produce paralysis and are structurally similar to acetylcholine. These drugs can be divided into depolarizing and nondepolarizing agents. Neuromuscular blocking agents are potentially hazardous medications and should be administered only by highly trained clinicians in a setting where respiratory and cardiovascular resuscitation are immediately available; therefore, they are not used routinely in the dental office.

This chapter provides a summary of neuromuscular blocking agents; however, these drugs are to be used only by clinicians trained in sedation and general anesthesia. Those administering any kind of general anesthetic or sedative should be well-versed in the drug's applications and contraindications. This text is not intended to be comprehensive in terms of information on sedative/general anesthetic agents. General prescribing information for these drugs can be found in Appendix N; for more specific details, consult anesthesia texts.

Depolarizing Neuromuscular Blockers

Succinylcholine is an example of a depolarizing neuromuscular blocker and is the only one used clinically. It provides rapid induction of paralysis to facilitate intubation of the trachea during induction of anesthesia. The most common use of succinylcholine in dental practice is to break a laryngospasm that occurs in a patient undergoing conscious sedation. The intravenous dose of succinylcholine to treat laryngospasm is 0.2-0.5mg/kg. If intravenous access is unavailable, 2-5mg/kg can be given sublingually or intramuscularly. Neuromuscular blocking agents are administered parenterally.

See Tables 22.1 and 22.2 for general information on succinylcholine.

Special Dental Considerations

The sustained depolarization produced by initial administration of succinylcholine is manifested initially by transient generalized skeletal muscle contractions known as fasciculations. Various degrees of increased muscle tension in the masseter muscles may develop with succinylcholine, especially in pediatric patients. In extreme cases, trismus can occur and make it difficult to open the mouth for intubation of the trachea. Patients who develop trismus with succinylcholine administration are prone to developing malignant hyperthermia.

Head, neck, abdomen and back myalgia can occur postoperatively owing to muscle fasciculation associated with depolarization.

Succinylcholine is a general anesthetic agent and should be used only by clinicians trained in sedation and general anesthesia.

Drug interactions of dental interest

Succinylcholine causes paralysis and does not have anesthetic or analgesic effects. Therefore, the dentist must ensure that not only paralysis but also adequate anesthesia has been achieved before performing procedures.

No interactions/contraindications are reported regarding the use of succinylcholine with general anesthetic for dental procedures performed in a surgical setting.

Laboratory value alterations

- Hyperkalemia sufficient to cause cardiac arrest may follow administration of succinylcholine; patients at risk include those with denervation of skeletal muscle, major burns, multiple trauma or upper motor neuron injury.

Pharmacology

Succinylcholine is an example of a depolarizing neuromuscular blocker and is the only one used clinically. It binds to the acetylcholine receptor and causes a prolonged depolarization of the postsynaptic membrane. This initial depolarization causes muscle contraction, which is seen clinically as muscle fasciculations throughout the patient's body. The duration of these initial contractions is short. The sustained depolarization of the postsynaptic membrane does not allow the function of acetylcholine to take place, because a depolarized membrane cannot respond to the release of acetylcholine.

These agents are metabolized by plasma cholinesterase, an enzyme found in the bloodstream but not in the synaptic cleft. Therefore, the duration of a depolarizing muscle relaxant is related to the rate of diffusion from the neuromuscular junction. In rare cases, a patient may have an atypical plasma cholinesterase that is not as effective in metabolizing the drug. In such patients, the action of depolarizing agents may be significantly prolonged. The function of a patient's plasma cholinesterase activity can be evaluated according to his or her dibucaine number. Dibucaine is an amide local anesthetic that reduces the function of normal cholinesterase to a greater degree than it diminishes atypical cholinesterase. This number reflects the quality, but not the quantity, of plasma cholinesterase. Any dentist administering a drug metabolized by plasma cholinesterase to a patient with a suspected history of plasma cholinesterase deficiency should obtain a dibucaine number to assess the quality of the patient's plasma cholinesterase enzyme system.

Adverse Effects, Precautions and Contraindications

Succinylcholine mimics acetylcholine at the cardiac postganglionic muscarinic receptors and induces cardiac dysrhythmias. Cardiac dysrhythmias including sinus bradycardia, junctional rhythm, and sinus arrest have occurred after administration of succinylcholine.

Many medications used for general anesthesia are potential triggers for malignant hyperthermia, and clinicians should be aware of this potentially fatal hypermetabolism of skeletal muscle.

Transient increases in ocular pressure are seen 2-4 minutes after injection of succinylcholine. Theoretically, succinylcholine may contribute to extrusion of intraocular contents in patients with open eye injuries.

Fasciculations induced by succinylcholine lead to unpredictable increases in gastric pressure and may cause gastric fluid to pass into the esophagus and pharynx, thus resulting in pulmonary aspiration.

Table 22.1 presents adverse effects and precautions/contraindications associated with succinylcholine.

Nondepolarizing Neuromuscular Blockers

Nondepolarizing neuromuscular blockers act through competitive inhibition of acetylcholine. They are useful for prolonged muscle relaxation in the operating room and intensive care units due to their long duration of action. Nondepolarizing neuromuscular blockers are categorized based on the duration of action as long-acting, intermediate-acting and short-acting. Examples include gallamine, atracurium, and vecuronium. The use of these drugs is primarily limited to muscle relaxation for general anesthesia.

Special Dental Considerations

Drug interactions of dental interest

No special consideration or drug intersctions/contraindications are reported regarding the use of nondedepolarizing neuromuscular blockers with general anesthetic for dental procedures. Nondepolarizing neuromuscular blockers have limited ability to cross lipid membrane barriers. Therefore, this class of drugs does not affect the fetus.

Pharmacology

Nondepolarizing neuromuscular blockers have structure similar to that of acetylcholine, which enables them to bind at the same receptor as that neurotransmitter. When the majority of acetylcholine receptors are bound by neuromuscular blockers, acetylcholine can no longer bind to the receptor. This mechanism produces the profound muscle relaxation characteristic of this class of skeletal muscle relaxants. The use of these drugs is primarily limited to muscle relaxation for general anesthesia.

The majority of nondepolarizing drugs are eliminated through renal excretion; however, some also undergo metabolism in the liver, ester hydrolysis or Hoffman elimination. Regardless of how these agents are metabolized, their duration of action is determined primarily by how rapidly they are redistributed to the peripheral tissues.

Adverse Effects, Precautions and Contraindications

Nondepolarizing neuromuscular blockers cause cardiovascular effects, and the dentist should take into consideration these agents' specific cardiovascular manifestations when selecting the appropriate agents for a patient. These cardiac effects usually are transient and vary because of these agents' interactions with other medications. Many drugs used in anesthetic practice can trigger malignant hyperthermia; clinicians should consider this when obtaining the patient's medical history before beginning treatment. Skeletal muscle fasciculations do not occur with onset of action of nondepolarizing neuromuscular blocking agents.

This category of medications is highly ionized at physiologic pH and has limited lipid solubility, resulting in a small volume of distribution primarily in the extracellular fluid. They have limited ability to cross lipid membrane barriers. Therefore, this class of drugs has few central nervous system effects and minimal oral and renal absorption; it also does not affect the fetus.

Spasmolytics

Spasmolytics are drugs which eliminate muscular spasms. The primary use of spasmolytics in the dental office is to relieve anxiety, postprocedural trismus, and muscle spasms of the head and neck including temporomandibular disorders. These agents often are used in conjunction with heat, physical therapy, rest and analgesics. Some of these agents have anxiolytic properties that may help reduce muscle tension.

Spasmolytics may be used to manage spasticity owing to systemic disease. Spasticity refers to abnormalities of regulation of skeletal muscle tone that result from lesions in the central nervous system (CNS). The most effective agents for control of spasticity include two that act directly on the CNS (benzodiazepines and baclofen) and one that acts directly on skeletal muscle (dantrolene).

Tables 22.1 and 22.2 present general information on spasmolytics.

Benzodiazepines

More than 2,000 benzodiazepines have been synthesized. Among these, several are recommended as spasmolytics: chlordiazepoxide, clonazepam, diazepam, lorazepam and midazolam. Although benzodiazepines exert similar clinical effects, differences in their pharmacokinetic properties have led to varying therapeutic applications. Chlordiazepoxide and diazepam are considered the prototypic drugs of their class.

Benzodiazepines have sedative-hypnotic, muscle relaxant, anxiolytic and anticonvulsant effects. The antianxiety effects of this class of drugs make them an excellent choice for preoperative oral sedation in the fearful dental patient.

Most benzodiazepines reduce sleep latency and reduce the number of awakenings. They can be used for insomnia, but prescribing for this purpose should be done only by a clinician who is an expert in sleep disorders. Prolonged use of benzodiazepines for insomnia can have serious detrimental effects on the sleep cycle. When administered intravenously, diazepam can be used to break status epilepticus in patients who suffer from grand mal seizures.

Chlordiazepoxide. Chlordiazepoxide is the original prototype for the benzodiazepines. It has been demonstrated to have sedative, anxiolytic and weak analgesic properties. Chlordiazepoxide is used for treatment of anxiety disorders, short-term anxiety and preoperative anxiety. It is not recommended for the management of stress associated with everyday life. Paradoxical reactions, including excitement and rage, have been reported, especially in psychiatric patients and hyperactive pediatric patients.

Clonazepam. General medical use of clonazepam includes use for treatment of seizures and panic disorders. In dentistry, it has been used for treatment of acute myofascial pain and burning mouth syndrome. No formal recommendations of dosage have been made for its use in this area, and it is usually given in doses similar to those used for panic disorders.

Diazepam. Diazepam is useful as an anxiolytic and as a spasmolytic. When administered intravenously, diazepam can be used to break status epilepticus in patients who suffer from grand mal seizures.

Lorazepam. Lorazepam produces excellent amnesia. Unfortunately, its peak onset can occur as long as 2-4 hours after oral administration. Its long duration and slow onset make it impractical as an oral sedative for outpatient procedures.

Midazolam. Midazolam is a rapid-onset, short-acting benzodiazepine that is commonly used intravenously for conscious sedation in an outpatient environment. It has good anxiolytic and amnesic effects, making it an excellent choice for IV sedation.

Special Dental Considerations

Benzodiazepines in general do not have any adverse interactions with dental materials. No special precautions are required for local anesthetic administration in conjunction with their use. Xerostomia is a common side effect that reverses itself when use of the medication is discontinued.

Drug interactions of dental interest

CNS depressants (alcohol, barbiturates, opioids) may enhance sedation and respiratory depression.

Patients with convulsant disorders may experience an increase in grand mal seizure activity with benzodiazepines; therefore, an increase in their standard anticonvulsant medication may be indicated.

Theophylline may antagonize the sedative effects of midazolam. Cimetidine may increase midazolam's serum concentrations.

Laboratory value alterations

- Isolated reports of benzodiazepine-associated neutropenia and jaundice exist, so periodic blood counts and liver function tests are recommended during long-term benzodiazepine therapy.

Pharmacology

The action of benzodiazepines is the result of potentiating the neural inhibition that is mediated by aminobutyric acid (GABA) resulting in relaxation of skeletal muscles.

Benzodiazepines are metabolized by the cytochrome p-450 system in the liver and then are excreted by the kidney. The rate of elimination depends on the drug's half-life. The duration of action of specific benzodiazepines ranges from short to very long.

Benzodiazepines with long half-lives accumulate during repeated dosages and even with a single dose. This is of particular concern in elderly people, in whom half-life may be increased two- to fourfold. Several benzodiazepines, such as diazepam (see below), produce active metabolites when they are metabolized. Metabolites of lorazepam and oxazepam are inactive and, therefore, make these drugs safer than diazepam for patients with liver disease.

Chlordiazepoxide. Chlordiazepoxide's mechanism of action is not known. Animal studies suggest that it acts on the limbic system of the brain (which is involved with emotional response).

Clonazepam. The mechanism of action of clonazepam is not fully understood. Its proposed pharmacologic effects are related to its ability to increase GABA activity. Peak concentrations of clonazepam are reached 1-4 hours after oral administration. The elimination half-life is about 30-40 hours.

Diazepam. The metabolism of diazepam warrants special attention. Diazepam is metabolized into desmethyldiazepam, an active metabolite. Desmethyldiazepam can reenter the bloodstream through the enterohepatic circulation and produce delayed-onset sedation. Therefore, even after the initial effects of diazepam have disappeared, the patient must not engage in any potentially dangerous activity for 24 hours. Diazepam is known to act on the limbic system and induce a calming effect. The peak onset of diazepam occurs 30-60 minutes after oral administration.

Lorazepam. Lorazepam acts on the CNS, resulting in a tranquilizing effect. IM onset of hypnosis is 20-30 minutes. Duration of action is 6-8 hours.

Midazolam. Midazolam is a short-acting, water-soluble benzodiazepine that depresses the CNS.

Adverse Effects, Precautions and Contraindications

Benzodiazepines may cause varying degrees of lightheadedness, motor incoordination, ataxia, impaired psychomotor and mental function, confusion, amnesia, dry mouth and bitter taste. Other side effects include headache, blurred vision, vertigo, nausea, vomiting, epigastric distress, joint pain, chest pain and incontinence. Anticonvulsant benzodiazepines can increase the frequency of seizures in patients with epilepsy. Benzodiazepines can have paradoxical effects such as nightmares, restlessness, hallucinations, paranoia, depression, unusual uninhibited behavior and occasional suicidal ideation. When the drug is administered in oral doses at the intended time of sleep, weakness and other previously mentioned side effects may not be noticed. It is considered undesirable if the drug was administered at bedtime and side effects persist during waking hours.

Benzodiazepines have a low incidence of abuse and dependence; however, the possibility must not be overlooked. Mild dependence may occur in patients who have taken benzodiazepines for a prolonged period. Tolerance to benzodiazepines can develop.

Benzodiazepines slightly reduce alveolar ventilation in preanesthetic doses. This group of drugs may cause CO_2 narcosis in patients with chronic obstructive pulmonary disease. Apnea can occur when benzodiazepines are given during general anesthesia or in combination with opioids. Cases have been reported in which respiratory distress has occurred when patients have combined benzodiazepines with other CNS depressants such as alcohol. Patients should be warned of potentially serious interactions with ethanol. Because their cognitive and motor function may be impaired, patients should be advised not to drive or participate in other potentially dangerous activities. Long-acting benzodiazepines have been associated with falls in elderly people and should be avoided in this patient population.

A specific benzodiazepine should be avoided if a patient has a known hypersensitivity to it. It should be noted that a cross-sensitivity between various benzodiazepines may exist. Benzodiazepines should be administered with caution to patients with liver disease or impaired renal function. They should not be used in patients who have CNS or respiratory depression or who are comatose. Benzodiazepines should not be administered to pregnant or nursing women. An increased risk of congenital malformations is associated with the use of tranquilizers during the first trimester of pregnancy. Patients with narrow-angle glaucoma should not receive benzodiazapines.

Clonazepam. Clonazepam should not be used in patients with a history of adverse reactions to benzodiazepines. It should be administered with caution to patients with liver disease or impaired renal function. Clonazepam may increase the incidence or precipitate the onset of grand mal seizures. It has not been shown to interfere with the pharmacokinetics of phenytoin, carbamazepine or phenobarbital. Valproic acid administered concomitantly with clonazepam may produce absence status.

Hypersalivation has been reported with the use of clonazepam; the dentist should consider this when selecting a medication for a patient who has difficulty controlling salivary flow. However, xerostomia is a more common complaint.

Diazepam. Diazepam should not be given to any patient with acute narrow-angle glaucoma. Precautions should be taken when it is administered to patients with a history of seizure disorders, chronic obstructive pulmonary disease or liver failure.

Midazolam. Theophylline may antagonize the sedative effects of midazolam. Cimetidine may increase serum concentrations. CNS depressants increase sedation and respiratory depression.

Benzodiazepine Antagonist: Flumazenil

Flumazenil is a benzodiazepine antagonist that binds to the GABA/benzodiazepine receptor in the CNS. This antagonist has been shown to reverse the effects of sedation, amnesia and respiratory depression in humans. If a benzodiazepine overdose is observed, flumazenil can be administered IV to reverse the effects of the benzodiazepine. Onset of reversal will occur in 1-2 minutes, with peak reversal occurring 6-10 minutes after administration. If a long-acting benzodiazepine has been given, the patient should be re-evaluated about every 20-30 minutes to see if repeat doses of flumazenil are necessary.

Special Dental Considerations

Drug interactions of dental interest
CNS depressants (alcohol, barbiturates, opioids), if used concurrently, may enhance sedation and respiratory depression.

Adverse Effects, Precautions and Contraindications

Side effects of the benzodiazepine antagonists include dizziness, drowsiness, somnolence, confusion and respiratory depression. Cardiovascular effects include palpitations, chest pain and syncope.

Patients may experience anorexia, xerostomia, vomiting and diarrhea.

Other Spasmolytics

Baclofen. Baclofen, a derivative of the inhibitory neurotransmitter GABA, functions as a GABA agonist in the brain as well as in the spinal cord. Baclofen may reduce substance P and, therefore, pain; it also may function as a spasmolytic. It is most effective for spasticity associated with multiple sclerosis and traumatic spinal cord lesions. In dentistry, it can be used for temporomandibular dystonia and is helpful in some cases of trigeminal neuralgia.

Baclofen is especially helpful in alleviating the spasticity of multiple sclerosis and spinal cord injury when administered intrathecally. Baclofen is as effective as, but much less sedating than, diazepam in reducing spasticity. It also does not reduce general muscle strength, as happens with other spasmolytics such as dantrolene.

Dantrolene. Dantrolene is indicated for spasticity secondary to upper motor neuron disease (multiple sclerosis, stroke, cerebral palsy) and is not indicated for spasms caused by rheumatic disorders. Treatment for chronic spasticity requires gradual titration until the patient experiences maximum effect. Dantrolene also is used for the management of malignant hyperthermia. This is a rare, dominantly inherited syndrome that is precipitated by the use of inhalation anesthetics or neuromuscular blocking agents. Vigorous muscle contraction occurs, leading to a rapid and dangerous rise in body temperature, renal failure and rhabdomyolysis. Dantrolene is administered IV immediately during an attack, or it may be administered prophylactically to patients who are susceptible to this syndrome.

Metaxalone. This drug is indicated as an adjunct to rest and physical therapy for the treatment of acute painful musculoskeletal conditions.

Tizanidine. This drug is used for the management of spasticity associated with multiple sclerosis and spinal cord injury. Tizanidine has a short-acting duration and administration should be reserved for daily activities when relief of spasticity is most important.

Special Dental Considerations

Baclofen. No information has been reported indicating the need for special precaution when baclofen is used with local anesthetics and vasoconstrictors.

Dantrolene. The safety of long-term use of dantrolene in humans has not been established.

Metaxalone. Patients with liver damage should undergo liver function tests before surgical procedures.

Tizanidine. Tizanidine has been associated with visual hallucinations or delusions. Before beginning dental treatment, the clinician should assess the psychological status of a patient taking tizanidine.

Drug interactions of dental interest

Baclofen. Lithium decreases the effect of baclofen. Benzodiazepines, antihypertensive agents and opioid analgesics increase baclofen's effect. Increased toxicity is noted when baclofen is administered concomitantly with CNS depressants, alcohol and monoamine oxidase inhibitors. Increased short-term memory loss is noted when baclofen is taken with tricyclic antidepressants.

Dantrolene. Hepatotoxicity has occurred more frequently in women older than 35 years of age who are receiving estrogen therapy while taking dantrolene. The exact interaction is unclear, and caution must be exercised when estrogen and dantrolene are given together.

Cardiovascular collapse has been reported on rare occasion in patients taking both dantrolene and verapamil; therefore, this combination is not recommended. Dantrolene potentiates vecuronium-induced neuromuscular blocking.

Increased toxicity also occurs with concomitant administration of CNS depressants (sedation), MAO inhibitors, phenothiazines, clindamycin (which increase neuromuscular blockade), verapamil (associated with hyperkalemia and cardiac depression), warfarin, clofibrate and tolbutamide.

Metaxalone. No drug interactions are reported. However, this drug is a possible CNS depressant and, therefore, it is suggested that prescribing clinicians follow the precautions for CNS depressant drugs.

Tizanidine. It has been shown that tizanidine and CNS depressants have an additive effect. The effects of tizanidine may be additive when it is taken with other muscle relaxants and sedatives. Oral contraceptives reduce the clearance of tizanidine by approximately 50%. Tizanidine interacts with antihypertensives and may increase levels of antihypertensive drugs.

Laboratory value alterations

- Liver function tests should be obtained on a regular basis to monitor for hepatotoxicity with dantrolene.
- Leukopenia, throbocytopenia and aplastic anemia also have been reported with dantrolene, and patients should be monitored for hematologic abnormalities.

Special patients

Dantrolene. Dantrolene's safety in women who are pregnant or may become pregnant has not been established. Its long-term side effects in the pediatric population younger than 5 years of age have not been established.

Pharmacology

Baclofen. Baclofen is rapidly absorbed and has a half-life of 3-4 hours.

Dantrolene. Dantrolene acts directly on the skeletal muscle by reducing the amount of calcium released from the sarcoplasmic reticulum.

Metaxalone. The mechanism of action for metaxalone is not known at this time, but it is believed it may be due to general CNS depression. It has been established that no direct action takes place at the contractile mechanism of the striated muscle, motor end plate or nerve fiber.

Tizanidine. Tizanidine hydrochloride is an agonist at the α_2-adrenergic receptor site and, therefore, increases the presynaptic inhibition of motor neurons.

Adverse Effects, Precautions and Contraindications

Baclofen. Side effects include dizziness, drowsiness, somnolence, confusion and respiratory depression. Cardiovascular effects include palpitations, chest pain and syncope.

Patients taking baclofen may experience anorexia, xerostomia, vomiting and diarrhea.

Dantrolene. Dantrolene has a serious side effect of hepatotoxicity; therefore, hepatic function should be monitored after this drug is administered. Active hepatic disease, such as hepatitis and cirrhosis, is a contraindication for use of dantrolene. Long-term use should be discontinued if clear benefits are not evident. This agent should be used with caution in patients with impaired pulmonary and cardiac function resulting from myocardial disease. Cardiovascular side effects may include pleural effusion with pericarditis.

Other side effects include weakness, confusion, lightheadedness, drowsiness, severe diarrhea, abdominal cramps, urinary retention, erectile dysfunction, blurred vision and fatigue. These side effects usually are temporary and can be reduced by using a small

initial dose and slowly increasing the dose until the optimal amount is reached. Diarrhea can be severe and require discontinuation of use of dantrolene.

Patients should be cautioned against driving or participating in potentially hazardous activities while taking dantrolene.

Photosensitivity has been associated with dantrolene, and patients taking it should be cautioned to avoid sun exposure.

Taste changes have been noted with dantrolene.

No information has been reported indicating the need for special precautions when dantrolene is used concomitantly with local anesthetics and vasoconstrictors.

Metaxalone. Adverse reactions have included leukopenia and hemolytic anemia. Metaxalone has been associated with false positive results in Benedict's test. It should be used with caution in patients with impaired liver and kidney function and is contraindicated for use with patients who have severe damage.

This drug is contraindicated for patients with a history of drug-induced, hemolytic or other anemias.

Tizanidine. Adverse reactions have included orthostatic hypotension, liver damage, hallucinations and psychotic-like symptoms. Clinicians should use tizanidine with caution in patients who have liver or kidney damage. They should caution patients that limited clinical trials exist with regard to duration of use and use of higher dosages to reduce muscle tone.

Tizanidine should never be used with other α_2-adrenergic agonists.

Spasmolytics for Acute Local Spasm

Many spasmolytic drugs are indicated for the treatment of temporary relief of muscle spasm caused by trauma. Cyclobenzaprine is considered the prototype of this group of drugs. It is structurally related to the tricyclic antidepressants and has similar properties. It is believed to act at the brainstem. Other drugs in this category include carisoprodol, chlorzoxazone, methocarbamol and orphenadrine. These medications are not helpful in the treatment of muscle spasm that is caused by spinal cord injury, CNS disease or systemic disease.

Carisoprodol. Carisoprodol is used for acute skeletal muscle pain in conjunction with rest, physical therapy and other measures used to manage acute skeletal muscle spasm.

Chlorzoxazone. Chlorzoxazone is indicated as an adjunct to rest, physical therapy and other measures for the relief of acute, painful musculoskeletal conditions.

Cyclobenzaprine. Cyclobenzaprine relieves muscle spasm of local origin without interfering with muscle function. It is used as an adjunct to rest and physical therapy for relief of acute painful muscle spasms.

Methocarbamol. Methocarbamol is recommended as an adjunct to rest, physical therapy and other measures to manage acute skeletal muscle spasm.

Orphenadrine. Orphenadrine is used with rest and physical therapy for the treatment of acute skeletal muscle spasms. It is intended for short-term use only, and no studies of its long-term efficacy and safety have been published.

Special Dental Considerations
No complications have been reported with dental treatment of patients taking spasmolytics used for acute local spasm.

Cyclobenzaprine. It is recommended that cyclobenzaprine be used only for short periods (2 weeks), as research demonstrating its effectiveness and safety for prolonged use has not been conducted. This is not likely to be an issue, as the drug is indicated for the treatment of acute painful muscle spasm of short duration.

Drug interactions of dental interest
Cyclobenzaprine. Cyclobenzaprine is closely related to tricyclic antidepressants; it also may interact with monoamine oxidase inhibitors and potentially can lead to hyperpyretic crisis, convulsions and death. It should not be used concomitantly with, or within 14 days of use of, MAO inhibitors. It should be used with caution in patients taking anticholinergic medications.

Laboratory value alterations
- Chlorzoxazone: Liver enzyme changes may occur with use, suggesting hepatic toxicity. Therefore, the dentist should consider monitoring the patient's liver function.
- Cyclobenzaprine: This drug is indicated for short-term use and significant laboratory value changes are not expected. Thrombocytopenia and leukopenia have been reported only rarely, and no causal relationship has been established.
- Methocarbamol may cause inaccurate results in screening tests for 5-hydroxyindoleacetic acid and vanillylmandelic. The dentist should inform the patient's physician when prescribing methocarbamol.

Special patients
Carisoprodol. No reports have been published of studies testing this drug's effect on pregnant or nursing women; therefore, it is suggested that use of carisoprodol be avoided in such patients. The drug is not recommended for use in children.

Chlorzoxazone. No reports have been published of studies testing this drug's effect on pregnant or nursing women; therefore, it is suggested that use of chlorzoxazone be avoided in such patients. There are no established guidelines for its use in children, so it should not be administered to pediatric patients.

Cyclobenzaprine. Animal studies have not demonstrated that cyclobenzaprine poses a risk to the fetus or affects fertility. It has not been determined if this drug is excreted in breast milk; therefore, it should be used cautiously in nursing women.

Methocarbamol. Methocarbamol's safety in pregnant and lactating women has not been established, and it is not known if methocarbamol is excreted in breast milk. Safety in children younger than 12 years has not been established.

Orphenadrine. No studies have been conducted testing orphenadrine's safety in pregnant and nursing women. Neither have pediatric safety and efficacy studies been performed. This agent should be used with caution in patients with coronary insufficiency, cardiac decompensation, tachycardia, palpitations and dysrhythmia.

Pharmacology

Carisoprodol. Carisoprodol is centrally acting and blocks interneuronal activity in the spinal cord. Its onset is rapid and lasts 6 hours. Its exact mechanism of action is not clear, but it is known that carisoprodol does not directly act on skeletal muscle.

Chlorzoxazone. Chlorzoxazone acts primarily at the spinal cord and the subcortical areas of the brain, where it inhibits multisynaptic reflex arcs involved in producing skeletal muscle spasm of varying etiology. Its exact mode of action has not been identified. This drug does not directly relax tense skeletal muscles. Peak blood levels of chlorzoxazone are detected 1-2 hours after oral administration.

Cyclobenzaprine. Cyclobenzaprine primarily acts within the CNS at the brainstem, as opposed to the spinal cord levels. It does not act at the neuromuscular junction or directly on skeletal muscle.

Methocarbamol. The drug's mechanism of action has not been determined, but it may be linked to the drug's CNS depressive abilities.

Orphenadrine. The mode of action of orphenadrine is not clear, but it may be related to its analgesic action. Orphenadrine has mild anticholinergic activity and analgesic properties. It does not directly relax skeletal muscles.

Adverse Effects, Precautions and Contraindications

Table 22.1 presents adverse effects and precautions/contraindications associated with spasmolytics.

Carisoprodol. Carisoprodol is metabolized by the liver and secreted by the kidneys and should be used with caution in patients with impaired liver or kidney function. Other adverse reactions may include drowsiness, malaise, dizziness, lightheadedness, epigastric distress, tachycardia, postural hypotension, facial flushing and, occasionally, idiosyncratic reaction. Seizure threshold may be lowered in patients with convulsive disorders. Patients should be advised of CNS effects and avoid driving and drinking alcohol.

Chlorzoxazone. Cardiovascular side effects include tachycardia and chest pain. Syncope, depression, dizziness, lightheadedness, headaches, trembling, hiccups and shortness of breath have been reported. Angioedema is a noted side effect. Serious and potentially fatal hepatotoxity has been reported with the use of this drug. The mechanism of this is not known, and factors predisposing patients to hepatotoxity have not been identified. Patients should be instructed to report early signs of toxicity such as dark urine, anorexia or upper-right-quadrant pain. Liver enzymes should be monitored if this drug is administered on a long-term basis. Other adverse reactions may include drowsiness, malaise, lightheadedness and, occasionally, overstimulation. Idiosyncratic reactions have been manifested as severe muscle weakness, confusion and ataxia. Patients may note a discoloration of the urine as a result of a phenolic metabolite of chlorzoxazone. This discoloration has no clinical significance.

Cyclobenzaprine. Cyclobenzaprine's potential side effects include drowsiness, malaise, tachycardia and dysrhythmia. Cyclobenzaprine may enhance the effects of alcohol, barbiturates and other CNS depressants. Cyclobenzaprine should be used with caution in patients who have a history of urinary retention, closed-angle glaucoma and increased intraocular pressure. It is contraindicated in patients who are taking MAO inhibitors or who have hyperthyroidism, congestive heart failure or dysrhythmias. This drug has no reported interactions with dental materials. No information has been reported indicating the need for special precautions with concomitant use of local anesthetics/vasoconstrictors. Patients may experience xerostomia while taking cyclobenzaprine.

Methocarbamol. Methocarbamol has CNS depressant effects. Patients taking CNS depressants should be cautioned not to combine methocarbamol with alcohol or other CNS depressants. Renal impairment has occurred on rare occasions as a side effect of methocarbamol use. Lightheadedness, dizziness, drowsiness, nausea, blurred vision, headache and fever are common side effects. The drug should be used with caution in patients with renal disease, hepatic disease, seizure disorders, myasthenia gravis and addictive personality.

Orphenadrine. As with all spasmolytic agents, orphenadrine may cause lightheadedness, drowsiness and syncope. This medication contains sodium bisulfate and may cause severe allergic reactions in patients with sulfite sensitivity. Sulfite sensitivity is seen more frequently in asthmatic patients. On rare occasions, aplastic anemia has been reported with orphenadrine use. It has mild anticholinergic effects, which may result in dry mouth and constipation. Other side effects include urinary retention, tachycardia, palpitations, blurred vision, dilation of pupils or gastric irritation. This drug can cause increased ocular tension and is contraindicated in patients with glaucoma. Orphenadrine also is contraindicated in people with pyloric or duodenal obstruction, prostate hypertrophy or obstruction of the bladder, cardiospasm and myasthenia gravis.

Suggested Readings

Drug Facts and Comparisons 2006. 60th ed. St. Louis: Facts and Comparisons; 2006.

Beebe FA, Barkin RL, Barkin S. A clinical and pharmacologic review of skeletal muscle relaxants for musculoskeletal conditions. Am J Ther. 2005;12:151-71.

Neidle EA, Yagiela JA. Pharmacology and therapeutics for dentistry. 4th ed. Philadelphia: C.V. Mosby Co.; 1998.

Physicians' Desk Reference. 60th ed. Montvale, N.J.: Thomson PDR; 2006.

Table 22.1: PRESCRIBING INFORMATION FOR SKELETAL MUSCLE RELAXANTS

NAME	FORM/ STRENGTH	DOSAGE	WARNINGS/PRECAUTIONS & CONTRAINDICATIONS	ADVERSE EFFECTS†
NEUROMUSCULAR BLOCKERS				
Mivacurium Chloride (Mivacron)	**Inj:** 2mg/mL	***Adults:*** Individualize dose. **Initial:** 0.15mg/kg over 5-15 seconds, 0.2mg/kg over 30 seconds, or 0.25mg/kg in divided doses (0.15mg/kg followed in 30 seconds by 0.1mg/kg. **Continuous Infusion: Initial:** 9-10mcg/kg/min. If initiated simultaneously with administration of initial dose, use lower rate (eg, 4mcg/kg/min). **Maint:** 5-7mcg/kg/min. ***Pediatrics:*** Individualize dose. **2-12 years: Initial:** 0.2mg/kg over 5-15 seconds. **Continuous Infusion: Average:** 14mcg/kg/min. **Range:** 5-31mcg/kg/min.	**W/P:** Employ peripheral nerve stimulator to measure neuromuscular function. Neuromuscular block should not be induced before unconscious- ness. Use with great caution, if at all, in patients known to be or suspected of being homozygous for the atypical plasma cholinesterase gene. May not be compatible with alkaline solutions having a pH >8.5. Multiple dose vials contain benzyl alcohol. May cause possible histamine release. Caution with cardiovascular disease. Use ideal body weight to determine initial dose in obese patients. May have a profound effect with neuromuscular diseases (eg, myasthenia gravis and myasthenic syndrome). Actions may be potentiated or antagonized by acid- base and/or serum electrolyte abnor- malities. Neuromuscular block may be prolonged with renal/hepatic disease, or reduced plasma cholinesterase. **Contra:** (MDV) Benzyl alcohol allergy. **P/N:** Category C, caution in nursing.	Flushing, hypotension, tachycardia, bradycar- dia, cardiac arrhythmia, phlebitis, bronchospasm, wheezing, hypoxemia, rash, urticaria, erythema, injection site reactions, dizziness, muscle spasms.
Pancuronium Bromide	**Inj:** 1mg/mL, 2mg/mL	***Adults:*** Individualize dose. **Initial:** 0.04-0.1mg/kg IV. Late incremental doses of 0.01mg/kg may be used. **Skeletal Muscle Relaxation For Endotracheal Intubation:** 0.06-0.1mg/kg bolus. ***Pediatrics:*** Individualize dose. **Initial:** 0.04-0.1mg/kg IV. Late incremental doses of 0.01mg/kg may be used. **Skeletal Muscle Relaxation For Endotracheal Intubation:** 0.06-0.1mg/kg bolus. **Neonates:** Use test dose of 0.02mg/kg.	**Administer by adequately trained individuals familiar with actions, characteristics, and hazards.** **W/P:** May have profound effect in myasthenia gravis or myasthenic (Eaton Lambert) syndrome; use small test dose and monitor closely. Contains benzyl alcohol; caution in neonates. Use peripheral nerve stimu- lator to monitor neuromuscular block- ing effect. Caution with pre-existing pulmonary, hepatic, or renal disease. Conditions associated with slower circulation time in cardiovascular dis- ease, old age, and edematous states may delay onset time; dosage should not be increased. Possible slower onset, higher total dosage, and prolon- gation of neuromuscular blockade with hepatic and/or biliary tract disease. In ICU, long-term use may be associated with prolonged paralysis and/or skel- etal muscle weakness; monitor closely. Severe obesity and neuromuscular disease may pose airway or ventilatory problems. Electrolyte imbalances may alter neuromuscular blockade. **P/N:** Category C, safety in nursing not known.	Skeletal muscle weakness and paralysis, **salivation**, rash.
Rocuronium Bromide (Zemuron)	**Inj:** 10mg/mL	***Adults:*** Individualize dose. **Rapid Sequence Intubation:** 0.6-1.2mg/kg; **Tracheal Intubation:** **Initial:** 0.6mg/kg. **Maint:** 0.1, 0.15, or 0.2mg/kg. **Continous Infusion: Initial:** 10-12mcg/kg/min. **Range:** 4-16mcg/kg/min. ***Pediatrics:* 3 months-14 yrs:** Individualize dose. **Initial:** 0.6mg/kg.	**W/P:** Employ peripheral nerve stimulator to monitor drug response. May have profound effects with myasthenia gravis or myasthenic (Eaton-Lambert) syndrome; use small test dose and monitor closely. Do not mix with alkaline solutions (eg, barbi- turate solutions) in the same syringe or administer simultaneously during IV infusion through the same needle. Anaphylactic reactions reported. Tolerance may develop during chronic	Arrhythmia, abnormal ECG, tachycardia, nausea, vomiting, asthma, **hiccup**, rash, injection site edema, pruritus.

*Scored.   †Bold entries denote special dental considerations.

Table 22.1: PRESCRIBING INFORMATION FOR SKELETAL MUSCLE RELAXANTS *(cont.)*

NAME	FORM/ STRENGTH	DOSAGE	WARNINGS/PRECAUTIONS & CONTRAINDICATIONS	ADVERSE EFFECTS†
NEUROMUSCULAR BLOCKERS *(cont.)*				
Rocuronium Bromide *(cont.)*			Anaphylactic reactions reported. Tolerance may develop during chronic administration. Not recommended for rapid sequence induction in Cesarean section. Caution with clinically significant hepatic disease. Conditions associated with slower circulation time (eg, cardiovascular disease or advanced age) may delay onset time. Electrolyte imbalances may enhance neuromuscular blockade. **P/N:** Category C, safety in nursing not known.	
Succinylcholine Chloride (Anectine)	**Inj:** 20mg/mL	**Adults: Short Surgical Procedure: Average Dose:** 0.6mg/kg IV. **Range:** 0.3-1.1mg/kg IV. Blockade develops in 1 minute, may persist up to 2 minutes. **Long Surgical Procedure:** 2.5-4.3mg/min IV; or 0.3-1.1mg/kg initial IV injection, then 0.04-0.07mg/kg IV at appropriate intervals. **IM (if vein not accessible):** Up to 3-4mg/kg IM. **Max:** 150mg/total dose. Effect observed in 2-3 minutes. **Pediatrics: Procedure to Secure Airway: Infants/Small Children:** 2mg/kg IV. **Older Children/Adolescents:** 1mg/kg IV. **IM (if vein not accessible): Infants/Older Children:** Up to 3-4mg/kg IM. **Max:** 150mg/total dose. Effect observed in 2-3 minutes.	**Rare reports of acute rhabdomyolysis with hyperkalemia followed by ventricular dysrhythmias, cardiac arrest, and death in children with undiagnosed skeletal muscle myopathy. Reserve in children for emergency intubation where securing airway is necessary.** **W/P:** Avoid administration before unconsciousness has been induced. May induce arrhythmias or cardiac arrest in electrolyte abnormalities or massive digitalis toxicity. Caution with chronic abdominal infection, subarachnoid hemorrhage, conditions causing degeneration of central and peripheral nervous system, fractures, muscle spasms, reduced plasma cholinesterase activity, and acute phase of injury following major burns, multiple trauma, extensive skeletal muscle denervation, upper motor neuron injury. Malignant hyperthermia reported. Higher incidence of bradycardia progressing to asystole with 2nd dose. May increase IOP, intracranial or intragastric pressure. With prolonged therapy, Phase I block will progress to Phase II block associated with prolonged respiratory paralysis and weakness. Confirm Phase II block before therapy. Hypokalemia or hypocalcemia prolong neuromuscular blockade. **Contra:** Personal or familial history of malignant hyperthermia, skeletal muscle myopathies. Acute phase of injury following major burns, multiple trauma, extensive skeletal muscle denervation, upper motor neuron injury. **P/N:** Category C, caution in nursing.	Respiratory depression, cardiac arrest, malignant hyperthermia, arrhythmia, bradycardia, tachycardia, HTN, hypotension, hyperkalemia, increased IOP, muscle fasciculation, **jaw rigidity**, post-op muscle pains.
Vecuronium Bromide	**Inj:** 10mg, 20mg	**Adults:** Individualize dose. **Initial:** 0.08-0.1mg/kg IV bolus. **Maint:** 0.01-0.015mg/kg IV within 25-40 minutes of initial dose. Administer subsequent doses at 12-15 minute intervals under balanced anesthesia and slightly longer with inhalation agents. **Max:** 0.15-0.28mg/kg. **Prior Succinylcholine:** Reduce dose to 0.04-0.06mg/kg with inhalation anesthesia and	**Administer by adequately trained individuals familiar with actions, characteristics, and hazards.** **W/P:** May have profound effect in myasthenia gravis or myasthenic (Eaton Lambert) syndrome; use small test dose and monitor closely. Prolongation of neuromuscular blockade may occur in anephric patients; consider lower initial dose. Conditions associated with slower circulation time in cardiovascular disease, old age, and edematous states may delay onset	Skeletal muscle weakness and paralysis.

*Scored. †Bold entries denote special dental considerations.

NAME	FORM/ STRENGTH	DOSAGE	WARNINGS/PRECAUTIONS & CONTRAINDICATIONS	ADVERSE EFFECTS†
Vecuronium Bromide *(cont.)*		0.05-0.06mg/kg with balanced anesthesia. **Continuous Infusion: Initial:** 1mcg/kg/min administered 20-40 minutes after intubating dose of 80-100mcg/kg. Administer infusion after evidence of recovery from bolus. Adjust infusion rate to maintain 90% suppression of twitch response. **Maint:** 0.8-1.2mcg/kg/min. **Concurrent Steady-State Enflurane/Isoflurane:** Reduce rate 25-60%, 45-60 minutes after intubating dose. *Pediatrics:* **10-17 yrs:** Individualize dose. **Initial:** 0.08-0.1mg/kg IV bolus. **Maint:** 0.01-0.015mg/kg IV within 25-40 minutes of initial dose. Administer subsequent dose at 12-15 minute intervals under balanced anesthesia and slightly longer with inhalation agents. **Max:** 0.15-0.28mg/kg. **Prior Succinylcholine:** Reduce dose to 0.04-0.06mg/kg with inhalation anesthesia and 0.05-0.06mg/kg with balanced anesthesia. **Continuous Infusion: Initial:** 1mcg/kg/min administered 20-40 minutes after intubating dose of 80-100mcg/kg. Administer infusion after evidence of recovery from bolus. Adjust infusion rate to maintain 90% suppression of twitch response. **Maint:** 0.8-1.2mcg/kg/min. **Concurrent Steady-State Enflurane/Isoflurane:** Reduce rate 25-60%, 45-60 minutes after intubating dose. **1-10 yrs:** May require a slightly higher initial dose and may also require supplementation slightly more often than adults.	time; dosage should not be increased. Prolonged recovery time reported with cirrhosis or cholestasis. In ICU, long-term use may be associated with prolonged paralysis and/or skeletal muscle weakness. Monitor neuromuscular transmission of ICU patients continuously with a nerve stimulator. Severe obesity and neuromuscular disease may pose airway or ventilatory problems. Electrolyte imbalances may alter neuromuscular blockade. **P/N:** Category C, safety in nursing not known.	

SPASMOLYTICS

BENZODIAZEPINES

NAME	FORM/ STRENGTH	DOSAGE	WARNINGS/PRECAUTIONS & CONTRAINDICATIONS	ADVERSE EFFECTS†
Chlordiazepoxide Hydrochloride[CIV] (Librium)	**Cap:** 5mg, 10mg, 25mg; **Inj:** 100mg	*Adults:* **Mild-Moderate Anxiety:** 5-10mg PO tid-qid. **Severe Anxiety:** 20-25mg PO tid-qid or 50-100mg IM/IV initially, then 25-50mg tid-qid as needed. **Alcohol Withdrawal:** 50-100mg IM/IV initially, may repeat in 2-4 hrs or 50-100mg PO, repeated until agitation is controlled. **Preoperative Anxiety:** 5-10mg PO tid-qid on days prior to surgery or 50-100mg IM 1 hr prior to surgery. **Max:** 300mg/24 hrs for above indications.	**W/P:** Avoid in pregnancy. Paradoxical reactions reported in psychiatric patients and in hyperactive aggressive pediatrics. Caution with porphyria, renal or hepatic dysfunction. Reduce dose in elderly, debilitated. Avoid abrupt withdrawal after extended therapy. Observe patients up to 3 hrs after IM/IV use. **P/N:** Not for use in pregnancy, safety in nursing not known.	Drowsiness, ataxia, confusion, skin eruptions, edema, nausea, constipation, extrapyramidal symptoms, libido changes, EEG changes.

Table 22.1: PRESCRIBING INFORMATION FOR SKELETAL MUSCLE RELAXANTS *(cont.)*

NAME	FORM/ STRENGTH	DOSAGE	WARNINGS/PRECAUTIONS & CONTRAINDICATIONS	ADVERSE EFFECTS†
SPASMOLYTICS *(cont.)*				
Chlordiazepox-ide Hydrochlo-rideCIV *(cont.)*		**Elderly/Debilitated:** Reduce dose (25-50mg IM/IV) or 5mg PO bid-qid. *Pediatrics:* **PO: ≥6 yrs:** 5mg bid-qid. May increase to 10mg bid-tid for all conditions except acute alcohol withdrawal. **Acute Alcohol Withdrawal:** 50-100mg followed by repeated doses until agitation is controlled. **Max:** 300mg/day. **IM/IV: ≥12 yrs: Withdrawal Symptoms of Acute Alcoholism: Initial:** 25-50mg; repeat in 2 to 4hrs. prn. **Acute/Severe Anxiety: Initial:** 25-50mg, then 12.5-50mg tid-qid prn. **Preoperative Anxiety:** 25-50mg 1 hr prior to surgery.		
ClonazepamCIV (Klonopin)	**Tab:** 0.5mg*, 1mg, 2mg; **Tab, Disintegrating (Wafer):** 0.125mg, 0.25mg, 0.5mg, 1mg, 2mg	*Adults:* **Seizure Disorders: Initial:** Not to exceed 1.5mg/day given tid. **Titrate:** May increase by 0.5-1mg every 3 days. **Max:** 20mg qd. **Panic Disorder: Initial:** 0.25mg bid. **Titrate:** Increase to 1mg/day after 3 days, then may increase by 0.125-0.25mg bid every 3 days. **Max:** 4mg/day. **Wafer:** Dissolve in mouth with or without water. *Pediatrics:* **<10 yrs or 30kg: Seizure Disorders: Initial:** 0.01-0.03mg/kg/day up to 0.05mg/kg/day bid-tid. **Titrate:** Increase by no more than 0.25-0.5mg every 3 days. **Maint:** 0.1-0.2mg/kg/day tid. **Wafer:** Dissolve in mouth with or without water.	**W/P:** May increase incidence of generalized tonic-clonic seizures. Monitor blood counts and LFTs periodically with long-term therapy. Caution with renal dysfunction, chronic respiratory depression. Increased fetal risks during pregnancy. Avoid abrupt withdrawal. Hypersalivation reported. **Contra:** Significant liver disease, acute narrow angle glaucoma, untreated open angle glaucoma. **P/N:** Category D, not for use in nursing.	Somnolence, depression, ataxia, CNS depression, upper respiratory tract infection, fatigue, dizziness, sinusitis, colpitis.
DiazepamCIV (Valium)	**Tab:** 2mg*, 5mg*, 10mg*	*Adults:* **Anxiety:** 2-10mg bid-qid. **Alcohol Withdrawal:** 10mg tid-qid for 24 hours. **Maint:** 5mg tid-qid prn. **Skeletal Muscle Spasm:** 2-10mg tid-qid. **Seizure Disorders:** 2-10mg bid-qid. **Elderly/Debilitated:** 2-2.5mg qd-bid initially; may increase gradually as needed and tolerated. *Pediatrics:* **≥6 months:** 1-2.5mg tid-qid initially; may increase gradually as needed and tolerated. *Pediatrics:* **≥6 months:** 1-2.5mg tid-qid initially; may increase gradually as needed and tolerated.	**W/P:** Monitor blood counts and LFTs in long-term use. Neutropenia and jaundice reported. Increase in grand mal seizures reported. Avoid abrupt withdrawal. Caution with kidney or hepatic dysfunction. **Contra:** Acute narrow angle glaucoma, untreated open angle glaucoma, patients <6 months. **P/N:** Not for use during pregnancy, safety in nursing not known.	Drowsiness, fatigue, ataxia, paradoxical reactions, minor EEG changes.

*Scored.   †Bold entries denote special dental considerations.

NAME	FORM/ STRENGTH	DOSAGE	WARNINGS/PRECAUTIONS & CONTRAINDICATIONS	ADVERSE EFFECTS[†]
Lorazepam[CIV] (Ativan, Ativan Injection)	**Inj:** 2mg/mL, 4mg/mL; **Tab:** 0.5mg, 1mg*, 2mg*	**Adults: (Inj)** ≥18 yrs: **Status Epilepticus:** 4mg IV (given slowly at 2mg/min); may repeat 1 dose after 10-15 minutes if seizures recur or fail to cease. **Preanesthetic Sedation: Usual:** 0.05mg/kg IM; 2mg or 0.044mg/kg IV (whichever is smaller). **Max:** 4mg IM/IV. **(Tab) Initial:** 2-3mg/day given bid-tid. Usual: 2-6mg/day in divided doses. **Insomnia:** 2-4mg qhs. **Elderly/Debilitated:** 1-2mg/day in divided doses. **Pediatrics: >12 yrs: Initial:** 2-3mg/day given bid-tid. **Usual:** 2-6mg/day in divided doses. **Insomnia:** 2-4mg qhs.	**W/P:** (Inj) Monitor all parameters to maintain vital function. Risk of respiratory depression or airway obstruction in heavily sedated patients. May cause fetal damage during pregnancy. Increased risk of CNS and respiratory depression in elderly. Avoid with hepatic/renal failure. Caution with mild to moderate hepatic/renal disease. Avoid outpatient endoscopic procedures. Possible propylene glycol toxicity in renal impairment. (Tab) Avoid with primary depression or psychosis. Withdrawal symptoms with abrupt discontinuation. Careful supervision if addiction-prone. Caution with elderly, and renal or hepatic dysfunction. Monitor for GI disease with prolonged therapy. Periodic blood counts and LFTs with long-term therapy. **Contra:** Acute narrow-angle glaucoma, sleep apnea syndrome, severe respiratory insufficiency. Not for intra-arterial injection. **P/N:** (Inj) Category D, not for use in nursing. (Tab) Not for use in pregnancy or nursing.	Sedation, dizziness, weakness, unsteadiness, transient amnesia, memory impairment, respiratory depression/failure, hypotension, somnolence, headache, hypoventilation.
Midazolam Hydrochloride[CIV] (Versed)	**Inj:** 1mg/mL, 5mg/mL **Syrup:** 2mg/mL	**Adults: IV: Sedation/ Anxiolysis/Amnesia Induction:** <60 yrs: **Initial:** 1-2.5mg IV over 2 min. **Max:** 5mg. **Titrate:** In small increments at 2 min intervals if needed. **Concomitant Narcotics/Other CNS Depressants:** Reduce by 30%. **≥60 yrs/Debilitated/ Chronically Ill: Initial:** 1-1.5mg IV over 2 min. **Max:** 3.5mg. **Titrate:** In small increments at 2 min intervals if needed. **Concomitant Narcotics/Other CNS Depressants:** Reduce by 50%. **Maint:** 25% of sedation dose by slow titration. **IM: Preoperative Sedation/ Anxiolysis/Amnesia: <60 yrs:** 0.07-0.08mg/kg IM up to 1 hr before surgery. **≥60 yrs/Debilitated:** 1-3mg IM. **Anesthesia Induction: Unpremedicated: <55 yrs: Initially:** 0.3-0.35mg/kg IV over 20-30 seconds. May give additional doses of 25% of initial dose to complete induction. **≥55 yrs: Initial:** 0.3mg/kg IV. **Debilitated: Initial:** 0.15-0.25mg/kg IV. **Premedicated: <55 yrs: Initial:** 0.25mg/kg IV over 20-30 seconds.	**Associated with respiratory depression and respiratory arrest especially when used for sedation in noncritical care settings. Do not administer by rapid injection to neonates. Continuous monitoring required.** **W/P:** Agitation, involuntary movements, hyperactivity, and combativeness reported. Caution with CHF, chronic renal failure, pulmonary disease, uncompensated acute illnesses (eg, severe fluid or electrolyte disturbances), elderly or debilitated. Avoid use with shock or coma, or in acute alcohol intoxication with depression of vital signs. Contains benzyl alcohol. **Contra:** Acute narrow-angle glaucoma, untreated open-angle glaucoma, intrathecal or epidural use. **P/N:** Category D, caution in nursing.	Decreased tidal volume and/or respiratory rate, BP/HR variations, apnea, hypotension, pain and local reactions at injection site, **hiccups,** nausea, vomiting, **desaturation.**

Table 22.1: PRESCRIBING INFORMATION FOR SKELETAL MUSCLE RELAXANTS *(cont.)*

NAME	FORM/ STRENGTH	DOSAGE	WARNINGS/PRECAUTIONS & CONTRAINDICATIONS	ADVERSE EFFECTS†
SPASMOLYTICS *(cont.)*				
Midazolam Hydrochloride^{CIV} *(cont.)*		**≥55 yrs: Initial:** 0.2mg/kg IV. **Debilitated:** 0.15mg/kg IV. **Maintenance Sedation:** LD: 0.01-0.05mg/kg IV. May repeat dose at 10-15 min intervals until adequate sedation. **Maint:** 0.02-0.1mg/kg/hr. Titrate to desired level of sedation using 25-50% adjustments. Infusion rate should be decreased 10-25% every few hrs to find minimum effective infusion rate. *Pediatrics:* 0.25-1mg/kg single dose. **Max:** 20mg.		
BENZODIAZEPINE ANTAGONIST				
Flumazenil (Romazicon)	**Inj:** 0.1mg/mL	*Adults:* **Reversal of Conscious Sedation/General Anesthesia:** Give IV over 15 seconds. **Initial:** 0.2mg. May repeat dose after 45 seconds and again at 60 second intervals up to a max of 4 additional times until reach desired level of consciousness. **Max Total Dose:** 1mg. In event of resedation, repeated doses may be given at 20-min intervals. **Max:** 1mg/dose (0.2mg/min) and 3mg/hr. **BZD Overdose:** Give IV over 30 seconds. **Initial:** 0.2mg. May repeat with 0.3mg after 30 seconds and then 0.5mg at 1-min intervals until reach desired level of consciousness. **Max Total Dose:** 3mg. In event of resedation, repeated doses may be given at 20-min intervals. **Max:** 1mg/dose (0.5mg/min); 3mg/hr. *Pediatrics:* **>1yr:** Give IV over 15 seconds. **Initial:** 0.01mg/kg (up to 0.2mg). May repeat dose after 45 seconds and again at 60-second intervals up to a max of 4 additional times until reach desired level of consciousness. **Max Total Dose:** 0.05mg/kg or 1mg, whichever is lower.	**W/P:** Caution in overdoses involving multiple drug combinations. Risk of seizures, especially with long-term BZD-induced sedation, cyclic antidepressant overdose, concurrent major sedative-hypnotic drug withdrawal, recent therapy with repeated doses of parenteral BZDs, myoclonic jerking or seizure prior to flumazenil administration. Monitor for resedation, respiratory depression, or other residual BZD effects (up to 2 hrs). Avoid use in the ICU; increased risk of unrecognized BZD dependence. Caution with head injury, alcoholism, and other drug dependencies. Does not reverse respiratory depression/hypoventilation or cardiac depression. May provoke panic attacks with history of panic disorder. Adjust subsequent doses in hepatic dysfunction. Not for use as treatment for BZD dependence or for management of protracted abstinence syndromes. May trigger dose-dependent withdrawal syndromes. **Contra:** Patients given BZDs for life-threatening conditions (eg, control of intracranial pressure or status epilepticus), signs of serious cyclic antidepressant overdose. **P/N:** Category C, caution in nursing.	Nausea, vomiting, dizziness, injection site pain, increased sweating, headache, abnormal or blurred vision, agitation.
MISCELLANEOUS				
Baclofen (Kemstro)	**Tab: (Generic)** 10mg, 20mg; **Tab, Disintegrating (ODT): (Kemstro)** 10mg, 20mg	*Adults:* **Initial:** 5mg tid for 3 days. **Titrate:** May increase dose by 5mg tid every 3 days. **Usual:** 40-80mg/day. **Max:** 80 mg/day (20mg qid). **Renal Impairment:** Reduce dose. *Pediatrics:* **≥12 yrs: Initial:** 5mg tid for 3 days.	**W/P:** Caution with psychosis, schizophrenia, confusional states; may exacerbate conditions. Caution with bladder sphincter hypertonia, peptic ulceration, seizures, elderly, cerebrovascular disorder, respiratory failure, hepatic or renal failure. Abnormal AST, alkaline phosphatase and blood glucose reported. Caution when used to maintain locomotion or to obtain increased function.	Drowsiness, dizziness, weakness, fatigue, confusion, daytime sedation, headache, insomnia, hypotension, nausea, constipation, urinary frequency.

*Scored.   †Bold entries denote special dental considerations.

NAME	FORM/ STRENGTH	DOSAGE	WARNINGS/PRECAUTIONS & CONTRAINDICATIONS	ADVERSE EFFECTS†
Baclofen (cont.)		**Titrate:** May increase dose by 5mg tid every 3 days. **Usual:** 40-80mg/day. **Max:** 80 mg/day (20mg qid). **Renal Impairment:** Reduce dose.	Decreased alertness with operating machinery. Has not significantly benefited stroke patients. Avoid abrupt discontinuation; reduce dose slowly over 1-2 weeks. **P/N:** Category C, caution in nursing.	
Carisoprodol (Soma)	**Tab:** 350mg	**Adults:** 350mg tid and hs. **Pediatrics:** ≥12 yrs: 350mg tid and hs.	**W/P:** First-dose idiosyncratic reactions reported (rare). Caution in addiction-prone patients. Caution with liver or renal dysfunction. **Contra:** Acute intermittent porphyria. **P/N:** Safety in pregnancy and nursing not known.	Drowsiness, dizziness, nausea, vomiting, tachycardia, postural hypotension, idiosyncratic reactions.
Chlorzoxazone (Parafon Forte DSC)	**Tab:** 500mg*	**Adults:** Usual: 500mg tid-qid. **Titrate:** May increase to 750mg tid-qid.	**W/P:** Serious (including fatal) hepato-cellular toxicity reported. Discontinue if develop signs of hepatotoxicity. Caution with history of drug allergies. **P/N:** Safety in pregnancy and nursing not known.	Drowsiness, dizziness, malaise, lightheadedness, overstimulation.
Cyclobenza-prine Hydrochloride (Flexeril)	**Tab:** 5mg, 10mg	**Adults:** Usual: 5mg tid. **Titrate:** May increase to 10mg tid. **Mild Hepatic Dysfunction/ Elderly: Initial:** 5mg qd, then slowly increase. **Moderate/Severe Hepatic Dysfunction:** Avoid use. Treatment should not exceed 2-3 weeks. **Pediatrics:** ≥15 yrs: Usual: 5mg tid. **Titrate:** May increase to 10mg tid. **Mild Hepatic Dysfunction/ Elderly: Initial:** 5mg qd, then slowly increase. **Moderate/Severe Hepatic Dysfunction:** Avoid use. Treatment should not exceed 2-3 weeks.	**W/P:** Caution with history of urinary retention, angle-closure glaucoma, increased IOP, hepatic dysfunction. Caution in elderly due to increased risk of CNS effects. May produce arrhythmias, sinus tachycardia and conduction time prolongation. May impair ability to drive. **Contra:** Acute recovery phase of MI, arrhythmias, heart block or conduction disturbances, CHF, hyperthyroidism, MAOI use during or within 14 days. **P/N:** Category B, caution in nursing.	Drowsiness, **dry mouth**, headache, fatigue.
Dantrolene Sodium (Dantrium)	**Cap:** 25mg, 50mg, 100mg	**Adults: Chronic Spasticity: Initial:** 25mg qd for 7 days. **Titrate:** Increase to 25mg tid for 7 days, then 50mg tid for 7 days, then 100mg tid. **Max:** 100mg qid. If no further benefit at next higher dose, decrease to previous lower dose. **Malignant Hyperthermia: Pre-Op:** 4-8mg/kg/day given tid-qid for 1-2 days before surgery, with last dose given 3-4 hrs before surgery. **Post-Op Following Malignant Hyperthermia Crisis:** 4-8mg/kg/day given qid for 1-3 days. **Pediatrics:** ≥5 yrs: Chronic Spasticity: Initial: 0.5mg/kg qd for 7 days. **Titrate:** Increase to 0.5mg/kg tid for 7 days, then 1mg/kg tid for 7 days, then 2mg/kg tid. **Max:** 100mg qid. If no further benefit at next higher dose, decrease to previous lower dose.	**W/P:** Monitor LFTs at baseline, then periodically. Increased risk of hepatocellular disease in females and patients >35 yrs. Caution with pulmonary, cardiac, and liver dysfunction. Photosensitivity reaction may occur; limit sunlight exposure. **Contra:** Active hepatic disease, where spasticity is utilized to sustain upright posture and balance in locomotion, when spasticity is utilized to obtain or maintain increased function. **P/N:** Category C; not for use in nursing.	Drowsiness, dizziness, weakness, malaise, fatigue, diarrhea, hepatitis, tachycardia, aplastic anemia, thrombocytopenia, depression, seizure.

Table 22.1: PRESCRIBING INFORMATION FOR SKELETAL MUSCLE RELAXANTS *(cont.)*

NAME	FORM/ STRENGTH	DOSAGE	WARNINGS/PRECAUTIONS & CONTRAINDICATIONS	ADVERSE EFFECTS†
MISCELLANEOUS *(cont.)*				
Metaxalone (Skelaxin)	**Tab:** 800mg*	***Adults:*** 800mg tid-qid. ***Pediatrics:*** **>12 yrs:** 800mg tid-qid	**W/P:** Caution with pre-existing liver damage. Monitor hepatic function. False-positive Benedict's test reported. **Contra:** Tendency for drug-induced, hemolytic, and other anemias. Significant renal or hepatic impairment. **P/N:** Not for use in pregnancy or nursing.	Nausea, vomiting, GI upset, drowsiness, dizziness, headache, nervousness, leukopenia, hemolytic anemia, jaundice.
Methocarbamol (Robaxin)	**Inj:** 100mg/mL; **Tab:** 500mg, 750mg	***Adults:*** **(PO) Initial:** (500mg tab) 1500mg qid for 2-3 days. **Maint:** 1000mg qid. **Initial:** (750mg tab) 1500mg qid for 2-3 days. **Maint:** 750mg q4h or 1500mg tid. **Max:** 6gm/d for 2-3 days; 8gm/d if severe. **(Inj) Moderate Symptoms:** 10mL IV/IM. **IV Max Rate:** 3mL undiluted drug/min. **IM Max:** 5mL into each gluteal region. **Severe/Post-Op Condition: Max:** 20-30mL/day up to 3 consecutive days. If feasible, continue with PO. **Tetanus:** 10-20mL up to 30mL. May repeat q6h until NG tube can be inserted. Continue with crushed tabs. **Max:** 24g/day PO. ***Pediatrics:*** **Tetanus: Initial:** 15mg/kg. Repeat q6h prn. Administer through tubing or IV. Safety and effctiveness in pediatric patients have not been established except tetanus.	**W/P:** May cause color interference in certain screening tests for 5-hydroxy-indoleacetic acid (5-HIAA) and vanillylmandelic acid (VMA). Caution in epilepsy with the injection. Injection rate should not exceed 3mL/min. Avoid extravasation with injection. **Contra:** (Inj) Renal pathology with injection due to propylene glycol content. **P/N:** Category C, caution in nursing.	Lightheadedness, dizziness, drowsiness, nausea, urticaria, pruritus, rash, conjunctivitis, nasal congestion, blurred vision, headache, fever, seizures, syncope, flushing.
Orphenadrine Citrate (Norflex)	**Inj:** 30mg/mL; **Tab, Extended Release:** 100mg	***Adults:*** **(Tab)** 100mg bid am and pm. **(Inj)** 60mg IM/IV q12h.	**W/P:** Caution with tachycardia, cardiac decompensation, coronary insufficiency, cardiac arrhythmias. Monitor blood, urine, and LFTs periodically with prolonged use. Injection contains sodium bisulfite. **Contra:** Glaucoma, pyloric or duodenal obstruction, stenosing peptic ulcers, prostatic hypertrophy, bladder neck obstruction, cardiospasm, myasthenia gravis. **P/N:** Category C, safety in nursing not known.	**Dry mouth**, tachycardia, palpitation, urinary hesitancy/retention, blurred vision, pupil dilation, increased ocular tension, weakness, dizziness, constipation.
Tizanidine Hydrochloride (Zanaflex)	**Cap:** 2mg, 4mg, 6mg; **Tab:** 2mg*, 4mg*	***Adults:*** **Initial:** 4mg single dose q6-8h. **Titrate:** Increase by 2-4mg. **Usual:** 8mg single dose q6-8h. **Max:** 3 doses/24h or 36mg/day.	**W/P:** May prolong QT interval. May cause liver damage; monitor baseline LFTs at 1, 3, and 6 months. Retinal degeneration and corneal opacities reported. Caution with renal impairment or elderly. May cause hypotension; caution with antihypertensives. **P/N:** Category C, caution in nursing.	**Dry mouth**, somnolence, asthenia, dizziness, UTI, urinary frequency, flu-like syndrome, rhinitis.

*Scored.   †Bold entries denote special dental considerations.

Table 22.2: DRUG INTERACTIONS FOR SKELETAL MUSCLE RELAXANTS

BENZODIAZEPINES

Chlordiazepoxide Hydrochloride[CIV] (Librium)

Alcohol	May produce additive CNS depression with alcohol.
CNS depressants	May produce additive CNS depression with other CNS depressants.
Psychotropic agents	Avoid other psychotropic agents.

Clonazepam[CIV] (Klonopin)

Alcohol	Alcohol potentiate CNS-depressant effects.
Antianxiety agents	Antianxiety agents potentiate CNS-depressant effects.
Anticonvulsant drugs	Anticonvulsant drugs potentiate CNS-depressant effects.
Barbiturates	Barbiturates potentiate CNS-depressant effects.
Butyrophenone antipsychotics	Butyrophenone antipsychotics potentiate CNS-depressant effects.
CYP3A inhibitors	Caution with CYP3A inhibitors (eg, oral antifungals).
CYP450 inducers	Decreased serum levels with CYP450 inducers (eg, phenytoin, carbamazepine, phenobarbital).
MAOIs	MAOIs potentiate CNS-depressant effects.
Narcotics	Narcotics potentiate CNS-depressant effects.
Nonbarbiturate hypnotics	Nonbarbiturate hypnotics potentiate CNS-depressant effects.
Phenothiazines	Phenothiazines potentiate CNS-depressant effects.
Thioxanthene	Thioxanthene potentiate CNS-depressant effects.
Tricyclic-antidepressants	TCAs potentiate CNS-depressant effects.

Diazepam[CIV] (Valium)

Alcohol	Avoid alcohol and other CNS-depressants.
Antidepressants	Antidepressants may potentiate effects.
Barbiturates	Barbiturates may potentiate effects.
Cimetidine	Delayed clearance with cimetidine.
CNS-depressants	Avoid CNS-depressants.
Flumazenil	Risk of seizure with flumazenil.
MAOIs	MAOIs may potentiate effects.
Narcotics	Narcotics may potentiate effects.
Phenothiazines	Phenothiazines may potentiate effects.

Table 22.2: DRUG INTERACTIONS FOR SKELETAL MUSCLE RELAXANTS (cont.)

BENZODIAZEPINES (cont.)

Lorazepam[CIV] (Ativan)

Alcohol	CNS-depressant effects with alcohol and diminished tolerance to alcohol.
Barbiturates	CNS-depressant effects with barbiturates.
CNS depressants	Diminished tolerance to CNS depressants.

Midazolam Hydrochloride[CIV] (Versed)

Alcohol	Avoid use with acute alcohol intoxication.
CNS depressants	Increased sedative effects with CNS depressants.
CYP450 3A4 inhibitors	Prolonged sedation with CYP450 3A4 inhibitors (eg, erythromycin, diltiazem, verapamil, ketoconazole, itraconazole, saquinavir, cimetidine).
Droperidol	Increased sedative effects with droperidol.
Fentanyl	Increased sedative effects with fentanyl. May cause severe hypotension with concomitant use of fentanyl in neonates.
Halothane	Decreases concentration of halothane required for anesthesia.
Meperidine	Increased sedative effects with meperidine.
Morphine	Increased sedative effects with morphine.
Secobarbital	Increased sedative secobarbital.
Thiopental	Decreases concentration of halothane and thiopental required for anesthesia.

BENZODIAZEPINE ANTAGONIST

Flumazenil (Romazicon)

Flumazenil	Avoid use until neuromuscular blockade effects are reversed.
Mixed drug overdose	Toxic effects (eg, convulsions, cardiac dysrhythmias) may occur with mixed drug overdose (eg, cyclic antidepressants).

MUSCLE RELAXANTS

Baclofen

Alcohol	Additive CNS effects with alcohol.
Antidiabetic agents	May increase blood glucose and require dosage adjustment of antidiabetic agents.
Antihypertensives	May potentiate antihypertensives.
CNS depressants	Additive CNS effects with CNS depressants.
Levodopa plus Carbidopa	Mental confusion, hallucinations and agitation with levodopa plus carbidopa therapy.
Magnesium sulfate	Synergistic effects with magnesium sulfate and other neuromuscular blockers.
MAO inhibitors	May increase CNS depressant effects with MAO inhibitors.

MUSCLE RELAXANTS *(cont.)*

Baclofen *(cont.)*

Neuromuscular blockers	Synergistic effects with magnesium sulfate and other neuromuscular blockers.
Tricyclic Antidepressants	Potentiated by TCAs.

Carisoprodol (Soma)

Alcohol	Additive effects with alcohol.
CNS depressants	Additive effects with CNS depressants.
Psychotropic drugs	Additive effects with psychotropic drugs.

Chlorzoxazone (Parafon Forte DSC)

Alcohol	Additive effects with alcohol.
CNS depressants	Additive effects with CNS depressants.

Cyclobenzaprine Hydrochloride (Flexeril)

Alcohol	Enhances effects of alcohol.
Anticholinergic medication	Caution with anticholinergic medication.
Barbiturates	Enhances effects of barbiturates.
CNS depressants	Enhances effects of CNS depressants.
Guanethidine	May block antihypertensive action of guanethidine and similar compounds.
MAOIs	Contraindicated with MAOIs.
Tramadol	May enhance seizure risk with tramadol.

Dantrolene Sodium (Dantrium)

Calcium channel blockers	Avoid with calcium channel blockers; risk of cardiovascular collapse.
CNS depressants	Increased drowsiness with CNS depressants.
Estrogens	Caution with estrogens; risk of hepatotoxicity.
Vecuronium	May potentiate vecuronium-induced neuromuscular block.

Metaxalone (Skelaxin)

Alcohol	May enhance the effects of alcohol.
Barbiturates	May enhance the effects of barbiturates.
CNS depressants	May enhance the effects of CNS depressants.

Methocarbamol (Robaxin)

Alcohol	Additive adverse effects with alcohol.

Table 22.2: DRUG INTERACTIONS FOR SKELETAL MUSCLE RELAXANTS *(cont.)*

MUSCLE RELAXANTS *(cont.)*

Methocarbamol (Robaxin) *(cont.)*

Anticholinergics	Caution in patients with myasthemia gravis receiving anticholinergics.
CNS depressants	Additive adverse effects with CNS depressants.
Pyridostigmine	May inhibit effect of pyridostigmine.

Mivacurium Chloride (Mivacron)

Anesthetics, local	Enhanced neuromuscular blocking action possible with local anesthetics.
Antibiotics	Enhanced neuromuscular blocking action possible with certain antibiotics (eg, aminoglycosides, tetracyclines, bacitracin, polymyxins, lincomycin, clindamycin, colistin, and sodium colistimethate).
Carbamazepine	Resistance to neuromuscular blocking action possible with chronically administered phenytoin or carbamazepine.
Enflurane	Enhanced neuromuscular blocking action possible with enflurane.
Halothane	Enhanced neuromuscular blocking action possible with halothane.
Isoflurane	Enhanced neuromuscular blocking action possible with isoflurane.
Lithium	Enhanced neuromuscular blocking action possible with lithium.
Magnesium salts	Enhanced neuromuscular blocking action possible with magnesium salts.
Phenytoin	Resistance to neuromuscular blocking action possible with chronically administered phenytoin.
Plasma cholinesterase inhibitors	Enhanced neuromuscular blocking action possible with drugs that reduce plasma cholinesterase activity (eg, chronically administered oral contraceptives, glucocorticoids, or certain MAOIs), or drugs that irreversibly inhibit plasma cholinesterase.
Procainamide	Enhanced neuromuscular blocking action possible with procainamide.
Quinidine	Enhanced neuromuscular blocking action possible with quinidine.
Succinylcholine	Prior administration of succinylcholine may potentiate neuromuscular blocking effect.

Orphenadrine Citrate (Norflex)

Propoxyphene	Confusion, anxiety, and tremors reported with propoxyphene.

Rocuronium Bromide (Zemuron)

Anesthetics, inhalation	Use of inhalation anesthetics has been shown to enhance the activity of other neuromuscular blocking agents.
Antibiotics	Certain antibiotics (eg, aminoglycosides, vancomycin; tetracyclines, bacitracin, polymyxins, colistin, and sodium colistimethate) may cause prolongation of neuromuscular block.
Anticonvulsant therapy, chronic	Resistance observed with chronic anticonvulsant therapy.
Magnesium salts	Magnesium salts may enhance neuromuscular blockade.
Quinidine	Quinidine injection during recovery from use of other muscle relaxants suggests that recurrent paralysis may occur.

MUSCLE RELAXANTS *(cont.)*

Succinylcholine Chloride (Anectine)

Anesthetics, volatile	Increased risk of malignant hyperthermia with volatile anesthetics.
Antibiotics, non-penicillin	Enhanced effects with certain non-penicillin antibiotics.
Aprotinin	Enhanced effects with aprotinin.
β-blockers	Enhanced effects with β-blockers.
Chloroquine	Enhanced effects with chloroquine.
Desflurane	Enhanced effects with desflurane.
Diethylether	Enhanced effects with diethylether.
Isoflurane	Enhanced effects with isoflurane.
Lidocaine	Enhanced effects with lidocaine.
Lithium carbonate	Enhanced effects with lithium carbonate.
Magnesium salts	Enhanced effects with magnesium salts.
Metoclopramide	Enhanced effects with metoclopramide.
Oxytocin	Enhanced effects with oxytocin.
Plasma cholinesterase inhibitors	Enhanced effects with drugs that reduce plasma cholinesterase activity (eg, chronically administered oral contraceptives, glucocorticoids, certain MAOIs) or inhibit plasma cholinesterase.
Procainamide	Enhanced effects with procainamide.
Promazine	Enhanced effects with promazine.
Quinine	Enhanced effects with quinine.
Terbutaline	Enhanced effects with terbutaline.
Trimethaphan	Enhanced effects with trimethaphan.

Tizanidine Hydrochloride (Zanaflex)

Alcohol	Potentiated depressant effect with alcohol.
Alpha-adrenergic agonists	Avoid alpha-adrenergic agonists.
Contraceptives, oral	Potentiated by oral contraceptives.
Aminoglycosides	Enhanced neuromuscular blockade with aminoglycosides.
Atracurium	Avoid use with atracurium.
Bacitracin	Enhanced neuromuscular blockade with bacitracin.
Colistin	Enhanced neuromuscular blockade with colistin.
D-tubocurarine	Avoid use with d-tubocurarine.

Table 22.2: DRUG INTERACTIONS FOR SKELETAL MUSCLE RELAXANTS *(cont.)*

MUSCLE RELAXANTS *(cont.)*

Tizanidine Hydrochloride (Zanaflex) *(cont.)*

Enflurane	Enhanced neuromuscular blockade with enflurane.
Gallamine	Avoid use with gallamine.
Halothane	Enhanced neuromuscular blockade with halothane.
Isoflurane	Enhanced neuromuscular blockade with isoflurane.
Magnesium salts	Enhanced neuromuscular blockade with magnesium salts.
Metocurine	Avoid use with metocurine.
Polymyxin B	Enhanced neuromuscular blockade polymyxin B.
Quinidine	Quinidine injection during recovery from use of other muscle relaxants suggests that recurrent paralysis may occur.
Sodium colistimethate	Enhanced neuromuscular blockade with sodium colistimethate.
Succinylcholine	Prior administration of succinylcholine may enhance neuromuscular blocking effect.
Tetracyclines	Enhanced neuromuscular blockade with tetracyclines.
Vercuronium	Avoid use with vercuronium.

Vecuronium Bromide

Aminoglycosides	Enhanced neuromuscular blocking action with aminoglycosides.
Bacitracin	Enhanced neuromuscular blocking action with bacitracin.
Colistin	Enhanced neuromuscular blocking action with colistin.
D-tubocurarine	Enhanced neuromuscular blocking action with pancuronium, d-tubocurarine, metocurine, gallamine, enflurane, isoflurane, halothane, aminoglycosides, tetracyclines, bacitracin, polymyxin B, colistin, sodium colistimethate, and magnesium salts.
Enflurane	Enhanced neuromuscular blocking action with enflurane.
Gallamine	Enhanced neuromuscular blocking action with gallamine.
Halothane	Enhanced neuromuscular blocking action with halothane.
Isoflurane	Enhanced neuromuscular blocking action with isoflurane.
Magnesium salts	Enhanced neuromuscular blocking action with magnesium salts.
Metocurine	Enhanced neuromuscular blocking action with metocurine.
Muscle relaxants	Possible synergistic or antagonistic effects with other muscle relaxants.
Pancuronium	Enhanced neuromuscular blocking action with pancuronium.
Polymyxin B	Enhanced neuromuscular blocking action with polymyxin B.
Sodium colistimethate	Enhanced neuromuscular blocking action with sodium colistimethate.
Succinylcholine	Prior administration of succinylcholine may enhance neuromuscular blocking effect.
Tetracyclines	Enhanced neuromuscular blocking action with tetracyclines.

Chapter 23

Drugs for Neoplastic Disorders

Sol Silverman Jr., M.A., D.D.S.; Alan M. Kramer, M.D.

More than 1.3 million new cases of cancer are diagnosed in the United States each year. In spite of improvements in surgical techniques and radiation therapy, only about half of these people will survive their disease. To diminish this high rate of mortality, chemotherapeutic drugs have become an increasingly important part of treatment regimens. These agents are used as single agents or in combination with other treatments. The intent of using these agents with many neoplasms is cure; however, they are more often used for palliation, to gain partial control over the growths and thus prolong life, or as adjuvants to improve response rates in radiation and surgical approaches. Additionally, highly cytotoxic levels of chemotherapeutic drugs are being used increasingly for persistent and recurrent cancers followed by rescue with bone-marrow and stem-cell transplantations.

The drugs used for neoplastic disorders can create cytotoxicity-induced immunosuppression, which can lead to significant symptoms and affect survival. Because the oral mucosae and microbial flora are extremely sensitive to immunosuppression, maintaining optimal oral and dental health becomes a key factor in patient management and outcomes.

Many agents are used to attack neoplastic cells through a variety of biochemical processes. They have efficacies for both solid and hematopoietic cancers.

Response rates depend on the type of neoplasm, the combination of antineoplastic drugs, and the patient's physical status and tolerance. Because these agents are detoxified either in the liver or kidneys, these organs must be functional.

For oral and pharyngeal malignancies, these agents are used primarily as adjuvants to radiation, with the aim of improving responses to radiation. By far the best results for control of nasopharyngeal carcinomas have been achieved by the combination of radiation therapy and chemotherapy. However, in such cases, chemotherapy also accentuates the adverse effects of radiation.

The choice of drug(s) and dosage regimen(s) depends on response rates derived from multi-institutional and group cooperative studies. The toxic side effects of these agents, as well as response rates, are the factors that limit their application. These effects often limit dental procedures required for optimal oral health and create oral problems that lead to dysfunction and pain and require professional help (see box on next page, "Guidelines for Dental Care of Patients Undergoing Chronic or Periodic Drug Treatment for Neoplastic Disorders"). Adverse side effects vary from patient to patient. Management by altering treatment, prescribing medications or instituting empirical procedures depends on the severity and the effects of patient outcomes.

Classification of Antineoplastic Drugs

Alkylating Agents

Alkylating agents are the oldest and most widely used class of anticancer drugs, being the major components of the combination chemotherapy regimens for disseminated solid tumors and for high-dose/stem-cell-support treatment regimens. Aklyating agents interfere with DNA synthesis by causing cross-linking, which can lead to cell death via several pathways. Examples of alkylating agents are cyclophosphamide, cisplatin and nitrogen mustard.

Antibiotics

Antibiotics are a class of cytotoxic agents naturally derived from microbial fermentation broths that include bacteria, fungi and related organisms. Their mechanisms involve intercalation with DNA base pairs, thereby interfering with DNA synthesis. Examples of antibiotics are bleomycin and doxorubicin.

Antimetabolites

Antimetabolites are one of the more diversified and best characterized types of the chemotherapeutic agents in use. Both RNA and DNA syntheses are interrupted by competitive inhibition of purine and pyrimidine nucleosides and of folic acid. Examples are methotrexate, hydroxyurea, 5-fluorouracil, cytarabine and gemcitabine.

Biologic agents

Targeted Therapy in Head and Neck Cancer

Target therapy implies a new method to treat cancer, exploiting unique molecular targets highly expressed in cancer cells. There has recently been a development of both small molecules and monoclonal antibodies that targets receptors involved with tumorgenesis.

Epidermal growth factor-receptor (EGF-R) is one such target highly expressed in squamous cell carcinoma of the head and neck. Cetuximab (IMC-C225, Ertbitux)

GUIDELINES FOR DENTAL CARE OF PATIENTS UNDERGOING CHRONIC OR PERIODIC DRUG TREATMENT FOR NEOPLASTIC DISORDERS

Dental, clinical and radiographic evaluation

- Dental caries, periapical lesions, periodontal disease, bone abnormalities
- Oral mucosal lesions

Consultation with primary care physician/oncologist

- Tumor site, type, stage
- Prognosis
- Medication(s)
- Other systemic diseases
- Suggested premedications
- Past treatment, next treatment

Dental treatment plan

- Immediate: Remove all sources of infection to prevent pain and bacteremia
- Long-term: Promote optimal function and esthetics and prevent infections

Optimal oral hygiene

- Pretreatment prophylaxis
- Initiation of fluoride applications
- Mouthrinses as tolerated (such as chlorhexidine)
- Home care instructions
- Orient patient to the side effects of treatment (such as mucositis) and hygiene modifications (such as soft brushes)

Limitations of treatment

- Infection risk: Leukopenia when white blood cell counts are <1,500 mm^3 (if procedure necessary, use antibiotics)
- Bleeding risk: Thrombocytopenia when platelet count is <100,000 mm^3 (extractions, cutting, invasive procedures)
- Candidiasis (yeast overgrowth): Use of topical/systemic antifungal drugs
- Herpes simplex virus reactivation: Use of systemic antiviral drugs
- Hyposalivation: Use of moisturizing agents and sialogogues
- Mucositis: Use of moisturizing agents, sialogogues, antimicrobial agents, and inflammatory agents

is a monoclonal antibody directed at the EGF-binding domain on the outer portion of the cell membrane. It has been shown to reduce cellular growth and to potentiate chemotherapy (cisplatin, taxanes) as well as radiotherapy in preclinical Models. Cetuximab has gone through Phase I, II and III testing with both chemotherapy and radiotherapy and has been recently FDA-approved for use with radiotherapy and in platinum-refractory disease in patients with head and neck cancer.

The internal domain of the EGF-R contains tyrosine kinase, which has also been targeted in an effort to block cell growth. Gefitinib (Iressa) and erlotinib (Tarceva, OSI-774) are two such tyrosine kinase inhibitors that have gone through clinical testing. Response rate remains modest for patients with head and neck cancer, but stable disease can be observed in 30%-40% of patients for up to 6 months.

The side effect profile that accompanies all the EGF-R targeted therapies remains consistent, usually in the form of tolerable skin rashes and mild diarrhea.

The future of targeted therapy remains in finding additional targets that exploit unique pathways to cancer growth. Combination targeted therapy with and without radiotherapy and chemotherapy are the challenge for the future.

Other examples of biologic agents that produce antitumor effects include interferons, interleukin-2, tumor vaccines, and retinoids.

Hormonal Agents

Hormonal agents are used in the hormonally responsive cancers, such as breast, prostate and endometrial carcinomas. As a group they have both cytostatic and cytocidal activity, which is largely mediated by secondary messengers via cytoplasmic and nuclear receptors. Examples of hormonal agents are tamoxifen, prednisone, androgens and estrogens, letrozole and flutamide.

Miscellaneous Antineoplastic Agents

There are miscellaneous other antineoplastic agents. Taxanes are novel agents that promote the formation of microtubules and stabilize them by preventing depoly merization. Examples are paclitaxel and docetaxel, which are used in breast, lung and ovarian cancers. Topoisomerase I inhibitors are a group of agents derived from cantothecin. They kill cancer cells by inhibiting the production of the enzyme topoisomerase I, which is essential to DNA replication. Examples are topotecan and irinotecan, used in refractory colon and ovarian cancers. Vinca alkaloids are part of a group of agents that interfere with microtubule assembly, thereby inhibiting the mitosis phase of the cell cycle. Examples are vinblastine, vincristine and a new agent, vinorelbine. These agents are used in patients with lymphomas, Kaposi's sarcoma, lung cancer and breast cancer.

Agents Under Investigation

Researchers have studied the use of vitamin A analogues (for example, 13-cis retinoic acid [Accutane]), as well as the use of antioxidants beta carotene or vitamin A ester, combined with vitamins C (ascorbic acid) and E (alpha-tocopherol). Daily ingestion may help control precancerous oral lesions (leukoplakia). While antioxidant vitamins have no evident clinical adverse side effects, 13-cis retinoic acid may cause skin dryness, pruritus, rash, angular cheilitis, photosensitivity and an increase in blood triglycerides. Optimal dosages and combinations have not yet been established and are presently not recommended. Clinical trials with cox-2 (cyclooxygenase) inhibitors have been discontinued because of the associated risk for cardiovascular disease. Table 23.1 provides general information on selected antineoplastic drugs in several commonly used categories: alkylating agents, antibiotics, antimetabolites, biologic agents and hormonal agents, as well as miscellaneous agents also used in cancer therapy.

Special Dental Considerations

The patient's response to chemotherapeutic agents, many of which suppress white blood cells and platelets, influences the timing and types of dental procedures. The dentist's main concern before providing care to a patient receiving chemotherapy relates to adequate numbers of white blood cells (because of concerns about infection) and blood platelets (because of concerns about excessive bleeding). The marrow suppression usually is cyclical, and there are periods during which the risks of infection and bleeding are minimal.

Before the dentist undertakes any dental procedure involving a patient with cancer, he or she should contact the patient's primary care physician or oncologist regarding the need for any premedication. This includes the use of antibiotics to protect against bacteremias.

Because many medications used by dental clinicians to control oral complaints (signs and symptoms) may put an extra burden on a patient's ability to detoxify drugs, the dentist should notify the physician before using such medications. It is important to coordinate medical and dental treatment to minimize complications for the patient.

Careful clinical and radiographic examination followed by any indicated corrective procedure are essential to minimize subsequent complications of dental pain, abscesses, poor hygiene and periodontal disease that may occur during cancer therapy. This is an important step in prevention, because dental infections that occur when the patient is temporarily compromised while undergoing chemotherapy can create critical problems in patient care and recovery.

Nausea and vomiting often complicate patient progress because of poor hygiene, inadequate food and liquid intake, pain and discomfort, malaise and depression. However, it is essential that patients maintain optimal oral hygiene by using appropriate brushing and flossing techniques as well as mouthrinses. If mouthrinses that contain alcohol cause discomfort, then blander mouthrinses (such as baking soda rinses) should be used. Alcohol-free mouthrinses are available, e.g., chlorhexidine (prescription) and Biotene (OTC). Some reports have stated that a daily rinse with chlorhexidine may reduce the risk of developing candidiasis (candidal overgrowth) and mucositis. Because of frequent instances of gingival sensitivity, soft toothbrushes or even gelfoam-type applicators are needed to apply a baking soda slurry or a flavor-free toothpaste, e.g., Biotene toothpaste, that also contains fluoride and an enzyme system that help control oral flora proliferation.

Oral Conditions Associated With Cancer Therapy

Mucositis

Mucositis, or stomatitis, is a complex pathologic process of inflammation and ulceration probably caused by a combination of suppression of epithelial growth, mucosal erosion, abnormal connective tissue cytokine signaling, and bacterial overgrowth. It is a common manifestation of induced leukopenia. The oral mucosal reaction usually is associated with pain, which interferes with nutrition and hydration. This can significantly alter a patient's course of recovery and become a major complaint and therapeutic problem.

Mucositis is best managed by maintaining optimal oral hygiene and waiting for the critical white blood cell recovery.

During this period, controlling pain with medication is important for maintaining the patient's comfort and nutritional intake. Antibiotics, antifungal drugs and antiviral agents are often necessary. These medications are administered by the medical team. Short-course glucocorticoid therapy (using agents such as prednisone 40-80 mg daily as needed) is often helpful in reducing inflammation and discomfort. If tolerated, topical corticosteroids may be helpful (e.g., elixir of dexamethasone 5 mg/5 mL). Fluocinonide (Lidex) ointment 0.05% as a gel or mixed with equal parts Orabase B can be administered topically for possible relief. Sometimes a mild mouthwash made up of anti-inflammatory, antifungal and antihistamine solutions is helpful. Administration of granulocyte-stimulating factors may help accelerate white cell proliferation and recovery. Studies have indicated that some mouth rinses may help prevent or accelerate the recovery from mucositis, e.g., L-glutamine, an amino acid associated with healing; and benzydamine, a nonsteroidal analgesic. Palifermin, an epithelial growth agent administered intravenously, has shown efficacy, as well as amifostine (Ethyol), an organic thiophosphate cytoprotective agent, administered intravenously or subcutaneously.

When utilizing bone marrow/stem cell transplantation to aid recovery from cytotoxic therapy and immunosuppression, graft versus host (GVH) disease can mimic mucositis and cause considerable chronic discomfort. Management is similar to approaches for mucositis.

Xerostomia

Because many antineoplastic drugs affect the salivary glands and suppress saliva production, subsequent oral dryness can be bothersome and interfere with eating, speech and hygiene. If hyposalivation is prolonged, it can also cause dental caries and promote candidiasis.

Fortunately, this hyposalivation is almost always transient. Therefore, conservative approaches are usually sufficient. These approaches include sucking on ice chips, taking frequent sips of water, sucking on sugarless candy, chewing sugarless gum and using saliva substitutes that provide temporary lubrication. More severe or longer-lasting xerostomia can be palliated by the use of systemic sialogogues (such as pilocarpine 5 mg tid or qid, bethanechol 25-50 mg tid or qid, or cevimeline 30 mg tid) (see Chapter 8). Topical lubricants, e.g., Gelclair gel (prescription) or Oral Balance liquid or gel (OTC) may be of some help. Nonalcohol Biotene mouthwash (OTC) contains ingredients (glucose oxidase, lactoperoxidase, lysozyme, and lactoferrin) that help control the oral microbial flora and are soothing.

Taste

Some agents used to control neoplastic growth affect the sensitive taste buds. Use of these agents often forms the basis for patients' complaints of altered food tastes (dysgeusia), or a "bad taste in the mouth." In some patients, this may even cause food aversion and further complicate their maintenance of adequate caloric intake. This complaint usually is a transient, direct response to a drug or combination of drugs.

Infections

Bone-marrow suppression is a common response to many antineoplastic drugs. This response often will reduce a normal white blood cell count of more than 4,000 cells/mm^3 to less than 2,000, and sometimes even to zero. The ensuing leukopenia lowers a patient's ability to control the proliferation of micro-organisms.

Overgrowth of bacteria, viruses and fungi that stems from drug-induced leukopenia can complicate patient care and the course of the disease. The main concern with bacterial overgrowth is the possibility of bacteremia, fevers of undetermined origin and patient morbidity and mortality.

Reactivation of the herpes simplex virus commonly occurs in the patient who is immunocompromised. The diagnosis is based on clinical suspicion combined with smears or cultures. Because of the acute nature of the viral infection, diagnosis and treatment are combined by instituting an antiviral drug along with the selected diagnostic technique.

Fungal overgrowth is usually caused by leukopenia, xerostomia and poor hygiene. The organism is candidal, most often *Candida albicans*. Different species of the organism may have implications regarding responses to antifungal drugs. As with bacteria and foci of infection, the possibility of candidemia exists.

Identifying a causative agent of the infection is important. The medical team will prescribe the appropriate medications. It is important to rule out dental sources by examining the teeth, gingiva and mucosal surfaces.

Bleeding
Bleeding may be the result of a reduction of blood platelets, which occurs along with the marrow suppression and leukopenia. As platelet levels decrease to below 100,000/mm³, the patient's risk of experiencing hemorrhage, either spontaneous or in response to trauma, increases. Therefore, it is important that the clinician have knowledge of a patient's blood status before beginning dental procedures. Bleeding in addition to marrow suppression often results in anemia. This in turn contributes to patient malaise and weakness.

Osteonecrosis
Bisphosphonates, such as zoledronic acid (Zometa) or pamidronate (Aredia), are widely used by medical oncologists as a preventive measure in malignancies that have a predilection for bone metastases and osteoporosis. It is estimated that up to 15% of patients treated with bisphosphonates given intravenously will develop associated osteonecrosis of the mandible or maxilla, most commonly following an invasive dental procedure, e.g., extraction. There is no reproducibly effective curative treatment. Conservative supportive measures, utilizing antibiotics and analgesic agents, or smoothing sharp bone spicules, are helpful. Surgery, hyperbaric oxygen, and discontinuing the bisphosphonate have not been effective in controlling the problem.

Dental anomalies
In children, antineoplastic drug therapy may result in various dental anomalies. When a drug is given during tooth development, it may result in delayed eruption, noneruption, malformations of crowns and/or roots, and discolorations of the crown. While the clinical features and the patient's history can be fairly conclusive as to the cause of such conditions, the differential diagnosis still must include genetic dental dysplasia, hypoparathyroidism, and adverse influences of excess fluoride and broad-spectrum antibiotics.

Drug Interactions of Dental Interest
Because combinations of drugs, dosage ranges and patient profiles and responses differ so greatly, it is necessary to maintain contact with the patient's physician to determine palliation and therapeutic dosages, expected side effects and potential drug interactions. Interactions, if they do occur, are most commonly related to detoxification and elimination of drug products, resulting in high and potentially toxic drug levels in the blood. In turn, the blood levels required

for effective pharmacologic response are balanced against potential adverse side effects.

Significant Laboratory Value Alterations

- Values for leukocytes in leukopenia: less than 2,000 cells/mm³ as opposed to the normal values, 5,000-10,000 cells/mm³.
- Values for platelets in thrombocytopenia: less than 50,000 platelets/mm³ as opposed to the normal values, 150,000-350,000 platelets/mm³.

Special Patients

Pregnant and nursing women
Chemotherapy is contraindicated in pregnant and nursing women.

Pediatric, geriatric and other special patients
In children, depending on the type of tumor and the patient's age and size, neoplastic drugs might affect tooth development.

In some geriatric patients and patients with disabilities, the dental treatment plan depends on the patient's overall prognosis, the type of tumor, the patient's medical status (in terms of general well-being) and the patient's ability to comply with protocols and self-care regimens.

Adverse Effects, Precautions and Contraindications

Table 23.1 lists adverse effects related to antineoplastic drugs.

The following precautions and contraindications apply to all antineoplastic agents: concerns of myelosuppression, hepatotoxicity, nephrotoxicity, ototoxicity and gastrointestinal upset. All antineoplastic drugs are classified in pregnancy risk category D.

Pharmacology

In general, aklylating agents, intercalators and antibiotics damage or disrupt DNA, block activity of topoisomerases or alter resistance gene nucleotide binding site (RNBS) structure. Antimetabolites block or decrease synthesis of both RNA and DNA. Steroids interfere with transcription, while plant alkaloids disrupt mitosis. Biologic agents stimulate natural host defense mechanisms. Taxanes are considered spindle poisons—but, unlike the vinca alkaloids, the taxanes allow microtubular assembly to occur and block disassociations.

Suggested Readings

Antonadou D, Pepelassi M, Synodinou M, et al. Prophylactic use of amifostine to prevent radiochemotherapy-induced mucositis and xerostomia in head-and-neck cancer. Int J Radiat Oncol Biol Phys 2002;52:739-47.

Bonner JA, Harari PM, Giralt J, et al. Radiotherapy plus cetuximab for squamous-cell carcinoma of the head and neck. N Engl J Med 2006;354:567-78.

Imanguli MM, Pavletic SZ, Guadagnini J-P, et al. Chronic graft versus host disease of oral mucosa: Review of available therapies. Oral Surg Oral Med Oral Pathol Oral Radiol Endod 2006;101:177-85.

Migliorati CA, Casiglia J, Epstein J, et al. Managing the care of patients with bisphosphonate-associated osteonecrosis. JADA 2005;136:1658-68.

Physicians' Desk Reference. 60th ed. Montvale, N.J.: Thomson PDR; 2006.

Saba NF, Khuri FR, Shin DM. Targeting the epidermal growth factor receptor. Oncology 2006;20:153-61.

Silverman S Jr. Complications of treatment. In: Silverman S Jr., ed. Oral Cancer. 5th ed. Hamilton,Ontario, Canada: BC Decker; 2003:113-28.

Sonis ST, Elting LS, Keefe D, et al. Perspectives on cancer therapy-induced mucosal injury: Pathogenesis, measurement, epidemiology, and consequences for patients. Cancer 2004;100(9 Suppl):1995-2025.

Tsao AS, Kim ES, Hong WK. Chemoprevention of cancer. CA Cancer J Clin 2004;54:150-80.

Table 23.1: PRESCRIBING INFORMATION FOR HEAD AND NECK CANCER AGENTS

NAME	FORM/ STRENGTH	DOSAGE	WARNINGS/PRECAUTIONS & CONTRAINDICATIONS	ADVERSE EFFECTS†
ALKYLATING AGENTS				
Cyclophosphamide (Cytoxan, Cytoxan Lyophilized)*	Inj (Lyophi-lized): 100mg, 200mg, 500mg, 1g, 2g; Tab: 25mg, 50mg	*Adults/Pediatrics*: **Malignant Diseases (Without Hematologic Deficiency): Monotherapy: Initial:** 40-50mg/kg IV in divided doses over 2-5 days, or 10-15mg/kg IV given every 7-10 days, or 3-5mg/kg twice weekly. **Oral Dosing: Initial/Maint:** 1-5mg/kg/day PO. Adjust dose according to antitumor activity and/or leukopenia. May need to reduce dose when combined with other cytotoxic drugs. *Pediatrics*: **Nephrotic Syndrome:** 2.5-3mg/kg/day PO for 60-90 days.	**W/P:** Second malignancies, cardiac dysfunction, and hemorrhagic cystitis reported. May cause fetal harm in pregnancy. Serious, fatal infections may develop if severely immunosuppressed. Monitor for toxicity with leukopenia, thrombocytopenia, tumor cell infiltration of bone marrow, previous x-ray therapy or cytotoxic therapy, and impaired hepatic and/or renal function. Monitor hematologic profile for hematopoietic suppression. Examine urine for red blood cells. Anaphylactic reactions reported. Possible cross-sensitivity with other alkylating agents. May cause sterility. May interfere with normal wound healing. Consider dose adjustment with adrenalectomy. **Contra:** Severely depressed bone marrow function. **P/N:** Category D, not for use in nursing.	Impairment of fertility, amenorrhea, nausea, vomiting, anorexia, abdominal discomfort, diarrhea, alopecia, leukopenia, thrombocytopenia, hemorrhagic ureteritis, interstitial pneumonitis, malaise, asthenia, renal tubular necrosis.
Ifosfamide (Ifex)*	Inj: 1g, 3g	*Adults*: 1.2g/m²/day slow IV infusion over a minimum of 30 minutes for 5 consecutive days. Repeat treatment every 3 weeks or after recovery from hematologic toxicity (platelets ≥100,000/µL, WBC ≥4000/µL). Give with extensive hydration (eg, 2L fluid/day) and protector (eg, mesna) to prevent bladder toxicity/hemorrhagic cystitis.	**Risk of urotoxic side effects, especially hemorrhagic cystitis, and CNS toxicities (eg, confusion, coma); may require discontinuation of therapy. Severe myelosuppression reported. W/P:** Obtain urinalysis before each dose. Withhold dose until complete resolution of microscopic hematuria. Monitor WBCs, platelets, Hgb before each dose and at appropriate intervals. Avoid with WBC <2000/µl and/or platelets <50,000/µl. Discontinue if somnolence, confusion, hallucinations, and/or coma occur. Caution with impaired renal function, compromised bone marrow reserve, prior radiation therapy. May interfere with normal wound healing. **Contra:** Severely depressed bone marrow function. **P/N:** Category D, not for use in nursing.	Alopecia, nausea, vomiting, hematuria, CNS toxicity, infection, renal impairment, liver dysfunction.
ANTHRACYCLINES				
Daunorubicin Citrate Liposome (DaunoXome)*	Inj: 2mg/mL	*Adults*: 40mg/m² IV infusion; repeat every 2 weeks until evidence of progressive disease or until other complications of HIV preclude continuation.	**Monitor for cardiac toxicity. Severe myelosuppression may occur. Reduce dose with hepatic dysfunction. A triad of back pain, flushing, and chest tightness reported during 1st 5 minutes of infusion; resume infusion at slower rate. W/P:** Primary toxicity is myelosuppression; careful hematologic monitoring (prior to each dose) required. Evaluate cardiac function before each course and determine left ventricular ejection fraction (LVEF) at total cumulative dose of 320mg/m², and every 160mg/m² thereafter. Monitor LVEF at cumulative doses prior to therapy and every 160mg/m² in those with prior anthracycline therapy, pre-existing cardiac disease, or previous radiotherapy. Avoid extravasation. Can cause fetal harm during pregnancy. **P/N:** Category D, safety in nursing not known.	Myelosuppression, alopecia, cardiomyopathy with CHF, nausea, vomiting, fatigue, fever, diarrhea, cough, dyspnea, abdominal pain, anorexia, rigors, back pain, increased sweating, rhinitis, neuropathy.

*Used as single or combination agents for head and neck cancer. †Bold entries denote special dental considerations.

NAME	FORM/ STRENGTH	DOSAGE	WARNINGS/PRECAUTIONS & CONTRAINDICATIONS	ADVERSE EFFECTS†
Daunorubicin Hydrochloride (Cerubidine)*	**Inj:** 20mg	***Adults:* ANLL: Combination Therapy: <60 yrs:** 45mg/m²/day IV on days 1, 2, 3 of 1st course and on days 1, 2 of subsequent courses. **≥60 yrs:** 30mg/m²/day IV on days 1, 2, 3 of 1st course and on days 1, 2 of subsequent courses. **ANLL: Combination Therapy:** 45mg/m²/day IV on days 1, 2, 3. **Renal Impairment:** If SCr >3mg%, reduce dose by 50%. Hepatic Impairment: If serum bilirubin 1.2-3mg%, reduce dose by 25%. If >3mg%, reduce dose by 50%. ***Pediatrics:* ANLL: Combination Therapy:** 25mg/m² IV on day 1 every week. If complete remission not obtained after 4 courses, may give additional 1-2 courses. If <2 yrs or <0.5m² BSA, calculate dose based on weight (1mg/kg) instead of BSA.	**Avoid IM/SC route. Severe local tissue necrosis with extravasation. Myocardial toxicity may occur during or after terminate therapy; increased risk if cumulative dose >400-550mg/m² in adults, >300mg/ m² in pediatrics >2yrs, or >10mg/m² in pediatrics <2yrs. Severe myelo-suppression may occur. Reduce dose with impaired hepatic or renal function. W/P:** Avoid if pre-existing drug-induced bone marrow suppression occurs unless benefit warrants the risk. May cause fetal harm during pregnancy. May impart red color to urine. Monitor blood uric acid levels. Determine CBC frequently. Evaluate cardiac, renal, and hepatic function before each course. **P/N:** Category D, not for use in nursing.	Cardiotoxicity, myelosuppression, alopecia, nausea, vomiting, diarrhea, abdominal pain, hyperuricemia, mucositis (3-7 days after therapy).
Doxorubincin Hydrochloride (Adriamycin)*	**Inj:** 2mg/mL, 10mg, 20mg, 50mg	***Adults/Pediatrics:* Monotherapy:** 60-75mg/m² IV every 21 days. Use the lower dose with inadequate bone marrow reserves due to old age, prior therapy, or neoplastic marrow infiltration. **Concomitant Chemotherapy:** 40-60mg/m² IV every 21-28 days. **Hyperbilirubinemia:** Reduce dose by 50% if 1.2-3mg/dL; reduce dose by 75% if 3.1-5mg/dL.	**Severe local tissue necrosis will occur if extravasation occurs. Do not give IM/SC route. Myocardial toxicity may occur during or after therapy. Increased risk of CHF with high cumulative doses, previous anthracycline/ anthracenedione therapy, pre-existing heart disease, radiotherapy to mediastinal/pericardial area, concomitant cardiotoxic drugs. Increased risk of delayed cardiotoxicity in pediatrics. Secondary acute myelogenous leukemia reported. Reduce dose in hepatic impairment. Severe myelosuppression may occur. W/P:** Irreversible myocardial toxicity may occur. Bone marrow depression and arrhythmias reported. Enhanced toxicity with hepatic impairment; evaluate hepatic function before dosing. Imparts a red coloration to urine for 1-2 days after administration. May induce tumor lysis syndrome and hyperuricemia with rapidly growing tumors. Periodically monitor CBC, hepatic function, and radionuclide left ventricular ejection fraction. May cause prepubertal growth failure and gonadal impairment. **Contra:** Marked myelosuppression induced by previous treatment with other antitumor agents or radiotherapy. Previous therapy with complete cumulative doses of doxorubicin, daunorubicin, idarubicin, or other anthracyclines and anthracenes. **P/N:** Category D, not for use in nursing.	Myelosuppression, cardiotoxicity, alopecia, nausea, vomiting, mucositis, ulceration and necrosis of colon, fever, chills, urticaria, phleboscierosis, facial flushing.
Doxorubicin Hydrochloride Liposome (Doxil)*	**Inj:** 2mg/mL	***Adults:* KS:** 20mg/m² IV over 30 minutes, once every 3 weeks. **Ovarian Cancer:** 50mg/m² IV once every 4 weeks. Initiate at 1mg/mL to minimize infusion reactions; may increase rate if no reactions to complete infusion at 1 hr. Minimum 4 courses is recommended. **Hepatic Dysfunction:** If serum bilirubin 1.2-3mg/dL, give	**Myocardial damage may lead to CHF when cumulative doses approach 550mg/m². May lead to cardiac toxicity, consider prior use of anthracyclines or anthracenediones in cumulative dose calculations. Cardiac toxicity may occur at lower cumulative doses with prior mediastinal irradiation or cyclophosphamide therapy. Acute infusion-associated**	Neutropenia, leukopenia, anemia, thrombocytopenia, stomatitis, nausea, asthenia, vomiting, rash, alopecia, diarrhea, constipation, PPE.

Table 23.1: PRESCRIBING INFORMATION FOR HEAD AND NECK CANCER AGENTS *(cont.)*

NAME	FORM/ STRENGTH	DOSAGE	WARNINGS/PRECAUTIONS & CONTRAINDICATIONS	ADVERSE EFFECTS†
ANTHRACYCLINES *(cont.)*				
Doxorubicin Hydrochloride Liposome *(cont.)*		50% of normal dose. If serum bilirubin >3mg/dL, give 25% of normal dose. **Stomatitis/PPE Toxicity: Grade 1:** Redose unless patient had previous Grade 3 or 4 toxicity. If so, delay up to 2 weeks and decrease dose by 25%. Return to original dose interval. **Grade 2:** Delay dose up to 2 weeks or until resolved to Grade 0-1. If no resolution after 2 weeks, discontinue. **Grade 3 or 4:** Delay dose up to 2 weeks or until resolved to Grade 0-1. Decrease dose by 25% and return to original dose interval. If no resolution after 2 weeks, discontinue. **Hematological Toxicity: Grade 1:** Resume therapy with no dose reduction. **Grade 2 or 3:** Wait until ANC ≥1500 and platelets ≥75,000; redose with no dose reduction. **Grade 4:** Wait until ANC ≥1500 and platelets ≥75,000; redose at 25% dose reduction or continue full dose with cytokine support.	reactions reported. **Severe myelosuppression, myocardial toxicity may occur. Reduce dose with hepatic dysfunction. Severe side effects reported with accidental substitution for doxorubicin Hydrochloride. Only administer to cardiovascular disease patients when benefit outweighs risk. W/P:** Monitor cardiac function. Cardiac toxicity may occur after discontinuation. Recall of skin reaction due to radiotherapy reported. Obtain CBC, including platelets, frequently and at a minimum before each dose. Secondary AML reported with anthracyclines. Evaluate hepatic function before therapy. Avoid extravasation. Can cause fetal harm. Palmar-plantar erythrodysestheia (PPE) reported. **Contra:** Nursing mothers. **P/N:** Category D, not for use in nursing.	
ANTIMETABOLITES				
Fluorouracil (Adrucil)*	**Inj:** 50mg/mL	***Adults:*** 12mg/kg IV qd for 4 days. **Max:** 800mg/day. If no toxicity, give 6mg/kg IV on 6th, 8th, 10th, and 12th days. Skip days 5, 7, 9, and 11. **Inadequate Nutritional State:** 6mg/kg IV for 3 days. If no toxicity, give 3mg/kg IV on 5th, 7th, and 9th days. **Max:** 400mg/day. Skip days 4, 6, and 8. **Maint (Use Schedule 1 or Schedule 2): Schedule 1:** If no toxicity, repeat 1st course every 30 days after last day of previous course. **Schedule 2:** When toxic signs from initial course subside, give 10-15mg/kg/week IV single dose; do not exceed 1g/week.	**Hospitalize patient during initial therapy due to possible severe toxic reactions. W/P:** Extreme caution in poor risk patients with history of high-dose irradiation, previous use of alkylating agents, hepatic/renal dysfunction, widespread bone marrow involvement by metastatic tumors. Dipyrimidine dehydrogenase deficiency prolongs 5-fluorouracil clearance; can cause severe toxicity. May cause fetal harm in pregnancy. Other therapy interfering with nutrition or depressing bone marrow function increases toxicity. Discontinue with stomatitis, esophagopharyngitis, leukopenia, intractable vomiting, diarrhea, GI ulceration or bleeding, thrombocytopenia, or hemorrhage from any site. Palmar-plantar erythrodysesthesia syndrome (hand-foot syndrome) reported. Perform WBC with differential before each dose. Narrow margin of safety; monitor patients very closely. **Contra:** Poor nutritional state, depressed bone marrow function, potentially serious infection. **P/N:** Category D, not for use in nursing.	Stomatitis, esophagopharyngitis, diarrhea, anorexia, nausea, emesis, leukopenia, alopecia, dermatitis.
Gemcitabine Hydrochloride (Gemzar)*	**Inj:** 200mg, 1g	***Adults:* Pancreatic Cancer:** 1000mg/m² IV weekly up to 7 weeks, then 1 week off. Give subsequent cycles as weekly infusions for 3 out of every 4 weeks. **Lung Cancer: 4 Week Cycle:** 1000mg/m² IV days 1, 8, and 15 of each 28-day cycle. Give cisplatin 100mg/m² IV on day 1 after infusion. **3 Week Cycle:** 1250mg/m² on	**W/P:** Increased toxicity with infusion time >60 minutes and more than once weekly dosing. Hemolytic-Uremic Syndrome, hepatotoxicity, pulmonary toxicity, renal failure, leukopenia, thrombocytopenia, and anemia reported. Myelosuppression is dose-limiting toxicity. Discontinue if severe lung toxicity occurs. Caution with significant renal or hepatic	Myelosuppression, nausea, vomiting, diarrhea, stomatitis, elevated serum transaminases, proteinuria, hematuria, fever, rash, dyspnea, edema, flu-syndrome, infection, alopecia, paresthesia.

*Used as single or combination agents for head and neck cancer.   †Bold entries denote special dental considerations.

NAME	FORM/ STRENGTH	DOSAGE	WARNINGS/PRECAUTIONS & CONTRAINDICATIONS	ADVERSE EFFECTS[†]
Gemcitabine Hydrochloride (cont.)		days 1 and 8 of each 21-day cycle. Give cisplatin 100mg/m^2 IV on day 1 after infusion. **Breast Cancer:** 1250mg/m^2 IV on days 1 and 8 of each 21-day cycle. Give paclitaxel 175mg/m^2 IV on day 1 before gemcitabine. Adjust dose based on hematologic toxicity.	impairment.Greater tendency for older women to not preceed to next cycle and experience grade 3/4 neutropenia and thrombocytopenia. Perform CBC, differential, and platelets before each dose. Decreased clearance in women and elderly. **P/N:** Category D, not for use in nursing.	

ANTIMICROTUBULE AGENTS

NAME	FORM/ STRENGTH	DOSAGE	WARNINGS/PRECAUTIONS & CONTRAINDICATIONS	ADVERSE EFFECTS[†]
Docetaxel (Taxotere)*	**Inj:** 20mg/0.5mL	***Adults/Pediatrics:*** **≥16 yrs:** Pre-medicate with oral corticosteroids. **Breast Cancer:** 60-100mg/m^2 IV over 1 hr every 3 weeks. Decrease dose from 100mg/m^2 to 75mg/m^2 with febrile neutropenia, neutrophils <500 cells/mm^3 for >1 week, or severe/cumulative cutaneous reactions. Decrease to 55mg/m^2 or discontinue if reactions continue. Discontinue if ≥grade 3 peripheral neuropathy occurs. **NSCLC:** 75mg/m^2 IV over 1 hr every 3 weeks. **NSCLC Monotherapy:** Withhold therapy with febrile neutropenia, neutrophils <500 cells/mm^3 for >1 week, severe/cumulative cutaneous reactions, or other grade 3/4 non-hematological toxicities. Resume with 55mg/m^2 when toxicities resolve. Discontinue if ≥grade 3 peripheral neuropathy occurs. **NSCLC Combination Therapy With Cisplatin:** Decrease dose to 65mg/m^2 with nadir of platelet count during previous course of therapy of <25,000 cells/mm^3, febrile neutropenia, and serious non-hematologic toxicities. May decrease to 50mg/m^2 if needed. **Prostate Cancer:** 75mg/m^2 every 3 weeks over 1 hr with prednisone 5mg bid. Reduce dose to 60mg/m^2 with febrile neutropenia, neutrophils <500 cells/mm^3 for >1 week, severe/cumulative cutaneous reactions or moderate neurosensory signs/symptoms. Discontinue treatment if reactions continue.	**Increased treatment-related mortality reported with hepatic dysfunction, high-dose therapy, and in non-small cell lung carcinoma previously treated with platinum-based chemotherapy with docetaxel 100mg/m^2. Severe hypersensitivity reactions, severe fluid retention reported. Avoid if neutrophils <1500 cells/mm^3, bilirubin >ULN, or SGOT/SGPT >1.5X ULN with alkaline phosphatase >2.5X ULN. W/P:** Toxic deaths, febrile neutropenia, neutropenia, localized erythema of extremities with edema and desquamation, severe neurosensory symptoms, severe asthenia reported. Monitor for hypersensitivity reactions. Can cause fetal harm. Caution in elderly. Monitor CBC frequently; avoid subsequent cycles until neutrophils recover to >1500 cells/mm^3 and platelets recover to >100,000 cells/mm^3. **Contra:** Neutrophils <1500 cells/mm^3, hypersensitivity to polysorbate 80. **P/N:** Category D, not for use in nursing.	Arthralgia, myalgia, alopecia, stomatitis, nausea, vomiting, diarrhea, nail changes, cutaneous and neurosensory reactions, fluid retention, hypersensitivity reaction, leukopenia, thrombocytopenia, anemia, neutropenia, fever.
Paclitaxel (Taxol)*	**Inj:** 6mg/mL	***Adults:*** **IV: Ovarian Carcinoma: Previously Untreated:** 175mg/m^2 over 3 hrs or 135mg/m^2 over 24 hrs every 3 weeks followed by cisplatin. **Previous Treatment:** 135mg/m^2 or 175mg/m^2 over 3 hrs every 3 weeks. **Breast Cancer:** 175mg/m^2 over 3 hrs every 3 weeks. **Non-small Cell Lung Cancer:** 135mg/m^2 over 24 hrs every 3 weeks followed by cisplatin. **Kaposi's Sarcoma:** 135mg/m^2 over 3 hrs every 3 weeks or 100mg/m^2 over 3 hrs every 2 weeks. Reduce dose of subsequent courses by 20% if neutrophils <500 cells/mm^3	**Anaphylaxis, severe hypersensitivity reactions reported. Pretreat with corticosteroids, diphenhydramine, and H$_2$ antagonists. Do not rechallenge if severe hypersensitivity reaction occurs. Monitor CBC frequently. W/P:** Severe conduction abnormalities, injection site reactions, peripheral neuropathy (more common in elderly) reported. Bone marrow suppression is dose dependent, dose limiting, and more common in elderly. Can cause fetal harm. Hypotension, bradycardia, and HTN may occur during administration. Toxicity enhanced with elevated liver enzymes. Contains dehydrated alcohol. **Contra:** Hypersensitivity	Neutropenia, leukopenia, thrombocytopenia, anemia, infections, bleeding, bradycardia, hypotension, peripheral neuropathy, myalgia/arthralgia, nausea, vomiting, diarrhea, mucositis, alopecia.

Table 23.1: PRESCRIBING INFORMATION FOR HEAD AND NECK CANCER AGENTS *(cont.)*

NAME	FORM/ STRENGTH	DOSAGE	WARNINGS/PRECAUTIONS & CONTRAINDICATIONS	ADVERSE EFFECTS[†]
ANTIMICROTUBULE AGENTS *(cont.)*				
Paclitaxel *(cont.)*		for ≥1 week or severe peripheral neuropathy occurs.	to drugs formulated in Cremophor® EL (eg, cyclosporine for injection concentrate, teniposide for injection concentrate), solid tumor patients with baseline neutrophils <1500 cells/mm³, AIDS-related Kaposi's sarcoma patients with baseline neutrophils <1000 cells/mm³. **P/N:** Category D, not for use in nursing.	
Paclitaxel Protein-Bound (Abraxane)*	Inj: 100mg	*Adults:* 260mg/m² IV over 30 minutes every 3 weeks. Severe neutropenia (neutrophil <500 cells/mm³ for a week or longer) or severe sensory neuropathy: Reduce to 220mg/m², if recurrence reduce to 180mg/m².	**Do not administer to patients with metastatic breast cancer who have baseline neutrophil counts of less than 1,500 cells/mm³. Perform peripheral blood cell counts on all patients to monitor occurence of bone marrow suppression, primarily neutropenia. Should only be administered under the supervision of a physician experienced in the use of cancer chemotherapeutic agents. Do not substitute for or with other paclitaxel formulations.** **W/P:** Men should be advised to not father a child while receiving treatment. Remote risk for transimission of viral diseases; theoretical risk for transmission of Creutzfeldt-Jacob disease. Sensory neuropathy occurs frequently. Reports of injection sites reactions. **Contra:** Patients with baseline neutrophil counts of <1,500 cells/mm³. **P/N:** Category D, not for use in nursing.	Neutropenia, infectious episodes, anemia, hypotension, ECG abnormalities, dyspnea, cough, sensory neuropathy, ocular/visual disturbances, arthralgia, myalgia, nausea, vomiting, asthenia, abnormal liver function test.
CYTOTOXIC GLYCOPEPTIDE ANTIBIOTICS				
Bleomycin sulfate (Blenoxane)*	Inj: 15U, 30U	*Adults:* **Squamous Cell Carcinoma/Non-Hodgkin's Lymphoma/Testicular Carcinoma:** 0.25-0.5U/kg IV/IM/SC weekly or twice weekly. For lymphoma patients, give ≤2U for the 1st two doses; continue with regular dosage schedule if no acute reaction occurs. **Hodgkin's Disease:** 0.25-0.5U/kg IV/IM/SC weekly or twice weekly. **Maint:** After 50% response, give 1U/day or 5U weekly IV/IM. **Malignant Pleural Effusion:** 60U as a single dose bolus intrapleural injection.	**Pulmonary fibrosis is the most severe toxicity reported (usually presents as pneumonitis occasionally progressing to pulmonary fibrosis); higher occurrence in elderly and if receiving >400 units total dose. A severe idiosyncratic reaction including hypotension, mental confusion, fever, chills, and wheezing reported in lymphoma patients.** **W/P:** Extreme caution with significant renal impairment or compromised pulmonary function. Pulmonary toxicity (dose and age related) may occur; frequent roentgenograms are recommended. Monitor for severe idiosyncratic reactions, especially after 1st and 2nd doses. Renal and hepatic toxicity reported. Can cause fetal harm during pregnancy. Risk of pulmonary toxicity with total dose >400U. Caution with dose selection in elderly. **Contra:** Status asthmaticus or other acute asthma or COPD episodes. **P/N:** Category D, not for use in nursing.	Pneumonitis, erythema, rash, striae, vesiculation, hyperpigmentation, skin tenderness, hyperkeratosis, nail changes, alopecia, pruritus, stomatitis, pulmonary toxicity.

*Used as single or combination agents for head and neck cancer.   †Bold entries denote special dental considerations.

NAME	FORM/ STRENGTH	DOSAGE	WARNINGS/PRECAUTIONS & CONTRAINDICATIONS	ADVERSE EFFECTS†
EPIDERMAL GROWTH FACTOR-RECEPTOR (EGFR) ANTAGONISTS				
Cetuximab (Erbitux)*	**Inj:** 2mg/mL [50mL]	**Adults: LD:** 400mg/m² IV infusion over 120 minutes. **Maint:** 250mg/m² IV infusion over 60 minutes once weekly. **Max Infusion Rate:** 5mL/min. Pre-medication with H1 antagonist (eg, diphenhydramine 50mg IV) is recommended. **Mild-moderate (Grade 1 or 2) Infusion Reactions:** Reduce rate by 50%. **Severe (Grade 3 or 4) Infusion Reactions:** Discontinue. **Development of Severe Acneform Rash:** Delay infusion 1-2 weeks for first three occurrences. **First Occurrence:** If improvement seen, continue at 250mg/m². **Second Occurrence:** If improvement seen, reduce dose to 200mg/m². **Third Occurrence:** If improvement seen, reduce dose to 150mg/m². **Fourth Occurrence/No improvement After Delaying Therapy:** Discontinue.	**Severe infusion reactions have occurred; discontinue if these reactions develop. W/P:** Infusion reactions reported; observe closely for 1 hr post-infusion. Dermatologic (eg, acneform rash, skin drying/fissuring, inflammatory and infectious sequelae) or pulmonary toxicities may occur. Discontinue if interstitial lung disease is confirmed. Adjust dose in cases of severe acneform rash. Apply sunscreen and limit sun exposure. Caution with hypersensitivity to murine proteins. Potential for immunogenicity. **P/N:** Category C, not for use in nursing.	Acneform rash, asthenia/malaise, diarrhea, nausea, abdominal pain, vomiting, fever, constipation, infusion reactions, dermatologic toxicities.
Erlotinib (Tarceva)*	**Tab:** 25mg, 100mg, 150mg	**Adults: NSCLC:** 150mg ≥1 hr before or 2 hrs after ingestion of food. **Pancreatic Cancer:** 100mg at least 1 hr before or 2 hrs after ingestion of food, in combination with gemcitabine. Continue until disease progression or unacceptable toxicity.	**W/P:** Serious interstitial disease (ILD) including fatalities reported. Discontinue if ILD is diagnosed. Asymptomatic increases in liver transaminases observed. Dose reduction or interruption should be considered if changes in liver function are severe. Elevations in INR and infrequent reports of bleeding have been reported. Monitor closely with concomitant anticoagulants. **P/N:** Category D, not for use in nursing.	Rash, diarrhea, anorexia, fatigue, dyspnea, cough, nausea, infection, vomiting, stomatitis, pruritus, dry skin, conjunctivitis, keratoconjunctivitis sicca, abdominal pain.
NUCLEOSIDE ANALOGS				
Dacarbazine (DTIC-DOME)*	**Inj:** 200mg	**Adults: Malignant Melanoma:** 2-4.5mg/kg/day for 10 days. May repeat every 4 weeks. **Alternate Dosage:** 250mg/m²/day IV for 5 days. May repeat every 3 weeks. **Hodgkin's Disease:** 150mg/m²/day for 5 days. May repeat every 4 weeks. **Alternate Dosage:** 375mg/m²/day on day 1. May repeat every 15 days.	**Hemopoietic toxicity and hepatotoxicity reported. W/P:** Hematopoietic depression, anemia, anaphylactic reactions reported. Hepatotoxicity with hepatic vein thrombosis and hepatocellular necrosis may result in death. Extravasation may result in tissue damage and severe pain. **P/N:** Category C, safety in nursing not known.	Nausea, vomiting, anorexia, diarrhea, flu-like syndromes, alopecia, renal or hepatic dysfunction, rash.
PLATINUM COORDINATION COMPOUNDS				
Carboplatin (Paraplatin)*	**Inj:** 10mg/mL	**Adults: Monotherapy:** 360mg/m² IV on day 1 every 4 weeks. **Concomitant Cyclophosphamide:** 300mg/m² IV on day 1 every 4 weeks for 6 cycles, with cyclophosphamide 600mg/m² IV on day 1 every 4 weeks for 6 cycles. **If platelets >100,000 or neutrophils >2000:** Give 125% of dose. **If platelets <50,000 or neutrophils <500:** Give 75% of dose. **Renal Impairment: Initial:** CrCl 41-59mL/min: 250mg/m². CrCl 16-40mL/min: 200mg/m². Subsequent dose adjustments based on the degree of bone marrow suppression.	**Bone marrow suppression, resulting in infection or bleeding reported. Anemia and anaphylactic-like reactions reported. W/P:** Bone marrow suppression is dose-dependent and is the dose-limiting toxicity. May need transfusion for anemia. Bone marrow suppression increased in patients who recieved prior therapy. Neurotoxicity increased if ≥65 yrs and previous cisplatin treatment. LFT abnormalities and temporary loss of vision with high doses. Emesis reported. **Contra:** Severe bone marrow depression, significant bleeding. History of severe allergic reactions to cisplatin, platinum-containing compounds, or mannitol. **P/N:** Category D, not for use in nursing.	Blood dyscrasias, infection, bleeding, nausea, vomiting, peripheral neuropathies, ototoxicity, elevated LFTs/bilirubin/serum creatinine, electrolyte loss, allergic reactions, alopecia, mucositis.

Table 23.1: PRESCRIBING INFORMATION FOR HEAD AND NECK CANCER AGENTS *(cont.)*

NAME	FORM/ STRENGTH	DOSAGE	WARNINGS/PRECAUTIONS & CONTRAINDICATIONS	ADVERSE EFFECTS†
RETINOIDS				
Bexarotene (Targretin)*	**Cap:** 75mg	***Adults:*** **Initial:** 300mg/m² qd with a meal. If toxicity occurs, adjust to 200mg/m²/day then to 100mg/ m²/day, or temporarily suspend. Readjust upward if toxicity controlled. If no response after 8 weeks and 300mg/m² is tolerated, increase to 400mg/m²/day.	**Retinoids are associated with birth defects. Avoid in pregnancy.** **W/P:** May induce lipid and LFT abnormalities, pancreatitis, hypothyroidism, leukopenia, cataracts. Perform fasting lipid levels before therapy, then weekly until lipid response to bexarotene (2-4 weeks), then at 8-week intervals. May need dose reduction or suspension if develop elevated triglycerides. Obtain baseline LFT; then monitor at 1, 2, and 4 weeks after initial therapy; then periodically if stable. Obtain WBC with differential at baseline, periodically thereafter. Minimize exposure to sunlight and artificial UV light. Great caution with hepatic dysfunction. Avoid if risk factors present for pancreatitis. **Contra:** Pregnancy. **P/N:** Category X, not for use in nursing.	Lipid abnormalities, anemia, nausea, headache, asthenia, infection, abdominal pain, chills, fever, flu syndrome, hypothyroidism, rash, dry skin, leukopenia, peripheral edema.
MISCELLANEOUS				
Bevacizumab (Avastin)*	**Inj:** 25mg/mL [4mL, 16mL]	***Adults:*** 5mg/kg IV infusion over 90 minutes, given once every 14 days until disease progression is detected. If 1st infusion is well tolerated, give 2nd infusion over 60 minutes and subsequent doses over 30 minutes.	**Gastrointestinal perforation, wound dehiscence, some fatal, have been reported. Permanently discontinue if such cases require medical intervention. Serious hemoptysis reported (primarily in non-small cell lung cancer patients). Avoid use with recent hemoptysis. W/P:** Discontinue with GI perforation, wound dehiscence, nephrotic syndrome or serious hemorrhage. Increased risk of HTN; permanently discontinue if hypertensive crisis occurs. Monitor BP every 2-3 weeks during treatment. Increased incidence/severity of proteinuria. Potential for immunogenicity. CHF reported. Avoid initiation of therapy for at least 28 days following major surgery; surgical incision must be fully healed prior to start of therapy. Suspend treatment prior to elective surgery. **P/N:** Category C, not for use in nursing.	Asthenia, pain, abdominal pain, headache, HTN, diarrhea, nausea, vomiting, anorexia, stomatitis, constipation, upper respiratory infection, epistaxis, dyspnea, exfoliative dermatitis, proteinuria.
Capecitabine (Xeloda)*	**Tab:** 150mg, 500mg	***Adults:*** Take with water within 30 minutes after meals. Usual: 1250mg/m² bid for 2 weeks, then 1 week off. Give as 3-week cycles. For adjuvant treatment of Dukes' C colon cancer give as 3-week cycles for a total of 8 cycles (24 weeks). **CrCl 30-50mL/min:** Reduce to 75% of starting dose. Interrupt and/or reduce dose if toxicity occurs. Re-adjust according to adverse effects (see labeling for details).	**Altered coagulation parameters and/or bleeding, including death, reported with coumarin-derivative anticoagulants (eg, warfarin). Monitor PT/INR frequently to adjust anticoagulant dose. W/P:** Reduce dose with moderate renal dysfunction. Carefully monitor for adverse events with mild to moderate renal dysfunction. Carefully monitor with severe diarrhea fluid/electrolyte balance; may need dose adjustment. Patients ≥80 yrs may experience increased grade 3 and 4 adverse events (see full prescribing info). Possible fetal harm with pregnancy. Monitor for hand-and-foot syndrome. Cardiotoxicity reported; more common with history of CAD. Carefully monitor with mild to	Diarrhea, hand and foot syndrome, pyrexia, anemia, nausea, fatigue, vomiting, dermatitis, neutropenia, thrombocytopenia, stomatitis, anorexia, hyperbilirubinemia, abdominal pain, paresthesia.

*Used as single or combination agents for head and neck cancer.   †Bold entries denote special dental considerations.

NAME	FORM/ STRENGTH	DOSAGE	WARNINGS/PRECAUTIONS & CONTRAINDICATIONS	ADVERSE EFFECTS†
Capecitabine *(cont.)*			moderate hepatic dysfunction due to hepatic metastases. Hyperbilirubine-mia, neutropenia, thrombocytopenia, and decrease in hemoglobin reported. **Contra:** Hypersensitivity to 5-FU, dihy-dropyrimidine dehydrogenase (DPD) deficiency, severe renal impairment (CrCl <30mL/min). **P/N:** Category D, not for use in nursing.	
Gefitinib (Iressa)*	**Tab:** 250mg	***Adults:*** 250mg qd. **Poorly Tolerated Diarrhea/Skin Adverse Reactions:** Provide brief (up to 14 days) therapy interruption fol-lowed by reinstatement of 250mg daily dose. **Concomitant Potent CYP3A4 Inducers (eg, rifampin, phenytoin):** Consider increasing dose to 500mg qd, in the absence of severe adverse reactions.	**W/P:** Interstitial lung disease reported; discontinue with acute onset or worsening of pulmonary symptoms (dyspnea, cough, fever). May cause fetal harm. Asymptomatic increases in liver transaminases observed; consider periodic liver function testing. Hepatic dysfunction may increase gefitinib exposure. Caution with severe renal impairment. **P/N:** Category D, not for use in nursing.	Diarrhea, rash, acne, dry skin, nausea, vomiting, pruritus, anorexia, asthenia, weight loss, eye pain, corneal erosion/ulcer.
Hydroxyurea (Hydrea)	**Cap:** 500mg	***Adults:*** **Solid Tumors: Intermit-tent:** 80mg/kg single dose every 3rd day. **Continuous:** 20-30mg/kg qd. **Head and Neck Carcinoma:** 80mg/kg single dose every 3rd day. Start at least 7 days before irradiation. **Resistant CML:** 20-30mg/kg qd. **Elderly/Renal Impairment:** May need dose reduction.	**W/P:** Patients with previous irradiation therapy may have exacerbation of post-irradiation erythema. Bone marrow suppression, erythrocytic abnormalities may occur. Correct severe anemia before initiating therapy. Caution with marked renal dysfunction. **May develop secondary leukemia with long-term therapy for myeloproliferative disorders. Monitor CBC, bone marrow, hepatic and kidney function before therapy and repeatedly thereafter. Inter-rupt therapy if WBC <2500/mm³ or platelets <100,000/mm³. Contra:** Marked bone marrow depression (leukopenia, thrombocytopenia or severe anemia). **P/N:** Category D, not for use in nursing.	Bone marrow depression, GI effects, maculopapular rash, skin ulceration, dermatomyositis-like skin changes, peripheral and facial erythema.
Imatinib Mesylate (Gleevec)*	**Tab:** 100mg, 400mg	***Adults:*** ≥18 yrs: **CML: Chronic Phase:** 400mg qd, may increase to 600 mg qd. **Accelerated Phase/ Blast Crisis:** 600mg qd, may increase to 400 mg bid. See label-ing for dose increase with CML. **GIST:** 400mg qd or 600mg qd. **Hepatotoxicity/Non-Hematologic Adverse Reaction:** If bilirubin >3X ULN or transaminases >5X ULN, hold drug until bilirubin >1.5X ULN and transaminases >2.5X ULN. Continue at reduced dose. **Neu-tropenia/Thrombocytopenia:** See labeling for dose adjustment. Take with food and water. ***Pediatrics:*** ≥3 yrs: **CML: Chronic Phase:** 260mg/ m²/day given qd or split into 2 doses (morning and evening). **Neutropenia/Thrombocytopenia:** See labeling for dose adjustment. Take with food and water.	**W/P:** Fluid retention/edema reported; monitor weight. Neutropenia/throm-bocytopenia reported; monitor CBC weekly during 1st month, biweekly during 2nd month, and periodically thereafter. May be hepatotoxic; moni-tor LFTs at baseline, then monthly or as needed. Avoid becoming pregnant. Interrupt treatment if severe non-hematologic adverse reaction develops (eg, severe hepatotoxicity or severe fluid retention); resume if appropriate. GI bleeds reported. **P/N:** Category D, not for nursing.	Nausea, vomiting, fluid retention, neutropenia, thrombocytopenia, diarrhea, hemorrhage, pyrexia, rash, headache, fatigue, abdominal pain, elevated transaminases or bilirubin, edema, muscle cramps, musculoskeletal pain, flatulence, nasopharyn-gitis, insomnia.
Megestrol Acetate (Megace ES)	**Sus:** 40mg/mL [240mL], (ES) 125mg/mL [150mL]	***Adults:*** **(Megace) Initial:** 800mg/ day (20mL/day). **Usual:** 400-800mg/day. Shake well before use. **Elderly:** Start at lower end of	**W/P:** May cause fetal harm; avoid in pregnancy. New onset or exacerbation of diabetes or Cushing's syndrome reported. Risk of adrenal suppression	Abdominal pain, chest pain, cardiomyopathy, palpitation, constipation, **dry mouth**, edema, confusion, convulsion,

Table 23.1: PRESCRIBING INFORMATION FOR HEAD AND NECK CANCER AGENTS (cont.)

NAME	FORM/ STRENGTH	DOSAGE	WARNINGS/PRECAUTIONS & CONTRAINDICATIONS	ADVERSE EFFECTS†
MISCELLANEOUS (cont.)				
Megestrol Acetate (cont.)		dosing range. **(Megace ES) Initial/ Usual:** 625mg/day (5mL/day).	if taking or withdrawing from chronic therapy; monitor for hypotension, nausea, vomiting, dizziness, or weakness. Caution with history of thromboembolic diseases. Experience is limited in HIV-infected women. Do not use as prophylactic to avoid weight loss. **Contra:** Pregnancy. **P/N:** Category X, not for use in nursing.	dyspnea, cough, alopecia, pruritus, thromboembolic phenomena.
Methotrexate Sodium (Rheumatrex)*	**Inj:** (Generic) 20mg, 25mg/mL, 1g; **Tab: (Rheumatrex)** 2.5mg* [Dose Pack 15mg, 4 x 6 tabs; 12.5mg, 4 x 5 tabs; 10mg, 4 x 4 tabs; 7.5mg, 4 x 3 tabs; 5mg, 4 x 2 tabs]	***Adults:* Choriocarcinoma/Tropho-blastic disease:** 15-30mg qd PO/IM for 5 days. May repeat 3-5 times as required with rest period of ≥1 week. **Leukemia: Induction:** 3.3mg/m² with prednisone 60mg/m² qd. **Remission Maintenance:** 15mg/m² PO/IM twice weekly or 2.5mg/kg IV every 14 days. **Burkitt's Tumor: Stages I-II:** 10-25mg/day PO for 4-8 days. Administer several courses with rest periods of 7-10 days in between. **Lymphosarcoma: Stage III:** 0.625-2.5mg/kg/day with other antitumor agents. **Mycosis Fungoides:** 5-50mg once weekly. If poor response, give 15-37.5mg twice weekly. Adjust dose based on response and hematologic monitoring. **Osteosarcoma: Initial:** 12g/m² IV, increase to 15g/m² if peak serum levels of 1000 micromolar not reached at end of infusion. **Meningeal Leukemia:** Dilute preservative free MTX to 1mg/mL. Give 12mg intrathecally at 2-5 day intervals. **Psoriasis: Initial:** 10-25mg weekly until response or use divided oral dose schedule, 2.5mg at 12 hr intervals for 3 doses. **Titrate:** Increase gradually until optimal response. **Maint:** Reduce to lowest effective dose. **Max:** 30mg/week. **Rheumatoid Arthritis: Initial:** 7.5mg PO once weekly, or 2.5mg q12h for 3 doses given as a course once weekly. **Titrate:** Gradual increase. **Max:** 20mg weekly. After response, reduce dose to lowest effective amount of drug. ***Pediatrics:* Meningeal Leukemia:** Dilute preservative free MTX to 1mg/mL. **<1 yr:** 6mg. **1 yr:** 8mg. **2 yrs:** 10mg. **≥3 yrs:** 12mg. Give intrathecally at 2-5 day intervals. **JRA: 2-16 yrs: Initial:** 10mg/m² once weekly. Adjust dose gradually to achieve optimal response.	**Only for life-threatening neoplastic disease, or in severe RA, and psoriasis unresponsive to other therapies. Death, fetal death/congenital anomalies, lung disease, tumor lysis syndrome, fatal skin reactions, PCP reported. Monitor for bone marrow, liver, lung, and kidney toxicities. Bone marrow suppression, aplastic anemia and GI toxicity reported with NSAIDs. Hepatotoxicity, fibrosis, and cirrhosis with prolonged use. Interrupt therapy with diarrhea, ulcerative stomatitis. Reduced elimination with renal dysfunction, ascites, or pleural effusion. Increased risk of soft tissue necrosis and osteonecrosis with radiotherapy. Malignant lymphoma may occur. Extreme caution with high dose regimen for osteosarcoma. Do not use formulations/diluents with preservatives for intrathecal or high dose therapy. W/P:** Monitor closely; toxicity may be related to dose and frequency of administration. When reactions do occur, doses should be reduced or discontinued and corrective measures should be taken. Avoid pregnancy if either partner is receiving therapy. Avoid intrathecal administration or high-dose therapy. Injection contains benzyl alcohol; avoid use in neonates (<1 month), may cause gasping syndrome. **Contra:** Pregnancy, nursing. Psoriasis or RA patients with alcoholism, alcoholic liver disease, chronic liver disease, immunodeficiency syndrome, and pre-existing blood dyscrasias. **P/N:** Category X, contraindicated in nursing.	Ulcerative stomatitis, leukopenia, nausea, abdominal distress, malaise, fatigue, chills, fever, dizziness, decreased resistance to infection.
Mitomycin (Mutamycin)*	**Inj:** 5mg, 20mg, 40mg	***Adults:* Usual:** (after full hematological recovery): 20mg/m² IV single dose q6-8 weeks. **Dosage Adjustments:** Leukocytes 2000-2999mm³/Platelets 25,000-74,999mm³: Give 70% of prior	**Bone marrow suppression (eg, thrombocytopenia, leukopenia) is the most common and severe toxic effects that may contribute to infections. Hemolytic-uremic syndrome (HUS) has been reported, mostly**	Bone marrow toxicity, fever, anorexia, nausea, vomiting, integument and mucous membrane toxicity, cellulitis, stomatitis, alopecia, necrosis, hemolytic uremic syndrome.

*Used as single or combination agents for head and neck cancer.   †Bold entries denote special dental considerations.

NAME	FORM/ STRENGTH	DOSAGE	WARNINGS/PRECAUTIONS & CONTRAINDICATIONS	ADVERSE EFFECTS†
Mitomycin *(cont.)*		dose. **Leukocytes <2000mm³/ Platelets <25,000mm³:** Give 50% of prior dose. No repeat dosage until leukocyte count has returned to 4000/mm³ and platelet counts to 100,000/mm³.	with high doses (≥60mg). Blood product transfusion may exacerbate HUS. **W/P:** Monitor platelets, WBCs, differential and Hgb repeatedly during therapy and for at least 8 weeks after. May cause renal toxicity, avoid if serum creatinine is >1.7 mg%. **Contra:** Thrombocytopenia, coagulation disorder, increased bleeding tendency due to other causes. **P/N:** Safety in pregnancy unknown, not for use in nursing.	
Pemetrexed (Alimta)	**Inj:** 500mg	*Adults:* **Premedication: Dexamethasone:** 4mg bid day before, day of, and day after pemetrexed. **Folic Acid:** At least 5 daily doses (350-1000µg) during 7 days prior to pemetrexed. Continue for 21 days after last pemetrexed dose. **Vitamin B12:** 1000µg IM once during week preceding first pemetrexed dose and every 3 cycles thereafter. **Treatment: Mesothelioma:** 500mg/m² IV over 10 minutes on Day 1 of each 21 day cycle with cisplatin 75mg/m² infused over 2 hours beginning 30 minutes after pemetrexed. **NSCLC:** 500mg/m² IV over 10 minutes on Day 1 of each 21 day cycle. **Hematologic Toxicity: Nadir ANC <500mm³/Nadir Platelets ≥50,000/mm³:** 75% of previous dose (both drugs). **Nadir Platelets <50,000/mm³:** 50% of previous dose (both drugs). **Nonhematologic Toxicity: Grade 3/4 (except Grade 3 transaminase elevation or mucositis)/Diarrhea Requiring Hospitalization:** 75% of previous dose (both drugs). **Grade 3/4 Mucositis:** 50% of previous pemetrexed dose. **Neurotoxicity: CTC Grade 2:** 50% of previous cisplatin dose. Discontinue with Grade 3/4 neurotoxicity; Grade 3/4 hematologic or nonhematologic toxicities after 2 dose reductions (except Grade 3 transaminase elevations). Avoid with CrCl <45mL/min.	**W/P:** May suppress bone marrow function. With pleural effusions, ascites, consider draining prior to therapy. Monitor CBCs, for nadir and recovery before each dose and on days 8 and 15 of each cycle. Do not begin new cycle unless ANC ≥1500 cells/mm³, platelets ≥100,000 cells/mm³, CrCl ≥45mL/min. **P/N:** Category D, not for use in nursing.	Nausea, fatigue, dyspnea, vomiting, hematologic effects, constipation, chest pain, anorexia, fever, infection, stomatitis, pharyngitis, rash/desquamation.
Vinorelbine tartrate (Navelbine)*	**Inj:** 10mg/mL	*Adults:* **Single-Agent:** 30mg/m² IV weekly over 6-10 minutes. **With Cisplatin:** 25mg/m² weekly with cisplatin 100mg/m² every 4 weeks, or 30mg/m² weekly with cisplatin 120mg/m² on days 1 and 29, then every 6 weeks. **Adjustments Based on Granulocytes:** If 1000-1499 cells/mm³ give 50% starting dose. If <1000 cells/mm³, hold dose and repeat count in 1 week. Discontinue if hold 3 consecutive weekly doses because granulocyte <1000 cells/mm³. If fever and/or sepsis occurs while	**For IV use only; fatal if given intrathecally. Severe granulocytopenia may occur; granulocyte counts should be ≥1000 cells/mm³ prior to administration. Use extreme caution to prevent extravasation; if this occurs, discontinue and restart in another vein. W/P:** Monitor for myelosuppression during and after therapy, and for infection and/or fever with developing severe granulocytopenia. Interstitial pulmonary changes, ARDS, acute shortness of breath and severe bronchospasm reported. Extreme caution with compromised bone marrow	Granulocytopenia, leukopenia, thrombocytopenia, anemia, asthenia, injection site reactions/pain, phlebitis, peripheral neuropathy, nausea, vomiting, diarrhea, severe constipation, paralytic ileus, intestinal obstruction, necrosis, and/or perforation, dyspnea, alopecia, chest pain, fatigue.

Table 23.1: PRESCRIBING INFORMATION FOR HEAD AND NECK CANCER AGENTS *(cont.)*

NAME	FORM/ STRENGTH	DOSAGE	WARNINGS/PRECAUTIONS & CONTRAINDICATIONS	ADVERSE EFFECTS†
MISCELLANEOUS *(cont.)*				
Vinorelbine tartrate *(cont.)*		granulocytopenic or if hold 2 consecutive weekly doses due to granulocytopenia; give 75% of the starting dose if granulocytes ≥1500 cells/mm³, and 37.5% of the starting dose if granulocytes 1000-1499 cells/mm³. **Hepatic Insufficiency:** (bilirubin 2.1-3mg/dL) 50% of the starting dose or (bilirubin >3mg/dL) 25% of the starting dose. If both hematologic toxicity and hepatic insufficiency, use lowest dose. **Neurotoxicity:** Discontinue if Grade ≥2 develops.	reserve due to prior irradiation or chemotherapy. Radiation recall reactions may occur. Monitor for new or worsening signs/symptoms of neuropathy. Discontinue if moderate or severe neurotoxicity develops. Avoid contact with skin, mucosa, and eyes. Avoid pregnancy. **Contra:** Pretreatment granulocytes <1000 cells/mm³. **P/N:** Category D, not for use in nursing.	
MUCOSITIS TREATMENTS				
Chlorhexidine (Peridex★, PerioGard)	**Oral Liquid:** 0.12%	***Adults***: **Gingivitis:** Swish 15mL for 30 sec then spit out. Use a.m. and p.m. after brushing teeth. Do not swallow liquid. Do not rinse, brush, or eat for several hours after use.	**W/P:** Anterior tooth restorations having rough surfaces or margins may develop permanent discoloration from chlorhexidine, necessitating replacement for cosmetic reasons. Should not be used as sole treatment of gingivitis. Use with caution in patients with hypersensitivity to chlorhexidine disinfectant skin cleansers. **P/N:** Category B, safety in nursing unknown.	Allergic reaction (skin rash, hives, swelling of face); **taste alteration; increase in calculus formation; staining of teeth, mouth, tooth fillings, and dentures or other mouth appliances; mouth irritation**; swollen glands on side of face or neck; **irritation to lips or tongue**.
Gelclair	**Gel:** 15mL/ packet [21ˢ]	***Adults***: Mix one packet with 1-3 tbsp of water. Gargle for 1 min then spit out. Use tid or prn. Avoid eating or drinking for 1 hr after use. May be used undiluted. No adverse effects anticipated if accidentally swallowed.	**P/N:** Safety not known in pregnancy or nursing.	None reported.
Rincinol P.R.N.	**Sol:** 120mL	***Adults/Pediatrics***: Swish 10mL for 60 sec then spit out; use prn. Avoid eating or drinking for 1 hr after use. No adverse effects anticipated if accidentally swallowed.	None reported.	None reported.

★ indicates a product bearing the ADA Seal of Acceptance.   †Bold entries denote special dental considerations.

Table 23.2: DRUG INTERACTIONS FOR HEAD AND NECK CANCER AGENTS

ALKYLATING AGENTS

Cyclophosphamide (Cytoxan, Cytoxan Lyophilized)

Doxorubicin	Potentiates succinylcholine chloride effects and doxorubicin-induced cardiotoxicity.
Phenobarbital	Chronic, high doses of phenobarbital increase metabolism and leukopenic activity.

Ifosfamide (Ifex)

Chemotherapeutic agents	Severe myelosuppression with other chemotherapeutic agents.
Cytotoxic agents	Caution with other cytotoxic agents.

ANTHRACYCLINES

Daunorubicin Hydrochloride (Cerubidine)

Antineoplastics	Possible secondary leukemias with other antineoplastics or radiation therapy.
Cyclophosphamide	Increased risk of cardiotoxicity with previous doxorubicin therapy or with concomitant cyclophosphamide.
Doxorubicin	Increased risk of cardiotoxicity with previous doxorubicin therapy.
Hepatotoxic agents	Hepatotoxic agents (eg, high dose MTX) may increase risk of toxicity.
Myelosuppres-sants	May need dose reduction with other myelosuppressants.

Doxorubincin Hydrochloride (Adriamycin)

6-mercaptopurine	May enhance hepatotoxicity of 6-mercaptopurine.
Actinomycin-D	Acute recall pneumonitis in pediatrics with actinomycin-D.
Anticancer therapies	May potentiate toxicity of other anticancer therapies.
Cardiotoxic drugs	Increased risk of CHF with radiotherapy to mediastinal/pericardial area or cardiotoxic drugs.
Calcium channel blockers	Possible increased risk of cardiotoxicity with calcium channel blockers.
Cisplatin	Seizures and coma reported with cisplatin.
Cyclophosphamide	May exacerbate cyclophosphamide-induced hemorrhagic cystitis.
Cyclosporine	Cyclosporine may prolong and exacerbate hematologic toxicity, seizures and coma reported with cyclosporine.
Cytarabine	Necrotizing colitis reported with cytarabine.
Cytotoxic chemotherapy	Live vaccines may be hazardous in those undergoing cytotoxic chemotherapy.
Paclitaxel	Paclitaxel infused before doxorubicin may decrease clearance of doxorubicin and increase neutropenia and stomatitis episodes, than the reverse sequence of administration.
Phenobarbital	Phenobarbital increases elimination.

Table 23.2: DRUG INTERACTIONS FOR HEAD AND NECK CANCER AGENTS *(cont.)*

ANTHRACYCLINES *(cont.)*

Doxorubincin Hydrochloride (Adriamycin) *(cont.)*

Phenytoin	May decrease phenytoin levels.
Progesterone, IV	Enhanced neutropenia and thrombocytopenia reported with IV progesterone.
Radiation-induced toxicity	May increase radiation-induced toxicity of the myocardium, mucosae, skin, and liver.
Streptozocin	Streptozocin may inhibit hepatic metabolism.
Vincristine	Seizures and coma reported with vincristine.

Doxorubicin Hydrochloride Liposome (Doxil)

Anticancer therapies	May potentiate toxicity of other anticancer therapies.
6-mercaptopurine	May enhance hepatotoxicity of 6-mercaptopurine.
Radiation-induced toxicity	May increase radiation-induced toxicity of the myocardium, mucosae, skin, and liver.
Cyclophosphamide	May exacerbate cyclophosphamide-induced hemorrhagic cystitis.

ANTIMETABOLITES

Fluorouracil (Adrucil)

Leucovorin	Leucovorin calcium may enhance toxicity.

Gemcitabine Hydrochloride (Gemzar)

Cisplatin	Monitor serum creatinine, K^+, calcium, and magnesium with cisplatin.
Hepatotoxic drugs	Serious hepatotoxicity reported with hepatotoxic drugs.

ANTIMICROTUBULE AGENTS

Docetaxel (Taxotere)

CYP450 3A4	Caution with agents that induce, inhibit, or are metabolized by CYP450 3A4 (eg, ketoconazole, erythromycin, terfenadine, astemizole, cyclosporine).

Paclitaxel (Taxol)

Cisplatin	Myelosuppression more profound with cisplatin.
CYP450 2C8/3A4	Caution with CYP450 2C8 and 3A4 substrates or inhibitors (eg, ritonavir, saquinavir, indinavir, nelfinavir).
Doxorubicin	Increases doxorubicin levels.

EPIDERMAL GROWTH FACTOR-RECEPTOR (EGFR) ANTAGONIST

Erlotinib (Tarceva)

CYP3A4 inhibitor	Co-treatment with potent CYP3A4 inhibitor ketoconazole increases erlotinib AUC by two thirds. Caution should be used when administering or taking erlotinib with ketoconazole and other strong CYP3A4 inhibitors such as atazanavir, clarithromycin, indinavir, itraconazole, nefazodone, nelfinavir, ritonavir, saquinavir, telithromycin, troleandomycin, and voriconazole.

PLATINUM COORDINATION COMPOUNDS

Carboplatin (Paraplatin)

Aminoglycosides	Aminoglycosides may increase ototoxic or nephrotoxic effects.
Nephrotoxic compounds	Nephrotoxic compounds may potentiate renal adverse effects.

RETINOIDS

Bexarotene (Targretin)

Contraceptives	May increase metabolism of hormonal contraceptives.
CYP3A4 inducers	CYP3A4 inducers (eg, rifampin, phenytoin, phenobarbital) may decrease levels.
CYP3A4 inhibitors	CYP3A4 inhibitors (eg, ketoconazole, itraconazole, erythromycin, gemfibrozil, grapefruit juice) may increase levels.
Gemfibrozil	Avoid gemfibrozil.
Insulin	May enhance hypoglycemia with insulin, sulfonylureas, or insulin sensitizers.
Sulfonylureas	May enhance hypoglycemia with insulin, sulfonylureas, or insulin sensitizers.
Tamoxifen	May increase metabolism of tamoxifen, hormonal contraceptives.
Vitamin A	Limit vitamin A intake to ≤1500 IU/day.

MISCELLANEOUS

Bevacizumab (Avastin)

Chemotherapy	Increased risk of thromboembolic events when coadministered with chemotherapy; discontinue if severe arterial thromboembolic event occurs.

Capecitabine (Xeloda)

Phenytoin	May increase phenytoin levels; reduce phenytoin dose.
Leucovorin	Leucovorin may increase levels and toxicity of 5-FU
Anticoagulants	Altered coagulation parameters and/or bleeding reported with anticoagulants (eg, coumarin, phenprocoumon); monitor PT/INR frequently.
Antacids	Aluminum and/or magnesium antacids may increase levels.
CYP2C9	Caution with CYP2C9 substrates.

Gefitinib (Iressa)

Cimetidine	Drugs causing significant sustained elevation in gastric pH (eg, ranitidine, cimetidine) may reduce efficacy.
CYP3A4 inducers	CYP3A4 inducers (eg, rifampicin, phenytoin) may decrease levels.
CYP3A4 inhibitors	Caution with potent CYP3A4 inhibitors (eg, ketoconazole, itraconazole); may increase levels.
Ranitidine	Drugs causing significant sustained elevation in gastric pH (eg, ranitidine, cimetidine) may reduce efficacy.

Table 23.2: DRUG INTERACTIONS FOR HEAD AND NECK CANCER AGENTS *(cont.)*

MISCELLANEOUS *(cont.)*

Gefitinib (Iressa) *(cont.)*

Warfarin	INR increases and/or bleeding reported with warfarin.

Hydroxyurea (Hydrea)

Antiretrovirals	Hepatotoxicity and hepatic failure reported in HIV patients with antiretrovirals (eg, stavudine, didanosine).
Didanosine	Pancreatitis and peripheral neuropathy reported in HIV patients with concomitant didanosine.
Myelosuppressants	Increased risk of bone marrow depression with other myelosuppressants or radiation therapy.
Radiation therapy	Increased risk of bone marrow depression with other myelosuppressants or radiation therapy.
Uricosurics	Uricosurics may need dose adjustments.

Imatinib Mesylate (Gleevec)

CYP3A4 inducers	Decreased levels with CYP3A4 inducers (eg, dexamethasone, phenytoin, carbamazepine, rifampin, phenobarbital, St. John's wort).
CYP3A4 inhibitors	Increased levels with CYP3A4 inhibitors (eg, ketoconazole, erythromycin, clarithromycin, itraconazole).
CYP3A4 substrates	Caution with CYP3A4 substrates with narrow therapeutic windows (eg, cyclosporine, pimozide). Increases levels of drugs metabolized by CYP3A4 (eg, dihydropyridines, triazolo-benzodiazepines, HMG-CoA reductase inhibitors).
Warfarin	Switch patients on warfarin to low molecular weight or standard heparin.

Megestrol Acetate (Megace ES)

Indinavir	Decrease in pharmacokinetic parameters of indinavir, higher dose should be considered.
Insulin	May increase insulin requirements.

Methotrexate Sodium (Rheumatrex)

Antibiotics	Oral antibiotics (eg, tetracycline, chloramphenicol) may decrease absorption or interfere with enterohepatic circulation.
Folic acid	Folic acid may decrease response to MTX.
Hepatotoxins	Closely monitor with hepatotoxins (eg, azathioprine, retinoids, sulfasalazine).
Nephrotoxic agents	Caution with nephrotoxic agents (eg, cisplatin).
NSAIDs	Avoid NSAIDs with high doses.
Penicillins	Penicillins may decrease clearance.
Phenylbutazone	Caution with highly protein bound drugs (eg, sulfonamides, phenytoin, phenylbutazone, salicylates).
Phenytoin	Caution with highly protein bound drugs (eg, sulfonamides, phenytoin, phenylbutazone, salicylates).

MISCELLANEOUS *(cont.)*

Methotrexate Sodium (Rheumatrex) *(cont.)*

Probenecid	Caution with probenecid, and highly protein bound drugs (eg, sulfonamides, phenytoin, phenylbutazone, salicylates).
Protein bound drugs	Caution with highly protein bound drugs (eg, sulfonamides, phenytoin, phenylbutazone, salicylates).
Salicylates	Caution with highly protein bound drugs (eg, sulfonamides, phenytoin, phenylbutazone, salicylates).
Sulfonamides	Caution with highly protein bound drugs (eg, sulfonamides, phenytoin, phenylbutazone, salicylates).
Theophylline	Decreased theophylline clearance.
TMP/SMZ	TMP/SMZ may increase bone marrow suppression.

Mitomycin (Mutamycin)

Chemotherapy	Adult respiratory distress syndrome reported with concomitant chemotherapy; monitor oxygen and fluid balance.
Mitomycin	Acute shortness of breath and bronchospasm reported following vinca alkaloids and mitomycin use.
Vinca alkaloids	Acute shortness of breath and bronchospasm reported following vinca alkaloids and mitomycin use.

Pemetrexed (Alimta)

Ibuprofen	Reduced clearance with ibuprofen; caution with CrCl <80mL/min.
Nephrotoxic agents	Delayed clearance with nephrotoxic or tubularly secreted drugs (eg, probenecid).
NSAIDs	In mild-to-moderate renal insufficiency, avoid NSAIDs with short elimination half-lives from 2 days prior to 2 days following therapy. Interrupt NSAID dosing with longer half-lives from at least 5 days before to 2 days following therapy.

Vinorelbine tartrate (Navelbine)

Cisplatin	Increased incidence of granulocytopenia with cisplatin.
CYP450 3A inhibitors	Caution with CYP450 3A inhibitors, or with hepatic dysfunction; earlier onset and/or increased severity of side effects may occur.
Mitomycin	Risk of acute pulmonary reactions with mitomycin.
Paclitaxel	Monitor for signs/symptoms of neuropathy with paclitaxel, either concomitantly or sequentially.
Radiation therapy	Radiosensitizing effects may occur with prior or concomitant radiation therapy.

Table 23.3: DRUG INFORMATION FOR OTHER TYPES OF CANCER AGENTS*

NAME	ADVERSE EFFECTS	DRUG INTERACTIONS
ALKYLATING AGENTS		
Busulfan (Myleran)	Myelosuppression, pulmonary fibrosis, cardiac tamponade, hyperpigmentation, weakness, fatigue, weight loss, nausea, vomiting, melanoderma, hyperuricemia, myasthenia gravis, hepatic veno-occlusive disease.	**Cyclophosphamide:** Reduced clearance with cyclophosphamide. **Itraconazole:** Reduced clearance with itraconazole; monitor for signs of toxicity. **Myelosuppressive drugs:** Additive myelosuppression with myelosuppressive drugs. **Myelotoxic drugs:** Additive pulmonary toxicity with myelotoxic drugs.
Carmustine (BiCNU)	Delayed myelosuppression, pulmonary infiltrates/fibrosis, nausea, vomiting, hepatic toxicity, azotemia, renal failure, neuroretinitis, chest pain, headache, allergic reaction, hypotension, tachycardia.	**Cimetidine:** Potentiates marrow toxicity of carmustine. **Digoxin:** Serum digoxin levels may decrease. **Pentostatin:** Acute pulmonary edema and hypotension reported when used in combination with carmustine, etoposide, and high dose cyclophosphamide as part of ablative regimen for bone marrow transplant. **Phenytoin:** Serum phenytoin levels may decrease.
Chlorambucil (Leukeran)	Bone marrow suppression, nausea, vomiting, diarrhea, tremors, muscular twitching, confusion, agitation, ataxia, urticaria, angioneurotic syndrome, pulmonary fibrosis, hepatotoxicity, jaundice.	**Alkylating agents:** Cross-hypersensitivity may occur with other alkylating agents.
Estramustine (Emcyt)	Edema, dyspnea, leg cramps, nausea, diarrhea, GI upset, breast tenderness/enlargement, increased hepatic enzymes.	**Anesthesia:** Alert anesthesiologist if treated within 10 days of general anesthesia. **Calcium-rich foods:** Milk, milk products, and calcium-rich foods or drugs may impair absorption.
Lomustine (CeeNU)	Delayed myelosuppression, pulmonary infiltrates/fibrosis, nausea, vomiting, hepatotoxicity, azotemia, renal failure, stomatitis, alopecia, optic atrophy, visual disturbances, lethargy, ataxia.	**Cimetidine:** May potentiate marrow toxicity of lomustine.
Mechlorethamine Hydrochloride (Mustargen)	Thrombosis, thrombophlebitis, hypersensitivity reactions, nausea, vomiting, lymphocytopenia, granulocytopenia, thrombocytopenia, maculopapular skin eruption, erythema multiforme, herpes zoster infection, oligomenorrhea, amenorrhea, impaired spermatogenesis, azoospermia.	Not available.
Melphalan (Alkeran)	Bone marrow suppression, alopecia, hemolytic anemia, pulmonary fibrosis, interstitial pneumonitis. (Inj) Hypersensitivity reactions (eg, urticaria, pruritus, edema, tachycardia). (Tab) Hepatic disorders (eg, abnormal LFTs, hepatitis, jaundice).	**Cisplatin:** Cisplatin may alter melphalan clearance from inducing renal dysfunction. **Cyclosporine:** (Inj) Severe renal failure reported with oral cyclosporine. **Nalidixic acid:** Nalidixic acid may increase incidence of severe hemorrhagic necrotic enterocolitis in pediatrics.
Streptozocin (Zanosar)	Nausea, vomiting, diarrhea, hepatic and renal toxicity, glucose tolerance abnormality.	**Cytotoxic drugs:** Additive toxicity with other cytotoxic drugs. **Nephrotoxins:** Avoid other potential nephrotoxins. **Doxorubicin:** May prolong doxorubicin half-life and lead to severe bone marrow suppression; consider reducing doxorubicin dose.
Temozolomide (Temodar)	Headache, fatigue, myelosuppression (thrombocytopenia, neutropenia), nausea, vomiting, convulsions, hemiparesis, asthenia, fever, peripheral edema, constipation, dizziness, diarrhea.	**Valproic acid:** Valproic acid may decrease clearance.
ANTHRACYCLINES		
Epirubicin Hydrochloride (Ellence)	Hematologic abnormalities, amenorrhea, hot flashes, lethargy, fever, GI disturbances, infection, conjunctivitis/keratitis, alopecia, local toxicity, rash/itch, skin changes.	**Anthracycline/anthracenedione:** Increased risk of cardiotoxicity with previous anthracycline or anthracenedione therapy, prior or concomitant radiotherapy to mediastinal/pericardial area, or with concomitant cardiotoxic drugs. **Cytotoxic drugs:** Increased risk of refractory secondary leukemia with concurrent DNA-damaging antineoplastics, heavy pretreatment with cytotoxic drugs, or escalated doses of anthracyclines. **Fluorouracil:** Fluorouracil may cause severe leukopenia, neutropenia, thrombocytopenia, and anemia. **Cyclophosphamide:** Cyclophosphamide may cause severe leukopenia, neutropenia, thrombocytopenia, and anemia. **Calcium channel blockers:** Monitor closely with cardioactive compounds that could cause heart failure (eg, calcium channel blockers). **Cimetidine:** Caution with agents that cause changes in hepatic function. AUC increased with cimetidine; stop cimetidine during therapy. **Radiation therapy:** Previous radiation therapy may induce inflammatory recall reaction at irradiation site.

*Agents *not* used for head and neck cancer.

NAME	ADVERSE EFFECTS	DRUG INTERACTIONS
Idarubicin (Idamycin PFS)	Infection, nausea, vomiting, alopecia, abdominal pain/diarrhea, hemorrhage, mucositis, rash, urticaria, bullous erythrodermatous rash of palms/soles of feet, fever, headache, cardiac toxicity (CHF, arrhythmia), pulmonary effects, mental status effects.	**Anthracycline:** Increased risk of idarubicin-induced cardiac toxicity with pre-existing heart disease, and previous therapy with high cumulative dose anthracycline therapy. **Cardiotoxic agents:** Increased risk of idarubicin-induced cardiac toxicity with other potentially cardiotoxic agents. **Radiation therapy:** Increased risk of idarubicin-induced cardiac toxicity with radiation to the mediastinal-pericardial area.

ANTIMETABOLITES

NAME	ADVERSE EFFECTS	DRUG INTERACTIONS
Clofarabine (Clolar)	Vomiting, nausea, diarrhea, anemia, leukopenia, thrombocytopenia, neutropenia, febrile neutropenia, and infection.	Not available.
Cytarabine (Cytosar-U)	Anorexia, nausea, vomiting, diarrhea, oral/anal inflammation or ulceration, hepatic dysfunction, fever, rash, thrombophlebitis, bleeding (all sites).	**Gentamicin:** Antagonizes susceptibility of gentamicin for K.pneumoniae. **Flucytosine:** May inhibit efficacy of flucytosine. **L-asparaginase treatment:** Acute pancreatitis reported in patients receiving prior L-asparaginase treatment. **Digoxin:** Monitor digoxin. **Cyclophosphamide:** Cardiomyopathy and death reported during high dose therapy with cyclophosphamide.
Cytarabine Liposome (Depocyt)	Chemical arachnoiditis (headache, fever, back pain, nausea, vomiting), confusion, somnolence, abnormal gait, peripheral edema, neutropenia, thrombocytopenia, urinary incontinence.	**Chemotherapeutic agents:** Intrathecal cytarabine in combination with other chemotherapeutic agents or with cranial/spinal irradiation may increase risk of neurotoxicity and other adverse events. **Radiation therapy:** Intrathecal cytarabine in combination with other chemotherapeutic agents or with cranial/spinal irradiation may increase risk of neurotoxicity and other adverse events.
Floxuridine (FUDR)	Nausea, vomiting, diarrhea, enteritis, stomatitis, localized erythema, anemia, leukopenia, thrombocytopenia, LFT elevation, alopecia.	Not available.
Fludarabine (Fludara)	Myelosuppression, fever, chills, infection, nausea, vomiting, malaise, fatigue, anorexia, weakness, serious opportunistic infections.	**Pentostatin:** Avoid pentostatin due to the risk of severe pulmonary toxicity.

AROMATASE INHIBITORS

NAME	ADVERSE EFFECTS	DRUG INTERACTIONS
Anastrozole (Arimidex)	Diarrhea, asthenia, nausea, headache, hot flushes, dyspnea, vomiting, cough, pain, dizziness, rash, edema.	**Estrogen-containing therapies:** Avoid tamoxifen, estrogen-containing therapies.
Exemestane (Aromasin)	Fatigue, nausea, hot flashes, pain, depression, insomnia, anxiety, dyspnea, dizziness, headache, vomiting, increased sweating, edema, HTN, anorexia.	**CYP3A4 inducers:** Potent CYP3A4 inducers (eg, rifampin, phenytoin, carbamazepine, phenobarbital, St. John's wort) may decrease plasma levels. **Estrogen-containing agents:** Avoid coadministration with estrogen-containing agents.
Letrozole (Femara)	Bone pain, back pain, nausea, arthralgia, dyspnea, fatigue, chest pain, decreased weight, hot flushes, peripheral edema, HTN, vomiting, constipation, diarrhea, musculoskeletal pain, insomnia, cough, alopecia.	**Tamoxifen:** Co-administration with tamoxifen may reduce letrozole plasma levels; if co-administered, give letrozole immediately after tamoxifen.
Testolactone (Teslac)	Maculopapular erythema, increased BP, paresthesia, malaise, aches, peripheral edema, glossitis, anorexia, nausea, vomiting.	**Anticoagulants:** May increase effects of anticoagulants; monitor/adjust anticoagulant dosage.

CYTOTOXIC GLYCOPEPTIDE ANTIBIOTICS

NAME	ADVERSE EFFECTS	DRUG INTERACTIONS
Mitotane (Lysodren)	GI disturbances, depression, lethargy, somnolence, dizziness, vertigo, skin toxicity.	**Anticoagulants:** May increase dosage requirements with warfarin; monitor with coumarin-type anticoagulants. **Hepatic enzyme induction:** Caution with drugs susceptible to hepatic enzyme induction.

DNA FRAGMENTATION AGENT

NAME	ADVERSE EFFECTS	DRUG INTERACTIONS
Arsenic (Trisenox)	Fatigue, pyrexia, edema, chest pain, injection site pain, nausea, vomiting, abdominal pain, constipation, hypokalemia, hypomagnesemia, hyperglycemia, increased ALT, headache, insomnia, dyspnea.	**Antiarrhythmics:** Caution with agents that prolong the QT interval, such as certain antiarrhythmics. **Amphotericin B:** Caution with agents that lead to electrolyte abnormalities, such as amphotericin B. **Diuretics:** Caution with agents that lead to electrolyte abnormalities, such as diuretics. **Thioridazine:** Caution with agents that prolong the QT interval, such as thioridazine.

Table 23.3: DRUG INFORMATION FOR OTHER TYPES OF CANCER AGENTS* *(cont.)*

NAME	ADVERSE EFFECTS	DRUG INTERACTIONS
ENZYMES		
Asparaginase (Elspar)	Allergic reactions, acute anaphylaxis, hyperthermia, pancreatitis, hyperglycemia, depression, fatigue, somnolence, coma, confusion, agitation, hallucinations, azotemia, liver function abnormalities.	**Methotrexate:** May diminish/abolish effects of methotrexate. **Prednisone:** Concurrent IV administration with or immediately before a course of vincristine and prednisone may increase toxicity. **Vincristine:** Concurrent IV administration with or immediately before a course of vincristine and prednisone may increase toxicity.
Denileukin (Ontak)	Chills/fever, asthenia, hypotension, nausea, vomiting, infection, pain, headache, anorexia, diarrhea, hypoalbuminemia, anemia, transaminase increase, myalgia, dizziness, dyspnea, cough increase, rash, infusion-associated reactions.	Not available.
ESTROGEN-RECEPTOR ANTAGONISTS		
Fulvestrant (Faslodex)	Gastrointestinal symptoms, headache, back pain, vasodilatation (hot flushes), pharyngitis, injection site reactions, asthenia, pain, dyspnea, increased cough.	**Anticoagulants:** Avoid with concurrent anticoagulants.
Tamoxifen Citrate (Nolvadex)	Hot flashes, increased bone and tumor pain, vaginal discharge, irregular menses, (men) loss of libido, impotence.	**Aminoglutethimide:** Decreased levels with aminoglutethimide. **Anticoagulants:** Increases effects of coumarin-type anticoagulant; monitor PT. **Bromocriptine:** Increased levels with bromocriptine. **Cytotoxic agents:** Increased risk of thromboembolic events with cytotoxic agents. **Letrozole:** May decrease letrozole levels. **Medroxyprogesterone:** Decreased plasma levels of major metabolite, N-desmethyl tamoxifen with medroxyprogesterone. **Rifampin:** Decreased levels with rifampin.
MONOCLONAL ANTIBODIES		
Alemtuzumab (Campath)	Infusion reactions (eg, rigors, fever, nausea, vomiting, hypotension), infections, hematologic toxicity (eg, neutropenia, anemia, pancytopenia), fatigue, skeletal pain, anorexia, asthenia, peripheral edema, back pain, chest pain, HTN, tachycardia, headache, diarrhea, stomatitis, myalgias, dyspnea, cough.	**Vaccines:** Avoid live viral vaccines.
Ibritumomab Tiuxetan (Zevalin)	Neutropenia, thrombocytopenia, anemia, nausea, vomiting, diarrhea, increased cough, dyspnea, arthralgia, anorexia, anxiety, ecchymosis.	**Anticoagulants:** Increased risk of bleeding and hemorrhage with drugs that interfere with platelet function or coagulation; monitor for thrombocytopenia more frequently. **Antiplatelet agents:** Increased risk of bleeding and hemorrhage with drugs that interfere with platelet function or coagulation; monitor for thrombocytopenia more frequently. **Vaccines:** Safety of immunization with live viral vaccines not studied.
Tositumomab (Bexxar)	Neutropenia, thrombocytopenia, anemia, asthenia, fever, infection, cough, pain, chills, headache, GI effects, myalgia, arthralgia, pharyngitis, dyspnea, rash.	**Anticoagulants:** Weigh risks vs. benefits of concomitant agents that interfere with platelet function and/or anticoagulation. **Antiplatelet agents:** Weigh risks vs. benefits of concomitant agents that interfere with platelet function and/or anticoagulation.
NONSTEROIDAL ANTIANDROGENS		
Bicalutamide (Casodex)	Hot flashes, back pain, asthenia, constipation, nausea, diarrhea, peripheral edema, dyspnea, pain, pelvic pain, infection, hematuria, nocturia.	**Anticoagulants:** Potentiates warfarin and other anticoagulants; monitor PT.
Flutamide (Eulexin)	Hot flashes, loss of libido, impotence, diarrhea, nausea, vomiting, gynecomastia, other GI disturbances, anemia, edema, hepatitis, jaundice, skin rash.	**Warfarin:** May increase PT; monitor warfarin.
Nilutamide (Nilandron)	Hot flushes, decreased libido, abnormal vision, increased LFTs, interstitial pneumonitis, dyspnea, GI effects, dry skin, sweating.	**Alcohol:** Intolerance to alcohol (eg, hypotension, malaise). **Phenytoin:** May potentiate vitamin K antagonists, phenytoin, and theophylline. **Theophylline:** May potentiate vitamin K antagonists, phenytoin, and theophylline. **Vitamin K antagonists:** May potentiate vitamin K antagonists, phenytoin, and theophylline.
NUCLEOSIDE ANALOGS		
Azacitidine (Vidaza)	Nausea, anemia, thrombocytopenia, vomiting, pyrexia, leukopenia, diarrhea, fatigue, injection site erythema, constipation, neutropenia, ecchymosis, cough, dyspnea, weakness.	Not available.

*Agents *not* used for head and neck cancer.

NAME	ADVERSE EFFECTS	DRUG INTERACTIONS
Cladribine (Leustatin)	Bone marrow suppression, neutropenia, fever, infection, fatigue, nausea, rash, headache, injection site reactions.	**Immunosuppression agents:** Caution with drugs that cause immunosuppression or myelosuppression. **Myelosuppression agents:** Caution with drugs that cause immunosuppression or myelosuppression. **Nephrotoxic agents:** Acute nephrotoxicity with nephrotoxic agents.

PLATINUM COORDINATION COMPOUNDS

NAME	ADVERSE EFFECTS	DRUG INTERACTIONS
Cisplatin (Platinol-AQ)	Nephrotoxicity, ototoxicity, vestibular toxicity, myelosuppression, Coombs' positive hemolytic anemia, immediate or delayed nausea and vomiting, serum electrolyte disturbances, hyperuricemia, neurotoxicity, hepatotoxicity.	**Aminoglycosides:** Cumulative nephrotoxicity potentiated with aminoglycosides. **Anticonvulsant:** Anticonvulsant levels may become subtherapeutic. **Pyridoxine:** Response duration adversely affected with pyridoxine and altretamine.
Oxaliplatin (Eloxatin)	Neuropathy, fatigue, nausea, neutropenia, emesis, diarrhea.	**5-FU:** Increased 5-FU plasma levels with doses of 130mg/m2 oxaliplatin dosed every 3 weeks; clearance may be decreased with nephrotoxic agents. **Nephrotoxic agents:** clearance may be decreased with nephrotoxic agents.

RETINOIDS

NAME	ADVERSE EFFECTS	DRUG INTERACTIONS
Tretinoin (Vesanoid)	Malaise, shivering, hemorrhage, infections, peripheral edema, pain, chest discomfort, edema, disseminated intravascular coagulation, weight change, injection site reactions, dyspnea, pleural effusion, respiratory insufficiency, pneumonia.	**Antifibrinolytic agents:** Cases of fatal thrombotic complications with antifibrinolytic agents (eg, tranexamic acid, aminocaproic acid). **CYP450:** Possible interactions with drugs that affect CYP450 system. **Vitamin A:** Aggravated symptoms of hypervitaminosis A with vitamin A.

SYNTHETIC GONADOTROPIN-RELEASING HORMONE ANALOGUES

NAME	ADVERSE EFFECTS	DRUG INTERACTIONS
Goserelin Acetate (Zoladex)	Males: hot flashes, sexual dysfunction, decreased erections, lower urinary tract symptoms, lethargy, pain (worsened in the first 30 days), edema, upper respiratory infection, rash, sweating. Females: hot flashes, vaginitis, emotional lability, decreased libido, sweating, depression, headache, acne, breast atrophy.	**Gonadotropins:** Ovarian hyperstimulation syndrome reported when used concomitantly with other gonadotropins.
Goserelin Acetate (Zoladex 3-Month)	Hot flashes, sexual dysfunction, decreased erections, osteoporosis, pain, asthenia, gynecomastia.	**Gonadotropins:** Ovarian hyperstimulation syndrome reported when used concomitantly with other gonadotropins.
Leuprolide (Eligard, Lupron Depot)	Hot flashes, pain/burning/stinging/erythema/bruising at injection site, malaise/fatigue, atrophy of testes.	Not available.

MISCELLANEOUS

NAME	ADVERSE EFFECTS	DRUG INTERACTIONS
Abarelix/ Sodium Chloride (Plenaxis)	Hot flashes, sleep disturbance, pain, breast enlargement, breast pain/nipple tenderness, back pain, constipation, peripheral edema, dizziness, headache, upper respiratory tract infection, diarrhea, dysuria, fatigue, micturition frequency.	**Antiarrhythmics:** Caution with Class IA (eg, quinidine, procainamide) or Class III (eg, amiodarone, sotalol) antiarrhythmics.
Aldesleukin (Proleukin)	Chills, fever, malaise, infection, hypotension, abdominal pain, tachycardia, vasodilation, arrhythmia, diarrhea, vomiting, nausea, stomatitis, anorexia, anemia, bilirubinemia, edema, weight gain, confusion, dyspnea.	**Antihypertensives:** Antihypertensives can potentiate hypotension. **Antineoplastics:** Hypersensitivity reactions reported with high dose antineoplastics. **Cardiotoxic drugs:** Cardiotoxic drugs may increase toxicity to that organ system. Increased risk of MI, myocarditis, ventricular hypokinesia, and severe rhabdomyolysis. **Glucocorticoids:** Glucocorticoids decrease antitumor effects. **Hepatotoxic drugs:** Hepatotoxic drugs may increase toxicity to that organ system. Increased risk of MI, myocarditis, ventricular hypokinesia, and severe rhabdomyolysis. **Iodinated contrast media:** Iodinated contrast media may cause hypersensitivity reactions up to several months after therapy. **Myelotoxic drugs:** Myelotoxic drugs may increase toxicity to that organ system. Increased risk of MI, myocarditis, ventricular hypokinesia, and severe rhabdomyolysis. **Nephrotoxic drugs:** Nephrotoxic drugs may increase toxicity to that organ system. Increased risk of MI, myocarditis, ventricular hypokinesia, and severe rhabdomyolysis **Psychotropics:** Increased CNS effects with psychotropics (eg, narcotics, analgesics, antiemetics, sedatives, and tranquilizers).

Table 23.3: DRUG INFORMATION FOR OTHER TYPES OF CANCER AGENTS* *(cont.)*

NAME	ADVERSE EFFECTS	DRUG INTERACTIONS
MISCELLANEOUS *(cont.)*		
Altretamine (Hexalen)	Nausea, vomiting, peripheral neuropathy, CNS symptoms (mood disorders, consciousness disorders, ataxia, dizziness, vertigo), leukopenia, thrombocytopenia, anemia, increased alkaline phosphatase.	**Cimetidine:** Cimetidine may increase levels. **MAOIs:** Severe orthostatic hypotension may occur with MAOIs. **Pyridoxine:** Avoid pyridoxine; possible adverse response duration effects.
BCG Live (TheraCys)	Malaise, fever, chills, uveitis, conjunctivitis, iritis, keratitis, granulomatous choreoretinitis, arthritis, arthralgia, urinary symptoms, skin rash.	**Antimicrobials:** Antimicrobials may interfere with efficacy. **Antituberculosis drugs:** Avoid antituberculosis drugs (eg, INH) to prevent or treat the local, irritative toxicities of BCG Live. **Bone marrow depressants:** Immunosuppressants, bone marrow depressants, and radiation may interfere with immune response; avoid concomitant use. **Immunosuppressants:** Immunosuppressants, bone marrow depressants, and radiation may interfere with immune response; avoid concomitant use. **Radiation:** Immunosuppressants, bone marrow depressants, and radiation may interfere with immune response; avoid concomitant use.
Bortezomib (Velcade)	Fatigue, malaise, weakness, nausea, diarrhea, decreased appetite, anorexia, constipation, thrombocytopenia, peripheral neuropathy, pyrexia, vomiting, anemia, headache, insomnia.	**Amiodarone:** Caution with concomitant use of medications associated with peripheral neuropathy (eg, amiodarone, antivirals, isoniazid, nitrofurantoin, statins) or hypotension. **Antidiabetic agents:** Oral antidiabetic agents may require dosage adjustment. **Antivirals:** Caution with concomitant use of medications associated with peripheral neuropathy (eg, amiodarone, antivirals, isoniazid, nitrofurantoin, statins) or hypotension. **Isoniazid:** Caution with concomitant use of medications associated with peripheral neuropathy (eg, amiodarone, antivirals, isoniazid, nitrofurantoin, statins) or hypotension. **Nitrofurantoin:** Caution with concomitant use of medications associated with peripheral neuropathy (eg, amiodarone, antivirals, isoniazid, nitrofurantoin, statins) or hypotension. **Statins:** Caution with concomitant use of medications associated with peripheral neuropathy (eg, amiodarone, antivirals, isoniazid, nitrofurantoin, statins) or hypotension.
Carmustine (Gliadel)	Fever, pain, abnormal healing, nausea, vomiting, brain edema, confusion, somnolence, UTI, seizures, headache, intracranial infection.	Not available.
Dactinomycin (Cosmegen)	Nausea, vomiting, fatigue, lethargy, fever, cheilitis, esophagitis, abdominal pain, liver toxicity, anemia, blood dyscrasias, skin eruptions, acne, alopecia.	**Radiation:** Increased GI toxicity, marrow suppression, and incidence of secondary tumors with radiation. May reactivate erythema from previous radiation therapy. **Radiotherapy:** Caution if used within 2 months of irradiation for treatment of right-sided Wilms' tumor; hepatomegaly and elevated AST levels reported. Only use with radiotherapy for Wilms' tumor if benefit outweighs risks.
Etoposide (Etopophos, Vepesid)	Myelosuppression, nausea, vomiting, anaphylactic-like reactions, BP changes, alopecia, anorexia.	**Cyclosporine:** High dose oral cyclosporine reduces clearance. **Levamisole:** Caution with drugs known to inhibit phosphatase activities (eg, levamisole).
Gemtuzumab Ozogamicin (Mylotarg)	Chills, fever, nausea, vomiting, headache, hypotension, HTN, hypoxia, dyspnea, hyperglycemia, antibody formation, myelosuppression, anemia, thrombocytopenia, sepsis, pneumonia, epistaxis, mucositis, hepatotoxicity.	Not available.
Hydroxyurea (Droxia)	Neutropenia, low reticulocyte and platelet levels, hair loss, skin rash, fever, GI disturbances, weight gain, bleeding, parvovirus B-19 infection, melanonychia.	**Didanosine:** Monitor for hepatoxicity and pancreatitis with didanosine, stavudine. **Stavudine:** Monitor for hepatoxicity and pancreatitis with didanosine, stavudine.
Irinotecan Hydrochloride (Camptosar)	Nausea, vomiting, diarrhea, abdominal pain, blood dyscrasias, asthenia, mucositis, anorexia, alopecia, fever, pain, constipation, infection, dyspnea, increased bilirubin.	**Anticonvulsants:** Decreased levels with CYP3A4 inducing anticonvulsants and St. John's wort. Consider substituting non-enzyme inducing anticonvulsants 2 weeks prior to and during treatment. **Antineoplastic agents:** Exacerbated myelosuppression and diarrhea with antineoplastic agents having similar adverse effects. **Dexamethasone:** Possible hyperglycemia and lymphocytopenia with dexamethasone. **Diuretics:** Consider withholding diuretics with irinotecan therapy. **Irradiation therapy:** Avoid concurrent irradiation therapy. **Ketoconazole:** Increased levels with ketoconazole. Discontinue ketoconazole at least 1 week prior to and during therapy. **Laxatives:** Laxatives may worsen diarrhea. **Prochlorperazine:** Akathisia reported with prochlorperazine. **St. John's wort:** Decreased levels with CYP3A4 inducing anticonvulsants and St. John's wort.

*Agents *not* used for head and neck cancer.

NAME	ADVERSE EFFECTS	DRUG INTERACTIONS
Mercaptopurine (Purinethol)	Bone marrow toxicity, hepatotoxicity, hyperuricemia (reduce incidence by prehydration, urine alkalinization, prophylactic allopurinol), intestinal ulceration, rash, hyperpigmentation, alopecia, transient oligospermia.	**Allopurinol:** Reduce to one-third to one-fourth of usual dose with allopurinol to avoid toxicity. **Myelosuppressants:** Reduce dose with myelosuppressants. **Thioguanine:** Cross-resistance with thioguanine. **Trimethoprim-sulfamethoxazole:** Bone marrow suppression reported with trimethoprim-sulfamethoxazole.
Mitoxantrone Hydrochloride (Novantrone)	Nausea, alopecia, menstrual disorder, upper respiratory infection, UTI, stomatitis, arrhythmia, diarrhea, constipation, back pain, abnormal ECG, asthenia, headache, cardiac toxicity.	**Anthracyclines:** Possible danger of cardiac toxicity if previously treated with anthracyclines. **Antineoplastics:** Development of acute leukemia associated with other concomitant antineoplastics.
Pegaspargase (Oncaspar)	Allergic reactions, SGPT increase, nausea, vomiting, fever, malaise.	**Anticoagulants:** Caution with concomitant anticoagulants (eg, coumadin, heparin, dipyridamole, aspirin or NSAIDs), hepatotoxic agents. **Hepatotoxic agents:** Caution with concomitant anticoagulants (eg, coumadin, heparin, dipyridamole, aspirin or NSAIDs), hepatotoxic agents. **Methotrexate:** May interfere with the action of drugs which require cell replication for their lethal effects (eg, methotrexate), and the enzymatic detoxification of other drugs, particularly in the liver. **Protein bound drugs:** May increase toxicity of protein bound drugs.
Pentostatin (Nipent)	Nausea, vomiting, fever, rash, fatigue, leukopenia, pruritus, cough, myalgia, chills, headache, diarrhea, abdominal pain, anorexia, upper respiratory infection.	**Anticoagulants:** Caution with concomitant anticoagulants (eg, coumadin, heparin, dipyridamole, aspirin or NSAIDs), hepatotoxic agents. **Hepatotoxic agents:** Caution with concomitant anticoagulants (eg, coumadin, heparin, dipyridamole, aspirin or NSAIDs), hepatotoxic agents. **Methotrexate:** May interfere with the action of drugs which require cell replication for their lethal effects (eg, methotrexate), and the enzymatic detoxification of other drugs, particularly in the liver. **Protein bound drugs:** May increase toxicity of protein bound drugs.
Porfimer Sodium (Photofrin)	Anemia, pleural effusion, fever, nausea, constipation, chest pain, abdominal pain, dyspnea, photosensitivity, vomiting, insomnia.	**Allopurinol:** Allopurinol may interfere with treatment. **Anticoagulants:** Decreased PDT activity with concomitant drugs that decrease clotting. **β-carotene:** Decreased PDT activity with concomitant DMSO, b-carotene. **Calcium channel blockers:** calcium channel blockers may interfere with treatment. **DMSO:** Decreased PDT activity with concomitant DMSO. Ethanol: Decreased PDT activity with concomitant ethanol. **Glucocorticoid hormones:** Decreased PDT activity with concomitant glucocorticoid hormones. **Mannitol:** Decreased PDT activity with concomitant mannitol. **Photosensitizing agents:** Increased photosensitivity with other photosensitizing agents (tetracyclines, sulfonamides, phenothiazines, thiazide diuretics, sulfunylureas, fluoroquinolones, griseofulvin). **Prostaglandin synthesis inhibitors:** Prostaglandin synthesis inhibitors may interfere with treatment. **Thromboxane A2 inhibitors:** Decreased PDT activity with concomitant platelet aggregation (eg, thromboxane A2 inhibitors). **Vasoconstriction:** Decreased PDT activity with concomitant vasoconstriction.
Procarbazine Hydrochloride (Matulane)	Leukopenia, anemia, thrombopenia, nausea, vomiting.	**Alcohol:** Avoid alcohol (may cause disulfiram-type reaction). **Antihistamines:** Caution with antihistamines. **Barbiturates:** Caution with barbiturates. **Hypotensives:** Caution with hypotensives. **Narcotics:** Caution with narcotics. **Phenothiazines:** Caution with phenothiazines. **Sympathomimetics:** Avoid sympathomimetics. **TCAs:** Avoid TCAs. **Tobacco:** Avoid tobacco. **Tyramine-containing drugs/foods:** Avoid tyramine-containing drugs/foods.
Rituximab (Rituxan)	Infusion reactions, TLS, mucocutaneous reactions, hypersensitivity reactions, arrhythmia, angina, renal failure, fever, chills, infection, asthenia, nausea, lymphopenia.	**Cisplatin:** Renal toxicity reported with cisplatin.
Teniposide (Vumon)	Myelosuppression, leukopenia, neutropenia, thrombocytopenia, anemia, mucositis, diarrhea, nausea, vomiting, infection, alopecia, bleeding, hypersensitivity reactions, rash, fever.	**Antiemetics:** Risk of CNS depression with antiemetics and high dose teniposide. **Methotrexate:** Increased plasma clearance of methotrexate. **Sodium salicylate:** sodium salicylate displace protein-bound teniposide; may potentiate toxicity **Sulfamethizole**: Sulfamethizole displaces protein-bound teniposide; may potentiate toxicity. **Tolbutamide:** Tolbutamide displace protein-bound teniposide; may potentiate toxicity.
Topotecan Hydrochloride (Hycamtin)	Neutropenia, leukopenia, thrombocytopenia, anemia, sepsis/fever/infection, nausea, vomiting, diarrhea, constipation, abdominal pain, anorexia, fatigue, pain, asthenia, alopecia.	**Carboplatin:** Increased severity of myelosuppression with carboplatin. **Cisplatin:** Increased severity of myelosuppression with cisplatin. **G-CSF:** Concomitant G-CSF can prolong duration of neutropenia; should not initiate until day 6 of therapy course, 24 hrs after treatment completion with topotecan.

Table 23.3: DRUG INFORMATION FOR OTHER TYPES OF CANCER AGENTS* *(cont.)*

NAME	ADVERSE EFFECTS	DRUG INTERACTIONS
MISCELLANEOUS *(cont.)*		
Toremifene Citrate (Fareston)	Hot flashes, sweating, nausea, vaginal discharge, dizziness, edema, vomiting, vaginal bleeding.	**Anticoagulants:** Increased PT with coumarin-type anticoagulants. **CYP450 3A4 inducers:** CYP450 3A4 inducers (eg, phenobarbital, phenytoin, carbamazepine) decrease serum levels. CYP450 3A4-6 inhibitors: **CYP450 3A4-6 inhibitors** (eg, ketoconazole, erythromycin) may inhibit metabolism. **Thiazide diuretics:** Increased risk of hypercalcemia with drugs that decrease calcium excretion (eg, thiazide diuretics).
Tositumomab (Bexxar)	Neutropenia, thrombocytopenia, anemia, asthenia, fever, infection, cough, pain, chills, headache, GI effects, myalgia, arthralgia, pharyngitis, dyspnea, rash.	**Anticoagulation:** Weigh risks vs. benefits of concomitant agents that interfere with platelet function and/or anticoagulation.
Trastuzumab (Herceptin)	Pain, asthenia, fever, nausea, chills, headache, increased cough, diarrhea, vomiting, abdominal pain, back pain, dyspnea, infection, rash.	**Anthracyclines:** Concomitant anthracyclines may increase incidence/severity of cardiac dysfunction. **Cyclophosphamide:** Concomitant cyclophosphamide may increase incidence/severity of cardiac dysfunction. **Paclitaxel:** Paclitaxel may increase serum levels.
Triptorelin Pamoate (Trelstar)	Hot flashes, HTN, headache, skeletal pain, dysuria, leg edema, pain, impotence.	**Hyperprolactinemic drugs:** Avoid hyperprolactinemic drugs.
Valrubicin (Valstar)	Urinary frequency, dysuria, urinary urgency, hematuria, bladder spasm and pain, urinary incontinence, cystitis, urinary tract infections.	Not available.
Vinblastine Sulfate	Leukopenia (granulocytopenia), anemia, thrombocytopenia, alopecia, constipation, anorexia, nausea, vomiting, abdominal pain, diarrhea, HTN, paresthesis.	**CYP3A inhibitors:** Caution with CYP3A inhibitors (eg, erythromycin, doxorubicin, etoposide), or with hepatic dysfunction; may cause earlier onset and/or an increased severity of side effects. **Mitomycin-C:** Increased risk of acute shortness of breath and severe bronchospasm with mitomycin-C. **Phenytoin:** May increase phenytoin metabolism/elimination, or decrease phenytoin absorption.

*Agents *not* used for head and neck cancer.

Section III.

Drug Issues in Dental Practice

Chapter 24

Oral Manifestations of Systemic Agents

B. Ellen Byrne, R.Ph., D.D.S., Ph.D.

Many commonly prescribed medications are capable of causing adverse oral drug reactions. The oral manifestations of drug therapy are often nonspecific and vary in significance. These undesirable effects can mimic many disease processes, such as erythema multiforme. They may also be very characteristic of a particular drug reaction (as in the case of phenytoin and gingival enlargement).

Oral Manifestations

Oral manifestations can be divided into several broad categories: abnormal hemostasis, altered host resistance, angioedema, coated tongue (black hairy tongue), dry socket, dysgeusia (altered taste), erythema multiforme, gingival enlargement, leukopenia and neutropenia, lichenoid lesions, movement disorders, salivary gland enlargement, sialorrhea (increased salivation), soft-tissue reactions and xerostomia. Table 24 lists systemic drugs that are associated with these side effects, as well as other oropharyngeal manifestations.

Abnormal Hemostasis

Abnormal hemostasis is seen with drugs that interfere with platelet function or that decrease coagulation by depressing prothrombin synthesis in the liver. Patients using such medications require a bleeding profile before undergoing extensive dental procedures.

Altered Host Resistance

Altered host resistance occurs when the microflora of the mouth is altered, resulting in an overgrowth of organisms that are part of the normal oral flora. Bacterial, fungal and viral superinfections all occur as a result of drug therapy. Broad-spectrum antibiotics and corticosteroids, as well as xerostomia, radiation and side effects of cancer chemotherapy (and AIDS), can elicit episodes of oral candidiasis. Oropharyngeal candidiasis or thrush has been associated with the use of orally inhaled and oral systemic corticosteroids, while pharyngeal candidiasis has been associated with the use of nasally inhaled and oral systemic corticosteroids. Treatment includes elimination of the causative factor, if possible, combined with use of an antifungal agent, such as nystatin suspension, clotrimazole troche or ketoconazole tablets. Various conditions such as diabetes, leukemia, lymphomas and AIDS can also render a patient more susceptible to oral candidal infections.

Angioedema

Angioedema is the result of drug-induced hypersensitivity reactions and can be life-threatening when it involves the mucosal and submucosal layers of the upper aerodigestive tract. Mild angioedema is treated with antihistamines. In more severe cases where the airway is threatened, the emergency treatment is managed the same way as in the case of an anaphylactic reaction. It may occur at any time during treatment with a drug; however, many times it will follow the first dose of a drug.

Coated Tongue (Black Hairy Tongue)

The most common discoloration of the tongue is a condition known as black hairy tongue. This results from hypertrophy of the filiform papillae. This condition is asymptomatic. The color is usually black, but may be various shades of brown. The exact mechanism by which this condition is produced is unknown and there is no effective treatment for this condition.

Dry Socket

Dry socket, or alveolar osteitis, is the result of lysis of a fully formed blood clot before the clot is replaced with granulation tissue. The incidence of dry socket seems to be higher in patients who smoke and in female patients who take oral contraceptives. Dry socket can be minimized in patients taking oral contraceptives if extractions are performed during days 23-28 of the tablet cycle.

Dysgeusia

Dysgeusia is manifested in taste alterations; medication taste; unusual taste; bitter, peculiar and metallic taste; taste perversion; and changes in taste and distaste for food. Xerostomia, malnutrition, neurological deficiencies and olfactory deficiencies also can be responsible for taste changes. Although the operative mechanism is unclear, there is some evidence that medications alter taste by affecting trace metal ions, which interact with the cell membrane proteins of the taste pores. There is no treatment other than withdrawal of the drug.

Erythema Multiforme

Erythema multiforme is a syndrome consisting of symmetrical mucocutaneous lesions that have a predilection for the oral mucosa, hands and feet. It presents initially as erythema, and vesicles and erosions develop within hours. Erythema multiforme usually has its onset from 1-3 weeks after the person begins taking the offending drug. Skin lesions can have concentric rings of erythema, producing the "target" or "bull's-eye" appearance that is associated with this condition. The lesions are normally self-limiting but will persist if the patient continues to take the offending drug. Oral lesions heal without scarring.

Gingival Enlargement

Gingival enlargement has been associated with numerous types of systemic drug therapy, and usually becomes apparent in the first 3 months after drug therapy begins. Clinically, the overgrowth starts as a diffuse swelling of the interdental papillae, which then coalesces for a nodular appearance. Many theories have been suggested to explain the overgrowth. The most attractive theory is that it is a direct effect of the drug or its metabolites on certain subpopulations of fibroblasts, which are capable of greater synthesis of protein and collagen. Many studies have shown a clear relationship between a patient's oral hygiene status and the extent of overgrowth. Also, mouth breathing and other local factors, such as crowding of teeth, significantly relate to the occurrence of gingival enlargement.

Leukopenia and Neutropenia

Many drugs can alter a patient's hematopoietic status. These effects can take the form of leukopenia, agranulocytosis and neutropenia. These conditions can have a variety of effects in the mouth: increased infections, ulcerations, nonspecific inflammation, bleeding gingiva and significant bleeding after a dental procedure. Treatment includes discontinuing use of the suspected offending drug and replacing it with a structurally dissimilar agent if continued therapy is indicated.

Lichenoid Lesions

Lichenoid lesions seen with systemic use of drugs differ from actual lichen planus in that the condition resolves when the patient discontinues taking the offending drug. Patients have pain after ulcerations have developed.

Buccal mucosa and lateral borders of the tongue are most often involved, and characteristic white striations (Wickham's striae) usually occur.

Movement Disorders

Movement disorders in the muscles of facial expression and mastication can be brought on by systemic drug therapy. These side effects include pseudoparkinsonism (rigidity, bradykinesia, tremor), akathisia (restlessness) and involuntary dystonic movements such as tardive dyskinesia. Tardive dyskinesia is characterized by repetitive, involuntary movements, usually of the mouth and tongue, secondary to long-term neuroleptic drug treatment. This type of movement, once developed, cannot be controlled and is usually irreversible. Tardive dyskinesia occurs in approximately 20% of all patients who take neuroleptic medications regularly. These patients may find it difficult to communicate, eat and use removable oral prostheses.

Osteonecrosis

Osteonecrosis of the jaw has been reported in cancer patients receiving IV bisphosphonate therapy. The majority of cases have been diagnosed after dental procedures such as tooth extraction. Less commonly, bisphosphonate-associated osteonecrosis of the jaw (BON) appears to occur spontaneously in patients taking these drugs. Rare cases of BON have also been reported in individuals taking orally administered nitrogen-containing bisphosphonates, used for the treatment of osteoporosis. See Appendix P for ADA recommendations on the dental management of patients on bisphosphonate therapy.

Typical signs and symptoms of osteonecrosis of the jaw include pain, soft-tissue swelling and infection, loosening of teeth, drainage, and exposed bone, which may occur spontaneously or, more commonly, at the site of previous tooth extraction. Some patients may present with atypical complaints, such as numbness, the feeling of a "heavy jaw," and various dysesthesias. Signs and symptoms that may occur before the development of clinical osteonecrosis include a sudden change in the health of periodontal or mucosal tissues, failure of the oral mucosa to heal, undiagnosed oral pain, loose teeth, or soft-tissue infection.

Salivary Gland Enlargement

Salivary gland problems can appear as salivary gland swelling or pain and can resemble mumps. Differential diagnosis must include salivary gland infections, obstructions and neoplasms. The mechanism of salivary gland enlargement is unknown, and the treatment is discontinuing the use of the offending drug.

Sialorrhea

Any drug that works by increasing cholinergic stimulation by directly stimulating parasympathetic receptors (such as pilocarpine) or by inhibiting the action of cholinesterase (such as neostigmine) may cause sialorrhea or increased salivation.

Soft-Tissue Reactions

Soft-tissue problems include discoloration, ulcerations, stomatitis and glossitis. Gingivitis is inflammation of the gingiva, while gingival enlargement is an overgrowth of fibrous gingival tissue.

Xerostomia

Xerostomia, defined as dry mouth or a decrease in salivation, is a frequently reported side effect. This effect may be exaggerated during prolonged drug use by elderly people and may be even more pronounced when several drugs causing dry mouth are taken simultaneously. Possible nondrug causes of xerostomia include dehydration, salivary gland infection, neoplasm, obstruction, radiation to the mouth, diabetes mellitus, nutritional deficiencies, Sjögren's syndrome and drugs that either stimulate sympathetic activity or depress parasympathetic activity.

Suggested Readings

Ackerman BH, Kasbekar N. Disturbances of taste and smell induced by drugs. Pharmacotherapy 1997;17(3):482-96.

Doty RL, Philip S, Reddy K, Kerr K-L. Influences of antihypertensives and antihyperlipidemic drugs on the senses of taste and smell: a review. J Hypertension 2003;21:1805-13.

Felder RS, Millar SB, Henry RH. Oral manifestations of drug therapy. Spec Care Dentist 1988;8(3):119-24.

Lewis IK, Hanlon JT, Hobbins MJ, Beck JD. Use of medications with potential oral adverse drug reactions in community-dwelling elderly. Spec Care Dentist 1993; 13(4):171-6.

Marx RE, Sawatari Y, Fortin M, Broumand V. Bisphosphonate-induced exposed bone (osteonerosis/osteopetrosis) of the jaws: risk factors, recognition, prevention, and treatment. J Oral Maxillofac Surg 2005;63:1567-75.

Migliorati CA, Schubert MM, Peterson DE, Seneda LM. Bisphosphonate-associated osteonecrosis of mandibular and maxillary bone: an emerging oral complication of supportive cancer therapy. Cancer 2005 Jul 1;104(1):83-93.

Mott AE, Grushka M, Sessle BJ. Diagnosis and management of taste disorders and burning mouth syndrome. Dent Clin North Am 1993;37(1):33-71.

Walton JG. Dental disorders. In: Davies DM, ed. Textbook of adverse drug reactions. 4th ed. Oxford, England: Oxford University Press; 1991:205-29.

Zelickson BD, Rogers RS. Oral drug reactions. Dermatol Clin North Am 1987;5(4):695-708.

Table 24: ORAL MANIFESTATIONS OF SYSTEMIC AGENTS

Abscess, periodontal/peritonsillar

Alefacept (Amevive)	Fentanyl Citrate (Actiq)	Pergolide Mesylate (Permax)
Aripiprazole (Abilify)	Fluoxetine Hydrochloride/Olanzapine	Ritonavir (Norvir)
Bicalutamide (Casodex)	(Symbyax)	Rosuvastatin Calcium (Crestor)
Cilostazol (Pletal)	Gabapentin (Neurontin)	Tacrolimus (Protopic)
Clindamycin Phosphate (Clindesse)	Glatiramer Acetate (Copaxone)	Tiagabine Hydrochloride (Gabitril)
Delavirdine Mesylate (Rescriptor)	Hydrochlorothiazide (Uniretic)	Valproate Sodium (Depacon)
Divalproex Sodium (Depakote)	Modafinil (Provigil)	Valproic Acid (Depakene)
Donepezil Hydrochloride (Aricept)	Olanzapine (Zyprexa)	
Doxorubicin Hydrochloride	Oseltamivir Phosphate (Tamiflu)	
Liposome (Doxil)	Pantoprazole Sodium (Protonix)	

Aftertaste

Disulfiram (Antabuse)	Etoposide Phosphate (Etopophos)	
Etoposide (Vepesid)	Flunisolide (Nasarel)	

Ageusia

Acitretin (Soriatane)	Diclofenac Sodium/Misoprostol	Paroxetine Hydrochloride (Paxil)
Alemtuzumab (Campath)	(Arthrotec)	Pregabalin (Lyrica)
Amitriptyline Hydrochloride (Elavil)	Dicyclomine Hydrochloride (Bentyl)	Rifaximin (Xifaxan)
Amlodipine Besylate/Atorvastatin	Doxorubicin Hydrochloride	Riluzole (Rilutek)
(Caduet)	Liposome (Doxil)	Rimantadine Hydrochloride
Amoxicillin/Clarithromycin/Lanso-	Esomeprazole Magnesium (Nexium)	(Flumadine)
prazole (PREVPAC)	Etidronate Disodium (Didronel)	Ritonavir (Norvir)
Aspirin/Dipyridamole (Aggrenox)	Flunisolide (Aerobid, Nasalide)	Rivastigmine Tartrate (Exelon)
Atorvastatin Calcium (Lipitor)	Fluoxetine Hydrochloride (Prozac,	Sodium Oxybate (Xyrem)
Atropine Sulfate/Hyoscyamine	Sarafem)	Sulindac (Clinoril)
Sulfate/Phenobarbital/Scopol-	Fluticasone Propionate (Flonase)	Tamoxifen Citrate (Nolvadex)
amine Hydrobromide (Donnatal)	Fluvoxamine Maleate (Luvox)	Terbinafine Hydrochloride (Lamisil)
Azelastine Hydrochloride (Astelin)	Gabapentin (Neurontin)	Tiagabine Hydrochloride (Gabitril)
Beclomethasone Dipropionate	Gatifloxacin (Tequin)	Topiramate (Topamax)
(Beclovent)	Glatiramer Acetate (Copaxone)	Valrubicin (Valstar)
Betaxolol Hydrochloride (Kerlone)	Glycopyrrolate (Robinul)	Venlafaxine Hydrochloride (Effexor)
Capecitabine (Xeloda)	Grepafloxacin Hydrochloride (Raxar)	Voriconazole (VFEND)
Captopril (Captopril)	Hyoscyamine Sulfate (Levbid, Nulev)	Zaleplon (Sonata)
Cefpodoxime Proxetil (Vantin)	Hyoscyamine Sulfate (Nulev)	
Cetirizine Hydrochloride (Zyrtec)	Interferon Alfa-2b, Recombinant	
Ciprofloxacin (Cipro)	(Intron)	
Cisplatin (Platinol-AQ)	Lamotrigine (Lamictal)	
Citalopram Hydrobromide (Celexa)	Lansoprazole (Prevacid)	
Clonazepam (Klonopin)	Mirtazapine (Remeron)	
Cyclobenzaprine Hydrochloride	Moxifloxacin Hydrochloride	
(Flexeril)	(Avelox)	

Table 24: ORAL MANIFESTATIONS OF SYSTEMIC AGENTS *(cont.)*

Airway obstruction

Calfactant (Infasurf)	Lisinopril (Prinivil, Zestril)	Propofol (Diprivan, Propofol)
Captopril (Captopril)	Lorazepam (Ativan)	Ramipril (Altace)
Enalapril Maleate (vaseretic, vasotec)	Midazolam Hydrochloride (Versed)	Sevoflurane (Ultane)
Enalaprilat	Muromonab-Cd3 (Orthoclone)	
Hydrochlorothiazide	Naratriptan Hydrochloride (Amerge)	
Levofloxacin (Levaquin)	Ofloxacin (Floxin)	

Angioedema, glottis

Amlodipine Besylate/Benazepril Hydrochloride (Lotrel)	Fosinopril Sodium (Monopril)	Ramipril (Altace)
Benazepril Hydrochloride (Lotensin)	Hydrochlorothiazide	Trandolapril (Mavik, Tarka)
Captopril (Captopril)	Lisinopril (Prinivil, Zestril)	
Enalapril Maleate (Vaseretic, Vasotec)	Losartan Potassium (Cozaar)	
	Perindopril Erbumine (Aceon)	

Angioedema, larynx

Alteplase (Activase)	Fosinopril Sodium (Monopril)	Ramipril (Altace)
Benazepril Hydrochloride (Lotensin)	Hydrochlorothiazide	Trandolapril (Mavik)
Captopril (Captopril)	Levofloxacin (Levaquin)	
Enalapril Maleate (Vaseretic, Vasotec)	Lisinopril (Prinivil, Zestril)	
	Perindopril Erbumine (Aceon)	

Angioedema, lips

Amlodipine Besylate/Benazepril Hydrochloride (Lotrel)	Fosinopril Sodium (Monopril)	Losartan Potassium (Cozaar)
Benazepril Hydrochloride (Lotensin)	Hydrochlorothiazide (Avalide)	Perindopril Erbumine (Aceon)
Captopril (Captopril)	Ipratropium Bromide (Atrovent)	Ramipril (Altace)
Enalapril Maleate (Vaseretic, Vasotec)	Irbesartan (Avapro)	Tamsulosin Hydrochloride (Flomax)
	Lisinopril (Prinivil, Zestril)	Trandolapril (Mavik)

Angioedema, mucous membranes of the mouth

Alteplase (Activase)	Captopril (Captopril)

Angioedema, oropharyngeal

Hydrochlorothiazide	Losartan Potassium (Cozaar)
Irbesartan (Avapro)	Nifedipine (Adalat)

Angioedema, throat

Levofloxacin (Levaquin)

Angioedema, tongue

Amlodipine Besylate/Benazepril Hydrochloride (Lotrel)	Benazepril Hydrochloride (Lotensin)	Clonidine (Catapres-TTS)
	Captopril (Captopril)	Enalapril Maleate (Vaseretic, Vasotec)

Angioedema, tongue *(cont.)*

Fosinopril Sodium (Monopril)
Hydrochlorothiazide
Ipratropium Bromide (Atrovent)
Irbesartan (Avapro)
Levofloxacin (Levaquin)

Lisinopril (Prinivil, Zestril)
Losartan Potassium (Cozaar)
Ofloxacin (Floxin)
Perindopril Erbumine (Aceon)
Ramipril (Altace)

Tamsulosin Hydrochloride (Flomax)
Trandolapril (Mavik)

Bleeding, dental

Acitretin (Soriatane)
Alteplase (Activase)
Amoxicillin/Clarithromycin/
  Lansoprazole (PREVPAC)
Amphotericin B, Liposomal
  (Ambisome)
Anistreplase (Eminase)
Aripiprazole (Abilify)
Aspirin
Atorvastatin Calcium (Lipitor)
Bevacizumab (Avastin)
Bupropion Hydrochloride
  (Wellbutrin, Zyban)
Cilostazol (Pletal)
Citalopram Hydrobromide (Celexa)
Clofarabine (Clolar)
Cyclosporine (Gengraf, Neoral)
Delavirdine Mesylate (Rescriptor)
Divalproex Sodium (Depakote)

Doxorubicin Hydrochloride
  Liposome (Doxil)
Fentanyl Citrate (Actiq)
Fluoxetine Hydrochloride
  (Prozac, Sarafem)
Gabapentin (Neurontin)
Glatiramer Acetate (Copaxone)
Indinavir Sulfate (Crixivan)
Interferon Alfa-2a, Recombinant
  (Roferon-A)
Interferon Alfa-2b, Recombinant
  (Intron)
Isotretinoin (Accutane)
Lamotrigine (Lamictal)
Lansoprazole (Prevacid)
Mechlorethamine Hydrochloride
  (Mustargen)
Mirtazapine (Remeron)
Oxcarbazepine (Trileptal)

Pentosan Polysulfate Sodium
  (Elmiron)
Propafenone Hydrochloride
  (Rythmol)
Quetiapine Fumarate (Seroquel)
Riluzole (Rilutek)
Topiramate (Topamax)
Venlafaxine Hydrochloride (Effexor)
Voriconazole (VFEND)
Warfarin Sodium (Coumadin)
Zaleplon (Sonata)
Zidovudine (Retrovir)
Ziprasidone Hydrochloride (Geodon)
Zonisamide (Zonegran)

Bleeding, gums

Amlodipine Besylate/Atorvastatin
  (Caduet)
Efalizumab (Raptiva)

Fluoxetine Hydrochloride/Olanzapine
  (Symbyax)
Gemtuzumab Ozogamicin (Mylotarg)

Lansoprazole (Prevacid)
Nifedipine (Adalat)

Bleeding, lip

Gabapentin (Neurontin)

Bleeding, mouth

Abciximab (Reopro)
Anistreplase (Eminase)
Cevimeline Hydrochloride (Evoxac)

Interferon Alfa-2b, Recombinant
  (Intron)
Rapacuronium Bromide (Raplon)

Bleeding, mucosal

Sodium Phosphate (Visicol)

Venlafaxine Hydrochloride (Effexor)

Table 24: ORAL MANIFESTATIONS OF SYSTEMIC AGENTS *(cont.)*

Bleeding, oropharyngeal

Eptifibatide (Integrilin)	Tenecteplase (Tnkase)	

Bleeding tendency, increased

Cilostazol (Pletal)	Montelukast Sodium (Singulair)	

Bleeding time, prolongation

Acitretin (Soriatane)	Diltiazem Hydrochloride (Cardizem, Tiazac)	Paroxetine Hydrochloride (Paxil)
Antihemophilic Factor (Recombinant) (Advate)	Divalproex Sodium (Depakote)	Pentosan Polysulfate Sodium (Elmiron)
Aspirin	Fentanyl Citrate (Actiq)	Piperacillin Sodium/Tazobactam (Zosyn)
Clavulanate Potassium (Timentin)	Gabapentin (Neurontin)	Tolmetin Sodium (Tolectin)
Diclofenac Potassium (Cataflam, Voltaren, Voltaren-XR)	Ketorolac Tromethamine (Acular)	Voriconazole (VFEND)
Diflunisal (Dolobid)	Mefenamic Acid (Ponstel)	
	Naproxen (EC-Naprosyn)	

Buccoglossal syndrome

Aripiprazole (Abilify)	Olanzapine (Zyprexa)	
Fluoxetine Hydrochloride (Prozac, Sarafem)	Quetiapine Fumarate (Seroquel)	
Fluoxetine Hydrochloride/Lanzapine (Symbyax)	Venlafaxine Hydrochloride (Effexor)	
	Ziprasidone Hydrochloride (Geodon)	

Candidiasis, oral

Amoxicillin/Clavulanate Potassium (Augmentin)	Dalfopristin/Quinupristin (Synercid)	Megestrol Acetate (Megace)
Amoxicillin/Clarithromycin/Lansoprazole (PREVPAC)	Delavirdine Mesylate (Rescriptor)	Meropenem (Merrem)
Anti-Thymocyte Globulin (Thymoglobulin)	Doxorubicin Hydrochloride Liposome (Doxil)	Mometasone Furoate (Asmanex)
Aripiprazole (Abilify)	Ertapenem (Invanz)	Mometasone Furoate Monohydrate (Nasonex)
Arsenic Trioxide (Trisenox)	Fentanyl Citrate (Actiq)	Moxifloxacin Hydrochloride (Avelox)
Atovaquone (Mepron)	Fluticasone Propionate (Flovent)	Mycophenolate Mofetil (Cellcept)
Azithromycin (Zmax)	Fluticasone Propionate/Salmeterol Xinafoate (Advair)	Mycophenolic Acid (Myfortic)
Azithromycin Dihydrate (Zithromax)	Gabapentin (Neurontin)	Olanzapine (Zyprexa)
Budesonide (Pulmicort)	Gatifloxacin (Tequin)	Oprelvekin (Neumega)
Capecitabine (Xeloda)	Glatiramer Acetate (Copaxone)	Palivizumab (Synagis)
Cefazolin Sodium (Ancef)	Griseofulvin (Fulvicin, Grifulvin, Gris-PEG)	Pantoprazole Sodium (Protonix)
Cefditoren Pivoxil (Spectracef)	Haemophilus B Conjugate Vaccine (Comvax)	Piperacillin Sodium/Tazobactam (Zosyn)
Cefepime Hydrochloride (Maxipime)	Hyoscyamine (Cystospaz)	Pneumococcal Vaccine, Diphtheria Conjugate (Prevnar)
Cefpodoxime Proxetil (Vantin)	Lansoprazole (Prevacid)	Salmeterol Xinafoate (Serevent)
Ceftazidime (Ceptaz, Fortaz)	Leflunomide (Arava)	Sirolimus (Rapamune)
Ciprofloxacin (Cipro)	Linezolid (Zyvox)	Sparfloxacin (Zagam)
Clofarabine (Clolar)		Tacrolimus (Prograf)

Candidiasis, oral *(cont.)*

Telithromycin (Ketek)	Tinidazole (Tindamax)	Venlafaxine Hydrochloride (Effexor)
Thalidomide (Thalomid)	Triamcinolone Acetonide (Azmacort)	

Candidiasis, pharynx

Beclomethasone Dipropionate (Vancenase)	Salmeterol Xinafoate (Serevent) Triamcinolone Acetonide (Azmacort)	

Carcinoma, laryngeal

Amoxicillin/Clarithromycin/ Lansoprazole (PREVPAC)	Lansoprazole (Prevacid)	

Cheek puffing

Amitriptyline Hydrochloride	Pimozide (Orap)	Trifluoperazine Hydrochloride
Chlorpromazine (Thorazine)	Prochlorperazine (Compazine,	(Stelazine)
Haloperidol (Haldol)	Compro)	
Molindone Hydrochloride (Moban)	Thiothixene (Thiothixene)	

Cheilitis

Acitretin (Soriatane)	Frovatriptan Succinate (Frova)	Saquinavir Mesylate (Invirase)
Amlodipine Besylate/Atorvastatin	Gatifloxacin (Tequin)	Tacrolimus (Protopic)
(Caduet)	Grepafloxacin Hydrochloride (Raxar)	Venlafaxine Hydrochloride (Effexor)
Atorvastatin Calcium (Lipitor)	Hydrochlorothiazide	Voriconazole (VFEND)
Bexarotene (Targretin)	Isotretinoin (Accutane, Amnesteem)	Zaleplon (Sonata)
Dactinomycin (Cosmegen)	Penicillamine (Cuprimine)	
Edetate Calcium Disodium	Riluzole (Rilutek)	
Fentanyl Citrate (Actiq)	Ritonavir (Norvir)	

Chewing movements

Amitriptyline Hydrochloride	Pimozide (Orap)	Thiothixene (Thiothixene)
Chlorpromazine (Thorazine)	Prochlorperazine (Compazine,	Trifluoperazine Hydrochloride
Haloperidol (Haldol)	Compro)	(Stelazine)
Molindone Hydrochloride (Moban)	Thioridazine Hydrochloride	
Perphenazine (Trilafon)	(Thioridazine)	

Clotting time, prolongation

Cefditoren Pivoxil (Spectracef)	Pegaspargase (Oncaspar)	Testosterone (Testim)
Diclofenac Sodium/Misoprostol	Piperacillin Sodium/Tazobactam	
(Arthrotec/)	(Zosyn)	
Oxymetholone (Anadrol-50)	Sertraline Hydrochloride (Zoloft)	

Table 24: ORAL MANIFESTATIONS OF SYSTEMIC AGENTS *(cont.)*

Coagulation dysfunction

Aldesleukin (Proleukin)
Alemtuzumab (Campath)
Aminocaproic Acid (Amicar)
Amiodarone Hydrochloride
  (Pacerone)
Amphotericin B Lipid Complex
  (Abelcet)
Amphotericin B, Liposomal
  (Ambisome)
Antihemophilic Factor,
  Recombinant (Novoseven)
Asparaginase (Elspar)
Bcg, Live (Intravesical) (Tice)
Capecitabine (Xeloda)
Cefdinir (Omnicef)

Citalopram Hydrobromide (Celexa)
Clopidogrel Bisulfate (Plavix)
Divalproex Sodium (Depakote)
Estrogens, Conjugated (Premarin)
Estrogens, Esterified (Estratest)
Ethinyl Estradiol/Norgestrel (Lo/
  Ovral-28, Ovral)
Fluoxetine Hydrochloride/Olanzapine
  (Symbyax)
Gabapentin (Neurontin)
Interferon Alfa-2a, Recombinant
  (Roferon-A)
Lomefloxacin Hydrochloride
  (Maxaquin)
Muromonab-Cd3 (Orthoclone)

Mycophenolate Mofetil (Cellcept)
Nimodipine (Nimotop)
Pegaspargase (Oncaspar)
Propofol (Diprivan, Propofol)
Rituximab (Rituxan)
Sargramostim (Leukine)
Tacrolimus (Prograf)
Trastuzumab (Herceptin)
Valproate Sodium (Depacon)
Valproic Acid (Depakene)

Coagulopathy

Aspirin
Aspirin/Dipyridamole (Aggrenox)

Etanercept (Enbrel)
Micafungin Sodium (Mycamine)

Sodium Benzoate (Ammonul)

Cold sore, nonherpetic

Interferon Alfa-2b, Recombinant
  (Intron)

Naltrexone Hydrochloride
  (Revia)

Varicella Virus Vaccine, Live
  (Varivax)

Cough

Abacavir Sulfate (Ziagen)
Abacavir Sulfate/Lamivudine/
  Zidovudine (Trizivir)
Acamprosate Calcium (Campral)
Acebutolol Hydrochloride (Sectral)
Acitretin (Soriatane)
Adefovir Dipivoxil (Hepsera)
Adenosine (Adenoscan)
Albuterol Sulfate (Proventil,
  Ventolin)
Albuterol Sulfate/Ipratropium
  Bromide (Combivent)
Aldesleukin (Proleukin)
Alefacept (Amevive)
Alemtuzumab (Campath)
Alosetron Hydrochloride (Lotronex)
Alpha1-Proteinase Inhibitor
  (Human) (Aralast, Zemaira)
Alprostadil (Caverject)

Amiloride Hydrochloride (Midamor)
Amiloride Hydrochloride/
  Hydrochlorothiazide (Moduretic)
Amiodarone Hydrochloride
  (Pacerone)
Amlodipine Besylate/Atorvastatin
  (Caduet)
Amlodipine Besylate/Benazepril
  Hydrochloride (Lotrel)
Amlodipine Besylate (Norvasc)
Amoxicillin/Clarithromycin/
  Lansoprazole (PREVPAC)
Amphotericin B, Liposomal
  (Ambisome)
Anagrelide Hydrochloride (Agrylin)
Anastrozole (Arimidex)
Antihemophilic Factor (Recombinant,
  Advate, Benefix, Refacto)
Aprepitant (Emend)

Argatroban (Argatroban)
Aripiprazole (Abilify)
Arsenic Trioxide (Trisenox)
Aspirin/Dipyridamole (Aggrenox)
Atazanavir Sulfate (Reyataz)
Atomoxetine Hydrochloride
  (Strattera)
Atovaquone/Proguanil
  Hydrochloride (Malarone)
Azelastine Hydrochloride (Astelin)
Azithromycin Dihydrate (Zithromax)
Balsalazide Disodium (Colazal)
Basiliximab (Simulect)
BCG Live, Intravesical (TICE BCG)
Beclomethasone Dipropionate
  (Vancenase, Vanceril)
Benazepril Hydrochloride (Lotensin)
Bendroflumethiazide (Corzide)
Bepridil Hydrochloride (Vascor)

Cough *(cont.)*

Betaxolol Hydrochloride (Kerlone)
Bexarotene (Targretin)
Bicalutamide (Casodex)
Bitolterol Mesylate (Tornalate)
Bortezomib (Velcade)
Botulinum Toxin Type A (Botox)
Brimonidine Tartrate (Alphagan)
Budesonide (Pulmicort, Rhinocort)
Buprenorphine Hydrochloride (Suboxone)
Bupropion Hydrochloride (Wellbutrin, Zyban)
Busulfan (I.V.)
Calcitonin-Salmon (Fortical, Miacalcin)
Candesartan Cilexetil (Atacand)
Capecitabine (Xeloda)
Captopril (Captopril)
Carbidopa (Lodosyn)
Carbidopa/Levodopa (Parcopa, Sinemet)
Carbidopa/Entacapone/Levodopa (Stalevo)
Carteolol Hydrochloride (Cartrol)
Carvedilol (Coreg)
Cefaclor (Ceclor)
Cefpodoxime Proxetil (Vantin)
Cefuroxime Axetil (Ceftin)
Celecoxib (Celebrex)
Cerivastatin Sodium (Baycol)
Cetirizine Hydrochloride (Zyrtec)
Cetirizine Hydrochloride/ Pseudoephedrine (Zyrtec-D)
Cetuximab (Erbitux)
Cevimeline Hydrochloride (Evoxac)
Chlorambucil (Leukeran)
Choriogonadotropin Alfa (Ovidrel)
Cilostazol (Pletal)
Cisapride (Propulsid)
Citalopram Hydrobromide (Celexa)
Cladribine (Leustatin)
Clindamycin Phosphate (Clindesse)
Clofarabine (Clolar)
Clonazepam (Klonopin)
Clopidogrel Bisulfate (Plavix)
Clozapine (Clozaril, Fazaclo)

Colesevelam Hydrochloride (Welchol)
Cromolyn Sodium (Intal)
Cyclosporine (Gengraf, Neoral)
Daclizumab (Zenapax)
Daptomycin (Cubicin)
Darbepoetin Alfa (Aranesp)
Delavirdine Mesylate (Rescriptor)
Denileukin Diftitox (Ontak)
Desflurane (Suprane)
Desloratadine (Clarinex)
Desmopressin Acetate (DDAVP, Desmopressin)
Diazepam (Diastat, Valium)
Diazoxide (Hyperstat)
Diclofenac Sodium/Misoprostol (Arthrotec)
Diltiazem Hydrochloride (Cardizem, Tiazac)
Divalproex Sodium (Depakote)
Dornase Alfa (Pulmozyme)
Dorzolamide Hydrochloride (Cosopt)
Doxapram Hydrochloride (Dopram)
Doxercalciferol (Hectorol)
Doxorubicin Hydrochloride Liposome (Doxil)
Dronabinol (Marinol)
Duloxetine Hydrochloride (Cymbalta)
Efavirenz (Sustiva)
Eletriptan Hydrobromide (Relpax)
Emtricitabine (Emtriva)
Emtricitabine/Tenofovir Disoproxil Fumarate (Truvada)
Enalapril Maleate/Hydrochlorothiazide (Vaseretic)
Enalapril Maleate (Vasotec)
Enfuvirtide (Fuzeon)
Enoxacin (Penetrex)
Epinastine Hydrochloride (Elestat)
Eplerenone (Inspra)
Epoetin Alfa (Epogen, Procrit)
Epoprostenol Sodium (Flolan)
Eprosartan Mesylate (Teveten)
Erlotinib (Tarceva)
Ertapenem (Invanz)
Escitalopram Oxalate (Lexapro)
Esomeprazole Magnesium (Nexium)

Estazolam (Prosom)
Estradiol (Prefest, Vivelle, Vivelle-Dot)
Estrogens, Conjugated (Premarin, Prempro)
Estrogens, Conjugated, Synthetic A (Cenestin)
Etanercept (Enbrel)
Etoposide (Vepesid)
Etoposide Phosphate (Etopophos)
Exemestane (Aromasin)
Ezetimibe/Simvastatin (Vytorin)
Ezetimibe (Zetia)
Felodipine (Plendil)
Fenofibrate (Antara, Lofibra, Tricor)
Fentanyl (Duragesic, Actiq)
Fexofenadine Hydrochloride (Allegra)
Filgrastim (Neupogen)
Flunisolide (Aerobid, Nasarel)
Fluoxetine Hydrochloride (Prozac, Sarafem)
Fluticasone Propionate/Salmeterol Xinafoate (Advair)
Fluticasone Propionate (Cutivate, Flonase, Flovent)
Fluvastatin Sodium (Lescol)
Fluvoxamine Maleate (Luvox)
Follitropin Alfa (Gonal-F)
Fondaparinux Sodium (Arixtra)
Foscarnet Sodium (Foscavir)
Fosinopril Sodium (Monopril)
Fulvestrant (Faslodex)
Gabapentin (Neurontin)
Galantamine Hydrobromide (Razadyne)
Ganciclovir (Cytovene)
Gemcitabine Hydrochloride (Gemzar)
Gemtuzumab Ozogamicin (Mylotarg)
Glatiramer Acetate (Copaxone)
Globulin, Immune (Human) (Iveegam)
Goserelin Acetate (Zoladex)
Graftskin (Apligraf)
Grepafloxacin Hydrochloride (Raxar)
Guanadrel Sulfate (Hylorel)
Haemophilus B Conjugate Vaccine (Comvax, Omnihib)
Hepatitis A Vaccine, Inactivated (Vaqta)

Table 24: ORAL MANIFESTATIONS OF SYSTEMIC AGENTS *(cont.)*

Cough *(cont.)*

Hepatitis B Vaccine, Recombinant
(Recombivax)
Hydrochlorothiazide
Hydrocodone Bitartrate/Ibuprofen
(Vicoprofen)
Ibritumomab Tiuxetan (Zevalin)
Iloprost (Ventavis)
Imatinib Mesylate (Gleevec)
Imiglucerase (Cerezyme)
Imiquimod (Aldara)
Immune Globulin Intravenous
(Human, Gammagard, Gamunex)
Indapamide
Indinavir Sulfate (Crixivan)
Infliximab (Remicade)
Influenza Virus Vaccine (Flumist)
Interferon Alfa-2a, Recombinant
(Roferon-A)
Interferon Alfa-2b, Recombinant
(Intron)
Interferon Alfa-N3 (Human
Leukocyte Derived) (Alferon)
Iodine I 131 Tositumomab (Bexxar)
Ipratropium Bromide (Atrovent)
Irbesartan (Avapro)
Irinotecan Hydrochloride
(Camptosar)
Isosorbide Mononitrate (Imdur)
Isradipine (Dynacirc)
Itraconazole (Sporanox)
Lamivudine/Zidovudine (Combivir)
Lamivudine (Epivir, Epivir-HBV)
Lamotrigine (Lamictal)
Lansoprazole (Prevacid)
Laronidase (Aldurazyme)
Leflunomide (Arava)
Lepirudin (Refludan)
Letrozole (Femara)
Levalbuterol Hydrochloride
(Xopenex)
Levetiracetam (Keppra)
Levobupivacaine Hydrochloride
(Chirocaine)
Levocarnitine (Carnitor)
Levofloxacin (Levaquin)

Levomethadyl Acetate Hydrochloride
(Orlaam)
Linezolid (Zyvox)
Lisinopril (Prinivil, Zestril)
Lomefloxacin Hydrochloride
(Maxaquin)
Loratadine (Claritin)
Loratadine/Pseudoephedrine
(Claritin-D)
Losartan Potassium (Cozaar)
Lyme Disease Vaccine, Recombinant
OspA, (LYMErix)
Measles Virus Vaccine, Live
(Attenuvax)
Measles, Mumps & Rubella Virus
Vaccine, Live (M-M-R)
Megestrol Acetate (Megace)
Meloxicam (Mobic)
Melphalan Hydrochloride (Alkeran)
Memantine Hydrochloride
(Namenda)
Menotropins (Menopur)
Meropenem (Merrem)
Mesalamine (Asacol)
Metaproterenol Sulfate (Alupent)
Methotrexate Sodium (Methotrexate)
Methylphenidate Hydrochloride
(Concerta)
Midazolam Hydrochloride (Versed)
Minocycline Hydrochloride
(Minocin)
Mirtazapine (Remeron)
Mitomycin (Mitomycin-C)
(Mutamycin)
Modafinil (Provigil)
Moexipril Hydrochloride (Univasc)
Mometasone Furoate Monohydrate
(Nasonex)
Montelukast Sodium (Singulair)
Moricizine Hydrochloride
(Ethmozine)
Moxifloxacin Hydrochloride
(Vigamox)
Mumps Virus Vaccine, Live
(Mumpsvax)

Mupirocin Calcium (Bactroban)
Mycophenolate Mofetil (Cellcept)
Mycophenolic Acid (Myfortic)
Nabumetone (Relafen)
Nadolol (Nadolol)
Naltrexone Hydrochloride (Revia)
Naratriptan Hydrochloride (Amerge)
Nateglinide (Starlix)
Nedocromil Sodium (Tilade)
Nesiritide (Natrecor)
Nicotine (Nicotrol)
Nifedipine (Adalat)
Nisoldipine (Sular)
Nitrofurantoin (Furadantin)
Nizatidine (Axid)
Ofloxacin (Floxin)
Olanzapine (Zyprexa)
Omega-3-Acid Ethyl Esters (Omacor)
Omeprazole (Prilosec, Zegerid)
Oprelvekin (Neumega)
Oseltamivir Phosphate (Tamiflu)
Oxaliplatin (Eloxatin)
Oxcarbazepine (Trileptal)
Oxybutynin Chloride (Ditropan)
Oxycodone Hydrochloride
(Oxycontin)
Palivizumab (Synagis)
Pamidronate Disodium (Aredia)
Pancrelipase (Cotazym)
Pantoprazole Sodium (Protonix)
Paroxetine Hydrochloride (Paxil)
Pegaspargase (Oncaspar)
Peginterferon Alfa-2a (Pegasys)
Peginterferon Alfa-2b (PEG-Intron)
Pemirolast Potassium (Alamast)
Penbutolol Sulfate (Levatol)
Pentostatin (Nipent)
Perindopril Erbumine (Aceon)
Pimecrolimus (Elidel)
Piperacillin Sodium/Tazobactam
(Zosyn)
Pirbuterol Acetate (Maxair)
Porfimer Sodium (Photofrin)
Pramipexole Dihydrochloride
(Mirapex)

Cough (cont.)

Pravastatin Sodium (Pravachol)
Procarbazine Hydrochloride
  (Matulane)
Progesterone (Prometrium)
Propafenone Hydrochloride
  (Rythmol)
Propofol (Diprivan, Propofol)
Quetiapine Fumarate (Seroquel)
Raloxifene Hydrochloride (Evista)
Ramipril (Altace)
Rapacuronium Bromide (Raplon)
Ribavirin (Copegus, Rebetol)
Riluzole (Rilutek)
Rimantadine Hydrochloride
  (Flumadine)
Risedronate Sodium (Actonel)
Risperidone (Risperdal)
Ritonavir (Norvir)
Rituximab (Rituxan)
Rivastigmine Tartrate (Exelon)
Rizatriptan Benzoate (Maxalt-MLT)
Ropinirole Hydrochloride (Requip)
Ropivacaine Hydrochloride
  (Naropin)
Rosuvastatin Calcium (Crestor)
Rotavirus Vaccine, Live, Oral,
  Tetravalent (Rotashield)
Rubella Virus Vaccine, Live (Meruvax)
Salmeterol Xinafoate (Serevent)
Saquinavir Mesylate (Invirase)
Sertraline Hydrochloride (Zoloft)
Sevelamer Hydrochloride (Renagel)

Sevoflurane (Ultane)
Sibutramine Hydrochloride
  Monohydrate (Meridia)
Sildenafil Citrate (Viagra)
Sirolimus (Rapamune)
Sodium Ferric Gluconate (Ferrlecit)
Solifenacin Succinate (Vesicare)
Somatropin (Humatrope, Serostim)
Sparfloxacin (Zagam)
Succimer (Chemet)
Sulfamethoxazole/Trimethoprim
  (Bactrim, Septra)
Sumatriptan (Imitrex)
Tacrolimus (Prograf, Protopic)
Tamoxifen Citrate (Nolvadex)
Tamsulosin Hydrochloride (Flomax)
Telmisartan (Micardis)
Temozolomide (Temodar)
Terazosin Hydrochloride (Hytrin)
Teriparatide (Forteo)
Thalidomide (Thalomid)
Tiagabine Hydrochloride (Gabitril)
Tigecycline (Tygacil)
Timolol Maleate (Blocadren,
  Timoptic, Timoptic-XE)
Tiotropium Bromide (Spiriva)
Tipranavir (Aptivus)
Tobramycin (TOBI)
Tolcapone (Tasmar)
Tolterodine Tartrate (Detrol)
Topiramate (Topamax)
Topotecan Hydrochloride (Hycamtin)

Trandolapril (Mavik)
Trandolapril/Verapamil
  Hydrochloride (Tarka)
Trastuzumab (Herceptin)
Triamcinolone Acetonide (Azmacort,
  Nasacort)
Triptorelin Pamoate (Trelstar)
Valganciclovir Hydrochloride
  (Valcyte)
Valproate Sodium (Depacon)
Valproic Acid (Depakene)
Valsartan (Diovan)
Varicella Virus Vaccine, Live
  (Varivax)
Venlafaxine Hydrochloride (Effexor)
Verteporfin (Visudyne)
Vinorelbine Tartrate (Navelbine)
Voriconazole (VFEND)
Zanamivir (Relenza)
Zidovudine (Retrovir)
Ziprasidone Hydrochloride (Geodon)
Zoledronic Acid (Zometa)
Zolmitriptan (Zomig)
Zolpidem Tartrate (Ambien)

Cough reflex, depression

Chlorpromazine (Thorazine)
Fluoxetine Hydrochloride (Prozac)
Morphine Sulfate (Astramorph/PF,
  Kadian)

Prochlorperazine (Compazine,
  Compro)
Trifluoperazine Hydrochloride
  (Stelazine)

Craniofacial deformities

Amlodipine Besylate/
  Benazepril Hydrochloride
  (Lotrel)
Captopril (Captopril)

Enalapril Maleate/Hydrochlorothia-
  zide (Vaseretic)
Enalapril Maleate (Vasotec)
Hydrochlorothiazide

Lisinopril (Prinivil, Zestril)
Losartan Potassium (Cozaar)
Ramipril (Altace)

Table 24: ORAL MANIFESTATIONS OF SYSTEMIC AGENTS *(cont.)*

Dental caries

Aripiprazole (Abilify)	Hyoscyamine (Cystospaz)	Sertraline Hydrochloride (Zoloft)
Fentanyl Citrate (Actiq)	Lithium Carbonate (Eskalith,	Tiagabine Hydrochloride (Gabitril)
Fluoxetine Hydrochloride/Olanzapine	Lithobid)	Zolpidem Tartrate (Ambien)
(Symbyax)	Loratadine (Claritin)	
Fluvoxamine Maleate (Luvox)	Paroxetine Hydrochloride (Paxil)	
Glatiramer Acetate (Copaxone)	Pergolide Mesylate (Permax)	
Hydrochlorothiazide	Quetiapine Fumarate (Seroquel)	

Dermatitis, perioral

Alclometasone Dipropionate	Clobetasol Propionate (Clobevate,	Fluticasone Propionate (Cutivate)
(Aclovate)	Clobex, Cormax, Embeline, Olux,	Halobetasol Propionate (Ultravate)
Bacitracin Zinc/Hydrocortisone/	Temovate)	Hydrocortisone Acetate (Analpram,
Neomycin Sulfate/Polymyxin B	Clocortolone Pivalate (Cloderm)	Epifoam, Pramosone, Procto-
Sulfate (Cortisporin)	Desonide (Desowen, Tidesilon)	foam-HC)
Benzoyl Peroxide (Vanoxide-HC)	Desoximetasone (Topicort)	Hydrocortisone Butyrate (Locoid)
Betamethasone Dipropionate	Diflorasone Diacetate (Psorcon)	Hydrocortisone Probutate (Pandel)
(Diprolene, Diprosone)	Fluocinolone Acetonide (Synalar)	Hydrocortisone/Neomycin Sulfate/
Betamethasone Dipropionate/	Fluocinolone Acetonide/Hydroqui-	Polymyxin B Sulfate (Pediotic)
Clotrimazole (Lotrisone)	none/Tretinoin (Tri-Luma)	Mometasone Furoate (Elocon)
Betamethasone Valerate (Luxiq)	Fluocinonide (Vanos)	Prednicarbate (Dermatop)

Drooling

Chlorpromazine (Thorazine)	Prochlorperazine (Compazine,	Trifluoperazine Hydrochloride
Dantrolene Sodium (Dantrium)	Compro)	(Stelazine)
Donepezil Hydrochloride (Aricept)	Thioridazine Hydrochloride	
Metyrosine (Demser)	(Thioridazine)	
Midazolam Hydrochloride (Versed)	Thiothixene (Thiothixene)	

Dryness, mucous membrane

Azatadine Maleate (Trinalin)	Chlorpheniramine Tannate/	Pravastatin Sodium (Pravachol)
Busulfan (Myleran)	Phenylephrine Tannate/Pyrilamine	Thiabendazole (Mintezol)
Carbetapentane Tannate (Tussi-12)	Tannate (Atrohist, Rynatan-S)	Tretinoin (Vesanoid)
Carbetapentane Tannate/Chlor-	Diflunisal (Dolobid)	
pheniramine Tannate/Ephedrine	Ezetimibe/Simvastatin (Vytorin)	
Tannate/Phenylephrine Tannate	Hydrochlorothiazide (Timolide)	
(Rynatuss)	Lovastatin/Niacin (Advicor)	

Dysphagia

Acamprosate Calcium (Campral)	Amitriptyline Hydrochloride	Amphotericin B, Liposomal
Acetaminophen/Tramadol (Ultracet)	Amlodipine Besylate/Atorvastatin	(Ambisome)
Alendronate Sodium (Fosamax)	(Caduet)	Aprepitant (Emend)
Alprazolam (Xanax)	Amlodipine Besylate (Norvasc)	Aripiprazole (Abilify)
Amantadine Hydrochloride	Amoxicillin/Clarithromycin/	Atorvastatin Calcium (Lipitor)
(Symmetrel)	Lansoprazole (PREVPAC)	Betaxolol Hydrochloride (Kerlone)

Dysphagia *(cont.)*

Bicalutamide (Casodex)
Botulinum Toxin Type A (Botox)
Bupropion Hydrochloride
  (Wellbutrin, Zyban)
Capecitabine (Xeloda)
Carbidopa (Atamet, Lodosyn)
Carbidopa/Levodopa (Parcopa,
  Sinemet)
Carbidopa/Entacapone/Levodopa
  (Stalevo)
Celecoxib (Celebrex)
Cevimeline Hydrochloride (Evoxac)
Ciprofloxacin (Cipro)
Citalopram Hydrobromide (Celexa)
Clozapine (Clozaril, Fazaclo)
Cyclosporine (Gengraf, Neoral)
Dactinomycin (Cosmegen)
Delavirdine Mesylate (Rescriptor)
Denileukin Diftitox (Ontak)
Dexrazoxane (Zinecard)
Diclofenac Sodium/Misoprostol
  (Arthrotec)
Dihydroergotamine Mesylate
  (Migranal)
Divalproex Sodium (Depakote)
Doxorubicin Hydrochloride
  Liposome (Doxil)
Doxycycline Monohydrate
  (Monodox)
Duloxetine Hydrochloride
  (Cymbalta)
Eletriptan Hydrobromide (Relpax)
Ertapenem (Invanz)
Esomeprazole Magnesium (Nexium)
Eszopiclone (Lunesta)
Ethacrynate Sodium (Edecrin)
Etoposide (Vepesid)
Etoposide Phosphate (Etopophos)
Fentanyl Citrate (Actiq)
Fluoxetine Hydrochloride (Prozac,
  Sarafem)
Fluvoxamine Maleate (Luvox)
Foscarnet Sodium (Foscavir)
Fosinopril Sodium (Monopril)
Frovatriptan Succinate (Frova)
Gabapentin (Neurontin)

Galantamine Hydrobromide
  (Razadyne)
Gatifloxacin (Tequin)
Glatiramer Acetate (Copaxone)
Grepafloxacin Hydrochloride (Raxar)
Hydrochlorothiazide
Hydrocodone Bitartrate/Ibuprofen
  (Vicoprofen)
Infliximab (Remicade)
Interferon Alfa-2b, Recombinant
  (Intron)
Itraconazole (Sporanox)
Lamotrigine (Lamictal)
Lansoprazole (Prevacid)
Leuprolide Acetate (Lupron)
Levofloxacin (Levaquin)
Lomefloxacin Hydrochloride
  (Maxaquin)
Lopinavir/Ritonavir (Kaletra)
Memantine Hydrochloride
  (Namenda)
Mesalamine (Pentasa)
Minocycline Hydrochloride (Minocin)
Moricizine Hydrochloride
  (Ethmozine)
Morphine Sulfate (Avinza, Kadian)
Moxifloxacin Hydrochloride (Avelox)
Mycophenolate Mofetil (Cellcept)
Nabumetone (Relafen)
Nifedipine (Adalat)
Nisoldipine (Sular)
Norfloxacin (Noroxin)
Octreotide Acetate (Sandostatin)
Olanzapine (Zyprexa)
Omega-3-Acid Ethyl Esters (Omacor)
Oxcarbazepine (Trileptal)
Oxycodone Hydrochloride
  (Oxycontin)
Oxytetracycline (Terramycin)
Pantoprazole Sodium (Protonix)
Paroxetine Hydrochloride (Paxil)
Pemetrexed (Alimta)
Pentostatin (Nipent)
Pergolide Mesylate (Permax)
Perphenazine (Trilafon)
Pimozide (Orap)

Porfimer Sodium (Photofrin)
Pramipexole Dihydrochloride
  (Mirapex)
Pregabalin (Lyrica)
Procarbazine Hydrochloride
  (Matulane)
Propafenone Hydrochloride
  (Rythmol)
Quetiapine Fumarate (Seroquel)
Rabeprazole Sodium (Aciphex)
Ramipril (Altace)
Riluzole (Rilutek)
Rimantadine Hydrochloride
  (Flumadine)
Risedronate Sodium (Actonel)
Risperidone (Risperdal)
Ritonavir (Norvir)
Rivastigmine Tartrate (Exelon)
Rizatriptan Benzoate (Maxalt-MLT)
Ropinirole Hydrochloride (Requip)
Saquinavir Mesylate (Invirase)
Sargramostim (Leukine)
Selegiline Hydrochloride (Eldepryl)
Sermorelin Acetate (Geref)
Sertraline Hydrochloride (Zoloft)
Sildenafil Citrate (Viagra)
Sirolimus (Rapamune)
Sumatriptan Succinate (Imitrex)
Tacrolimus (Prograf)
Tadalafil (Cialis)
Thalidomide (Thalomid)
Tiagabine Hydrochloride (Gabitril)
Tocainide Hydrochloride (Tonocard)
Tolcapone (Tasmar)
Topiramate (Topamax)
Vardenafil Hydrochloride (Levitra)
Venlafaxine Hydrochloride (Effexor)
Vinorelbine Tartrate (Navelbine)
Voriconazole (VFEND)
Zaleplon (Sonata)
Zidovudine (Retrovir)
Ziprasidone Hydrochloride (Geodon)
Zoledronic Acid (Zometa)
Zolmitriptan (Zomig)
Zolpidem Tartrate (Ambien)
Zonisamide (Zonegran)

Table 24: ORAL MANIFESTATIONS OF SYSTEMIC AGENTS *(cont.)*

Edema, laryngeal

Alteplase (Activase)
Amifostine (Ethyol)
Amitriptyline Hydrochloride
Amlodipine Besylate/Benazepril
  Hydrochloride (Lotrel)
Antihemophilic Factor
  (Recombinant) (Benefix)
Aspirin
Cefdinir (Omnicef)
Ceftazidime (Ceptaz, Fortaz)
Chloroprocaine Hydrochloride
  (Nesacaine)
Chlorpromazine (Thorazine)
Ciprofloxacin (Cipro)
Codeine Phosphate (Phenergan)
Cromolyn Sodium (Intal)
Diclofenac Sodium/Misoprostol
  (Arthrotec)
Dipyridamole (Persantine)
Enalapril Maleate/Hydrochlorothia-
  zide (Vaseretic)
Enalapril Maleate (Vasotec)
Enoxacin (Penetrex)
Esomeprazole Magnesium
  (Nexium)

Fluoxetine Hydrochloride (Prozac,
  Sarafem)
Gentamicin Sulfate (Garamycin)
Grepafloxacin Hydrochloride
  (Raxar)
Hydrochlorothiazide/Lisinopril
  (Prinzide, Zestoretic)
Infliximab (Remicade)
Ketoprofen (Orudis)
Lisinopril (Prinivil, Zestril)
Lomefloxacin Hydrochloride
  (Maxaquin)
Menotropins (Pergonal, Repronex)
Mepivacaine Hydrochloride
  (Polocaine)
Metoclopramide (Reglan)
Moxifloxacin Hydrochloride (Avelox)
Muromonab-Cd3 (Orthoclone)
Nalbuphine Hydrochloride (Nubain)
Nizatidine (Axid)
Ofloxacin (Floxin)
Ondansetron Hydrochloride (Zofran)
Oprelvekin (Neumega)
Oxymorphone Hydrochloride
  (Numorphan)

Penicillin G Benzathine (Permapen)
Pentostatin (Nipent)
Pergolide Mesylate (Permax)
Perphenazine (Trilafon)
Prochlorperazine (Compazine,
  Compro)
Rapacuronium Bromide (Raplon)
Ropivacaine Hydrochloride
  (Naropin)
Sparfloxacin (Zagam)
Tenecteplase (Tnkase)
Thioridazine Hydrochloride
Thiotepa (Thioplex)
Thyrotropin Alfa (Thyrogen)
Trandolapril/Verapamil
  Hydrochloride (Tarka)
Tretinoin (Vesanoid)
Trifluoperazine Hydrochloride
  (Stelazine)
Urofollitropin (Bravelle)
Vardenafil Hydrochloride (Levitra)
Venlafaxine Hydrochloride (Effexor)
Zolmitriptan (Zomig)

Edema, lips

Agalsidase Beta (Fabrazyme)
Albuterol Sulfate/Ipratropium
  Bromide (Combivent)
Ciprofloxacin (Cipro)
Delavirdine Mesylate (Rescriptor)
Finasteride (Propecia)

Infliximab (Remicade)
Losartan Potassium (Cozaar)
Moricizine Hydrochloride
  (Ethmozine)
Muromonab-Cd3 (Orthoclone)
Pegaspargase (Oncaspar)

Sumatriptan Succinate (Imitrex)
Trandolapril/Verapamil
  Hydrochloride (Tarka)
Zidovudine (Retrovir)

Edema, mouth

Alemtuzumab (Campath)
Cevimeline Hydrochloride (Evoxac)

Frovatriptan Succinate (Frova)
Gatifloxacin (Tequin)

Edema, oropharyngeal

Albuterol (Proventi, Ventolin,
  Vospire)
Albuterol Sulfate/Ipratropium
  Bromide (Combivent)
Ciprofloxacin (Cipro)

Diclofenac Sodium/Misoprostol
  (Arthrotec)
Fluticasone Propionate/Salmeterol
  Xinafoate (Advair)
Fluticasone Propionate Hfa (Flovent)

Ipratropium Bromide (Atrovent)
Penciclovir (Denavir)
Zanamivir (Relenza)

Edema, pharyngeal

Candesartan Cilexetil (Atacand)	Losartan Potassium (Cozaar)	
Ciprofloxacin (Cipro)	Moxifloxacin Hydrochloride (Avelox)	
Grepafloxacin Hydrochloride (Raxar)	Nalidixic Acid (Neggram)	
Infliximab (Remicade)	Norfloxacin (Noroxin)	
Lomefloxacin Hydrochloride	Omalizumab (Xolair)	
(Maxaquin)	Rizatriptan Benzoate (Maxalt-MLT)	

Edema, tongue

Acetaminophen/Tramadol (Ultracet)	Fluticasone Propionate (Flonase)	Quetiapine Fumarate (Seroquel)
Albuterol Sulfate/Ipratropium	Gatifloxacin (Tequin)	Risperidone (Risperdal)
Bromide (Combivent)	Grepafloxacin Hydrochloride (Raxar)	Rizatriptan Benzoate (Maxalt-MLT)
Amitriptyline Hydrochloride (Elavil)	Hydrochlorothiazide	Ropinirole Hydrochloride (Requip)
Aripiprazole (Abilify)	Interferon Beta-1a (Avonex)	Sertraline Hydrochloride (Zoloft)
Budesonide (Entocort)	Interferon Beta-1b (Betaseron)	Sibutramine Hydrochloride
Bupropion Hydrochloride	Lamotrigine (Lamictal)	Monohydrate (Meridia)
(Wellbutrin, Zyban)	Levofloxacin (Levaquin)	Topiramate (Topamax)
Cetirizine Hydrochloride (Zyrtec)	Losartan Potassium (Cozaar)	Trandolapril/Verapamil
Cetirizine Hydrochloride/	Metoclopramide (Reglan)	Hydrochloride (Tarka)
Pseudoephedrine (Zyrtec-D)	Mirtazapine (Remeron)	Trimipramine Maleate (Surmontil)
Cilostazol (Pletal)	Moricizine Hydrochloride	Venlafaxine Hydrochloride (Effexor)
Cyclobenzaprine Hydrochloride	(Ethmozine)	Voriconazole (VFEND)
(Flexeril)	Olanzapine (Zyprexa)	Zaleplon (Sonata)
Donepezil Hydrochloride (Aricept)	Omalizumab (Xolair)	Zidovudine (Retrovir)
Eletriptan Hydrobromide (Relpax)	Oprelvekin (Neumega)	Ziprasidone Hydrochloride (Geodon)
Esomeprazole Magnesium (Nexium)	Paroxetine Hydrochloride (Paxil)	Zolmitriptan (Zomig)
Eszopiclone (Lunesta)	Polyethylene Glycol/Potassium Chlo-	Fluticasone Propionate/Salmeterol
Etoposide (Vepesid)	ride/Sodium Bicarbonate/ Sodium	Xinafoate (Advair)
Etoposide Phosphate (Etopophos)	Chloride/Sodium Sulfate/ Sodium	
Fluoxetine Hydrochloride (Prozac,	Sulfate (Colyte)	
Sarafem)	Pregabalin (Lyrica)	

Gagging

Escitalopram Oxalate (Lexapro)	Midazolam Hydrochloride (Versed)	

Gingival disorder, unspecified

Nifedipine (Adalat)	Orlistat (Xenical)	Rifaximin (Xifaxan)

Gingival hyperplasia

Acitretin (Soriatane)	Basiliximab (Simulect)	Diltiazem Hydrochloride (Cardizem,
Amlodipine Besylate/Atorvastatin	Cevimeline Hydrochloride	Tiazac)
(Caduet)	(Evoxac)	Felodipine (Plendil)
Amlodipine Besylate	Cyclosporine (Gengraf, Neoral,	Interferon Alfa-2b, Recombinant
(Norvasc)	Sandimmune)	(Intron)

Table 24: ORAL MANIFESTATIONS OF SYSTEMIC AGENTS *(cont.)*

Gingival hyperplasia *(cont.)*

Lamotrigine (Lamictal)	Phenytoin Sodium (Phenytek)	Trandolapril/Verapamil Hydrochloride (Tarka)
Mycophenolate Mofetil (Cellcept)	Pimozide (Orap)	Verapamil Hydrochloride (Covera-HS, Verelan)
Mycophenolic Acid (Myfortic)	Sertraline Hydrochloride (Zoloft)	Voriconazole (VFEND)
Nifedipine (Adalat)	Sirolimus (Rapamune)	Zonisamide (Zonegran)
Nisoldipine (Sular)	Tiagabine Hydrochloride (Gabitril)	
Oxcarbazepine (Trileptal)	Topiramate (Topamax)	

Gingivitis

Acitretin (Soriatane)	Gatifloxacin (Tequin)	Pergolide Mesylate (Permax)
Alemtuzumab (Campath)	Glatiramer Acetate (Copaxone)	Probenecid (Benemid)
Aripiprazole (Abilify)	Gold Sodium Thiomalate (Myochrysine)	Quetiapine Fumarate (Seroquel)
Aurothioglucose (Solganal)	Grepafloxacin Hydrochloride (Raxar)	Rabeprazole Sodium (Aciphex)
Bexarotene (Targretin)	Homeopathic Formulations (Iscar)	Risperidone (Risperdal)
Bupropion Hydrochloride (Wellbutrin, Zyban)	Hydrochlorothiazide (Uniretic)	Ritonavir (Norvir)
Cevimeline Hydrochloride (Evoxac)	Interferon Alfa-2b, Recombinant (Intron)	Rivastigmine Tartrate (Exelon)
Citalopram Hydrobromide (Celexa)	Isotretinoin (Accutane)	Ropinirole Hydrochloride (Requip)
Clonazepam (Klonopin)	Lamotrigine (Lamictal)	Saquinavir Mesylate (Invirase)
Colchicine	Leflunomide (Arava)	Sildenafil Citrate (Viagra)
Cyclosporine (Gengraf, Neoral)	Leuprolide Acetate (Lupron)	Sirolimus (Rapamune)
Delavirdine Mesylate (Rescriptor)	Levetiracetam (Keppra)	Sparfloxacin (Zagam)
Donepezil Hydrochloride (Aricept)	Methotrexate Sodium (Methotrexate)	Testosterone (Striant)
Doxorubicin Hydrochloride Liposome (Doxil)	Modafinil (Provigil)	Tiagabine Hydrochloride (Gabitril)
Duloxetine Hydrochloride (Cymbalta)	Mycophenolate Mofetil (Cellcept)	Topiramate (Topamax)
Eletriptan Hydrobromide (Relpax)	Nabumetone (Relafen)	Venlafaxine Hydrochloride (Effexor)
Eprosartan Mesylate (Teveten)	Octreotide Acetate (Sandostatin)	Voriconazole (VFEND)
Fentanyl Citrate (Actiq)	Olanzapine (Zyprexa)	Zaleplon (Sonata)
Fluoxetine Hydrochloride/Olanzapine (Symbyax)	Oxaliplatin (Eloxatin)	Zolmitriptan (Zomig)
Fluvoxamine Maleate (Luvox)	Pantoprazole Sodium (Protonix)	Zonisamide (Zonegran)
Gabapentin (Neurontin)	Paroxetine Hydrochloride (Paxil)	
	Pentostatin (Nipent)	

Glossitis

Acitretin (Soriatane)	Bacampicillin Hydrochloride (Spectrobid)	Cevimeline Hydrochloride (Evoxac)
Amlodipine Besylate/Atorvastatin (Caduet)	Balsalazide Disodium (Colazal)	Cilastatin (Primaxin)
Amoxicillin/Clavulanate Potassium (Augmentin)	Betaxolol Hydrochloride (Betoptic)	Citalopram Hydrobromide (Celexa)
Amoxicillin/Clarithromycin/ Lansoprazole (PREVPAC)	Budesonide (Entocort)	Clarithromycin (Biaxin)
Aripiprazole (Abilify)	Bupropion Hydrochloride (Wellbutrin, Zyban)	Cyclosporine (Gengraf, Neoral)
Atorvastatin Calcium (Lipitor)	Calcium Carbonate (Actonel)	Diclofenac Potassium (Cataflam)
Aurothioglucose (Solganal)	Captopril (Captopril)	Diclofenac Sodium/Misoprostol (Arthrotec)
Azelastine Hydrochloride (Astelin)	Carbamazepine (Carbatrol, Equetro, Tegretol)	Diclofenac Sodium (Voltaren, Voltaren-XR)
		Divalproex Sodium (Depakote)

Glossitis *(cont.)*

Doxorubicin Hydrochloride
Liposome (Doxil)
Doxycycline Monohydrate (Monodox)
Eletriptan Hydrobromide (Relpax)
Enalapril Maleate/Hydrochlorothia-
zide (Vaseretic)
Enalapril Maleate (Vasotec)
Etidronate Disodium (Didronel)
Fentanyl Citrate (Actiq)
Flunisolide (Aerobid)
Fluoxetine Hydrochloride (Prozac,
Sarafam)
Fluvoxamine Maleate (Luvox)
Gabapentin (Neurontin)
Gatifloxacin (Tequin)
Gold Sodium Thiomalate
(Myochrysine)
Grepafloxacin Hydrochloride (Raxar)
Guanadrel Sulfate (Hylorel)
Hydrochlorothiazide
Hydrocodone Bitartrate/Ibuprofen
(Vicoprofen)
Isosorbide Mononitrate (Imdur)
Lamotrigine (Lamictal)

Lansoprazole (Prevacid)
Leuprolide Acetate (Lupron)
Mecamylamine Hydrochloride
(Inversine)
Mefenamic Acid (Ponstel)
Meropenem (Merrem)
Minocycline Hydrochloride (Dynacin,
Miniocin)
Mirtazapine (Remeron)
Moxifloxacin Hydrochloride (Avelox)
Nabumetone (Relafen)
Naproxen
Nisoldipine (Sular)
Octreotide Acetate (Sandostatin)
Olanzapine (Zyprexa)
Oxytetracycline (Terramycin)
Pantoprazole Sodium (Protonix)
Paroxetine Hydrochloride (Paxil)
Penicillamine (Cuprimine)
Pentostatin (Nipent)
Pergolide Mesylate (Permax)
Pirbuterol Acetate (Maxair)
Propafenone Hydrochloride (Rythmol)
Pyrimethamine (Daraprim)

Quetiapine Fumarate (Seroquel)
Rabeprazole Sodium (Aciphex)
Riluzole (Rilutek)
Rivastigmine Tartrate (Exelon)
Ropinirole Hydrochloride (Requip)
Saquinavir Mesylate (Invirase)
Sertraline Hydrochloride (Zoloft)
Sildenafil Citrate (Viagra)
Sulfamethoxazole/Trimethoprim
(Bactrim, Septra)
Sulindac (Clinoril)
Telithromycin (Ketek)
Testolactone (Teslac)
Tetracycline Hydrochloride
Tiagabine Hydrochloride (Gabitril)
Tolmetin Sodium (Tolectin)
Topiramate (Topamax)
Valproate Sodium (Depacon)
Valproic Acid (Depakene)
Venlafaxine Hydrochloride (Effexor)
Vitamin B_{12} (Nascobal)
Voriconazole (VFEND)
Zaleplon (Sonata)
Zonisamide (Zonegran)

Glossodynia

Adenosine (Adenoscan)
Amitriptyline Hydrochloride
(Etrafon)
Chlorothiazide (Aldoclor)

Clozapine (Clozaril)
Hydrochlorothiazide (Aldoril)
Methyldopa Hydrochloride
(Aldomet)

Perphenazine (Trilafon)
Propafenone Hydrochloride
(Rythmol)
Sumatriptan Succinate (Imitrex)

Glossoncus

Aurothioglucose (Solganal)
Calcitonin-Salmon (Fortical,
Miacalcin)
Cefuroxime Axetil (Ceftin)
Flecainide Acetate (Tambocor)

Gold Sodium Thiomalate
(Myochrysine)
Influenza Virus Vaccine
(Fluvirin)
Oseltamivir Phosphate (Tamiflu)

Ramipril (Altace)
Rizatriptan Benzoate (Maxalt-MLT)

Glossoplegia

Risperidone (Risperdal)

Glossotrichia

Amitriptyline Hydrochloride
Amoxicillin/Clavulanate Potassium
(Augmentin)

Amoxicillin/Clarithromycin/Lanso-
prazole (PREVPAC)

Bacampicillin Hydrochloride
(Spectrobid)

Table 24: ORAL MANIFESTATIONS OF SYSTEMIC AGENTS *(cont.)*

Glossotrichia *(cont.)*

Clonazepam (Klonopin)	Protriptyline Hydrochloride (Vivactil)	
Methyldopa Hydrochloride (Aldomet)	Trimipramine Maleate (Surmontil)	

Gums, sore

Bupropion Hydrochloride (Wellbutrin)	Propafenone Hydrochloride (Rythmol)	Testosterone (Striant)

Halitosis

Amoxicillin/Clarithromycin/Lanso-prazole (PREVPAC)	Lamotrigine (Lamictal)	Tiagabine Hydrochloride (Gabitril)
Eletriptan Hydrobromide (Relpax)	Lansoprazole (Prevacid)	Venlafaxine Hydrochloride (Effexor)
Eszopiclone (Lunesta)	Ofloxacin (Floxin)	
Gatifloxacin (Tequin)	Pantoprazole Sodium (Protonix)	
Interferon Alfa-2b, Recombinant (Intron)	Propafenone Hydrochloride (Rythmol)	
	Rivastigmine Tartrate (Exelon)	

Herpes simplex

Acitretin (Soriatane)	Ertapenem (Invanz)	Paroxetine Hydrochloride (Paxil)
Alefacept (Amevive)	Estradiol (Vivelle, Vivelle-Dot)	Pegaspargase (Oncaspar)
Alemtuzumab (Campath)	Fenofibrate (Antara, Lofibra, Tricor)	Pentostatin (Nipent)
Amphotericin B, Liposomal (Ambisome)	Fluorouracil (Efudex)	Pergolide Mesylate (Permax)
Anti-Thymocyte Globulin (Thymoglobulin)	Fluticasone Propionate (Cutivate)	Perindopril Erbumine (Aceon)
Arsenic Trioxide (Trisenox)	Gabapentin (Neurontin)	Pimecrolimus (Elidel)
Azelastine Hydrochloride (Astelin)	Gemtuzumab Ozogamicin (Mylotarg)	Prednisolone Acetate
Basiliximab (Simulect)	Glatiramer Acetate (Copaxone)	Progesterone (Prometrium)
Budesonide (Pulmicort, Rhinocort)	Goserelin Acetate (Zoladex)	Rivastigmine Tartrate (Exelon)
Celecoxib (Celebrex)	Grepafloxacin Hydrochloride (Raxar)	Ropinirole Hydrochloride (Requip)
Cevimeline Hydrochloride (Evoxac)	Hydrochlorothiazide	Saquinavir Mesylate (Invirase)
Clindamycin Phosphate (Clindesse)	Imatinib Mesylate (Gleevec)	Sibutramine Hydrochloride Monohy-drate (Meridia)
Clofarabine (Clolar)	Imiquimod (Aldara)	Sildenafil Citrate (Viagra)
Clonazepam (Klonopin)	Interferon Alfa-2b, Recombinant (Intron)	Somatropin (Serostim)
Cyclosporine (Gengraf, Neoral)	Leflunomide (Arava)	Sparfloxacin (Zagam)
Delavirdine Mesylate (Rescriptor)	Levofloxacin (Levaquin)	Tacrolimus (Prograf, Protopic)
Dihydroergotamine Mesylate (Migranal)	Methotrexate Sodium (Methotrexate)	Thalidomide (Thalomid)
Donepezil Hydrochloride (Aricept)	Mirtazapine (Remeron)	Tiagabine Hydrochloride (Gabitril)
Doxorubicin Hydrochloride Liposome (Doxil)	Modafinil (Provigil)	Tipranavir (Aptivus)
	Mycophenolate Mofetil (Cellcept)	Tolcapone (Tasmar)
Enfuvirtide (Fuzeon)	Mycophenolic Acid (Myfortic)	Trastuzumab (Herceptin)
Eprosartan Mesylate (Teveten)	Nisoldipine (Sular)	Venlafaxine Hydrochloride (Effexor)
	Paclitaxel (Taxol)	Voriconazole (VFEND)
	Pantoprazole Sodium (Protonix)	Zolpidem Tartrate (Ambien)

Hoarseness

Albuterol (Proventil, Ventolin)	Enalapril Maleate (Vasotec)	Medroxyprogesterone Acetate
Beclomethasone Dipropionate	Estramustine Phosphate Sodium	(Depo-Provera, Depo-Subq)
(Beclovent, Vanceril)	(Emcyt)	Methyltestosterone (Android)
Budesonide (Rhinocort)	Flunisolide (Aerobid, Nasarel)	Naltrexone Hydrochloride (Revia)
Capecitabine (Xeloda)	Fluticasone Propionate/Salmeterol	Nicotine (Nicotrol)
Captopril (Captopril)	Xinafoate (Advair)	Oxandrolone (Oxandrin)
Carbidopa (Atamet, Lodosyn)	Fluticasone Propionate (Flonase,	Perindopril Erbumine (Aceon)
Carbidopa/Levodopa (Parcopa,	Flovent)	Procarbazine Hydrochloride
Sinemet)	Fluvoxamine Maleate (Luvox)	(Matulane)
Carbidopa/Entacapone/Levodopa	Gabapentin (Neurontin)	Rizatriptan Benzoate (Maxalt-MLT)
(Stalevo)	Hydrocodone Bitartrate/Ibuprofen	Triamcinolone Acetonide (Azmacort)
Clonazepam (Klonopin)	(Vicoprofen)	Zidovudine (Retrovir)
Cromolyn Sodium (Intal)	Ipratropium Bromide	
Enalapril Maleate/Hydrochlorothia-	(Atrovent)	
zide (Vaseretic)	Levofloxacin (Levaquin)	

Hyperesthesia, tongue

Interferon Alfa-N3 (Human Leukocyte Derived, Alferon)		

Hypertrophy, gum

Ethotoin (Peganone)	Isotretinoin (Amnesteem)	

Hypertrophy, tonsillar

Mecasermin [rDNA origin] (Increlex)		

Infection, pharyngeal

Alosetron Hydrochloride (Lotronex)	Lamivudine (Epivir-HBV)	

Irritation, oral

Almotriptan Malate (Axert)	Furosemide	Pancrelipase (Cotazym)
Cyclosporine (Sandimmune)	Naratriptan Hydrochloride (Amerge)	Sumatriptan (Imitrex)
Flunisolide (Aerobid)	Nystatin (Mycostatin)	Testosterone (Striant)

Irritation, oropharynx

Albuterol (Proventil, Ventolin, Vospire)	Salmeterol Xinafoate (Serevent)	

Laryngismus

Acamprosate Calcium (Campral)	Almotriptan Malate (Axert)	Delavirdine Mesylate (Rescriptor)

Table 24: ORAL MANIFESTATIONS OF SYSTEMIC AGENTS *(cont.)*

Laryngismus *(cont.)*

Fluoxetine Hydrochloride/Olanzapine (Symbyax)	Iodine I 131 Tositumomab (Bexxar)	Sertraline Hydrochloride (Zoloft)
Fluvoxamine Maleate (Luvox)	Oxcarbazepine (Trileptal)	Sparfloxacin (Zagam)
Glatiramer Acetate (Copaxone)	Paroxetine Hydrochloride (Paxil)	Venlafaxine Hydrochloride (Effexor)
Grepafloxacin Hydrochloride (Raxar)	Pregabalin (Lyrica)	
	Rapacuronium Bromide (Raplon)	

Laryngitis

Acitretin (Soriatane)	Fluoxetine Hydrochloride/Olanzapine (Symbyax)	Rabeprazole Sodium (Aciphex)
Agalsidase Beta (Fabrazyme)	Fluticasone Propionate/Salmeterol Xinafoate (Advair)	Raloxifene Hydrochloride (Evista)
Albuterol Sulfate (Ventolin)		Riluzole (Rilutek)
Almotriptan Malate (Axert)	Fluticasone Propionate (Flovent)	Rivastigmine Tartrate (Exelon)
Alosetron Hydrochloride (Lotronex)	Fosinopril Sodium (Monopril)	Ropinirole Hydrochloride (Requip)
Aripiprazole (Abilify)	Frovatriptan Succinate (Frova)	Salmeterol Xinafoate (Serevent)
Azelastine Hydrochloride (Astelin)	Gabapentin (Neurontin)	Saquinavir Mesylate (Invirase)
Botulinum Toxin Type A (Botox)	Glatiramer Acetate (Copaxone)	Sertraline Hydrochloride (Zoloft)
Capecitabine (Xeloda)	Hydrochlorothiazide	Sibutramine Hydrochloride Monohydrate (Meridia)
Celecoxib (Celebrex)	Leuprolide Acetate (Lupron)	
Cevimeline Hydrochloride (Evoxac)	Lisinopril (Prinivil, Zestril)	Sildenafil Citrate (Viagra)
Citalopram Hydrobromide (Celexa)	Loratadine (Claritin)	Somatropin (Norditropin)
Clozapine (Clozaril, Fazaclo)	Loratadine/Pseudoephedrine (Claritin-D)	Tacrolimus (Protopic)
Dornase Alfa (Pulmozyme)		Tiagabine Hydrochloride (Gabitril)
Doxorubicin Hydrochloride Liposome (Doxil)	Mirtazapine (Remeron)	Tiotropium Bromide (Spiriva)
	Montelukast Sodium (Singulair)	Tolcapone (Tasmar)
Eletriptan Hydrobromide (Relpax)	Nisoldipine (Sular)	Trastuzumab (Herceptin)
Escitalopram Oxalate (Lexapro)	Olanzapine (Zyprexa)	Venlafaxine Hydrochloride (Effexor)
Estazolam (Prosom)	Omega-3-Acid Ethyl Esters (Omacor)	Zaleplon (Sonata)
Eszopiclone (Lunesta)	Pantoprazole Sodium (Protonix)	Zolmitriptan (Zomig)
Fenofibrate (Antara, Lofibra, Tricor)	Pergolide Mesylate (Permax)	Zolpidem Tartrate (Ambien)
Flunisolide (Aerobid)		

Laryngospasm

Acebutolol Hydrochloride (Sectral)	Dorzolamide Hydrochloride (Cosopt)	Lidocaine (Lidoderm)
Albuterol Sulfate/Ipratropium Bromide (Combivent)		Metoclopramide (Reglan)
	Doxapram Hydrochloride (Dopram)	Metoprolol Succinate (Toprol-XL)
Aripiprazole (Abilify)	Efalizumab (Raptiva)	Midazolam Hydrochloride (Versed)
Atenolol/Chlorthalidone (Tenoretic)	Etoposide (Vepesid)	Morphine Sulfate (MSIR)
Atenolol (Tenormin)	Etoposide Phosphate (Etopophos)	Muromonab-Cd3 (Orthoclone)
Atracurium Besylate (Tracrium)	Fluticasone Propionate/Salmeterol Xinafoate (Advair)	Nadolol (Nadolol)
Bendroflumethiazide (Corzide)		Ondansetron Hydrochloride (Zofran)
Benzonatate (Tessalon)	Haloperidol (Haldol)	Oxymorphone Hydrochloride (Numorphan)
Betaxolol Hydrochloride (Kerlone)	Hydrochlorothiazide (Timolide)	
Carteolol Hydrochloride (Cartrol)	Hydromorphone Hydrochloride (Dilaudid, Dilaudid-HP)	Penbutolol Sulfate (Levatol)
Desflurane (Suprane)		Propofol (Diprivan, Propofol)
Diazepam (Valium)	Ipratropium Bromide (Atrovent)	

Laryngospasm *(cont.)*

Propranolol Hydrochloride (Inderal, Innopran) Salmeterol Xinafoate (Serevent)	Sevoflurane (Ultane) Sucralfate (Carafate)	Timolol Maleate (Blocadren, Timoptic, Timoptic-XE)

Laryngotracheobronchitis

Hepatitis A Vaccine, Inactivated (Vaqta)	Influenza Virus Vaccine (Flumist) Palivizumab (Synagis)	Pneumococcal Vaccine, Diphtheria Conjugate (Prevnar)

Lesions, oral

Cefpodoxime Proxetil (Vantin) Fluticasone Propionate/Salmeterol Xinafoate (Advair)	Irbesartan (Avapro) Nevirapine (Viramune) Testosterone (Striant)	

Leukoplakia, oral

Doxorubicin Hydrochloride Liposome (Doxil)	Interferon Alfa-2b, Recombinant (Intron)	Ziprasidone Hydrochloride (Geodon)

Lips, cracked

Acyclovir (Zovirax)		

Lips, enlargement

Lithium Carbonate (Eskalith)	Phenytoin Sodium (Phenytek)	

Lips, swelling

Finasteride (Propecia, Proscar) Flecainide Acetate (Tambocor)	Influenza Virus Vaccine (Fluvirin) Levofloxacin (Levaquin)	Lithium Carbonate (Lithobid) Ramipril (Altace)

Mouth, burning

Acetaminophen/Butalbital/Caffeine/ Codeine Phosphate (Phrenilin)	Selegiline Hydrochloride (Eldepryl)	

Mouth, discoloration

Palifermin (Kepivance)		

Mouth, fissuring in corner of

Tranylcypromine Sulfate (Parnate)		

Mouth, puckering

Amitriptyline Hydrochloride	Chlorpromazine (Thorazine)	Haloperidol (Haldol)

Table 24: ORAL MANIFESTATIONS OF SYSTEMIC AGENTS *(cont.)*

Mouth, puckering *(cont.)*

Molindone Hydrochloride (Moban) Perphenazine (Trilafon) Pimozide (Orap)	Prochlorperazine (Compazine, Compro)	Trifluoperazine Hydrochloride (Stelazine)

Mouth, sore

Anisindione (Miradon) Aurothioglucose (Solganal) Cyclosporine (Gengraf, Neoral)	Fluticasone Propionate (Flovent) Interferon Alfa-N3 (Human Leukocyte Derived) (Alferon)	Pegaspargase (Oncaspar) Sumatriptan Succinate (Imitrex)

Mouth, thickening of

Palifermin (Kepivance)		

Mouth ulceration

Doxorubicin Hydrochloride Liposome (Doxil)	Pregabalin (Lyrica)	

Mucosal pigmentation, changes

Interferon Alfa-2b, Recombinant (Intron)	Minocycline Hydrochloride (Dynacin, Minocin)	

Mucositis

Alemtuzumab (Campath) Allopurinol Sodium (Aloprim) Amlexanox (Aphthasol) Amphotericin B, Liposomal (Ambisome) Azithromycin Dihydrate (Zithromax) Busulfan (Myleran) Cevimeline Hydrochloride (Evoxac) Daunorubicin Hydrochloride (Cerubidine) Doxorubicin Hydrochloride (Adriamycin, Rubex)	Epirubicin Hydrochloride (Ellence) Etoposide Phosphate (Etopophos) Filgrastim (Neupogen) Gabapentin (Neurontin) Gemtuzumab Ozogamicin (Mylotarg) Hydroxyurea (Hydrea, Mylocel) Idarubicin Hydrochloride (Idamycin) Interferon Alfa-2b, Recombinant (Intron) Interferon Alfa-N3 (Human Leukocyte Derived) (Alferon)	Irinotecan Hydrochloride (Camptosar) Oprelvekin (Neumega) Oxaliplatin (Eloxatin) Paclitaxel (Taxol) Pegaspargase (Oncaspar) Pegfilgrastim (Neulasta) Rasburicase (Elitek) Teniposide (Vumon) Tretinoin (Vesanoid) Vinorelbine Tartrate (Navelbine) Zoledronic Acid (Zometa)

Mucous membrane, abnormalities

Aprepitant (Emend) Atropine Sulfate/Chlorpheniramine Maleate/Hyoscyamine Sulfate/Phenylephrine Hydrochloride/Phenylpropanolamine Hydrochloride/Scopolamine Hydrobromide (Atrohist) Captopril (Captopril)	Cerivastatin Sodium (Baycol) Fentanyl Citrate (Actiq) Fluvastatin Sodium (Lescol) Gabapentin (Neurontin) Lovastatin (Altoprev, Mevacor) Minocycline Hydrochloride (Minocin) Mirtazapine (Remeron)	Perindopril Erbumine (Aceon) Sargramostim (Leukine) Simvastatin (Zocor) Sparfloxacin (Zagam) Sulindac (Clinoril) Thiabendazole (Mintezol)

Mucus, excess

Naltrexone Hydrochloride (Revia)		

Necrosis, buccal

Ketoprofen (Orudis)		

Neoplasm, laryngeal, malignant

Ropinirole Hydrochloride (Requip)		

Numbness, buccal mucosa

Clozapine (Clozaril, Fazaclo)	Nicotine (Nicotrol)	Sumatriptan Succinate (Imitrex)
Lidocaine Hydrochloride (Xylocaine)	Propafenone Hydrochloride (Rythmol)	

Numbness, lips

Dipotassium Phosphate/Disodium Phosphate/Sodium Phosphate (Uro-KP-Neutral)	Methenamine Mandelate (Uroqid-Acid) Pegaspargase (Oncaspar)	Potassium Phosphate (K-Phos)

Osteonecrosis, jaw

Alendronate Sodium (Fosamax)	Ibandronate sodium (Boniva)	Risedronate Sodium/Calcium Car-
Alendronate Sodium-Cholecalciferol	Pamidronate disodium	bonate (Actonel with Calcium)
(Fosamax Plus D)	(Aredia)	Tiluronate disodium (Skelid)
Etidronate Disodium (Didronel)	Risedronate Sodium (Actonel)	Zoledronic Acid (Zometa)

Pain, dental

Aripiprazole (Abilify)	Estradiol (Vivelle, Vivelle-Dot)	Olanzapine (Zyprexa)
Atazanavir Sulfate (Reyataz)	Fluticasone Propionate/Salmeterol	Oxcarbazepine (Trileptal)
Bupropion Hydrochloride (Well-	Xinafoate (Advair)	Pimecrolimus (Elidel)
butrin)	Fluticasone Propionate (Flovent)	Risperidone (Risperdal)
Cefpodoxime Proxetil (Vantin)	Frovatriptan Succinate (Frova)	Ropinirole Hydrochloride (Requip)
Cevimeline Hydrochloride (Evoxac)	Hydrochlorothiazide	Sumatriptan (Imitrex)
Clonazepam (Klonopin)	Interferon Alfacon-1 (Infergen)	Telmisartan (Micardis)
Eprosartan Mesylate (Teveten)	Losartan Potassium (Cozaar)	Thalidomide (Thalomid)
Escitalopram Oxalate (Lexapro)	Montelukast Sodium (Singulair)	Triamcinolone Acetonide (Azmacort)

Pain, facial

Botulinum Toxin Type A (Botox)	Ritonavir (Norvir)	Sumatriptan Succinate (Imitrex)
Fluorouracil (Carac)	Saquinavir Mesylate (Invirase)	Tazarotene (Tazorac)

Pain, jaw

Aripiprazole (Abilify)	Clonazepam (Klonopin)	Estazolam (Prosom)
Ciprofloxacin (Cipro)	Epoprostenol Sodium (Flolan)	Nicotine (Nicotrol)

Table 24: ORAL MANIFESTATIONS OF SYSTEMIC AGENTS *(cont.)*

Pain, jaw *(cont.)*

Pergolide Mesylate (Permax) Propafenone Hydrochloride (Rythmol)	Vinorelbine Tartrate (Navelbine) Zolmitriptan (Zomig)	

Pain, oral mucosa

Ciprofloxacin (Cipro) Fluticasone Propionate/Salmeterol Xinafoate (Advair)	Fluticasone Propionate (Flovent) Lomefloxacin Hydrochloride (Maxaquin)	Ofloxacin (Floxin) Sparfloxacin (Zagam)

Pain, pharyngolaryngeal

Alprazolam (Xanax) Dexmethylphenidate Hydrochloride (Focalin)	Mycophenolic Acid (Myfortic) Rifaximin (Xifaxan) Tegaserod Maleate (Zelnorm)	

Pain, pharynx

Antihemophilic Factor (Recombinant, Advate) Carbidopa/Levodopa (Sinemet) Carbidopa/Entacapone/Levodopa (Stalevo)	Cilastatin (Primaxin) Estradiol (Vivelle, Vivelle-Dot) Hydrochlorothiazide/Lisinopril (Prinzide, Zestoretic) Lisinopril (Prinivil, Zestril)	Omeprazole (Prilosec, Zegerid)

Pain, salivary gland

Cevimeline Hydrochloride (Evoxac)	Frovatriptan Succinate (Frova)	

Pain, throat

Alosetron Hydrochloride (Lotronex) Aripiprazole (Abilify)	Desmopressin Acetate (DDAVP)	Zolmitriptan (Zomig)

Pain, tongue

Iloprost (Ventavis)		

Paralysis, facial

Amlodipine Besylate/Atorvastatin (Caduet) Atorvastatin Calcium (Lipitor) Bivalirudin (Angiomax) Botulinum Toxin Type A (Botox) Fentanyl Citrate (Actiq) Fluvastatin Sodium (Lescol) Gabapentin (Neurontin)	Glatiramer Acetate (Copaxone) Hydrochlorothiazide Lopinavir/Ritonavir (Kaletra) Lovastatin (Altoprev) Medroxyprogesterone Acetate (Depo-Provera) Olanzapine (Zyprexa) Omega-3-Acid Ethyl Esters (Omacor)	Riluzole (Rilutek) Sumatriptan Succinate (Imitrex) Tretinoin (Vesanoid) Venlafaxine Hydrochloride (Effexor) Zaleplon (Sonata) Zonisamide (Zonegran)

Paralysis, tongue

Frovatriptan Succinate (Frova)	Rizatriptan Benzoate (Maxalt-MLT)	Topiramate (Topamax)

Paresthesia, oral

Amprenavir (Agenerase) Fosamprenavir Calcium (Lexiva)	Indinavir Sulfate (Crixivan)	Nicotine (Nicotrol)

Periodontitis

Carvedilol (Coreg) Eprosartan Mesylate (Teveten) Lopinavir/Ritonavir (Kaletra)	Pantoprazole Sodium (Protonix) Ropinirole Hydrochloride (Requip) Thalidomide (Thalomid)	Venlafaxine Hydrochloride (Effexor) Voriconazole (VFEND)

Pharyngeal discomfort

Clozapine (Fazaclo) Ertapenem (Invanz)	Esomeprazole Magnesium (Nexium) Hydrochlorothiazide	Losartan Potassium (Cozaar)

Pharyngitis

Abacavir Sulfate (Ziagen) Abacavir Sulfate/Lamivudine/ Zidovudine (Trizivir) Acamprosate Calcium (Campral) Acebutolol Hydrochloride (Sectral) Acitretin (Soriatane) Adefovir Dipivoxil (Hepsera) Agalsidase Beta (Fabrazyme) Albuterol Sulfate/Ipratropium Bromide (Combivent) Albuterol Sulfate (Duoneb, Proventil, Ventolin) Alefacept (Amevive) Alemtuzumab (Campath) Alfuzosin Hydrochloride (Uroxatral) Allopurinol Sodium (Aloprim) Almotriptan Malate (Axert) Alpha1-Proteinase Inhibitor [Human] (Aralast) Amlodipine Besylate/Atorvastatin (Caduet) Amlodipine Besylate/Benazepril Hydrochloride (Lotrel) Amoxicillin/Clarithromycin/Lanso- prazole (PREVPAC)	Amphotericin B, Liposomal (Ambisome) Anagrelide Hydrochloride (Agrylin) Anastrozole (Arimidex) Antihemophilic Factor (Recombinant, Refacto) Aprepitant (Emend) Aripiprazole (Abilify) Atorvastatin Calcium (Lipitor) Aurothioglucose (Solganal) Azelastine Hydrochloride (Astelin, Optivar) Azithromycin Dihydrate (Zithromax) Balsalazide Disodium (Colazal) Basiliximab (Simulect) Beclomethasone Dipropionate (Qvar, Vancenase, Vanceril) Bepridil Hydrochloride (Vascor) Betaxolol Hydrochloride (Kerlone) Bexarotene (Targretin) Bicalutamide (Casodex) Botulinum Toxin Type A (Botox) Brimonidine Tartrate (Alphagan) Brinzolamide (Azopt) Budesonide (Pulmicort, Rhinocort)	Buprenorphine Hydrochloride (Suboxone) Bupropion Hydrochloride (Wellbutrin, Zyban) Calcitonin-Salmon (Fortical, Miacalcin) Candesartan Cilexetil (Atacand) Carbamazepine (Equetro) Carteolol Hydrochloride (Cartrol) Cefaclor (Ceclor) Cefditoren Pivoxil (Spectracef) Celecoxib (Celebrex) Cerivastatin Sodium (Baycol) Cetirizine Hydrochloride (Zyrtec) Cetirizine Hydrochloride/Pseudo- ephedrine (Zyrtec-D) Cevimeline Hydrochloride (Evoxac) Cilostazol (Pletal) Cisapride (Propulsid) Citalopram Hydrobromide (Celexa) Clindamycin Phosphate (Clindesse) Clonazepam (Klonopin) Colesevelam Hydrochloride (Welchol) Cyclosporine (Gengraf, Neoral)

Table 24: ORAL MANIFESTATIONS OF SYSTEMIC AGENTS *(cont.)*

Pharyngitis *(cont.)*

Daclizumab (Zenapax)
Dactinomycin (Cosmegen)
Darifenacin (Enablex)
Delavirdine Mesylate (Rescriptor)
Denileukin Diftitox (Ontak)
Desflurane (Suprane)
Desloratadine (Clarinex)
Desloratadine/Loratadine/Pseudo-
ephedrine Sulfate (Clarinex-D)
Dihydroergotamine Mesylate
(Migranal)
Diltiazem Hydrochloride (Tiazac)
Diltiazem Hydrochloride/Estradiol/
Ursodiol (Dilacor)
Divalproex Sodium (Depakote)
Donepezil Hydrochloride (Aricept)
Dornase Alfa (Pulmozyme)
Dorzolamide Hydrochloride
(Cosopt)
Doxorubicin Hydrochloride
Liposome (Doxil)
Drospirenone (Yasmin)
Eletriptan Hydrobromide (Relpax)
Epinastine Hydrochloride (Elestat)
Epoetin Alfa (Epogen)
Epoprostenol Sodium (Flolan)
Eprosartan Mesylate (Teveten)
Ertapenem (Invanz)
Escitalopram Oxalate (Lexapro)
Esomeprazole Magnesium (Nexium)
Estazolam (Prosom)
Estradiol (Climara, Prefest, Vivelle,
Vivelle-Dot)
Estradiol/Norethindrone Acetate
(Combipatch)
Estrogens, Conjugated (Premarin,
Prempro)
Estrogens, Conjugated, Synthetic A
(Cenestin)
Eszopiclone (Lunesta)
Etanercept (Enbrel)
Exemestane (Aromasin)
Ezetimibe/Simvastatin (Vytorin)
Ezetimibe (Zetia)
Famciclovir (Famvir)

Felodipine (Plendil)
Fenofibrate (Antara, Lofibra, Tricor)
Fentanyl (Duragesic, Actiq)
Flunisolide (Aerobid, Nasarel)
Fluoxetine Hydrochloride (Prozac,
Sarafem)
Fluoxetine Hydrochloride/Olanzapine
(Symbyax)
Fluticasone Propionate/Salmeterol
Xinafoate (Advair)
Fluticasone Propionate (Flonase,
Flovent)
Fluvastatin Sodium (Lescol)
Fluvoxamine Maleate (Luvox)
Follitropin Alfa (Gonal-F)
Formoterol Fumarate (Foradil)
Foscarnet Sodium (Foscavir)
Fosinopril Sodium (Monopril)
Frovatriptan Succinate (Frova)
Fulvestrant (Faslodex)
Gabapentin (Neurontin)
Gatifloxacin (Tequin)
Gemifloxacin Mesylate (Factive)
Gemtuzumab Ozogamicin
(Mylotarg)
Glatiramer Acetate (Copaxone)
Goserelin Acetate (Zoladex)
Graftskin (Apligraf)
Grepafloxacin Hydrochloride (Raxar)
Hepatitis A Vaccine, Inactivated
(Havrix, Vaqta)
Hepatitis B Vaccine, Recombinant
(Recombivax)
Hydrochlorothiazide
Hydrocodone Bitartrate/Ibuprofen
(Vicoprofen)
Ibandronate Sodium (Boniva)
Ibuprofen/Oxycodone Hydrochloride
(Combunox)
Imatinib Mesylate (Gleevec)
Imiquimod (Aldara)
Immune Globulin Intravenous
(Human) (Gamunex)
Indapamide
Indinavir Sulfate (Crixivan)

Infliximab (Remicade)
Interferon Alfa-2b, Recombinant
(Intron)
Interferon Alfacon-1 (Infergen)
Interferon Alfa-N3 (Human
Leukocyte Derived) (Alferon)
Iodine I 131 Tositumomab (Bexxar)
Ipratropium Bromide (Atrovent)
Irbesartan (Avapro)
Isosorbide Mononitrate (Imdur)
Itraconazole (Sporanox)
Ketoprofen (Orudis)
Ketotifen Fumarate (Zaditor)
Lamotrigine (Lamictal)
Lansoprazole (Prevacid)
Leflunomide (Arava)
Levalbuterol Hydrochloride
(Xopenex)
Levetiracetam (Keppra)
Levocarnitine (Carnitor)
Levofloxacin (Levaquin, Quixin)
Linezolid (Zyvox)
Lisinopril (Prinivil, Zestril)
Lomefloxacin Hydrochloride
(Maxaquin)
Lopinavir/Ritonavir (Kaletra)
Loratadine/Pseudoephedrine
(Claritin-D)
Losartan Potassium (Cozaar)
Lyme Disease Vaccine
(Recombinant Ospa, Lymerix)
Medroxyprogesterone Acetate
(Depo-Subq)
Megestrol Acetate (Megace)
Meloxicam (Mobic)
Meropenem (Merrem)
Mesalamine (Asacol)
Metformin Hydrochloride/Piogli-
tazone Hydrochloride (Actoplus
Met)
Methotrexate Sodium (Methotrexate)
Methylphenidate Hydrochloride
(Concerta)
Modafinil (Provigil)
Moexipril Hydrochloride (Univasc)

Pharyngitis *(cont.)*

Mometasone Furoate (Asmanex)
Mometasone Furoate Monohydrate
  (Nasonex)
Montelukast Sodium (Singulair)
Moricizine Hydrochloride (Ethmozine)
Moxifloxacin Hydrochloride
  (Vigamox)
Mupirocin Calcium (Bactroban)
Mycophenolate Mofetil (Cellcept)
Nedocromil Sodium (Tilade)
Nelfinavir Mesylate (Viracept)
Nicotine (Nicotrol)
Nifedipine (Adalat)
Nisoldipine (Sular)
Nitazoxanide (Alinia)
Nizatidine (Axid)
Octreotide Acetate (Sandostatin)
Ofloxacin (Floxin)
Olanzapine (Zyprexa)
Olopatadine Hydrochloride (Patanol)
Omalizumab (Xolair)
Omega-3-Acid Ethyl Esters (Omacor)
Omeprazole (Prilosec, Zegerid)
Oprelvekin (Neumega)
Oxaliplatin (Eloxatin)
Oxcarbazepine (Trileptal)
Oxybutynin Chloride (Ditropan)
Oxycodone Hydrochloride
  (Oxycontin)
Palivizumab (Synagis)
Pancrelipase (Cotazym)
Pantoprazole Sodium (Protonix)
Paroxetine Hydrochloride (Paxil)
Peginterferon Alfa-2b (PEG-Intron)
Pemetrexed (Alimta)
Pentosan Polysulfate Sodium
  (Elmiron)
Pentostatin (Nipent)
Pergolide Mesylate (Permax)
Perindopril Erbumine (Aceon)

Pimecrolimus (Elidel)
Pioglitazone Hydrochloride (Actos)
Piperacillin Sodium/Tazobactam
  (Zosyn)
Pneumococcal Vaccine, Diphtheria
Conjugate (Prevnar)
Porfimer Sodium (Photofrin)
Pramipexole Dihydrochloride
  (Mirapex)
Progesterone (Crinone, Prochieve,
  Prometrium)
Propofol (Diprivan, Propofol)
Propranolol Hydrochloride (Inderal,
  Innopran)
Quetiapine Fumarate (Seroquel)
Raloxifene Hydrochloride (Evista)
Rapacuronium Bromide (Raplon)
Ribavirin (Rebetol)
Rifaximin (Xifaxan)
Risedronate Sodium (Actonel)
Risperidone (Risperdal)
Ritonavir (Norvir)
Rivastigmine Tartrate (Exelon)
Rizatriptan Benzoate (Maxalt-MLT)
Ropinirole Hydrochloride (Requip)
Rosuvastatin Calcium (Crestor)
Rotavirus Vaccine, Live, Oral, Tetra-
  valent (Rotashield)
Salmeterol Xinafoate (Serevent)
Saquinavir Mesylate (Invirase)
Sargramostim (Leukine)
Sertraline Hydrochloride (Zoloft)
Sevoflurane (Ultane)
Sibutramine Hydrochloride Monohy-
  drate (Meridia)
Sildenafil Citrate (Viagra)
Sirolimus (Rapamune)
Sodium Ferric Gluconate (Ferrlecit)
Sodium Oxybate (Xyrem)
Solifenacin Succinate (Vesicare)

Somatropin (Humatrope, Serostim)
Sparfloxacin (Zagam)
Tacrolimus (Prograf, Protopic)
Tadalafil (Cialis)
Tamsulosin Hydrochloride (Flomax)
Tegaserod Maleate (Zelnorm)
Telmisartan (Micardis)
Temozolomide (Temodar)
Terazosin Hydrochloride (Hytrin)
Teriparatide (Forteo)
Thalidomide (Thalomid)
Tiagabine Hydrochloride (Gabitril)
Tinidazole (Tindamax)
Tiotropium Bromide (Spiriva)
Tobramycin (TOBI)
Tolcapone (Tasmar)
Tolterodine Tartrate (Detrol)
Topiramate (Topamax)
Trastuzumab (Herceptin)
Triamcinolone Acetonide (Azmacort,
  Nasacort)
Triptorelin Pamoate (Trelstar)
Troglitazone (Rezulin)
Valganciclovir Hydrochloride
  (Valcyte)
Valproate Sodium (Depacon)
Valproic Acid (Depakene)
Valsartan (Diovan)
Vardenafil Hydrochloride (Levitra)
Varicella Virus Vaccine, Live
  (Varivax)
Venlafaxine Hydrochloride (Effexor)
Verapamil Hydrochloride (Verelan)
Verteporfin (Visudyne)
Voriconazole (VFEND)
Zidovudine (Retrovir)
Ziprasidone Hydrochloride (Geodon)
Zolmitriptan (Zomig)
Zolpidem Tartrate (Ambien)
Zonisamide (Zonegran)

Pharyngolaryngeal pain

Duloxetine Hydrochloride
  (Cymbalta)

Imatinib Mesylate (Gleevec)

Table 24: ORAL MANIFESTATIONS OF SYSTEMIC AGENTS *(cont.)*

Pharyngoxerosis

Carbamazepine (Carbatrol, Tegretol)		

Prothrombin time, decrease

Ciprofloxacin (Cipro)	Estrogens, Conjugated (Premarin, Prempro)	

Prothrombin time, deviation

Cefepime Hydrochloride (Maxipime)	Moxifloxacin Hydrochloride (Avelox)	Thrombin (Thrombin-JMI)

Prothrombin time, elevation

Aspirin	Caspofungin Acetate (Cancidas)	Lovastatin/Niacin (Advicor)

Prothrombin time, prolongation

Amoxicillin/Clarithromycin/Lanso-prazole (PREVPAC)	Cilastatin (Primaxin)	Niacin (Niaspan)
Aspirin/Dipyridamole (Aggrenox)	Ciprofloxacin (Cipro)	Norfloxacin (Noroxin)
Aspirin	Clarithromycin (Biaxin)	Ofloxacin (Floxin)
Balsalazide Disodium (Colazal)	Clavulanate Potassium (Timentin)	Oxandrolone (Oxandrin)
Cefadroxil (Duricef)	Delavirdine Mesylate (Rescriptor)	Oxymetholone (Anadrol-50)
Cefixime (Suprax)	Enoxacin (Penetrex)	Pegaspargase (Oncaspar)
Cefotetan Disodium (Cefotan)	Ertapenem (Invanz)	Pentosan Polysulfate Sodium (Elmiron)
Cefoxitin Sodium (Mefoxin)	Ethinyl Estradiol	Piperacillin Sodium/Tazobactam (Zosyn)
Cefpodoxime Proxetil (Vantin)	Interferon Alfacon-1 (Infergen)	Sertraline Hydrochloride (Zoloft)
Cefprozil (Cefzil)	Levofloxacin (Levaquin)	Sparfloxacin (Zagam)
Ceftazidime (Ceptaz, Fortaz, Tazicef)	Lomefloxacin Hydrochloride (Maxaquin)	Sulindac (Clinoril)
Ceftriaxone Sodium (Rocephin)	Meropenem (Merrem)	Testosterone (Testim)
Cefuroxime (Zinacef)	Moxifloxacin Hydrochloride (Avelox)	Tigecycline (Tygacil)
Cefuroxime Axetil (Ceftin)	Mycophenolate Mofetil (Cellcept)	
Cephalexin Hydrochloride	Netilmicin Sulfate (Netromycin)	

Saliva, discoloration

Carbidopa (Lodosyn)	Carbidopa/Levodopa (Parcopa, Sinemet)	Carbidopa/Entacapone/Levodopa (Stalevo)

Salivary gland enlargement

Cevimeline Hydrochloride (Evoxac)	Glatiramer Acetate (Copaxone)	Rabeprazole Sodium (Aciphex)
Clozapine (Clozaril, Fazaclo)	Leflunomide (Arava)	Riluzole (Rilutek)
Cyclosporine (Gengraf, Neoral)	Lithium Carbonate (Lithobid)	Sumatriptan (Imitrex)
Fluoxetine Hydrochloride (Prozac, Sarafem)	Mirtazapine (Remeron)	
Gabapentin (Neurontin)	Nitazoxanide (Alinia)	
	Pergolide Mesylate (Permax)	

Sialadenitis

Amiloride Hydrochloride/Hydrochlorothiazide (Moduretic)
Benazepril Hydrochloride (Lotensin)
Bendroflumethiazide (Corzide)
Candesartan Cilexetil (Atacand)
Cevimeline Hydrochloride (Evoxac)
Chlorothiazide Sodium (Diuril)
Delavirdine Mesylate (Rescriptor)
Efalizumab (Raptiva)

Enalapril Maleate/Hydrochlorothiazide (Vaseretic)
Eprosartan Mesylate (Teveten)
Fosinopril Sodium (Monopril)
Hydrochlorothiazide
Hydroflumethiazide (Diucardin)
Indapamide
Lopinavir/Ritonavir (Kaletra)
Methyclothiazide (Enduron)

Methyldopate Hydrochloride (Aldomet)
Naratriptan Hydrochloride (Amerge)
Nitrofurantoin (Furadantin)
Oxcarbazepine (Trileptal)
Paroxetine Hydrochloride (Paxil)
Pergolide Mesylate (Permax)
Zolmitriptan (Zomig)

Stomatitis

Abacavir Sulfate (Epzicom)
Abacavir Sulfate/Lamivudine/Zidovudine (Trizivir)
Acitretin (Soriatane)
Aldesleukin (Proleukin)
Alemtuzumab (Campath)
Amitriptyline Hydrochloride (Elavil)
Amlodipine Besylate/Atorvastatin (Caduet)
Amoxicillin/Clavulanate Potassium (Augmentin)
Amoxicillin (PREVPAC)
Amphotericin B, Liposomal (Ambisome)
Aripiprazole (Abilify)
Atorvastatin Calcium (Lipitor)
Aurothioglucose (Solganal)
Azithromycin Dihydrate (Zithromax)
Bacampicillin Hydrochloride (Spectrobid)
Bevacizumab (Avastin)
Bleomycin Sulfate (Blenoxane)
Bupropion Hydrochloride (Wellbutrin, Zyban)
Capecitabine (Xeloda)
Carbamazepine (Carbatrol, Equetro, Tegretol)
Cefdinir (Omnicef)
Cefditoren Pivoxil (Spectracef)
Cefpodoxime Proxetil (Vantin)
Celecoxib (Celebrex)
Cetirizine Hydrochloride (Zyrtec)
Cetirizine Hydrochloride/Pseudoephedrine (Zyrtec-D)

Cetuximab (Erbitux)
Cevimeline Hydrochloride (Evoxac)
Citalopram Hydrobromide (Celexa)
Clarithromycin (Biaxin)
Clavulanate Potassium (Timentin)
Clofibrate (Atromid-S)
Clopidogrel Bisulfate (Plavix)
Cyclobenzaprine Hydrochloride (Flexeril)
Cyclosporine (Gengraf, Neoral)
Cytarabine (Cytosar-U)
Dalfopristin (Synercid)
Daptomycin (Cubicin)
Delavirdine Mesylate (Rescriptor)
Dexrazoxane (Zinecard)
Diclofenac Potassium (Cataflam)
Diclofenac Sodium/Misoprostol (Arthrotec)
Diclofenac Sodium (Voltaren, Voltaren-XR)
Diflunisal (Dolobid)
Divalproex Sodium (Depakote)
Docetaxel (Taxotere)
Doxorubicin Hydrochloride (Adriamycin, Rubex)
Doxorubicin Hydrochloride Liposome (Doxil)
Eletriptan Hydrobromide (Relpax)
Enalapril Maleate/Hydrochlorothiazide (Vaseretic)
Enalapril Maleate (Vasotec)
Enoxacin (Penetrex)

Epirubicin Hydrochloride (Ellence)
Erlotinib (Tarceva)
Ertapenem (Invanz)
Estrogens, Esterified (Estratest)
Eszopiclone (Lunesta)
Ethionamide (Trecator)
Etoposide (Vepesid)
Etoposide Phosphate (Etopophos)
Fentanyl Citrate (Actiq)
Filgrastim (Neupogen)
Fluorouracil (Efudex)
Fluoxetine Hydrochloride (Prozac)
Fluoxetine Hydrochloride/Olanzapine (Symbyax)
Fluvoxamine Maleate (Luvox)
Frovatriptan Succinate (Frova)
Gabapentin (Neurontin)
Gatifloxacin (Tequin)
Gemcitabine Hydrochloride (Gemzar)
Gemtuzumab Ozogamicin (Mylotarg)
Gentamicin Sulfate (Garamycin)
Glatiramer Acetate (Copaxone)
Gold Sodium Thiomalate (Myochrysine)
Grepafloxacin Hydrochloride (Raxar)
Hydrochlorothiazide
Hydroxyurea (Droxia, Hydrea, Mylocel)
Interferon Alfa-2a, Recombinant (Roferon-A)
Interferon Alfa-2b, Recombinant (Intron)

Table 24: ORAL MANIFESTATIONS OF SYSTEMIC AGENTS *(cont.)*

Stomatitis *(cont.)*

Interferon Alfa-N3 (Human Leuko-
  cyte Derived) (Alferon)
Irinotecan Hydrochloride
  (Camptosar)
Ketoprofen (Orudis)
Lamivudine/Zidovudine (Combivir)
Lamivudine (Epivir, Epivir-HBV)
Lamotrigine (Lamictal)
Lansoprazole (Prevacid)
Leflunomide (Arava)
Leucovorin Calcium (Leucovorin)
Levofloxacin (Levaquin)
Lomefloxacin Hydrochloride
  (Maxaquin)
Lomustine (Ccnu) (Ceenu)
Lopinavir/Ritonavir (Kaletra)
Loratadine (Claritin)
Loratadine/Pseudoephedrine
  (Claritin-D)
Mefenamic Acid (Ponstel)
Mesalamine (Asacol)
Methotrexate Sodium
  (Methotrexate)
Minocycline Hydrochloride (Minocin)
Mirtazapine (Remeron)
Mitomycin (Mitomycin-C)
  (Mutamycin)
Mitoxantrone Hydrochloride
  (Novantrone)
Moxifloxacin Hydrochloride (Avelox)
Mycophenolate Mofetil (Cellcept)
Nabumetone (Relafen)

Naproxen (EC-Naprosyn)
Nicotine (Nicotrol)
Norfloxacin (Noroxin)
Octreotide Acetate (Sandostatin)
Olanzapine (Zyprexa)
Oxaliplatin (Eloxatin)
Oxcarbazepine (Trileptal)
Oxycodone Hydrochloride
  (Oxycontin)
Pamidronate Disodium (Aredia)
Pantoprazole Sodium (Protonix)
Paroxetine Hydrochloride (Paxil)
Pegfilgrastim (Neulasta)
Peginterferon Alfa-2b (PEG-Intron)
Pemetrexed (Alimta)
Pentostatin (Nipent)
Pirbuterol Acetate (Maxair)
Procarbazine Hydrochloride
  (Matulane)
Protriptyline Hydrochloride (Vivactil)
Quetiapine Fumarate (Seroquel)
Rabeprazole Sodium (Aciphex)
Riluzole (Rilutek)
Rimantadine Hydrochloride
  (Flumadine)
Risperidone (Risperdal)
Ropinirole Hydrochloride (Requip)
Saquinavir Mesylate (Invirase)
Sargramostim (Leukine)
Sertraline Hydrochloride (Zoloft)
Sildenafil Citrate (Viagra)
Sirolimus (Rapamune)

Sodium Oxybate (Xyrem)
Sparfloxacin (Zagam)
Sulfamethoxazole/Trimethoprim
  (Bactrim)
Sulfamethoxazole (Septra)
Sulindac (Clinoril)
Tacrolimus (Prograf)
Telithromycin (Ketek)
Temozolomide (Temodar)
Testosterone
Thalidomide (Thalomid)
Thioguanine (Tabloid)
Tiagabine Hydrochloride (Gabitril)
Tinidazole (Tindamax)
Tiotropium Bromide (Spiriva)
Tocainide Hydrochloride (Tonocard)
Tolmetin Sodium (Tolectin)
Topiramate (Topamax)
Topotecan Hydrochloride
  (Hycamtin)
Trastuzumab (Herceptin)
Trimipramine Maleate (Surmontil)
Valproate Sodium (Depacon)
Valproic Acid (Depakene)
Venlafaxine Hydrochloride (Effexor)
Vinorelbine Tartrate (Navelbine)
Voriconazole (VFEND)
Zaleplon (Sonata)
Zidovudine (Retrovir)
Zoledronic Acid (Zometa)
Zolmitriptan (Zomig)
Zonisamide (Zonegran)

Stomatitis, ulcerative

Acitretin (Soriatane)
Alemtuzumab (Campath)
Amlodipine Besylate/Atorvastatin
  (Caduet)
Amoxicillin/Clarithromycin/Lanso-
  prazole (PREVPAC)
Amphotericin B, Liposomal
  (Ambisome)
Anagrelide Hydrochloride (Agrylin)
Atazanavir Sulfate (Reyataz)
Atorvastatin Calcium (Lipitor)

Azelastine Hydrochloride (Astelin)
Balsalazide Disodium (Colazal)
Basiliximab (Simulect)
Cetirizine Hydrochloride (Zyrtec)
Cetirizine Hydrochloride/Pseudo-
  ephedrine (Zyrtec-D)
Cevimeline Hydrochloride
  (Evoxac)
Dactinomycin (Cosmegen)
Diclofenac Sodium/Misoprostol
  (Arthrotec)

Doxorubicin Hydrochloride
  Liposome (Doxil)
Duloxetine Hydrochloride (Cymbalta)
Esomeprazole Magnesium (Nexium)
Eszopiclone (Lunesta)
Fluoxetine Hydrochloride (Prozac,
  Sarafem)
Fluoxetine Hydrochloride/Olanzapine
  (Symbyax)
Follitropin Alfa (Gonal-F)
Foscarnet Sodium (Foscavir)

Stomatitis, ulcerative *(cont.)*

Gabapentin (Neurontin)
Ganciclovir (Cytovene)
Glatiramer Acetate (Copaxone)
Indomethacin (Indocin)
Interferon Alfa-2b, Recombinant
 (Intron)
Itraconazole (Sporanox)
Lansoprazole (Prevacid)
Lopinavir/Ritonavir (Kaletra)
Meloxicam (Mobic)
Methotrexate Sodium (Methotrexate)

Mirtazapine (Remeron)
Mupirocin Calcium (Bactroban)
Naproxen
Nevirapine (Viramune)
Olanzapine (Zyprexa)
Oxcarbazepine (Trileptal)
Pantoprazole Sodium (Protonix)
Paroxetine Hydrochloride (Paxil)
Pergolide Mesylate (Permax)
Piperacillin Sodium/Tazobactam
 (Zosyn)

Pregabalin (Lyrica)
Risperidone (Risperdal)
Rivastigmine Tartrate (Exelon)
Ropinirole Hydrochloride (Requip)
Sertraline Hydrochloride (Zoloft)
Tiagabine Hydrochloride (Gabitril)
Tiotropium Bromide (Spiriva)
Zaleplon (Sonata)
Zonisamide (Zonegran)

Swallowing, impairment

Aprepitant (Emend)
Aurothioglucose (Solganal)
Captopril (Captopril)
Chlorpromazine (Thorazine)
Cyclosporine (Gengraf, Neoral,
 Sandimmune)
Dantrolene Sodium (Dantrium)
Enalapril Maleate/Hydrochlorothia-
 zide (Vaseretic)
Enalapril Maleate (Vasotec)
Escitalopram Oxalate (Lexapro)

Fosinopril Sodium (Monopril)
Gold Sodium Thiomalate (Myochry-
 sine)
Hydrochlorothiazide/Lisinopril
 (Prinzide, Zestoretic)
Levofloxacin (Levaquin)
Lidocaine Hydrochloride (Xylocaine)
Lisinopril (Prinivil, Zestril)
Muromonab-Cd3 (Orthoclone)
Prochlorperazine (Compazine,
 Compro)

Sumatriptan Succinate (Imitrex)
Thioridazine Hydrochloride
 (Thioridazine)
Trandolapril (Mavik)
Trifluoperazine Hydrochloride
 (Stelazine)
Warfarin Sodium (Coumadin)

Swelling, mouth

Diphtheria & Tetanus Toxoids
 And Acellular Pertussis Vaccine
 Adsorbed (Acel-Imune. Adacel,
 Boostrix, Infanrix)

Diphtheria & Tetanus Toxoids
 And Acellular Pertussis Vaccine
 Adsorbed/Hepatitis B Vaccine,
 Recombinant/Poliovirus Vaccine
 Inactivated (Pediarix)

Diphtheria & Tetanus Toxoids And
 Pertussis With Haemophilus B
 Conjugate Vaccine (Tetramune)
Flecainide Acetate (Tambocor)

Swelling, oropharyngeal

Duloxetine Hydrochloride (Cymbalta)

Swelling, salivary gland

Cyclobenzaprine Hydrochloride
 (Flexeril)

Lithium Carbonate (Eskalith)

Tardive dyskinesia

Amitriptyline Hydrochloride (Elavil)
Aripiprazole (Abilify)

Bupropion Hydrochloride (Wellbutrin, Zyban)

Buspirone Hydrochloride (Buspar)
Chlorpromazine (Thorazine)

Table 24: ORAL MANIFESTATIONS OF SYSTEMIC AGENTS *(cont.)*

Tardive dyskinesia *(cont.)*

Clozapine (Clozaril, Fazaclo)
Divalproex Sodium (Depakote)
Fluvoxamine Maleate (Luvox)
Haloperidol (Haldol)
Loxapine Hydrochloride (Loxitane)
Memantine Hydrochloride
   (Namenda)
Metoclopramide (Reglan)
Molindone Hydrochloride (Moban)
Olanzapine (Zyprexa)

Perphenazine (Trilafon)
Pimozide (Orap)
Prochlorperazine (Compazine,
   Compro)
Quetiapine Fumarate (Seroquel)
Risperidone (Risperdal)
Selegiline Hydrochloride (Eldepryl)
Thioridazine Hydrochloride
   (Thioridazine)
Thiothixene (Thiothixene)

Trifluoperazine Hydrochloride
   (Stelazine)
Valproate Sodium (Depacon)
Valproic Acid (Depakene)
Venlafaxine Hydrochloride (Effexor)
Ziprasidone Hydrochloride (Geodon)
Zolmitriptan (Zomig)

Taste, altered

Acamprosate Calcium (Campral)
Acitretin (Soriatane)
Albuterol Sulfate/Ipratropium
   Bromide (Combivent)
Albuterol Sulfate (Duoneb, Proven-
   til, Ventolin, Vospire)
Aldesleukin (Proleukin)
Alendronate Sodium (Fosamax)
Almotriptan Malate (Axert)
Alosetron Hydrochloride (Lotronex)
Alprazolam (Niravam)
Amiodarone Hydrochloride
   (Pacerone)
Amitriptyline Hydrochloride (Triavil)
Amlodipine Besylate/Atorvastatin
   (Caduet)
Amlodipine Besylate (Norvasc)
Amoxicillin/Clarithromycin/Lanso-
   prazole (PREVPAC)
Amprenavir (Agenerase)
Antihemophilic Factor (Recombi-
   nant, Benefix, Kogenate, Refacto)
Aprepitant (Emend)
Aripiprazole (Abilify)
Atazanavir Sulfate (Reyataz)
Atorvastatin Calcium (Lipitor)
Atovaquone (Mepron)
Azithromycin (Zithromax, Zmax)
Balsalazide Disodium (Colazal)
Beclomethasone Dipropionate
   (Vanceril)
Benazepril Hydrochloride (Lotensin)
Bepridil Hydrochloride (Vascor)

Betaxolol Hydrochloride (Kerlone)
Bevacizumab (Avastin)
Bitolterol Mesylate (Tornalate)
Brimonidine Tartrate (Alphagan)
Budesonide (Pulmicort)
Bupropion Hydrochloride
   (Wellbutrin, Zyban)
Buspirone Hydrochloride (Buspar)
Calcitonin-Salmon (Fortical,
   Miacalcin)
Captopril (Captopril)
Carbidopa (Lodosyn)
Carbidopa/Levodopa (Parcopa,
   Sinemet)
Carbidopa/Entacapone/Levodopa
   (Stalevo)
Cefditoren Pivoxil (Spectracef)
Cefpodoxime Proxetil (Vantin)
Celecoxib (Celebrex)
Cerivastatin Sodium (Baycol)
Cetirizine Hydrochloride (Zyrtec)
Cetirizine Hydrochloride/Pseudo-
   ephedrine (Zyrtec-D)
Cevimeline Hydrochloride (Evoxac)
Cilastatin (Primaxin)
Ciprofloxacin (Cipro)
Ciprofloxacin/Dexamethasone
   (Ciprodex)
Citalopram Hydrobromide (Celexa)
Clarithromycin (Biaxin)
Clavulanate Potassium (Timentin)
Clonidine (Catapres-TTS)
Clopidogrel Bisulfate (Plavix)

Cyclosporine (Gengraf, Neoral)
Dantrolene Sodium (Dantrium)
Daptomycin (Cubicin)
Delavirdine Mesylate (Rescriptor)
Diazoxide (Hyperstat)
Diclofenac Sodium/Misoprostol
   (Arthrotec)
Dihydroergotamine Mesylate
   (Migranal)
Diltiazem Hydrochloride (Dilacor)
Disulfiram (Antabuse)
Divalproex Sodium (Depakote)
Docetaxel (Taxotere)
Dolasetron Mesylate (Anzemet)
Dorzolamide Hydrochloride
   (Cosopt)
Doxepin Hydrochloride (Prudoxin)
Doxorubicin Hydrochloride
   Liposome (Doxil)
Efavirenz (Sustiva)
Eletriptan Hydrobromide (Relpax)
Enalapril Maleate/Hydrochlorothia-
   zide (Vaseretic)
Enalapril Maleate (Vasotec)
Enfuvirtide (Fuzeon)
Enoxacin (Penetrex)
Entacapone (Comtan)
Ertapenem (Invanz)
Escitalopram Oxalate (Lexapro)
Esmolol Hydrochloride (Brevibloc)
Esomeprazole Magnesium (Nexium)
Estazolam (Prosom)
Etanercept (Enbrel)

Taste, altered *(cont.)*

Etidronate Disodium (Didronel)
Etoposide Phosphate (Etopophos)
Ezetimibe/Simvastatin (Vytorin)
Famotidine (Pepcid)
Fentanyl Citrate (Actiq)
Flecainide Acetate (Tambocor)
Fluconazole (Diflucan)
Fluoxetine Hydrochloride (Prozac,
    Sarafem)
Fluoxetine Hydrochloride/Olanzapine
    (Symbyax)
Fluticasone Propionate/Salmeterol
    Xinafoate (Advair)
Fluticasone Propionate (Flonase)
Fluvastatin Sodium (Lescol)
Fluvoxamine Maleate (Luvox)
Foscarnet Sodium (Foscavir)
Fosinopril Sodium (Monopril)
Frovatriptan Succinate (Frova)
Gabapentin (Neurontin)
Ganciclovir (Cytovene)
Gatifloxacin (Tequin, Zymar)
Gemifloxacin Mesylate (Factive)
Glatiramer Acetate (Copaxone)
Granisetron Hydrochloride (Kytril)
Grepafloxacin Hydrochloride (Raxar)
Hydrochlorothiazide
Hydromorphone Hydrochloride
    (Dilaudid, Dilaudid-HP)
Ibuprofen/Oxycodone Hydrochloride
    (Combunox)
Imatinib Mesylate (Gleevec)
Indinavir Sulfate (Crixivan)
Interferon Alfa-2a, Recombinant
    (Roferon-A)
Interferon Alfa-2b, Recombinant
    (Intron, Rebetron)
Interferon Alfacon-1 (Infergen)
Interferon Alfa-N3 (Human
    Leukocyte Derived, Alferon)
Ipratropium Bromide (Atrovent)
Iron Dextran (Infed)
Itraconazole (Sporanox)
Ketoprofen (Orudis)
Labetalol Hydrochloride
    (Normodyne)

Lamotrigine (Lamictal)
Lansoprazole (Prevacid)
Leflunomide (Arava)
Leuprolide Acetate (Eligard,
    Lupron)
Levocarnitine (Carnitor)
Levofloxacin (Levaquin)
Lidocaine (Lidoderm)
Linezolid (Zyvox)
Lisinopril (Prinivil, Zestril)
Lithium Carbonate (Eskalith,
    Lithobid)
Lomefloxacin Hydrochloride
    (Maxaquin)
Lopinavir/Ritonavir (Kaletra)
Loratadine (Claritin)
Loratadine/Pseudoephedrine
    (Claritin-D)
Losartan Potassium (Cozaar)
Lovastatin (Altoprev, Mevacor)
Meloxicam (Mobic)
Mesalamine (Asacol)
Metformin Hydrochloride
    (Glucophage)
Metoprolol Succinate (Toprol-XL)
Metronidazole (Metrogel-Vaginal)
Mezlocillin Sodium (Mezlin)
Modafinil (Provigil)
Moexipril Hydrochloride (Univasc)
Mometasone Furoate Monohydrate
    (Nasonex)
Morphine Sulfate (Avinza, MSIR)
Moxifloxacin Hydrochloride (Avelox)
Mupirocin Calcium (Bactroban)
Nabumetone (Relafen)
Naratriptan Hydrochloride (Amerge)
Nicotine (Nicotrol)
Nifedipine (Adalat)
Nisoldipine (Sular)
Octreotide Acetate (Sandostatin)
Ofloxacin (Floxin)
Olanzapine (Zyprexa)
Olopatadine Hydrochloride (Patanol)
Omega-3-Acid Ethyl Esters (Omacor)
Omeprazole (Prilosec, Zegerid)
Oxaliplatin (Eloxatin)

Oxcarbazepine (Trileptal)
Oxycodone Hydrochloride
    (Oxycontin)
Palifermin (Kepivance)
Pancrelipase (Cotazym)
Pantoprazole Sodium (Protonix)
Paricalcitol (Zemplar)
Paroxetine Hydrochloride (Paxil)
Pegfilgrastim (Neulasta)
Peginterferon Alfa-2b (PEG-Intron)
Penciclovir (Denavir)
Penicillamine (Cuprimine)
Pentostatin (Nipent)
Pergolide Mesylate (Permax)
Pimozide (Orap)
Piperacillin Sodium/Tazobactam
    (Zosyn)
Pirbuterol Acetate (Maxair)
Pramipexole Dihydrochloride
    (Mirapex)
Pravastatin Sodium (Pravachol)
Pregabalin (Lyrica)
Propafenone Hydrochloride
    (Rythmol)
Propofol (Diprivan, Propofol)
Quetiapine Fumarate (Seroquel)
Ramipril (Altace)
Ranitidine Bismuth Citrate (Tritec)
Ribavirin (Rebetol)
Rimantadine Hydrochloride
    (Flumadine)
Ritonavir (Norvir)
Rituximab (Rituxan)
Rivastigmine Tartrate (Exelon)
Saquinavir Mesylate (Invirase)
Selegiline Hydrochloride (Eldepryl)
Sevoflurane (Ultane)
Sibutramine Hydrochloride Monohy-
    drate (Meridia)
Simvastatin (Zocor)
Sodium Phenylbutyrate (Buphenyl)
Sparfloxacin (Zagam)
Sumatriptan Succinate (Imitrex)
Tacrolimus (Protopic)
Temozolomide (Temodar)
Terbinafine Hydrochloride (Lamisil)

Table 24: ORAL MANIFESTATIONS OF SYSTEMIC AGENTS *(cont.)*

Taste, altered *(cont.)*

Testosterone (Testim)	Topiramate (Topamax)	Voriconazole (VFEND)
Tiagabine Hydrochloride (Gabitril)	Triamcinolone Acetonide (Tri-Nasal)	Warfarin Sodium (Coumadin)
Tigecycline (Tygacil)	Trimipramine Maleate (Surmontil)	Zaleplon (Sonata)
Tinidazole (Tindamax)	Valproate Sodium (Depacon)	Zidovudine (Retrovir)
Tobramycin (TOBI)	Valproic Acid (Depakene)	Zinc Nasal Gel (Zicam)
Tocainide Hydrochloride (Tonocard)	Venlafaxine Hydrochloride (Effexor)	Zolmitriptan (Zomig)
Tolcapone (Tasmar)	Vinorelbine Tartrate (Navelbine)	Zolpidem Tartrate (Ambien)
Tolterodine (Detrol)	Vitamin K_1 (Aquamephyton)	Zonisamide (Zonegran)

Taste, bad

Albuterol Sulfate (Ventolin)	Ciprofloxacin (Cipro, Ciloxan)	Mesna (Mesnex)
Amiloride Hydrochloride/Hydrochlorothiazide (Moduretic)	Cromolyn Sodium (Intal)	Metaproterenol Sulfate (Alupent)
	Donepezil Hydrochloride (Aricept)	Protirelin (Thyrel)
Antithrombin Iii (Thrombate)	Hydrocodone Bitartrate/Ibuprofen (Vicoprofen)	Sodium Phenylbutyrate (Buphenyl)
Budesonide (Rhinocort)		Sumatriptan Succinate (Imitrex)

Taste, bitter

Azelastine Hydrochloride (Astelin, Optivar)	Dorzolamide Hydrochloride (Cosopt, Trusopt)	Nalbuphine Hydrochloride (Nubain)
		Norfloxacin (Noroxin)
Brinzolamide (Azopt)	Flurazepam Hydrochloride (Dalmane)	Risperidone (Risperdal)
Cefuroxime Axetil (Ceftin)		Sulindac (Clinoril)
Clozapine (Clozaril, Fazaclo)	Isosorbide Mononitrate (Monoket)	Tinidazole (Tindamax)
	Moricizine Hydrochloride (Ethmozine)	

Taste, metallic

Adenosine (Adenocard, Adenoscan)	Etidronate Disodium (Didronel)	Methocarbamol (Robaxin)
Aurothioglucose (Solganal)	Fenoprofen Calcium (Nalfon)	Metronidazole (Metrogel)
Calcitriol (Calcijex)	Gold Sodium Thiomalate (Myochrysine)	Potassium Iodide (Pima)
Disulfiram (Antabuse)		Succimer (Chemet)
Doxercalciferol (Hectorol)	Lidocaine (Lidoderm)	Sulindac (Clinoril)
Escitalopram Oxalate (Lexapro)	Lithium Carbonate (Eskalith, Lithobid)	Tinidazole (Tindamax)
Ethionamide (Trecator)		

Taste, salty

Calcitonin-Salmon (Miacalcin)		

Taste, unpleasant

Amitriptyline Hydrochloride (Elavil)	Brinzolamide (Azopt)	Dextroamphetamine Sulfate (Dexedrine, Dextrostat)
Amphetamine Aspartate/Amphetamine Sulfate/Dextroamphetamine Saccharate/Dextroamphetamine Sulfate (Adderall)	Cefuroxime Axetil (Ceftin)	Eszopiclone (Lunesta)
	Ciprofloxacin (Cipro)	Flunisolide (Aerobid)
	Clotrimazole (Mycelex)	Fluorouracil (Efudex)
	Cyclobenzaprine Hydrochloride (Flexeril)	Fluticasone Propionate (Flonase)
Beclomethasone Dipropionate (Beclovent, Beconase)		

Taste, unpleasant *(cont.)*

Methamphetamine Hydrochloride (Desoxyn) Moxifloxacin Hydrochloride (Avelox)	Nedocromil Sodium (Tilade) Phentermine Hydrochloride (Adipex-P, Fastin)	Protriptyline Hydrochloride (Vivactil) Vitamin K$_1$ (Mephyton)

Teeth grinding

Citalopram Hydrobromide (Celexa)	Sertraline Hydrochloride (Zoloft)

Throat burning

Azelastine Hydrochloride (Astelin) Budesonide (Rhinocort) Estramustine Phosphate Sodium (Emcyt)	Propofol (Diprivan, Propofol) Selegiline Hydrochloride (Eldepryl)	

Throat dryness

Azatadine Maleate (Trinalin) Beclomethasone Dipropionate (Beclovent, Beconase) Brompheniramine Cefpodoxime Proxetil (Vantin) Chlorpheniramine Maleate Clonidine (Catapres-TTS) Clozapine (Clozaril, Fazaclo) Cromolyn Sodium (Intal)	Enoxacin (Penetrex) Flunisolide (Aerobid) Fluticasone Propionate (Flonase) Gabapentin (Neurontin) Glycopyrrolate (Robinul) Guanadrel Sulfate (Hylorel) Ipratropium Bromide (Atrovent) Levalbuterol Hydrochloride (Xopenex)	Metaproterenol Sulfate (Alupent) Mometasone Furoate (Asmanex) Propafenone Hydrochloride (Rythmol) Rifaximin (Xifaxan) Rizatriptan Benzoate (Maxalt-MLT) Triamcinolone Acetonide (Azmacort) Trospium Chloride (Sanctura)

Throat irritation

Albuterol Sulfate (Ventolin) Bitolterol Mesylate (Tornalate) Budesonide (Rhinocort) Cabergoline (Dostinex) Clozapine (Clozaril) Cromolyn Sodium (Intal) Dorzolamide Hydrochloride (Cosopt, Trusopt) Fexofenadine Hydrochloride (Allegra)	Fexofenadine Hydrochloride/ Pseudoephedrine (Allegra-D) Flunisolide (Aerobid) Fluticasone Propionate/Salmeterol Xinafoate (Advair) Fluticasone Propionate (Flonase, Flovent) Ibritumomab Tiuxetan (Zevalin) Interferon Alfa-2a, Recombinant (Roferon-A)	Lamivudine (Epivir-HBV) Metaproterenol Sulfate (Alupent) Nicotine (Nicotrol) Pamidronate Disodium (Aredia) Paroxetine Hydrochloride (Paxil) Ritonavir (Norvir) Rituximab (Rituxan) Triamcinolone Acetonide (Azmacort)

Throat soreness

Acebutolol Hydrochloride (Sectral) Adenosine (Adenoscan) Albuterol Sulfate (Duoneb) Alpha1-Proteinase Inhibitor (Human) (Zemaira)	Amitriptyline Hydrochloride (Etrafon) Anisindione (Miradon) Antihemophilic Factor (Recombinant) (Kogenate)	Arsenic Trioxide (Trisenox) Atenolol/Chlorthalidone (Tenoretic) Atenolol (Tenormin) Atomoxetine Hydrochloride (Strattera)

Table 24: ORAL MANIFESTATIONS OF SYSTEMIC AGENTS (cont.)

Throat soreness (cont.)

Bendroflumethiazide (Corzide)	Guanidine Hydrochloride	Propafenone Hydrochloride (Rythmol)
Betaxolol Hydrochloride (Kerlone)	(Guanidine)	Propranolol Hydrochloride (Inderal,
Buspirone Hydrochloride (Buspar)	Hydrochlorothiazide	Innopran)
Capecitabine (Xeloda)	Imatinib Mesylate (Gleevec)	Ramipril (Altace)
Captopril (Captopril)	Infliximab (Remicade)	Rubella & Mumps Virus Vaccine,
Carbamazepine (Carbatrol, Tegretol)	Influenza Virus Vaccine (Flumist)	Live (Biavax)
Carteolol Hydrochloride (Cartrol)	Lisinopril (Prinivil, Zestril)	Rubella Virus Vaccine, Live
Clofarabine (Clolar)	Measles & Rubella Virus Vaccine,	(Meruvax)
Clozapine (Clozaril, Fazaclo)	Live (M-R-VAX)	Salmeterol Xinafoate (Serevent)
Cytarabine (Cytosar-U)	Measles, Mumps & Rubella Virus	Succimer (Chemet)
Dapsone (Dapsone)	Vaccine, Live (M-M-R)	Sulfamethoxazole (Septra)
Daptomycin (Cubicin)	Metoprolol Succinate (Toprol-XL)	Sumatriptan Succinate (Imitrex)
Desmopressin Acetate (DDAVP)	Mirtazapine (Remeron)	Ticlopidine Hydrochloride (Ticlid)
Diazepam (Valium)	Mycophenolic Acid (Myfortic)	Timolol Maleate (Blocadren, Timop-
Donepezil Hydrochloride (Aricept)	Nadolol (Nadolol)	tic, Timoptic-XE)
Dorzolamide Hydrochloride (Cosopt)	Naltrexone Hydrochloride (Revia)	Tocainide Hydrochloride (Tonocard)
Enalapril Maleate/Hydrochlorothia-	Nifedipine (Adalat)	Trandolapril (Mavik)
zide (Vaseretic)	Paclitaxel (Taxol)	Trifluoperazine Hydrochloride
Enalapril Maleate (Vasotec)	Penbutolol Sulfate (Levatol)	(Stelazine)
Filgrastim (Neupogen)	Perindopril Erbumine (Aceon)	Vitamin B$_{12}$ (Nascobal)
Flunisolide (Aerobid, Nasalide)	Pimecrolimus (Elidel)	Zoledronic Acid (Zometa)
Fluticasone Propionate/Salmeterol	Pirbuterol Acetate (Maxair)	
Xinafoate (Advair)	Prochlorperazine (Compazine,	
Fluticasone Propionate (Flovent)	Compro)	

Throat swelling

Budesonide (Rhinocort)	Fluticasone Propionate (Cutivate)	
Calcitonin-Salmon (Fortical, Miacalcin)	Ofloxacin (Floxin)	

Throat tightness

Adenosine (Adenocard)	Etoposide (Vepesid)	Paroxetine Hydrochloride (Paxil)
Alemtuzumab (Campath)	Etoposide Phosphate (Etopophos)	Perphenazine (Trilafon)
Amitriptyline Hydrochloride	Interferon Alfa-N3 (Human Leuko-	Propafenone Hydrochloride (Rythmol)
Aripiprazole (Abilify)	cyte Derived) (Alferon)	Protirelin (Thyrel)
Doxorubicin Hydrochloride	Levofloxacin (Levaquin)	Rizatriptan Benzoate (Maxalt-MLT)
Liposome (Doxil)	Oprelvekin (Neumega)	Zolmitriptan (Zomig)

Tightness, tongue

Aripiprazole (Abilify)		

Tongue, burning

Buspirone Hydrochloride (Buspar)	Carbidopa/Levodopa (Sinemet)	Fenoprofen Calcium (Nalfon)
Carbidopa (Lodosyn)	Carbidopa/Entacapone/Levodopa	Sumatriptan Succinate (Imitrex)
Carbidopa/Levodopa (Parcopa)	(Stalevo)	

Tongue discoloration

Amitriptyline Hydrochloride
Amoxicillin/Clarithromycin/Lanso-
 prazole (PREVPAC)
Balsalazide Disodium (Colazal)
Bismuth Subsalicylate (Pepto-
 Bismol)
Cetirizine Hydrochloride (Zyrtec)
Cetirizine Hydrochloride/Pseudo-
 ephedrine (Zyrtec-D)
Cevimeline Hydrochloride (Evoxac)
Cilastatin (Primaxin)
Clarithromycin (Biaxin)

Glatiramer Acetate (Copaxone)
Grepafloxacin Hydrochloride (Raxar)
Hydrochlorothiazide (Uniretic)
Linezolid (Zyvox)
Lomefloxacin Hydrochloride
 (Maxaquin)
Methyldopate Hydrochloride
 (Aldomet)
Mirtazapine (Remeron)
Moxifloxacin Hydrochloride (Avelox)
Olanzapine (Zyprexa)
Omeprazole (Prilosec, Zegerid)

Palifermin (Kepivance)
Pantoprazole Sodium (Protonix)
Paroxetine Hydrochloride (Paxil)
Perphenazine (Trilafon)
Ranitidine Bismuth Citrate (Tritec)
Riluzole (Rilutek)
Risperidone (Risperdal)
Thalidomide (Thalomid)
Tinidazole (Tindamax)
Venlafaxine Hydrochloride (Effexor)
Zaleplon (Sonata)

Tongue disorder, unspecified

Acitretin (Soriatane)
Amoxicillin/Clarithromycin/Lanso-
 prazole (PREVPAC)
Cevimeline Hydrochloride
 (Evoxac)
Cyclosporine (Gengraf, Neoral)

Eletriptan Hydrobromide (Relpax)
Esomeprazole Magnesium (Nexium)
Fluticasone Propionate (Flovent)
Gabapentin (Neurontin)
Grepafloxacin Hydrochloride
 (Raxar)

Lansoprazole (Prevacid)
Sparfloxacin (Zagam)
Tolcapone (Tasmar)

Tongue, fine vermicular movements

Amitriptyline Hydrochloride
Chlorpromazine (Thorazine)
Haloperidol (Haldol)
Lithium Carbonate (Eskalith,
 Lithobid)

Metoclopramide (Reglan)
Molindone Hydrochloride (Moban)
Pimozide (Orap)
Prochlorperazine (Compazine,
 Compro)

Thioridazine Hydrochloride
 (Thioridazine)
Thiothixene (Thiothixene)
Trifluoperazine Hydrochloride
 (Stelazine)

Tongue, furry

Tinidazole (Tindamax)

Tongue, mucosal atrophy

Omeprazole (Prilosec, Zegerid)

Tongue, protrusion

Amitriptyline Hydrochloride
Chlorpromazine (Thorazine)
Fluoxetine Hydrochloride (Sarafem)
Haloperidol (Haldol)
Loxapine Hydrochloride (Loxitane)
Metoclopramide (Reglan)
Molindone Hydrochloride (Moban)

Perphenazine (Trilafon)
Pimozide (Orap)
Prochlorperazine (Compazine,
 Compro)
Promethazine Hydrochloride
 (Phenergan)

Thioridazine Hydrochloride
 (Thioridazine)
Thiothixene (Thiothixene)
Trifluoperazine Hydrochloride
 (Stelazine)

Table 24: ORAL MANIFESTATIONS OF SYSTEMIC AGENTS *(cont.)*

Tongue, rounding

Amitriptyline Hydrochloride	Perphenazine (Trilafon)	

Tongue, thickening of

Palifermin (Kepivance)		

Tonsillitis

Cyclosporine (Gengraf, Neoral) Fluticasone Propionate (Flovent)	Formoterol Fumarate (Foradil) Montelukast Sodium (Singulair)	Pimecrolimus (Elidel)

Tooth discoloration

Amoxicillin (Amoxil) Amoxicillin/Clarithromycin/Lanso- prazole (PREVPAC) Amoxicillin/Clavulanate Potassium (Augmentin)	Cilastatin (Primaxin) Clarithromycin (Biaxin) Doxycycline Monohydrate (Monodox) Gabapentin (Neurontin)	Minocycline Hydrochloride (Dynacin, Minocin) Oxytetracycline (Terramycin) Tetracycline Hydrochloride

Tooth disorder

Amphetamine Aspartate/Amphet- amine Sulfate/Dextroamphetamine Saccharate/Dextroamphetamine Sulfate (Adderall) Benazepril Hydrochloride (Lotensin) Botulinum Toxin Type A (Botox) Budesonide (Entocort) Bupropion Hydrochloride (Wellbutrin) Cefpodoxime Proxetil (Vantin) Celecoxib (Celebrex) Cetirizine Hydrochloride (Zyrtec) Cetirizine Hydrochloride/Pseudo- ephedrine (Zyrtec-D) Cevimeline Hydrochloride (Evoxac) Cyclosporine (Gengraf, Neoral, Sangcya) Delavirdine Mesylate (Rescriptor) Diltiazem Hydrochloride (Dilacor) Divalproex Sodium (Depakote) Eletriptan Hydrobromide (Relpax) Estradiol (Prefest, Vivelle, Vivelle-Dot) Estradiol/Norethindrone Acetate (Combipatch)	Fenofibrate (Antara, Lofibra, Tricor, Triglide) Fentanyl Citrate (Actiq) Fluoxetine Hydrochloride/Olanzapine (Symbyax) Fluticasone Propionate (Flovent) Fluvastatin Sodium (Lescol) Fluvoxamine Maleate (Luvox) Follitropin Alfa (Gonal-F) Gabapentin (Neurontin) Ibandronate Sodium (Boniva) Interferon Alfa-2a, Recombinant (Roferon-A) Isosorbide Mononitrate (Ismo) Lamotrigine (Lamictal) Leflunomide (Arava) Loratadine/Pseudoephedrine (Claritin-D) Metformin Hydrochloride (Actoplus) Modafinil (Provigil) Nicotine (Nicotrol) Nizatidine (Axid) Olanzapine (Zyprexa) Orlistat (Xenical) Paroxetine Hydrochloride (Paxil)	Pentostatin (Nipent) Pioglitazone Hydrochloride (Actos) Pramipexole Dihydrochloride (Mirapex) Progesterone (Prometrium) Rapacuronium Bromide (Raplon) Repaglinide (Prandin) Riluzole (Rilutek) Risedronate Sodium (Actonel) Risperidone (Risperdal) Saquinavir Mesylate (Invirase) Sibutramine Hydrochloride Monohydrate (Meridia) Sparfloxacin (Zagam) Tacrolimus (Protopic) Tamsulosin Hydrochloride (Flomax) Teriparatide (Forteo) Thalidomide (Thalomid) Tolcapone (Tasmar) Topiramate (Topamax) Ziprasidone Mesylate (Geodon)

Toothache

Bupropion Hydrochloride (Wellbutrin, Zyban)	Eprosartan Mesylate (Teveten)	Progesterone (Crinone, Prochieve)
Cabergoline (Dostinex)	Escitalopram Oxalate (Lexapro)	Risperidone (Risperdal)
Cefpodoxime Proxetil (Vantin)	Estradiol (Vivelle, Vivelle-Dot)	Ropinirole Hydrochloride (Requip)
Cevimeline Hydrochloride (Evoxac)	Follitropin Alfa (Gonal-F)	Telmisartan (Micardis)
Clonazepam (Klonopin)	Frovatriptan Succinate (Frova)	Testosterone
Delavirdine Mesylate (Rescriptor)	Interferon Beta-1a (Avonex)	Triamcinolone Acetonide (Azmacort)
Donepezil Hydrochloride (Aricept)	Oxcarbazepine (Trileptal)	
	Pimecrolimus (Elidel)	

Trismus

Amitriptyline Hydrochloride	Fluvoxamine Maleate (Luvox)	Riluzole (Rilutek)
Carbidopa (Lodosyn)	Iloprost (Ventavis)	Thioridazine Hydrochloride
Carbidopa/Levodopa (Parcopa, Sinemet)	Metoclopramide (Reglan)	(Thioridazine)
	Metyrosine (Demser)	Trifluoperazine Hydrochloride
Carbidopa/Entacapone/Levodopa (Stalevo)	Paroxetine Hydrochloride (Paxil)	(Stelazine)
	Perphenazine (Trilafon)	Venlafaxine Hydrochloride (Effexor)
Cefuroxime Axetil (Ceftin)	Pregabalin (Lyrica)	Zaleplon (Sonata)
Chlorpromazine (Thorazine)	Prochlorperazine (Compazine, Compro)	Ziprasidone Hydrochloride (Geodon)
Etidocaine Hydrochloride (Duranest)		

Ulceration, tongue

Acitretin (Soriatane)	Delavirdine Mesylate (Rescriptor)	Saquinavir Mesylate (Invirase)
Aurothioglucose (Solganal)	Loratadine/Pseudoephedrine (Claritin-D)	Sertraline Hydrochloride (Zoloft)
Cevimeline Hydrochloride (Evoxac)		

Ulcers, oral mucosal

Abacavir Sulfate (Ziagen)	Bupropion Hydrochloride (Wellbutrin, Zyban)	Estazolam (Prosom)
Abacavir Sulfate/Lamivudine/ Zidovudine (Trizivir)	Carbamazepine (Carbatrol, Tegretol)	Eszopiclone (Lunesta)
Acamprosate Calcium (Campral)		Etanercept (Enbrel)
Albuterol Sulfate/Ipratropium Bromide (Combivent)	Cefpodoxime Proxetil (Vantin)	Fenoprofen Calcium (Nalfon)
	Cefuroxime Axetil (Ceftin)	Fentanyl Citrate (Actiq)
Amlodipine Besylate/Atorvastatin (Caduet)	Chlorambucil (Leukeran)	Fluoxetine Hydrochloride (Prozac, Sarafem)
	Ciprofloxacin (Cipro)	
Amoxicillin/Clarithromycin/Lanso- prazole (PREVPAC)	Clozapine (Clozaril)	Fluticasone Propionate/Salmeterol Xinafoate (Advair)
	Cyclophosphamide (Cytoxan)	
Anisindione (Miradon)	Cytarabine (Cytosar-U)	Fluticasone Propionate (Flovent)
Aripiprazole (Abilify)	Delavirdine Mesylate (Rescriptor)	Gabapentin (Neurontin)
Atazanavir Sulfate (Reyataz)	Denileukin Diftitox (Ontak)	Gatifloxacin (Tequin)
Atorvastatin Calcium (Lipitor)	Divalproex Sodium (Depakote)	Gefitinib (Iressa)
Atovaquone (Malarone)	Doxorubicin Hydrochloride Liposome (Doxil)	Glatiramer Acetate (Copaxone)
Aurothioglucose (Solganal)		Gold Sodium Thiomalate (Myochrysine)
Betaxolol Hydrochloride (Kerlone)	Ertapenem (Invanz)	Grepafloxacin Hydrochloride (Raxar)

Table 24: ORAL MANIFESTATIONS OF SYSTEMIC AGENTS *(cont.)*

Ulcers, oral mucosal *(cont.)*

Hydrocodone Bitartrate/Ibuprofen (Vicoprofen)	Nelfinavir Mesylate (Viracept)	Sirolimus (Rapamune)
Imatinib Mesylate (Gleevec)	Nisoldipine (Sular)	Sodium Oxybate (Xyrem)
Interferon Alfa-2b, Recombinant (Intron)	Norfloxacin (Noroxin)	Sparfloxacin (Zagam)
Lamotrigine (Lamictal)	Olanzapine (Zyprexa)	Tiagabine Hydrochloride (Gabitril)
Lansoprazole (Prevacid)	Pantoprazole Sodium (Protonix)	Tolcapone (Tasmar)
Leflunomide (Arava)	Paroxetine Hydrochloride (Paxil)	Trimetrexate Glucuronate (Neutrexin)
Lopinavir/Ritonavir (Kaletra)	Penicillamine (Cuprimine)	Venlafaxine Hydrochloride (Effexor)
Melphalan Hydrochloride (Alkeran)	Pentosan Polysulfate Sodium (Elmiron)	Voriconazole (VFEND)
Mesalamine (Asacol, Pentasa)	Propafenone Hydrochloride (Rythmol)	Zaleplon (Sonata)
Midodrine Hydrochloride (Proamatine)	Quetiapine Fumarate (Seroquel)	Zidovudine (Retrovir)
Modafinil (Provigil)	Rabeprazole Sodium (Aciphex)	Zonisamide (Zonegran)
Mycophenolate Mofetil (Cellcept)	Ritonavir (Norvir)	
	Sibutramine Hydrochloride Monohydrate (Meridia)	

Ulcers, oropharyngeal

Alendronate Sodium (Fosamax)	Aurothioglucose (Solganal)	Gold Sodium Thiomalate (Myochrysine)

Xerochilia

Acyclovir (Zovirax)	Escitalopram Oxalate (Lexapro)	Saquinavir Mesylate (Invirase)
Doxepin Hydrochloride (Prudoxin)	Rifaximin (Xifaxan)	

Xerostomia

Abciximab (Reopro)	Amiloride Hydrochloride/Hydrochlorothiazide (Moduretic)	Anastrozole (Arimidex)
Acamprosate Calcium (Campral)	Amitriptyline Hydrochloride	Aripiprazole (Abilify)
Acetaminophen/Tramadol (Ultracet)	Amlodipine Besylate/Atorvastatin (Caduet)	Arsenic Trioxide (Trisenox)
Acetaminophen/Butalbital/Caffeine/Codeine Phosphate (Phrenilin)	Amlodipine Besylate/Benazepril Hydrochloride (Lotrel)	Aspirin/Caffeine/Orphenadrine Citrate (Norgesic)
Adenosine (Adenoscan)	Amlodipine Besylate (Norvasc)	Atenolol/Chlorthalidone (Tenoretic)
Albuterol Sulfate/Ipratropium Bromide (Combivent)	Amoxicillin/Clarithromycin/Lansoprazole (PREVPAC)	Atenolol (Tenormin)
Albuterol Sulfate (Proventil, Ventolin)	Amphetamine Aspartate/Amphetamine Sulfate/Dextroamphetamine Saccharate/Dextroamphetamine Sulfate (Adderall)	Atomoxetine Hydrochloride (Strattera)
Almotriptan Malate (Axert)		Atorvastatin Calcium (Lipitor)
Alprazolam (Niravam, Xanax)		Atropine Sulfate (Motofen)
Alprostadil (Caverject)		Atropine Sulfate/Benzoic Acid/Hyoscyamine/Methenamine/Methylene Blue/Phenyl Salicylate (Urised)
Amantadine Hydrochloride (Symmetrel)	Amphotericin B, Liposomal (Ambisome)	Atropine Sulfate/Hyoscyamine Sulfate/Phenobarbital/Scopolamine Hydrobromide (Donnatal)
Amiloride Hydrochloride (Midamor)		

Xerostomia *(cont.)*

Azatadine Maleate (Trinalin)
Azelastine Hydrochloride (Astelin)
Balsalazide Disodium (Colazal)
Beclomethasone Dipropionate
(Beclovent, Vanceril)
Belladonna Alkaloids/Hyoscyamine
Sulfate/Methenamine/Methylene
Blue/Phenyl Salicylate/Sodium
Biphosphate (Urimax)
Benazepril Hydrochloride
(Lotensin)
Bendroflumethiazide (Corzide)
Benztropine Mesylate (Cogentin)
Bepridil Hydrochloride (Vascor)
Betaxolol Hydrochloride (Kerlone)
Bevacizumab (Avastin)
Bexarotene (Targretin)
Bicalutamide (Casodex)
Biperiden Hydrochloride (Akineton)
Brimonidine Tartrate (Alphagan)
Brinzolamide (Azopt)
Brompheniramine Maleate
(Bromfed)
Budesonide (Pulmicort, Rhinocort)
Bupropion Hydrochloride
(Wellbutrin, Zyban)
Buspirone Hydrochloride (Buspar)
Butabarbital/Fluoxetine Hydrochlo-
ride/Hyoscyamine Hydrobromide/
Phenazopyridine Hydrochloride
(Pyridium)
Cabergoline (Dostinex)
Calcitonin-Salmon (Fortical,
Miacalcin)
Calcitriol (Calcijex)
Capecitabine (Xeloda)
Captopril (Captopril)
Carbamazepine (Carbatrol, Equetro,
Tegretol)
Carbidopa (Lodosyn)
Carbidopa/Levodopa (Parcopa,
Sinemet)
Carbidopa/Entacapone/Levodopa
(Stalevo)

Carbinoxamine Maleate/Dextro-
methorphan Hydrobromide/
Pseudoephedrine Hydrochloride
(Balamine)
Carvedilol (Coreg)
Cefdinir (Omnicef)
Cefditoren Pivoxil (Spectracef)
Cefpodoxime Proxetil (Vantin)
Celecoxib (Celebrex)
Cetirizine Hydrochloride (Zyrtec)
Cetirizine Hydrochloride/Pseudo-
ephedrine (Zyrtec-D)
Cevimeline Hydrochloride (Evoxac)
Chlorothiazide Sodium (Diuril)
Chlorpheniramine Maleate
Chlorpromazine (Thorazine)
Chlorthalidone
Ciprofloxacin (Cipro)
Cisapride (Propulsid)
Citalopram Hydrobromide (Celexa)
Clonazepam (Klonopin)
Clonidine (Catapres, Catapres-TTS)
Clorazepate Dipotassium
(Tranxene-SD)
Clozapine (Clozaril, Faxaclo)
Cyclobenzaprine Hydrochloride
(Flexeril)
Cyclosporine (Gengraf, Neoral)
Darifenacin (Enablex)
Delavirdine Mesylate (Rescriptor)
Desloratadine (Clarinex)
Desloratadine/Loratadine/Pseudo-
ephedrine Sulfate (Clarinex-D)
Dexmethylphenidate Hydrochloride
(Focalin)
Dextroamphetamine Sulfate
(Dexedrine, Dextrostat)
Diazoxide (Hyperstat)
Diclofenac Potassium (Cataflam)
Diclofenac Sodium/Misoprostol
(Arthrotec)
Diclofenac Sodium (Voltaren,
Voltaren-XR)
Dicyclomine Hydrochloride (Bentyl)

Dihydroergotamine Mesylate
(Migranal)
Diltiazem Hydrochloride (Cardizem,
Dilacor, Tiazac)
Divalproex Sodium (Depakote)
Donepezil Hydrochloride (Aricept)
Dorzolamide Hydrochloride (Cosopt,
Trusopt)
Doxepin Hydrochloride (Prudoxin)
Doxercalciferol (Hectorol)
Doxorubicin Hydrochloride
Liposome (Doxil)
Duloxetine Hydrochloride
(Cymbalta)
Eletriptan Hydrobromide (Relpax)
Enalapril Maleate/Hydrochlorothia-
zide (Vaseretic)
Enalapril Maleate (Vasotec)
Enalaprilat
Enfuvirtide (Fuzeon)
Enoxacin (Penetrex)
Entacapone (Comtan)
Ephedrine Sulfate/Hydroxyzine
Hydrochloride/Theophylline
(Marax)
Eprosartan Mesylate (Teveten)
Escitalopram Oxalate (Lexapro)
Esmolol Hydrochloride (Brevibloc)
Esomeprazole Magnesium (Nexium)
Estazolam (Prosom)
Eszopiclone (Lunesta)
Etanercept (Enbrel)
Famotidine (Pepcid)
Felodipine (Plendil)
Fenofibrate (Antara, Lofibra, Tricor)
Fenoprofen Calcium (Nalfon)
Fentanyl (Duragesic)
Fentanyl Citrate (Actiq)
Fexofenadine Hydrochloride
(Allegra-D)
Flecainide Acetate (Tambocor)
Fluocinolone Acetonide/Hydroqui-
none/Tretinoin (Tri-Luma)
Fluoxetine Hydrochloride (Prozac)

Table 24: ORAL MANIFESTATIONS OF SYSTEMIC AGENTS *(cont.)*

Xerostomia *(cont.)*

Fluoxetine Hydrochloride/Olanzapine (Symbyax)	Ketoprofen (Orudis)	Metyrosine (Demser)
Flurazepam Hydrochloride (Dalmane)	Ketotifen Fumarate (Zaditor)	Midodrine Hydrochloride (Proamatine)
Fluticasone Propionate/Salmeterol Xinafoate (Advair)	Lamotrigine (Lamictal)	Mirtazapine (Remeron)
	Lansoprazole (Prevacid)	Modafinil (Provigil)
	Leflunomide (Arava)	Moexipril Hydrochloride (Univasc)
Fluvoxamine Maleate (Luvox)	Leuprolide Acetate (Lupron, Viadur)	Molindone Hydrochloride (Moban)
Formoterol Fumarate (Foradil)	Levalbuterol Hydrochloride (Xopenex)	Mometasone Furoate (Elocon)
Foscarnet Sodium (Foscavir)		Moricizine Hydrochloride (Ethmozine)
Fosinopril Sodium (Monopril)	Levofloxacin (Levaquin)	
Frovatriptan Succinate (Frova)	Levomethadyl Acetate Hydrochloride (Orlaam)	Morphine Sulfate (Avinza, Kadian, MSIR, Roxanol)
Furosemide	Levorphanol Tartrate (Levorphanol)	Moxifloxacin Hydrochloride (Avelox)
Gabapentin (Neurontin)	Lisinopril (Prinivil, Zestril)	Mupirocin Calcium (Bactroban)
Galantamine Hydrobromide (Razadyne)	Lithium Carbonate (Eskalith, Lithobid)	Mycophenolate Mofetil (Cellcept)
		Nabumetone (Relafen)
Ganciclovir (Cytovene)	Lomefloxacin Hydrochloride (Maxaquin)	Nadolol (Nadolol)
Gemifloxacin Mesylate (Factive)		Nalbuphine Hydrochloride (Nubain)
Grepafloxacin Hydrochloride (Raxar)	Loperamide Hydrochloride (Imodium)	Naltrexone Hydrochloride (Revia)
Glatiramer Acetate (Copaxone)		Naproxen
Glycopyrrolate (Robinul)	Lopinavir/Ritonavir (Kaletra)	Nedocromil Sodium (Tilade)
Goserelin Acetate (Zoladex)	Loratadine/Pseudoephedrine (Claritin-D)	Niacin (Niaspan)
Guanadrel Sulfate (Hylorel)	Losartan Potassium (Cozaar)	Nicotine (Nicotrol)
Guanidine Hydrochloride (Guanidine)	Lovastatin/Niacin (Advicor)	Nifedipine (Adalat)
	Lovastatin (Altoprev, Mevacor)	Nisoldipine (Sular)
Haloperidol (Haldol)	Loxapine Hydrochloride (Loxitane)	Nizatidine (Axid)
Hydrochlorothiazide	Mecamylamine Hydrochloride (Inversine)	Norfloxacin (Noroxin)
Hydrocodone Bitartrate/Ibuprofen (Vicoprofen)		Octreotide Acetate (Sandostatin)
	Meclizine Hydrochloride (Bonine)	Ofloxacin (Floxin)
Hydromorphone Hydrochloride (Dilaudid, Dilaudid-HP)	Mefenamic Acid (Ponstel)	Olanzapine (Zyprexa)
	Megestrol Acetate (Megace)	Omega-3-Acid Ethyl Esters (Omacor)
Hyoscyamine (Cystospaz, Levbid, Nulev)	Meloxicam (Mobic)	Omeprazole (Prilosec, Zegerid)
	Meperidine Hydrochloride (Mepergan)	Ondansetron (Zofran)
Ibuprofen/Oxycodone Hydrochloride (Combunox)		Orphenadrine Citrate (Norflex)
	Mesalamine (Asacol)	Oxaliplatin (Eloxatin)
Interferon Alfa-2b, Recombinant (Intron)	Metaproterenol Sulfate (Alupent)	Oxcarbazepine (Trileptal)
	Methadone Hydrochloride (Dolophine, Methadone)	Oxybutynin (Oxytrol)
Interferon Alfacon-1 (Infergen)		Oxybutynin Chloride (Ditropan)
Interferon Alfa-N3 (Human Leukocyte Derived) (Alferon)	Methamphetamine Hydrochloride (Desoxyn)	Oxycodone Hydrochloride (Oxycontin)
Interferon Beta-1a (Rebif)	Methyldopate Hydrochloride (Aldomet)	Oxymorphone Hydrochloride (Numorphan)
Ipratropium Bromide (Ipratropium)		
Isosorbide Mononitrate (Imdur, Monoket)	Metoprolol Succinate (Toprol-XL)	Palonosetron Hydrochloride (Aloxi)
	Metronidazole (Metrogel-Vaginal, Noritate)	Pantoprazole Sodium (Protonix)
Isotretinoin (Accutane, Amnesteem)		Paricalcitol (Zemplar)
Isradipine (Dynacirc)		

Xerostomia *(cont.)*

Paroxetine Hydrochloride (Paxil)
Peginterferon Alfa-2a (Pegasys)
Peginterferon Alfa-2b (PEG-Intron)
Pemetrexed (Alimta)
Pergolide Mesylate (Permax)
Perindopril Erbumine (Aceon)
Perphenazine (Trilafon)
Phendimetrazine Tartrate (Bontril)
Phentermine Hydrochloride
  (Adipex-P, Fastin)
Pimozide (Orap)
Pirbuterol Acetate (Maxair)
Pramipexole Dihydrochloride
  (Mirapex)
Pregabalin (Lyrica)
Procarbazine Hydrochloride
  (Matulane)
Prochlorperazine (Compazine,
  Compro)
Progesterone (Crinone, Prochieve,
  Prometrium)
Promethazine Hydrochloride
  (Phenergan)
Propafenone Hydrochloride
  (Rythmol)
Propofol (Diprivan, Propofol)
Protirelin (Thyrel)
Protriptyline Hydrochloride (Vivactil)
Quetiapine Fumarate (Seroquel)
Rabeprazole Sodium (Aciphex)
Ramipril (Altace)
Rescinnamine (Moderil)
Ribavirin (Copegus, Rebetol)
Riluzole (Rilutek)
Rimantadine Hydrochloride
  (Flumadine)
Risedronate Sodium (Actonel)
Risperidone (Risperdal)

Ritonavir (Norvir)
Rivastigmine Tartrate (Exelon)
Rizatriptan Benzoate (Maxalt-MLT)
Ropinirole Hydrochloride (Requip)
Salmeterol Xinafoate (Serevent)
Saquinavir Mesylate (Invirase)
Scopolamine (Transderm)
Selegiline Hydrochloride (Eldepryl)
Sertraline Hydrochloride (Zoloft)
Sevoflurane (Ultane)
Sibutramine Hydrochloride
  Monohydrate (Meridia)
Sildenafil Citrate (Viagra)
Sodium Ferric Gluconate (Ferrlecit)
Solifenacin Succinate (Vesicare)
Sparfloxacin (Zagam)
Sucralfate (Carafate)
Sulindac (Clinoril)
Sumatriptan Succinate (Imitrex)
Tadalafil (Cialis)
Telithromycin (Ketek)
Telmisartan (Micardis)
Terazosin Hydrochloride (Hytrin)
Terbutaline Sulfate (Brethine)
Testosterone
Thalidomide (Thalomid)
Thiabendazole (Mintezol)
Thioridazine Hydrochloride
  (Thioridazine)
Thiothixene (Thiothixene)
Tiagabine Hydrochloride (Gabitril)
Tigecycline (Tygacil)
Timolol Hemihydrate (Betimol)
Timolol Maleate (Timoptic,
  Timoptic-XE)
Tinidazole (Tindamax)
Tiotropium Bromide (Spiriva)
Tocainide Hydrochloride (Tonocard)

Tolcapone (Tasmar)
Tolterodine Tartrate (Detrol)
Topiramate (Topamax)
Trandolapril/Verapamil
  Hydrochloride (Tarka)
Tranylcypromine Sulfate (Parnate)
Triamcinolone Acetonide (Azmacort,
  Nasacort)
Triamterene (Dyrenium)
Trifluoperazine Hydrochloride
  (Stelazine)
Trihexyphenidyl Hydrochloride
  (Artane)
Trimipramine Maleate (Surmontil)
Trospium Chloride (Sanctura)
Valproate Sodium (Depacon)
Valproic Acid (Depakene)
Valsartan (Diovan)
Vardenafil Hydrochloride (Levitra)
Venlafaxine Hydrochloride (Effexor)
Verapamil Hydrochloride (Covera-
  HS, Verelan)
Voriconazole (VFEND)
Zaleplon (Sonata)
Ziprasidone Hydrochloride (Geodon)
Zolmitriptan (Zomig)
Zolpidem Tartrate (Ambien)
Zonisamide (Zonegran)

Chapter 25

Herbs and Dietary Supplements

Adriane Fugh-Berman, M.D.; Maria Salnik, M.S. candidate

Herbs and Dental Health

Many drugs used in dentistry have their origins in the plant world, including lidocaine and novacaine, derived from the coca plant *(Erythroxylum coca)*; opioids, derived from the poppy *(Papaver somniferum)*; and several antibiotics derived from fungi, including penicillin from *Penicillium notatum* and cephalosporins from a marine fungus *(Cephalosporium acremonium)*. Clove oil, which contains eugenol, is the essential oil of *Eugenia caryophyllus*.[1] In fact, the best-selling herbal products in the United States may well be oral hygiene products, which rely heavily on essential oils (or their components), including eucalyptol, derived from eucalyptus *(E. globulus)*; thymol, derived from thyme *(Thymus vulgaris)*; menthol, derived from peppermint *(Mentha piperita)*; and sanguinarine, derived from bloodroot *(Sanguinaria canadensis)*.

Chewing sticks, used in African and Southern Asian communities, are oral hygiene products made from a variety of plants, including neem *(Azadirachta indica)*, salvadora *(S. persica)* and species of *Garcinia* and *Diospyros*.[1] Chewing sponges made from *Hibiscus* species and other plants are popular in Ghana. A study comparing periodontal status of Sudanese miswak and toothbrush users found the two comparable for oral hygiene.[2] One hundred nine men who used miswak sticks prepared from the roots or twigs of *S. persica* were compared with 104 toothbrush users (all had ≥ 18 teeth). Attachment level was measured, and gingival

bleeding, supragingival dental calculus, and probing pocket depth of teeth were scored by the Community Periodontal Index.

Gingival bleeding and dental calculus were common in the study population, especially among those aged > 40 years. Compared to toothbrush users, miswak users had significantly lower numbers of posterior sextants with dental calculus and ≥ 4 mm probing depth. However, miswak use demonstrated no advantage over toothbrush use in the anterior teeth, and probing depth ≥ 4 mm was more common in the anterior teeth of miswak users. The results did not show a significant benefit of miswak use versus toothbrush use in gingival bleeding. Camellia and other plants are rich in fluoride; the chewing stick with the highest fluoride content is from a plant related to persimmon *(Diospyros tricolor)*. *Fagara zanthoxyloides* and *Massularia acuminata* reduce both acid production and bacterial growth. Extracts from *Rhus natalensis* and *Euclea divinorum*, used in Kenya as chewing sticks, inhibited the proteolytic activity of *Bacteroides gingivalis, B. intermedius* and *Treponema denticola*.[3]

A recent study compared the antibacterial properties of aqueous extracts from 17 plants used as chewing sticks in Nigeria and the fruit of *Cnestis ferruginea* used in oral hygiene.[4] *C. ferruginea* fruit and *Terminalia glaucescens* were active against cultures of *Staphylococcus aureus, Bacillus subtilis, Escherichia coli*, and *Pseudomonas aeruginosa*; nine other extracts showed some activity. When tested against clinical isolates from orofacial infections, three extracts (*Bridellia ferruginea, Terminalia glaucescens,* and *Anogeissus leiocarpus*) were active against facultative gram-negative rods (*Escherichia, citrobacter,* and *Enterobacter* species). Ten of eleven extracts tested were active against obligate anaerobes; the most active were *Phyllanthus, muellerianus, Anogeissus leiocarpus,* and *C. ferruginea* fruit.

Commercial toothpastes have been made from neem (*Azadirachta indica*) and arak (*Salvadora persica,* one of several plants called "toothbrush tree"). Powdered plants used in abrasive dentrifices include sweet flag root (*Acorus calamus*), gum-resin of myrrh (*Commiphora myrrha*), yellow dock root (*Rumex crispus*), toothbrush tree (*Gouania lupuloides*) and ashes from the branches of the European grape (*Vitis vinifera*). Essential oils of plants are commonly used in commercial mouthwashes; Listerine, for example, contains thymol, menthol, eucalyptol and methyl salicylate, all derived from botanicals.[1]

The sugar substitute xylitol (birch sugar) is as sweet as sucrose; sorbitol, another sugar alcohol, is less sweet but less expensive and easier to formulate into products. Both stimulate saliva production; xylitol is not fermented by oral microbes, while sorbitol is very slowly fermented. An analysis of published double-blind trials of sorbitol and xylitol (usually in the form of chewing gums administered 3-5 times daily) found that xylitol was superior to sorbitol in two longer, secondary dentition trials but not in two primary dentition trials.[5]

The acidity of herbal teas

Herbal teas are perceived to be healthful, but many are as acidic as orange juice (pH 3.73). An in vitro study found that the pH of one chamomile, apple, and cinnamon herbal tea was 7.08, but the pH of nine other mixed herbal teas ranged from 3.15 to 3.78, significantly lower than traditional black tea (*Camellia sinensis,* pH 5.67).[6] Compared to black tea, all herbal teas tested except for the chamomile/cinnamon tea caused

significantly higher enamel loss in a molar immersion test. It bears noting that all herbal teas in this experiment were mixed herbals, so effects cannot be attributed to specific herbs. Further research should be done on single-herb teas.

Herbs and Oral bacteria

Several herbs have been tested against pathogenic oral bacteria. Licorice (*Glycyrrhiza glabra*) and glycyrrhizin (a component of licorice) both inhibit bacterial adherence. In the presence of sucrose, glycyrrhizin did not affect growth of *Streptococcus mutans* but did reduce plaque formation; inhibition was almost complete at concentrations of 0.5-1% glycyrrhizin or 5-10% licorice.[7]

A high–molecular-weight constituent of cranberry (*Vaccinium macrocarpon*) juice reversed the coaggregation of 58% of 84 coaggregating bacterial pairs tested.[8] This effect was strongest when at least one species was a gram-negative anaerobe; thus, it may alter subgingival microflora. Most cranberry juice, however, contains large amounts of sugar.

An in vitro study found no effect of an infant dentifrice containing calendula (*Calendula officinalis*) nor a dentifrice containing lactoperoxidase, glucose oxidase and lactoferrin against microorganisms in biofilms from saliva or dental plaque; the calendula preparation also had no significant effect on any microorganism evaluated. Compared to controls, only a dentifrice containing sodium fluoride and sodium lauryl sulfate significantly reduced viable microorganisms.[9]

Adverse Effects of Herbs

Bleeding

Several herbs can increase the risk of bleeding, especially when combined with anticoagulants. Both ginkgo (*G. biloba*) and garlic (*Allium sativum*) have been associated with bleeding episodes. Other herbs associated with increased anticoagulant effect when combined with warfarin include the Chinese herbs dong quai *(Angelica sinensis)* and danshen *(Salvia miltiorrhiza)*. It is prudent to discontinue the use of herbs and dietary supplements a week before surgery.[10]

Cancer and Precancerous Conditions

Betel nut *(Areca catechu)*, a masticant with mild stimulatory effects, has been linked to oral and esophageal cancers.[11] Oral squamous cell carcinoma usually occurs in parts of the mouth directly contacted by betel quid (primarily in the midbuccal mucosa and the lateral borders of the tongue). Betel use also causes oral submucous fibrositis, a precancerous condition.[12] The addition of tobacco clearly increases carcinogenic risk.[11] The addition of lime may increase the generation of reactive oxygen species; oral squamous cell cancers were noted to correspond to the site of lime application in 77% of 169 cases in Papua New Guinea.[13]

Although betel traditionally is thought of as beneficial to the teeth and gums, it is difficult to assess its possible benefits because populations that chew betel have a high rate of caries and periodontal disease. Some evidence suggests that chewing betel helps to prevent dental caries, possibly via mechanical cleansing or altering salivary pH. It also is possible that the darkened layer on the teeth forms a barrier to cariogenic agents.[12]

Betel stains the saliva a reddish color and can stain the teeth, gingiva and oral mucosa red or black. Another stimulatory masticant, khat *(Catha edulis)*, also can stain teeth, as well as cause caries, thickened oropharyngeal mucosa and dependence.[14]

Colloidal Silver

Colloidal silver, which has a long history as an antibacterial agent, is marketed as a "natural" antibiotic. Argyria (discoloration caused by silver deposition) often manifests first in the mouth, causing a slate-blue or silver line in the gingiva. Deposits in the skin or mucosa cause a permanent gray-blue discoloration. Although proponents claim that colloidal silver is not associated with argyria, colloidal silver protein does in fact cause argyria.[15,16]

Vitamins and Minerals

Nutrition is important in craniofacial and oral tissue development. Prolonged vitamin A deficiency during tooth development can result in enamel hypoplasia. Deficiencies of vitamin D or phosphorus can cause incomplete calcification of teeth. Deficiency of calcium, vitamin D, magnesium or copper can cause defects in alveolar bone. Iodine deficiency can delay the eruption of both primary and secondary teeth and can cause malocclusion.[17]

Many nutritional deficiencies manifest first in the oral cavity. Glossitis can occur from multiple nutritional deficiencies; vitamin E appears to be particularly important in papillary health. Angular cheilosis can be caused by too little vitamin B_2 (riboflavin), B_3 (niacin), B_6 (pyridoxine), B_{12} (cobalamin), folic acid or iron. Burning mouth syndrome may be the result of deficiency of vitamin B complex, protein or iron.[17]

Vitamin C deficiency causes impaired wound healing, inflamed gingiva and swollen interdental papillae. Inadequate calcium can cause increased tooth mobility and premature loss; too little magnesium or vitamin A can cause gingival hypertrophy. Vitamin A deficiency also increases the risk of candidiasis and can cause desquamation of oral mucosa, leukoplakia and xerostomia. Excessive or inadequate vitamin A intake can impair healing. Zinc deficiency can cause distortions of taste and smell, delayed wound healing, atrophic oral mucosa, xerostomia and increased susceptibility to periodontal disease.[17]

Magnesium deficiency may cause tooth loss, decreased alveolar crestal bone height and other manifestations of low bone mass.

An epidemiologic study of 4290 subjects aged 20-80 in northeastern Germany found that about a third had low serum (<0.75 mmol/L) magnesium levels. Magnesium regulates cell functions; physiologically, it antagonizes calcium so the ratio between the two minerals was assessed. In a subset study, no influence of the Mg/Ca ratio on periodontal status was found in subjects younger than 40 years old. However, in subjects over 40, a statistically significant inverse association was noted between Mg/Ca ratio and level of periodontitis. Additionally, a higher Mg/Ca ratio was associated with more remaining teeth. A matched pairs analysis found that subjects who used magnesium-containing drugs had fewer signs of periodontal disease than matched controls.[18]

A case-control study of 54 female adolescents (aged 17-19 years) found that low intakes of riboflavin, calcium and fiber were correlated with gingivitis risk. Milk was the main dietary source of both calcium and riboflavin.[19]

Clinical Trials of Herbs and Dietary Supplements for Treatment of Dental Conditions

Aphthous Ulcers

Acemannan, a component of *Aloe vera* gel, may be effective for aphthous stomatitis.[20] A double-blind randomized trial of 60 patients with recurrent aphthae compared acemannan hydrogel to an over-the-counter product as an active control. Lesions treated with acemannan hydrogel healed in 5.89 days, while those treated with control healed in 7.8 days.

Caries and Oral Microbial Growth

Propolis

Propolis, or "bee glue," is an adhesive, resinous substance used by honeybees in building and sealing a hive. A double-blind study comparing a propolis-containing mouthwash with a positive control (chlorhexidine) and a negative control found that the chlorhexidine mouthrinse was best; there was no significant difference between the propolis-containing mouthrinse and the negative control.[21] Another study in 10 volunteers tested propolis and honey against oral bacteria; propolis reduced streptococci counts both in vitro and clinically.[22]

Calcium

A calcium-fortified chewing gum ameliorated the cariogenic effects of sucrose more than a conventional gum, as measured by increased pH, calcium and phosphate concentrations in plaque fluid and saliva.[23]

Lactic bacteria

A clinical trial in 245 7-year-olds compared chewable tablets containing vitamin B_6 and heat-killed lactic bacteria (streptococci and lactobacilli) against placebo (vitamin B_6 only) to prevent caries.[24] Treatments were given once weekly for 16 weeks. Permanent teeth were evaluated four times during 24 months of follow-up using the Decayed, Missing and Filled Surfaces (DMFS) Index. The incidence of dental caries in the lactic bacteria group was reduced at all time points; compared to controls, the experimental group had a 42% reduction in incidence of caries at the end of the study.

Labial Herpes

A study in 16 adults with recurrent herpes (eight genital, eight labial; viral type unspecified) compared the effects of topical honey with 5% acyclovir on duration of outbreaks, pain and healing time.[25] For labial herpes outbreaks, topical honey was more effective than acyclovir for all parameters measured, including mean duration of attacks (35%), mean duration of pain (39%), occurrence of crusting (28%), and mean healing time (43%). Results were similar for genital herpes. No side effects associated with the application of honey were reported; three patients reported itching with acyclovir.

Oral Candidiasis

Uncontrolled trials have claimed a benefit for oral solutions of tea tree (*Melaleuca alternifolia*)[26] or cinnamon (*Cinnamomum* species) oral solution to treat oral candidiasis in patients with HIV[27]; however, no controlled trials were identified.

Oral Leukoplakia

A placebo-controlled trial of 87 tobacco chewers with oral leukoplakia tested 1 gram daily of a blue-green alga, *Spirulina fusiformis*, against placebo for 12 months.[28] Complete regression of lesions was noted in 20 of 44 (45%) subjects in the *Spirulina*-treated group, vs. 3 of 43 (7%) subjects in the placebo group. No effect was seen in those with ulcerated or nodular lesions. Within 1 year of discontinuing use of *Spirulina fusiformis*, 9 of 20 subjects experienced complete regression of lesions. No toxicity was noted. These results could be explained by the high vitamin A content of *Spirulina*, but, interestingly, no increase in serum concentrations of retinol or β-carotene were seen.

Oral Mucositis

Honey

A randomized controlled trial compared the incidence and severity of mucositis in 40 patients undergoing radiation for head and neck cancer. Twenty patients were instructed to swish and swallow 20 mL of raw honey from tea flowers (*Camellia sinensis*) before, after, and 6 hours following radiotherapy, while the remaining patients received no such instructions. There was no difference between groups in overall incidence of mucositis, but the incidence of grade 3 or 4 mucositis was significantly lower in the experimental group. While treatment was interrupted because of mucositis in four

controls, no interruptions occurred in the honey-treated group.[29]

Chamomile

A randomized, double-blind, placebo-controlled trial of chamomile mouthwash in 164 patients entering their first cycle of 5-fluorouracil (5FU)-based chemotherapy tested chamomile mouthwash three times daily for 2 weeks against placebo. All patients also received oral cryotherapy.[30] Physicians and patients each scored stomatitis severity on a scale from 1 to 4. Daily mean mucositis scores were similar between the chamomile group and the placebo group. No toxicity was noted.

Vitamin E

A randomized double-blind study of 18 patients receiving chemotherapy tested vitamin E against placebo oil for treatment of oral mucositis. After 5 days of topical application (1 mL of 400 mg/mL vitamin E oil twice daily), six of nine patients had complete resolution of lesions; only one of nine subjects in the placebo group had complete resolution.[31]

A substudy of 409 male cigarette smokers in a study of vitamin E and β-carotene found gingival bleeding on probing to be more common in those with a high prevalence of dental plaque assigned to α-tocopherol (50 mg daily), especially when combined with aspirin (aspirin alone did not increase bleeding significantly).[32]

However, a study specifically designed to address the risk of bleeding with vitamin E supplementation found no effect of all-rac-α-tocopherol (60, 200 or 800 IU for 4 months) on bleeding time in 88 healthy subjects > 65 years old.[33]

Periodontal Disease

Herbal mixtures

An herbal extract containing a mixture of equal parts juniper (*Juniperus communis*), nettle *(Urtica dioca)* and yarrow *(Achillea mille-folium)* was tested in 45 subjects with moderate gingival inflammation, randomized to treatment or control in a 2:1 ratio.[34] All were asked to rinse with 10 mL of mouthwash twice a day for 3 months. Plaque index, modified gingival index and angulated bleeding index were assessed at baseline, at 6 weeks and at 3 months. There was no difference between the treated group and the control group. Another recent study found no benefit of an herbal rinse over a placebo rinse on the gingival health in 63 participants over 3 months.[35]

A randomized, double-blind, placebo-controlled clinical trial compared a toothpaste containing *P. vulgaris* (0.5%) and *M. conrata* (0.005%) extracts to a placebo toothpaste for gingivitis in 40 subjects. Compared to placebo, the treated group showed a statistically significant improvement in inflammation, assessed by the Papillary Bleeding Index and the Community Periodontal Index of Treatment Needs. There was no difference between groups in plaque reduction, measured by the Plaque Index.[36]

Folate
A randomized, double-blind, placebo-controlled study tested folate mouthwash against established gingivitis in 60 subjects who had > 20 teeth and visible gingival inflammation around >6 teeth.[37] Subjects rinsed with 5 mL of placebo or folate-containing mouthwash (5 mg folate/5 mL) for 1 minute twice daily for 4 weeks. Oral examination was done at baseline and at 4 weeks. Compared with the control group, the treated group showed a significant decrease in mean number of color change sites (from 70.17 ± 12.89 to 56.62 ± 17.42) and in bleeding sites (from 48.59 ± 24.28 to 29.28 ± 19.64).

Topical vitamin E
A double-blind trial compared the effect of a topical vitamin E gel (5%), a placebo gel and a chlorhexidine rinse on established and developing plaque and periodontal disease in 48 adults.[38] The first two groups applied either 12 mL of placebo or vitamin E gel (containing 800 mg α-tocopherol) daily; the chlorhexidine group rinsed with 0.5 oz of 0.12% chlorhexidine gluconate. Plaque index, gingival index and periodontal probing depth were assessed at baseline and at 2 weeks; root planing and scaling was done at 2 weeks, with additional data collection at 4 and 6 weeks. Only chlorhexidine significantly reduced plaque; vitamin E had no significant effects on plaque or gingivitis, compared with placebo.

Coenzyme Q10
A review of coenzyme Q10 (involved in electron transport in mitochondria) to treat periodontal disease identified two controlled trials, neither published in the periodontal literature, and found that both trials were methodologically deficient.[39]

Gingival enlargement
Two controlled trials assessed the effect of folic acid (3 mg for 4 months and 5 mg for 1 year) on phenytoin-induced gingival enlargement.[40,41] Neither found an effect. A third small study of eight institutionalized disabled residents tested 5 mg folic acid for 6 months in an effort to reduce recurrence of phenytoin-induced gingival enlargement after gingivectomy. The treatment group had significantly less recurrence of gingival enlargement, but the mean difference was only 7% at 6 months.[42]

Xerostomia
Yohimbine, an α_2 antagonist used to treat impotence, has been tested for its effect on salivary secretion in 11 healthy volunteers and in volunteers treated with tricyclic anti-depressants.[43] A regimen of yohimbine (4 mg three times daily for 3 weeks) did not affect resting salivary secretion levels (tested at baseline and weekly thereafter) in either group; acute administration, however,

significantly increased salivary volume within 1 hour in both groups.

Conclusion

Herbs and dietary supplements are used commonly by the general public and may have both beneficial and adverse effects relevant to dentistry. (Table 25 shows adverse effects—those described previously as well as others[10,17,44-46]—of herbs and dietary supplements.) Nutritional deficiencies can manifest first in the mouth; stained gingiva can indicate the use of betel, khat or silver; garlic, ginkgo, danshen and other herbs can increase bleeding after an invasive procedure. Therefore, it is worthwhile to include questions about the use of herbs and dietary supplements in the patient's health history, and to be aware of possible adverse effects or interactions. Several herbs may hold promise in dental treatment and should be researched further.

Editor's note: Because herbs and dietary supplements are not regulated as drugs by the U.S. Food and Drug Administration, claims regarding their therapeutic benefit should not be accepted without support from extensive, well-controlled studies published in peer-reviewed journals. Only a limited number of controlled clinical trials have been conducted with these agents; more are needed. However, in light of these agents' potential adverse effects as discussed here, the practitioner is encouraged to include information about use of these agents in each patient's health history.

1. Lewis WH, Elvin-Lewis PF. Medical botany: plants affecting man's health. New York: John Wiley and Sons; 2003:379-459.
2. Darout IA, Albandar JM, Skaug N. Periodontal status of adult Sudanese habitual users of miswak chewing sticks or toothbrushes. Acta Odontol Scand 2000;58(1):25-30.
3. Homer KA, Manji F, Beighton D. Inhibition of protease activities of periodontopathic bacteria by extracts of plants used in Kenya as chewing sticks (mswaki). Arch Oral Biol 1990;35:421-4.
4. Biswal BM, Zakaria A, Ahmad NM. Topical application of honey in the management of radiation mucositis: a preliminary study. Support Care Cancer 2003;11(4):242-8.
5. Gales MA, Nguyen T-M. Sorbitol compared with xylitol in prevention of dental caries. Ann Pharmacother 2000;34:98-100.
6. Phelan J, Rees J. The erosive potential of some herbal teas. J Dent 2003;31(4):241-6.
7. Segal R, Pisanti S, Wormser R, et al. Anticariogenic activity of licorice and glycyrrhizin inhibition of in vitro plaque formation by Streptococcus mutans. J Pharm Sci 1985;74(1):79-81.
8. Weiss EI, Lev-Dor R, Kashamn Y, et al. Inhibiting interspecies coaggregation of plaque bacteria with a cranberry juice constituent. JADA 1998;129:1719-23.
9. Modesto A, Lima KC, de Uzeda M. Effects of three different infant dentifrices on biofilms and oral microorganisms. J Clin Pediatr Dent 2000;24(3):237-43.
10. Fugh-Berman A, Ernst E. Herb-drug interactions: review and assessment of report reliability. Br J Clin Pharm 2001;52:587-95.
11. Morton JF. Widespread tannin intake via stimulants and masticatories, especially guarana, kola nut, betel vine, and accessories. In: Hemingway RW, Laks PE, eds. Plant polyphenols. New York: Plenum Press; 1992:739-65.
12. Norton SA. Betel: consumption and consequences. J Am Acad Dermatol 1998;38(1):81-8.
13. Thomas SJ, MacLenna R. Slaked lime and betel nut cancer in Papua New Guinea. Lancet 1992;340:577-8.
14. D'Arcy PF. Adverse reactions and interactions with herbal medicines. Adverse Drug React Toxicol Rev 1991;10:189-208.
15. Kim CS. Argyria secondary to chronic ingestion of colloidal silver (abstract 121). Clin Tox 2000;38(5):552.
16. Gulbranson SH, Hud JA, Hansen RC. Argyria following the use of dietary supplements containing colloidal silver protein. Cutis 2000;66:373-4.
17. Depaola DP, Faine MP, Palmer CA. Nutrition in relation to dental medicine. In: Shils ME, Olson JA, Shike M, Ross AC, eds. Modern nutrition in health and disease. 9th ed. Baltimore: Williams & Wilkins; 1999:1099-1124.
18. Meisel P, Schwahn C, Luedemann J, et al. Magnesium deficiency is associated with periodontal disease. J Dent Res 2005;84(10):937-41.
19. Petti S, Cairella G, Tarsitani G. Nutritional variables related to gingival health in adolescent girls. Community Dent Oral Epidemiol 2000;28(6):407-13.
20. Plemons JM, Rees TD, Binnie WH, et al. Evaluation of acemannan in the treatment of recurrent aphthous stomatitis. Wounds 1994;6(2):40-5.
21. Murray MC, Worthington HV, Blinkhorn AS. A study to investigate the effect of a propolis-containing mouthrinse on the inhibition of de novo plaque formation. J Clin Periodontol 1997;24:796-8.
22. Steinberg D, Kaine G, Gedalia I. Antibacterial effect of propolis and honey on oral bacteria. Am J Dent 1996;9(6):236-9.
23. Vogel GL, Zhang Z, Carey CM, et al. Composition of plaque and saliva following a sucrose challenge and use of an α-tricalcium-phosphate-containing chewing gum. J Dent Res 1998;77(3):518-24.
24. Bayona-Gonzalez A, Lopez-Camara V, Gomez-Castellanos A. Final results of a dental caries clinical trial using heat killed lactic acid bacteria (streptococci and lactobacilli) orally. Pract Odontol 1990;11(6):41-7.
25. Al-Waili NS. Topical honey application vs. acyclovir for the treatment of recurrent herpes simplex lesions. Med Sci Monit 2004;10(8):MT94-8.)

26. Jandourek A, Vaishapayan JK, Vazquez JA. Efficacy of melaleuca oral solution for the treatment of fluconazole refractory oral candidiasis in AIDS patients. AIDS 1998;12:1033-7.

27. Quale JM, Landman D, Zaman MM, et al. In vitro activity of *Cinnamomum zeylanicum* against azole resistant and sensitive *Candida* species and a pilot study of cinnamon for oral candidiasis. Am J Chin Med 1996;24(2):103-9.

28. Mathew B, Sankaranarayanan R, Nair PP, et al. Evaluation of chemoprevention of oral cancer with *Spirulina fusiformis*. Nutr Cancer 1995;24(2):197-202.

29. Biswal BM, Zakaria A, Ahmad NM. Topical application of honey in the management of radiation mucositis: a preliminary study. Support Care Cancer 2003;11(4):242-8.

30. Fidler P, Loprinzi CL, O'Fallon JR, et al. Prospective evaluation of a chamomile mouthwash for prevention of 5-FU-induced oral mucositis. Cancer 1996;77:522-5.

31. Wadleigh RG, Redman RS, Graham ML, et al. Vitamin E in the treatment of chemotherapy-induced mucositis. Am J Med 1992;92:481-4.

32. Liede KE, Haukka JK, Saxen LM, et al. Increased tendency towards gingival bleeding caused by joint effect of α-tocopherol supplementation and acetylsalicylic acid. Ann Med 1998;30:542-6.

33. Meydani SN, Meydani M, Blumberg JB, et al. Assessment of the safety of supplementation with different amounts of vitamin E in healthy older adults. Am J Clin Nutr 1998;68:311-8.

34. Van der Weijden GA, Timmer CJ, Timmerman MF, et al. The effect of herbal extracts in an experimental mouthrinse on established plaque and gingivitis. J Clin Periodontol 1998;25:399-403.

35. Southern EN, McCombs GB, Tolle SL, et al. The comparative effects of 0.12% chlorhexidine and herbal oral rinse on dental plaque-induced gingivitis. J Dent Hyg 2006;80(1):12.

36. Adámková H, Vicar J, Palasová J, et al. *Macleya cordata* and *Prunella vulgaris* in oral hygiene products – their efficacy in the control of gingivitis. Biomed Pap Med Fac Univ Palacky Olomouc Czech Repub 2004;148(1):103-5.

37. Pack AR. Folate mouthwash: effects on established gingivitis in periodontal patients. J Clin Periodontol 1984;11:619-28.

38. Cohen RE, Ciancio SG, Mather ML, et al. Effect of vitamin E gel, placebo gel and chlorhexidine on periodontal disease. Clin Prev Dent 1991;13(5):20-4.

39. Watts TLP. Coenzyme Q10 and periodontal treatment: is there any beneficial effect? Br Dent J 1995;178:209-13.

40. Brown RS, Di Stanislao PT, Beaver WT, et al. The administration of folic acid to institutionalized epileptic adults with phenytoin-induced gingival hyperplasia. A double-blind, randomized, placebo-controlled, parallel study. Oral Surg Oral Med Oral Pathol 1991;71:565-8.

41. Backman N, Holm AK, Hanstrom L, et al. Folate treatment of diphenylhydantoin-induced gingival hyperplasia. Scand J Dent Res 1989;97:222-32.

42. Poppell TD, Keeling SD, Collins JF, et al. Effect of folic acid on recurrence of phenytoin-induced gingival overgrowth following gingivectomy. J Clin Periodontol 1991;18(2):134-9.

43. Bagheri H, Schmitt L, Berlan M, et al. Effect of 3 weeks' treatment with yohimbine on salivary secretion in healthy volunteers and in depressed patients treated with tricyclic antidepressants. Br J Clin Pharmacol 1992;34:555-8.

44. Ernst E. Harmless herbs? A review of the recent literature. Am J Med 1998;104:170-8.

45. Garty BZ. Garlic burns. Pediatrics 1993;91(3):658-9.

46. D'Arcy PF. Adverse reactions and interactions with herbal medicines. Adverse Drug React Toxicol Rev 1991;10:189-208.

Table 25: USAGE INFORMATION FOR HERBS AND DIETARY SUPPLEMENTS

COMMON USE(S)	ADVERSE EFFECTS/INTERACTIONS
Aloe *(A. vera)*	
Burns, skin/mucosal irritation	Diarrhea from anthraquinones in leaf (not gel)[44]
Betel nut *(Areca catechu)*	
Masticatory stimulant	Oral leukoplakia; oral cancer; stained teeth and gingiva; bronchoconstriction; can interact with the antipsychotics flupenthixol and fluphenazine, causing bradykinesia, jaw tremor, rigidity[45]
Chaparral *(Larrea tridentata)*	
Cancer	Hepatotoxicity[45]
Coltsfoot *(Tussilago farfara)*	
Cough	Hepatotoxicity[10]
Comfrey *(Symphytum officinale)*	
Ulcers, wound healing	Hepatotoxicity[10]
Danshen *(Salvia miltiorrhiza)*	
Cardiovascular disease	Potentiates warfarin[10]
Dong quai *(Angelica sinensis)*	
Gynecologic conditions	Potentiates warfarin[40]
Ephedra *(E. sinica)*	
Respiratory conditions, weight loss	Hypertension, cardiac dysrhythmias, anxiety; can potentiate sympathomimetic drugs[10]
Feverfew *(Tanacetum parthenium)*	
Migraine	Aphthous ulcers[10]
Garlic *(Allium sativum)*	
Cardiovascular health	Anticoagulant effects[44]; topical garlic may cause a chemical burn[46]
Germander *(Teucrium chamaedrys)*	
Weight control	Hepatotoxicity[45]
Ginkgo *(G. biloba)*	
Memory, circulatory problems	Anticoagulant effects[44]
Khat *(Catha edulis)*	
Masticatory stimulant	Caries, stained teeth, thickened oropharyngeal mucosa, psychosis, dependence[46]

Table 25: USAGE INFORMATION FOR HERBS AND DIETARY SUPPLEMENTS *(cont.)*

COMMON USE(S)	ADVERSE EFFECTS/INTERACTIONS
Licorice *(Glycyrrhiza glabra)*	
Oral or gastrointestinal ulcers, inflammation	Hypokalemia, hypertension, edema; may potentiate glucocorticoids[10] *Note*: Deglycyrrhizinated licorice (DGL) preparations will not cause these effects.
St. John's wort *(Hypericum perforatum)*	
Depression	Phototoxic reactions; decreases levels of many drugs; increases serotonergic effects when combined with sertraline, trazodone or nefazodone[44]
Silver	
Antibiotic	Argyria (slate-blue or silver line in the gingiva)[16]
Vitamin A	
Acne	Excessive vitamin A can cause hepatotoxicity and delay wound healing; in early pregnancy, excess can cause severe craniofacial and oral clefts and other birth defects[17]
Vitamin D	
Osteoporosis	Excessive vitamin D can cause pulp calcification and enamel hypoplasia[17]

Chapter 26

Legal Implications of Using Drugs in Dental Practice

ADA Division of Legal Affairs

Dentists often fear that they need a law license to practice their profession successfully in today's climate of excessive federal regulation and burgeoning litigation. This fear is sometimes manifested when doctors face difficult choices about the types of drugs they prescribe in their practices.

Two types of approval processes can assist dentists in making difficult choices: the federal Food, Drug, and Cosmetic Act approval process, and the American Dental Association's Seal of Acceptance Program. Overall, a dentist who prescribes a drug approved by the U.S. Food and Drug Administration in a manner that is consistent with the label approved by the FDA—according to the approved directions for dosage, indications for usage and so forth—can feel relatively confident that the drug is safe and effective for its approved uses. Similarly, products that bear the ADA's Seal have been found by the ADA Council on Scientific Affairs to meet ADA guidelines for safety and effectiveness. An FDA-approved, ADA-accepted drug is a wise choice.

However, the wise choice may not always be the reasonable choice. In court, a doctor will be judged according to the applicable standard of care. Generally, doctors are judged according to a reasonableness standard; in a malpractice action, courts look to see how a reasonably prudent doctor would have acted in the same or similar circumstances. This means the doctor must be able to show at all times that his or her decision about which drug to prescribe was reasonable.

For example, it may be unreasonable to prescribe a drug approved for pain relief to a patient who has no pain. Although the safety and efficacy of the drug may be well established by the FDA, prescribing the drug for a pain-free patient could be inappropriate and might well constitute a breach of the standard of care.

Conversely, there may be instances in which it is reasonable for a doctor to prescribe an approved drug for a nonapproved use or even to prescribe a non–FDA-approved drug. In this situation, in the absence of state regulations that might prohibit the use of a non–FDA-approved drug, the doctor's actions will be judged primarily by the same standard of reasonableness that would be used in a typical dental or medical malpractice action. However, the analysis is trickier, because some jurisdictions have found that use of nonapproved drugs or use of approved drugs in nonapproved ways is prima facie negligence—in other words, negligence on the face of it. Such a finding does not end the inquiry, but it does place the burden on the doctor to justify the scientific basis for his or her decision, to show that a reasonably prudent doctor acting in the same or similar circumstances would have made the same decision. In some situations, it may be appropriate to obtain specific informed consent for the use prescribed.

Overall, the law defers to the doctor's need and ability to exercise independent professional judgment in the prescription of all drugs but holds doctors accountable for the results of negligent decisions. This chapter will discuss the legal ramifications of various decisions that are made in the context of making difficult prescription choices.

Use of FDA-Approved Drugs for Unapproved Uses

Generally, the FDA does not regulate dentists and physicians.[2] Thus, if an approved drug is shipped in interstate commerce with an approved package insert, and neither the shipper nor the recipient intends that it be used for an unapproved purpose, all requirements of the Food, Drug, and Cosmetic Act (the Act) are satisfied. Once the drug is in a local pharmacy, a dentist or physician may lawfully prescribe a different dosage for his or her patient, or may otherwise vary the conditions of use from those approved in the package insert, without informing or obtaining the approval of the FDA.[2,3]

The FDA has itself explained that Congress did not intend the FDA to interfere with medical practice or to regulate the practice of medicine between the doctor and the patient. Congress recognized that patients have the right to seek civil damages in the courts if there should be evidence of malpractice and declined to place any legislative restrictions on the medical profession.[4,5] (The FDA stated in an issue of FDA Drug Bulletin, "Accepted medical practice often includes drug use that is not reflected in approved drug labeling."[4] And in Chaney vs. Heckler, the court stated, "Congress would have created havoc in the medical profession had it required physicians to follow the expensive and time-consuming procedure of obtaining FDA approval before putting drugs to new uses."[5]) These pronouncements also should apply to

the practice of dentistry, although the FDA has not made any specific statements to that effect.

In 1997, Congress adopted sweeping reforms of the Food Drug and Cosmetic Act via the Food and Drug Administration Modernization Act (FDAMA).[6] The FDAMA was approved in part because Congress recognized that the "prompt approval of safe and effective new drugs and other therapies is critical to the improvement of the public health so that patients may enjoy the benefits provided by these therapies to treat and prevent illness and disease."[7]

Nothing in the FDAMA changes the FDA's fundamental position on noninterference in the doctor-patient relationship. However, the Act does make it easier for drug manufacturers to at least discuss, if not promote, off-label or unapproved uses for their drug products by abolishing the previous prohibition on dissemination of information about unapproved uses of drugs and medical devices. It allows, among other things, a manufacturer to disseminate certain written information (primarily a reprint or copy of a peer-reviewed article) concerning the safety, effectiveness or benefit of a use not described in the approved labeling of a drug or device if the manufacturer meets the specific requirements set forth in the Act.[8] The manufacturer must include with the information to be disseminated a prominently displayed statement disclosing that the information concerns a use of a drug or device that has not been approved or cleared by the Food and Drug Administration.

The FDA's policy on dissemination of information on off-label uses was the subject of long-standing litigation initiated by the Washington Legal Foundation. In July 1999, the U.S. District Court of the District of Columbia ruled that the FDAMA was unconstitutional to the extent that it impermissibly restrained a manufacturer's First Amendment right to disseminate truthful and non-misleading information about its product.[9] The FDA appealed to the U.S. Court of Appeals for the District of Columbia. In February 2000, the appeals court dismissed the FDA's appeal after FDA attorneys assured the court during oral argument that the agency did not interpret the FDAMA to give the agency new powers to prohibit or sanction constitutionally protected speech. In dismissing the appeal, the court vacated a district court injunction against FDA enforcement of the act. However, the appellate court did not disturb the district court's opinion about the limits the First Amendment places on the FDA's ability to regulate manufacturers' communications about off-label uses of drugs and devices.[10]

Determining Liability in Malpractice Cases

Although FDA does not regulate the prescription by doctors of FDA-approved drugs, doctors are subject to civil liability for their actions. Thus, while it is not uncommon for doctors to prescribe approved drugs for unapproved purposes, in doing so they take upon themselves the burden of justifying their actions and assume potential liability if a mistake is made. In a typical dental or medical malpractice case, the plaintiff must prove these elements[11]:

- the existence of a duty, created by a doctor-patient relationship between the plaintiff and defendant;
- evidence of the standard of care owed by the defendant doctor to the plaintiff;
- evidence that the standard of care was violated or breached;
- proof that the breach of the standard of care was the proximate cause of the plaintiff's injury.

Generally, the standard of care in a malpractice case is determined under state law and must be established through the use of expert testimony. The rationale for the rule requiring expert testimony is that laypeople (in other words, jurors) cannot comprehend technical information without expert assistance.[12-14]

Courts have relied heavily on FDA-approved uses for approved drugs as evidence of the standard of care. In a malpractice action involving administration of a drug, some courts have gone so far as to hold that a drug manufacturer's clear and explicit instructions regarding the proper manner of administering a drug, accompanied by specific warnings of the hazards encountered in its improper administrations, are prima facie evidence of the standard of care. Under these decisions, no expert testimony is needed for the plaintiff to show the standard of care.

For example, in Haught vs. Maceluch,[15] the *Physicians' Desk Reference®* (PDR), which publishes drug manufacturers' instructions and package inserts, was cited as independent evidence of the medical standard for the administration of the drug oxytocin (Pitocin). This drug induces or augments labor. In the Haught case, the plaintiff claimed the defendant physician was negligent for failing to recognize well-established signs of fetal distress and to take appropriate action, and that the defendant negligently administered Pitocin. At trial, the court accepted evidence directly from the PDR that specifically contraindicated the use of Pitocin when fetal distress is suspected. The court held that the PDR established the standard because the physician ignored two important indicators of fetal distress.

In another case, a physician was found to have ignored the manufacturer's instructions for the intravenous injection of promazine hydrochloride (Sparine), as well as the warnings about complications that would arise from its improper administration.[16] The court relied directly on the FDA-approved manufacturer's instructions as evidence of the standard of care. The court held that where a drug manufacturer recommends to the medical profession the conditions under which its drug should be prescribed, the disorders it is designed to relieve, and the precautionary measures that should be observed and warns of the dangers inherent in its use, a doctor's deviation from such recommendations is prima facie evidence of negligence.[16,17] This evidence creates a rebuttable presumption that the doctor acted negligently and requires the doctor to come forward at trial with evidence as to why he or she was not negligent in deviating from the instructions.

Is it sufficient to follow manufacturer's instructions?

These cases represent an extreme view.[18] Other cases, even from the same jurisdictions as the cases discussed above, have been careful to require that the manufacturer's instructions be absolutely clear and explicit before the courts will presume negligence. In Young vs. Cerniak,[19] for example, the defendant physicians were accused of deviating from the standard of care in failing to administer a proper dosage of the anticoagulant heparin. The plaintiff had an expert witness who relied at trial not on the manufacturer's instructions about the appropriate dosage, but on texts and treatises of experts in the field. The manufacturer's instructions were not, in the appellate court's opinion, explicit about the proper dosage and method of administration of the drug, and did not contain warnings about undesirable results if the physician deviated from the precise instructions. Moreover, the defendant physicians' experts testified that the manufacturer's recommendations contained one acceptable procedure for determining dosage, but the defendants followed an equally acceptable alternative method. The appellate court held that the manufacturer's instructions were not evidence of the standard of care, and the trial court had erred by telling the jury that the drug company's recommendations were a standard against which defendant's conduct was to be measured.

Similarly, in Nicolla vs. Fasulo,[20] an oral surgeon was sued for injuries allegedly resulting from his prescribing the drug oxycodone and acetaminophen (Percodan). The plaintiff asked the court to instruct the jury that the defendant would be prima facie negligent if the defendant deviated from the manufacturer's recommendations contained in the PDR. The appellate court held that the trial judge acted appropriately by refusing the request, because there was no clear and explicit contraindication or warning about Percodan in the PDR from which the defendant deviated.[21]

In any case, even in those jurisdictions that do not treat departure from PDR recommendations as prima facie evidence of malpractice, manufacturer recommendations will undoubtedly still be cited as some evidence of the standard of care.

Product inserts and expert testimony

An even more common approach is to allow product inserts and their parallel PDR references into evidence to show the standard of care, but only if expert testimony is also presented to explain the standard to the jury. This rule was followed in the case of Morlino vs. Medical Center of Ocean County.[22,23] In Morlino, a physician prescribed the antibiotic ciprofloxacin hydrochloride to the plaintiff, who was 8 months pregnant and suffering from acute pharyngitis. Earlier treatment with another antibiotic had been ineffective. The plaintiff's fetus died 1 day after she ingested the drug. Experts for the plaintiff testified that a reasonable and prudent physician would not have used ciprofloxacin in a pregnant patient and pointed to the explicit warning in the PDR against such use. The defendant physician acknowledged that he was familiar with the PDR warning but produced an expert who testified that the suspected infectious agent (*Haemophilus influenzae*) was much more risky to the mother and the developing fetus than ciprofloxacin. The defendant argued that it was reasonable for him to prescribe ciprofloxacin in these circumstances.

The jury rendered a verdict for the defendant, and the plaintiff appealed. On appeal, the plaintiff argued that the jury should have been allowed to find that the physician was prima facie negligent for deviating from the PDR warning, without reference to conflicting expert testimony. The appellate court disagreed. It reasoned that to have allowed the jury to find that failure to follow the PDR warning alone was negligence would force a physician to follow the PDR directives or automatically suffer the consequences of a malpractice action. The court pointed out the differences between a package insert and accepted medical practice. The former is based on the rigorous proof a regulatory agency demands, the latter on the clinical judgment of a doctor based on the doctor's training, experience and skill and the specific needs of the individual patient. The court (quoting Peter H. Rheinstein, Drug Labeling as Standard for Medical Care, 4 J. Legal Med. 22, 24 [1976]) held that one cannot be taken as a standard for the other.[22]

The cases discussed above deal with the use of FDA-approved drugs for unapproved purposes, or the simple use of drugs in a manner inconsistent with the manufacturer's instructions. There appear to be no reported cases discussing the legal effect of a dentist's use of an ADA-accepted drug. It is logical to assume, however, that if the dentist used the drug in the manner recommended by the manufacturer, the dentist would certainly try to introduce testimony about the product's acceptance by the ADA as evidence of the reasonableness of the dentist's action. When the ADA accepts a dental product, all of the packaging claims made by the manufacturer about the product are also reviewed and approved. In fact, attorneys representing dentists frequently contact the ADA to find out whether a product used by a dentist bears the ADA Seal.

In summary, dentists and physicians may prescribe and use FDA-approved drugs in ways that differ from the uses approved by the FDA. Doctors should always base these decisions on sound professional judgment and should recognize that the decisions may need to be justified if the doctor is accused of malpractice.

Failure to Obtain Adequate Informed Consent

A related issue that needs to be considered is whether a doctor must obtain a special informed consent from a patient if the doctor prescribes an FDA-approved drug for a nonapproved purpose. A doctor's failure to obtain adequate informed consent can form a basis of liability to a patient that is separate and distinct from a negligence claim.

Traditionally, the standard of disclosure has been based on the customary practice of the community. Thus, courts look at what risks of treatment a reasonably prudent doctor would disclose in similar circumstances.[24,25] A more contemporary approach focuses on a lay standard of disclosure. While the details of this patient-centered approach vary by jurisdiction, courts generally look at what information a reasonable patient would consider material to the decision about whether or not to undergo treatment or diagnosis.[26-30]

The case of Reinhardt vs. Colton[31] is informative on the issue of informed consent in the context of using FDA-approved drugs for unapproved uses. In this case, the plaintiff's physician prescribed the drug penicillamine for the treatment of rheumatoid arthritis. At the time the drug was prescribed for her, it was used by other doctors to treat rheumatoid arthritis, but it was not approved by the FDA for this purpose. Penicillamine has the potential to cause many side effects, including destruction of the capacity to make red blood cells, which causes aplastic anemia. The plaintiff developed aplastic anemia after using penicillamine and brought suit against her physician.

One of the theories on which she based her lawsuit was a theory of "negligent non-disclosure of risk." Under this theory (a contemporary version of lack of informed consent), the plaintiff was required to prove that the physician had a duty to know of a risk or alternative treatment plan, that the physician had a duty to disclose the risk or alternative, that the duty was breached and that the plaintiff was harmed because of the nondisclosure of the risk. The standard used to judge the duty to disclose was based on the significance that a reasonable person in the plaintiff's position would have attached to the risk or the alternative in deciding whether to consent to treatment.

At trial, there was conflicting testimony about whether the plaintiff was informed that the use of penicillamine for rheumatoid arthritis was not approved by the FDA. However, the important testimony was the doctor's own statement about the risks of aplastic anemia associated with using the drug, the wide recognition of this risk in the medical community and other testimony about whether the patient had been sufficiently warned about this risk. The court held that this testimony was sufficient to create an issue that had to be decided by the jury.

In addition to informed consent for using drugs for unapproved purposes, there has recently been a flurry of litigation involving the use of unapproved medical devices. In the case of Blazoski vs. Cook, 787 A.2d 910 (N.J. Super. A.D., 2002), the appeals court of New Jersey held that an orthopedic surgeon who performed spinal-fusion surgery on a patient need not disclose to the patient prior to surgery that the pedicle screws were not approved by the Food and Drug Administration (FDA) for use on lumbar spine. The Blazoski case was representative of a majority view that the FDA status of a medical device is not a material fact that must be disclosed

to a patient to get informed consent. See Southard vs. Temple University Hospital, 781 A.2d 101, 107 (Pa. 2001). However, this case is not binding precedent throughout the United States.

These cases show that standard principles of informed consent, just like standard principles of negligence, govern the doctor's treatment decisions. It may not be necessary always to disclose whether a particular drug or device has been approved by the FDA. The overall analysis will focus on the total circumstances, as well as on whether the doctor acted within the applicable standard of care and informed the patient of risks and alternatives in a manner consistent with the standard applicable in the doctor's jurisdiction.

Use of Drugs Not Approved by the FDA

As discussed in the previous section, the FDA does not generally have jurisdiction over the practice of dentistry or medicine. Therefore, the FDA cannot, as a general rule, take action against a dentist or physician who prescribes drugs that do not have FDA approval.

Pharmacy as Manufacturer

An exception to this general principle arises if a dentist or physician places bulk orders from a pharmacy for unapproved prescription drugs. In this situation, the doctor may not be exempt from regulation by the FDA. For example, the FDA has stated that the dental drug called Sargenti Paste, Sargenti Compound, or N2 is an unapproved new drug (letter from Carl C. Peck, M.D., director, Center for Drug Evaluation and Research, Food and Drug Administration, to Newell Yaple, D.D.S., secretary, Ohio State Dental Board, Aug. 12, 1991).[32] Single prescriptions for individual patients may be lawfully prepared by pharmacies according to the Food, Drug, and Cosmetic Act, but bulk shipments by pharmacists to dentists are not permitted.

The maximum amount of the formulation that the FDA permits to be dispensed is five grams (letter from Carl C. Peck, M.D., to Newell Yaple, D.D.S., Aug. 12, 1991). Conceivably, the FDA could take enforcement action against a dentist who ordered Sargenti Paste in bulk from a pharmacy.

A note about the above situation: Under the "pharmacy" exception to the Act, pharmacies are exempt from regulation under the Act if they are regularly engaged in dispensing prescription drugs or devices for prescriptions of practitioners licensed to administer such drugs or devices to patients under the care of such practitioners in the course of their professional practice; and if they do not manufacture, prepare, propagate, compound, or process drugs or devices for sale other than in the regular course of their business of dispensing or selling drugs or devices at retail. On the other hand, where a pharmacy compounds drugs in bulk, and sells them at wholesale prices with nationwide distribution, the pharmacy becomes a "manufacturer" under the act and is subject to FDA regulation. Relevant factors used to determine whether a pharmacy qualifies for the "pharmacy" exception to the Act are:

- whether particular drugs are being compounded on a regular basis, as opposed to periodic compounding of different drugs;
- whether drugs are being compounded primarily for individual patient prescriptions as opposed to orders contemplating larger amounts for office use;
- the geographic area of distribution;
- whether any form of advertising or promotion is being used;
- the percentage of gross income received from sales of particular compounded drugs;
- whether particular compounded drugs are being offered at wholesale prices.[33]

A dentist's use of non–FDA-approved drugs could conceivably also be limited by state law or by rules issued by a state licensing board. Some years ago, the Ohio State Dental Board considered a rule that would have prohibited dentists in that state from using any drug or medication not approved by the FDA in the treatment of patients. The rule was not adopted.

Use of Drugs Not Accepted by the ADA

The American Dental Association does not require its members to use only products that bear the ADA Seal of Acceptance. This policy reflects the voluntary nature of the ADA's Seal Program. While the Seal is an important indicator that a product meets ADA guidelines, the fact that a product has not been evaluated by the ADA Council on Scientific Affairs does not necessarily mean the product is unsafe or ineffective. Manufacturers of many safe and effective products may simply not have submitted those products to the ADA Seal Program.

Therefore, lack of the Seal should not be used to create any presumptions about the safety or efficacy of the unaccepted product.

Unproven Reliability and Effectiveness

Potential civil liability in a malpractice suit remains the most significant legal consequence of using a non–FDA-approved drug. In this area of inquiry, the existence of informed consent can be crucial, but will not always be enough to protect a doctor from later claims of negligence. Another crucial fact is whether alternative drugs of known effectiveness and proven reliability were available. In some cases, the outcome seems to depend upon the apparent egregiousness of the doctor's conduct.

The case of Sullivan vs. Henry illustrates the problems that can arise when a doctor prescribes a non–FDA-approved drug.[34] Sullivan involved a general physician who diagnosed his patient with cancer, determined it could not be treated with conventional cancer therapies and suggested that the patient try amygdalin (Laetrile). Use of Laetrile was not approved by the FDA except for investigational use by experts qualified by scientific training and experience to investigate the safety and efficacy of the drug. The doctor in this case was not participating in such an investigation.

The patient was informed about the experimental nature of her treatment with Laetrile and knew that the drug was not approved by the FDA. The key issue was whether the physician acted negligently in choosing this course of treatment. The defendant asserted that he should win as a matter of law because he acted reasonably and within the standard of care. In opposition to that claim, the plaintiffs (the patient's family) produced affidavits from expert witnesses stating that Laetrile was not listed in the PDR, was a known poison with no known benefits and was unsafe at any dosage. Another expert for the plaintiffs expressed the opinion that the defendant doctor did not fully explore the nature of the patient's malignancy. This raised questions about the doctor's conclusion that conventional cancer therapies, such as chemotherapy and radiotherapy, were not suitable for this patient's cancer. These facts created a jury question as to whether the defendant was negligent.

It is interesting to note that the plaintiffs' expert in Sullivan focused on the potential that experimental treatment was unnecessary. Failure to prescribe a drug of known effectiveness and proven reliability, which could have been used instead of a non–FDA-approved drug, may constitute a breach of the standard of care. This occurred in Blanton vs. U.S.,[35] in which the plaintiff was asked to participate in an experiment to test whether the drug $Rh_o(D)$ immune globulin (HypRho-D) had effectiveness beyond its FDA-approved shelf life. The plaintiff, a hospital patient, refused to participate in the experiment, but she received the drug anyway by mistake.

The court noted that this was not a simple case of the plaintiff receiving one drug that was inaccurately represented as another. Rather, the drug was in effect a "new drug" that was not FDA-approved, and "it was administered despite the availability of a drug of known effectiveness and proven reliability." The court held that the hospital, by administering the drug to plaintiff without her consent, violated "accepted medical standards."[35 (at 362)] While this case involved a hospital's conduct, not that of a physician or dentist, the rationale could be extended to a health professional as well.

Duty of Disclosure

In truly egregious cases, courts may look beyond a negligence theory to impose liability on doctors who act improperly in prescribing non–FDA-approved therapies. For example, in Nelson vs. Gaunt, the plaintiff received from the defendant a series of silicone injections for breast augmentation.[36] The uncontested evidence showed that at the time the plaintiff received the injections, the FDA considered silicone injections dangerous for use in human body tissues, and only persons who obtained a special permit to administer the injections under scientific circumstances could use silicone for this purpose. The defendant physician not only had no such permit, but he told the plaintiff that the substance was safe, inert and had absolutely no side effects. He did not tell her the name of the substance, the fact that it could be used only for the purposes of scientific research, that even under those conditions its use required state or federal approval, and that he did not have a permit to perform the injections.

These facts, the court found, went beyond an ordinary negligence theory and even beyond a claim of battery, which would exist if, for example, a doctor performed an operation without the patient's consent. The theory applicable on these facts was fraud, based on the physician's fiduciary duty to disclose information to the patient that may be relevant to a meaningful decision-making process and necessary to form the basis of an intelligent consent by the patient to the proposed treatment. In this case, the court found, the doctor provided the patient with false and misleading information and knowingly concealed information that was material to the cause of the plaintiff's injuries.[36]

The fact that a doctor is participating in an FDA-approved clinical investigation is not in itself sufficient to protect the doctor from claims of negligence. In a case involving use of a medical device, Daum vs. Spinecare Medical Group, Inc.,[37] a physician was required to defend himself against the charge that he failed to obtain the patient's informed consent to use the investigational device—a metal screw—in spinal fusion surgery. Applicable federal and state laws incorporated in the manufacturer's protocol for clinical trials required that patients be informed of the device's investigational status, give written consent to participate in the trial and be provided with a copy of their consent form.

The patient claimed that he was not told that the device was investigational or provided with the consent form until he was sedated and on a gurney being wheeled to the operating room; this raised an issue of whether the patient's consent was truly informed. However, the immediate question for the appellate court was whether the jury could find that simple failure to comply with the rules for conduct of the clinical trial, including the rule on informed consent, was negligence per se. The court held that it could, reasoning that the physician was not required to participate in the clinical trials but that once he did, he was required to abide by its rules. The jury was entitled to consider the physician's failure to comply with the rules on informed consent

as evidence of negligence per se, shifting to the physician the burden of proving that he did what might reasonably be expected of a person of ordinary prudence, acting under similar circumstances who desired to comply with the law. There is no reason to believe that the court would not apply the same rule to a new drug.

Conclusion

Dentists, in using drugs in their practices, need to be cognizant of the status of those agents within the FDA and the ADA. However, the more important concern is to exercise sound professional judgment in making choices and to be sure that patients are fully cognizant of material information concerning their treatments and the alternatives available to them.

Editor's note: This chapter was originally based on a 1992 article by Linda M. Wakeen, J.D., that appeared in the *Journal of Public Health Dentistry*[1] and was edited by Kathleen M. Todd, J.D., and Jill Wolowitz, J.D., LL.M. The chapter has since been further edited for this publication.

1. Wakeen LM. Legal implications of using drugs and devices in the dental office. J Public Health Dent 1992;52(6):403-8.
2. See 21 CFR Part 130, Legal Status of Approved Labeling for Prescription Drugs; Prescribing for Uses Unapproved by the Food and Drug Administration, Aug. 15, 1972.
3. Beck JM, Azari ED. FDA, off-label use, and informed consent: debunking myths and misconceptions. Food and Drug Law J 1998;53:71-104.
4. See also "Use of Approved Drugs for Unlabeled Indications," 12 FDA Drug Bulletin 4 (April 1982).
5. See also Chaney vs. Heckler, 718 F.2d 1174, 1180 (D.C. App. 1983), rev'd on other grounds, 470 U.S. 821 (1985).
6. Pub L No. 105-115, 111 Stat. 2296 (1997).
7. 21 U.S.C.A. 279g.
8. 21 U.S.C.A. 360aaa, et seq., Requirements for dissemination of treatment information on drugs or devices.
9. Washington Legal Foundation vs. Henney, 56 F.Supp.2d 81 (D.D.C. 1999).
10. Washington Legal Foundation v. Henney, 202 F.3d 331 (D.C. Cir., 2000).
11. See, e.g., Nold v. Binyon, 272 Kan. 87 (Kan. 2001); and Winkjer vs. Herr, 277 N.W.2d 579, 583 (N.D. 1979).
12. See, e.g., Olivier v. Robert L. Yeager Mental Health Center, 398 F.3d 183, 190 (2d Cir. 2005) ("we note that

a jury composed of non-experts typically cannot discern generally accepted medical standards for itself. In order to demonstrate an objective violation of those standards, therefore, a plaintiff ordinarily must introduce expert testimony to establish the relevant medical standards that were allegedly violated."); and, Blackwell vs. Hurst, 46 Cal.App.4th 939, 942 (Cal. App. 1996).

13. See, e.g., Rallings vs. Evans, 930 S.W.2d 259, 262 (Texas Ct. App. 1996).

14. See, e.g., Ellis vs. Oliver, 323 S.C. 121, 125 (1996).

15. Haught vs. Maceluch, 681 F.2d 291 (5th Cir. 1982).

16. Ohligschlager vs. Proctor Community Hospital, 303 N.E.2d 392 (Ill. 1973).

17. See also Mulder vs. Parke Davis & Company, 181 N.W.2d 882 (Minn. 1970).

18. See, e.g., Spensieri v. Lasky, 94 N.Y.2d 231 (N.Y. 1999) (holding that a PDR by itself cannot be used to establish a standard of care for prescribing of drugs) (declining to follow Ohligschlager vs. Proctor Community Hospital, 303 N.E.2d 392 [Ill. 1973]).

19. See Young vs. Cerniak, 467 N.E.2d 1045 (Ill. App. 1984).

20. See Nicolla vs. Fasulo, 557 N.Y.S.2d 539 (App. Div. 1990).

21. See, e.g., Ramon By and Through Ramon v. Farr, 770 P.2d 131 (Utah. 1991), for a case distinguishing Mulder.

22. Morlino vs. Medical Center of Ocean County, 295 N.J.Super. 113, 122 (1996).

23. See also Ramon vs. Farr, 770 P.2d 131 (Utah 1989).

24. See, e.g., Ross vs. Hodges, 234 So.2d 905 (Miss. 1970).

25. See, e.g., Aiken vs. Clary, 396 S.W.2d 668 (Mo. 1965).

26. See, e.g., Howard v. University of Medicine and Dentistry of New Jersey, 172 N.J. 537, 547 (N.J.. 2002); and Cobbs vs. Grant, 502 P.2d 1 (Cal. 1972).

27. See, e.g., Wilkinson vs. Vesey, 295 A.2d 676 (R.I. 1972).

28. See also Pa. Stat. Ann. Tit. 40, §1301.103 (Purdon Supp. 1997).

29. See also R.I. Gen. Laws §9–19–32 (1996).

30. See also Wash. Rev. Code Ann.§7.70.050(1)(c) (West Supp. 1997).

31. Reinhardt vs. Colton, 337 N.W.2d 88 (Minn. 1983).

32. See 21 U.S.C. §360(g)(1).

33. See Cedars North Towers Pharmacy, Inc. vs. United States of America, 824 CCH Food-Drug-Cosmetics Law Reporter par 38,200 (S.D.Fla. 1978).

34. Sullivan vs. Henry, 287 S.E.2d 652 (Ga.App. 1982).

35. Blanton vs. United States, 428 F.Supp. 360 (D.D.C. 1977).

36. Nelson vs. Gaunt, 125 Cal.App.3d 623 (1981).

37. Daum vs. Spinecare Medical Group, Inc., 52 Cal. App.4th 1285 (Cal.App.1997).

Appendices

U.S. Schedules for Controlled Substances

U.S. CLASSIFICATIONS

Schedule I	No recognized legal medical use; used in research with appropriate registration.
Schedule II	Most stringent classification for drugs; these drugs have legitimate medical use and very high abuse potential; inventory and distribution are tightly controlled; prescriptions not refillable.
Schedule III	Significant abuse potential, but less than Schedule II; up to 5 authorized refills within 6 months.
Schedule IV	Abuse potential lower than Schedule III; up to 5 authorized refills within 6 months.
Schedule V	Lowest abuse potential; prescriber may authorize as many refills as desired; some drugs in this class may be available without a prescription.

SCHEDULES FOR CONTROLLED SUBSTANCES

Heroin, LSD, peyote, marijuana, mescaline, phencyclidine	Schedule I (CI)
Opium, fentanyl, morphine, meperidine, methadone, oxycodone (and combinations), hydromorphone, codeine (single-drug entity), cocaine	Schedule II (CII)
Short-acting barbiturates	Schedule II (CII)
Amphetamine, methylphenidate	Schedule II (CII)
Codeine combinations, hydrocodone combinations, glutethimide, paregoric, phendimetrazine, thiopental, testosterone, other androgens	Schedule III (CIII)
Benzodiazepines (e.g., diazepam, midazolam), chloral hydrate, meprobamate, phenobarbital, propoxyphene (and combinations), pentazocine (and combinations), methohexital	Schedule IV (CIV)
Antidiarrheals and antitussives with opioid derivatives	Schedule V (CV)

U.S. Food and Drug Administration Pregnancy Classifications

FDA USE-IN-PREGNANCY CLASSIFICATIONS

CLASSIFICATION	DEFINITION
A	No risk demonstrated to the fetus in any trimester.
B	No adverse effects in animals; no human studies available.
C	Only given after risks to the fetus are considered; animal studies have shown adverse reactions; no human studies available.
D	Definite fetal risks; may be given in spite of risks if needed in life-threatening situations.
X	Absolute fetal abnormalities; not to be used at any time during pregnancy.

Agents That Affect the Fetus and Nursing Infant

Angelo J. Mariotti, D.D.S., Ph.D.

A teratogen is a drug or chemical that induces alterations in the formation of cells, tissues and organs and thus creates physical defects in a developing embryo or fetus. Teratogens act via a number of diverse mechanisms to ultimately damage the developing fetus. Drug-induced teratogenic changes can occur only during organogenesis; however, drug-induced toxicological changes affect the fetus after completion of tissue or organ formation because these drugs induce degenerative changes in formed tissue or organs. Unfortunately, the teratogenic or toxicological potential of many drugs has not been evaluated in utero.

To be safe, drugs that are known to be innocuous to the embryo or fetus should be the drugs of choice in the dental management of pregnant women. Drugs with unknown teratogenic or toxicological potential should be prescribed in consultation with the patient's obstetrician and used sparingly. Drugs with known teratogenic or toxicological effects should not be considered for use during dental procedures.

To aid health care providers, the U.S. Food and Drug Administration has developed a rating system for drugs that affect the fetus. The five categories the FDA uses to evaluate drug effects during pregnancy are shown in Appendix B.

The first list on the following page contains examples of drugs that require special precautions when used during pregnancy. Many of these drugs are not teratogenic, but the potential side effect of each agent may affect the embryo or fetus; therefore, each drug should be carefully investigated. If you have questions about any drug that might cause problems during pregnancy, contact an obstetrician or the Organization of Teratology Information Services (1-888-285-3410 or "http://www.otispregnancy.org") for agencies in your region that deal with potential harmful drugs to pregnant women.

The second list contains example of drugs that are excreted in breast milk. Please keep in mind that neither list is meant to be comprehensive. For further pregnancy and nursing precautions, consult the prescribing information tables within each chapter.

PREGNANCY CAUTION INFORMATION LIST

Alprazolam (systemic)
Amitriptyline (systemic)
Amobarbital (systemic)
Aprobarbital (systemic)
Ascorbic acid (systemic)
Aspirin, alone and in combination
  (systemic)
Atropine (systemic)
Clorazepate (systemic)
Clotrimazole
Codeine
Cortisone (systemic)
Cyanocobalamin Co 57 (systemic)
Demeclocycline (systemic)
Desoximetasone
Dexamethasone
Diclofenac (systemic)
Diflunisal
Epinephrine
Erythromycin estolate
Ethchlorvynol (systemic)
Etidocaine (parenteral-local)
Etodolac (systemic)
Fenoprofen (systemic)
Fentanyl (systemic)
Fluconazole (systemic)
Flurazepam (systemic)
Flurbiprofen (systemic)
Griseofulvin (systemic)
Halazepam (systemic)
Haloperidol (systemic)
Halothane (systemic)
Hydralazine (systemic)
Hydrocodone (systemic)
Hydrocortisone (systemic)
Bupivacaine (parenteral-local)

Butabarbital, alone and in
  combinations (systemic)
Butorphanol (systemic)
Caffeine (systemic)
Calcium carbonate (oral-local)
Carbamazepine (systemic)
Cefoxitin (systemic)
Hydromorphone (systemic)
Hyoscyamine (systemic)
Ibuprofen (systemic)
Indomethacin (systemic)
Iodine (topical)
Ketazolam (systemic)
Ketoprofen (systemic)
Ketorolac (systemic)
Labetalol (systemic)
Lidocaine (parenteral-local)
Lorazepam (systemic)
Meclizine (systemic)
Meclofenamate (systemic)
Mefenamic acid (systemic)
Meperidine (systemic)
Methadone (systemic)
Metronidazole (systemic)
Miconazole (vaginal)
Minocycline (systemic)
Morphine (systemic)
Naproxen (systemic)
Neomycin (oral-local)
Nicotine (systemic)
Nitrous oxide (systemic)
Nitrous oxide (systemic)
Norfloxacin (systemic)
Ofloxacin (ophthalmic)
Orphenadrine, aspirin and caffeine
  (systemic)

Chloral hydrate (systemic)
Chloramphenicol (systemic)
Chlordiazepoxide, alone and in
  combination (systemic)
Ciprofloxacin (ophthalmic)
Clarithromycin (systemic)
Clonazepam (systemic)
Clonidine (systemic)
Oxazepam (systemic)
Oxycodone (systemic)
Oxytetracycline (systemic)
Paregoric (systemic)
Penbutolol (systemic)
Pentazocine (systemic)
Phenobarbital (systemic)
Phenylbutazone (systemic)
Prednisone (systemic)
Procaine (parenteral-local)
Promazine (systemic)
Promethazine (systemic)
Propoxyphene (systemic)
Pseudoephedrine (systemic)
Rifampin (systemic)
Salicylic acid (topical)
Salsalate (systemic)
Secobarbital (systemic)
Sufentanil (systemic)
Sulindac (systemic)
Tetracaine (parenteral-local)
Tetracycline (systemic)
Triamcinolone (systemic)
Triazolam (systemic)
Vitamin A (systemic)

DRUGS EXCRETED IN BREAST MILK

Ampicillin
Antihistamines*
Aspirin
Atropine
Barbiturates
Cephalexin*
Cephalothin*
Chloral hydrate
Chloramphenicol
Codeine
Corticosteroids
Demeclocycline*

Diazepam
Diphenhydramine*
Erythromycin*
Fluorides*
Lincomycin*
Meperidine
Meprobamate
Methacycline
Methadone
Morphine
Narcotics
Oxacillin*

Penicillins*
Pentazocine*
Phenobarbital
Propantheline bromide*
Propoxyphene
Salicylates
Scopolamine*
Streptomycin
Tetracyclines*
Thiopental sodium*

*No adverse effects reported.

Prevention of Bacterial Endocarditis

Prevention of Bacterial Endocarditis: A Statement for the Dental Profession

ADA Council on Scientific Affairs

The current American Heart Association (AHA) recommendations for the prevention of bacterial endocarditis adopted in 1997 represent a substantial departure from past guidelines. The 1997 recommendations reflect a better understanding of the disease and its potential prevention. Major changes from past guidelines involve the indications for prophylaxis, antibiotic choice and dosing, ancillary procedures that may reduce bacteremic risk, a detailed discussion of mitral valve prolapse and greater attention to the medicolegal aspects of endocarditis.

Previously, antibiotic prophylaxis was suggested for dental procedures associated with any amount of bleeding. Now, only those that are associated with significant bleeding are recommended for prophylaxis as dictated by clinical judgment. This allows for a substantial number of dental procedures to be eliminated from the prophylaxis recommendation. A table is provided that delineates dental treatment procedures into those that may be associated with significant bleeding and those that pose negligible or no bacteremic risk. Recommended antibiotic prophylaxis regimens consist of a single preprocedural dose; no second dose is recommended. If the clinical decision is made not to premedicate and significant unanticipated bleeding occurs, the dental professional may then begin the antibiotic and continue the procedure. (Note: Some have interpreted the 1997 recommendations as saying it is acceptable to premedicate at the time of treatment. The AHA continues to recommend that patients be premedicated 1 hour prior to treatment.) A gentle prerinse with chlorhexidine can be employed, but gingival (subgingival) irrigation is not recommended due to conflicting data on efficacy in bacteremia reduction, the lack of data establishing that gingival irrigation will reduce endocarditis, its own potential for causing bacteremias and the lack of any standardized regimen.

It is recommended that all identified at-risk patients be strongly encouraged to maintain good oral health via professional and home care and plaque control procedures. This is particularly true for patients prior to cardiovascular surgical procedures. It is acknowledged that plaque control may induce bacteremias, but with much less or negligible risk as compared to a mouth with ongoing inflammation. The recommendations identify at-risk patients both medically and dentally.

Importantly, the medicolegal aspects of bacterial endocarditis are thoroughly addressed in the new recommendations, particularly regarding causation. The incubation period for most cases of endocarditis is defined, as are several factors that must be considered before attempting to attribute cause and effect to a given invasive procedure. It is acknowledged that most endocarditis is not associated with invasive procedures and that professional dental care is responsible for only a small percentage of endocarditis cases. However, antibiotic prophylaxis is still recommended prior to dental procedures associated with significant bleeding in high- and moderate-risk patients who are at a much greater risk of endocarditis than the general population. These recommendations are not intended as the standard of care, and practitioners should use their own clinical judgment in individual cases or special circumstances.

The new AHA recommendations for the prevention of bacterial endocarditis better define at-risk patients and the dental procedures to be covered by antibiotic prophylaxis. As a result, these new recommendations should aid in both patient and practitioner compliance, and diminish the adverse effects of prophylaxis including its role in promoting the development of microbial antibiotic resistance.

Prevention of Bacterial Endocarditis: Recommendations by the American Heart Association

The following tables are reprinted with permission of the publisher from Dajani AS, Taubert KA, Wilson W, et al. Prevention of Bacterial Endocarditis: Recommendations by the American Heart Association. JAMA 1997;277:1794-801.

CARDIAC CONDITIONS ASSOCIATED WITH ENDOCARDITIS[1-21]

ENDOCARDITIS PROPHYLAXIS RECOMMENDED

HIGH-RISK CATEGORY

Prosthetic cardiac valves, including bioprosthetic and homograft valves
Previous bacterial endocarditis
Complex cyanotic congenital heart disease (e.g., single ventricle states, transposition of the great arteries, tetralogy of Fallot)
Surgically constructed systemic pulmonary shunts or conduits

MODERATE-RISK CATEGORY

Most other congenital cardiac malformations (other than above and below)
Acquired valvar dysfunction (e.g., rheumatic heart disease)
Hypertrophic cardiomyopathy
Mitral valve prolapse with valvar regurgitation and/or thickened leaflets

ENDOCARDITIS PROPHYLAXIS NOT RECOMMENDED

NEGLIGIBLE-RISK CATEGORY (NO GREATER THAN THE GENERAL POPULATION)

Isolated secundum atrial septal defect
Surgical repair of atrial septal defect, ventricular septal defect, or patent ductus arteriosus (without residua beyond 6 mo)
Previous coronary artery bypass graft surgery
Mitral valve prolapse without valvar regurgitation
Physiologic, functional or innocent heart murmurs
Previous Kawasaki disease without valvar dysfunction
Previous rheumatic fever without valvar dysfunction
Cardiac pacemakers (intravascular and epicardial) and implanted defibrillators

DENTAL PROCEDURES AND ENDOCARDITIS PROPHYLAXIS[22-25]

ENDOCARDITIS PROPHYLAXIS RECOMMENDED*

Dental extractions
Periodontal procedures including surgery, scaling and root planing, probing and recall maintenance
Dental implant placement and reimplantation of avulsed teeth
Endodontic (root canal) instrumentation or surgery only beyond the apex
Subgingival placement of antibiotic fibers or strips
Initial placement of orthodontic bands but not brackets
Intraligamentary local anesthetic injections
Prophylactic cleaning of teeth or implants where bleeding is anticipated

ENDOCARDITIS PROPHYLAXIS NOT RECOMMENDED

Restorative dentistry[†] (operative and prosthodontic) with or without retraction cord[‡]
Local anesthetic injections (nonintraligamentary)
Intracanal endodontic treatment; post placement and buildup
Placement of rubber dams
Postoperative suture removal
Placement of removable prosthodontic or orthodontic appliances
Taking of oral impressions
Fluoride treatments
Taking of oral radiographs
Orthodontic appliance adjustment
Shedding of primary teeth

* Prophylaxis is recommended for patients with high- and moderate-risk cardiac conditions.
† This includes restoration of decayed teeth (filling cavities) and replacement of missing teeth.
‡ Clinical judgment may indicate antibiotic use in selected circumstances that may create significant bleeding.
Reprinted with permission of the publisher from Dajani AS, Taubert KA, Wilson W, et al. Prevention of Bacterial Endocarditis: Recommendations by the American Heart Association. JAMA 1997;277:1794-801.

PROPHYLACTIC REGIMENS FOR DENTAL, ORAL, RESPIRATORY TRACT, OR ESOPHAGEAL PROCEDURES[26-29]

SITUATION	AGENT	REGIMEN*
Standard general prophylaxis	Amoxicillin	*Adults:* 2.0g orally 1 hr before procedure. *Pediatrics:* 50mg/kg orally 1 hr before procedure.
Unable to take oral medications	Ampicillin	*Adults:* 2.0g IM or IV within 30 min before procedure. *Pediatrics:* 50mg/kg IM or IV within 30 min before procedure.
Allergic to penicillin	Clindamycin OR Cephalexin[†] or cefadroxil[†] OR Azithromycin or clarithromycin	**(Clindamycin)** *Adults:* 600mg orally 1 hr before procedure. *Pediatrics:* 20mg/kg orally 1 hr before procedure. **(Cephalexin or cefadroxil)** *Adults:* 2.0g orally 1 hr before procedure. *Pediatrics:* 50mg/kg orally 1 hr before procedure. **(Azithromycin or clarithromycin)** *Adults:* 500mg orally 1 hr before procedure. *Pediatrics:* 15mg/kg orally 1 hr before procedure.
Allergic to penicillin and unable to take oral medications	Clindamycin OR Cefazolin[†]	**(Clindamycin)** *Adults:* 600mg IV within 30 min before procedure. *Pediatrics:* 20mg/kg IV within 30 min before procedure. **(Cefazolin)** *Adults:* 1.0g IM or IV within 30 min before procedure. *Pediatrics:* 25mg/kg IM or IV within 30 min before procedure.

*Total children's dose should not exceed adult dose.
† Do not use cephalosporins in patients with a history of hypersensitivity reaction (urticaria, angioedema, or anaphylaxis) to penicillins.
Reprinted with permission of the publisher from Dajani AS, Taubert KA, Wilson W, et al. Prevention of Bacterial Endocarditis: Recommendations by the American Heart Association. JAMA. 1997;277:1794-801.

1. Steckelberg JM, Wilson WR. Risk factors for infective endocarditis. Infect Dis Clin North Am. 1993;7:9-9.
2. Saiman L, Prince A, Gersony WM. Pediatric infective endocarditis in the modern era. J Pediatr. 1993;122: 847-853.
3. Gersony WM, Hayes CJ, Driscoll DJ, et al. Bacterial endocarditis in patients with aortic stenosis, pulmonary stenosis, or ventricular septal defect. Circulation. 1993;87(suppl I):121-126.
4. Prabhu SD, O'Rourke RA. Mitral valve prolapse. In: Braunwald E, series ed, Rahimtoola SH, volume ed. Atlas of Heart Diseases: Valvular Heart Disease Vol XI. St. Louis, Mo: Mosby-Year Book Inc;1997:10.1-10.18.
5. Boudoulas H, Wooley CF. Mitral valve prolapse. In: Emmanouilides GC, Riemenschneider TA, Allen HD, Gutgesell HP, eds. Moss and Adams Heart Disease in Infants, Children, and Adolescents Including the Fetus and Young Adult. 5th ed. Baltimore, Md: Williams & Wilkins; 1995; 1063-1086.
6. Carabello BA. Mitral valve disease. Curr Probl Cardiol. 1993;7:423-478.
7. Devereux RB, Hawkins I, Kramer-Fox R, et al. Complications of mitral valve prolapse: disproportionate occurrence in men and older patients. Am J Med. 1986; 81:751-758.
8. Danchin N, Briancon S, Mathieu P, et al. Mitral valve prolapse as a risk factor for infective endocarditis. Lancet. 1989;1:743-745.
9. MacMahon SW, Roberts JK, Kramer-Fox R, et al. Mitral valve prolapse and infective endocarditis. Am Heart J. 1987;113:1291-1298.
10. Marks AR, Choong CY, Sanfilippo AJ, Ferre M, Weyman AE. Identification of high-risk and low-risk subgroups of patients with mitral-valve prolapse. N Engl J Med. 1989;320:1031-1036.
11. Devereux RB, Frary CJ, Kramer-Fox R, Roberts RB, Ruchlin HS. Cost-effectiveness of infective endocarditis prophylaxis for mitral valve prolapse with or without a mitral regurgitant murmur. Am J Cardiol. 1994;74:1024-1029.
12. Zuppiroli A, Rinaldi M, Kramer-Fox R, Favili S, Roman MJ, Devereux RB. Natural history of mitral valve prolapse. Am J Cardiol. 1995;75:1028-1032.
13. Wooley CF, Baker PB, Kolibash AJ, et al. The floppy, myxomatous mitral valve, mitral valve prolapse, and mitral regurgitation. Prog Cardiovasc Dis. 1991;33: 397-433.
14. Morales AR, Romanelli R, Boucek RJ, Tate LG, Alvarez RT, Davis JT. Myxoid heart disease: an assessment of extravalvular cardiac pathology in severe mitral valve prolapse. Human Pathol. 1992;23:129-137.
15. Weissman NJ, Pini R, Roman MJ, Kramer-Fox R, Andersen HS, Devereux RB. In vivo mitral valve morphology and motion in mitral valve proplapse. Am J Cardiol. 1994;73:1080-1088.
16. Nishimura RA, McGoon MD, Shub C, et al. Echocardiographically documented mitral-valve prolapse. N Engl J Med. 1985;313:1305-1309.
17. McKinsey DS, Ratts TE, Bisno AL. Underlying cardiac lesions in adults with infective endocarditis. Am J Med. 1987;82:681-688.
18. Devereux RB, Kramer-Fox R, Kligfield P. Mitral valve prolapse: causes, clinical manifestations, and management. Ann Intern Med. 1989;111:305-317.
19. Stoddard MF, Prince CR, Dillon S, Longaker RA, Morris GT, Liddell NE. Exercise-induced mitral regurgitation is a predictor of morbid events in subjects with mitral valve prolapse. J Am Coll Cardiol. 1995;25: 693-699.
20. Awadallah SM, Kavey REW, Byrum CJ, Smith FC, Kveselis DA, Blackman MS. The changing pattern of infective endocarditis in childhood. Am J Cardiol. 1991;68:90-94.
21. Durack DT. Prevention of infective endocarditis. N Engl J Med 1995;332:38-44.
22. Cheitlin MD, Alpert JS, Armstrong WF, et al. ACC/AHA guidelines for the clinical application of echocardiography: a report of the American College of Cardiology/American Heart Association Task Force on Practice Guidelines (Committee on Clinical Application of Echocardiography). Circulation. 1997;95:1686-1744.
23. Pallasch TJ, Slots J. Antibiotic prophylaxis and the medically compromised patient. Periodontol 2000. 1996;10:107-138.
24. Bender IB, Naidorf IJ, Garvey GJ. Bacterial endocarditis: a consideration for physicians and dentists. J Am Dent Assoc. 1984;109:415-420.
25. Guntheroth WG. How important are dental procedures as a cause of infective endocarditis? Am J Cardiol. 1984;54:797-801.
26. Dajani AS, Bisno AL, Chung KJ, et al. Prevention of bacterial endocarditis. JAMA. 1990;264:2919-2922.
27. Durack DT. Prevention of infective endocarditis. N Engl J Med 1995;332:38-44.
28. Dajani AS, Bawdon RE, Berry MC. Oral amoxicillin as prophylaxis for endocarditis: what is the optimal dose? Clin Infect Dis. 1994;18:157-160.
29. Rouse MS, Steckelberg JM, Brandt CM, Patel R, Miro JM, Wilson WR. Efficacy of azithromycin or clarithromycin for the prophylaxis of viridans group streptococcus experimental endocarditis. Antimicrob Agents Chemother. 1997; 41:1673-6.

Antibiotic Prophylaxis for Dental Patients With Total Joint Replacements

Advisory Statement: Antibiotic Prophylaxis for Dental Patients With Total Joint Replacements

American Dental Association; American Academy of Orthopaedic Surgeons

Approximately 450,000 total joint arthroplasties are performed annually in the United States. Deep infections of these total joint replacements usually result in failure of the initial operation and the need for extensive revision. Due to the use of perioperative antibiotic prophylaxis and other technical advances, deep infection occurring in the immediate postoperative period resulting from intraoperative contamination has been markedly reduced in the past 20 years.

Patients who are about to have a total joint arthroplasty should be in good dental health prior to surgery and should be encouraged to seek professional dental care if necessary. Patients who already have had a total joint arthroplasty should perform effective daily oral hygiene procedures to remove plaque (for example, by using manual or powered toothbrushes, interdental cleaners or oral irrigators) to establish and maintain good oral health. The risk of bacteremia is far more substantial in a mouth with ongoing inflammation than in one that is healthy and employing these home oral hygiene devices.[1]

Bacteremias can cause hematogenous seeding of total joint implants, both in the early postoperative period and for many years following implantation.[2] It appears that the most critical period is up to 2 years after joint placement.[3] In addition, bacteremias may occur in the course of normal daily life[4-6] and concurrently with dental and medical procedures.[6] It is likely that many more oral bacteremias are spontaneously induced by daily events than are dental treatment-induced.[6] Presently, no scientific evidence supports the position that antibiotic prophylaxis to prevent hematogenous infections is required prior to dental treatment in patients with total joint prostheses.[1] The risk/benefit[7,8] and cost/effectiveness[7,9] ratios fail to justify the administration of routine antibiotic prophylaxis. The analogy of late prosthetic joint infections with infective endocarditis is invalid, as the anatomy, blood supply, microorganisms and mechanisms of infection are all different.[10]

It is likely that bacteremias associated with acute infection in the oral cavity,[11,12] skin, respiratory, gastrointestinal and urogenital systems and/or other sites can and do cause late implant infection.[12] Any patient with a total joint prothesis with acute orofacial infection should be vigorously treated as any other patient with elimination of the source of the infection (incision and drainage, endodontics, extraction) and appropriate therapeutic antibiotics when indicated.[1,12] Practitioners should maintain a high index of suspicion for any unusual signs and symptoms (such as fever, swelling, pain, joint that is warm to touch) in patients with total joint prostheses.

Antibiotic prophylaxis is not indicated for dental patients with pins, plates and screws, nor is it routinely indicated for most dental patients with total joint replacements. This position agrees with that taken by the ADA Council on Dental Therapeutics[13] and the American Academy of Oral Medicine,[14] and is similar to that taken by of the British Society for Antimicrobial Chemotherapy.[15] There is limited evidence that some immunocompromised patients with total joint replacements (Box 1) may be at higher risk for hematogenous infections.[12,16-23] Antibiotic prophylaxis for such patients undergoing dental procedures with a higher bacteremic risk (as defined in Box 2) should be considered using an empirical regimen (Box 3). In addition, antibiotic prophylaxis may be considered when the higher-risk dental procedures (again, as defined in Box 2) are performed on dental patients within 2 years post-implant surgery,[3] on those who have had previous prosthetic joint infections and on those with some other conditions (Box 1).

Occasionally, a patient with a total joint prosthesis may present to the dentist with a recommendation from his or her physician that is not consistent with these guidelines. This could be due to lack of familiarity with the guidelines or to special considerations about the patient's medical condition that are not known to the dentist. In this situation, the dentist is encouraged to consult with the physician to determine if there are any special considerations that might affect the dentist's decision on whether or not to premedicate, and may wish to share a copy of these guidelines with the physician if appropriate. After this consultation, the dentist may decide to follow the physician's recommendation or, if in the dentist's professional judgment antibiotic prophylaxis is not indicated, may decide to proceed without antibiotic prophylaxis. The dentist is ultimately responsible for making treatment recommendations for his or her patients based on the dentist's professional judgment. Any perceived potential benefit of antibiotic prophylaxis must be weighed against the known risks of antibiotic toxicity; allergy; and development, selection and transmission of microbial resistance.

This statement provides guidelines to supplement practitioners in their clinical judgment regarding antibiotic prophylaxis for dental patients with a total joint prosthesis. It is not intended as the standard of care nor as a substitute for clinical judgment as it is impossible to make recommendations for all conceivable clinical situations in which bacteremias originating from the oral cavity may occur. Practitioners must exercise their own clinical judgment in determining whether or not antibiotic prophylaxis is appropriate.

BOX 1: PATIENTS AT POTENTIAL INCREASED RISK OF HEMATOGENOUS TOTAL JOINT INFECTION*

All patients during first 2 years following joint replacement

Immunocompromised/immunosuppressed patients

Inflammatory arthropathies such as rheumatoid arthritis or systemic lupus erythematosus
Drug- or radiation-induced immunosuppression

Examples of patients with comorbidities

Previous prosthetic joint infections	HIV infection
Malnourishment	Insulin-dependent (type 1) diabetes
Hemophilia	Malignancy

*Based on Ching and colleagues,[12] Brause,[16] Murray and colleagues,[17] Poss and colleagues,[18] Jacobson and colleagues,[19] Johnson and Bannister,[20] Jacobson and colleagues[21] and Berbari and colleagues.[22]

BOX 2: INCIDENCE STRATIFICATION OF BACTEREMIC DENTAL PROCEDURES*

Higher incidence[†]

Dental extractions
Periodontal procedures including surgery, subgingival placement of antibiotic fibers/strips, scaling and
    root planing, probing, recall maintenance
Dental implant placement and replantation of avulsed teeth
Endodontic (root canal) instrumentation or surgery only beyond the apex
Initial placement of orthodontic bands but not brackets
Intraligamentary and intraosseous local anesthetic injections
Prophylactic cleaning of teeth or implants where bleeding is anticipated

Lower incidence[‡§]

Restorative dentistry** (operative and prosthodontic) with/without retraction cord
Local anesthetic injections (nonintraligamentary and nonintraosseous)
Intracanal endodontic treatment; post placement and buildup
Placement of rubber dam
Postoperative suture removal
Placement of removable prosthodontic/orthodontic appliances
Taking of oral impressions
Fluoride treatments
Taking of oral radiographs
Orthodontic appliance adjustment

* Adapted with permission of the publisher from Dajani AS, Taubert KA, Wilson W, et al.[23]
† Prophylaxis should be considered for patients with total joint replacement who meet the criteria in Box 1. No other patients with
    orthopedic implants should be considered for antibiotic prophylaxis prior to dental treatment/procedures.
‡ Prophylaxis not indicated.
§ Clinical judgment may indicate antibiotic use in selected circumstances that may create significant bleeding.
** This includes restoration of carious (decayed) or missing teeth.

BOX 3: SUGGESTED ANTIBIOTIC PROPHYLAXIS REGIMENS*

PATIENT TYPE	REGIMEN
Patients not allergic to penicillin: cephalexin, cephradine or amoxicillin	2g orally 1 hr prior to dental procedure
Patients not allergic to penicillin and unable to take oral medications: cefazolin or ampicillin	Cefazolin 1g or ampicillin 2g intramuscularly or intravenously 1 hr prior to the dental procedure
Patients allergic to penicillin: clindamycin	600mg orally 1 hr prior to the dental procedure
Patients allergic to penicillin and unable to take oral medications: clindamycin	600mg IV 1 hr prior to the dental procedure

* No second doses are recommended for any of these dosing regimens.

The ADA/AAOS Expert Panel that developed the original of this statement consisted of Robert H. Fitzgerald Jr., M.D.; Jed J. Jacobson, D.D.S., M.S., M.P.H.; James V. Luck Jr., M.D.; Carl L. Nelson, M.D.; J. Phillip Nelson, M.D.; Douglas R. Osmon, M.D.; and Thomas J. Pallasch, D.D.S. The staff liaisons were Clifford W. Whall Jr., Ph.D., for the ADA, and William W. Tipton Jr., M.D., for the AAOS. The ADA and the AAOS reviewed and updated this statement in 2003.

Dentists and physicians are encouraged to reproduce the above Advisory Statement for distribution to colleagues. Permission to reprint the Advisory Statement is hereby granted by ADA and AAOS, provided that the Advisory Statement is reprinted in its entirety including citations and that such reprints contain a notice stating "Copyright © 2003 American Dental Association and American Academy of Orthopaedic Surgeons. Reprinted with permission." If you wish to use the Advisory Statement in any other fashion, written permission must be obtained from ADA and AAOS.

1. Pallasch TJ, Slots J. Antibiotic prophylaxis and the medically compromised patient. Periodontology 2000 1996;10:107-38.
2. Rubin R, Salvati EA, Lewis R. Infected total hip replacement after dental procedures. Oral Surg Oral Med Oral Pathol 1976;41(1):13-23.
3. Hansen AD, Osmon DR, Nelson CL. Prevention of deep prosthetic joint infection. Am J Bone Joint Surg 1996;78-A (3):458-71.
4. Bender IB, Naidorf IJ, Garvey GJ. Bacterial endocarditis: a consideration for physicians and dentists. JADA 1984;109:415-20.
5. Everett ED, Hirschmann JV. Transient bacteremia and endocarditis prophylaxis: a review. Medicine 1977; 56:61-77.
6. Guntheroth WG. How important are dental procedures as a cause of infective endocarditis? Am J Cardiol 1984; 54:797-801.
7. Jacobsen JJ, Schweitzer SO, DePorter DJ, Lee JJ. Antibiotic prophylaxis for dental patients with joint prostheses? A decision analysis. Int J Technol Assess Health Care 1990; 6:569-87.
8. Tsevat J, Durand-Zaleski I, Pauker SG. Cost-effectiveness of antibiotic prophylaxis for dental procedures in patients with artificial joints. Am J Public Health 1989;79:739-43.
9. Norden CW. Prevention of bone and joint infections. Am J Med 1985;78(6B):229-32.
10. McGowan DA. Dentistry and endocarditis. Br Dent J 1990;169:69.
11. Bartzokas CA, Johnson R, Jane M, Martin MV, Pearce PK, Saw Y. Relation between mouth and haematogenous infections in total joint replacement. Br Med J 1994;309:506-8.
12. Ching DWI, Gould IM, Rennie JAN, Gibson PII. Prevention of late haematogenous infection in major prosthetic joints. J Antimicrob Chemother 1989;23: 676-80.
13. Council on Dental Therapeutics. Management of dental patients with prosthetic joints. JADA 1990; 121: 537-8.
14. Eskinazi D, Rathbun W. Is systematic antimicrobial prophylaxis justified in dental patients with prosthetic joints? Oral Surg Oral Med Oral Pathol 1988;66:430-1.
15. Cawson RA. Antibiotic prophylaxis for dental treatment: for hearts but not for prosthetic joints. Br Dent J 1992;304:933-4.
16. Brause BD. Infections associated with prosthetic joints. Clin Rheum Dis 1986;12:523-35.
17. Murray RP, Bourne MH, Fitzgerald RH Jr. Metachronous infection in patients who have had more than one total joint arthroplasty. J Bone Joint Surg [Am] 1991;73(10):1469-74.
18. Poss R, Thornhill TS, Ewald FC, Thomas WH, Batte NJ, Sledge CB. Factors influencing the incidence and outcome of infection following total joint arthroplasty. Clin Orthop 1984;182:117-26.
19. Jacobson JJ, Millard HD, Plezia R, Blankenship JR. Dental treatment and late prosthetic joint infections. Oral Surg Oral Med Oral Pathol 1986;61:413-17.
20. Johnson DP, Bannister GG. The outcome of infected arthroplasty of the knee. J Bone Joint Surg [Br] 1986;68(2):289-91.
21. Jacobson JJ, Patel B, Asher G, Wooliscroft JO, Schaberg D. Oral *Staphylcoccus* in elderly subjects with rheumatoid arthritis. J Am Geriatr Soc 1997;45:1-5.
22. Berbari EF, Hanssen AD, Duffy MC, Ilstrup DM, Harmsen WS, Osmon DR. Risk factors for prosthetic joint infection: case-control study. Clin Infectious Dis 1998;27:1247-54.
23. Dajani AS, Taubert KA, Wilson W, et al. Prevention of bacterial endocarditis: Recommendations by the American Heart Association. From the Committee on Rheumatic Fever, Endocarditis and Kawasaki Disease, Council on Cardiovascular Disease in the Young. JAMA 1997;277:1794-1801.

A Legal Perspective on Antibiotic Prophylaxis

ADA Division of Legal Affairs

The Advisory Statement on Antibiotic Prophylaxis for Dental Patients with Total Joint Replacements reflects growing concern about the development of microbial resistance owing to the inappropriate use of antibiotics and recognizes that there are risks as well as benefits involved in the use of antibiotics. It delineates the limited circumstances in which antibiotic prophylaxis should be considered for dental patients who have had total joint replacements and cautions physicians and dentists to weigh the perceived potential benefits of antibiotic prophylaxis against the known risks of antibiotic toxicity, allergies and the development of microbial resistance.

But what should the dentist do if the patient brings to the appointment a recommendation for premedication from his or her physician with which the dentist disagrees? Should the dentist ignore the physician's recommendation or simply defer to the physician's judgment?

Neither approach is prudent from a risk management perspective. On the one hand, the physician's recommendation may be based on facts about the patient's medical condition that are not known to the dentist.

On the other, the physician may not be familiar with this advisory statement or that premedication may be indicated for some dental procedures but not for others. The careful dentist will attempt to ascertain the basis for the physician's recommendation and to acquaint the physician with the reasons why the dentist disagrees. Ideally, consensus can be reached. Most dentists would be uncomfortable with the thought of the physician's testifying in a malpractice suit that the dentist failed to follow the physician's treatment recommendation. However, the dentist who blindly follows the physician's recommendation, even though it conflicts with the dentist's professional judgment, will not be able to defend himself or herself by claiming "the devil made me do it" if the patient sues. The courts recognize that each independent professional is ultimately responsible for his or her own treatment decisions.

The answer to this dilemma may lie in the concept of informed consent, which acknowledges the patient's right to autonomous decision making. Informed consent usually can be relied on to protect from legal liability the practitioner who respects the patient's wishes, as long as the practitioner is acting within the standard of care. However, for informed consent to be legally binding, it is incumbent on the practitioner to inform the patient of all reasonable treatment options and the risks and benefits of each. In the situation in question, the dentist would be prudent to inform the patient when the dentist's treatment recommendations differ from those of the patient's physician and even encourage the patient to discuss the treatment options with his or her physician before making a decision. All discussions with the patient and the patient's physician should be well-documented. Of course, allowing the patient to choose assumes that both the dentist's and the physician's treatment recommendations are acceptable.

Dentists are not obligated to render treatment that they deem not to be in the patient's best interest, simply because the patient requests it. In such circumstances, referral to another practitioner may be the only solution.

The above information should not be construed as legal advice or a standard of care. A dentist should always consult his or her own attorney for answers to the dentist's specific legal questions.

The material in this appendix first appeared in the following two sources:

American Dental Association and American Academy of Orthopaedic Surgeons. Advisory statement: antibiotic prophylaxis for dental patients with total joint replacements.

Todd K. A legal perspective on antibiotic prophylaxis. JADA 1997;128:1004-7.

Antibiotic Use in Dentistry

ADA Council on Scientific Affairs

Microbial resistance to antibiotics is increasing at an alarming rate. In the last few years, penicillin resistance in *Streptococcus pneumoniae* has risen from virtually zero to 25-60% of all isolates. Such penicillin resistance is increasing in viridans streptococci, and a significant number of *Prevotella* and *Porphyromonas* isolates exhibit β-lactamase production. Hospital epidemics of vancomycin-aminoglycoside-methicillin–resistant staphylococci and vancomycin-resistant, β-lactamase–producing enterococci contribute significantly to the 150,000 annual deaths in United States hospitals that result from nosocomial septicemias.

The major cause of this public health problem is the use of antibiotics in an inappropriate manner, leading to the selection and dominance of resistant microorganisms and/or the increased transfer of resistance genes from antibiotic-resistant to antibiotic-susceptible microorganisms. Inappropriate antibiotic use includes faulty dosing (too low a dose, too long a duration), wrong choice of antibiotic (microorganisms not likely to be sensitive), improper combination of antibiotics and therapeutic or prophylactic use in unwarranted and unproven clinical situations.

Antibiotics are properly employed only for the management of active infectious disease or the prevention of metastatic infection (such as infective endocarditis) in medically high-risk patients. Antibiotic prophylaxis to prevent medical perioperative surgical infections is documented effective in high-risk surgical procedures (cardiovascular, neurological, orthopedic) when the antibiotics are employed intraoperatively (begun shortly before and terminated shortly after the surgery). The use of antibiotics after routine dental treatment to prevent infection has generally not been proven effective. However, the use of antimicrobial therapy may be of benefit in selective surgical procedures and their postoperative management on an empirical basis, and further research in this area is encouraged.

Dentistry has been relatively conservative with antibiotic use and has likely not contributed greatly to the worldwide problems of antibiotic microbial resistance. Adherence to the above principles of antibiotic use will continue and even improve our record of judicious use of antibiotics. Antibiotics are one of the few kinds of drugs that affect not only a single patient but entire populations of individuals through their collective effects on microbial ecology. Our responsibility lies not only with our own patients but with a world of such patients.

This statement was adopted by the Council on Scientific Affairs in September 1996. It first appeared in ADA Council on Scientific Affairs. Antibiotic use in dentistry. JADA 1997; 128:648.

Nitrous Oxide in the Dental Office

ADA Council on Scientific Affairs; ADA Council on Dental Practice

The safe use of nitrous oxide in the dental office has been an issue the ADA has monitored for many years. In 1977, an ad hoc committee convened by the Association published a report on the potential health hazards of trace anesthetics in dentistry.[1] Also in 1977, the National Institute of Occupational Safety and Health (NIOSH) reported that, by using several control measures, nitrous oxide levels of approximately 50 parts per million were achievable in dental operatories during routine dental anesthesia/analgesia.[2] A few years later, in 1980, the ADA Council on Dental Materials, Instruments and Equipment recommended that effective scavenging devices be installed and monitoring programs be instituted in dental offices in which nitrous oxide is used, and the council indicated that using these methods or devices would assist in keeping the levels of nitrous oxide at the lowest possible level.[3]

NIOSH continued its activities relating to nitrous oxide concentrations in the dental office and, in 1994, published an alert called "Request for Assistance in Controlling Exposures to Nitrous Oxide During Anesthetic Administration."[4] In the same year, NIOSH also reported on field evaluations and laboratory studies evaluating nitrous oxide scavenging systems and modifications in attempts to achieve the current NIOSH recommended exposure limit of 25 ppm during administration. NIOSH concluded that nitrous oxide levels may be controlled to about 25 ppm by maintaining leak-free delivery systems and using proper exhaust rates, better-fitting masks and auxiliary exhaust ventilation.[5]

In 1995 the ADA Council on Scientific Affairs convened an expert panel to review scientific literature on nitrous oxide and to revise recommendations on controlling nitrous oxide concentrations in the dental office. What follows is an overview of the conclusions reached by that panel.

Conclusions and Recommendations of the Expert Panel

Nitrous oxide continues to be a valuable agent for the control of pain and anxiety. However, chronic occupational exposure to nitrous oxide in offices not using scavenging systems may be associated with possible deleterious neurological and reproductive effects on dental personnel. Limited studies show that as little as three to five hours per week of unscavenged nitrous oxide exposure could result in adverse reproductive effects. In contrast, in dental offices using nitrous oxide scavenging systems, there has been no evidence of adverse health effects.[6] It is strongly recommended, therefore, that while there is no consensus on a recommended exposure limit to nitrous oxide, appropriate scavenging systems and methods of administration should be adopted. A protocol for controlling nitrous oxide is outlined below.

Recommendations for Controlling Nitrous Oxide Exposure

The expert panel identified a number of recommendations that are important to consider in the safe and effective use of nitrous oxide:

- The dental office should have a properly installed nitrous oxide delivery system. This includes appropriate scavenging equipment with a readily visible and accurate flow meter (or equivalent measuring device), a vacuum pump with the capacity for up to 45 L of air per min per workstation, and a variety of sizes of masks to ensure proper fit for individual patients.
- The vacuum exhaust and ventilation exhaust should be vented to the outside (for example, through the vacuum system) and not in close proximity to fresh-air intake vents.
- The general ventilation should provide good room air mixing.
- Each time the nitrous oxide machine is first turned on and every time a gas cylinder is changed, the pressure connections should be tested for leaks. High-pressure–line connections should be tested for leaks on a quarterly basis. A soap solution may be used to test for leaks. Alternatively, a portable infrared spectrophotometer can be used to diagnose an insidious leak.
- Prior to first daily use, all nitrous oxide equipment (reservoir bag, tubings, mask, connectors) should be inspected for worn parts, cracks, holes or tears. Replace as necessary.
- The mask may then be connected to the tubing and the vacuum pump turned on. All appropriate flow rates (that is, up to 45 L/min or per manufacturer's recommendations) should be verified.
- A properly sized mask should be selected and placed on the patient. A good, comfortable fit should be ensured. The reservoir (breathing) bag should not be over- or underinflated while the patient is breathing oxygen (before administering nitrous oxide).

- The patient should be encouraged to minimize talking and mouth breathing while the mask is in place.
- During administration, the reservoir bag should be periodically inspected for changes in tidal volume and the vacuum flow rate should be verified.
- On completing administration, 100% oxygen should be delivered to the patient for 5 minutes before removing the mask. In this way, both the patient and the system will be purged of residual nitrous oxide. Do not use an oxygen flush.
- Periodic (semiannual interval is suggested) personal sampling of dental personnel, with emphasis to chairside personnel exposed to nitrous oxide, should be conducted (for example, use of diffusive sampler [dosimeters] or infrared spectrophotometer).

Research Priorities

The expert panel identified a number of areas that require high-priority research:

- The elucidation of biological mechanisms that result in the adverse health effects associated with exposure to nitrous oxide.
- Studies to gain a full understanding of the potential health effects of chronic low-level exposure to nitrous oxide, with emphasis on prospective studies that use direct nitrous oxide exposure measurement.
- The investigation of possible cognitive effects related to exposure to low levels of nitrous oxide.
- The development of equipment to evaluate and control exposure to nitrous oxide.
- The study of ventilation systems and air-exchange mechanisms for dental office designs.
- The evaluation of advantages associated with the use of nitrous oxide in combination with other sedative drugs.

The councils will continue to work with industry and the research community to address research and development needs that will further reduce occupational exposure to nitrous oxide.

1. ADA Ad Hoc Committee on Trace Anesthetics as Potential Health Hazard in Dentistry. Reports of subcommittees of the ADA Ad Hoc Committee on Trace Anesthetics as Potential Health Hazard in Dentistry: review and current status of survey. JADA 1977;95(10):787-90.
2. Whitcher CE, Zimmerman DC, Piziali RL. Control of occupational exposure to N2O in the dental operatory. Cincinnati: National Institute of Occupational Safety and Health, 1977; DHEW publication no. (NIOSH) 77-171.
3. Council on Dental Materials, Instruments and Equipment. Council position on nitrous oxide scavenging and monitoring devices. JADA 1980;101(1):62.
4. Alert: request for assistance in controlling exposures to nitrous oxide during anesthetic administration. Cincinnati: U.S. Department of Health and Human Services, Public Health Service, Centers for Disease Control, National Institute of Occupational Safety and Health, 1994; DHHS publication no. (NIOSH) 94100.
5. Technical report: control of nitrous oxide in dental operatories. Cincinnati: U.S. Department of Health and Human Services, Public Health Service, Centers for Disease Control and Prevention, National Institute of Occupational Safety and Health, Division of Physical Sciences and Engineering, Engineering Control Technology Branch, 1994; DHHS publication no. (NIOSH) 94-129.
6. Rowland AS, Baird DD, Weinberg CR, Shore DL, Shy CM, Wilcox AJ. Reduced fertility among women employed as dental assistants exposed to high levels of nitrous oxide. N Engl J Med 1992;327:993-7.

This material first appeared in ADA Council on Scientific Affairs and ADA Council on Dental Practice. Nitrous oxide in the dental office. JADA 1997; 128:864-5.

Normal Laboratory Values for Adults

HEMATOLOGIC EXAMINATIONS

EXAMINATION	RANGE
BLOOD CELLS	
Erythrocytes (RBC) (per mm^3)	
Men	4,100,000-5,900,000
Women	3,800,000-5,500,000
Leukocytes (WBC) (per mm^3)	4,100-12,300
Differential leukocytes (per mm^3)	
Segmented neutrophils	2,500-6,000 (40-60%)
Band neutrophils	0-500 (0-5%)
Juvenile neutrophils	0-100 (0-1%)
Myelocytes	0 (0%)
Lymphocytes	1,000-4,000 (15.5-46.6%)
Monocytes	200-800 (2.8-12.9%)
Eosinophils	50-300 (0-6%)
Basophils	0-100 (0-2.3%)
Platelets (Plt) (per mm^3)	140,000-450,000
Hemoglobin (Hgb) (g/100 mL)	
Men	13-17.5
Women	11.6-16.2
Hemoglobin, total glycolated (percentage)	4.0-8.0
Hematocrit (HcT) (percentage)	
Men	40-52
Women	35-47
Erythrocyte sedimentation rate (ESR) (mm/h)	
Men	1.0-13
Women	1.0-20
Mean corpuscular volume (MCV) (mm^3)	86-98
Mean corpuscular hemoglobin (MCH) (pg/cell)	28-33
Mean corpuscular hemoglobin concentration (MCHC) (g/dL)	32-36

HEMATOLOGIC EXAMINATIONS *(cont.)*

EXAMINATION	RANGE
COAGULATION SCREENING TESTS	
Bleeding time	3-9 min
Coagulation time (Lee-White) (glass)	5-15 min
International normalized ratio (INR)	1
Prothrombin time	less than 2 s deviation from control
Activated partial thromboplastin time (aPTT)	25-37 s
Thrombin time (TT)	± 5 s of control

CHEMICAL CONSTITUENTS OF BLOOD

CONSTITUENT	RANGE
PROTEINS (g/100 mL)	
Total serum protein	6.0-8.4
Albumin, serum	3.5-5.0
Globulin, serum	2.3-3.5
A/G ratio	1.5:1-3.1
LIPIDS (mg/dL)	
Cholesterol, total	
Men	140-284
Women	140-252
HDL cholesterol	40-60
LDL cholesterol	65-170
Triglycerides	30-170
ENZYMES	
Amylase	4-25 U/mL
Creatine phosphokinase—CPK (mU/mL)	
Men	5.0-55
Women	5.0-35
Lactate dehydrogenase—LDH (IU/L)	
Men	86-272
Women	82-249
Phosphatase (alkaline)	31-121 IU/L
Transaminases	

CHEMICAL CONSTITUENTS OF BLOOD *(cont.)*

CONSTITUENT	RANGE
ENZYMES *(cont.)*	
Aspartate transaminase (AST) (SGOT) (IU/L)	
Men	6.0-37
Women	5.0-37
Alanine transaminase (ALT) (SGPT) (IU/L)	
Men	6.0-46
Women	6.0-37
UREA NITROGEN (BUN)	
Urea nitrogen (BUN)	4-24 mg/100 mL
URIC ACID	
Men	2.4-8.7
Women	2.1-6.9
CREATININE (mg/100 mL)	
Men	0.5-1.3
Women	0.4-1.2
BUN/CREATININE	
BUN/creatinine	7.0-20
OXYGEN SATURATION (ARTERIAL)	
Oxygen saturation (arterial)	96-100%
PO_2	
PO_2	75-100 mm Hg
PCO_2	
PCO_2	35-45 mm Hg
CO_2 COMBINING POWER	
CO_2 combining power	24-34 mEq/L
pH	
pH	7.35-7.45
ELECTROLYTES AND INORGANIC CONSTITUENTS	
Chloride (Cl-serum)	94-111 mEq/L
Sodium (serum)	135-145 mEq/L
Potassium (serum)	3.5-5.0 mEq/L
Calcium (serum)	9-11 mg/100 mL

CHEMICAL CONSTITUENTS OF BLOOD (cont.)

CONSTITUENT	RANGE
ELECTROLYTES AND INORGANIC CONSTITUENTS (cont.)	
Phosphorus (serum) (mg/100 mL)	
Adults	2.3-5.1
Children	4-6.5
Iron, total	50-150 µg/100 mL
Total base	143-155 mEq/L
GLUCOSE, FASTING	
Glucose, fasting	70-110 mg/100 mL
BILIRUBIN (mg/100 mL)	
Total	0.3-1.2
Direct	0.0-0.2
Bromsulfalein (BSP)	Less than 5% retention (45 min)

URINE ANALYSIS

COMPONENT	RANGE
MACROSCOPIC (FRESH SPECIMEN)	
Color	clear yellow
Specific gravity	1.010-1.025
pH	.4.8-7.5
MICROSCOPIC	
Bacteria	0 (single specimen)
Leukocytes	0-few (single specimen) up to 1,800,000/24 hrs
Erythrocytes	0-few (single specimen) up to 500,000/24 hrs
Casts (hyaline)	0 (single specimen) up to 5,000/24 hrs
CHEMICAL COMPONENTS	
Glucose	0 (single specimen) less than 100 mg/100 mL (24-hr specimen)
Albumin	0 (single specimen) 10-150 mg/24 hrs
Ketones	0 (single specimen) less than 50 mg/24 hrs
Creatinine clearance	150-180 L/day/1.73 m^2 surface area

Weights and Measures

COMMON METRIC MEASUREMENTS AND THEIR ABBREVIATIONS

METRIC MEASUREMENTS	ABBREVIATIONS
WEIGHT	
gram	g
kilogram	kg
milligram	mg
microgram	µg
VOLUME	
Liter	L
Milliliter	mL
Microliter	µL

COMMON METRIC EQUIVALENTS

METRIC MEASUREMENTS	EQUIVALENTS
WEIGHT	
0.000001 gram (g)	1 microgram (µg)
0.001 g	1 milligram (mg)
1 g	1,000 milligrams (mg) 1,000,000 µg
1 kg	1,000 g
VOLUME	
0.001 milliliter (mL)	1 microliter (µL)
1 mL	0.001 liter (L)
1,000 mL	1 L

MEASURES OF VOLUME

METRIC MEASUREMENTS	APOTHECARY
—	1 dram
5 milliliters (mL)	1 teaspoonful
30 mL	1 fluid ounce
480 mL	1 pint
960 mL	1 quart

MEASURES OF WEIGHT

METRIC MEASUREMENTS	APOTHECARY
1 gram (g)	15 grains (gr)
—	60 gr
4 g	1 dram
30 g	1 ounce (oz)
1 kilogram (kg)	2.2 pounds (lb)
60 milligram (mg)	1 gr

Calculation of Local Anesthetic and Vasoconstrictor Dosages

LOCAL ANESTHETIC DOSAGES

PERCENTAGE CONCENTRATION	= mg/mL	× 1.8 = mg/CARTRIDGE
0.5	5	9
1.5	15	27
3	30	54
1	10	18
2	20	36
4	40	72

VASOCONSTRICTOR CONCENTRATIONS (EQUIVALENCY FORMULA AND USE)

DILUTION OR	mg/mL × 1.8	= mg/CARTRIDGE	RECOMMENDED USE
1:1,000	1	—	Anaphylaxis (IM, SC)
1:10,000	0.1	—	Cardiac arrest (IV)
1:20,000	0.05	0.09	Local anesthesia; levonordefrin
1:50,000	0.02	0.036	Local anesthesia; epinephrine
1:80,000	0.0125	0.0225	Local anesthesia; epinephrine (UK)
1:100,000	0.01	0.018	Local anesthesia; epinephrine
1:200,000	0.005	0.009	Local anesthesia; epinephrine

HIV and Common Antiretroviral Medications

Lida Radfar, D.D.S., M.S.

Treatment regimens for human immunodeficiency virus (HIV) disease include prophylactic and maintenance medications. Prophylactic medications usually are indicated when the patient's immune system has deteriorated to a point at which opportunistic infections can be expected. The more common medications include anti–*Pneumocystis-carinii*-pneumonia (PCP) agents such as trimethoprim sulfamethoxazole; antifungal medications such as fluconazole; and antimycobacterial agents such as rifampin and isoniazid. Many of these medications interact with other medications commonly used in dentistry.

Approximately 21 antiretroviral medications, representing five drug classes, have been approved by the FDA for treatment of HIV disease, with many more in development. These medications directly or indirectly inhibit HIV replication through different mechanisms. Nucleoside reverse transcriptase inhibitors (NRTIs) and non-nucleoside reverse transcriptase inhibitors (NNRTIs) act as competitive inhibitors to an enzyme, reverse transcriptase, that the virus carries for the purpose of transcribing the viral RNA into viral DNA. One of the newer antiretroviral classes is protease inhibitors, which prevent the breakdown of proteins produced by the HIV-infected cell into appropriate sizes for viral production. The latest group of antiretroviral drugs, which received FDA approval in early 2003, is fusion inhibitors. These medications prevent entry of HIV into a target cell.

To maximize the treatment effect, a combination of several antiretroviral medications is recommended. This approach has been named highly active antiretroviral therapy, or HAART. This combination regimen has been shown to suppress the plasma viral load titer to less than 50 copies per milliliter in 60% of patients and raise CD4 cell counts to 175-200 per cubic milliliter after 48 weeks of treatment.

Continuous development of antiretroviral medications will challenge all health care workers treating HIV-infected patients to keep apprised of new agents that are often associated with a high degree of toxicity, including liver toxicity, hyperglycemia and lipid dystrophy.

The table on the following page presents antiretroviral medications used for HIV disease, which may interact with a number of drugs prescribed by dentists.

COMMON ANTIRETROVIRAL MEDICATIONS: DENTAL CONSIDERATIONS

GENERIC NAME	BRAND NAME(S)	INTERACTIONS WITH DRUGS IN DENTISTRY	ADVERSE EFFECTS RELEVANT TO DENTISTRY
FUSION INHIBITOR			
Enfuvirtide (T-20)	Fuzeon	Not available.	None noted.
NUCLEOSIDE REVERSE TRANSCRIPTASE INHIBITORS (NRTIs)			
Abacavir (ABC)	Ziagen	Not available.	Xerostomia.
Abacavir/lamivudine/zidovudine	Trizivir	Not available.	Anemia, neutropenia.
Didanosine (ddI)	Videx	Reduces efficacy of itraconazole and ketoconazole, so these drugs should be administered more than 2 hrs apart from ddI administration. Reduces efficacy of quinolone and tetracyclines, so these drugs should be administered 2 hrs before or 6 hrs after ddI administration.	Peripheral neuropathy, xerostomia.
Lamivudine (3TC)	Epivir	Not available.	None noted.
Stavudine (d4T)	Zerit	Not available.	Peripheral neuropathy.
Zalcitabine (ddC)	Hivid	Not available.	Peripheral neuropathy, oral ulcerations.
Zidovudine (AZT, ZDV)	Retrovir	Not available.	Anemia, neutropenia.
Zidovudine/lamivudine	Combivir	Not available.	Anemia, neutropenia.
NON-NUCLEOSIDE REVERSE TRANSCRIPTASE INHIBITORS (NNRTIs)			
Delavirdine (DLV)	Rescriptor	Inhibits cytochrome p-450 enzymes. Levels decreased by phenobarbitol. Increases levels of clarithromycin, dapsone. Administration of buffered medications should be avoided within 2 hrs of delavirdine administration. Contraindicated for concomitant administration with midazolam.	Stevens-Johnson syndrome (rare).
Efavirenz (EFV)	Sustiva	Induces cytochrome p-450 enzymes. Increases levels of clarithromycin. Concurrent use with midazolam, triazolam and clarithromycin should be avoided.	Hallucinations, xerostomia.
Nevirapine (NVP)	Viramune	Induces cytochrome p-450 enzymes.	Stevens-Johnson syndrome (rare).
NUCLEOTIDE REVERSE TRANSCRIPTASE INHIBITORS			
Adefovir	Preveon	Not available.	Anemia.
Tenofovir (TDF)	Viread	Not available.	None noted.

*Protease inhibitors have been associated with reactivation of hepatitis, diabetes mellitus and diminished response to narcotics.

GENERIC NAME	BRAND NAME(S)	INTERACTIONS WITH DRUGS IN DENTISTRY	ADVERSE EFFECTS RELEVANT TO DENTISTRY
PROTEASE INHIBITORS*			
Amprenavir (APV)	Agenerase	Not available.	Perioral paresthesia, Stevens-Johnson syndrome (rare).
Indinavir (IDV)	Crixivan	Inhibits cytochrome p-450 enzymes. Avoid concurrent use with midazolam and triazolam. Levels increased by ketoconazole.	Thrombocytopenia, chapped lips, metallic taste, dry mouth.
Lopinavir/ritonavir	Kaletra	Not available.	None noted.
Nelfinavir (NFV)	Viracept	Inhibits cytochrome p-450 enzymes. Avoid concurrent use with midazolam and triazolam. Levels increased by ketoconazole.	None noted.
Ritonavir (RTV)	Norvir	Inhibits cytochrome p-450 enzymes (potent). Increases levels of clarithromycin. Decreases levels of trimethoprim-sulfamethoxazole. Contraindicated for concomitant administration with diazepam, meperidine, midazolam, piroxicam, propoxyphene.	Dysgeusia, perioral parasthesia.
Saquinavir (SQV)	Fortovase, Invirase	Inhibits cytochrome p-450 enzymes. Levels decreased by dexamethasone.	None noted.
RIBONUCLEOTIDE REDUCTASE INHIBITOR			
Hydroxyurea	Hydrea	Not available.	Bone marrow suppression, oral ulcerations.

Sample Prescriptions and Prescription Abbreviations

Sample Prescriptions

The following prescriptions are not all-inclusive; they are provided only as examples of prescriptions commonly written by dentists. Drugs are listed by generic name in these examples. Those listed as drug combinations are available under a variety of brand names. Selection of any particular drug for inclusion in these examples in no way indicates recommendation of that agent over another.

The last table in this appendix shows abbreviations for prescription directions. However, if in doubt, write out the full directions.

ANTIBIOTICS FOR PATIENTS REQUIRING ANTIBIOTIC PREMEDICATION

DRUG	NUMBER	DIRECTIONS	ABBREVIATED DIRECTIONS
Penicillin			
Amoxicillin 500 mg	4	Sig: 4 capsules 1 hour before procedure	Sig: 4 caps 1 h ā procedure
For patients allergic to penicillins			
Clindamycin HCl 150 mg	4	Sig: 4 capsules 1 hour before procedure	Sig: 4 caps 1 h ā procedure
Cephalexin 500 mg*	4	Sig: 4 capsules 1 hour before procedure	Sig: 4 caps 1 h ā procedure
Azithromycin 250 mg	2	Sig: 2 capsules 1 hour before procedure	Sig: 2 caps 1 h ā procedure
Clarithromycin 500 mg	1	Sig: 1 tablet 1 hour before procedure	Sig: 1 tab 1 h ā procedure

*Do not use cephalosporins in patients with a history of recent, severe or immediate-type hypersensitivity reaction (urticaria, angioedema, or anaphylaxis) to penicillins.

TO REDUCE EXCESS SALIVATION

DRUG	NUMBER	DIRECTIONS	ABBREVIATED DIRECTIONS
Atropine sulfate 0.4 mg	9	Sig: 1-2 tablets 1 hour before procedure	Sig: 1-2 tab 1 h ā procedure
Propantheline bromide 15 mg	6	Sig: 1-2 tablets 1 hour before procedure	Sig: 1-2 tab 1 h ā procedure

TO INCREASE SALIVATION

DRUG	NUMBER	DIRECTIONS	ABBREVIATED DIRECTIONS
Cevimeline HCl 30 mg	90	Sig: 1 tab three times daily	Sig: 1 tab tid
Pilocarpine 5 mg	30	Sig: 1-2 tablets three times daily	Sig: 1-2 tab tid

TO REDUCE PATIENT ANXIETY BEFORE A DENTAL PROCEDURE

DRUG	NUMBER	DIRECTIONS	ABBREVIATED DIRECTIONS
Diazepam 5 mg	V	Sig: 1-2 tablets 1 hour before sleep; 1-2 tablets 1 hour before procedure	Sig: 1-2 tab 1 hs; 1-2 tab 1 h ā procedure
Lorazepam 1 mg	V	Sig: 1-2 tablets 1 hour before sleep; 1-2 tablets 1-2 hours before procedure	Sig: 1-2 tab 1 hs; 1-2 tab 1-2 h ā procedure
Triazolam 0.25 mg	V	Sig: 1 tablet ½ hour before sleep; 1 tablet ½-1 hour before procedure	Sig: 1 tab ½ hs; 1 tab ½-1 h ā procedure
Hydroxyzine pamoate 50 mg	V	Sig: 2 tablets 1 hour before sleep; 1-2 tablets 1 hour before procedure	Sig: 2 tabs 1 hs; 1-2 tab 1 h ā procedure

V: Varies with number of appointments.

FOR ANALGESIA

DRUG	NUMBER	DIRECTIONS	ABBREVIATED DIRECTIONS
For mild-to-moderate pain			
Ibuprofen 400 mg	18	Sig: 1 tablet every 4-6 hours as needed; maximum daily dose 8 tablets	Sig: 1 tab q 4-6 h for pain; MDD 8 tab
Acetaminophen with codeine #3 (30 mg)	24	Sig: 1-2 tablets every 4 hours as needed for pain; maximum daily dose 12 tablets, acetaminophen 4,000 mg	Sig: 1-2 tab q 4 h for pain; MDD 12 tab, acetaminophen 4,000 mg
Ketoprofen 25 mg or 50 mg	12	Sig: 1 tablet every 6-8 hours as needed; maximum daily dose 300 mg	Sig: 1 tab q 6-8 h for pain; MDD 300 mg
For moderate-to-severe pain (unresponsive to NSAIDs)			
Hydrocodone bitartrate 5 mg and acetaminophen 500 mg, 650 mg or 750 mg	18	Sig: 1-2 tablets every 4-6 hours; maximum daily dose 8 tablets, acetaminophen 4,000 mg	Sig: 1-2 tab q 4-6 h; MDD 8 tab, acetaminophen 4,000 mg
Oxycodone HCl 5 mg and acetaminophen 325 mg or 500 mg	18	Sig: 1-2 tablets every 6 hours; maximum daily dose 8 tablets, acetaminophen 4,000 mg	Sig: 1-2 tab q 6 h; MDD 8 tab, acetaminophen 4,000 mg
For severe pain (unresponsive to opioid combinations)			
Hydromorphone HCl 2 mg	30	Sig: 1-2 tablets every 4-6 hours as needed for pain; maximum daily dose 8 tablets	Sig: 1-2 tab q 4-6 h for pain; MDD 8 tab

FOR INFECTIONS IN THE MOUTH AND ADJACENT TISSUES

DRUG	NUMBER	DIRECTIONS	ABBREVIATED DIRECTIONS
Penicillin V potassium 500 mg	30	Sig: 2 tablets at once, then 1 tablet every 6 hours until gone	Sig: 2 tabs stat, then 1 tab q 6 h until gone
Amoxicillin 500 mg	30	Sig: 1 capsule every 8 hours until gone	Sig: 1 cap q 8 h until gone
Metronidazole 250 mg	28	Sig: Take 1 tablet every 6 hours until gone	Sig: 1 tab q 6 h until gone
Clindamycin HCl 150 mg	28	Sig: Take 1 capsule every 6 hours until gone	Sig: 1 cap q 6 h until gone
Erythromycin stearate 250 mg	30	Sig: 1 tablet every 6 hours until gone	Sig: 1 tab q 6 h until gone
Doxycycline HCl 100 mg	15	Sig: 1 capsule twice on day one; 1 capsule once daily until gone	Sig: 1 cap bid day one; 1 cap d until gone
Tetracycline HCl 250 mg	40	Sig: 1 capsule every 6 hours until gone	Sig: 1 cap q 6 h until gone
Cephalexin 250 mg	30	Sig: 1 capsule every 6 hours until gone	Sig: 1 cap q 6 h until gone

FOR ORAL CANDIDIASIS

DRUG	NUMBER	DIRECTIONS	ABBREVIATED DIRECTIONS
Nystatin oral suspension 100,000 units/mL	480 mL	Sig: Rinse for 2 minutes and swallow one teaspoonful four times daily until symptoms disappear	Sig: one teaspoonful qid, rinse 2 min and swallow
Chlorhexidine 0.12 %	16 oz	Sig: 0.5 oz twice a day as a rinse until symptoms disappear	Sig: 0.5 oz bid as rinse
Clotrimazole troche 10mg	70	Sig: 1 troche by mouth five times daily until symptoms disappear	Sig: 1 troche po 5 times d

FOR ANGULAR CHEILITIS (FUNGAL ETIOLOGY)

DRUG	NUMBER	DIRECTIONS	ABBREVIATED DIRECTIONS
Nystatin 100,000 units/g ointment	15-g tube	Sig: Apply to lesion 4 times a day until healing occurs	Sig: Apply to lesion qid until healing occurs
Nystatin 100,000 units/g and triamcinolone 0.1% ointment	15-g tube	Sig: Apply to lesion 2-3 times a day until healing occurs	Sig: Apply to lesion bid-tid until healing occurs

FOR MILD-TO-MODERATE LICHEN PLANUS, PEMPHIGUS VULGARIS, OR MUCOUS MEMBRANE PEMPHIGOID

DRUG	NUMBER	DIRECTIONS	ABBREVIATED DIRECTIONS
Fluocinonide gel 0.05%	15 g	Sig: Apply with cotton swab to affected areas twice daily	Sig: Apply c̄ cotton swab bid

FOR MILD ALLERGIC REACTIONS

DRUG	NUMBER	DIRECTIONS	ABBREVIATED DIRECTIONS
Diphenhydramine HCl 50 mg	30	Sig: 1 capsule every 6 hours as needed	Sig: 1 cap qid prn

FOR HERPETIC INFECTIONS

DRUG	NUMBER	DIRECTIONS	ABBREVIATED DIRECTIONS
Penciclovir 1% cream	2-g tube	Sig: Apply to affected area every 2 hours while awake	Sig: Apply q 2 h while awake

PRESCRIPTION ABBREVIATIONS

ABBREVIATION	TERM
$\bar{a}$	before
ac	before meals
aq, H_2O	water
bid	2 times a day
$\bar{c}$, c	with
cap	capsule
d	day
gtt	drops
h	hour
hs, HS, hor som	at bedtime
non rep, nr, NR	do not repeat
pc	after eating
po	by mouth
prn	as needed
qh	each hour
qid	4 times a day
$\bar{s}$, sine	without
sig	write on the label
$\overline{ss}$, ss	one-half
stat	immediately
tab	tablet
tid	3 times a day

Drugs That Cause Photosensitivity

B. Ellen Byrne, R.Ph., D.D.S., Ph.D.

Photosensitivity reactions may be caused by systemic or topical drugs, perfumes, cosmetics or sunscreens. Even brief exposures to sunlight in warm or cold weather can cause intense cutaneous reactions in patients with drug-induced photosensitivity. Individual sensitivity varies widely.

Suggested Readings

Allen JE. Drug-induced photosensitivity. Clin Pharm 1993;12:580-7.

Anderson PO, Knoben JE, Troutman WG. Handbook of clinical drug data 1997-1998. 8th ed. New York: McGraw-Hill Professional Publishing; 1999.

Drugs that may cause photosensitivity. Pharmacist's Letter PHARM-FaxBACK document no. 120617. Available from: Pharmacist's Letter, 2453 Grand Canal Blvd., Suite A, P.O. Box 8190, Stockton, Calif. 95203, by subscription.

Physicians' Desk Reference. 60th ed. Montvale, NJ: Thomson PDR; 2006.

Moore DE. Drug-induced cutaneous photosensitivity: incidence, mechanism, prevention and management. Drug Saf 2002;25:345-72.

DRUGS THAT CAUSE PHOTOSENSITIVITY

BRAND NAME (GENERIC NAME)

Abilify (apripiprazole)	Altoprev (lovastatin)	Bactrim (sulfamethoxazole/ trimethoprim)
Accupril (quinapril)	Amaryl (glimepiride)	Benadryl (diphenhydramine)
Accuretic (quinapril/hydrochloro-thiazide)	Ambien (zolpidem)	Benicar HCT (olmesartan medoxomil/hydrochlorothiazide)
Accutane (isotretinoin)	Amerge (naratriptan)	Betapace (sotalol)
Aciphex (rabeprazole sodium)	Amnesteem (isotretinoin)	Betapace AF (sotalol)
Adalat CC (nifedipine)	Anaprox (naproxen sodium)	Betaseron (interferon beta-1b)
Advicor (lovastatin/niacin)	Ancobon (flucytosine)	Bextra (valdecoxib)
Agrylin (anagrelide)	Aralen (chloroquine)	Bromfed-DM (brompheniramine/ dextromethorphan/pseudoephed-rine)
Alacol DM (brompheniramine/ dextromethorphan/phenylephrine)	Arthrotec (diclofenac sodium/ misoprostol)	
Aldactazide (hydrochlorothiazide/ spironolactone)	Atacand HCT (candesartan/ hydrochlorothiazide)	Caduet (amlodipine/atorvastatin)
Aldara (imiquimod)	Avalide (irbesartan/hydrochloro-thiazide)	Campral (acamprosate)
Aldoril (methyldopa/hydrochloro-thiazide)	Avelox (moxifloxacin)	Capoten (captopril)
Alferon-N (interferon alfa-n3 [human leukocyte derived])	Avonex (interferon beta-1a)	Capozide (captopril/hydrochloro-thiazide)
Altace (ramipril)	Axert (almotriptan)	Carbatrol (carbamazepine)
	Azmacort (triamcinolone)	Cardizem (diltiazem)
	Azulfidine (sulfasalazine)	

DRUGS THAT CAUSE PHOTOSENSITIVITY *(cont.)*

BRAND NAME (GENERIC NAME) *(cont.)*

Cataflam (diclofenac potassium)
Celebrex (celecoxib)
Celexa (citalopram)
Cerebyx (fosphenytoin)
Cipro (ciprofloxacin)
Claritin (loratadine)
Claritin-D (loratadine/
    pseudoephedrine)
Clinoril (sulindac)
Clorpres (clonidine/chlorthalidone)
Clozaril (clozapine)
Compazine (prochlorperazine)
Compro (prochlorperazine)
Copaxone (glatiramer)
Cordarone (amiodarone)
Coreg (carvedilol)
Corzide (bendroflumethiazide/
    nadolol)
Corzide (nadolol/bendroflumethia-
    zide)
Cozaar (losartan)
Crestor (rosuvastatin)
Cymbalta (duloxetine)
Cyproheptadine (cyproheptadine)
D.H.E. 45 (dihydroergotamine)
Dantrium (dantrolene)
Daypro (oxaprozin)
Declomycin (demeclocycline)
Depacon (valproate)
Depakene (valproic acid)
Depakote (divalproex)
DiaBeta (glyburide)
Diabinese (chlorpropamide)
Diamox (acetazolamide)
Diovan HCT (valsartan/hydrochlo-
    rothiazide)
Dipentum (olsalazine)
Diuril (chlorothiazide)
Dolobid (diflunisal)
Doryx (doxycycline hyclate)
DTIC-Dome (dacarbazine)
Dyazide (triamterene/hydrochloro-
    thiazide)
Dynacin (minocycline)
Dyrenium (triamterene)
EC-Naprosyn (naproxen)
Effexor (venlafaxine)
Efudex (fluorouracil)

Elavil (amitriptyline)
Eldepryl (selegiline)
Ellence (epirubicin)
Elmiron (pentosan polysulfate)
Enduron (methyclothiazide)
Estrogel (estradiol)
Eulexin (flutamide)
Evoxac (cevimeline)
Factive (gemifloxacin mesylate)
Fazaclo (clozapine)
Felbatol (felbamate)
Feldene (piroxicam)
Flexeril (cyclobenzaprine)
Floxin (ofloxacin)
Fortovase (saquinavir)
Fosamax (alendronate)
Fulvicin P/G (griseofulvin)
Gabitril (tiagabine)
Garamycin (gentamicin)
Gastrocrom (cromolyn sodium)
Geodon (ziprasidone)
Gleevec (imatinib mesylate)
Glucotrol (glipizide)
Glucovance (glyburide/metformin
    HCl)
Glynase (glyburide)
Grifulvin (griseofulvin)
Gris-PEG (griseofulvin)
Gynodiol (estradiol)
Haldol (haloperidol)
Helidac (bismuth/metronidazole/
    tetracycline)
Hibistat (chlorhexidine gluconate)
Hivid (zalcitabine)
Hydra-zide (hydralazine/hydrochlo-
    rothiazide)
HydroDIURIL (hydrochlorothiazide)
Hydroflumethiazide (hydroflume-
    thiazide)
Hyzaar (losartan/hydrochlorothia-
    zide)
Imitrex (sumatriptan)
Inderide (hydrochlorothiazide/
    propranolol)
Intron A (interferon alfa-2b,
    recombinant)
Invirase (saquinavir mesylate)
Kerastick (aminolevulinic acid)

Kira (St. John's wort [*Hypericum*])
Lamictal (lamotrigine)
Lasix (furosemide)
Lescol (fluvastatin)
Levamisole (levamisole)
Levitra (vardenafil)
Levulan (aminolevulinic acid)
Lexxel (enalapril/felodipine)
Limbitrol (amitriptyline/chlordiaz-
    epoxide)
Lipitor (atorvastatin)
Lodine (etodolac)
Lofibra (fenofibrate)
Lopid (gemfibrozil)
Lotensin (benazepril)
Lotensin HCT (benazepril/
    hydrochlorothiazide)
Lozol (indapamide)
Lunesta (eszopiclone)
Lupron (leuprolide)
Luvox (fluvoxamine)
Malarone (atovaquone/proguanil)
Maprotiline (maprotiline)
Maxalt (rizatriptan)
Maxaquin (lomefloxacin)
Maxzide (triamterene/hydrochloro-
    thiazide)
Mellaril (thioridazine hydrochloride)
Meridia (sibutramine)
Mevacor (lovastatin)
Micardis HCT (telmisartan/
    hydrochlorothiazide)
Micronase (glyburide)
Microzide (hydrochlorothiazide)
Minizide (polythiazide/prazosin)
Minocin (minocycline)
Mobic (meloxicam)
Moduretic (amiloride/hydrochloro-
    thiazide)
Monodox (doxycycline
    monohydrate)
Monopril (fosinopril)
Monopril HCT (hydrochlorothiazide/
    fosinopril)
8-MOP (methoxsalen)
Motrin (ibuprofen)
Mykrox (metolazone)
Nalidixic acid (nalidixic acid)

BRAND NAME (GENERIC NAME) *(cont.)*

Naprelan (naproxen sodium)
Naprosyn (naproxen)
Navane (thiothixene)
Neurontin (gabapentin)
Nipent (pentostatin)
Noroxin (norfloxacin)
Norpramin (desipramine)
Norvir (ritonavir)
One-A-Day Tension & Mood (St. John's wort [*Hypericum*]/vitamin B₁/vitamin C/kava-kava)
Oretic (hydrochlorothiazide)
Orudis (ketoprofen)
Oruvail (ketoprofen)
Oxsoralen (methoxsalen)
Pacerone (amiodarone)
Palgic-D (carbinoxamine/ pseudoephedrine)
Palgic-DS (carbinoxamine/ pseudoephedrine)
Pamelor (nortriptyline)
Panretin (alitretinoin)
Parsnip (pastinaca sativa)
Paxil (paroxetine)
Pediatex-D (carbinoxamine/ pseudoephedrine)
Pediazole (erythromycin/ sulfisoxazole)
Pentasa (mesalamine)
Periostat (doxycycline hyclate)
Perphenazine (perphenazine)
Phenergan (promethazine)
pHisoHex (hexachlorophene)
Photofrin (porfimer sodium)
Plaquenil (hydroxychloroquine)
Ponstel (mefenamic acid)
Pravachol (pravastatin)
Pravigard PAC (buffered aspirin/ pravastatin)
Prinivil (lisinopril)
Prinivil (lisinorpil/hydrochlorothia- zide)
Prinzide (hydrochlorothiazide/ lisinopril)
Procardia (nifedipine)
Prograf (tacrolimus)
Prolixin (fluphenazine)
ProSom (estazolam)

Protonix (pantoprazole)
Protopic (tacrolimus)
Prozac (fluoxetine)
Pyrazinamide (pyrazinamide)
Quinidex (quinidine sulfate)
Quinidine (quinidine gluconate)
Relafen (nabumetone)
Remeron (mirtazapine)
Renese (polythiazide)
Requip (ropinirole)
Retin-A (tretinoin)
Reyataz (atazanavir)
Rifater (isoniazid/pyrazinamide/ rifampin)
Rilutek (riluzole)
Risperdal (risperidone)
Risperdal Consta (risperidone)
Roxicodone (oxycodone)
Rue (*Ruta graveolens*)
Rynatan (chlorpheniramine/ phenylephrine/pyrilamine)
Salagen (pilocarpine)
Sarafem (fluoxetine)
Septra (sulfamethoxazole/ trimethoprim)
Seroquel (quetiapine)
Serostim (somatropin)
Serzone (nefazodone)
Sinequan (doxepin)
Sonata (zaleplon)
Soriatane (acitretin)
Sporanox (itraconazole)
St. John's wort (*Hypericum*)
Sterile FUDR (floxuridine)
Sular (nisoldipine)
Sumycin (tetracycline)
Surmontil (trimipramine)
Symbyax (olanzapine/fluoxetine)
Targretin (bexarotene)
Tavist (clemastine)
Tazorac (tazarotene)
Tegretol (carbamazepine)
Tegretol-XR (carbamazepine)
Tenoretic (atenolol/chlorthalidone)
Tequin (gatifloxacin)
Terramycin (oxytetracycline)
Teveten HCT (eprosartan mesylate/ hydrochlorothiazide)

Thalitone (chlorthalidone)
Thalomid (thalidomide)
Thorazine (chlorpromazine)
Tiazac (diltiazem)
Timolide (hydrochlorothiazide/ timolol)
Tofranil (imipramine)
Tolazamide (tolazamide)
Tolbutamide (tolbutamide)
Topamax (topiramate)
Trecator-SC (ethionamide)
Trexall (methotrexate)
Triavil (amitriptyline/perphenazine)
Tricor (fenofibrate)
Trifluoperazine (trifluoperazine)
Trileptal (oxcarbazepine)
Trinalin (azatadine/pseudoephed- rine)
Trovan (trovafloxacin)
Tussend (chlorpheniramine/ hydrocodone/pseudoephedrine)
Uniretic (moexipril/hydrochloro- thiazide)
Univasc (moexipril)
Uvadex (methoxsalen)
Valtrex (valacyclovir)
Vaseretic (enalapril/hydrochloro- thiazide)
Vasotec (enalapril)
Vasotec I.V. (enalaprilat)
Vfend (voriconazole)
Viagra (sildenafil)
Vibramycin (doxycycline hyclate)
Vibra-Tabs (doxycycline hyclate)
Vinblastine (vinblastine)
Vistide (cidofovir)
Visudyne (verteporfin)
Vivactil (protriptyline)
Voltaren (diclofenac sodium)
Vytorin (simvastatin/ezetimibe)
Wellbutrin (bupropion)
Xeloda (capecitabine)
Zaroxolyn (metolazone)
Zestoretic (hydrochlorothiazide/ lisinopril)
Zestoretic (lisinorpil/hydrochloro- thiazide)
Zestril (lisinopril)

DRUGS THAT CAUSE PHOTOSENSITIVITY *(cont.)*

BRAND NAME (GENERIC NAME) *(cont.)*

Ziac (bisoprolol/hydrochlorothiazide)	Zomig (zolmitriptan)	Zyrtec (cetirizine)
Zithromax (azithromycin)	Zovirax (acyclovir)	Zyrtec-D (cetirizine/pseudoephedrine)
Zocor (simvastatin)	Zyban (bupropion)	
Zoloft (sertraline)	Zyprexa (olanzapine)	

General Anesthetics

Inhalation and general anesthetics are used to induce and maintain general anesthesia. Despite dentists' decreasing need to rely on general anesthesia, its use may be indicated for patients who:

- Are extremely anxious or fearful.
- Are mentally or physically challenged, or both.
- Are too young to cooperate with the dentist.
- Fail to respond to local anesthesia.
- Are undergoing stressful, traumatic procedures.

Selected agents have also been approved for use in providing sedation and analgesia for specific procedures that do not require general anesthesia. General anesthetics have a narrow margin of safety, and their administration must be individualized (titrated) according to the desired depth of anesthesia, the concomitant use of other medications and the patient's physical condition, age, size and body temperature.

The following tables provide dosing information and clinically significant drug interactions for general anesthetics.

PRESCRIBING INFORMATION FOR GENERAL ANESTHETICS

NAME	FORM/ STRENGTH	DOSAGE	WARNINGS/PRECAUTIONS & CONTRAINDICATIONS	ADVERSE EFFECTS
Etomidate (Amidate)	Inj: 2mg/mL	*Adults:* 0.2-0.6mg/kg IV. **Usual:** 0.3mg/kg IV, over 30 to 60 seconds. *Pediatrics:* **>10 yrs:** 0.2-0.6mg/kg IV. **Usual:** 0.3mg/kg IV, over 30 to 60 seconds.	**W/P:** Not for prolonged infusion. Reduction of plasma cortisol and aldosterone concentrations have occurred; consider exogenous replacement during severely stressful conditions. **P/N:** Category C, caution in nursing.	Transient venous pain, transient skeletal muscle movements, including myoclonus, hyper/hypoventilation, apnea of short duration, hyper/hypotension, tachycardia, bradycardia.
Methohexital Sodium (Brevital Sodium)	Inj: 500mg, 2.5g	*Adults:* **Individualize dose. Induction:** 1% solution administered at a rate of 1mL/5 seconds. **Range:** 50-120mg or more (average: 70mg). **Usual:** 1-1.5mg/kg. **Maint: Intermittent:** 20-40mg (2 to 4mL of a 1% solution) q 4-7 minutes. **Continuous Drip:** Average rate of administration is 3mL of a 0.2% solution/minute (1 drop/second). *Pediatrics:* **≥1 month: Individualize Dose: Induction: IM:** 6.6 to 10mg/kg IM of the 5% concentration. **Rectal:** 25mg/kg rectally of the 1% solution.	Should be used only in hospital or ambulatory care settings that provide for continuous monitoring of respiratory and cardiac function. Immediate avail ability of resuscitative drugs and age- and size-appropriate equipment for bag/valve/mask ventilation and intubation and personnel trained in their use and skilled in airway management should be assured. For deeply sedated patients, a designated individual other than the practitioner performing the procedure should be present to continuously monitor the patient. **W/P:** Seizures may be elicited in patients with previous history of convulsive activity. Caution in severe hepatic dysfunction, severe cardiovascular instability, shock-like condition, asthma, COPD, severe HTN or hypotension, MI, CHF, severe	Circulatory depression, thrombophlebitis, hypotension, tachycardia, respiratory depression, skeletal muscle hypersensitivity (twitching), emergence delirium.

PRESCRIBING INFORMATION FOR GENERAL ANESTHETICS *(cont.)*

NAME	FORM/STRENGTH	DOSAGE	WARNINGS/PRECAUTIONS & CONTRAINDICATIONS	ADVERSE EFFECTS
Methohexital Sodium *(cont.)*			anemia, status asthmaticus, extreme obesity, debilitated patients or those with impaired function of respiratory, circulatory, renal, hepatic, or endocrine system. Unintended intra-arterial injection may produce platelet aggregates and thrombosis at the site of injection. **Contra:** Patients with latent or manifest porphyria. **P/N:** Category B, caution in nursing.	
Propofol (Diprivan)	**Inj:** 10mg/mL	***Adults:* General Anesthesia: <55 yrs:** 40mg IV every 10 seconds until induction onset. **Maint:** 100-200µg/kg/min IV or 20-50mg intermittently by IV bolus prn. **Elderly/Debilitated/ASA III & IV:** 20mg IV every 10 seconds until induction onset. **Maint:** 50-100µg/kg/min IV. **Cardiac Anesthesia:** 20mg IV every 10 seconds until induction onset. **Maint:** 100-150µg/kg/min IV with secondary opioid or 50-100µg/kg/min IV with primary opioid. **Neurosurgical Patients:** 20mg IV every 10 seconds until induction onset. **Maint:** 100-200µg/kg/min IV. **MAC Sedation:** 100-150µg/kg/min IV infusion or 0.5mg/kg slow IV injection over 3-5 min followed immediately by maintenance infusion. **Maint:** 25-75µg/kg/min IV infusion or 10-20mg incremental IV boluses. **Elderly/Debilitated/ASA III & IV:** Use doses similar to healthy adults. Avoid rapid boluses. **Maint:** 80% of the usual adult dose. **ICU Sedation: Initial:** 5µg/kg/min IV infusion for 5 min. Increase 5-10µg/kg/min IV over 5-10 min. **Maint:** 5-50µg/kg/min IV or higher may be required. ***Pediatrics:* 3-16 yrs: General Anesthesia:** 2.5-3.5mg/kg IV over 20-30 seconds. **Maint: 2 months-16 yrs:** 125-300µg/kg/min IV.	**W/P:** Avoid rapid bolus administration in elderly, debilitated or ASA III/IV patients. Monitor oxygen saturation and for signs of significant hypotension, bradycardia, cardiovascular depression, apnea or airway obstruction. Caution with hyperlipoproteinemia, diabetic hyperlipemia, pancreatitis, epilepsy. Rare reports of anaphylaxis reactions, pulmonary edema, perioperative myoclonia, postoperative pancreatitis, bradycardia, asystole, cardiac arrest, rhabdomyolysis. Minimize transient local pain by using larger veins of forearm or antecubital fossa and/or prior lidocaine injection. May elevate serum TG. Do not infuse for >5 days without drug holiday to replace zinc losses; consider supplemental zinc with chronic use in those predisposed to zinc deficiency. In renal impairment, perform baseline urinalysis/urinary sediment then monitor on alternate days during sedation. (Neurosurgical Anesthesia) Use infusion or slow bolus to avoid significant hypotension and decreases in cerebral perfusion pressure. (Cardiac Anesthesia) Use slower rates of administration in premedicated and geriatric in premedicated and geriatric patients, patients with recent fluid shifts or those hemodynamically unstable. Correct fluid deficits prior to use. **P/N:** Category B, not for use in nursing.	Bradycardia, arrhythmia, hypotension, HTN, tachycardia nodal, decreased cardiac output, CNS movement, injection site burning/stinging/pain, hyperlipemia, apnea, rash, pruritus, respiratory acidosis during weaning.
Enflurane (Ethrane)	**Inhalation Sol:** 99.9 %	***Adults:* Analgesia for Labor/Delivery:** 0.25-1% concentration. **General Anesthesia: Initial:** 2-4.5% concentration via vaporizer; with oxygen or combination with oxygen-nitrous oxide mixtures. **Maint:** 0.5-3% concentration. **Max:** 3%. **Patients: General Anesthesia:** Dosage must be individualized; **(5-14 yr)** 2% concentration; (very young or very apprehensive) 3-4% concentration.	**W/P:** Patients considered more susceptible to cortical stimulation produced by enflurane, action of nondepolarizing relaxants augmented by influrane, caution in pregnancy, close monitoring of patients with renal or hepatic dysfunction, may cause decrease in intellectual function for 2-3 days following anesthesia, increasing depth of anesthesia associated with changes in EEG which may or may not be associated with motor movement. **Contra:** Malignant hyperthermia (history of or suspected genetic susceptibility), seizure disorders. **P/N:** Category B, safety in nursing not known.	Cardiac dysrhythmia, hypotension, seizure, nausea, vomiting, involuntary movement, shivering.
Isoflurane	**Liq:** 100mL, 250mL	***Adults:* Induction:** 1.5-3%. **Maint:** 1-2.5% with concomitant nitrous oxide or an additional 0.5-1% may be required when used with oxygen.	**W/P:** Hypotension and respiratory depression increase as anesthesia is deepened. Increased blood loss comparable to that seen with halothane reported	Respiratory depression, hypotension, arrhythmias, shivering, nausea, vomiting, ileus.

NAME	FORM/ STRENGTH	DOSAGE	WARNINGS/PRECAUTIONS & CONTRAINDICATIONS	ADVERSE EFFECTS
Isoflurane *(cont.)*			in patients undergoing abortions. May cause a reversible rise in CSF pressure. May cause sensitivity hepatitis in patients sensitized by previous exposure to halogenated anesthetics. May cause a slight decrease in intellectual function for 2-3 days post-anesthesia. May cause small mood changes and symptoms may persist for up to 6 days post-administration. Transient increases in BSP retention, blood glucose, and serum creatinine with decrease in BUN, serum cholesterol, and alkaline phosphatase reported. **Contra:** Genetic susceptibility to malignant hyperthermia. **P/N:** Category C, caution in nursing.	
Halothane	**Liq:** 125mL, 250mL	**Adults:** Individualize dose. **Maint:** 0.5-1.5%.	**W/P:** Not for use in women where pregnancy is possible and particularly during early pregnancy unless potential benefits outweigh unknown hazards to fetus. Increases CSF pressure; caution with raised intracranial pressure. **Contra:** Obstetrical anesthesia except when uterine relaxation is required. **P/N:** Safety in pregnancy and nursing not known.	Hepatic necrosis, cardiac arrest, hypotension, respiratory arrest, cardiac arrhythmias, hyperpyrexia, shivering, nausea, emesis.
Ketamine Hydrochloride	**Inj:** 50mg/mL	**Adults: Initial: IV:** 1-4.5mg/kg. Infuse slowly over 60 seconds. May administer with 2-5mg doses of diazepam over 60 seconds. **IM:** 6.5-13mg/kg. **Maint:** Adjust according to anesthetic needs. May increase in increments of one-half to full induction dose. **Pediatrics: Initial: IV:** 1-4.5mg/kg. Infuse slowly over 60 seconds. **IM:** 6.5-13mg/kg. **Maint:** Adjust according to anesthetic needs. May increase in increments of one-half to full induction dose.	**W/P:** Monitor cardiac function in patients with hypertension or cardiac dysfunction. Postoperative confusional states may occur during recovery. Respiratory depression may occur; maintain airway and respiration. Do not use alone in pharynx, larynx, or bronchial tree procedures. Use with caution in chronic alcoholics and acutely intoxicated patients. May increase cerebrospinal fluid pressure; use with extreme caution in patients with preanesthetic cerebrospinal fluid pressure. Use with agent that obtunds visceral pain when surgical procedure involving visceral pain. **Contra:** Patients in whom a significant elevation in blood pressure would constitute a serious hazard. **P/N:** Not recommended with pregnancy, use in nursing unknown.	Nausea, vomiting, anorexia, elevated blood pressure and pulse, hypotension, bradycardia, arrhythmia, respiratory depression, apnea, airway obstruction, diplopia, nystagmus, slight elevation of IOP, enhanced skeletal muscle tone.
Thiopental Sodium	**Inj:** 20mg/mL, 25mg/mL	**Adults: Individualize dose. IV: Test Dose:** 25-75mg. **Anesthesia:** 50-75mg at 20-40 second intervals. Once anesthesia is established, additional injections of 25-50mg may be given whenever patient moves. **Induction in Balanced Anesthesia: Initial:** 3-4mg/kg. **Convulsive States:** Following anesthesia, give 75-125mg as soon as possible after convulsion begins. Convulsions following use of local anesthetic may require 125-250mg over 10 minute period. **Neurosurgical Patients With Increased Intracranial Pressure:** 1.5-3.5mg/kg bolus. **Psychiatric Disorders:** After test dose, infuse at 100mg/min with patient counting backwards from 100;	**W/P:** Avoid extravasation or intra-arterial injection. May be habit forming. Reduce dose and administer slowly with relative contraindications. Caution with advanced cardiac disease, increased intracranial pressure, ophthalmoplegia plus, asthma, myasthenia gravis, and endocrine insufficiency (pituitary, thyroid, adrenal, pancreas). **Contra:** (Absolute) Absence of suitable veins for IV administration, variegate porphyria (South Africa) or acute intermittent porphyria. (Relative) Severe cardiovascular disease, hypotension, shock, conditions in which the hypnotic effect may be prolonged or potentiated (excessive premedication, Addison's disease, hepatic/renal dysfunction, myxedema, increased blood urea, severe anemia,	Respiratory/myocardial depression, cardiac arrhythmias, prolonged somnolence and recovery, sneezing, coughing, bronchospasm, laryngospasm, shivering, anaphylactic and anaphylactoid reactions.

PRESCRIBING INFORMATION FOR GENERAL ANESTHETICS *(cont.)*

NAME	FORM/ STRENGTH	DOSAGE	WARNINGS/PRECAUTIONS & CONTRAINDICATIONS	ADVERSE EFFECTS
Thiopental Sodium *(cont.)*		discontinue shortly after counting becomes confused but before actual sleep is produced.	asthma, and myasthenia gravis), and status asthmaticus. **P/N:** Category C, caution in nursing.	
Desflurane (Suprane)	**Liq:** 240mL	**Adults:** Individualize dose. **MAC Values: 70 yrs:** 5.2 with oxygen 100% or 1.7 with nitrous oxide 60%. **45 yrs:** 6 with oxygen 100% or 2.8 with nitrous oxide 60%. **25 yrs:** 7.3 with oxygen 100% or 4 with nitrous oxide 60%. **With Fentanyl or Midazolam: 31-65 yrs: No Fentanyl:** 6.3. **With 3mcg/kg Fentanyl:** 3.1. **With 6mcg/kg Fentanyl:** 2.3. **No Midazolam:** 5.9. **With Midazolam 25mcg/kg:** 4.9. **With Midazolam 50mcg/kg:** 4.9. **18-30 yrs: No Fentanyl:** 6.4. **With Fentanyl 3mcg/kg:** 3.5. **With Fentanyl 6mcg/kg:** 3. **No Midazolam:** 6.9. Pediatrics: **Individualize dose. MAC Values: 7 yrs:** 8.1 with oxygen 100%. **4 yrs:** 8.6 with oxygen 100%. **3 yrs:** 6.4 with nitrous oxide 60%. **2 yrs:** 9.1 with oxygen 100%. 9 months: 10 with oxygen 100% or 7.5 with nitrous oxide 60%. 10 weeks: 9.4 with oxygen 100%. **2 weeks:** 9.2 with oxygen 100%.	**W/P:** Not recommended for induction of general anesthesia via mask in infants or children. Produces dose-dependent decreases in BP. Concentrations >1 MAC may increase HR. Administer at 0.8 MAC or less, in conjunction with a barbiturate induction and hyperventilation. Maintain normal hemodynamics with coronary artery disease. May cause sensitivity hepatitis in patients who have been sensitized by previous exposure to halogenated anesthetics. May trigger malignant hyperthermia. May produce a dose-dependent increase in CSF pressure when administered to patients with intracranial space occupying lesions. **Contra:** Known or suspected susceptibility to malignant hyperthermia. **P/N:** Category B, caution in nursing.	Coughing, breathholding, apnea, laryngospasm, oxyhemoglobin desaturation, increased secretions, bronchospasm, nausea, vomiting.
Sevoflurane (Ultane)	**Liq:** 250mL	**Adults:** Individualize dose. **MAC Values: 40 yrs:** 2.1% sevoflurane in oxygen or 1.1% sevoflurane in 65% nitrous oxide/35% oxygen. **25 yrs:** 2.6% sevoflurane in oxygen or 1.4% sevoflurane in 65% nitrous oxide/35% oxygen. **Pediatrics:** Individualize dose. **MAC Values: 3-12 yrs:** 2.5% sevoflurane in oxygen. **6 months-<3 yrs:** 2.8% sevoflurane in oxygen or 2% sevoflurane in 65% nitrous oxide/35% oxygen. **1-<6 months:** 3% sevoflurane in oxygen. **0-1 month:** 3.3% sevoflurane in oxygen.	**W/P:** Potential for renal injury. May be associated with glycosuria and proteinuria. May cause malignant hyperthermia. May decrease BP. Rare cases of seizures have been reported. Transient changes in postoperative LFTs and very rare cases of post-operative hepatic dysfunction or hepatitis reported. Concomitant use of desiccated CO_2 absorbents (eg, potassium hydroxide) may result in rare cases of extreme heat, smoke, and/or spontaneous fire in anesthesia breathing circuit; replace CO_2 absorbent routinely. **Contra:** Susceptibility to malignant hyperthermia. **P/N:** Category B, caution in nursing.	Bradycardia, hypotension, agitation, laryngospasm, airway obstruction, breath holding, cough, tachycardia, shivering, somnolence, dizziness, increased salivation, nausea, vomiting.

DRUG INTERACTIONS FOR GENERAL ANESTHETICS

Methohexital Sodium (Brevital Sodium)

Anticoagulants	May influence the metabolism of other concomitantly used drugs, such as anticoagulants.
Barbiturates	Prior chronic administration of barbiturates may reduce the effectiveness of methohexital.
Corticosteroids	May influence the metabolism of other concomitantly used drugs, such as corticosteroids.
Ethyl alcohol	May influence the metabolism of other concomitantly used drugs, such as ethyl alcohol. Additive CNS effects with other CNS depressants.
Halothane	May influence the metabolism of other concomitantly used drugs, such as halothane.
Phenytoin	May influence the metabolism of other concomitantly used drugs, such as phenytoin. Phenytoin may reduce the effectiveness of methohexital.
Propylene alcohol	Additive CNS effects with other CNS depressants, including ethyl alcohol and propylene alcohol.
Propylene glycol	May influence the metabolism of solutions containing propylene glycol.

Propofol (Diprivan)

Fentanyl	Concomitant fentanyl may cause bradycardia in pediatrics.
Inhalational agents	Increased effects with potent inhalational agents (eg, isoflurane, enflurane, halothane).
Narcotics	Increased effects with narcotics (eg, morphine, meperidine, fentanyl).
Sedatives/ opioids	Increased effects with combinations of opioids and sedatives (eg, benzodiazepines, barbiturates, chloral hydrate, droperidol).

Enflurane (Ethrane)

Amiodarone	Increased risk of cardiotoxicity (QT prolongation, torsades de pointes, cardiac arrest).
Bretylium	Increased risk of cardiotoxicity (QT prolongation, torsades de pointes, cardiac arrest).
Cisapride	Increased risk of cardiotoxicity (QT prolongation, torsades de pointes, cardiac arrest).
Clarithromycin	Excessive prolongation of neuromuscular blocking effects of cisatracurium.
Desipramine	Increased risk of cardiotoxicity (QT prolongation, torsades de pointes, cardiac arrest) and an increased risk of seizure activity.
Doxacurium	Doxacurium toxicity (respiratory depression, apnea).
Doxepin	Increased risk of cardiotoxicity (QT prolongation, torsades de pointes, cardiac arrest) and an increased risk of seizure activity.
Imipramine	Increased risk of cardiotoxicity (QT prolongation, torsades de pointes, cardiac arrest) and an increased risk of seizure activity.
Labetalol	Hypotension and decreased cardiac output.
Nortriptyline	Increased risk of cardiotoxicity (QT prolongation, torsades de pointes, cardiac arrest) and an increased risk of seizure activity.
Octreotide	Increased risk of cardiotoxicity (QT prolongation, torsades de pointes, cardiac arrest).
Pancuronium	Prolongation of neuromuscular blockade.

DRUG INTERACTIONS FOR GENERAL ANESTHETICS *(cont.)*

Enflurane *(cont.)*

Pimozide	Increased risk of cardiotoxicity (QT prolongation, torsades de pointes, cardiac arrest).
St. John's wort	Increased risk of cardiovascular collapse and/or delayed emergence from anesthesia.
Trimipramine	Increased risk of cardiotoxicity (QT prolongation, torsades de pointes, cardiac arrest) and an increased risk of seizure activity.
Tubocurarine	Tubocurarine toxicity (respiratory depression, apnea).

Isoflurane

Muscle relaxants	May potentiate the muscle relaxant effect of all muscle relaxants, most notably nondepolarizing muscle relaxants.
Nitrous oxide	Minimum alveolar concentration is reduced by concomitant administration of nitrous oxide.

Halothane

Epinephrine/ norepinephrine	Simultaneous use with epinephrine or norepinephrine may induce ventricular tachycardia or fibrillation.
Muscle relaxants	May augment actions of nondepolarizing relaxants and ganglionic blocking agents; use with caution.
Succinylcholine	Use with succinylcholine may trigger malignant hyperthermic crisis in genetically susceptible individuals.

Ketamine Hydrochloride (Ketalar)

Barbiturates	Prolonged recovery time with barbiturates and/or narcotics.
Narcotics	Prolonged recovery time with barbiturates and/or narcotics.

Thiopental Sodium (Pentothal)

Aminophylline	Antagonism with aminophylline.
Diazoxide	Hypotension with diazoxide.
Midazolam	Synergism with midazolam.
Opioid analgesics	Decreased antinociceptive action with opioid analgesics.
Probenecid	Prolonged action with probenecid.
Zimelidine	Antagonism with zimelidine.

Desflurane (Suprane)

Benzodiazepines	Decreased MAC with benzodiazepines and opioids.
Neuromuscular blockers	May decrease the required dose of neuromuscular blocking agents.
Opioids	Decreased MAC with benzodiazepines and opioids.

Sevoflurane (Ultane)

Muscle relaxants	May increase both the intensity and duration of neuromuscular blockade induced by nondepolarizing muscle relaxants.
Nitrous oxide	Decreased anesthetic requirement with nitrous oxide.

Therapeutics in Renal and Hepatic Disease

The dosage of many drugs that are normally cleared by the kidneys or liver must be adjusted in patients with renal or liver disease. If such adjustments are not made, drug accumulation and toxicity are likely to occur. The goal of therapy in a patient with renal impairment is to achieve unbound drug serum concentrations similar to those that have been associated with optimal response in patients with normal renal function. In renal disease, creatinine serves as an endogenous marker to predict the clearance of renally eliminated drugs (abbreviated in clinical tests as CrCl).

Drug dosage adjustments for hepatically eliminated drugs in patients with liver disease or dysfunction are difficult to predict due to the complexity of hepatic metabolism. Unfortunately, there are no reliable endogenous markers to accurately predict a drug's hepatic clearance in patients with liver dysfunction. Because of this, unnecessary and potentially hepatotoxic medications are best avoided.

The following table lists drugs that often require dosage adjustments in patients with renal or hepatic impairment. For specific dosing information, refer to the index for page numbers of the prescribing tables where each drug can be found.

DRUGS REQUIRING DOSAGE ADJUSTMENTS DUE TO RENAL OR HEPATIC DYSFUNCTION

GENERIC NAME (BRAND NAME)

Acyclovir (Zovirax)	Atomoxetine (Strattera)	Candesartan (Atacand)
Almotriptan (Axert)	Atropine Sulfate/Hyoscyamine	Capreomycin Sulfate (Capastat
Amifostine (Ethyol)	Sulfate/Phenobarbital/Scopol-	Sulfate)
Amikacin (Amikin)	amine (Donnatal)	Captopril
Amlodipine (Norvasc)	Azacitidine (Vidaza)	Captopril/Hydrochlorothizide
Amlodipine/Atorvastatin Calcium	Azathioprine (Imuran)	(Capozide)
(Caduet)	Baclofen	Carboplatin (Paraplatin)
Amlodipine/Benazepril Hydrochlo-	Betaxolol	Caspofungin (Cancidas)
ride (Lotrel)	Bisoprolol (Zebeta)	Cefepime (Maxipime)
Amoxicillin (Amoxil, Trimox)	Bisoprolol Fumarate/Hydrochloro-	Cefoperazone (Cefobid)
Amphotericin B (Amphocin)	thiazide (Ziac)	Cefoxitin
Amprenavir (Agenerase)	Bivalirudin (Angiomax)	Ceftazidime (Ceptaz, Fortaz,
Anagrelide (Agrylin)	Bupropion (Wellbutrin SR,	Tazidime)
Argatroban	Wellbutrin XL, Zyban)	Ceftizoxime (Cefizox)
Atazanavir (Reyataz)	Butabarbital (Butisol)	Ceftriaxone (Rocephin)
Atenolol (Tenormin)	Butorphanol (Stadol)	Celecoxib (Celebrex)

DRUGS REQUIRING DOSAGE ADJUSTMENTS DUE TO RENAL OR HEPATIC DYSFUNCTION *(cont.)*

GENERIC NAME (BRAND NAME) *(cont.)*

Cetirizine (Zyrtec)
Cetirizine/Pseudoephedrine
    (Zyrtec-D)
Chlorpropamide (Diabinese)
Choline Magnesium Trisalicylate
    (Trilisate)
Citalopram (Celexa)
Cladribine (Leustatin)
Clavulanate Potassium/Ticarcillin
    Disodium (Timentin)
Clonidine (Catapres)
Colchicine/Probenecid
Cromolyn (Intal)
Cyclobenzaprine (Flexeril)
Cyclosporine (Neoral)
Dalfopristin/Quinupristin (Synercid)
Daptomycin (Cubicin)
Darifenacin (Enablex)
Daunorubicin (Cerubidine)
Demeclocycline (Declomycin)
Desloratadine (Clarinex)
Desloratadine/Pseudoephedrine
    sulfate (Clarinex D)
Dexrazoxane (Zinecard)
Digoxin (Lanoxin)
Disopyramide (Norpace)
Dofetilide (Tikosyn)
Doxorubicin (Doxil)
Duloxetine (Cymbalta)
Eletriptan (Relpax)
Enalapril/Felodipine (Lexxel)
Epirubicin (Ellence)
Eprosartan (Teveten)
Eprosartan/Hydrochlorothiazide
    (Teveten HCT)
Escitalopram (Lexapro)
Esomeprazole (Nexium)
Ethambutol (Myambutol)
Ezetimibe/Simvastatin (Vytorin)
Felbamate (Felbatol)
Felodipine (Plendil)
Fenofibrate (Antara,Tricor, Triglide)
Fexofenadine (Allegra)
Fexofenadine/Pseudoephedrine
    (Allegra-D)
Floxuridine
Flucytosine (Ancobon)

Fluoxetine (Prozac, Sarafem)
Fluoxetine/Olanzapine (Symbyax)
Fluvastatin (Lescol, Lescol XL)
Fluvoxamine
Fosamprenavir (Lexiva)
Foscarnet (Foscavir)
Fosinopril (Monopril)
Gabapentin (Neurontin)
Galantamine (Razadyne)
Ganciclovir (Cytovene)
Gemifloxacin (Factive)
Gentamicin
Glimepiride (Amaryl)
Glipizide (Glucotrol, Glucotrol XL)
Glyburide (DiaBeta, Glynase
    PresTab, Micronase)
Hydroxyurea (Hydrea)
Ibuprofen (Motrin)
Idarubicin (Idamycin PFS)
Imipenem/Cilastatin (Primaxin IV)
Indinavir (Crixivan)
Ketoprofen
Ketorolac
Lepirudin (Refludan)
Loratadine (Claritin)
Loratadine/Pseudoephedrine
    (Claritin-D)
Losartan (Cozaar)
Lymphocyte immune globulin,
    anti-thymocyte globulin (equine)
    (Atgam)
Melphalan (Alkeran)
Memantine (Namenda)
Mephobarbital (Mebaral)
Mercaptopurine (Purinethol)
Methyldopa
Methyldopate
Metronidazole (Flagyl, Flagyl ER)
Mexiletine
Midodrine (ProAmatine)
Minocycline (Dynacin, Minocin)
Minoxidil (Loniten)
Modafinil (Provigil)
Morphine (Avinza, Roxanol)
Mycophenolate (CellCept)
Naloxone (Suboxone)
Naratriptan (Amerge)

Nicardipine (Cardene)
Nisoldipine (Sular)
Nizatidine (Axid)
Octreotide (Sandostatin LAR)
Ofloxacin (Floxin,Floxin IV)
Olmesartan (Benicar)
Olmesartan/Hydrochlorothiazide
    (Benicar HCT)
Oxaprozin (Daypro)
Oxcarbazepine (Trileptal)
Pamidronate (Aredia)
Paroxetine (Paxil, Paxil CR,
    Pexeva)
Peginterferon alfa-2a (Pegasys)
Penicillin G (Pfizerpan)
Pentobarbital (Nembutal Sodium)
Perindopril (Aceon)
Phenobarbital
Piperacillin (Pipracil)
Pravastatin (Pravachol)
Pregabalin (Lyrica)
Probenecid
Procainamide (Procanbid)
Propafenone (Rythmol, Rythmol
    SR)
Propoxyphene (Darvon)
Propoxyphene/Acetaminophen
    (Darocet-N, DarvocetA500)
Quetiapine (Seroquel)
Ramipril (Altace)
Repaglinide (Prandin)
Rimantadine (Flumadine)
Risperidone (Risperdal)
Rosuvastatin (Crestor)
Secobarbital (Seconal Sodium)
Sertraline (Zoloft)
Sildenafil (Viagra)
Simvastatin (Zocor)
Sirolimus (Rapamune)
Sodium Oxybate (Xyrem)
Solifenacin (VESIcare)
Sotalol (Betapace AF)
Sulbactam/Ampicillin (Unasyn)
Sumatriptan (Imitrex)
Tacrolimus (Prograf)
Tadalafil (Cialis)
Telithromycin (Ketek)

GENERIC NAME (BRAND NAME) *(cont.)*

Telmisartan/Hydrochlorothiazide (Micardis HCT)	Topiramate (Topamax)	Verapamil (Calan, Calan SR, Covera-HS, Verelan, Verelan PM)
Tetracycline (Sumycin)	Topotecan (Hycamtin)	Vinorelbine (Navelbine)
Theophylline (Theo-24, Theo-Dur, Theolair, Uniphyl)	Torsemide (Demadex)	Voriconazole (Vfend)
Tigecycline (Tygacil)	Trandolapril (Mavik)	Zaleplon (Sonata)
Tobramycin (Nebcin)	Trimethoprim/Sulfamethoxazole (Bactrim, Septra)	Zidovudine (Retrovir)
Tocainide (Tonocard)	Valsartan (Diovan)	Zoledronic Acid (Zometa)
Tolazamide (Tolinase)	Vancomycin (Vancocin)	Zolmitriptan (Zomig)
Tolterodine (Detrol, Detrol LA)	Vardenafil (Levitra)	Zolpidem (Ambien, Ambien CR)
	Venlafaxine (Effexor, Effexor XR)	

Dental Management of Bisphosphonate-Associated Osteonecrosis of the Jaw

American Dental Association

Reports of bisphosphonate-associated osteo-necrosis of the jaw (BON) associated with the use of Zometa (zolendronic acid) and Aredia (pamidronate) began to surface in 2003. The majority of reported cases have been associated with dental procedures such as tooth extraction; however, less commonly BON appears to occur spontaneously in patients taking these drugs.[1] Zolendronic acid and pamidronate are intravenous IV bisphosphonates used to reduce bone pain, hypercalcemia and skeletal complications in patients with multiple myeloma, breast, lung and other cancers and Paget's disease of bone.

Several cases of BON have also been associated with the use of the oral bisphosphonates Fosamax (alendronate), Actonel (risedronate) and Boniva (ibandronate), which are used for the treatment of osteoporosis; however, it is not clear if these patients had other conditions that would put them at risk for developing BON.[2]

The tables at right list all oral and IV bisphosphonates currently on the market in the U.S. For prescribing information and drug interactions, see Chapter 20.

Clinical Presentation

The typical clinical presentation of BON includes pain, soft-tissue swelling and infection, loosening of teeth, drainage, and

ORALLY ADMINISTERED BISPHOSPHONATES

BRAND NAME	MANUFACTURER	GENERIC NAME
Actonel	Procter & Gamble Pharmaceuticals	risedronate
Boniva	Roche Laboratories	ibandronate
Didronel	Procter & Gamble Pharmaceuticals	etidronate
Fosamax	Merck & Co.	alendronate
Fosamax Plus D	Merck & Co.	alendronate
Skelid	Sanofi-Aventis	tiludronate

INTRAVENOUSLY ADMINISTERED BISPHOSPHONATES

BRAND NAME	MANUFACTURER	GENERIC NAME
Aredia	Novartis	pamidronate
Zometa	Novartis	zolendronic acid

exposed bone.[3] These symptoms may occur spontaneously, or more commonly, at the site of previous tooth extraction. Patients may also present with feelings of numbness, heaviness and dysesthesias of the jaw. However, BON may remain asymptomatic for weeks or months, and may only become evident after finding exposed bone in the jaw.

Dental Management

It is important to understand that, based on the information currently available, the risk for developing BON is much higher for cancer patients on IV bisphosphonate therapy than the risk for patients on oral bisphosphonate therapy. Therefore, there are different recommendations for dental management of these patients.

For Patients on Oral Bisphosphonate Therapy

The risk of developing BON in patients on oral bisphosphonate therapy appears to be very low;[4] however, though the risk is small, currently millions of patients take these drugs. Therefore, recommendations for dental management of patients on oral bisphosphonate therapy were developed by an expert panel assembled by the ADA's Council on Scientific Affairs[5] (available at: **http://www.ada.org/prof/resources/topics/topics_osteonecrosis_recommendations.pdf**). These panel recommendations focus on conservative surgical procedures, proper sterile technique, appropriate use of oral disinfectants and the principals of effective antibiotic therapy. There is currently no data from clinical trials evaluating dental management of patients on oral bisphosphonate therapy, and therefore, these recommendations are based on expert opinion only. A comprehensive oral evaluation is recommended for all patients about to begin therapy with oral bisphosphonates (or as soon as possible after beginning therapy). These recommendations do not address treatment of patients on IV bisphosphonate therapy or patients with BON. Refer to the information below regarding their treatment.

For Patients on IV Bisphosphonate Therapy

It is important for dentists to be aware that while on treatment, invasive dental procedures should be avoided in patients receiving IV bisphosphonates, if possible. Dentists need to exercise their professional judgment, perhaps after consultation with the patient's physician, in deciding whether invasive treatment is needed under the particular clinical situations.

The prescribing information for these drugs recommends that cancer patients:

- Receive a dental examination prior to initiating therapy with IV bisphosphonates (Aredia and Zometa); and
- Avoid invasive dental procedures while receiving bisphosphonate treatment. For patients who develop osteonecrosis of the jaw while on bisphosphonate therapy, dental surgery may exacerbate the condition. Clinical judgment by the treating physician should guide the management plan of each patient based on an individual benefit/risk assessment.

Among tools useful to the dentist is a patient's medical history, including medications. Dentists should be aware that patients may not relay information about receiving IV bisphosphonates, because these drugs are administered in oncology wards. Therefore, patients with a history of multiple myeloma, metastatic cancer, Paget's disease and osteoporosis may need to be questioned about receiving IV bisphosphonates. In addition, it may be important to know of any history of IV bisphosphonate administration, because these drugs have a long half-life (years).[6]

An expert panel convened by Novartis Pharmaceuticals Corporation (the manufacturer of Zometa and Aredia) in 2004, made the following recommendations for prevention, diagnosis and treatment of osteonecrosis of the jaw in patients on IV bisphosphonate therapy:[3,7]

- Patients should be educated on maintaining excellent oral hygiene to reduce the risk of infection.
- Dentists should check and adjust removable dentures to avoid soft-tissue injury.

- Routine dental cleanings should be performed with care not to inflict any soft-tissue injury.
- Dental infections should be managed aggressively and nonsurgically (when possible).

Endodontic therapy is preferable to extractions; and, when necessary, coronal amputation with root canal therapy on retained roots to avoid the need for extraction.

For Patients With BON

Recommendations for the treatment of patients with BON have been published in the *Journal of Oncology Practice.*[7]

Obtaining Informed Consent

The ADA has created a document designed to provide general information to patients and to guide dentists in fully and clearly explaining risks, benefits and treatment alternatives to patients[8] (available at: **http://www.ada.org/prof/resources/topics/topics_osteonecrosis_consent.pdf**). However, this document contains only a general discussion of issues surrounding treating patients taking oral bisphosphonates. It does not contain the specific information likely required to be in an informed consent form. The requirements for informed consent forms may vary from one jurisdiction to another. Dentists should consult with an attorney to develop a form which will be effective in a particular state.

1. Woo S-B, Hande K, Richardson PG. Osteonecrosis of the jaw and bisphosphonates. N Engl J Med 2005;353:100.
2. Ruggiero SL, Mehrotra B, Rosenberg TJ, Engroff SL. Osteonecrosis of the jaws associated with the use of bisphosphonates: A review of 63 cases. J Oral Maxillofac Surg 2004;62:527-34.
3. Expert Panel Recommendations for the Prevention, Diagnosis, and Treatment of Osteonecrosis of the Jaws: June 2004. Available at: http://www.ada.org/prof/resources/topics/topics_osteonecrosis_whitepaper.pdf
4. Migliorati CA, Casiglia J, Epstein J, Jacobsen PL, Siegel MA, Woo S-B. Managing the care of patients with bisphosphonate-associated osteonecrosis: An American Academy of Oral Medicine position paper. JADA 2005;136:1658-68.
5. ADA Council on Scientific Affairs. Expert Panel Recommendations: Dental Management of Patients on Oral Bisphosphonate Therapy. June 2006. Available at: http://www.ada.org/prof/resources/topics/topics_osteonecrosis_recommendations.pdf
6. Ott SM. Long-term safety of bisphosphonates. J Clin Endocrinol Metab 2005;90:1897-9.
7. Ruggiero S, Gralow J, Marx RE, Hoff AO, Schubert MM, Huryn JM, Toth B, Damato K, Valero V. Practical Guidelines for the Prevention, Diagnosis, and Treatment of Osteonecrosis of the Jaw in Patients With Cancer. J Oncol Prac 2006;2:7-14.
8. ADA. Obtaining Informed Consent Relating to Risks Associated with Oral Bisphosphonate Use. Available at: http://www.ada.org/prof/resources/topics/topics_osteonecrosis_consent.pdf

Substance Use Disorders

It is important that the dentist be aware of a patient's substance use history. Questions included in the ADA health history form will help the dentist do this. It should be noted that the use of this information will be subject to state confidentiality law, and possibly the federal Health Insurance Portability and Accountability Act (HIPAA) privacy regulations, and also may be subject to federal, state and local antidiscrimination laws. Information related to substance abuse treatment is subject to special federal confidentiality protection (under the U.S. Code of Federal Regulations, Title 42, Chapter 1, Part 2, Confidentiality of Alcohol and Drug Abuse Patient Records) and may not be redisclosed without express written permission of the patient.

Some patients may not reveal their history of substance abuse out of shame or fear of judgment or because they do not understand how important this information is to their dental treatment. Therefore, it is important that dentists are aware of the signs and symptoms of substance abuse. The tables on the following pages provide general information on commonly abused substances.

CONTROLLED SUBSTANCES: USES AND EFFECTS

DRUGS	CSA SCHEDULES	TRADE OR OTHER NAMES	MEDICAL USES	PHYSICAL DEPENDENCE
Anabolic Steroids				
Nandrolone (decanoate, phenpropionate)	III		Anemia, breast cancer	Unknown
Oxymetholone	III	Anadrol-50	Anemia	Unknown
Testosterone (cypionate, enanthate)	III	Depo-Testosterone, Delatestryl	Hypogonadism	Unknown
Cannabis				
Hashish and hashish oil	I	Hash, Hash Oil	None	Unknown
Marijuana	I	Pot, Acapulco Gold, Grass, Reefer, Sinsemilla, Thai Sticks	None	Unknown
Tetrahydrocannabinol	I,II	THC, Marinol	Antinauseant	Unknown
Depressants				
Barbiturates	II,III,IV	Fiorinal, Nembutal, Seconal, Pheno-barbital, Pentobarbital	Anesthetic, anticonvulsant, sedative hypnotic, veterinary euthanasia agent	High-Moderate
Benzodiazepines	IV	Ativan, Dalmane, Diazepam, Librium, Xanax, Serax, Valium, Tranxene, Verstran, Versed, Halcion, Restoril	Antianxiety, sedative, anticonvulsant, hypnotic	Low
Chloral hydrate	IV	Noctec, Somnos, Felsules	Hypnotic	Moderate
Other depressants	I,II,III,IV	Equanil, Miltown, Noludar, Placidyl, Valmid, Methaqualone	Antianxiety, sedative, hypnotic	Moderate
Hallucinogens				
Amphetamine variants	I	2, 5-DMA, STP, MDA (DOM), MDMA (Ecstasy), DOB	None	Unknown
LSD	I	Acid, Microdot	None	None
Mescaline and peyote	I	Mescal, Buttons, Cactus	None	None
Phencyclidine and analogs	I,II	PCE, PCPy, TCP, PCP, Hog, Loveboat, Angel Dust	None	Unknown
Other hallucinogens	I	Bufotenine, Ibogaine, DMT, DET, Psilocybin, Psilocyn	None	None

PSYCHOLOGICAL DEPENDENCE	TOLERANCE	DURATION (HOURS)	USUAL METHOD	POSSIBLE EFFECTS	EFFECTS OF OVERDOSE	WITHDRAWAL SYNDROME
Anabolic Steroids						
Unknown	Unknown	14-21 days	Injected	Virilization, acne, testicular atrophy, gynecomastia, aggressive behavior, edema	Unknown	Possible depression
Unknown	Unknown	24	Oral			
Unknown	Unknown	14-28 days	Injected			
Cannabis						
Moderate	Yes	2.0-4	Smoked, oral	Euphoria, relaxed inhibitions, increased appetite, disorientation	Fatigue, paranoia, possible psychosis	Occasional reports of insomnia, hyperactivity, decreased appetite
Moderate	Yes	2.0-4	Smoked, oral			
Moderate	Yes	2.0-4	Smoked, oral			
Depressants						
High-Moderate	Yes	1.0-16	Oral, injected	Slurred speech, disorientation, drunken behavior without odor of alcohol	Shallow respiration, clammy skin, dilated pupils, weak and rapid pulse, coma, possible death	Anxiety, insomnia, tremors, delirium, convulsions, possible death
Low	Yes	4.0-8	Oral, injected			
Moderate	Yes	5.0-8	Oral			
Moderate	Yes	4.0-8	Oral			
Hallucinogens						
Unknown	Yes	Variable	Oral, injected	Illusions and hallucinations, altered perception of time and distance	Longer, more intense "trip" episodes, psychosis, possible death	Unknown
Unknown	Yes	8.0-12	Oral			
Unknown	Yes	8.0-12	Oral			
High	Yes	Days	Smoked, oral			
Unknown	Possible	Variable	Smoked, oral, injected, sniffed			

CONTROLLED SUBSTANCES: USES AND EFFECTS *(cont.)*

DRUGS	CSA SCHEDULES	TRADE OR OTHER NAMES	MEDICAL USES	PHYSICAL DEPENDENCE
Narcotics				
Codeine	II,III,V	Tylenol w/Codeine, Empirin w/Codeine, Robitussin A-C, Fiorinal w/Codeine, APAP w/Codeine	Analgesic, antitussive	Moderate
Fentanyl and analogs	I,II	Sublimaze, Alfenta, Sufenta, Duragesic	Analgesic, adjunct to anesthesia, anesthetic	High
Heroin	I	Diacetylmorphine, Horse, Smack	None in U.S., analgesic, antitussive	High
Hydrocodone	II,III	Lorcet, Tussionex, Vicodin	Analgesic, antitussive	High
Hydromorphone	II	Dilaudid	Analgesic	High
Methadone and LAAM	I,II	Dolophine, Methadose, Levo-alphaacetylmethadol, Levomethadyl acetate	Analgesic, treatment of dependence	High
Morphine	II	Duramorph, MS-Contin, Roxanol, Oramorph SR	Analgesic	High
Oxycodone	II	Percodan, Percocet, Tylox, Roxicet, Roxicodone	Analgesic	High
Other narcotics	II,III,IV,V	Percodan, Percocet, Tylox, Opium, Darvon, Talwin*, Buprenorphine, Meperidine (Pethidine), Demerol	Analgesic, antidiarrheal	High-Low
Stimulants				
Amphetamine/methamphetamine	II	Desoxyn, Dexedrine, Obetrol, Ice	Attention deficit disorder, narcolepsy, weight control	Possible
Cocaine†	II	Coke, Flake, Snow, Crack	Local anesthetic	Possible
Methylphenidate	II	Ritalin	Attention deficit disorder, narcolepsy	Possible
Other stimulants	I,II,III,IV	Adipex, Didrex, Ionamin	Weight control	Possible

*Designated a narcotic under the Controlled Substances Act (CSA).
†Not designated a narcotic under the CSA.

PSYCHOLOGICAL DEPENDENCE	TOLERANCE	DURATION (HOURS)	USUAL METHOD	POSSIBLE EFFECTS	EFFECTS OF OVERDOSE	WITHDRAWAL SYNDROME
Narcotics						
Moderate	Yes	3.0-6	Oral, injected	Euphoria, drowsiness, respiratory depression, constricted pupils, nausea	Slow and shallow breathing, clammy skin, convulsions, coma, possible death	Watery eyes, runny nose, yawning, loss of appetite, irritability, tremors, panic, cramps, nausea, chills and sweating
High	Yes	10.0-72	Injected, transdermal patch			
High	Yes	3.0-6	Injected, sniffed, smoked			
High	Yes	3.0-6	Oral			
High	Yes	3.0-6	Oral, injected			
High	Yes	12.0-72	Oral, injected			
High	Yes	3.0-6	Oral, smoked, injected			
High	Yes	4.0-5	Oral			
High-Low	Yes	Variable	Oral, injected			
Stimulants						
High	Yes	2.0-4	Oral, injected, smoked	Increased alertness, excitation, euphoria, increased pulse rate & blood pressure, insomnia, loss of appetite	Agitation, increased body temperature, hallucination, convulsions, possible death	Apathy, long periods of sleep, irritability, depression, disorientation
High	Yes	1.0-2	Sniffed, smoked, injected			
High	Yes	2.0-4	Oral, injected			
High	Yes	2.0-4	Oral, injected			

SUBSTANCES OF ABUSE: DENTAL IMPLICATIONS

ABUSED SUBSTANCE	FACTS TO AID IN DIAGNOSIS	DRUGS THAT MAY INTERACT	DENTAL IMPLICATIONS
Alcohol			
	Patient may appear drunk or drowsy and have slurred speech. Odor of alcohol, heavy cologne, mouthwash, fruity acetone breath may be present. Patient may have difficulty maintaining position of head. Periodontal disease does not respond to therapy.	Other central nervous system (CNS) depressants (such as opioid analgesics) enhance alcohol-induced respiratory depression. Metronidazole interacts with alcohol to produce flushing, hypotension, nausea and vomiting.	Alcohol-containing mouthrinses and liquid medications that contain high concentrations of alcohol should be avoided in dental treatment of recovering alcoholics. Recovering alcoholics with liver disease may require a lower dose of medications containing acetaminophen. Periodontal disease does not respond to therapy.
Amphetamine/methamphetamines and derivatives (such as Ecstasy, MDMA)			
	Patient may act jittery, irritable, unable to sit still, extremely talkative, verbose, exaggerated behavior. Patient may exhibit tremors, dilated pupils, increased blood pressure and heart rate.	Intravascular injection of local anesthetics containing vasoconstrictors may enhance amphetamine-induced increase in blood pressure.	Measure blood pressure preoperatively; if high (systolic ≥180mm or diastolic ≥110mm), postpone treatment and refer to source of care. If patient is suspected of use of these drugs within 24 hrs, avoid local anesthetics containing vasoconstrictors; local anesthetics without vasoconstrictor may be used. Methamphetamine users have been reported to have high caries index; Ecstasy (MDMA, MDA, MDEA, PMA) users brux and may display wear facets and request fabrication of bite guard.
Barbiturates and gammahydroxybutyrates (GHB, Liquid X, Hug Drug)			
	Patient may appear drunk or drowsy and have slurred speech. Patient may have difficulty maintaining position of head.	Other CNS depressants (such as opioid analgesics) may enhance barbiturate-induced respiratory depression.	Dose of opioids should be reduced to avoid enhanced respiratory depression.
Benzodiazepines (alprazolam [Xanax], clonazepam [Klonopin])			
	These CNS depressants are favorites among drug abusers.	Benzodiazepines may enhance opioid-induced respiratory depression.	Dose of opioids should be reduced to avoid enhanced respiratory depression. Xerostomia is a frequent side effect and may lead to increased caries. Although carisoprodol (Soma) is not considered a benzodiazepine and is not classified as a controlled substance by the Drug Enforcement Administration, it is often requested by the drug abuser to enhance the opioid-induced euphoria or "high."
Cocaine			
	Patient may act jittery, irritable, unable to sit still. Patient may exhibit tremors, dilated pupils, increased blood pressure and heart rate.	Intravascular injection of local anesthetics containing vasoconstrictors may enhance cocaine-induced increase in blood pressure and heart rate; cardiac arrest.	Measure blood pressure preoperatively; if high (systolic ≥180mm or diastolic ≥110mm), postpone treatment and refer to source of care. If patient is suspected of use of these drugs within 6 h, avoid local anesthetics containing vasoconstrictors; local anesthetics without vasoconstrictor may be used.
Inhalants			
	Most, if not all, inhalants are excreted via the lungs. Patient who has abused an inhalant within a few hours will have an odor on breath.	Most inhalants are CNS depressants. Other CNS depressants (such as opioid analgesics) may enhance inhalant-induced respiratory depression.	Chronic inhalant abuse may cause liver damage, decreasing rate of inactivation of prescribed or over-the-counter drugs such as acetaminophen and thus increasing their toxicity.

ABUSED SUBSTANCE	FACTS TO AID IN DIAGNOSIS	DRUGS THAT MAY INTERACT	DENTAL IMPLICATIONS
Lysergic acid diethylamide (LSD)			
	Patient may appear disoriented and confused. Patient may exhibit dilated pupils, increased blood pressure and heart rate.	No confirmed interactions with dental drugs.	None of significance to dentistry.
Marijuana			
	Patient may appear sedated and lethargic and have bloodshot eyes. Heart rate may be increased but blood pressure will be decreased.	No confirmed interactions with dental drugs.	None of significance to dentistry.
Nicotine			
	Patient may have history of use. Patient may exhibit staining of teeth and oral tissues, malodor characteristic of smokers.	No confirmed interactions with dental drugs.	See Appendix R, Cessation of Tobacco Use.
Opioids			
	Patient may appear drowsy, lethargic, disoriented and confused. Pupils may be constricted. Arms may exhibit scars from previous injuries or needle marks.	Other CNS depressants (such as sedatives or hypnotics) may enhance opioid-induced respiratory depression. Patients taking naltrexone, an opioid antagonist, during recovery may exhibit decreased effect of opioid analgesics.	Opioid users in recovery or actively using drugs may require increased dose of opioid analgesics to achieve analgesia. Avoid prescribing opioid-type analgesics postoperatively in patients recovering from opioid addiction. Opioid users exhibit profound xerostomia with increased craving for sweets, resulting in rampant caries.
Phencyclidine hydrochloride (PCP, Angel Dust) and ketamine (Vitamin K, Ketalar, Cat Tranquilizer, K)			
	This anesthetic agent may program CNS depression with paradoxical CNS excitation accompanied by hallucinations.	Other CNS depressants may enhance PCP-induced respiratory depression.	None of significance to dentistry.

Note: As a general rule, patients in recovery from chemical dependency, including alcohol, should not be given any psychoactive drug, such as nitrous oxide or benzodiazepines.

Cessation of Tobacco Use

Dentists may be the first health care providers exposed to the signs and symptoms of oral cancer and other diseases that result from smoking or using smokeless tobacco. Signs and symptoms related to cancer may include oral sores that do not heal; lumps in the head and neck region; thickened white, red or mixed patches on the oral mucosa (oral leukoplakia); or difficulty in chewing, swallowing, or moving the tongue or jaw. The importance of a thorough dental examination for patients who use tobacco products cannot be overemphasized. Careful extra- and intraoral examination may lead to early detection and may decrease the chance for metastases to occur. Some forms of oral malignancies are aggressive, so prompt diagnosis is critical. Beyond this, the correlation between tobacco use in a variety of forms with a variety of oral diseases and nonoral diseases that are expressed in the mouth warrants careful evaluation of patients who use tobacco products.

Helping patients quit is practical in every clinical setting and can be done by any clinician. A few moments of assistance from a clinician can be significantly more effective than self-help methods. Minimum assistance includes identifying whether patients use tobacco; advising users to stop; strengthening their interest in quitting and, for those who make a commitment to quit, equipping them with coping skills needed during the quitting process; encouraging extra-treatment social support; and providing clinical follow-up support. Nicotine patches, polacrilex gum, polacrilex lozenges, nasal sprays, and oral inhalers used alone or together with a non-nicotine pharmacotherapy are to be used in combination with, not as substitutes for, support and follow-up programs. The tables on the following pages provide general usage and prescribing information for smoking cessation products.

PRESCRIBING INFORMATION FOR TOBACCO-USE CESSATION PRODUCTS

NAME	INDICATIONS/USES	DOSAGE	INTERACTIONS WITH OTHER AGENTS
CENTRALLY ACTING NON-NICOTINE AGENT			
Bupropion SR (Zyban)	As part of a comprehensive behavioral tobacco-use cessation program to relieve nicotine withdrawal symptoms	*Adults:* ≥ 18 yrs: **Initial:** 150mg qd for 3 days. **Usual:** 150mg bid; separate dose intervals by at 8 hrs. **Max:** 300mg/day. Initiate treatment while patient is still smoking. Patients should set a "target quit date" within the first 2 weeks. Treat for 7 to weeks; discontinue at 7 weeks if no progress seen. **Renal/Hepatic Dysfunction:** Reduce dose. **Severe Hepatic Cirrhosis:** 150mg every other day.	Contraindicated for simultaneous use with monoamine oxidase (MAO) inhibitors, other medications containing bupropion, alcohol, antipsychotic agents, hepatic enzyme inducers and inhibitors, levodopa; such agents may inhibit bupropion metabolism so that plasma levels increase, thereby increasing risk of seizures.
Varenicline (Chantix)	As part of a comprehensive behavioral tobacco-use cessation program to relieve nicotine withdrawal symptoms	*Adults:* ≥18 yrs: Days 1-3: 0.5mg daily. Days 4-7: 0.5mg bid. Day 8-End of treatment: 1mg bid. *Severe Renal Impairment:* **Initial:** 0.5mg daily. **Titrate: Max:** 0.5mg bid. **End-Stage Renal Disease: Max:** 0.5mg daily.	Reduced renal clearance with cimetidine. Tobacco-use cessation, with or without cessation aids, may require adjustment of doses of other medications (eg, theophylline, warfarin, insulin).
NICOTINE INHALATION SYSTEM			
Nicotine inhalation system (Nicotrol Inhaler)	As part of a comprehensive behavioral tobacco-use cessation program to relieve nicotine withdrawal symptoms	*Adults:* **Initial:** At least 6 cartridges/day for 3-6 weeks. **Usual:** 6-16 cartridges/day. **Max:** 16 cartridges/day for 12 weeks. Best effect achieved by frequent continuous puffing (20 minutes). Continue for 3 months. Wean by gradual reduction of daily dose over the following 6-12 weeks. Do not treat > 6 months.	Should not be used with tobacco products owing to risk of nicotine toxicity. Tobacco-use cessation, with or without nicotine replacement, may require adjustment of doses of other medications (eg, TCA, theophylline).
NICOTINE NASAL SPRAY			
Nicotine nasal spray (Nicotrol NS)	As part of a comprehensive behavioral tobacco-use cessation program to relieve nicotine withdrawal symptoms	*Adults:* **Initial:** 2-4 sprays/hr, up to 10 sprays/hr, for up to 8 weeks. **Minimum:** 16 sprays/day. **Max:** 80 sprays/day. Elderly: Start at low end of the dosing range. May discontinue abruptly or over 4-6 weeks. Do not treat >3 months. Do not sniff, swallow, or inhale through nose as spray is being administered and should wait 2-3 min before blowing nose. Tilt head back slightly to administer.	Should not be used with tobacco products owing to risk of nicotine toxicity. Tobacco-use cessation, with or without nicotine replacement, may require adjustment of doses of other medications.
NICOTINE POLACRILEX GUM			
Nicotine polacrilex gum (Nicorette, Nicorette DS, Nicorette Mint, Nicorette Mint DS, Nicorette Orange, Nicorette Orange DS)	As part of a comprehensive behavioral tobacco-use cessation program to relieve nicotine withdrawal symptoms	*Adults:* Stop smoking completely before use. **<25 Cigarettes/Day:** Use 2mg. **>25 Cigarettes/Day:** Use 4mg. Chew 1 piece for 30 minutes q1-2h for 6 weeks, then 1 piece q2-4h for 3 weeks, then 1 piece q4-8h for 3 weeks. Max 24 pieces/day and 12 weeks of therapy. Chew at least 9 pieces/day. Do not eat/drink for 15 minutes before or while chewing gum. Should be chewed until tingling is felt (which means nicotine is being released); when tingling stops, chewing can be resumed; do not swallow saliva when tingling is felt.	Should not be used with tobacco products owing to risk of nicotine toxicity. Tobacco-use cessation, with or without nicotine replacement, may require adjustment of doses of other medications. Coffee, wine, colas and fruit juices taken within 15 min before or during use of polacrilex may decrease salivary pH and thereby decrease absorption of nicotine; therefore, patient should rinse mouth with water before using nicotine gum and refrain from ingesting acidic foods or beverages while using the gum.
NICOTINE POLACRILEX LOZENGE			
Nicotine polacrilex lozenge (Commit)	As part of a comprehensive behavioral tobacco-use cessation program to relieve nicotine withdrawal symptoms	*Adults:* Stop smoking completely before use. Use 4mg loz if time to 1st cigarette is within 30 minutes of waking. Use 2mg loz if your time to 1st cigarette is >30 minutes after waking. **Weeks 1-6:** 1 loz q1-2h. **Weeks 7-9:** 1 loz q2-4h. **Weeks 10-12:** 1 loz q4-8h. Use at least 9 loz/day for first 6 weeks. **Max:** 5 loz/6 hrs or 20 loz/day. Dissolve loz in mouth for 20-30 minutes (minimize swallowing) moving it from one side of your mouth to the other; do not chew or swallow whole. Do not eat/drink for 15 minutes before or during use.	Should not be used concomitantly with tobacco products. Should not be used concomitantly with a nicotine patch or other nicotine-containing products. Tobacco-use cessation, with or without nicotine replacement, may require adjustment of doses of other medications.

NAME	INDICATIONS/USES	DOSAGE	INTERACTIONS WITH OTHER AGENTS
TRANSDERMAL NICOTINE SYSTEM			
Nicotine transdermal patches (Habitrol, Nico-Derm CQ, Nicotrol)	As part of a comprehensive behavioral tobacco-use cessation program to relieve nicotine withdrawal symptoms	Depending on stage of treatment and patient's health, weight and level of nicotine dependence, dosage can range from 7 to 22mg/day. Entire course of nicotine substitution and gradual withdrawal takes between 6 and 8 weeks, depending on brand and size of initial dose. See manufacturer's instructions.	Should not be used with tobacco products owing to risk of nicotine toxicity. Tobacco-use cessation, with or without nicotine replacement, may require adjustment of doses of other medications. Following agents may require decreased dose of nicotine on cessation of tobacco use: acetaminophen, adrenergic antagonists (for example, prazosin and labetalol), caffeine, imipramine, insulin, oxazepam, pentazocine, propranolol, theophylline. Adrenergic agonists (for example, isoproterenol and phenylephrine) may require increased dose on cessation of tobacco use.

ADVERSE EFFECTS OF TOBACCO-USE CESSATION DRUGS*

BODY SYSTEM	CENTRALLY ACTING NON-NICOTINE AGENT	NICOTINE INHALATION SYSTEM	NICOTINE NASAL SPRAY	NICOTINE POLACRILEX GUM AND LOZENGES	TRANSDERMAL NICOTINE SYSTEMS
CV	**Hypertension** (Zyban)	Edema, cardiac irritability, **hypertension**	Edema, cardiac irritability, **hypertension**	Edema, cardiac irritability, **hypertension**	**Hypertension**
CNS	**Insomnia** (Chantix and Zyban); **seizures** (Zyban, related to dose); **headache** and abnormal dreams (Chantix)	Anorexia, dizziness, **headache,** insomnia	Anorexia, dizziness, **headache,** insomnia	Anorexia, dizziness, **headache**, insomnia	Dizziness, **headache**, insomnia, abnormal dreams
EENT	None of significance to dentistry	**Pharyngitis**; during first week, **local irritant effects, including cough, mouth and throat irritation**	**Pharyngitis**; during first week, local irritant effects, including nasal irritation, runny nose, throat irritation, watering eyes, sneezing, coughing	**Pharyngitis,** hoarseness	None of significance to dentistry
Endoc	None of significance to dentistry	Dysmenorrhea	Dysmenorrhea	Dysmenorrhea	Dysmenorrhea
GI	Altered appetite (Zyban); **nausea,** abdominal pain, and constipation (Chantix)	**GI upset, nausea, vomiting, eructation, increased appetite**	**GI upset, nausea, vomiting, eructation, increased appetite**	**GI upset, nausea, vomiting, eructation, increased appetite**	Diarrhea, dyspepsia, nausea, GI upset, increased appetite
Integ	None of significance to dentistry	Erythema, flushing, itching, rash, hypersensitivity	Erythema, flushing, itching, rash, hypersensitivity	Erythema, flushing, itching, rash, hypersensitivity	Cutaneous hypersensitivity, rash, increased sweating, erythema
Musc	None of significance to dentistry	None of significance to dentistry	None of significance to dentistry	Gum only: Muscle pain	Arthralgia, back pain
Oral	**Altered taste** (Chantix); **xerostomia** (Zyban)	**Xerostomia, increased susceptibility to oral fungal infections**	None of significance to dentistry	**Aphthous ulcers, altered taste, excess salivation, glossitis, jaw ache (gum only), hiccups**	**Altered taste, xerostomia**
Resp	None of significance to dentistry	None of significance to dentistry	None of significance to dentistry	None of significance to dentistry	Chest pain, increased cough

* Bold entries denote special dental considerations.

PRECAUTIONS/CONTRAINDICATIONS FOR TOBACCO-USE CESSATION PRODUCTS

NAME	PRECAUTIONS	CONTRAINDICATIONS
Centrally acting non-nicotine agent: bupropion SR	Associated with dose-dependent risk of seizures; risk related to patient factors, clinical situation and concurrent medication, all of which should be considered before prescription is given. Dose should not be > 300mg/day for tobacco-use cessation.	Contraindicated for patients with anorexia or bulimia nervosa, bipolar disorders, CNS tumor, head trauma, history of drug abuse, hepatic or renal function impairment, recent history of myocardial infarct, unstable heart disease, psychosis, seizure disorders. Contraindicated for simultaneous use with monoamine oxidase inhibitors or within 14 days of monoamine oxidase inhibitor use. Contraindicated for patients with sensitivity to bupropion (Wellbutrin).
Nicotine inhalation system	Can be toxic and addictive. Should be kept out of reach of children and pets. Patient should stop smoking completely on initiating therapy. Should be used with caution and only when the benefits of use (including nicotine replacement in a smoking cessation program) outweigh risks for patients with following conditions: coronary heart disease, serious cardiac dysrhythmias, vasospastic disease, renal or hepatic impairment, hyperthyroidism, pheochromocytoma, insulin-dependent diabetes and active peptic ulcers. Not recommended for use with children; although not nicotine inhalation system–specific, smoking cessation may elicit or exacerbate depression among patients with a prior history of affective disorder.	Contraindicated for continuous use of > 6 mo. Contraindicated for patients who have asthma or chronic nasal disorders. Contraindicated for patients during immediate postmyocardial infarction period, patients with serious dysrhythmias or severe or worsening angina pectoris, pregnant women. Contraindicated for patients who have hypersensitivity or allergy to any component of therapeutic system.
Nicotine nasal spray	See note above. Although not specific to nicotine nasal spray, smoking cessation may elicit or exacerbate depression among patients with a prior history of affective disorder.	Contraindicated for continuous use of > 3 mo. Contraindicated for patients who have asthma or chronic nasal disorders. Contraindicated for patients during immediate postmyocardial infarction period, patients with serious dysrhythmias or severe or worsening angina pectoris, pregnant women. Contraindicated for patients who have hypersensitivity or allergy to any component of therapeutic system.
Nicotine polacrilex gum and lozenge	Can be toxic and addictive. Should be kept out of reach of children and pets. Patient should stop smoking completely on initiating therapy. Should be used with caution by patients having the following conditions: coronary heart disease, serious cardiac dysrhythmias, vasospastic disease, renal or hepatic impairment, hyperthyroidism, pheochromocytoma, insulin-dependent diabetes and active peptic ulcers. Not recommended for use with children. May have oral side effects, including interactions with restorative materials, xerostomia and pharyngeal and oral inflammation.	Contraindicated for patients who are nonsmokers, are in immediate postmyocardial infarction period, have severe or worsening angina pectoris, or are pregnant. Contraindicated for patients who have hypersensitivity or allergy to any component of therapeutic system. Contraindicated for patients with a history of GI disorders. Gum only: Contraindicated for patients with active temporomandibular joint disorders. Gum only:. Contraindicated for patients who wear dental prostheses if gum's sticking to dental work becomes a problem.
Transdermal nicotine system	See note above, with exception of paragraph on oral side effects. Treatment should be discontinued if patient experiences severe or persistent local skin reactions at the site of application.	Contraindicated for continuous use of > 3 mo. Contraindicated for patients during immediate postmyocardial infarction period, patients with serious dysrhythmias or severe or worsening angina pectoris, pregnant women. Contraindicated for patients who have hypersensitivity or allergy to any component of therapeutic system.

Index

In this index, dental indications are found in **boldface** type. Locators referring to usage and/or drug interaction tables are marked with "t" following the page number. Brand names are followed by the generic name or compounding ingredients in parentheses. Products that have the ADA Seal of Acceptance are indicated with a star (★).